Cardiovascular and Pulmonary Physical Therapy

An Evidence-Based Approach

Second Edition

William E. DeTurk, PT, PhD
Clinical Associate Professor
Doctor of Physical Therapy Program
School of Health Technology & Management
Stony Brook University
Stony Brook, New York

Lecturer, Doctor of Physical Therapy Program
School of Public Health
New York Medical College
Valhalla, New York

Consultant to Cardiac & Pulmonary
  Rehabilitation Program
Physical Medicine & Rehabilitation Services
Veterans Affairs Medical Center
Northport, New York

Lawrence P. Cahalin, PT, MS, CCS
Senior Clinical Professor
Department of Physical Therapy
Northeastern University
Bouve College of Health Sciences
Boston, Massachusetts

Clinical Research Physical Therapist
Heart Failure/Cardiac Transplantation Unit
Massachusetts General Hospital
Boston, Massachusetts

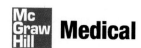

New York   Chicago   San Francisco   Lisbon   London   Madrid   Mexico City
Milan   New Delhi   San Juan   Seoul   Singapore   Sydney   Toronto

Cardiovascular and Pulmonary Physical Therapy: An Evidence-Based Approach, Second Edition

1 2 3 4 5 6 7 8 9 0 CTP/CTP 14 13 12 11 10

Book and CD
ISBN-13 978-0-07-159812-5
MHID 0-07-159812-X

Book
ISBN-13 978-0-07-159814-9
MHID 0-07-159814-6

CD
ISBN-13 978-0-07-159815-6
MHID 0-07-159815-4

This book was set in Minion by Aptara, Inc.
The editors were Joseph Morita and Cindy Yoo.
The production supervisor was Sherri Souffrance.
Project management was provided by Sandhya Joshi, Aptara, Inc.
The designer was Elise Lansdon; the cover designer was The Gazillion Group.
China Translation & Printing, Ltd. was printer and binder.

This book is printed on acid-free paper.

Library of Congress Cataloging-in-Publication Data

DeTurk, William E.
  Cardiovascular and pulmonary physical therapy : an evidence-based
approach / William E. DeTurk, Lawrence P. Cahalin.—2nd ed.
     p. ; cm.
  Includes bibliographical references and index.
  ISBN-13: 978-0-07-159814-9 (book)
  ISBN-10: 0-07-159814-6 (book)
  ISBN-13: 978-0-07-159812-5 (book and CD)
  ISBN-10: 0-07-159812-X (book and CD)
 1. Cardiopulmonary system—Diseases—Physical therapy. 2. Evidence-based medicine.
  I. Cahalin, Lawrence P. II. Title.
  [DNLM: 1. Cardiovascular Diseases—physiopathology. 2. Cardiovascular Diseases—rehabilitation.
 3. Evidence-Based Medicine. 4. Lung Diseases—physiopathology. 5. Lung Diseases—rehabilitation.
 6. Physical Therapy Modalities. WG 166 D479c 2010]
  RC702.D48 2010
  616.1'062—dc22   2010004820

Contents

PART **I**

INTRODUCTION   1

PART **II**

BASIC MEDICAL SCIENCE   35

PART **III**

CARDIOVASCULAR AND PULMONARY ASSESSMENT   243

Contributors

Kathy Lee Bishop, PT, MS, CCS [17]

Manager, Emory HeartWise^{SM} Risk Reduction Program; Assistant Professor, School of Medicine, Emory University, School of Physical Therapy, Atlanta, Georgia

Physical Therapy Associated with Airway Clearance Dysfunction

Dawn M. Blatt, PT, DPT [16]

Clinical Assistant Professor, Doctor of Physical Therapy Program, School of Health Technology and Management, Stony Brook University, Stony Brook, New York

Physical Therapy Associated with Obesity

Lawrence P. Cahalin, PT, MS, CCS [1, 2, 6, 9, 10–12, 18, 20]

Senior Clinical Professor, Department of Physical Therapy, Northeastern University, Bouve College of Health Sciences, Boston, Massachusetts; Clinical Research Physical Therapist, Heart Failure/Cardiac Transplantation Unit, Massachusetts General Hospital, Boston, Massachusetts

History of Cardiopulmonary Rehabilitation; History and Use of the Guide; Cardiovascular Pathophysiology; Pulmonary Evaluation; Cardiovascular Evaluation; Electrocardiography; Evaluation of Patient Intolerance to Exercise; Physical Therapy Associated with Cardiovascular Pump Dysfunction and Failure; Physical Therapy Associated with Ventilatory Pump Dysfunction and Failure

Sandra L. Cassady, PT, PhD, FAACVPR [6]

Professor and Director, Physical Therapy Department, St. Ambrose University, Davenport, Iowa

Cardiovascular Pathophysiology

Charles D. Ciccone, PT, PhD, FAPTA [8]

Professor, Department of Physical Therapy, Ithaca College, Ithaca, New York

Medications

Nancy D. Ciesla, PT [19]

Adjunct Faculty, Shenandoah University, Winchester, Virginia; Physical Therapy Supervisor, Johns Hopkins Hospital, Baltimore, Maryland

Physical Therapy Associated with Respiratory Failure

Jerome A. Dempsey, PhD [5]

John Robert Sutton Professor of Population Health Sciences, University of Wisconsin-Madison, Madison, Wisconsin

Physiology of the Cardiovascular and Pulmonary Systems

Barbara W. DeTurk, PT, MS [23]

Instructor, Physical Therapy Program, School of Health Technology and Management, SUNY Stony Brook, Stony Brook, New York; Clinical Manager-Therapy, Tender Loving Care Staff Builders Home Health care, Medford, New York

The Future of Cardiopulmonary Rehabilitation

William E. DeTurk, PT, PhD [1, 3, 10, 11, 12]

Clinical Associate Professor, Doctor of Physical Therapy Program, School of Health Technology & Management, Stony Brook University, Stony Brook, New York; Lecturer, DPT Program School of Public Health, New York Medical College, Valhalla, New York; Consultant to Cardiac & Pulmonary Rehabilitation Program, Physical Medicine & Rehabilitation Services, Veterans Affairs Medical Center, Northport, New York

History of Cardiopulmonary Rehabilitation; Essentials of Exercise Physiology; Cardiovascular Evaluation; Electrocardiography; Evaluation of Patient Intolerance to Exercise

Cheri L. Gostic, PT, DPT [16]

Clinical Assistant Professor, Doctor of Physical Therapy Program, School of Health Technology and Management, Stony Brook University, Stony Brook, New York

Physical Therapy Associated with Obesity

Lisa Johnson, PT, DPT, OCS, CSCS [3]

Clinical Assistant Professor, Health Policy and Management Master of Science Program, School of Health Technology and Management, Stony Brook University, Stony Brook, New York; Owner, Clinical Director, Body in Balance Physical Therapy, Hauppauge and East Setauket, New York

Essentials of Exercise Physiology

The numbers in brackets following each contributor's name indicates the chapter(s) written or cowritten by that contributor. An asterisk (*) next to a contributor's name in the chapter opener indicates the first edition of the chapter was written by that person.

Jill D. Kuramoto, MPT [19]

Advanced Physical Therapist, R Adams Cowley Shock Trauma Center, University of Maryland Medical Center, Baltimore, Maryland

Physical Therapy Associated with Respiratory Failure

Kimberly D. Leaird, PT, MEd, CLT-LANA [22]

Physical Therapist, Instructor, Lymphedema Consultant, Academy of Lymphatic Studies, Sebastian, Florida

Physical Therapy Associated with Lymphatic System Disorders

Mary Massery, PT, DPT [20]

Doctoral Student, Rocky Mountain University of Health Professions, Provo, Utah; Owner, Massery Physical Therapy, Genview, Illinois

Physical Therapy Associated with Ventilatory Pump Dysfunction and Failure

Anne Mejia-Downs, PT, MPH, CCS [17]

Assistant Professor, Krannert School of Physical Therapy University of Indianapolis, Indianapolis, IN; Cardiopulmonary Physical Therapist, Department of Rehabilitation Services, Clarian Health Partners, Indianapolis, IN

Physical Therapy Associated with Airway Clearance Dysfunction

Barbara J. Morgan, PT, PhD [5]

Associate Professor, Physical Therapy Program, Department of Orthopedics and Rehabilitation, University of Wisconsin-Madison, Madison, Wisconsin

Physiology of the Cardiovascular and Pulmonary Systems

Sue Ann Sisto, PT, MA, PhD [14]

Assistant Professor, Physical Medicine and Rehabilitation, University of Medicine and Dentistry of New Jersey/New Jersey Medical School (UMDNJ/NJMS), Newark, New Jersey; Clinical Assistant Professor of Physical Therapy, Department of Physical Therapy, UMDNJ, Newark, New Jersey; Assistant Clinical Professor of Physical Therapy, Department of Physical Therapy, Columbia University, New York, New York; Assistant Research Professor, Department of Biomedical Engineering, New Jersey Institute of Technology, Newark, New Jersey; Director, Human Performance and Movement Analysis Laboratory, Kessler Medical Rehabilitation Research and Education Corporation, West Orange, New Jersey

Cardiopulmonary Concerns in the Patient with Neurological Deficits: An Evidence-Based Approach

Chris L. Wells, PT, PhD, CCS, ATC [7, 13]

Adjunct Faculty, University of Pittsburgh, School of Nursing, Pittsburgh, Pennsylvania; Adjunct Assistant Professor, Department of Physical Therapy and Rehabilitation Sciences, University of Maryland, School

of Medicine, Baltimore, Maryland; Advanced Clinical Specialist, Department of Rehabilitation Services, University of Maryland Medical System, Baltimore, Maryland

Pulmonary Pathology; Cardiopulmonary Concerns in the Patient with Musculoskeletal and Integumentary Deficits: An Evidence-Based Approach

Contributors to the First Edition

Gary Brooks, PT, DrPH, CCS [2, 15]

Associate Professor, School of Health Professions, Grand Valley State University; Research Associate, Grand Rapids Medical Education and Research Center, Grand Rapids, Michigan

History and Use of the Guide; Physical Therapy Associated with Primary Prevention, Risk Reduction, and Deconditioning

Lori A. Buck, PT, MS, CCS [18]

Cardiopulmonary Advanced Clinician, New York Presbyterian Hospital Columbia Presbyterian Center, New York, New York

Physical Therapy Associated with Cardiovascular Pump Dysfunction and Failure

Catherine M. Certo, PT, ScD, FAPTA [1]

Chairman, Department of Physical Therapy, University of Hartford, West Hartford, Connecticut

History of Cardiopulmonary Rehabilitation

Barbara Cocanour, PhD [4]

Professor, Department of Physical Therapy, University of Massachusetts Lowell, Lowell, Massachusetts

Anatomy of the Cardiopulmonary System

Sean M. Collins, PT, ScD, CCS [4]

Assistant Professor, Department of Physical Therapy, University of Massachusetts Lowell, Lowell, Massachusetts

Anatomy of the Cardiopulmonary System

M. Kathleen Kelly, PT, PhD [21]

Assistant Professor and Vice Chair, Department of Physical Therapy, School of Health and Rehabilitation Sciences, University of Pittsburgh; Staff Physical Therapist, Children's Hospital of Pittsburgh, Pittsburgh, Pennsylvania

Physical Therapy Associated with Respiratory Failure in the Neonate

John S. Leard, PT, EdD, ATC [13]

Assistant Professor of Physical Therapy, University of Hartford, West Hartford, Connecticut

Cardiopulmonary Concerns in the Patient with Musculoskeletal and Integumentary Deficits: An Evidence-Based Approach

Foreword

With all the changes that are going on within physical therapy, this is an exciting time to be in the field!

I look back at my own career and PT practice as it was 40 years ago. There was no cardiopulmonary physical therapy service. We were not allowed to see patients with cardiac disease—they were "too sick." The only interventions that fell within our purview were pulse and an occasional blood pressure measurement.

I look forward with a sense of satisfaction at how far our profession has come. There is a new standard of care embodied in clinical specialization, an area of practice that began with my own efforts in 1966 with the development of the first specialist program in the nation at the University of Southern California. This was a Cardiopulmonary Specialization 2-year program terminating in an MS degree. Those first graduates included Ray Blessey, Randy Ice, and Scott Irwin.

Now there is a new standard of practice that is evidence-based. There is also a new standard of education embodied in entry into the profession as a Doctor of Physical Therapy. As we move into the 21st century, it is imperative that we have textbooks that reflect these developments. The text that professors DeTurk and Cahalin have put together incorporate these important practice trends. It is a comprehensive textbook that spans the entire scope of cardiovascular and pulmonary physical therapy practice and, most importantly, reflects current best practice. It also contains the latest and best available evidence that adds strength to our clinical decision making.

I believe you will find that this textbook will serve you well. Now go forth and practice your craft with confidence!
Oath of the physical therapist:

I pledge to hold faithful to my responsibility as a physical therapist;

To use the highest science and skills of my profession at all times;

To exercise judgment to the highest degree of which I am capable when determining treatment to be offered;

To refrain from treatment when it will not benefit the patient;

To always place the welfare of my patients above my own self-interest.

I pledge to uphold and preserve the rights and esteem of every person placed in my care;

To hold all confidences in trust;

To exercise all aspects of my calling with dignity and honor.

I commit myself to the highest ideal of service, learning, and the pursuit of knowledge.

These things I do swear.

Helen J. Hislop, PT, PhD, FAPTA
Emeritus Professor and Chair
Department of Biokinesiology and Physical Therapy
University of Southern California

Preface

"Knowledge comes, but wisdom lingers"—Alfred Tennyson

Welcome to the world of cardiovascular and pulmonary physical therapy! There are at least four things that we think you should know about this book:

- It reflects the broadest possible spectrum of cardiovascular and pulmonary physical therapy practice and draws upon the experience of the many experts who we recruited as chapter authors.
- The *Guide to Physical Therapist Practice*, second edition, is the framework we used for the description of tests, measures, and interventions. Our text links these tests, measures, and interventions with pathophysiologies in a case study format.
- This textbook provides an evidence base for many of the tests, measures, and interventions used by physical therapists.
- It is accompanied by a CD-ROM that provides the user with an interactive, visual workbook of case studies.

Why did we write this new second edition textbook for cardiovascular and pulmonary physical therapy? We believe that a fundamental paradigm shift has occurred in both the practice of physical therapy and the education of physical therapy students. These changes include health care cost containment, the introduction of the *Guide to Physical Therapist Practice*, and the utilization of the disablement model. Within the educational environment, these changes have moved the entry-level physical therapy degree to the doctoral level. This updated textbook reflects these dramatic changes.

Here are ways we believe our book helps physical therapists meet the challenges of this new environment:

- It integrates the *Guide to Physical Therapist Practice*. Chapter 2 describes both the history and use of the *Guide*.
- Preferred practice patterns for cardiovascular and pulmonary physical therapy form Chapters 15 through 22 and are used as springboards to describe interventions and outcomes.
- A case study in each practice pattern chapter permits the student to experience the proper application of the practice patterns.

- The patient–client management model is used in the case studies; appropriate tests, measures, and interventions are selected from the practice pattern and applied to the patient.
- Language has been standardized across chapters.
- "International Perspectives" provide ways to gain insight into the global practice of physical therapy. Prominant therapists from Australia, Canada, Japan, Singapore, and Colombia comment on physical therapy in their countries; these discussions allow comparison of clinical practice behaviors, which may differ from those in the United States.
- With the inclusion of an evidence base and peer-reviewed published research in this book, the physical therapist is able to "narrow the circle" and to develop more specific intervention regimens using hypothesis-oriented algorithms that clarify the use of the *Guide*. The limits of current knowledge are also provided as a stimulus to research.

Several chapters bear special mention:

- The newer ICF Model of Disablement is included in Chapter 2 of the second edition, with discussion of its utility.
- Exercise physiology coverage in Chapter 3 summarizes aspects of the field that are particularly applicable to physical therapy and applies it to patient care.
- Patients with orthopedic and neurological disease are addressed in Chapters 13 and 14, and the principles of cardiovascular and pulmonary physical therapy are applied to them.
- A new Chapter 16—Physical Therapy Associated with Obesity—recognizes this important area of medical practice and the expanding role of physical therapy services in its management.
- The history and future of cardiovascular and pulmonary physical therapy are addressed in Chapters 1 and 23 and provide the proper context for our craft.

The accompanying CD-ROM has a number of important features. It has been completely overhauled and updated, and includes

- a variety of multimedia interactive presentations complementing many of the textbook chapters;

- case study–driven exercises requiring the student to actively engage in problem-solving exercises using animations;
- demonstrations of cardiac and pulmonary physical exams, new for the second edition;
- video clips to illustrate technical psychomotor skills.

We hope that this textbook will meet the needs of our rapidly changing profession as we move forward in the new millennium. Students will find this text replete with evidence that supports our craft. Practicing clinicians will find that the application and utility of our second edition will advance their skills.

William E. DeTurk
Lawrence P. Cahalin

Acknowledgments

Many thanks to the following people who helped bring this book to fruition:

To Rick Johnson, Chair of the Doctor of Physical Therapy Program at Stony Brook, for giving me the time to write; I could not have asked for a more supportive environment.

To Craig Lehmann, Dean of the School of Health Technology & Management at Stony Brook, who has "been there and seen the elephant"—for all his guidance, encouragement, and advice on things great and small.

To Barbara Holton at McGraw-Hill and Patrick Geiger at Interactive Works who worked with us to replace the computer animations with real patients and clients and who made it possible for us to add new material, particularly the wonderful real-life blood pressure sequences.

To the chapter authors, from whom I have learned so much!

To Larry Cahalin, for his command of the literature.

To Catherine Johnson and Joe Morita, our editors at McGraw-Hill, who launched this second edition and who created an *esprit de corps* that made this undertaking a truly collaborative effort.

And to my own wonderful wife Barbara and son Alex who somehow managed to find the strength to go along with yet another project, who listened to a daily endless stream of textbook-related triumph and tragedy, and who baked the other half of a half-baked idea—how do you do it?

WED

Thanks to my parents (for so much); my wife (for everything); Sean, Brendan, and Alison (for putting up with me and my many absences from home); Irma Reubling (for a second chance); Ethel Freese, Randy Ice, Ray Blessey, Elizabeth Protas, Helen Hislop, Dave Nielson, Cindy Moore, Bill DeTurk, and the Massachusetts General Hospital Heart Failure and Transplantation team (for the mentoring and opportunities); all of my past patients (for teaching me how to question); all of my past students (for asking the questions you thought were "stupid," but were really the most important); and to all of my colleagues both here and abroad (thanks, gum xia, arigato, gracias).

LPC

Cardiovascular and Pulmonary Physical Therapy

An Evidence-Based Approach

History of Cardiopulmonary Rehabilitation

Catherine M. Certo*, William E. DeTurk, &
Lawrence P. Cahalin

INTRODUCTION

The relative importance of physical activity was first noted in 1772, when the famous physician William Heberden published a report describing a 6-month exercise program consisting of 30 minutes of daily sawing for a male patient with "chest disorder."[1] One can surmise that the diagnosis was coronary artery disease and that the patient was probably experiencing angina pain or recovering from a myocardial infarction (MI). In 1799, an English physician, C. H. Parry, independently noted the beneficial effects of physical activity in his patients who suffered from chest pain.[2] The reaction by the medical community to this notion met with much resistance and was not assimilated into practice. In 1912, Herrich gave the first clinical description of an acute MI and encouraged physicians to reevaluate the role of physical activity in the treatment of patients with coronary heart disease.[3] However, the medical community expressed fear that increased physical exertion could lead to increased risk of ventricular aneurysm, myocardial rupture, or heightened arterial hypoxemia. The conservative treatment approach of 6 to 8 weeks of bed rest for patients with MI continued to be the common protocol well into the 20th century.

The debate over the benefits of physical activity for patients with MI persisted and won small gains in the late 1930s when two physicians G. K. Mallory and P. D. White[3] found that the necrotic myocardial region was converted into scar tissue after approximately 6 weeks. Accordingly, they prescribed a minimum of only 3 weeks of bed rest for patients with uncomplicated MI and limited physical activity after hospital discharge. Stair climbing was prohibited, in some cases for up to a year. It was becoming clear, however, that, during the convalescent period, patients were becoming invalid due to either fear or lack of patient education. Follow-up medical management provided little advice regarding exercise tolerance, stress management, or education about the disability and its limitations. Typically, patients never returned to work and were put on long-term disability. This resulted in patients with MI being viewed as nonproductive members of society.

Most of the research performed during the first three decades of the 20th century centered both on identifying better methods of diagnosing and classifying cardiac disorders and on developing simple testing for "circulatory efficiency." Little attention was directed toward identifying the risk factors associated with coronary artery disease or to establishing its cause.[4]

WORK EVALUATION UNIT

By the late 1930s, significant numbers of the labor force had retired on disability due to cardiac problems. The New York

State Employment Service, concerned about the growing numbers of men on disability, decided to evaluate the reason for lack of return to work in patients with heart disease.[5] A state survey revealed that 80% of the individuals receiving disability benefits were patients with heart disease who had not returned to their jobs. Furthermore, only 10% had attempted either to be retrained or to seek a less strenuous position within their company.

In 1940, the New York State Employment Service sought assistance from the New York Heart Association in evaluating return-to-work status for workers with cardiac disease. The purpose of this evaluation was to determine a level of activity that would be safe and would allow recovered individuals to return to work and once again become productive members of society. This request eventually led to the establishment of the Work Classification Units or Work Evaluation Units.[5] These Work Evaluation Units were located in teaching hospitals, rehabilitation centers, and community hospitals all across the state.

The purpose of these units was threefold: (1) to provide a clinical service by using a team evaluation approach of the client's work capacity regardless of the type or severity of cardiac dysfunction and by offering an opportunity for appropriate job placement, (2) to serve as an educational instrument for training physicians and for informing the general public, and (3) to serve as a research opportunity for studying the effects of coronary artery disease on return to work. The cardiac Work Evaluation Units of the 1940s became the earliest approach to formalized cardiac rehabilitation programs.

As a result of the implementation of the Work Evaluation Units, many individuals were able to return to the labor force and once again become productive members of society. This reduced both the number of men receiving disability funds and the financial burden to the state. However, in spite of these positive results, by the 1950s, dissatisfaction over declining referrals to the units and the methods used to classify coronary artery disease disability caused many units to close. Additionally, the lack of any formal exercise intervention or follow-up evaluation led to client disinterest. Gradually, the effectiveness of the units dwindled and the programs closed.

DELETERIOUS EFFECTS OF PHYSICAL INACTIVITY

In 1952, Levine and Lown[6] openly questioned the need for enforced bed rest and prolonged inactivity after an uncomplicated MI. On the basis of earlier research,[6] they prescribed early sitting up at bedside and armchair exercises for patients recovering from MI. Their work concluded that long, continued bed rest ". . . decreases functional capacity, saps morale, and provokes complications."[6] Their highly acclaimed published report caught the attention of the medical community and elevated the level of investigation about the management of cardiovascular disease. Today, this article is recognized as a landmark article, demonstrating that early mobilization of patients with acute heart disease significantly reduces complications and mortality.[6]

At the 13th scientific session of the American Heart Association in 1953, the noted physician Louis Katz told the medical community, "Physicians must be ready to discard old dogma when they are proven false and accept new knowledge."[7] He recommended that new research findings on physical activity should be incorporated into the management of patients with cardiac disease. In 1958, two cardiologists, Turell and Hellerstein, urged physicians to provide a more positive and comprehensive approach to the treatment of coronary artery disease.[8] They recommended a graded step program (a prototype to contemporary cardiac rehabilitation) based on established energy requirements of physical activity and patient exercise tolerance while monitoring cardiovascular function, both founded on principles of work physiology. This set the stage for renewed interest concerning the effect of physical activity on patients with coronary artery disease.

This new approach, which incorporated exercise into the medical management of patients with coronary artery disease, was provided high visibility when President Dwight Eisenhower suffered a heart attack in the late 1950s, while in office. His physician Paul Dudley White, a man strongly committed to the positive effects of exercise, prescribed for his eminent patient a program of graded levels of activities, including swimming, walking, and golf. The results were so positive for the president that he created the President's Youth Fitness Council. In the 1960s, President John F. Kennedy renamed the council as the President's Fitness Council in order to encourage physical activity in individuals of all ages and foster an appreciation of its positive effects throughout the life span.

ADVANCEMENTS IN ACUTE CARDIAC CARE

The 1960s was a period of rapid advancement in the care of patients with coronary artery disease. The general public became better educated on the early warning signs of an impending heart attack. It was becoming clear that survival from MI was dependent on rapid transport to a hospital and immediate intervention to reduce the risk of sudden death and/or minimize the damage caused by the infarction. In 1966, Congress passed the Highway Safety Act. This landmark piece of legislation directed states to develop emergency medical service systems, whose mission was to provide emergency treatment in the field and rapid transportation to the hospital. The 1960s and 1970s saw improvement in prehospital emergency care, with emergency medical technician–paramedic personnel providing treatment in the field and in ambulances that were evolving into sophisticated mobile emergency units. The public was receiving instruction and certification in basic life support (BLS), whereas physicians, nurses, and allied health personnel were being trained in advanced cardiac life support (ACLS). Cardiac intensive care units (CICUs) were multiplying and flourishing: These units specialized in the acute care of patients in the early stage of evolving MI. In addition, the experience in the cardiac intensive care units made the diagnosis of sudden death, which was most likely to occur at the inception of a myocardial ischemic episode, perhaps reversible and/or preventable. The use of sophisticated diagnostic and monitoring equipment, like radionuclide imaging, Holter monitoring, and invasive hemodynamic pressure monitoring, was becoming the new standard of care in the management of patients in the acute phase of MI. Most recently, current outcomes research has confirmed that the likelihood of survival from MI increases when the earlier emergency treatment is instituted. "Every minute counts" and "time is muscle" are today's battle cries in the fight against heart disease.[9]

CARDIAC REHABILITATION

By the mid-1960s, numerous research studies had demonstrated the adverse effects of physical inactivity after an uncomplicated MI.[10-15] Saltin et al. reported that the functional capacity of normal subjects confined to bed for 3 weeks decreased approximately 33%. Equally important was the finding that, with physical training, subjects were able to achieve their pre–bed rest aerobic condition. After 3 months of twice-daily rigorous exercise programs, Saltin found that all subjects exceeded their control state.[13]

Cardiac Rehabilitation Programs as Formalized Interventions

As a result of the work of Wenger, Zohman, Hellerstein, and others, the concept of progressive supervised exercise for medically stable patients soon expanded to include more complicated patients with MI as well as patients following coronary artery bypass graft (CABG).[16-25] By the end of the 1970s, cardiac rehabilitation programs were stratified into four phases: phase 1—the hospital inpatient period; phase 2—the convalescent stage following hospital discharge; phase 3—the extended, supervised endurance training program; and phase 4—the ongoing maintenance period. Each phase had its own objectives for patient care and progression.[16-25]

Phases of Cardiac Rehabilitation from the Late 1960s to 1990s

Phase 1 Cardiac Rehabilitation

Many inpatient early mobilization hospital programs were originally 14 steps in length, which started in the cardiac intensive care units and continued through the step-down phase (approximately 24 days). Activities appropriate to phase 1 were generally low-level, rhythmic, isotonic exercises that were calisthenic in nature. Early mobilization programs were designed for uncomplicated patients with acute MI in order to progressively increase activity levels in three areas—active

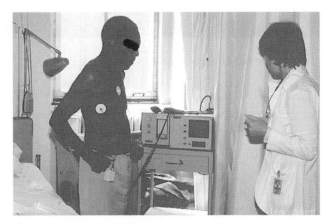

FIGURE 1-1   Physical therapist in a large metropolitan hospital helping a post–myocardial infarction patient to perform low-level exercises as part of a phase 1 cardiac rehabilitation program. Note the use of the portable bedside telemeter. Photograph taken in the late 1970s.

exercises, activities of daily living (ADL), and educational activities (Fig. 1-1).[17,18] A patient was eligible for phase 1 cardiac rehabilitation when his or her clinical condition stabilized. This structured plan greatly assisted the patient toward discharge and an early return to everyday activities. The favorable outcome of these formalized programs led to the development of similar programs across the country. Soon many hospitals were observing the positive economic implications of early mobilization. These included a hastened recovery time, which decreased hospital stay and improved functional status at discharge; a decrease in depression; and an early return to work.[22,23] As coronary artery bypass graft surgery became a routine intervention, many of these surgical patients were also included in the phase 1 programs. Eventually, the strong positive effects of these programs seemed appropriate for more complicated patients with coronary artery disease. See Box 1-1 for an example of an early mobilization phase 1 protocol dating from the late 1960s.

Phase 2 Cardiac Rehabilitation

Phase 2, the convalescent phase, followed hospital discharge and was originally referred to as the "home phase."[24] These early programs lasted 6 to 8 weeks, depending on the patient status. Physicians were acting on the notion that myocardial scar formation takes between 6 and 8 weeks. Thus, phase 2 allowed the heart muscle the time to heal. Patients were not allowed to return to work. They were discharged from the hospital and instructed to continue the exercises performed in the hospital and commence a walking or biking program. This transitional phase was often difficult for patients and families because they were each independently adjusting to the new diagnosis and were often uncomfortable with the implementation of progressive activities.[24]

In the early 1980s, many phase 2 programs were extended for up to 12 weeks. Family and physician consultation was done on a regular basis. Additionally, risk-factor modification and

BOX 1-1

Summary of the 14-Step Wenger Program

Step 1   *Exercise:* Passive range of motion exercises to the upper and lower extremities.

     Activities of daily living: Begin feeding self with trunk and arm support using pillows.

     Activities: Initial interview—explain program.

Step 2   *Exercise:* Same as step 1.

     Activities of daily living: Patient may wash hands and face and brush teeth in bed.

     Activities: Finger and wrist craft activity in bed (eg, lacing a coin purse).

Step 3   *Exercise:* Passive and active range of motion exercises in bed.

     Activities of daily living: Same as step 2.

     Activities: Complete craft activity.

Step 4   *Exercise:* Active range of motion exercises progressing to minimal resistive exercises in bed.

     Activities of daily living: Same as step 2. Add dressing self. Use bedside commode.

     Activities: Begin copper tooling project.

Step 5   *Exercise:* Minimal to moderate resistive exercises.

     Activities of daily living: Chair sitting with self-feeding 3× day.

     Activities: Continue copper tooling project. Use higher-energy–level tools.

Step 6   *Exercise:* Begin use of 1- to 5-lb weights for upper and lower extremitiy exercises.

     Activities of daily living: Self-care activities. Walk to bathroom. Bathe self in tub.

     Activities: Refinish a precut wood project.

Step 7   *Exercise:* Add walking 50 ft down the hall.

     Activities of daily living: Same as step 6.

     Activities: Continue wood project.

Step 8   *Exercise:* Add trunk exercise. Add walking down one flight of stairs.

     Activities of daily living: Self-care activities plus walking down stairs.

     Activities: Continue wood project.

Step 9   *Exercise:* Add walking 50 ft × 2.

     Activities of daily living: Self-care activities plus walking down stairs.

     Activities: Begin metal hammering project.

Step 10   *Exercise:* Add trunk exercises using 1-lb weight.

     Activities of daily living: Self-care activities plus walking down stairs.

     Activities: Continue metal hammering project.

Step 11   *Exercise:* Same as step 10.

     Activities of daily living: Self-care activities plus walking down stairs.

     Activities: Continue metal hammering project.

Step 12   *Exercise:* Same as step 10. Add walking down two flights of stairs.

     Activities of daily living: Begin homemaking activities. Introduce conservation of energy techniques.

     Activities: Cut out wood project using a table saw.

Step 13   *Exercise:* Same as step 10. Add trunk exercises using a 2-lb weight.

     Activities of daily living: Walk down stairs.

     Activities: Continue wood project.

Step 14   *Exercise:* Add seated toe touches and walking up one flight of stairs.

     Activities of daily living: Same as step 12.

     Activities: Complete all projects.

Modified from Zohman LR, Tobis JS. *Cardiac Rehabilitation*. Orlando, FL: Grune & Stratton; 1970, with permission from Elsevier.

psychological and vocational outcomes were established.[25–28] In the early 1990s, phase 2 programs actually decreased in length as a result of reimbursement, severity of disease, and patient need.[26]

Phase 3 Cardiac Rehabilitation

Phase 3 followed approximately 6 to 12 weeks of convalescence at home.[24] Patients were medically supervised and frequently located in hospital-based outpatient departments or private cardiac rehabilitation facilities. Entrance into phase 3 began with the performance of a maximum, symptom-limited exercise test. The results of the test were used to write an exercise prescription, which was characterized by elevating the patient's heart rate to a relatively high level and maintaining it in a "training zone" for a prescribed period of time. The goal of such programs was the induction of an aerobic endurance training effect, which would allow the patient to participate in higher levels of activities before the onset of symptoms.[24–32] Patients were closely monitored during training sessions. After induction of this training effect, patients became candidates for phase 4 cardiac rehabilitation.

Phase 4 Cardiac Rehabilitation

Phase 4 programs were frequently located in YMCAs, Jewish community centers, university settings, or physical therapy private practices where patients could exercise and have their vital signs monitored.[24] Patients in phase 4 were considered medically stable and only occasionally monitored during moderate levels of exercise, which often included recreational activities like noncompetitive basketball, kickball, and volleyball. An ECG monitor and crash cart were brought into the gym or other exercise area. Patients were instructed to monitor their own pulse and occasionally stop by the ECG station for an ECG check. These phase 4 programs had a significant impact on secondary prevention and were also used as primary intervention for individuals at high risk for coronary events.[24–32]

Use of Weiss and Karpovich Calisthenic Exercises in Cardiac Rehabilitation

Many exercises performed by patients in phase 1 and phase 2 cardiac rehabilitation programs appear to have been based on the work of Weiss and Karpovich,[33] who developed a series of progressive calisthenic exercises suitable for patients recovering from coronary events. The authors performed expired gas analysis on an Air Force pilot while he performed dozens of calisthenic exercises. These exercises were then rank ordered by MET (metabolic equivalent) requirement from low level to moderate level. Although their paper was based on a single subject who was free of disease, these exercises found their way into inpatient and outpatient cardiac rehabilitation programs in the 1970s and 1980s, where fairly precise calibration of exercise energy requirements was deemed important. The exercises were performed to a metronome and could be administered to the patient individually in the patient's room (phase 1) or later on in a group setting (phase 2 or phase 4). See Fig. 1-2.

Cardiac Rehabilitation Guideline

In the mid-1980s, a new national professional organization, the American Association of Cardiovascular and Pulmonary Rehabilitation (AACVPR), emerged as an organization dedicated to the improvement of clinical practice, promotion of scientific inquiry, and the advancement of education. The uniqueness of this organization was and continues to be the contributions of physicians, nurses, and allied health professionals, each of whom brings a unique set of practice patterns and educational perspectives to the area of cardiac and pulmonary rehabilitation.

In 1990, the AACVPR published a position paper on the scientific merits of exercise and risk factor modification in the management of patients with coronary artery disease.[34] This position paper was an important initial step in documenting the scientific basis of cardiac rehabilitation. However, over the next few years, managed care and the changes in health care reimbursement motivated the Agency for Health Care Policy and Research (AHCPR) to begin a reassessment of cardiac rehabilitation as an intervention.

The Agency for Health Care Policy and Research is the federal agency responsible for evaluating the quality, appropriateness, and effectiveness of health care services and access to these services. The Agency for Health Care Policy and Research carries out its mission by conducting and supporting general health services research, including medical effectiveness research, facilitating development of clinical practice guidelines, and disseminating research guidelines to health care providers, policymakers, and the public. The AACVPR saw an opportunity to promote a multidisciplinary approach to cardiopulmonary

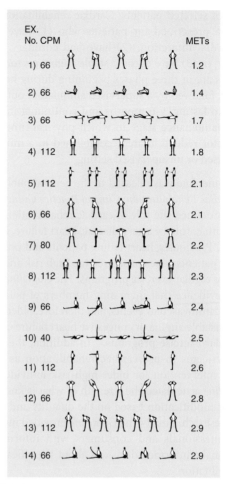

FIGURE 1-2   Example of a series of exercises from Weiss and Karpovich. Note the metronome cadence in CPM (counts per minute) and the energy requirements (in METS). (Reproduced with permission from Weiss RA, Karpovich PV. Energy cost of exercises for convalescents. *Arch Phys Med.* 1947;28:447.)

rehabilitation and submitted a proposal to the Health Care Finance Administration that would validate the scientific basis of cardiac rehabilitation and describe the current standards of practice. The contract was awarded to the AACVPR, which convened a private-sector multidisciplinary panel of experts that included physicians, nurses, physical therapists, other allied health professionals, and consumers. The panel based its conclusions and recommendations on scientific evidence from an extensive review of original research published in peer-reviewed medical and health science journals. The panel used the following definition of cardiac rehabilitation:

Cardiac rehabilitation services are comprehensive, long-term programs involving medical evaluation, prescribed exercise, cardiac risk factor modification, education, and counseling. These programs are designed to limit physiologic and psychological effects of cardiac illness, reduce the risk of sudden death or reinfarction, control cardiac symptoms, stabilize or reverse the atherosclerotic process, and enhance the psychological and vocational status of selected patients. Cardiac rehabilitation services are prescribed for patients who (1) have had a myocardial infarction; (2) have had coronary bypass surgery; or (3) have chronic stable angina pectoris. The services are in three phases beginning during hospitalization, followed by a supervised ambulatory outpatient program lasting 3–6 months and continuing in a lifetime maintenance stage in which physical fitness and risk factor reduction are accomplished in a minimally supervised or unsupervised setting.[35]

The guideline was released to the general public in 1995 as the *Cardiac Rehabilitation: Clinical Practice Guideline Number 17*.[35] It defined the role of cardiac rehabilitation for adult patients with coronary artery disease, heart failure, and transplantation. Previously, heart failure patients and post–cardiac transplant patients were considered too high risk and were not referred for regular exercise programs. The *Guideline* provided scientific evidence that increasing numbers of patients were surviving cardiovascular events, and therefore, older individuals with unstable angina or congestive heart failure can benefit from regular exercise programs.[35] In addition, the *Guideline* urged physicians to use cardiac rehabilitation as a regular treatment intervention for older high-risk individuals. Also, the *Guideline* articulated the strength of what is known about risk-factor modification based on the quantity and quality of available research. Finally, the *Guideline* provided medical and health professionals and consumers with information on which to make informed decisions about the efficacy of cardiac rehabilitation.

PULMONARY REHABILITATION

The history of pulmonary rehabilitation is not as clear-cut as that described for cardiac rehabilitation. The first real documentation of treatment for "chest conditions" was that of chest physical therapy performed at the famous Brompton Hospital in England in 1934. The basic techniques of breathing exercises and postural drainage were used with a wide variety of medical and surgical cardiothoracic conditions. In addition, artificial ventilation and intermittent positive pressure breathing were valuable adjuncts to "chest physiotherapy."

The polio epidemic in the 1950s caused a reevaluation of the use of chest physical therapy, not only for individuals with pulmonary dysfunction but also as an adjunct to preoperative and postoperative care. Prior to this, patients with pulmonary dysfunction were told to rest and to be physically inactive because it was thought that exercise was deleterious to their fragile condition. Like patients with heart disease, these individuals were treated as invalids and popularly called "respiratory cripples."[36-38] However, intervention options changed when, in 1964, Pierce et al.[37] demonstrated an improvement in exercise abilities in patients with chronic obstructive pulmonary disease (COPD) after a treadmill walking program. Patients showed a modest decrease in exercise heart rate, respiratory rate, and minute ventilation after training. The

impact of these findings on patients with chronic pulmonary disease indicated a need for further outcome evaluation. This came at a time when morbidity and mortality had increased dramatically in the United States and throughout the world. Early detection was and will continue to be an important step in the rehabilitation process because many of these individuals live with severe symptoms that limit physical activity and a productive lifestyle.

Most research in the area of COPD has demonstrated small gains in exercise capacity but not reversal of the progression of the disease process.[39,40] The creation of pulmonary rehabilitation as an intervention strategy has historically been attributed to Thomas Petty, who began extensive study of patients with COPD, participating in an inpatient and outpatient program in Denver, Colorado. However, Alvin Barach appears to have been just as instrumental in the development of pulmonary rehabilitation as it pertained first to patients with polio and then to patients with COPD. Over time, many studies suggested that pulmonary rehabilitation enhances the patient's sense of well-being, improves exercise capacity, decreases the need for hospitalization, and therefore, lowers overall health costs.[41-42] Today, many successful pulmonary rehabilitation programs are currently in existence and recognize the important interactions of psychological and emotional characteristics on physical work capacity.

In 1974, the American College of Chest Physician's Committee on Pulmonary Rehabilitation adopted a definition of pulmonary rehabilitation that is widely used today.[43] The American Thoracic Society also incorporated this definition into an official position statement on pulmonary rehabilitation in 1981[44]:

> Pulmonary Rehabilitation may be defined as an art of medical practice wherein an individually tailored multidisciplinary program is formulated which, through accurate diagnosis, therapy, emotional support, and education, stabilizes or reverses both the physio- and psychopathology of pulmonary disease, and attempts to return the patient to the highest possible functional capacity allowed by his pulmonary handicap and overall life situation.[44]

Inpatient Pulmonary Rehabilitation Programs

Chest physical therapy, ie, the use of chest percussion for the purpose of airway clearance, became an accepted and successful therapeutic intervention during the late 1950s, particularly with polio victims. The implementation of chest physical therapy expanded in the late 1960s and 1970s as a pre- and postoperative technique to minimize the complications of surgery and later expanded to all acute and chronic patients at risk for pulmonary complications due to medical conditions or surgical interventions.[45-49]

Upper respiratory infections are the most common complications for individuals with pulmonary impairment. These infections range in severity from colds to pneumonia. The goals of acute pulmonary care are focused around improvement of ventilation and gas exchange, improvement of secretion clearance, and the maintenance of functional capacity.[45] Patients may receive interventions from a number of allied health professionals including, but not limited to, physical therapists, respiratory therapists, and nurses. The limited length of hospital stay does not generally allow enough time for an exercise program geared toward improving functional capacity. However, a home program is usually developed that includes a combination of airway clearance techniques, breathing exercises, and a progressive exercise program. Inpatient pulmonary care programs have been shown to be effective for treating patients with pulmonary disease and/or reducing the risk of pneumonia postoperatively.[46] To that end, in the 1970s, many hospitals adopted preoperative and postoperative chest physical therapy programs as a means of reducing the deleterious effects of surgery and other complications seen with normal and high-risk surgical patients.[47] Preoperative examinations identified individuals with musculoskeletal limitations, an ineffective cough, or a high-risk profile. A preoperative patient education session informed the patient on what to expect postoperatively and often reduced the patient's anxiety about monitoring devices and postoperative management protocols. Most intensive care units today routinely refer patients to physical therapy for chest physical therapy. As a result of this intervention, outcome studies[48–50] have shown a reduction in length of hospital stay, a reduction in postsurgical complications, and a more immediate return to activities of daily living and work.

Outpatient Pulmonary Rehabilitation Programs

The success of acute care chest physical therapy in the 1970s was attributed to reduction of morbidity and mortality in both medical and surgical patients. It was also shown to reduce the economic costs associated with hospital stay.[47–53] On the basis of the same concepts as outpatient cardiac rehabilitation programs, formalized outpatient pulmonary rehabilitation programs began to emerge. As with cardiac rehabilitation programs, these programs were outpatient hospital-based programs and community-based programs. In addition, established cardiac rehabilitation programs expanded their program options to include patients with other chronic diseases such as pulmonary disease, renal disease, or metabolic disease.[42,52,54] Typically, referrals to these programs occurred posthospitalization after an acute exacerbation or when individuals with chronic diseases were diagnosed. Then, as now, most common referrals were due to symptoms such as dyspnea that interfere with the ability to maintain appropriate levels of physical activity. Most recently, rehabilitation research has emphasized functional outcomes as a means of evaluating efficacy in lieu of physiologic parameters.[51,52] As with cardiac rehabilitation, the goals of these expanded outpatient programs are aimed at restoring optimal physical and psychological functions that include exercise, education, and counseling.

The essential components of an effective pulmonary rehabilitation program are team assessment, patient training, exercise, psychological interventions, and follow-up. Each patient may not need all of these services, but an individualized comprehensive program is the key to success. The team may include a wide range of health care professionals such as the medical director, respiratory care practitioner, the nurse, the physical therapist, the psychologist, the vocational counselor, the social worker, and the nutritionist. The exercise component not only includes exercise conditioning, as well as a good home exercise program, but also builds on upper extremity and respiratory muscle strengthening. Patient training for functional independence may include breathing retraining, bronchial hygiene, nutrition, activities of daily living training, relaxation techniques, energy conservation, and warning signs of infection. Knowledge in these areas empowers the patient to manage his or her care. Finally, the support systems put in place directly influence the psychosocial aspect of care. Physical therapists played an important role in outpatient hospital-based pulmonary rehabilitation programs. The continuum of care from inpatient to outpatient services is often critical in reducing costs and maintaining functional independence of patients with chronic pulmonary dysfunction.

As managed care emerged, pulmonary rehabilitation was viewed as an appropriate intervention, but was not necessarily successful in improving pulmonary function or reversing pulmonary disease progression. Third-party payers reduced the benefits paid for pulmonary rehabilitation. Once again, health care professionals involved in the care of patients with pulmonary disease initiated a formal evaluation of pulmonary rehabilitation as a treatment intervention in order to document the validity of pulmonary rehabilitation as a successful intervention for third-party reimbursers.

In the 1990s, the AACVPR published a position paper on the scientific basis of pulmonary rehabilitation.[53,54] This position paper was written in response to the long-held view that pulmonary rehabilitation was not an effective intervention for patients with pulmonary disease, because many patients showed deteriorating function and eventual death in spite of program participation. Reimbursers continued to view pulmonary rehabilitation as a maintenance activity and therefore limited the benefits that they paid out for rehabilitation. This paper provided scientific evidence that most pulmonary rehabilitation programs ". . . have been developed based on sound preventative, therapeutic and rehabilitative principles with the goal of training patients in specific techniques and strategies to improve functional capacity and reduce the economic, medical and social burdens of their disease."[43,53–54]

Today, the importance of both cardiac and pulmonary rehabilitation has been well-documented and continues to play a role in the continuum of care. Although reimbursement for these programs has been reduced, modest benefits are still in existence to allow for short-term objectives to be met. The one critical element lost in this process is the time necessary for appropriate patient education. The ability of the physical therapist to ensure that the patient is able to follow the outlined program and progress effectively is still in question.

TURF WARS

The role of the physical therapist in cardiopulmonary rehabilitation has expanded over the last 30 years. Initially, the physical therapist was involved only with the inpatient phase of cardiac and pulmonary rehabilitation. Patients with coronary disease were not seen in the intensive care unit by physical therapy. Physical therapy involvement came only after the patient was stabilized and moved to a step-down unit. Progression of activity was at the discretion of the physician. Vital signs and all other monitoring were within the responsibilities of the nurse. Patients with pulmonary disease, particularly those individuals with pneumonia/atelectasis, were referred to physical therapy for examination and intervention including postural drainage, breathing exercises, and energy conservation techniques. Soon, however, physical therapists were performing all preoperative evaluations and instructions for surgical patients and then were following the patient postoperatively for chest physical therapy.

During the 1980s and 1990s, physical therapists were responsible for directing cardiopulmonary rehabilitation programs in a variety of settings. In states with direct access, examination and intervention procedures were performed by physical therapists in all phases of cardiopulmonary rehabilitation. During this period, health care professionals from other disciplines began to challenge the role of the physical therapist as a primary provider of cardiopulmonary rehabilitation services. Physical therapists, physicians, nurses, occupational therapists, respiratory therapists, and exercise physiologists—all participated in turf wars, in an effort to broaden the scope of their practice. Hospitals from all across the country became the battleground for these turf wars. When the smoke cleared, it became apparent that individual hospitals representing the peculiarities of their respective geographic regions were the primary determinant of which allied health professionals would be the primary providers of cardiopulmonary services. Coincidentally, from the 1960s through the 1980s health maintenance organizations (HMOs), preferred provider organizations (PPOs), and diagnosis-related groups (DRGs) were being developed.[55] Purchasers of medical care, both public and private, became increasingly concerned about the rising cost of health care and more reluctant to shoulder the cost of such care. Purchasers began to question the wide variations in practice patterns across

diverse geographic areas and the lack of uniformity in delivery systems.[55]

In the early 1980s, respiratory therapists and nurses were claiming "chest physical therapy" as their own intervention. Physical therapy took the lead in responding to the challenges of turf wars, the appearance of managed care groups, and rising health care costs by defining the role of the physical therapist in cardiopulmonary care. In 1982, the Cardiopulmonary Section of the American Physical Therapy Association (APTA) published a definition of chest physical therapy and validated this as "an array of treatment interventions unique to the physical therapist" that are included as part of the interdisciplinary team approach to cardiopulmonary rehabilitation.[56] Additionally, the December 1985 APTA journal devoted an entire issue to cardiac rehabilitation. This special issue further defined the role of the physical therapist in cardiac rehabilitation and reinforced the need for the development of clinical specialization.[57]

THE EMERGENCE OF SPECIALIZATION

In 1973, the APTA published a position paper on competence testing. In 1976, the House of Delegates of the APTA approved the concept of specialization and established the Task Force on Clinical Specialization. In 1977, a working document delineating competencies in physical therapy was published, titled, *Competencies in Physical Therapy: An Analysis of Practice.* In 1978, the House of Delegates recognized four specialty areas, including cardiopulmonary physical therapy. Each specialty council was asked to develop advanced-level competencies that would form the foundation for specialty certification. The Cardiopulmonary Section of the APTA completed this task in 1983 and submitted a Validation for Patient Care Competency in Cardiopulmonary Physical Therapy. These competencies were in the area of patient care, educational services, communications, research, administration, and consultation. Criteria for revalidation of those initial competencies were completed in 1987 and updated in 1996.[58] The Cardiopulmonary Specialty Examination was the first of the specialty examinations to be offered in 1985, resulting in three candidates receiving specialty certification. As of June 2003, 88 individuals have achieved specialty certification awarded by the American Board of Physical Therapy Specialties and 26 individuals have been recertified. This professional certification process has become widely accepted within the profession, and the creation of this credentialing process has garnered respect from other allied health professionals as they strive to define competencies in their own clinical care areas.

VALIDATION OF CARDIOPULMONARY CLINICAL COMPETENCIES

Validation of cardiopulmonary clinical competencies has been previously performed.[59–63] Two validations, or self-studies, have been performed in the cardiopulmonary physical therapy field: one that validates competencies that the entry-level practitioner should master and the other validates advanced clinical competencies appropriate to the cardiopulmonary clinical specialist.[59,62]

Entry-Level Competencies

When students graduate, become licensed, get their first job, and are assigned to a cardiopulmonary service, what should they be able to do? In an effort to guide entry-level professional-phase education programs, a Cardiovascular and Pulmonary Section Task Force was formed, and in 1985 it put forth a set of entry-level clinical competencies.[59] These competencies were updated in 1992.[60]

A task force was named in August 1993, with the intent to validate the entry-level competencies. The project was completed in 1994. Entry-level competency components prioritized as high included those that represented activity tolerance evaluation, general conditioning exercises and exercise prescription, and "evaluating the effects of therapeutic procedures and stating the relationship of those effects [to] the client." Advanced skills (ie, not entry level) included those that involved interpretation of special tests (eg, ECG, blood profiles), interacting with patients on mechanical ventilation, suctioning, and auscultation of heart sounds. Of moderate importance were appreciation of breath sounds and differentiation between chest wall and anginal pain. This survey and several presentations were the first of their kind to validate professional or entry-level competencies in physical therapy.[60,61]

Advanced Level Competencies: Cardiopulmonary Clinical Specialization

A physical therapist with clinical experience on a cardiopulmonary service may be eligible for board certification as a clinical specialist. What are the qualities and skills that separate the entry-level practitioner from the specialist? This issue is examined every 10 years through a process that revalidates existing advanced clinical competencies. The latest revalidation was begun in early 1994 and completed in mid-1996.[62] Like the entry-level process, the advanced competency process utilized a survey instrument. It identified selected tasks and skills and required the therapist to estimate the level of knowledge (entry level or advanced), importance, and frequency of use. It was sent out to members of the Cardiovascular and Pulmonary Section and to clinical specialists. The results of the survey were released in the summer of 1999.[62]

The survey suggested that most of the elements listed under assessment, therapeutic intervention, response to change, discharge, education, and communication were found to be of entry level. Advanced skills included research, administration, and consultation. Also identified as advanced skills were ECG interpretation, performance of exercise stress testing, heart auscultation, nasotracheal and endotracheal suctioning, and the treatment of patients on mechanical inotropic support. Treatment of patients in the intensive care unit and recovery unit were considered advanced clinical practice settings.[62] These advanced skills were analogous to those skills identified as advanced in the entry-level survey.

As a result of practice revalidation, a new specialist examination was created in order to more accurately reflect current best practice. All the questions were based on case studies, an approach that is different from the other six clinical specialty areas, which utilize free-standing multiple-choice questions. The content of the examination was changed to reflect the higher level of practice and training among entry-level therapists. Assessment was weighted 25% of the total examination, therapeutic intervention was 45%, and other activities like administration and research were weighted the remaining 30%. Another revalidation survey which was conducted in 2004 reflected more changes in cardiopulmonary patient care because of the dramatic changes brought about by health care reform.

THE 1990S: HEALTH CARE REFORM AND ITS CHALLENGES

The advent of managed care has had significant and far-reaching effects on providers of rehabilitation services. When the Clinton administration began its push for health care reform in 1994, the APTA praised these efforts as ". . . a bold step toward addressing the nation's health care problems."[64] However, the plan failed to incorporate the scope of physical therapy practice beyond the rehabilitative area and failed to extend it to such areas as work-related injury prevention, preventative services in musculoskeletal and cardiopulmonary areas, as well as fitness exercise and consumer education. Additionally, the plan contained inadequate provisions for the treatment of chronic or congenital conditions as well as coverage for patients with chronic conditions that affect functional independence. Finally, restrictions on self-referrals by health care providers needed to be expanded in light of the increasing number of states that had adopted "direct access" or the Independent Practice Acts for Physical Therapists.[64]

Making the transition to managed care by physical therapy has required a blend of well-timed and coordinated strategies. Inherent in this transition was the acceptance of a paradigm shift in the philosophy and practice of physical therapy and the inclusion of cost-containment efforts.[65] One of the most positive benefits arising from health care reform has been an increased emphasis on outcome management and evidence-based practice. Practitioners were urged to become more accountable and responsible for patient outcomes by providing cost-effective and efficient services that would meet consumers' needs and support the mission of the APTA.[65] One strategy that was developed to achieve this

Nursing Sisters Home Care   P. T.   COPD Pathway   PHASE I (Visit _____)

Patient Name _____ Town _____ PID# _____

ASSESSMENT ☐ Homebound status : 9 Bed bound   9 Blind   9 Cognitive impairment   9 Lost use of UEs   9 SOB or severe fatigue after amb. _____ feet   9 PWB/NWB requiring significant effort to get out   9 Considerable and taxing effort 9 Homebound due to medical condition restricted by M.D. **Specify** _____

☐ Vital signs prn B/P: _____ PR: _____ R: _____
After activity B/P _____ PR _____ R _____

☐ Assess barriers for learning: Medication _____

☐ Oxygen _____

☐ Assess pain level _____ (0-10) Location: _____

Intervention: Medication/Response: _____

☐ Subjective comments: _____

☐ Bed Mobility/Transfers: _____

☐ Balance: Static/Dynamic (circle) _____
_____

☐ Ambulation: Device _____ WB _____ Even _____

Uneven _____

☐ Endurance:_____

☐ Stairs: _____

☐ ROM/MMT:_____
_____

☐ Instruction to Pt./Family (circle) Specify:_____

☐ Self-care/ADL_____
_____

Narrative:_____
_____
_____
_____

KNOWLEDGE ☐ Instruct/assess for safe home environment/fall prevention education | **DISCHARGE** ☐ Discharge planning started
☐ Patient educated in safe use of equipment | **PLANNING**   Comments: _____
☐ Begin to teach HEP

Check all appropriate treatments:

97002	**Physical Therapy Re-Evaluation?**		97530	**Therapeutic activities, dynamic activities, TT, Bed Mob.**
97110	**Therapeutic Exercises?**		97535	**Self-care/home management training (ADL)**
97112	**Neuromuscular re-education, balance/coordination**		97542	**W/C management and training**
97116	**Gait Training/Stairs**		97139	**HEP instruction/progression**
97504	**Orthotic Training**		97139	**Unlisted Ther. Procedure(specify)**

PATIENT/CAREGIVER OUTCOMES/GOALS?	Met	Not Met	Comments	NA
1. Pt/caregiver demonstrates understanding of proper breathing technique?				
2. Pt beginning to verbalize understanding of energy conservation tech?				
3. Home environment assessed to be safe?				
4. Patient verbalizes understanding of fall prevention?				
5. Performs HEP with cueing?				
6. Pt/caregiver understands safe use of equipment?				

Plan:_____ ☐ **Progress to phase 2**

Communication/New Equipment or MD orders:_____
_____

Signature _____Title_____ Frequency _____Date _____
Patient Signature _____AT_____ DT_____

(Phase 1 – COPD Pathway PT)   3-2-01

FIGURE 1-3 An example of a clinical pathway, this one for chronic obstructive pulmonary disease. Developed in November 1999 with the cooperation of the Catholic Health Systems of Long Island and Long Island Health Network. Used with permission.

was the establishment of clinical pathways. Clinical pathways are algorithms that link interventions to expected outcomes for selected groups of patients. Clinical pathways allow health systems to standardize care and to improve the process and outcomes of care.[55] Figure 1-3 presents an example of a clinical pathway, developed in November 1999, with the cooperation of the Catholic Health Systems of Long Island Health Network. Another method to provide cost-effective and efficient services is to have a primary physician orchestrate all aspects of the individuals' health care. This, in combination with the introduction of a prospective payment system (PPS), where a standardized fee is paid per diagnosis, has made significant cuts in health care. All of these health care reforms have changed the scope of rehabilitation practice.

SUMMARY

The important message that underlies much of this chapter is that, as physical therapists, we must not relinquish the important clinical services that we provide to patients with cardiovascular and pulmonary disease. It is clear that as professionals we need to remain involved with our professional organization in order to protect the patient, and we need to support changes in health care management that have a positive influence on rehabilitation services. Managed care today assumes many forms, invokes multiple strategies, and influences choices of care, quality of care, and pricing of care. In such a rapidly changing environment, it is difficult to identify and respond to trends because today's trends are just that—"today's trends."[55] What is clear is the need to nurture and support the profession while continuing to educate the public on the vital role that physical therapy plays not only in cardiopulmonary care but also in all aspects of the health care market.

As a health care professional in the 21st century, the physical therapist must be competent in the area of assessment. Every patient/client has a cardiopulmonary system. The cardiopulmonary examination should be an integral component of every patient profile. Every physical therapist should have, at a minimum, the knowledge and skills identified as entry-level competencies in cardiopulmonary care. These skills will ensure a proper examination together with the recognition of indications for intervention, based on the identification of impairments, functional limitations, disabilities, or other special needs that may warrant further tests and measures. A thorough evaluation will ensure that interventions are both safe and effective and that goals are realistic and attainable.

It is imperative that the cardiopulmonary physical therapists of the 21st century acquire advanced knowledge in order to maintain quality of patient care. This can be achieved through membership in the Cardiovascular and Pulmonary Section of the APTA and other cardiovascular and pulmonary national organizations, enrollment in continuing education courses, attendance at national and state conferences, participation in in-services and case study presentations to peers, and provision of patient care in a wide variety of settings. The true strength of the profession resides in the strength of its constituency. The cardiopulmonary physical therapist who maintains his or her clinical competency and practices with integrity, care, and precision will serve both the profession and the patient well.

REFERENCES

1. Heberden W. Some accounts of a disorder of the chest. *Med Trans Coll Physicians.* 1772;2:59.
2. Parry CH. *An Inquiry into the Symptoms and Causes of Syncopy Anginosa Commonly Called Angina Pectoris.* London, UK: Cadwell and Davis; 1799.
3. Mallory GK, White PD, Salcedo-Salger J. The speed of healing of myocardial infarction: a study of the pathological anatomy of seventy-two cases. *Am Heart J.* 1939;18:647-671.
4. Masters AM, Oppenheimer ET. A simple exercise tolerance test for circulatory efficiency with standard tables for normal individuals. *Am J Med Sci.* 1929;177:223.
5. Zohman LR, Tobis JS. *Cardiac Rehabilitation.* Orlando, FL: Grune & Stratton; 1970.
6. Levine SA, Lown B. Armchair treatment of acute coronary thrombosis. *JAMA.* 1952;148:1365.
7. Katz LN. Symposium: unsettled clinical questions in the management of cardiovascular disease. *Circulation.* 1953;18:430-450.
8. Turell D, Hellerstein H. Evaluation of cardiac function in relation to specific physical activities following recovery from acute myocardial infarction. *Prog Cardiovasc Dis.* 1958;1(2):237.
9. Sanders MJ. *Mosby's Paramedic Textbook.* 2nd ed. Philadelphia, PA: Harcourt; 2001.
10. Wenger NK. *Coronary Care—Rehabilitation After Myocardial Infarction.* Dallas, TX: American Heart Association; 1973.
11. Moss AJ, DeCamilla J, Davis H. Cardiac death in the first six months after a myocardial infarction: potential for mortality reduction in the early post hospital period. *Am J Cardiol.* 1977;39:816.
12. Detrich H. Effects of immobilization upon various metabolic and physiologic functions of normal men. *Am J Med.* 1948;4:3.
13. Saltin B, Bloomquist G, Mitchel JH, et al. Response to exercise after bed rest and after training. *Circulation.* 1968;38(suppl VII):1-78.
14. Wenger N. The use of exercise in the rehabilitation of patients after myocardial infarction. *J S C Med Assoc.* 1969;65(suppl 1):66-68.
15. Zohman L, Tobis JS. A rehabilitation program for inpatients with recent myocardial infarction. *Arch Phys Med Rehabil.* 1968;49:443.
16. Bruce RA. Evaluation of functional capacity in patients with cardiovascular disease. *Geriatrics.* 1957;12:317.
17. Wenger NK, Gilbert CA, Siegel W. Symposium: the use of physical activity in the rehabilitation of patients after myocardial infarction. *South Med J.* 1970;63:891-897.
18. Zohman L. Early ambulation of post-myocardial infarction patients: Montefiore Hospital. In: Naughton J, Hellerstein HK, eds. *Exercise Testing and Exercise Training in Coronary Heart Disease.* Orlando, FL: Academic Press; 1973;329-335.

19. Kannel WB, Castelli WP, Gordon T, McNamara P. Serum cholesterol, lipoproteins and the risk of coronary heart disease: the Framingham study. *Ann Intern Med.* 1971;74:1.

20. Kannel WB, McGee D, Gordon T. A general cardiovascular risk profile: the Framingham study. *Am J Cardiol.* 1976;38:46.

21. Kannel WB, Castelli WP, Gordon P. Cholesterol in the prediction of atherosclerotic disease: new perspectives based on the Framingham study. *Ann Intern Med.* 1979;90:85.

22. Cohen BS, Grant A. Acute myocardial infarction: effect of a rehabilitation program on length of hospitalization and functional status at discharge. *Arch Phys Med Rehabil.* 1971;54:201-206.

23. Cohen BS. A program for rehabilitation after acute myocardial infarction. *South Med J.* 1975;68:145-148.

24. Hellerstein H. Exercise therapy in coronary disease. *Bull N Y Acad Med.* 1968;44:1028-1047.

25. Foster C, Pollock ML, Anholm JD, et al. Work capacity in left ventricular function during rehabilitation after myocardial revascularization surgery. *Circulation.* 1984;69:748-755.

26. American Association of Cardiovascular and Pulmonary Rehabilitation. *Guidelines for Cardiac Rehabilitation Programs.* Champaign, IL: Human Kinetics; 1991.

27. Health and Public Policy Committee, American College of Physicians. Cardiac rehabilitative services. *Ann Intern Med.* 1988;1098:671-673.

28. May GS, Eberlein KA, Furberg CD, Passamani ER, DeMets DL. Secondary prevention after myocardial infarction: a review of long-term trials. *Prog Cardiovasc Dis.* 1982;24:331-362.

29. Vermueulen A, Lie K, Derer D. Effects of cardiac rehabilitation after myocardial infarction: changes in coronary risk factors and long-term prognosis. *Am Heart J.* 1983;105:798-801.

30. Oldridge NB, Guyait GH, Fischer ME, Rimm AA. Cardiac rehabilitation after myocardial infarction. Combined experience of randomized clinical trials. *JAMA.* 1988;260:945-950.

31. Thompson PD. The benefits and risks of exercise training in patients with chronic coronary artery disease. *JAMA.* 1988;259:1537-1540.

32. O'Connor GT, Buring JE, Yusaf S, et al. An overview of randomized trials of rehabilitation with exercise after myocardial infarction. *Circulation.* 1989;80(2):234-244.

33. Weiss RA, Karpovich PV. Energy cost of exercises for convalescents. *Arch Phys Med Rehabil.* 1947;28:7.

34. Leon AS, Certo C, Comoss P, et al. Position paper of the American Association of Cardiovascular and Pulmonary Rehabilitation: scientific evidence of the value of cardiac rehabilitation services with emphasis on patients following myocardial infarction—section 1: exercise conditioning component. *J Cardiopulm Rehabil.* 1990;10:79-87.

35. Wenger NK, Froelicher ES, Smith LK, et al. *Cardiac Rehabilitation. Clinical Practice Guideline No. 17.* Rockville, MD: U.S. Department of Health and Human Services, Public Health Service, Agency for Health Care Policy and Research, and the National Heart, Lung, and Blood Institute; 1995. AHCPR Publication No. 96-0672.

36. Hughes R, Davidson R. Limitation of exercise reconditioning in cold. *Chest.* 1983;83(2):241-249.

37. Pierce A et al. Responses to exercise training in patients with emphysema. *Arch Intern Med.* 1964;114:28-36.

38. Hale T, Cumming G, Spriggs J. The effects of physical training in chronic obstructive pulmonary disease. *Bull Eur Physiopathol Respir.* 1978;14:593-608.

39. Bedout D, Hodgkin J, Zorn E, et al. Clinical and physiological outcomes of a university hospital pulmonary rehabilitation program. *Respir Care.* 1983;28(11):1468-1471.

40. Carter R, Nicotra B, Clark L, et al. Exercise conditioning in the rehabilitation of patients with chronic obstructive pulmonary disease. *Arch Phys Med Rehabil.* 1988;69:118-121.

41. Belman M, Wasserman K. Exercise training and testing in patients with chronic obstructive pulmonary disease. *Basic Respir Dis.* 1981;10:1-6.

42. Sneider R, O'Malley J, Kahn M. Trends in pulmonary rehabilitation at Eisenhower Medical Center: an 11-year experience (1976–1987). *J Cardiopulm Rehabil.* 1988;11:453-461.

43. American Association of Cardiovascular and Pulmonary Rehabilitation. *Guidelines for Pulmonary Rehabilitation Programs.* Champaign, IL: Human Kinetics; 1993.

44. American Thoracic Society. Pulmonary rehabilitation: official American Thoracic Society position statement. *Am Rev Respir Dis.* 1981;124:663-666.

45. Holden DA, Stelmach KD, Curtis PS, et al. The impact of a rehabilitation program on functional status of patients with chronic lung disease. *Respir Care.* 1990;35(4):332-341.

46. Oldenburg FA, Dolovica MB, Montgomery JM, et al. Effects of postural drainage, exercise and cough on mucus clearance in chronic bronchitis. *Am Rev Respir Dis.* 1979;120:739-745.

47. Jenkins SC. International perspectives in physical therapy 7: respiratory care. In: Pryor JA, ed. *Pre-operative and Postoperative Physiotherapy—Are They Necessary?* New York: Churchill Livingstone; 1991:62-67.

48. Forshag MS, Cooper AD. Clinics in chest medicine: thoracic surgical considerations for the pulmonologist. In: Buchalter SE, McElvein RB, eds. *Postoperative Care of the Thoracotomy Patient.* Philadelphia, PA: WB Saunders; 1992.

49. Sutton PP, Lopez-Vidriero MT, Pavia D, et al. Assessment of percussion, vibratory-shaking and breathing exercises in chest physiotherapy. *Eur J Respir Dis.* 1985;66:147-152.

50. Foster S, Thomas HM. Pulmonary rehabilitation in lung disease other than chronic obstructive pulmonary disease. *Am Rev Respir Dis.* 1990;141:601-604.

51. Moser KM, Bokinsky G, Savage RT, et al. Results of a comprehensive rehabilitation program: physiologic and functional effects of patients with chronic obstructive pulmonary disease. *Arch Intern Med.* 1980;140:1596-1601.

52. Swerts P. Kretzers L, Terpstra-Lindeman E, et al. Exercise reconditioning in the rehabilitation of patients with chronic obstructive pulmonary disease: a short- and long-term analysis. *Arch Phys Med Rehabil.* 1990;71:570-573.

53. Miller NH et al. Position paper of the American Association of Cardiovascular and Pulmonary Rehabilitation. *J Cardiopulm Rehabil.* 1990;10(6):198-209.

54. Reis A. Position paper of the American Association of Cardiovascular and Pulmonary Rehabilitation. Scientific basis of pulmonary rehabilitation. *J Cardiopulm Rehabil.* 1996;10:148-441.

55. Kongstvedt P. *The Managed Health Care Handbook.* 3rd ed. Gaithersburg, MD: Aspen Publishers; 1996.

56. Cardiopulmonary Section, American Physical Therapy Association. A definition of chest physical therapy. *Phys Ther Cardiopulm Sect Q.* 1982;3(3):14.

57. Cardiac rehabilitation. *Phys Ther.* 1995;65(12):1791-1865.

58. Cardiopulmonary Specialty Council. *Physical Therapy Advanced Clinical Competencies (cardiopulmonary).*

Alexandria, VA: Board for Certification of Advanced Clinical Competencies; 1988.

59. Cardiopulmonary Section, American Physical Therapy Association. Cardiopulmonary physical therapy entry-level competencies. *Phys Ther Cardiopulm Sect Q.* 1984:4-8.

60. Crane L. Cardiopulmonary entry-level competencies: then, now and in the future. *Phys Ther.* 1996;7(3):15-16.

61. Crane L. Testing validity of entry-level cardiopulmonary physical therapy competencies. Paper presented at: APTA Combined Sections Meeting; February 10, 1995; Reno, NV.

62. DeTurk W, Buck L, Cahalin L, et al. Revalidation of advanced clinical practice in cardiopulmonary physical therapy. *Cardiopulm Phys Therapy J.* 1999;10:105-108.

63. American Physical Therapy Association. *A Normative Model of Physical Therapist Professional Education.* Alexandria, VA: American Physical Therapy Association; 1997.

64. Moffat M. *Statement on Health Care Reform.* Alexandria, VA: American Physical Therapy Association; 1994.

65. Glickman L. An analysis of managed care—survival strategies for rehabilitation service providers: part four. *Resource.* 1998;28(3):1-7.

History and Use of the Guide

Gary Brooks* & Lawrence P. Cahalin

INTRODUCTION

The *Guide to Physical Therapist Practice* has been an important publication for the physical therapy community both nationally and internationally. It was developed out of a need to better define the role of the physical therapist (PT) in the changing health care arena.[1-8] Jules Rothstein, the editor of the journal *Physical Therapy,* presented his opinions about the role of the *Guide* in two separate editorials preceding the publication of the 1st and 2nd editions of the *Guide.*[3,4] Box 2-1 provides an overview of several of the comments made by Dr. Rothstein regarding the *Guide* including the definition of a guide (directions along a path): the fact that the *Guide,* to

its credit, is nonspecific (drawing large circles; practice patterns that are broadly defined) and that the *Guide* is a "very gross first approximation of what we do and what we should do . . . and possibly what we can do."[3,4] Dr. Rothstein concluded his editorial by stating that there is a need (1) for research to help narrow the circle (to develop practice patterns that are less broad and with more specificity) for future versions of the *Guide,* (2) for dialogue from all clinicians about whether the *Guide* helps or does not help them in their practice, and (3) to clarify particular items or change them in the future.[3]

Prior to the publication of the 2nd edition of the *Guide,* Dr. Rothstein made several statements similar to those mentioned previously, but it appeared that he was more cautious about the role of the *Guide* in physical therapy.[4] The following remarks, and others shown in Box 2-1, are examples of the apparent caution Dr. Rothstein has about the *Guide.* Some of the comments are that (1) the *Guide* should accurately convey what the tests, interventions, and preferred practice patterns are; (2) the *Guide* can greatly enhance practice—when it is properly used; (3) if the *Guide* is viewed as containing immutable truths, however, we will be using it incorrectly; and (4) the next edition of the *Guide* will be based primarily on evidence—and that PTs will use that evidence.[4] Related to the need for evidence and appropriate use of available evidence is the emphasis that Dr. Rothstein made on the Clinical Research Agenda, which likely has significant implications for both physical therapy practice and the future development of the *Guide.*[5]

One goal of this textbook is to use peer-reviewed published research to narrow the circle (to develop more specific practice patterns using hypothesis-oriented algorithms) and to clarify particular items, depending on peer-reviewed published research, published in the *Guide* (under the Cardiovascular and Pulmonary Practice Patterns). We hope that dialogue will ensue in physical therapy classrooms and clinics. It is also our hope that through such dialogue and evidence-based medicine, cardiovascular and pulmonary physical therapy examinations and managements will be (1) more easily taught and

understood, (2) more effective, and (3) justified to our patients, other health care providers, and health care payers.

DEVELOPMENT OF THE *GUIDE*

The *Guide* has been a work in progress for many years. Box 2-2 shows the chronological development of the *Guide.* The first step in the development of the *Guide* was a request from one of the American Physical Therapy Association's (APTA's) state components to develop practice parameters for physical therapy that could be provided to third-party payers and health care policymakers.[1,2,8]

Several other important steps in the development of the *Guide* included the development of *A Guide to Physical Therapist Practice, Volume I: A Description of Patient Management* ("Volume I") by an APTA board-appointed task force beginning in 1992, which included Roger Nelson, John Barbis, Eileen Hamby, Catherine Page, Robert Post, Gretchen Swanson, and Marilyn Moffat as the Practice Parameters Project Core Group; and Marilyn Moffat, Andrew Guccione, Roger Nelson, and Jayne Snyder as the task force to review practice parameters and taxonomy documents, the publication of Volume I in August of 1995, and the initiation of the process needed for the development of Volume II.[1,2,6-8]

As mentioned previously and documented in Box 2-2, following the acceptance of Part I by the APTA's board of

BOX 2-1

Editorial Comments Regarding the Preferred Practice Patterns

First Edition Comments

1. Definition of a guide as directions along a path.
2. The *Guide* is nonspecific and therefore good.
3. The *Guide* is not "intended to serve as clinical guidelines . . . and represents expert consensus."
4. The *Guide* draws large circles (practice patterns that are broadly defined).
5. The *Guide* is a "very gross first approximation of what we do and what we should do . . . and possibly what we can do."
6. The *Guide* has developed documents that will allow us to gain consensus on practice that can lead to the examination and refinement of that practice.
7. The *Guide* offers fodder for researchers and clinic managers.
8. The *Guide* begins to define the world of physical therapist practice.
9. There is a need for research to help narrow the circle (to develop practice patterns that are less broad with more specificity) for future versions of the *Guide*.
10. There is a need for dialogue from all clinicians about whether the *Guide* helps or does not help them in their practice.
11. There is a need to clarify particular items or change them in the future.

Second Edition Comments

1. The *Guide* forms a framework for describing and implementing practice.
2. The *Guide* has proven that it can be an invaluable adjunct to our literature.

3. Physical therapists need to understand what this new edition is—and what it is not.
4. The *Guide* contains the opinions of our colleagues on how to manage patients and clients—which is very different from evidence for practice.
5. The *Guide* is a work in progress.
6. It is hoped that the next edition of the *Guide* will appear soon—one that will be created not because of political necessity, but because of the need to codify a growing body of scientific knowledge.
7. We should look forward to a third edition of the *Guide* that relies less on personal views and more on evidence that becomes available in the public arena, evidence that deals directly with clinical practice and that has been published in peer-reviewed literature.
8. The *Guide* could never achieve the stated goal of ". . . standardizing terminology used in and related to physical therapist practice." The *Guide* instead contains an official or semiofficial version of how terms should be used. The journal *Physical Therapy* will continue to depend on scientific literature for the evolution of terms and definitions.
9. The *Guide* should accurately describe tests, interventions, and preferred practice patterns.
10. The *Guide* can greatly enhance practice—when it is properly used.
11. If the *Guide* is viewed as containing immutable truths, however, we will be using it incorrectly.
12. It is hoped that the next edition of the *Guide* will be based primarily on evidence—and that physical therapists will use that evidence.

Editorial comments made by Jules Rothstein in editorials preceding the publication of the 1st and 2nd editions of the *Guide*.[3,4]

directors, work began on Part II of the *Guide* in 1995. This effort was led by the Board Oversight Committee (BOC), made up of the current APTA president and two vice presidents, which appointed a six-member Project Advisory Group (PAG) to over see the development of preferred practice patterns for each of the four domains of practice. Together, the BOC and PAG chose 24 physical therapists with broad expertise in overall and specialty practice, familiarity with the scientific method and documentation procedures, and a willingness to work together to complete the project. These therapists formed the four panels of experts that created and revised the preferred practice patterns over the next 2 years. The cardiopulmonary panel of experts included Gary Brooks, Lawrence Cahalin, Dianne Carrio, Nancy Ciesla, and Ellen Hillegass.[2,8]

The pattern development process involved consensus of expert opinion as well as use of available scientific evidence to support or refute the examinations and interventions used in PT practice. Key concepts that guided the panelists during their deliberations included the Disablement Model, prevention and wellness considerations, the continuum of care across various practice settings and across the life span, and the influence of gender and culture. Each panel was charged with developing one primary prevention practice pattern.[2,8]

The development of the preferred practice patterns was an extensive process that included numerous consensus developing meetings among practice pattern specialty area panels; dialogue and feedback from the PAG and BOC; select reviews; suggestions; edits from APTA administration, components, and clinical specialists; and numerous field reviews from the APTA membership. After 2 years of meetings at APTA headquarters in Alexandria, VA (complete with floods, blizzards, and numerous other adventures), and countless phone calls and e-mails, the panels presented the PAG and BOC with a total of 34 preferred practice patterns. The patterns were meant to cover a broad array of patient/client problems, but were not intended to be totally inclusive. There are certainly patient/client situations that may not come under one of the preferred practice patterns; new features have been added and even new patterns have been proposed. Nor were the patterns meant to be prescriptive; in other words, they are not recipes in a cookbook. Rather, the patterns were meant to "describe

BOX 2-2

The Chronological Development of the Guide

1. Request from one of the APTA's state components to develop practice parameters for physical therapy which could be provided to third-party payers and health care policymakers in 1992.

2. Development of *A Guide to Physical Therapist Practice, Volume I: A Description of Patient Management* ("Volume I") by an APTA board-appointed task force from 1992 to 1995.

3. The publication of *A Guide to Physical Therapist Practice, Volume I: A Description of Patient Management* in August 1995.

4. Initiation of the process needed for the development of Volume II, which "was to be composed of descriptions of preferred physical therapist practice for patient groupings defined by common physical therapist management" in the fall of 1995.

5. APTA Board of Directors Oversight Committee, Project Advisory Group, and Panel members for the Musculoskeletal, Neuromuscular, Cardiopulmonary, and Integumentary Practices selected in the fall of 1995.

6. Development of the Practice Patterns by the Panel members for the Musculoskeletal, Neuromuscular, Cardiopulmonary, and Integumentary Practices from the fall of 1995 through 1996.

7. Field Review of the developed Practice Patterns late in 1996.

8. Analysis of the Field Review Results and editing of Practice Patterns through most of 1997.

9. Publication of Volume II as Part II of the *Guide* in November 1997.

10. APTA Board of Directors Oversight Committee, Project Editors for Parts I and II (consisting of three members of which two were members of the 1995–1997 Project Advisory Group and one was a member of the 1995–1997 APTA Board of Directors Oversight Committee), and a Task Force on Development of Part III of the *Guide* (consisting of 13 members of which 4 were members of one of the 1995–1997 practice panels and 2 were members of the 1995–1997 Project Advisory Group) were selected in 1998–1999.

11. Development of Part III of the *Guide* by two task forces (one task force to examine the available literature pertaining to tests and measures used in the assessment of the four primary areas of physical therapy [cardiovascular and pulmonary, integumentary, musculoskeletal, and neuromuscular] and one task force to retrieve and review the available literature on tests and measures of health status, health-related quality of life, and patient/client satisfaction) from 1998 to 2000.

12. Field reviews and presentations at APTA national meetings of comprehensive lists of tests and measures used by physical therapists throughout 1999–2000.

13. Revisions to the *Guide* in June 1999.

14. Revisions to the *Guide* in November 1999.

15. The *Guide* (Parts I and II) is edited and appears to undergo a limited field review in 1999–2000.

16. Publication of the 2nd edition of the *Guide to Physical Therapist Practice* in January 2001.

17. Part III of the *Guide* available on CD-ROM in the summer of 2001.

---

common sets of management strategies used by physical therapists for selected patient/client diagnostic groups."[2]

It is apparent from Box 2-1 that an important part of the development of the *Guide* is dialogue (in the form of both the written and the spoken word) from PTs about the *Guide*. Searches of MEDLINE and CINAHL identified only a few articles related to the practice patterns and the *Guide* (Box 2-3).[9–15] It is hoped that the profession will continue to critically appraise the clinical utility of this document.

This textbook will present numerous reviews of the literature with occasional research syntheses and meta-analyses when sufficient and adequate literature was available. The following sections will discuss particular aspects of Parts I and II of the *Guide* and will present methods to use the *Guide* and this textbook in an educational and clinical setting.

PART I OF THE *GUIDE TO PHYSICAL THERAPIST PRACTICE*

Part I of the 2nd edition of the *Guide to Physical Therapist Practice* consists of three chapters that specifically outline the roles of a PT. The majority of material in these three chapters was developed by expert consensus during the time period between 1992 and 1995 and was first published in the journal *Physical Therapy* in August 1995.[1]

Chapters 1 through 3 of the 2nd edition of the *Guide* follow a similar format to the original 1995 publication. However, major revisions and additions were made to the 2nd edition.[8,16] The majority of revisions made to Chapters 1 through 3 of Part I occurred during the time period between the publication of the 1st and 2nd editions (1997–2001).[2,6–8] The major revisions included the development of disablement within the realm of physical therapy, including risk reduction and prevention as well as health, wellness, and fitness interventions, as well as identifying the goals of many management techniques as outcomes.[8] For example, the role of disablement (as described by Nagi and others) in physical therapy examination and management has been extensively reviewed. As such, the specific pathologies, impairments, functional abilities or limitations, disabilities, and quality of life issues have been incorporated in all appropriate areas of the physical therapy examination and management process described in Chapters 2 and 3, respectively. Likewise, attempts were made to incorporate disablement into the role of the PT as described in Chapter 1.[8] Table 2-1 provides an overview of the manner in which this was accomplished. The examination and

BOX 2-3

Published Literature About the Guide to Physical Therapist Practice

1. Rothstein J. Editorial. *Phys Ther.* 1997;77:1-3.
2. Rothstein J. On the second edition of the *Guide. Phys Ther.* 2001;81:6-8.
3. Hillegass E. Applying the cardiopulmonary practice patterns: case study of a person with multisystem problems. *Cardiopulm Pher Ther J.* 1999;10(3):84-89.
4. Cahalin LP. Applying the cardiopulmonary practice patterns: heart failure. *Cardiopulm Phys Ther J.* 1999;10(3):90-97.
5. Bourgeois MC. Diagnosing pulmonary impairment: a lung volume reduction surgery case that uses the patient management model. *Cardiopulm Phys Ther J.* 1999;10(3): 98-100.
6. Schuster NB. Simultaneous implementation of two cardiopulmonary preferred practice patterns across the continuum of care. *Phys Ther Case Rep.* 1999;2(6):241-248.
7. Gordon J, Quinn L. *Guide* to physical therapist practice: a critical appraisal. *Neurol Rep.* 1999;23(3):122-128.
8. Focused issue: the *Guide* to physical therapist practice. *GeriNotes.* 1999;6(5):1-35.
9. Giallonardo L. *Guide* in action: patient with total hip replacement. *PT Magazine.* 2000;8(9):76-88.

TABLE 2-1   Revisions of Part I (Chapters 1–3) and Part II of the Guide: Several Key Differences and Effects on Physical Therapy

Part I Revisions	
Chapter 1	
Revision	*Effect on physical therapy*
1. Disablement added to PT role	Expands the role of the PT in all areas of health care
2. Addition of clients as recipients of PT	Expands the role of the PT in wellness/prevention
3. Discharge planning added to role	Increases the efficiency of PT care
4. Addition of PT role in prevention/wellness	Increases the role of the PT in wellness/prevention and diminishes the economic burden of disablement
Chapter 2	
Revision	*Effect on physical therapy*
1. Disablement added to PT role	Expands the role of the PT in all areas of health care
2. Addition of clinical indications for tests and measures within disablement	Improves the allocation of PT services to patients
Chapter 3	
Difference	*Effect on physical therapy*
1. Disablement added to PT role	Expands the role of the PT in all areas of health care
2. Expansion of clinical considerations, interventions, and anticipated goals and expected outcomes	Improves the allocation of PT services to patients
Part II Revisions	
Chapter 6	
Revision	*Effect on physical therapy*
1. Disablement added to PT role	Expands the role of the PT in all areas of health care
2. Practice patterns combined	Makes the distinction between practice patterns less apparent
3. Lymphatic practice pattern added	Identifies a patient population in need of PT care and research

management of various domains of disablement have now been identified to be an important aspect of physical therapy.

Disablement and Functioning

Much of the practice pattern design and language is based on the disablement schema developed by Nagi, in which pathology, impairment, functional limitations, and disabilities have

been identified as the key areas of disablement (Fig. 2-1).[17–20] Pathology has been defined as the interruption of normal processes of an organism to regain normalcy; impairment, as anatomical, physiological, mental or emotional abnormalities, or loss; functional limitations or functional abilities of a person, as limitations in performance of the person; and disability, as the limitation in the performance of socially defined roles or tasks.[17–20] Figure 2-1 shows that extra- and intraindividual

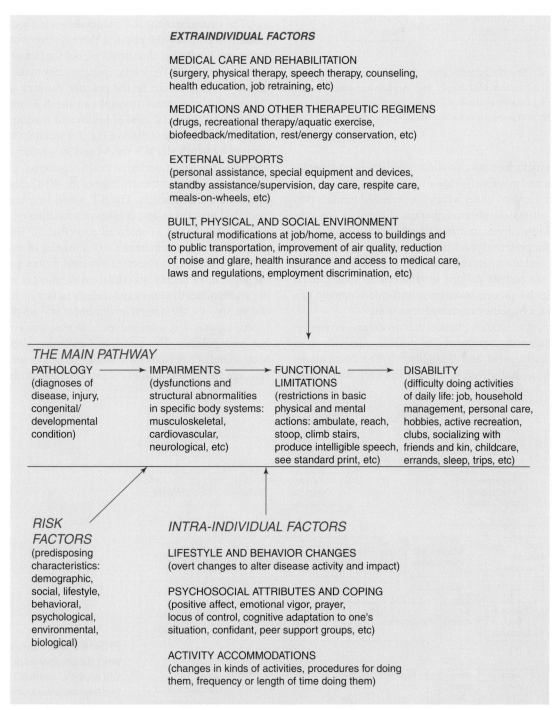

FIGURE 2-1   The influence of extraindividual factors, intraindividual factors, and risk factors on disablement. (Reprinted from *Social Science and Medicine*, Vol. 38. Verbrugge and Jette, "The Disablement Process," p. 4, 1994, with permission from Elsevier.)

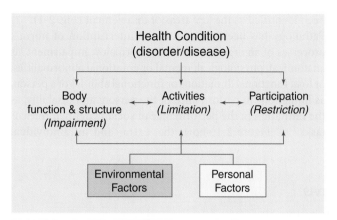

FIGURE 2-2 The WHO classification of disablement and disability via the ICF and interaction of concepts. (Reprinted from *International Classification of Functioning, Disability and Health; ICF.* Geneva, Switzerland: World Health Organization; 2001, with permission of the World Health Organization.)

factors and risk factors can also affect disablement and require examination and possibly therapeutic intervention.

The key domains under which the preferred practice patterns (and ultimately physical therapy diagnosis) are subsumed are impairments and functional abilities. In fact, the majority of the preferred practice patterns begin with the word *impairment* and are often clarified with a statement of function which are further defined in relationship to a specific pathology. Such a process is common in the development of a diagnosis and a hypothesis-oriented algorithm.[21,22]

Developing a complete physical therapy diagnosis requires a more detailed discussion of the possible methods used to classify disablement and disability.[21,22] The Nagi model described above and shown in Fig. 2-1 has been used exten-

sively in the development of the preferred practice patterns.[17–22] However, the more recent World Health Organization (WHO) classification of disablement and disability (International Classification of Functioning, Disability, and Health; ICF) has been considered to be a superior conceptual model because of a focus on functioning in health and disease (eliminating the distinctions between healthy and disabled persons) within a context of personal and environmental factors (Fig. 2-2).[23–25] Figure 2-3 further outlines the ICF model with several additional components, constructs, and categories.

The structure of the ICF model shown in Figs. 2-2 and 2-3 is likely to enhance the physical therapy diagnosis of impairments and functional abnormalities, but the lack of association with the current APTA practice patterns may make the application of the ICF model to the practice patterns difficult.[17–25] Despite this, the major strengths of the ICF model are the broad biopsychosocial view of health and subdomains shown in Fig. 2-3.[23–25] Examination of Fig. 2-3 will help to clarify the manner by which the ICF model and its subdomains may be applied to the APTA-preferred practice patterns.

Figure 2-3 shows the structure of the WHO classification of disablement and disability. The ICF model (moving downward from the top of the figure) consists of a functioning and disability part (Part 1) and a contextual part (Part 2). The contextual part contains two component parts consisting of environmental and personal factors. The environmental factors are defined as the physical, social, and attitudinal environment in which people live and conduct their lives and include factors such as products and technology, the natural environment and adapted environments, support and relationships, attitudes, and available services and policies. The personal factors are defined as the background of a person's life and include factors such as gender, race, age, habits, and a variety of psychological attributes.[23–25]

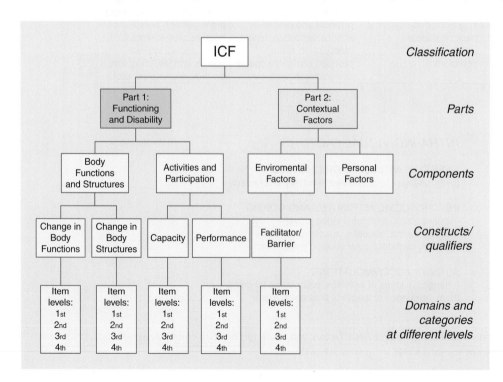

FIGURE 2-3 Structure of the WHO classification of disablement and disability via the ICF. (Reprinted from *International Classification of Functioning, Disability and Health; ICF.* Geneva, Switzerland: World Health Organization; 2001, with permission of the World Health Organization.)

The functioning and disability part of the ICF model contains two component parts consisting of (1) body functions and structures and (2) activities and participation. Constructs or qualifiers of each of the component parts delineate the manner by which the component parts may affect a patient and as shown in the fourth level of the ICF model in Fig. 2-3 include change in body functions, change in body structures, capacity, performance, and facilitator/barrier. A particular strength about the ICF is that a particular change in body function and body structure (both are qualifiers) can be quantified using a 5-point scale from no impairment to a severe impairment. Furthermore, the other two qualifiers under activities and participation (capacity and performance) provide quantifiable measures that represent individuals' ability to optimally function in their environment with assistive device or accommodations (performance) and without assistive device or accommodations (capacity).[23-25]

The bottom portion of Fig. 2-3 consists of domains and categories at different levels and represents a further delineation of each component and qualifier positioned above it. For example, the domains under both of the qualifiers capacity and performance, and thus the component "activities and participation" include learning and applying knowledge, general tasks and demands, communication, mobility, self-care, domestic life, interpersonal interactions and relationships, major life areas, and community life.[23-25] The above structure provides a broader, yet more specific assessment of function, disability, and health.

The ICF model has been reported to have substantial clinical utility with an important distinction between it and other models being the potential for multicultural application and comparability.[23-25] However, a better understanding of the ICF model and its application to physical therapy and the APTA practice patterns is needed to facilitate its full use in physical therapy. In fact, a major area in need of investigation is the measurement characteristics of ICF concepts and categories and their ability to discriminate between the two primary parts of the ICF as well as among the different vertical levels of the ICF.[23-25] It also appears that investigation of the ICF and the *Guide to Physical Therapist Practice* is needed.

Overview of Part 1 Chapters

The following section provides a brief overview of the three chapters in Part 1 of the *Guide to Physical Therapist Practice*. The specific sections of Chapter 1 include the education and qualifications of the PT; practice settings; types of patients and clients; scope of practice; the roles of the PT in primary, secondary, and tertiary care as well as prevention and wellness; elements of patient/client management, outcomes of PT care, discharge planning, other professional roles; and the direction and supervision of other health care personnel.[8] Important changes in Chapter 1, since the 1995 publication, include a more detailed description of the PT and the roles of a PT (including clients, not just patients as potential recipients of physical therapy care); expansion of the elements of patient or client management leading to optimal outcomes (with outcomes and discharge planning being important additions and significant expansion in the types of data that may be generated from a patient/client history); and minimal expansion of other professional roles of the PT in consultation, education, critical inquiry, and administration (but with a movement of prevention and wellness to a common rather than "other" professional role).[8]

Two of the previous sections worthy of further discussion include the distinction between patients and clients seen by the PT and the potential role of the PT in prevention and wellness. The distinction between patients and clients is important because prior to the publication of Part I of the *Guide*, most PT care was considered to be provided (whether true or not) to patients rather than to clients. Several of the main differences and effects on the PT are shown in Table 2-1. Likewise, the role of the PT in prevention and wellness reflects the vision of treating clients and actually preventing disablement. The emphasis on such a role and the necessary changes are also shown in Table 2-1. The five elements of patient/client management shown in Fig. 2-4 provide a foundation for the PT to participate and direct PT intervention and assume a variety of roles. The types of data that may be generated from a patient/client history are shown in Fig. 2-5.[8]

Chapter 2 describes the tests and measurements that a PT may use in the management of patients or clients. Twenty-four categories of tests and measures have been presented as in the 1st edition,[2] but there is now an attempt to include clinical indications for the tests and measures within particular domains of disablement.[8] An example of the integration of the tests and measures within the Disablement Model is shown in Table 2-2.

Chapter 3 lists different interventions that may be provided by the PT. Figure 2-6 identifies the three components of physical therapy intervention (Coordination, Communication, and Documentation; Patient/Client-Related Instruction; and Procedural Interventions) along with a listing of the nine specific procedural interventions.[8] All of the sections within Chapter 3 have been expanded including the clinical considerations, interventions, and anticipated goals and expected outcomes.

As in Chapter 2, an attempt to include clinical considerations for procedural interventions within particular domains of disablement has been made.[8] These changes are shown in Fig. 2-5. The breadth of PT is apparent in the variety of tests and measures as well as in the direct treatments that may be provided by a PT, which are listed in Chapters 2 and 3, respectively. These tests and measures and interventions are listed in the most appropriate domain of disablement. Examples of this are shown in Table 2-3. This is an important addition to the 2nd edition of the *Guide to Physical Therapist Practice*.[8] A major part of disablement and PT tests and measures and interventions are outcomes. Identification of appropriate and measurable outcomes for specific patient populations is needed in PT. Many of the goals listed in the intervention sections of the cardiopulmonary practice patterns of the 1st edition of the *Guide* are likely important outcomes for patients with cardiovascular and pulmonary disease. In fact, these goals have now been identified as expected outcomes in the 2nd edition.[8] Although the goals and expected outcomes of

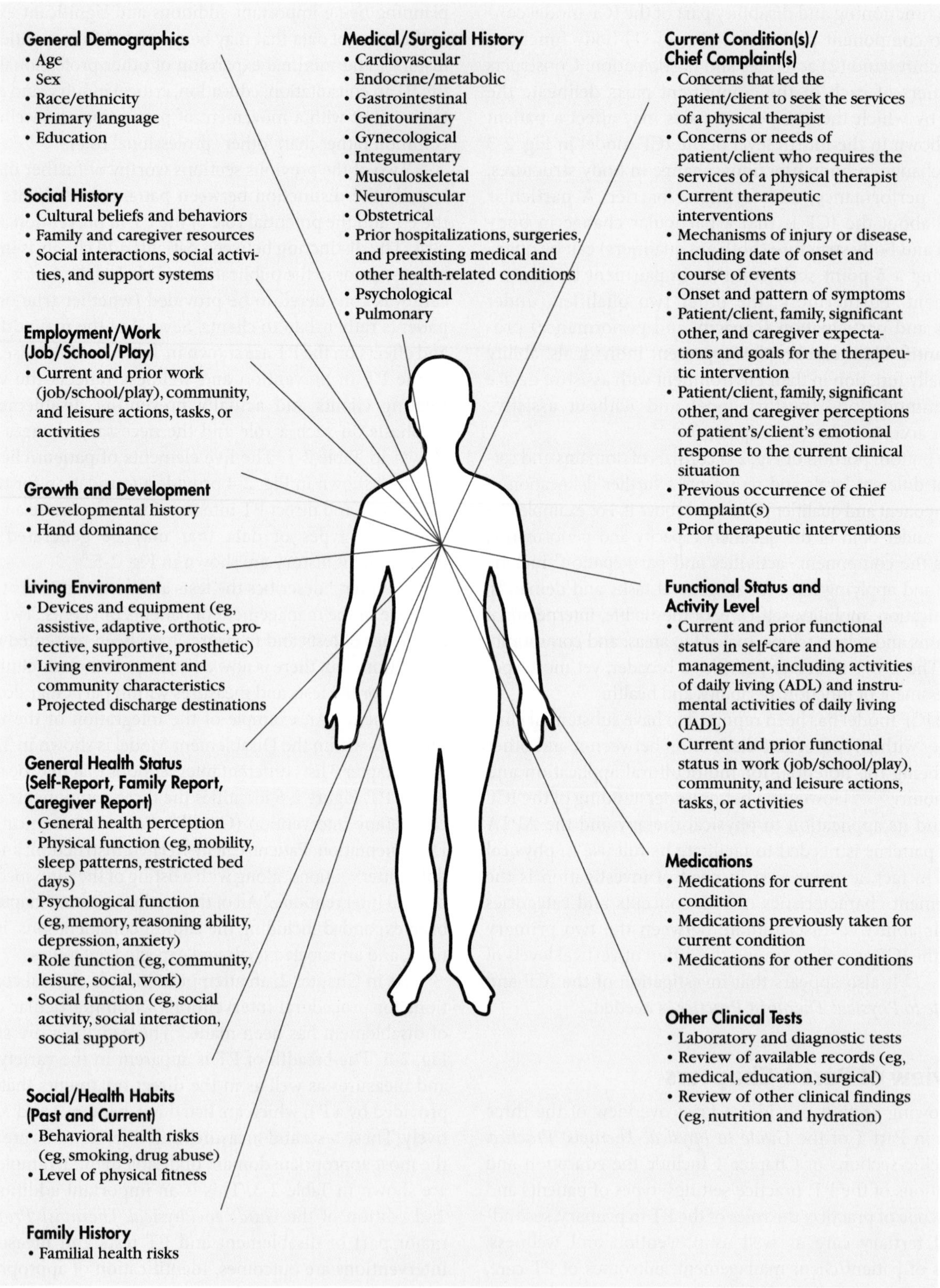

General Demographics
- Age
- Sex
- Race/ethnicity
- Primary language
- Education

Social History
- Cultural beliefs and behaviors
- Family and caregiver resources
- Social interactions, social activities, and support systems

Employment/Work (Job/School/Play)
- Current and prior work (job/school/play), community, and leisure actions, tasks, or activities

Growth and Development
- Developmental history
- Hand dominance

Living Environment
- Devices and equipment (eg, assistive, adaptive, orthotic, protective, supportive, prosthetic)
- Living environment and community characteristics
- Projected discharge destinations

General Health Status (Self-Report, Family Report, Caregiver Report)
- General health perception
- Physical function (eg, mobility, sleep patterns, restricted bed days)
- Psychological function (eg, memory, reasoning ability, depression, anxiety)
- Role function (eg, community, leisure, social, work)
- Social function (eg, social activity, social interaction, social support)

Social/Health Habits (Past and Current)
- Behavioral health risks (eg, smoking, drug abuse)
- Level of physical fitness

Family History
- Familial health risks

Medical/Surgical History
- Cardiovascular
- Endocrine/metabolic
- Gastrointestinal
- Genitourinary
- Gynecological
- Integumentary
- Musculoskeletal
- Neuromuscular
- Obstetrical
- Prior hospitalizations, surgeries, and preexisting medical and other health-related conditions
- Psychological
- Pulmonary

Current Condition(s)/Chief Complaint(s)
- Concerns that led the patient/client to seek the services of a physical therapist
- Concerns or needs of patient/client who requires the services of a physical therapist
- Current therapeutic interventions
- Mechanisms of injury or disease, including date of onset and course of events
- Onset and pattern of symptoms
- Patient/client, family, significant other, and caregiver expectations and goals for the therapeutic intervention
- Patient/client, family, significant other, and caregiver perceptions of patient's/client's emotional response to the current clinical situation
- Previous occurrence of chief complaint(s)
- Prior therapeutic interventions

Functional Status and Activity Level
- Current and prior functional status in self-care and home management, including activities of daily living (ADL) and instrumental activities of daily living (IADL)
- Current and prior functional status in work (job/school/play), community, and leisure actions, tasks, or activities

Medications
- Medications for current condition
- Medications previously taken for current condition
- Medications for other conditions

Other Clinical Tests
- Laboratory and diagnostic tests
- Review of available records (eg, medical, education, surgical)
- Review of other clinical findings (eg, nutrition and hydration)

FIGURE 2-4   The five elements of patient/client management. (Reprinted from American Physical Therapy Association. Guide to Physical Therapist Practice, 2nd ed. *Phys Ther.* 2001 Jan;81(1):9-746, with permission of the American Physical Therapy Association. This material is copyrighted, and any further reproduction or distribution is prohibited. All rights reserved.)

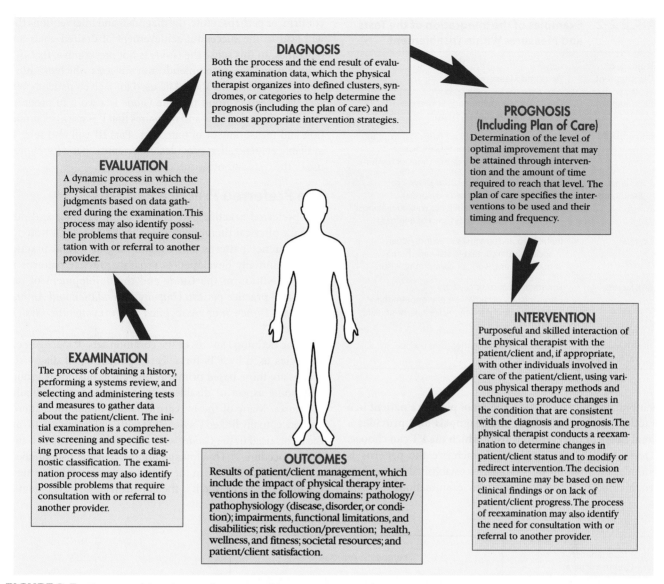

FIGURE 2-5   The types of data that may be generated from a patient/client history. (Reprinted from American Physical Therapy Association. Guide to Physical Therapist Practice, 2nd ed. *Phys Ther.* 2001 Jan;81(1):9-746, with permission of the American Physical Therapy Association. This material is copyrighted, and any further reproduction or distribution is prohibited. All rights reserved.)

specific cardiovascular and pulmonary PT outcomes have now been identified, the manner in which to attain these goals is not clear. The goals of the practice patterns are shown in Box 2-4.[8] It is important to note that the *Guide* is "not intended to serve as a clinical guideline" and that it at best represents expert consensus.[8] However, a more specific examination approach and treatment plan is needed in physical therapy. Fortunately, a substantial literature exists for cardiovascular and pulmonary care that provides an adequate evidence base for specific examination and treatment techniques in persons with cardiovascular and pulmonary diseases.

The purpose of this textbook is to identify specific tests and measures that are most appropriate and informative when examining and treating persons with cardiovascular and pulmonary diseases. Observation of particular test results can provide diagnostic, prognostic, and therapeutic direction. The special-

ized tests that can provide this information will be presented in the practice pattern chapters of this textbook (Chapters 15–20). The following section will review the material in Part II of the *Guide to Physical Therapist Practice.*

PART II OF THE *GUIDE TO PHYSICAL THERAPIST PRACTICE*

Although Part I of the *Guide* is meant to define PT for the profession, for other professionals, and for the public, the intent of Part II is to link the elements of Part I with recognizable groups of patients and clients.[2,8] In devising the preferred practice patterns, PT is staking a claim to a unique field of clinical management and inquiry. The patterns, in effect, establish PT *diagnoses* that give therapists a common framework on which to base

TABLE 2-2   **Examples of the Integration of the Tests and Measures Within Disablement**

Domain of Disablement	Tests and Measures
Pathology	Cardiovascular, pulmonary, endocrine/metabolic, multiple systems
Impairments	Circulation (abnormal heart rate, rhythm, or BP) Ventilation and respiration/gas exchange (abnormal respiratory pattern, rate, or rhythm)
Functional limitations	Self-care (inabililty to perform shower or overhead ADL because of dyspnea) Community/leisure (inability to walk to religious activities because of dyspnea or angina)
Disability	Inability to perform tasks in an individuals sociocultural context in self-care, home management, work, or community/leisure
Risk factors	For impaired aerobic capacity Family history of cardiovascular or pulmonary disease, obesity, sedentary lifestyle, or smoking history
Health, wellness, and fitness	Physical performance measures (exercise test results)

their practice. **As we shall see, the act of placing a patient in a practice pattern establishes the diagnosis and provides a broad range of interventions from which the PT can choose.** A term used by the *Guide* to characterize the patterns is "boundaries."[8] Within the boundaries established by the pattern, a clinician is free to choose any examinations that will confirm, or perhaps refute, the diagnosis and interventions that will lead to the successful achievement of desired goals and outcomes. In this sense the *Guide* is not prescriptive; that is, it neither mandates, recommends, nor suggests which examinations or interventions should be used for a given patient/client scenario. Keep in mind that the *Guide* is a work in progress. Part III will catalog tests and measures that PTs use in examination and measurement of outcomes. Part III will also refer to available evidence that provides the scientific basis for clinical use of the tests and measures cited.[16]

The Preferred Practice Patterns

The preferred practice patterns for cardiovascular and pulmonary physical therapy are listed in Table 2-4. Of note for these practice patterns is the combining of several practice patterns initially developed as separate practice patterns in the first edition of the *Guide* and the development of one additional practice pattern (*Impaired Circulation and Anthropometric Dimensions Associated with Lymphatic System Disorders*).[8]

The defining features of the common sets of management strategies used by PTs for selected patient/client diagnostic groups are those based primarily on patient diagnostic groups with some aspect of disablement associated with particular diagnoses. Many of the impairments that define the patterns are conceptually linked ("associated with" or "secondary to" are the terms used in the *Guide*) with a medical diagnosis or a surgical procedure.[2,8] This linkage implies that the patient/client conditions that PTs see in the clinic are closely related to medical diagnoses; however, it is the impairments and the potential

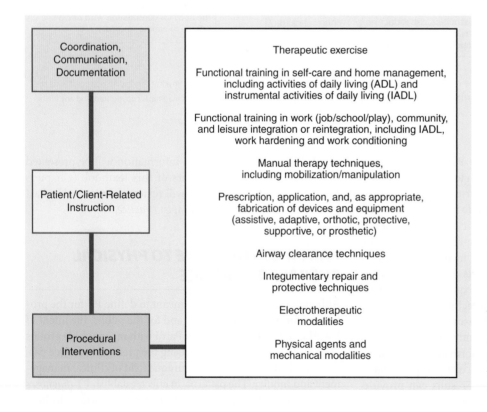

FIGURE 2-6   The three components of physical therapy intervention (coordination, communication, and documentation; patient-/client-related instruction; and procedural interventions) along with a listing of the nine specific procedural interventions. (Reprinted from American Physical Therapy Association. Guide to Physical Therapist Practice, 2nd ed. *Phys Ther.* 2001 Jan;81(1):9-746, with permission of the American Physical Therapy Association. This material is copyrighted, and any further reproduction or distribution is prohibited. All rights reserved.)

TABLE 2-3 **Major Revisions in Chapters 1–3 of Part I of the *Guide* to Physical Therapy: Development of Disablement Within Physical Therapy**

Domain of Disablement	Tests and Measures	Goals of Procedural Interventions
Pathology	Cardiovascular, pulmonary, endocrine/metabolic, multiple systems	Decreased pain and symptoms
Impairments	Circulation (abnormal heart rate, rhythm, or BP), ventilation and respiration/gas exchange (abnormal respiratory pattern, rate, or rhythm)	Decreased work of breathing increased endurance
Functional limitations	Self-care (inabililty to perform overhead ADL because of dyspnea) community/leisure (inability to walk to religious activities because of dyspnea or angina)	Improved ADL, increased tolerance of positions and activities, less supervision
Disability	Inability to perform tasks in an individual's sociocultural context in self-care, home management, work, or community/leisure	Improved self-care in home, work, or community
Risk factors	Impaired aerobic capacity, family history, obesity, sedentary lifestyle, and/or smoking history	Reduce risk factors and improve safety
Health, wellness, and fitness	Physical performance measures (exercise tests)	Improve fitness and health status

functional limitations and disabilities that are the focus of PT management. The Disablement Model reminds us that functional limitations pertain to the whole person and that disability pertains to the individual's role in society.

For every pattern, a *Patient/Client Diagnostic Classification* is listed. Under this heading is located a more detailed description of the features that define the pattern, including a list of *Inclusion* and *Exclusion* criteria. The *Inclusion* and *Exclusion* criteria refer to general categories of medical/surgical diagnoses or conditions that either qualify or disqualify an individual from each pattern. Also listed are *Findings That May Require Classification in Additional Patterns*. These, typically,

---

BOX 2-4

Goals of the Practice Patterns

1. To describe PT practice in general, using the disablement model as the basis.
2. To describe the roles of PTs in primary, secondary, and tertiary care; in prevention; and in the promotion of health, wellness, and fitness.
3. To describe the setting in which PTs practice.
4. To standardize terminology used in, and related to, PT practice.
5. To delineate the tests and measures and the interventions that are used in PT practice.
6. To delineate preferred practice patterns that will help PTs (1) improve quality of care, (2) enhance the positive outcomes of physical therapy services, (3) enhance patient/ client satisfaction, (4) promote appropriate utilization of health care services, (5) increase efficiency and reduce unwarranted variation in the provision of services, and (6) diminish the economic burden of disablement through prevention and the promotion of health, wellness, and fitness initiatives.

TABLE 2-4 **Cardiovascular and Pulmonary Preferred Practice Patterns**

Pattern A	Primary Prevention/Risk Reduction for Cardiovascular/Pulmonary Disorders
Pattern B	Impaired Aerobic Capacity/Endurance Associated with Deconditioning
Pattern C	Impaired Ventilation, Respiration/Gas Exchange, and Aerobic Capacity/Endurance Associated with Airway Clearance Dysfunction
Pattern D	Impaired Aerobic Capacity/Endurance Associated with Cardiovascular Pump Dysfunction or Failure
Pattern E	Impaired Ventilation and Respiration/Gas Exchange Associated with Ventilatory Pump Dysfunction or Failure
Pattern F	Impaired Ventilation and Respiration/Gas Exchange Associated with Respiratory Failure
Pattern G	Impaired Ventilation, Respiration/Gas Exchange, and Aerobic Capacity/Endurance Associated with Respiratory Failure in the Neonate
Pattern H	Impaired Circulation and Anthropometric Dimensions Associated with Lymphatic System Disorders

are diagnoses with features that are common to multiple practice patterns. The page immediately following the title page for each pattern supplies a list of *ICD-9-CM (International Classification of Diseases, Ninth Revision, Clinical Modification)* codes that may be present in patients/clients who qualify for each of the patterns. The *ICD-9-CM* codes are standard numeric codes corresponding to specific diagnoses and subcategories of diagnoses that are used for billing and research purposes.

The next part of each pattern is the *Examination* section. This section contains the *Patient/Client History, Systems Review,* and *Tests and Measures* that a PT might choose for patients/clients in the pattern. Following this is the section pertaining to *Evaluation, Diagnosis, and Prognosis.* Included in this section is a statement of the *Expected Range of Number of Visits Per Episode of Care,* which discloses the anticipated span of PT visits across all involved practice settings. An episode of care, for example, may begin when the patient/client is in the acute hospital, continues in a rehabilitation facility, and ends in a home care environment. Note the clause stating that the range covers 80% of persons in the diagnostic group. This covers patients or clients who may require more (or less) care beyond the published range for each pattern. Variables that may influence how often or how many times a patient/client may be seen are included under *Factors That May Require New Episode of Care or That May Modify Frequency of Visits/Duration of Episode.* These factors comprise many of the intra- and extraindividual factors that impact functional limitations according to the Disablement Model.[17]

Intervention comes next. This portion lays out all of the potential *Procedural Interventions* that may be used in clinical management as well as interventions related to *Coordination, Communication, and Documentation* and *Patient-/Client-Related Instruction.* The first three *Procedural Interventions* listed for most of the cardiovascular and pulmonary patterns are considered to be fundamental PT interventions. These are *Therapeutic Exercise (including aerobic conditioning), Functional Training in Self-Care and Home Management (including ADL and IADL),* and *Functional Training in Community and Work (job/school/play), Community, and Leisure Integration or Reintegration (including IADL, work hardening, and work conditioning).*[8]

The final section comprises *Reexamination, Global Outcomes for Patients/Clients in* (each) *Pattern* and *Criteria for Termination of Physical Therapy Services.* Potential outcomes of PT intervention span the range of elements in the Disablement Model—from *pathology/pathophysiology* to *disabilities*—and they also include *risk reduction/prevention,* improvements in *health, wellness, and fitness;* more efficient use of *societal resources* and *patient/client satisfaction.*[8]

The philosophy behind the *Guide* recognizes the importance of prevention in physical therapy practice. In the preferred practice patterns, the *Guide* encompasses all three types of prevention. Primary prevention seeks to prevent the occurrence of disease. The *Guide* includes primary prevention practice patterns in all four clinical domains. For the cardiovascular/pulmonary practice patterns, Pattern A is the primary prevention pattern. Its focus is on cardiovascular risk-factor reduc-

tion through aerobic training and lifestyle change. Secondary prevention involves prevention of disease progression and the development of related diseases. For example, PT interventions for persons with diabetes, such as aerobic conditioning, do not "cure" the patient of diabetes, but can and do prevent many of the undesirable complications of diabetes and may help the patient to control his or her blood glucose level. Tertiary prevention attempts to prevent disability resulting from disease. An example of tertiary prevention may be seen in pulmonary rehabilitation, where PT interventions that involve therapeutic exercise and patient/client instruction in breathing strategies may slow the progression of disability associated with chronic obstructive pulmonary disease.

LIMITATIONS OF PARTS I AND II OF THE *GUIDE*

Readers of the *Guide* expecting to find recipes for how to manage a patient with, for example, myocardial infarction or cystic fibrosis will be disappointed. Indeed, that the *Guide* is not a "cookbook" is not so much a limitation as it is a strength. Clinicians using their professional judgment may choose from a broad array of tests and measures as well as from interventions. Nonetheless, the *Guide* has been criticized for its lack of clarity with regard to an ordering or prioritizing of its components for specific practice patterns.[13] Although this criticism is not entirely unfounded, it should be kept in mind that the *Guide* was never meant to be prescriptive, that is, to delineate what PTs should or should not do in the management of their patients/clients. It will be up to future revisions of, and additions to, the *Guide,* as well as to publications such as this one, to color in the maps for each practice pattern as evidence becomes available.

There is also controversy regarding the concept of *diagnoses* that are unique to PT. Gordon and Quinn argue that the preferred practice patterns are largely pathology based, though their remarks are in reference to the neuromuscular patterns. However, the cardiovascular and pulmonary practice patterns are impairment based as well as pathology based. Each pattern, with the exception of the primary prevention pattern, focuses primarily on impairment in aerobic capacity and/or ventilation and secondarily on the associations with very broadly defined pathologic features. Both "impaired aerobic capacity," and "impaired ventilation"—two primary elements common to most of the cardiovascular and pulmonary practice patterns—are consistent with the definition of impairments in the Disability Model (see Fig. 2-1).

Remember, too, that the *Guide* is a work in progress. Revisions have been and will continue to be made. Not all patient groups seen by PTs are represented in the current revision, though the breadth of the practice patterns has increased by the addition of new patterns. As it evolves, the *Guide* will provide PTs with more clinically useful information and guidance. It is the purpose of this textbook to help provide some guidance to the PT caring for the disablement associated with cardiovascular and pulmonary disorders.

THE DISABLEMENT PROCESS MODEL

The *Guide to Physical Therapist Practice* is rooted in a theoretical model that is characterized as the disablement process. This model has been articulated by Verbrugge and Jette and is based on a classification framework that was developed by Nagi.[17] It is an attractive and useful model for physical therapy practice and research for several reasons. First, the Disablement Model contrasts with the traditional medical model in which a disease or diagnosis, rather than a person, is treated. The model recognizes that multiple pathologic conditions may, and often do, coexist in individuals, particularly in the elderly and in those who have disabling developmental or acquired conditions. There is not a straightforward, one-to-one relationship between a particular pathologic condition, for example, coronary heart disease, and its outcome in a given individual or population. Some individuals become limited in their activities as a result of the pathologic condition; others experience few or no limitations. The Disablement Model provides a means by which we can acknowledge the value of services that may not directly impact medical diagnoses but instead impact important personal and societal consequences of disease, namely, the development of disability.

Another attractive feature of the Disablement Model is that it recognizes the process inherent in the progression from disease to disability. Process implies a dynamic, potentially interactive continuum that may be affected at various points in positive or negative ways. The interventions provided by PTs are examples of actions that help to halt or slow the progression from disease to disability. The model helps clinicians to organize their thinking about what aspect of the disablement process an examination measures or how intervention will impact the slowing or prevention of disability. Figure 2-1 illustrates the main pathway of the Disablement Model, in addition to other factors that contribute to the process.

The *Guide* suggests that PTs are involved, primarily, in the management of impairments, functional limitations, and disability. Pathology may or may not be a management concern for the PT in the area of cardiovascular and pulmonary disorders. PTs may intervene in the presence of ". . . changes in physical function and health status resulting from injury, disease or other causes."[2,8] The degree to which "changes in health status" may reflect involvement in pathology needs further investigation and clarification.

Impairments, such as decreased range of motion and decreased strength and deconditioning, are features with which PTs are perhaps most familiar. Functional limitations are aspects of the patient/client that pertain to specific activities, for example, rolling over, sitting up from a supine position, or walking. According to Verbrugge and Jette, these activities may be necessary components of particular activities of daily living (ADL), but they are not, themselves, ADL.[17] In the Disability Model, ADL are classified in the disability domain, including tasks such as moving in bed, transferring from a bed to a chair, and ambulating across a room.

A clinical example may help to distinguish between a functional limitation and a disability. A PT visits a woman, who has a diagnosis of congestive heart failure at her home. The therapist observes members of the woman's family assisting her frequently with tasks such as moving in bed, sitting up and getting to a chair, and walking across the room to the bathroom. When the therapist examines the patient, however, she requires very little assistance to perform the same tasks. This illustrates the social context in which disabilities occur. The patient in this instance has a higher level of disability than her functional limitations would seem to indicate—the disability being exacerbated by the interaction of the patient with her family. Indeed, one of the key points of interest in both the Disablement Model and the *Guide* is that elements of the main pathway may or may not be causally related. In other words, having an impairment may or may not guarantee a functional limitation, nor does having a functional impairment guarantee a disability. As can be seen in the clinical example, the level of disability may exceed the level expected based solely on the degree of functional limitation present. Because of this, it is important to utilize specialized tests and measures that provide important information that can clarify the diagnosis and prognosis and provide direction for examination and management techniques. The information from such specialized tests and measures has been referred to as threshold behaviors and will be further discussed in the following section.[18] Threshold behaviors can be defined as measurable behaviors at the pathology, impairment, functional, disability, quality of life, intra- or extraindividual, or risk-factor level.

Figure 2-1 also shows the other inputs that may influence how impairments translate into functional limitations and how functional limitations translate into disabilities. To continue with the clinical example, the patient's family exacerbated the disability by helping too much (provided excessive external support), and the patient was willing to accept that assistance (perhaps an example of external locus of control). The PT would presumably mitigate the disability through rehabilitation interventions, the outcome of which would be independence in ADL. The line distinguishing functional limitations from disabilities can be quite blurry, which may be why the *Guide* combined the two concepts in its classification of outcomes. However, identification of threshold behaviors is necessary to determine specifics about the disablement associated with cardiovascular and pulmonary disorders.

DEVELOPMENT OF THRESHOLD BEHAVIORS WITHIN THE DISABLEMENT OF CARDIOVASCULAR AND PULMONARY DISORDERS: A PHYSICAL THERAPY PERSPECTIVE

Physical therapy is presently undergoing rapid and monumental change. Educational, clinical, and social aspects of physical therapy have recently been questioned and have resulted in different approaches to physical therapy education and clinical care. These changes have partly been responsible for the development of the preferred practice patterns for physical therapy just described. As mentioned, the preferred practice patterns for physical therapy "provide information about common management strategies for specific patient/client diagnostic groups."[2,8] The purpose of this last section is to describe how specific evidence-based objective observations and measurements of cardiovascular and pulmonary function can be used to (1) identify the appropriate preferred practice pattern for a patient with specific cardiovascular and pulmonary measurements, (2) direct further physical therapy examinations, and (3) direct physical therapy management interventions.

As previously stated, much of the practice pattern design and language is based on the disablement schema developed by Nagi and others in which pathologies, impairments, functional abilities or limitations, disabilities, and quality of life issues have been identified as important areas of physical therapy.[17-20] Recent, but limited research has demonstrated the important role that measurement of specific impairments, functional abilities, disabilities, and quality of life issues may have for physical therapy research and practice.[17-39] Measurement in these areas is important because with such measurements the success or failure of physical therapy interventions may be predicted. Improved predictive ability of physical therapy interventions will likely lead to more efficient care provided to the patients in greatest need of physical therapy and to the patients who will most likely benefit from particular therapeutic interventions. Predicting success or failure from medical or physical therapy appears to be dependent on identifying threshold levels. Test measurements, physical performance, or measured behaviors above or below a particular level frequently direct medical care to the most appropriate patients. Identifying similar threshold behaviors in physical therapy requires a clear definition of a threshold behavior. An extensive medical literature and limited physical therapy literature suggest that **threshold behaviors can be defined as measurable behaviors at the impairment, functional, disability, quality of life, intra- or extraindividual, or risk-factor level that identifies the specific need and type of physical therapy intervention to provide to a patient.**

A Physical Therapy Example of a Threshold Level

An example of allocating physical therapy to patients most likely to benefit from a particular intervention has been described by Jette,[38] who used data previously reported by Buchner et al.[39] They hypothesized that a curvilinear relationship exists between measures of muscle force (impairment) and the gait speed (functional status) of frail elderly persons.[39] This hypothetical relationship is shown in Fig. 2-7. The curvilinear shape shown in Fig. 2-7 suggests the possibility that a threshold level exists in regard to the relationship between muscle force and gait speed. Above a particular threshold level of muscle force and gait speed, disability is absent. Below the threshold level, disability is present. The presence of specific threshold levels of behavior in particular areas of physical therapy will likely result in some patient populations receiving physical therapy care, whereas other patient populations receive no treatment or at least education in the prevention of disability. Repeat patient examinations may find that an initial measured behavior above the threshold has decreased below the threshold level and will likely require physical therapy intervention to prevent disability. **Therefore, it appears that physical therapy interventions should be provided to those patients below a particular threshold behavior.**

In fact, Jette states that the "benefit from physical therapy (eg, exercise in frail older persons), in part, will depend on the status of the target group."[18] This can be further understood by again viewing Fig. 2-7 in which the frail and near-frail adults from studies 1 and 2, respectively, received benefit from exercise.[39] However, the asymptomatic adults of study 3 received no benefit from exercise. The asymptomatic adults of study 3 demonstrated no improvement in gait or muscle force production because the average relationship between gait speed and muscle force was far above the threshold level, whereas the average relationships of gait speed and muscle force of the frail and near-frail adults were below the threshold level. The average of the frail adults was lower than that of the near-frail adults and resulted in a larger improvement from exercise than that seen in the near-frail adults.[39]

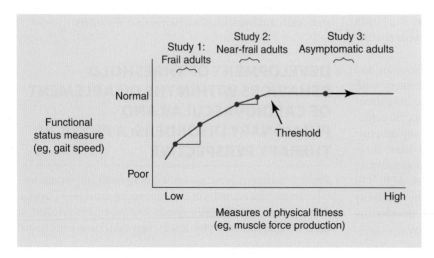

FIGURE 2-7   An example of a threshold behavior.

The allocation of physical therapy in this manner will likely result in more effective physical therapy care but will require more extensive tests and measures and, in particular, measurements of the relationships among physical therapy measurements, interventions, and patient outcomes. Furthermore, it appears that there is a need to measure the relationships within, between, and among pathologies, impairments, functional abilities, disabilities, and quality-of-life issues. Understanding these relationships will enable physical therapy care to be provided to the correct patients at the correct time and with a better understanding of the behaviors needed to amend or discontinue a physical therapy intervention.

A Cardiovascular and Pulmonary Physical Therapy Example of a Threshold Level

The clinical application of threshold behaviors to physical therapy can be exemplified with several measurements made in a research study investigating the clinical utility of the 6-minute walk test in persons with heart failure.[40] The purpose of this study was to investigate the relationship between the 6-minute walk test (a functional performance measure) and (1) peak oxygen consumption (an impairment measure) or (2) survival (an important measurement of health outcome) in persons with heart failure. These relationships were investigated to see whether a functional performance threshold behavior (walking) could help to evaluate patients' (1) appropriateness for cardiac transplantation and (2) response to physical therapy without measuring oxygen consumption.

Figure 2-8 shows long-term survival stratified by distance ambulated during the 6-minute walk test and by peak oxygen consumption. Patients ambulating less than 300 m had a poorer survival than those patients ambulating greater than 300 m, and patients with a peak oxygen consumption less than 14 mL/kg/min also had a poorer survival than those patients with a peak oxygen consumption greater than 14 mL/kg/min.[40] **These examples demonstrate the important role that the threshold value of 300 m has in determining survival in persons with heart failure.** Measurements of impairment, function, disability, and quality of life and the relationships among them can also be useful when examining patient status and the effectiveness of physical therapy intervention.

Ambulating a distance of 300 m during the 6-minute walk test provides a threshold behavior level that can be useful not only for the prediction of survival but also for the medical management of a person with heart failure and in directing physical therapy intervention.[40]

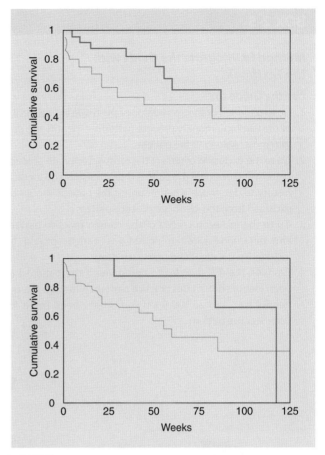

FIGURE 2-8 **(Top)** Long-term survival stratified by 6-minute walk test distance less than 300 m (light line) or greater than 300 m (dark line). **(Bottom)** Long-term survival stratified by peak oxygen consumption less than 14 mL/kg/min (light line) or greater than 14 mL/kg/min (dark line). (Used with permission from Hillegass E, Sadowsky S. *Essentials of Cardiopulmonary Physical Therapy.* 2nd ed. WB Saunders; 2001.)

Specific Methods to Integrate Threshold Behaviors with the Cardiovascular and Pulmonary Practice Patterns

An overview of the methods to use this textbook with the cardiovascular and pulmonary practice patterns is provided in Box 2-5. The information presented in this book should complement the use of the practice patterns and help to implement optimal examination and management techniques based on published literature. However, several recent changes in the 2nd edition of the *Guide* will be presented so that the application and integration of several threshold behaviors with the cardiovascular and pulmonary practice patterns can be better understood.[8]

Three major changes that have been made to the 2nd edition of the *Guide* in the cardiovascular and pulmonary practice patterns that are worthy of discussion include the grouping of several of the practice patterns and changes in the inclusion/exclusion criteria of several of the practice patterns from the 1st edition, as well as the addition of an additional practice pattern (impaired circulation and anthropometric dimensions associated with lymphatic system disorders).[8]

CLINICAL CORRELATE

Heart failure patients ambulating a threshold distance of less than 300 m are frequently provided more extensive medical and physical therapy management than patients ambulating a distance greater than 300 m.

BOX 2-5

Method to Integrate the Guide with the Textbook

Use the Guide to:

1. Go to page 471 of the 2nd edition of the *Guide* to find the list of the cardiopulmonary practice patterns—identify the pattern most likely to fit the patient.

2. Go to the exclusion criteria of the most appropriate practice pattern and examine the patient characteristics and medical history to determine whether or not the patient should be excluded from the identified practice pattern.

3. Go to the inclusion criteria of the chosen practice pattern and determine whether or not the patient should be included in the identified practice pattern.

4. Examine the *ICD-9* codes to determine if the patient has been identified to fit this practice pattern. Although this is a helpful step, not all *ICD-9-CM* codes have been listed for each practice pattern.

Use the Textbook to:

5. Go to the cardiovascular and pulmonary practice pattern chapters of this textbook (Chapters 15–20).

6. Use the specialized tests and measurements listed in the identified cardiovascular and pulmonary practice pattern chapters to either confirm or refute the choice of practice patterns, thus rendering a physical therapy diagnosis.

7. Use the results of the specialized tests and measurements to direct the specific physical therapy interventions listed in each chapter and in the hypothesis-oriented algorithms listed in each chapter.

8. Use the specialized tests and measurements to reexamine the patient and determine the results of the hypothesis-oriented algorithmic interventions.

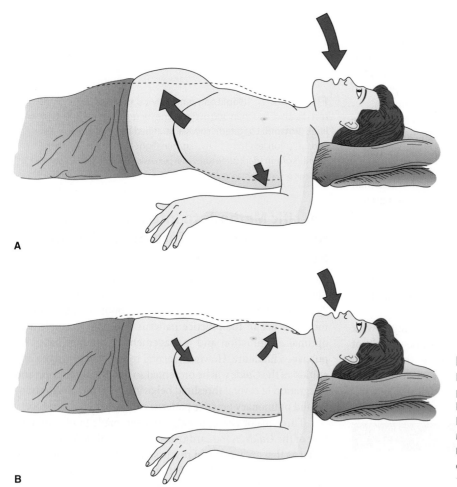

A

B

FIGURE 2-9 Two types of paradoxical breathing patterns suggestive of ventilatory pump failure. (**A**) Upper chest paradoxical breathing pattern. (**B**) Abdominal paradoxical breathing pattern. (Modified, with permission, from Massery M. The patient with neuromuscular or musculoskeletal dysfunction. In: Principles and Practice of Cardiopulmonary Physical Therapy. 3rd ed. Mosby Yearbook; 1996.)

In the 1st edition of the *Guide*, a distinction between cardiac pump dysfunction and failure was made. This was also true for ventilatory pump dysfunction and potential for failure. The 2nd edition found no useful distinction between cardiovascular dysfunction and failure, and they were combined into one practice pattern. Pulmonary dysfunction and failure were combined in a similar way.[3] The combination of these particular practice patterns is in keeping with the manner in which this textbook has been developed. By maintaining two separate identifiable conditions and treatment arms within several of the practice patterns, we believe that specific evidence-based tests and measurements can be used to identify the key pathology and area of disablement most affected by the primary pathology.

The other areas in need of further discussion are the inclusion/exclusion criteria for the new practice patterns related to ventilatory pump dysfunction/failure and respiratory failure. The *Guide* is unclear regarding into which of these practice patterns the patient requiring mechanical ventilation is to be placed. This placement issue is discussed in Chapters 18 and 19 of this textbook. Because dysfunction and failure have been combined, the utilization of specific tests and measures to differentiate them becomes of paramount importance. One example of the process used to distinguish between ventilatory pump dysfunction and failure involves examining the patient for the presence of paradoxical breathing (see Fig. 2-9). This is described in detail in Chapters 9 and 19 of this textbook.

USING THE *GUIDE* WITH THIS TEXTBOOK—A CLINICAL CASE STUDY

The abdominal paradoxical breathing pattern shown in Fig. 2-9B will be utilized in the following case study (Box 2-6). A 65-year-old male patient with a very long history of cigarette smoking and severe shortness of breath at rest and during exertion was referred to physical therapy for exercise training and patient education. The PT was provided several baseline measurements (Box 2-6). A quick glance at Box 2-6 reveals that the patient has been a long-time smoker, which has produced severe emphysema and many impairments and functional limitations.

BOX 2-6

A Patient with Chronic Obstructive Pulmonary Disease and "Some" Baseline Data—A Case Study Integrating the Use of the Guide with the Textbook

Patient History and Inclusion Criteria for Preferred Practice Pattern 6E of the Guide

- A 65-year-old male with a very long history of cigarette smoking and complaints of severe shortness of breath at rest and during self-care.
- Markedly abnormal pulmonary function test results revealing severe chronic obstructive pulmonary disease (COPD) and severe hyperinflation of the lungs due to **emphysema.**
- **Rapid respiratory rate and decreased movement of air in and out of the mouth (tidal volume).**
- **Markedly decreased breath sounds.**
- **Decreased strength and endurance of the ventilatory muscles.**
- **Decreased arterial oxygen and increased carbon dioxide levels.**
- **Observation of an abdominal paradoxical breathing pattern (Fig. 2-7B).**

Method to Integrate the Guide with the Textbook

1. Go to page 471 of the *Guide* to identify the most likely practice pattern under which the patient falls. Based on the previous information, the patient will best fit under Practice Patterns C, E, or F.
2. The exclusion criteria for Practice Pattern C exclude neonates with respiratory failure and patients with respiratory failure requiring mechanical ventilation, but include patients with COPD who have airway clearance dysfunction. The above patient does not have airway clearance dysfunction and so he is excluded from Practice Pattern C.
3. The exclusion criteria for Practice Pattern F also exclude neonates with respiratory failure and patients with cardiovascular pump failure, but include patients with COPD who have respiratory failure. The above patient does not have respiratory failure and so he is excluded from Practice Pattern F.
4. In view of the above exclusion/inclusion criteria, this patient best fits under Practice Pattern E. Several *ICD-9 CM* codes fit this patient under the *ICD-9-CM* codes of Practice Pattern E including Codes 492 (emphysema), 492.8 (other emphysema), and 786.0 (dyspnea and respiratory abnormalities).
5. Go to Chapter 19 of this textbook.
6. Find the hypothesis-oriented algorithm of Chapter 19 and identify the primary test directing the algorithm (observation of an abdominal paradoxical breathing pattern) and the secondary tests (eg, pulmonary function, arterial blood gas, and diaphragmatic excursion test results) further directing the examination and management of this patient.
7. Forward Lean Test: Note correction of abdominal paradoxical breathing pattern and
   a. decreased the respiratory rate, shortness of breath, and arterial carbon dioxide level.
   b. increased the tidal volume, arterial oxygen level, breath sounds, and strength/endurance of the ventilatory muscles.
8. Use Forward Lean as an intervention: Note improvement in ability to perform functional tasks.

---

*Bolded areas are inclusion criteria for Practice Pattern E.

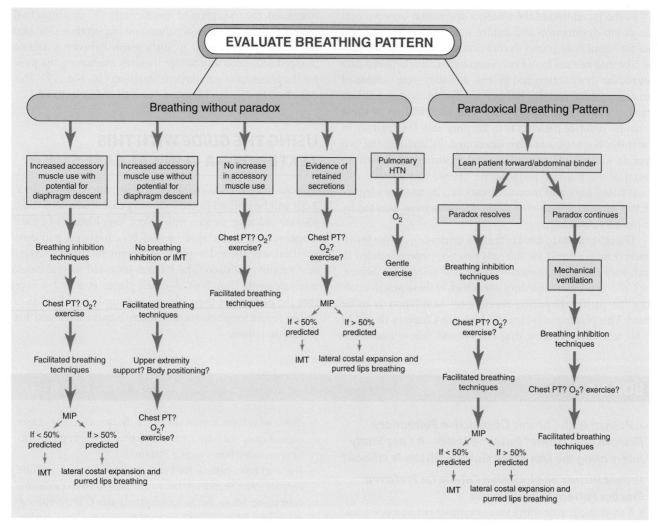

FIGURE 2-10   A brief example of a hypothesis-oriented algorithm for the examination and management of persons with impaired ventilation and respiration/gas exchange associated with ventilatory pump dysfunction or failure.

Much of the previous information is important as inclusion criteria listed for Practice Pattern E (ventilatory pump dysfunction or failure), but it does not provide much specificity about the pathology or other areas of disablement affected by the emphysema. Because of this, the use of a specialized test that has been shown to distinguish between ventilatory pump dysfunction and failure is necessary (Box 2-6).

Observation of an abdominal paradoxical breathing pattern can distinguish a failing ventilatory pump from a dysfunctional ventilatory pump. The specifics of this specialized test are briefly described in Box 2-6 and thoroughly discussed in Chapters 9 and 19 of this textbook as well as on the CD-ROM. The specific treatments provided to patients with ventilatory pump failure (breathing with paradox) and dysfunction (breathing without paradox, but demonstrating one of the problems in the second level on the left-hand side of Fig. 2-10) are presented in Fig. 2-10. Other specific interventions that can be provided to patients based on specific results from specialized tests are given in the practice pattern chapters of this textbook (Chapters 15–21).

SUMMARY

This overview of the practice patterns and threshold behaviors reveals that there is indeed an eminent paradigm shift in physical therapy research and clinical care. A modest number of investigations have demonstrated significant relationships between areas of disablement and physical therapy examination or intervention.[21–39] Similar investigations are likely to be performed, and more specific disablement measurements will likely be found. The results from these investigations will identify specific patient populations who will likely benefit from specific physical therapy interventions and allow physical therapy outcomes to be predicted. Specific interventions and outcomes will likely be determined and predicted by identifying "threshold behaviors." PTs have historically measured impairments, and some have focused on the functional abilities of patients. Recently, more PTs have begun to measure impairments, functional abilities, disabilities, and quality of life issues. These additional measurements of disablement are likely to improve patient examinations and the implementation of future physical therapy. Hopefully, the new evidence obtained from this paradigm shift will find its way into future editions of the *Guide*. An additional issue worthy of attention is the manner that the ICF conceptual model will be implemented within the *Guide* and the preferred practice patterns of physical therapy. Addressing the above issues will serve to make the *Guide* even more clinically useful.

REFERENCES

1. Guide to Physical Therapist Practice, Volume I: A Description of Patient Management. *Phys Ther.* 1995;75:707-764.
2. Guide to Physical Therapist Practice. *Phys Ther.* 1997;77:1163-1650.
3. Rothstein J. Editorial. *Phys Ther.* 1997;77:1160-1161.
4. Rothstein J. On the second edition of the *Guide. Phys Ther.* 2001;81:6-8.
5. Clinical Research Agenda. *Phys Ther.* 2000;80:499-513.
6. Guide to Physical Therapist Practice. Revisions. *Phys Ther.* 1999;623-629.
7. Guide to Physical Therapist Practice. Revisions. *Phys Ther.* 1999;1078-1081.
8. American Physical Therapy Association. Guide to Physical Therapist Practice. 2nd ed. *Phys Ther.* 2001 Jan;81(1):9-746.
9. Hillegass E. Applying the cardiopulmonary practice patterns: case study of a person with multisystem problems. *Cardiopulm Phys Ther J.* 1999;10(3):84-89.
10. Cahalin LP. Applying the cardiopulmonary practice patterns: heart failure. *Cardiopulm Phys Ther J.* 1999;10(3):90-97.
11. Bourgeois MC. Diagnosing pulmonary impairment: a lung volume reduction surgery case that uses the patient management model. *Cardiopulm Phys Ther J.* 1999;10(3):98-100.
12. Schuster NB. Simultaneous implementation of two cardiopulmonary preferred practice patterns across the continuum of care. *Phys Ther Case Rep.* 1999;2(6):241-248.
13. Gordon J, Quinn L. *Guide* to physical therapist practice: a critical appraisal. *Neurol Rep.* 1999;23(3):122-128.
14. Focused Issue: the *Guide* to Physical Therapist Practice. *GeriNotes.* 1999;6(5):1-35.
15. Giallonardo L. *Guide* in action: patient with total hip replacement. *PT Magazine.* 2000;8(9):76-88.
16. Bernhardt-Bainbridge D. What's new: *guide* to physical therapists practice, 2nd ed. *PT Magazine.* 2001;9(3):34-37.
17. Verbrugge L, Jette A. The disablement process. *Soc Sci Med.* 1994;38:1.
18. Jette AM. Outcomes research: shifting the dominant research paradigm in physical therapy. *Phys Ther.* 1995;75:965-970.
19. Nagi S. Some conceptual issues in disability and rehabilitation. In: Sussman M, ed. *Sociology and Rehabilitation.* Washington, DC: American Sociological Association; 1965:100-113.
20. Nagi S. Disability concepts revisited: implication for prevention. In: Pope A, Tarlov A, eds. *Disability in America: Toward a National Agenda for Prevention.* Washington, DC: National Academy Press; 1991:309-327.
21. Sahrmann SA. Diagnosis by the physical therapist. *Phys Ther.* 1988;68:1703-1706.
22. Jette AM. Diagnosis and classification by physical therapists. *Phys Ther.* 1989;69:967-969.
23. World Health Organization. *International Classification of Functioning, Disability and Health: ICF.* Geneva, Switzerland: World Health Organization; 2001.
24. Jette AM. The changing language of disablement. *Phys Ther.* 2005;85(2):118-119.
25. Jette AM. Toward a common language for function, disability, and health. *Phys Ther.* 2006;86:726-734.
26. Sahrmann SA. Commentary on: Dekker J, van Baar ME, Curfs EC, Kerssens JJ. Diagnosis and treatment in physical therapy: an investigation of their relationship. *Phys Ther.* 1993;73:578-579.
27. Guccione AA. Physical therapy diagnosis and the relationship between impairment and function. *Phys Ther.* 1991;71:499-504.
28. Rothstein JM. Editor's note: disability and our identity. *Phys Ther.* 1994;74:375-378.
29. Jette AM. Physical disablement concepts for physical therapy research and practice. *Phys Ther.* 1994;74:380-386.
30. Frontera WR, Meredith CN, O'Reilly KP, et al. Strength conditioning in older men: skeletal muscle hypertrophy and improved function. *J Appl Physiol.* 1988;64:1038-1044.
31. Fisher NM, Gresham GF, Abrams M, et al. Quantitative effects of physical therapy on muscular and functional performance in subjects with osteoarthritis of the knees. *Arch Phys Med Rehabil.* 1993;74:840-847.
32. Stratford PW, Blinkley J, Solomon P, et al. Assessing change over time in patients with low back pain. *Phys Ther.* 1994;74:528-533.
33. Erhard RE, Delitto A, Cibulka MT. Relative effectiveness of an extension program and combined program of manipulation and flexion and extension exercises in patients with acute low back syndrome. *Phys Ther.* 1994;74:1093-1100.
34. Tovin BJ, Wolf SL, Greenfield BH, et al. Comparison of the effects of exercise in water and on land on the rehabilitation of patients with intra-articular anterior cruciate ligament reconstructions. *Phys Ther.* 1994;74:710-719.
35. Physical disability. *Phys Ther.* 1994;74(special issue):375-505.
36. Delitto A, Erhard RE, Bowling RW. A treatment-based classification approach to low back syndrome: identifying and staging patients for conservative treatment. *Phys Ther.* 1995;75:470-489.
37. Jette DU, Downing J. The relationship of cardiovascular and psychological impairments to the health status of patients enrolled in cardiac rehabilitation programs. *Phys Ther.* 1996;76:130-139.
38. Jette DU, Manago D, Medved E, et al. The disablement process in patients with pulmonary disease. *Phys Ther.* 1997;77:385-394.
39. Buchner DM, Beresford SA, Larson EB, et al. Effects of physical activity on health status in older adults, II: intervention studies. *Ann Rev Public Health.* 1992;13:469-488.
40. Cahalin LP, Mathier MA, Semigran MJ, et al. The six-minute walk test predicts peak oxygen uptake and survival in patients with advanced heart failure. *Chest.* 1996;110:325-332.

Essentials of Exercise Physiology

William E. DeTurk & Lisa Johnson

INTRODUCTION

It is one of the great marvels and mysteries of life that simple elements like carbon, hydrogen, and oxygen can be combined with a life force to produce human existence and movement. These elements are found in carbohydrate, fat, and protein—the food substrates that we consume. This chapter begins with quantification of energy expenditure and then describes the formation of energy substrates and their subsequent breakdown. Nutrition for optimum health will be explored. Adenosine triphosphate (ATP) will be appreciated as the link between the breakdown of food and the ability to perform physical activity. Exercise states will be described as a function of metabolic pathways. Obesity and measurement of body composition will be discussed. The chapter concludes with components of a physical fitness program and principles of exercise prescription.

This chapter is not intended to be an in-depth examination of exercise physiology. Rather, it is an extraction of select basic principles of exercise that has meaning and application to patients with disease. Understanding the normal physiological response to exercise will provide a firm foundation to appreciate abnormal responses.

MEASURES OF ENERGY EXPENDITURE

The Calorie

The energy value of the food that we eat can be quantified in terms of calorie. A kilocalorie (kcal) is the amount of heat necessary to raise the temperature of 1.0 kg of water by 1.0°C. The energy value of food is determined by placing a known quantity of food in a *bomb calorimeter*. This device uses oxygen to completely burn the substrate and measure the amount of heat liberated. Thus, the energy value of 4.0 oz of cheesecake is almost 350 kcal. As you will see, it takes a lot of exercise to burn off a slice of cheesecake!

Oxygen Consumption: Rest

Oxygen is utilized as an adjunct to substrate *catabolism*, or breakdown, in all metabolically active tissues. Oxygen consumption may be abbreviated as $\dot{V}_{O_2}$, or the volume of oxygen consumed per minute, and expressed as either mL O_2/min or mL O_2/kg of body weight/min. The basal metabolic rate (BMR) is the minimal amount of oxygen utilized in order to support life. It is the sum total of cellular activity in all metabolically active tissues while under basal conditions. Skeletal muscle $\dot{V}_{O_2}$ accounts for approximately 20% of the total BMR. The BMR is measured under strictly controlled laboratory conditions. The resting metabolic rate (RMR) is a more easily acquired measurement. Patients are instructed to avoid strenuous exercise for at least 24 hours before testing. Measurements are obtained at least 4 hours after a light meal and no caffeine.[1] Its value is only slightly higher than the BMR. Measurement of the RMR was once costly and time-consuming and involved use of a metabolic cart or Douglas bag collection systems. Newer, handheld portable devices (eg, the *BodyGem*) are beginning to replace such instrumentation.[2] **There is considerable variation in BMR and RMR values across human subjects.** This variation is a function of overall body size, gender, age, fat-free mass (FFM), and endocrine function.[1,3–6] Normal measurements of BMR fall around 200 mL O_2/min for women and 250 mL O_2/min for men.

The BMR/RMR can also be measured indirectly using regression equations such as the revised Harris–Benedict equation[7] or the WHO/FAO/UNU regression equation.[8]

In general, the BMR and RMR tend to be 5% to 10% lower in women than in men.[9] This is not a true sex difference, but rather the presence of more adipose tissue in women, which has a lower level of metabolic activity than muscle and provides an increase in thermal insulation. The variation in BMR and RMR within subjects of the same gender is a function of differences in lean body mass (LBM) and endocrine function. There is a strong association between LBM and body surface area within gender; for this reason, body surface area is commonly used to reflect LBM and, by extension, to predict BMR. The BMR also varies as a function of age, such that there is a decline in BMR of 2% to 3% per decade of life.[10] This is most likely due to the reduction in physical activity associated with aging and the resultant decrease in LBM, change in endocrine function, and increase in body fat.[11,12]

Both kilocalories and $\dot{V}O_2$ are useful tools to measure the body's response to exercise. **Indeed, a relationship exists between kilocalories and $\dot{V}O_2$, such that, for every liter of oxygen consumed, approximately 5.0 kcal of energy is liberated.**

OXYGEN CONSUMPTION: EXERCISE

With progressive increases in submaximal workload, $\dot{V}O_2$ increases in a linear fashion. This relationship is sustained until a maximum exercise level is reached ($\dot{V}O_2$ *peak or functional capacity*), at which point a further increase in workload produces no further increase in $\dot{V}O_2$.

The MET

METs are defined as multiples of resting energy metabolism. One MET is, therefore, a close approximation of the RMR in the seated position. The value of 1 MET has been standardized as

$$1 \text{ MET} = 3.5 \text{ mL } O_2/\text{kg/min.}$$

This value is assumed to be approximately the same across all subjects—man, woman, young, or old. The derivation of the MET, and its relationship to the RMR, requires some comment.

It has been noted that the BMR varies as a function of body size, gender, age, FFM, and endocrine function and that its direct measurement normally falls between 200 mL O_2/min for women and 250 mL O_2/min for men. The BMR can be bet-

ter standardized by including the subject's individual body weight in the equation. Thus, for an "average" woman weighing 57 kg and an "average" man weighing 71 kg,

for women: 200 mL O_2/min/57 kg = 3.5 mL O_2/kg/min
= 1 MET.

for men: 250 mL O_2/min/71 kg = 3.5 mL O_2/kg/min
= 1 MET.

In order to standardize a MET value of 3.5 mL O_2/kg/min, the transformation noted in the equation assumes some sort of a reference, or idealized as woman weighing 57 kg (125 lb) and man weighing 71 kg (156 lb). Indeed, this is probably the case. Albert Behnke, a pioneer in body composition research, first defined a "reference man" and a "reference woman" in the 1970s.[13,14] His work paved the way for conceptualization of the MET and its application to exercise.

Acceptance of the value of 1 MET = 3.5 mL O_2/kg/min across individuals allows one to quantify exercise based on the number of METs required to perform the activity. **However, it must be noted that use of METs to quantify exercise assumes the following: (1) the exercise is primarily reliant on the oxygen transport system; (2) the activity is being performed at a steady state, that is, the amount of oxygen needed to perform the activity is matched by a supply of oxygen; (3) the subject is performing the activity with biomechanical efficiency.** An example of an activity that meets these requirements is that of a patient free from lower-extremity biomechanical impairment, walking at a moderate, comfortable pace down a hallway.

If 1 MET is defined as resting $\dot{V}O_2$ (ie, RMR), then 7.0 mL O_2/kg/min measured during a walk down the hall corresponds to 2 METs. Similarly, walking on a treadmill set at 1.7 miles per hour (mph) at a 10% grade requires approximately 5.0 METs of oxidative energy expenditure, a gross value that includes the resting energy expenditure. These values are assumed to be about the same for all biomechanically normal subjects irrespective of gender, age, or body composition—as long as the exercise is submaximal, utilizes the oxygen transport mechanism, and as long as the value is normalized to body weight and expressed on a per-kilogram basis. A useful analogy is that of the cost of a cheeseburger: It is the same for everyone, rich or poor. Similarly, the cost of walking on the treadmill using a normal gait pattern at a submaximal workload should be about the same for everyone. See Table 3-1 for standardized energy values in METs for treadmill work and relatively unstructured leisure time activities.

When calculating the amount of energy required to perform any given task, particularly as it relates to weight loss, resting energy metabolism should be removed from the equation, because this energy would have been utilized whether or not exercise was performed. Thus,

net energy expenditure = gross − resting energy expenditure.

TABLE 3-1 Energy Values for Select Leisure and Recreational Activities in METs

Activity	Mean	Range
Badminton	5.8	4–9+
Climbing hills	7.2	5–10
Fishing from bank	3.7	2–4
Football (touch)	7.9	6–10
Golf (walking)	5.1	4–7
Racquetball	9	8–12
Running (6-minute mile)	16.3	—[a]
Running (8-minute mile)	12.5	—
Running (10-minute mile)	10.2	—
Tennis	6.5	4–9+

[a]Insignificant range.

Modified with permission from American College of Sports Medicine. *ACSM's Guidelines for Exercise Testing and Prescription.* 6th ed. Philadelphia, PA: Lippincott Williams & Wilkins; 2000.

CLINICAL CORRELATE

Quantifying the amount of exercise that the physical therapist prescribes to a patient through the use of MET units allows exercises to be graded from lower intensity to higher intensity and provides a basis for comparisons between subjects. Use of MET units can also be used to plot individual patient progress. However, physical therapists should be aware that use of MET units to normalize work is referenced to a man and woman of "ideal" body weight and stature and that this person is free from biomechanical impairments. More importantly, the heart rate and blood pressure response to exercise is highly individualistic at any given MET level, which may make the use of MET units impractical, especially for patients with heart and lung disease and for patients with lower extremity impairments (eg, stroke, amputation).

NUTRIENTS/FOODSTUFFS

All nutrients consist of carbon, hydrogen, and oxygen. It is the ratio of one component to the other and their molecular structure that differentiates them. Nutrients used to power exercise include carbohydrates, fats, and proteins. These nutrients, together with vitamins, minerals, and water, are essential for the maintenance of optimum health. This section will describe the structural characteristics of these nutrients and current nutritional recommendations for health and the prevention of disease.

CLINICAL CORRELATE

Physical therapists should possess knowledge of basic nutrition, understand how diet and exercise may work together in helping patients achieve their ideal weight, and recognize when to refer patients to professionals trained in nutrition sciences.

Proper nutrition may improve the quality of life of our patients by improving their ability to carry out work and leisure time activity without fatigue.

Carbohydrates

Introduction

Carbohydrates consist of carbon, hydrogen, and oxygen, and the hydrogen-to-oxygen ratio is always 2:1. They are classified as *monosaccharides, oligosaccharides,* or *polysaccharides.* We will spend some time discussing the monosaccharide glucose because it is the principal substrate used to fuel exercise and the final common denominator that allows entrance into one of the main energy extraction pathways (see Fig. 3-1A).

Glucose is formed by plants during photosynthesis, but its relevance for us resides in the reverse equation called *cellular respiration,* which breaks down glucose and releases energy:

$$C_6H_{12}O_6 + 6O_2 \rightarrow 6CO_2 + 6H_2O + \text{energy}.$$

Circulating blood glucose is one element in a blood chemical analysis found in "panel tests" (SMA-6,12). Normal fasting levels are 70 to 110 mg/dL. **Glucose, or "blood sugar," is also known as dextrose, a 5% solution of water and glucose. In the intensive care unit, patients frequently have a bag of "D5W" running intravenously for nutrition and blood volume expansion to maintain blood pressure and thus peripheral perfusion.**

The storage form of glucose is *glycogen,* a polysaccharide polymer. It is stored in muscle and liver tissue. Glucose molecules are linked together in long helical chains to form glycogen (see Fig. 3-1B). Notice that it is very easy to move from glycogen to glucose because of the way that glucose molecules are strung together.

Each cell has its own glycogen store, limited by the size of the cell. Once maximum glycogen storage is reached and the cell can hold no more, glucose will not enter the cell; instead, excess glycogen is moved to the liver where it is reconverted, or stored, in adipose cells as fat.

When there is an increase in sugar intake, blood glucose levels go up as well. This triggers an increase in insulin secretion by the pancreas. The hormone *insulin* regulates the movement of glucose into cells, thereby decreasing blood glucose levels. When there is a decrease in blood glucose levels below the baseline level, glucagon, the "insulin antagonist," is secreted

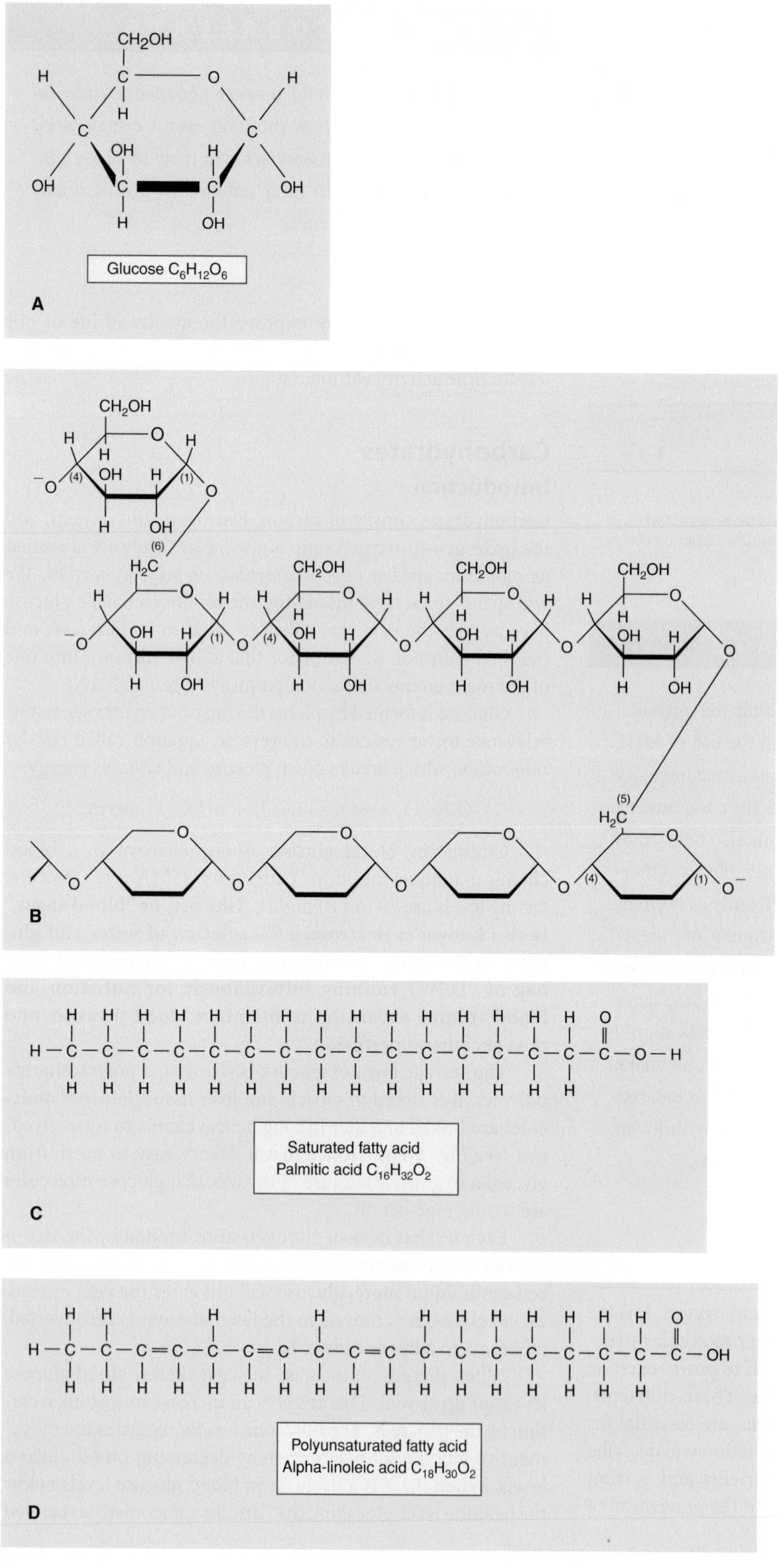

FIGURE 3-1 Chemical structure of fuel substrates—carbohydrate, fats, and protein. (**A**) Glucose; (**B**) glycogen; (**C**) saturated fatty acid, palmitic acid; (**D**) unsaturated fatty acid α-linoleic acid; *(continued)*

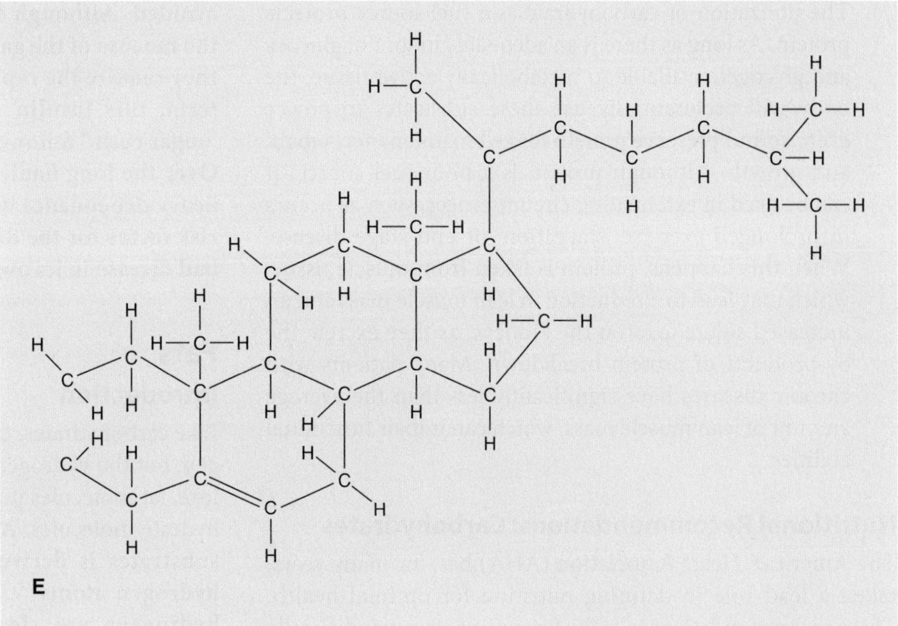

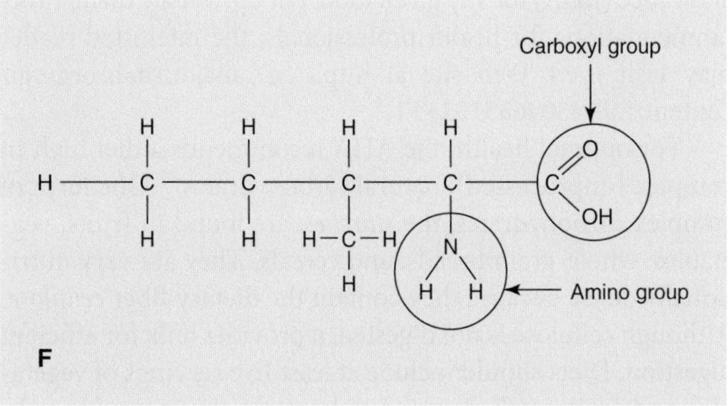

FIGURE 3-1 *(Continued)* (**E**) cholesterol; (**F**) protein isoleucine.
(Adapted with permission from Foss M, Keteyian S. *Fox's: Physiological Basis for Exercise and Sport.* 6th ed. Boston, MA: WCB McGraw-Hill; 1998.)

by the pancreas to increase blood glucose levels. Thus, the pancreas plays a pivotal role in maintaining normal circulating blood glucose levels. We will expand on control of glucose blood levels when diabetes is discussed in Chapter 15.

Role of Carbohydrates

Carbohydrates serve a variety of important roles in normal body function.

1. Carbohydrate is the primary fuel source of the body. The energy yield from the complete degradation of a mole of glucose is 686 kcal/mol, or approximately 4 kcal/g. **In fact, glucose is the *only* ingested foodstuff that can be used during efforts of high intensity.** Its availability in a wide range of foodstuffs makes it readily accessible. There are efficient metabolic processes in the human body that break carbohydrate down into molecular fragments that can be used to make adenosine triphosphate, or ATP, the "energy packets" that are used to power work. These processes break down $C_6H_{12}O_6$ into two pyruvic acid molecules during glycolysis; energy is extracted and captured in the form of ATP. The remaining energy is extracted in the citric acid (Kreb) cycle. More will be said about this later.

2. Carbohydrate is a necessary adjunct for the catabolism of fats. The correct breakdown of fats, particularly triglyceride, depends on the presence of glucose. Without glucose, the body will mobilize more lipid than can be broken down. Lipid will be incompletely catabolized, with the formation of lipid fragments consisting of acetone-like bodies called *ketone bodies.* These ketone bodies create an acid environment that decreases systemic pH, sometimes to dangerous levels. **Diabetic patients whose insulin levels are low and whose blood glucose levels are high may deteriorate into *diabetic ketoacidosis* with resultant diabetic coma.**

3. Carbohydrate is the principal fuel for the central nervous system (CNS). In healthy persons under normal conditions, glucose is the exclusive substrate of the CNS. The brain cannot store glucose; therefore, the only route for nutrition is through circulating blood glucose. Liver glycogenolysis maintains circulating blood glucose levels. When glycogen stores become depleted and blood glucose levels go down, most people start to feel weak and dizzy. Both healthy persons and patients alike may require a drink that is high in a readily absorbed simple sugar to keep them from becoming *hypoglycemic.*

4. The utilization of carbohydrate as a fuel source protects protein. As long as there is an adequate amount of glucose and glycogen available to metabolically active tissue, the body will preferentially use these substrates to power exercise and preserve protein for cell maintenance, repair, and growth. Although protein is a poor fuel source, it can be used in extenuating circumstances, such as occurs in prolonged exercise, starvation, or end-stage disease. When this happens, protein is taken from muscle tissue, which may lead to a reduction in lean muscle mass and an increased solute load on the kidneys, as they excrete the by-products of protein breakdown. Many patients with chronic diseases have significantly less than the average amount of lean muscle mass, which can impair functional abilities.

Nutritional Recommendations: Carbohydrates

The American Heart Association (AHA) has, for many years, taken a lead role in defining nutrition for optimal health. These recommendations take the form of a recommended daily allowance (RDA) for any given food. For up-to-date dietary recommendations for health professionals, the interested reader may visit their Web site at http://circ.ahajournals.org/cgi/content/full/4304635102#T1.

For optimal health, the AHA recommends a diet high in complex (unprocessed), natural carbohydrates.[15] One form of complex carbohydrates, the *starches,* are found in fruits, vegetables, whole-grain breads, and cereals. They are very nutritionally dense because they contain the dietary fiber *cellulose.* Although cellulose is not digested, it provides bulk for efficient digestion. Diets should include at least five servings of vegetables and fruits each day and at least six servings of breads, cereals, and/or legumes. Diets high in carbohydrates are usually low in saturated fats and are, therefore, linked with a lower incidence of lung, colon, esophageal, and stomach cancer and heart disease.

After ingestion, carbohydrates get absorbed into the bloodstream at different rates. This depends on particle size and degree of processing, amount of fiber, and fat and protein content, for example. The *glycemic index* measures the relative rise in blood glucose levels in the 2-hour period following ingestion of any given substrate, compared to a "reference food," usually 50 g of white bread or glucose. Glucose, as the reference food, has a glycemic index of 100. Kidney beans have a glycemic index of 27, which indicates that consuming 50 g of kidney beans provokes an increase in blood glucose that is 27% as great as ingesting 50 g of glucose. Foods may be rank ordered from those with a low glycemic index to those with a high glycemic index. Individuals can get a more stable and long-term rise in blood glucose levels by eating low glycemic-index foods (eg, whole-wheat bread, spaghetti, legumes). Individuals may choose to eat foods with a moderate-to-high glycemic index for a more rapid elevation in blood glucose levels (eg, instant rice, baked potatoes, honey).[16,17] **Unless specific events dictate otherwise, it may be said that simple processed sugars, like those in candy bars, should be avoided. Although they can be absorbed quickly through the mucosa of the gastrointestinal tract and taken into cells, they require the rapid mobilization of insulin. In the short term, this insulin dependence contributes to an initial "sugar rush," followed by feelings of low energy and fatigue. Over the long haul, consumption of processed sugars and heavy dependence on insulin may contribute to diabetes, a risk factor for the development of heart disease and a very bad disease in its own right.**

Fats

Introduction

Like carbohydrates, fats consist of carbon, hydrogen, and oxygen, but the hydrogen-to-oxygen ratio is much higher. Therefore, fat molecules possess many more hydrogens than carbohydrate molecules. **As we shall see, the energy value of fuel substrates is derived from the number and amount of hydrogen atoms "exposed" on their binding sites. When hydrogens are cleaved off their substrates, energy is released and then captured in the form of ATP.** There are three main groups of fats: simple lipids, compound lipids, and derived lipids.

Simple Lipids

Triglycerides are perhaps the best known of the simple lipids. Fat is stored in the body as triglyceride. A single molecule consists of three fatty acids and one glycerol unit. Fatty acid molecules may be either *saturated* or *unsaturated.* Saturated fatty acids have single bonds between carbon atoms, thus freeing up more binding sites for hydrogens. Unsaturated fatty acids possess double bonds between carbons, with proportionately less binding sites for hydrogen. Most saturated fats are derived from animal sources, whereas unsaturated fatty acids come from plant sources and liquify at room temperature (see Figs. 3-1C and 3-1D for examples of saturated and unsaturated fatty acids).

The unsaturated fatty acids may be subdivided into the *monounsaturated fatty acids* (MUFAs) and the *polyunsaturated fatty acids* (PUFAs). MUFAs contain one double bond along the main carbon chain; olive oil is an example of a MUFA. PUFAs contain multiple double bonds along the main carbon chain; corn oil and fish oils are examples of PUFAs.

Yet another type of fatty acids are the *trans fatty acids* (TFAs). TFAs are formed when a hydrogen atom is moved from its original naturally occurring position along a restructured carbon chain to a different position. This results in a modified fatty acid that contains no cholesterol. TFAs form the principal component of dietary margarine, which is derived from vegetable oil. Margarine has been promoted as a safe alternative to butter, because it is low in cholesterol. However, there is considerable debate about the health benefit of margarine ingestion. It has been found that margarine increases serum low-density lipoprotein (LDL) levels and that this increase is equivalent to a diet high in saturated fatty acids.[18] Margarine also decreases high-density lipoprotein (HDL) cholesterol.[19] These findings support the notion that ingestion of TFAs is dangerous to your health and actually increases the risk of heart disease.[20,21] In July 2003, the FDA required that the amount of TFAs appear on nutrition labels.

Compound Lipids

Important examples of the compound lipids are the *lipoproteins*. The lipoproteins are synthesized in the liver, although they are present in all cells. Lipoproteins consist of a hydrophobic protein core and an outer shell containing free cholesterol, phospholipid, and a regulatory protein called an *apolipoprotein* (apo). They function as the transport mechanism for lipids and are categorized according to their molecular weight. The HDLs possess the highest amount of protein (up to 50%) and the lowest amount of cholesterol (approximately 20%). They are popularly called the "good cholesterol" because they remove cholesterol from arterial walls and transport it to the liver, where it is excreted. The LDLs, or "bad cholesterol," contain large amounts of cholesterol, which they transport to arterial walls, thus contributing to atherosclerosis or "hardening of the arteries." Clearly it is in our best interest to maintain high levels of HDL and low levels of LDL. Although only a few studies to date have isolated exercise from multifactorial interventions aimed at reducing LDL and increasing HDL, **current best practice recognizes the appropriate use of exercise as an essential component in the nonpharmacologic treatment of elevated serum lipids.**[22] There is also convincing evidence that moderate consumption of alcohol elevates HDL levels and exerts a protective influence from heart disease.[23]

The apos form the shell of the lipoproteins. They help to keep the lipids in solution during circulation through the bloodstream. Apos regulate plasma lipid metabolism and direct lipids to their appropriate target organs. There are multiple isoforms of apos. Apo AI is of interest because it is the major apo of HDL. Similarly, apo B and apo E surround the LDL molecule.[24] Apos have come under scrutiny because of their association with the development of heart disease. Studies show that apo AI and apo B_{100} are better discriminators of individuals with coronary artery disease than the cholesterol of the corresponding protein.[25,26] Additionally, these two apos correlate better with the severity of coronary artery stenosis than LDL and HDL.[24,27]

Derived Lipids

Perhaps the best known of the derived fats is *cholesterol*. Serum cholesterol is a composite of the total cholesterol contained in each of the lipoproteins. Indeed, cholesterol distribution among the lipoproteins is a stronger predictor of heart disease than total serum cholesterol.[28] Cholesterol is found exclusively in animal tissue. It is both consumed in the food we eat and produced by the body, mainly in the liver (70%) but also in other areas (eg, arterial walls). A high cholesterol level in the blood is an independent risk factor for the development of heart disease. Cholesterol's bad reputation is balanced by the fact that it is an essential precursor for vitamin D production and is needed to synthesize hormones, especially estrogen, androgen, and progesterone. See Fig. 3-1E for the chemical composition of a cholesterol molecule.

Role of Fats

The presence of fat in our body *habitus* has become the source of intense investigation, as scientists weigh the positive role of body fat against excessive dietary intake. The benefits of fats in the maintenance of proper body function are listed as follows. (1) Fats have the highest energy yield of any of the substrates in the body. In fact, 1.0 g of fat yields over twice the energy compared to an equal amount of carbohydrate. The complete degradation of a mole of a typical lipid yields 9 kcal/g. Recall that energy is released when hydrogen is cleaved off food substrate. This high yield is due to the presence of the increased number of hydrogens referred to earlier. (2) Fat provides a layer of insulation for the body that helps maintain thermal homeostasis. (3) Fat surrounds body organs (eg, heart, kidneys) and protects them from injury. (4) Fat serves as a carrier for the fat-soluble vitamins A, D, E, and K, which are required for normal nerve propagation, menstruation, and reproduction as well as for growth and maturation during pubescence. Finally, the presence of at least a small amount of fat in the daily diet impacts on the satiety center found in the brainstem. Positive stimulation of this structure causes feelings of gastric fullness that can reduce the total daily caloric intake and helps retard weight gain.

Nutritional Recommendations: Fats

For the most part, body fat is inversely proportional to optimal health. A diet high in fat, especially saturated fat, increases the risk of atherosclerotic cardiovascular disease as well as breast, prostate, and colon cancer.[29] The AHA currently recommends that total dietary fat should comprise no more than 30% of the total daily caloric intake. Of this amount, saturated fat should make up no more than 7% to 10% of total calories, no more than 10% should be PUFA, and no more than 15% should be MUFA. PUFA and MUFA should be substituted for saturated fat because saturated fat augments endogenous cholesterol production. Dietary (exogenous) cholesterol should be limited to 300 mg/d. These values change frequently as more research data become available regarding true risk for the development of heart disease. Indeed, as of May 2003, the National Cholesterol Education Program branch of the National Institutes of Health now considers 7% to be the cutoff for the maximum number of calories that should be derived from saturated fat.

Elevated serum triglyceride levels have been associated with an increased risk for the development of heart disease. However, it has become apparent that this risk is confined to the presence of elevated saturated fatty acids and that this risk can be decreased by increasing intake of MUFAs and PUFAs. One such PUFA, omega-3, is of special interest because of its beneficial health effect. Omega-3 is a naturally occurring oil found in cold-water fish, such as cod, tuna, herring, and mackerel. Omega-3 reduces the risk of developing heart disease by preventing clot formation on arterial walls. Indeed, the ingestion of one fatty fish meal per week is associated with a 50% reduction in risk for primary cardiac arrest.[30] It also reduces the risk of developing chronic obstructive lung disease among smokers. The AHA recommends two servings of cold-water fish per week.

Currently, only 33% of Americans older than 2 years meet the goal of eating no more than 30% of the diet as fat. **Sensible restriction of fat intake should take into account the tremendous energy value of lipid and the need for essential fats like linoleic acid and fat-soluble vitamins.**

Proteins

Introduction

Proteins also contain the carbon, hydrogen, and oxygen found in carbohydrates and fats, but their chemical composition also includes phosphorus, nitrogen, iron, and minerals. The major components of proteins are the *amino acids.* Indeed, proteins are defined on the basis of their amino acid composition (see Fig. 3-1F).

Note that each amino acid contains an *amino* (NH_2) *radical* and an *organic acid carboxyl* (COOH) *group* that remain consistent across different amino acids. The third major component of the amino acid is the *side chain*. It is the structural characteristics of the side chain that define the amino acid. There are 20 different amino acids in the human body. This allows amino acids to combine in thousands of combinations to create over 50,000 different proteins that serve roles that range from cellular reproduction to muscular contraction.

There are nine *essential amino acids,* which are provided exclusively through ingestion. There are nine *nonessential amino acids,* which are made in the body. The two remaining are *derived amino acids,* those synthesized from the essential amino acids.

Protein is used primarily for tissue maintenance, repair, and growth. The largest amount of protein is found in skeletal muscle (65%). Protein is the primary constituent of actin and myosin, the contractile elements of skeletal muscle tissue. Amino acids form DNA and RNA and, in the process, encode our genetic characteristics.

Protein is a poor fuel source. There are few hydrogens available for energy conversion, and the process of breaking down protein into usable substrate is metabolically expensive, requiring the removal of nitrogen and its excretion from the body as urea.

Because nitrogen is a component of the amino radical, nitrogen is a useful marker for the presence of protein. When nitrogen intake (protein) equals nitrogen excretion (urea), a *nitrogen balance* exists. A *positive nitrogen balance* exists when intake exceeds excretion.

Excess protein, like carbohydrate, gets converted to fat.

CLINICAL CORRELATE

Patients who are very ill and confined to bed may be in a state of "negative nitrogen balance." This means that protein output exceeds protein intake and that protein is being used as a fuel source. Patients who demonstrate a negative protein balance frequently present with generalized muscle atrophy. Protein supplementation combined with muscle strengthening exercises can make these patients more functional.

Nutritional Recommendations: Proteins

Protein is a poor fuel source to power activities. Nevertheless, protein plays an important role in rebuilding tissue after strenuous exercise and, because there are no nutritional stores of protein in the body, is a vital component of the RDA. The AHA recommends a protein ingestion of 50 to 100 mg/d, or 0.8 to 1.2 g/kg of body weight. This represents 15% of the total daily energy expenditure and provides the body with adequate protein for cell maintenance, repair, and growth.[31] Vegetarians need to carefully select a combination of foods that assure adequate intake of the essential amino acids and supplement their diet with vitamin B_{12}, which humans cannot make and must obtain from the diet.

Some substrates are deemed *complete proteins* because they supply all the essential amino acids. Meat, fish, eggs, and milk fall into this category. Vegetables, grains, and fruits provide a rich source of high-quality protein, particularly nuts, legumes, and cereals. None of these sources are complete proteins in and of themselves, but a well-balanced diet of vegetables, grains, and fruits will provide all the essential amino acids.

CLINICAL CORRELATE

Protein supplementation enjoys widespread popularity among strength trainers and bodybuilders. However, there have been no controlled studies that show that high levels of protein ingestion in bodybuilders contribute to changes in metabolism or improved health.[32–34] Indeed, prolonged high-protein ingestion may lead to renal damage and a reduction in bone density.[31]

Similar to carbohydrates, excess proteins get converted to fat.

Vitamins

Vitamins are organic micronutrients that are necessary, in small amounts, for the normal metabolic functioning of the body. They play highly specific roles in energy transfer and tissue synthesis. Although adequate vitamin intake is necessary for health and wellness, excessive vitamin intake is unnecessary and may, in fact, be harmful. A balanced diet of foods containing the minimal RDA is essential for the prevention of disease. Some foods are associated with reducing the incidence of cancers because of the vitamins they contain. These foods, carotenoids and retinoids, include the green and yellow vegetables, which are rich in vitamin A; citrus fruits and vegetables, rich in vitamin C; and green leafy vegetables, rich in vitamin E. Recent studies have shown that vitamins C and E and carotenoid-rich foods act as *antioxidants*.[35,36] Beta-carotenes (plant products that convert to vitamin A in the body) are also included in this group. Antioxidants are believed to inactivate free radicals (activated oxygen molecules) that result from environmental pollution and cause cell damage that may lead to a variety of diseases. There is an emerging evidence that antioxidants may prevent the development of atherosclerosis. The top 10 antioxidant foods include broccoli, cantaloupe, carrots, kale, mango, pumpkin, red pepper, spinach, strawberries, and sweet potato. The adult RDA of 1.0 mg (vitamin A), 60 mg (vitamin C), and 10 mg (vitamin E) should be met with a diet that meets the RDA standards for carbohydrates, fats, and proteins.

Minerals

Minerals are nonorganic metallic elements that are found naturally in the earth's crust. They are constituents of hormones, vitamins, and enzymes. Similar to vitamins, adequate mineral intake is required for optimal health, but excessive mineral consumption is not necessary and may be harmful. Although minerals provide no calories or energy, they are important in regulating body function. Two important minerals are iron and calcium. Iron is necessary for the blood to carry oxygen, and calcium is necessary for the development and function of bone, muscle, nerve, and blood. Calcium may also decrease the risk of heart disease. Other key minerals include phosphorous, sodium, zinc, potassium, and chloride. Phosphorus builds teeth and bone, whereas sodium plays a key role in regulating body water. Zinc and potassium assist in healing and are important for muscle function. Minerals should be consumed in the diet in amounts equal to the RDAs. This can generally be accomplished with a diet containing the food servings recommended for carbohydrates, proteins, and fats. Salt should be limited to no more than 4 to 6 g/day. A calcium dietary supplement is not recommended for the general population but is recommended for adults with poor dietary habits, for postmenopausal women, and for individuals on very low-calorie diets.

Water and Fluids

Despite providing no energy or key nutrients, water is a critical component in a healthy diet. Water is in many foods that we eat, and more than half of all body tissues are composed of water. Regular water intake helps maintain the water balance that is critical to many important body functions. It has been popularly reported that lack of water (dehydration) can be the cause of many ailments, including excess body fat, decreased digestive efficiency and organ function, joint and muscle soreness, and water retention.[37] Recent research evidence suggests that drinking hard water (water with the minerals left in) may reduce the incidence of heart disease.[38] It is generally recommended that the average adult drink eight 8-oz glasses of water each day on top of the water present in the foods we eat.[39] It should be noted that more water is needed for more active individuals and for those with exposure to hot environments.[40]

Caffeine and Alcohol

Coffee, tea, and soft drinks should not be substituted for water. Consuming more than three beverages per day containing caffeine should be avoided, as high caffeine intake may have negative health consequences including dehydration and irregular heart rhythms.

Excessive alcohol intake can be harmful, as alcohol replaces nutrients and increases the risk of hypertension, stroke, heart disease, and osteoporosis. However, current research has provided convincing evidence that moderate daily alcohol ingestion is associated with lower risk of stroke and heart attack, independent of the level of physical fitness.[41,42]

Adults who choose to consume alcohol should do so in moderation. A "drink equivalent" is defined as either a 12-oz bottle of beer, a 4-oz glass of wine, or a 1.5-oz shot of 80-proof spirits. Each of these beverages contains the same amount of alcohol (1/2 oz). Current research has identified that the lowest all-cause mortality among middle-aged men and women occurs in individuals who consume one or two drinks per day.[43] Mortality rises rapidly beyond 3 drinks per day. Box 3-1 summarizes the deleterious effects of excessive alcohol consumption.

Total Recommended Daily Allowance

The total number of calories needed per day is a function of all the metabolic processes that sustain life. These processes reflect both synthesis and breakdown of biomolecules. The total daily energy expenditure is a function of three variables: the RMR, the thermogenic effect of food that is consumed, and the energy utilized during activities of daily living and other exercise states.[6,44,45]

Box 3-2 lists dietary recommendations derived from guidelines provided by the American Dietetic Association, the AHA, and the American Cancer Society for a healthy North American diet. Currently, poor eating habits span all age groups. As a nation, many Americans are overweight, eat foods that are too high in fat and salt, and eat too little complex carbohydrates and fiber. Many women and children do not eat enough foods rich in iron and calcium. Eating well can reduce an individual's risk of developing a variety of health problems.

BOX 3-1

Deleterious Effects of Chronic Alcohol Consumption

Central nervous system:	Kills brain cells; impairs judgment, learning ability, memory; prevents deep sleep; alters personality
Gastrointestinal system:	Cirrhosis of the liver, pancreatitis, esophagitis, gastritis, small–large-bowel bleeds; blockage of absorption of thiamine, folic acid, vitamins B_1 and B_{12}, and amino acids
Genitourinary system:	Women—infertility, spontaneous abortions, fetal alcohol syndrome; men—premature senility, sexual dysfunction
Musculoskeletal system:	Alterations in calcium metabolism, increased risk of fractures, alcoholic myopathy with painful, swollen muscles
Cardiovascular system:	Cardiomyopathy, heart failure, arrhythmia
Other:	Increased risk of cancer of the stomach, liver, pancreas, breast; decreased production of white blood cells

Reproduced with permission from Fauci A, Braunwald E, Isselbacher K, et al., eds. *Harrison's Principles of Internal Medicine.* 14th ed. New York: McGraw-Hill; 1998.

BOX 3-2

Recommendations for a Healthy North American Diet

Balance the food you eat with physical activity to maintain or improve your weight.

Eat a nutritionally adequate diet consisting of a wide variety of foods.

Choose a diet that is low in total fat, saturated fat, and cholesterol.

Choose a diet with plenty of whole-grain products, legumes, fruits, and vegetables that are rich in complex carbohydrates and fiber.

Choose a diet moderate in sugars.

Choose a diet moderate in salt and sodium.

If you drink alcoholic beverages, do so in moderation. Pregnant women should not drink any alcohol.

Maintain protein intake at a moderate, yet adequate level, obtaining much of your daily protein from plant sources.

Choose a diet adequate in calcium and iron.

Children and others susceptible to tooth decay should obtain adequate fluoride.

In general, avoid taking dietary supplements in excess of the RDA in any 1 day.

Eat fewer foods with questionable additives.

Many medical conditions including cardiovascular disease, stroke, diabetes, colon cancer, hypertension, and osteoporosis are affected by eating patterns. Figure 3-2 depicts some possible health problems associated with poor dietary habits.

$\dot{V}O_2$ and caloric expenditure vary over the course of a day depending on exercise state, ambient temperature, and mental status. On an average, a moderately active typical young man requires a total of approximately 3,000 kcal/day. A moderately active woman needs approximately 2,000 kcal/day.[28] It should be noted that these values are also a function of daily activity, lifestyle, and profession: A male athlete in training may burn 3,500 to 6,000 kcal/day, whereas a female athlete may expend 2,600 to 4,500 kcal/day.

Maintenance of Body Weight

For body weight to remain constant, caloric intake must equal energy output. If too much food is consumed, a positive energy balance results and the individual will gain weight. In contrast, if our energy needs are greater than the caloric intake, a negative energy balance occurs. In the latter example, the body utilizes stored fat for energy, resulting in a loss in body weight.

OVERWEIGHT AND OBESITY

Obesity is a serious health problem that reduces life expectancy by increasing one's risk of developing coronary artery disease, hypertension, type 2 diabetes mellitus, obstructive pulmonary disease, osteoarthritis, and certain types of cancer.[46–48] Having too little body fat also presents a health risk because body fat is required for normal physiological functions such as cell membrane formation, thermal insulation, and storage of free fatty acids. Further evidence tells us that the increased risks are not only related to the total amount of body fat but also to the way in which fat is distributed. Intra-abdominal or visceral fat is a stronger predictor of cardiovascular disease[49,50] and other metabolic disorders (type 2 diabetes) than overall body fat.

Being overweight is defined as having body weight in excess of a reference standard, usually a mean weight for a given height, skeletal frame size, grouped by sex.[51] When assessing the health status of a large population, a synthesis of mass and height—the *body mass index* (BMI)—is often computed. The BMI is a weight-to-height ratio using the metric formula:

$$BMI = \frac{\text{body weight in kilograms}}{(\text{height in meters})^2}.$$

When measurements are recorded in pounds and inches, the following equation may be used:

$$BMI = \frac{(\text{body weight in pounds}) \times 705}{(\text{height in inches})^2}.$$

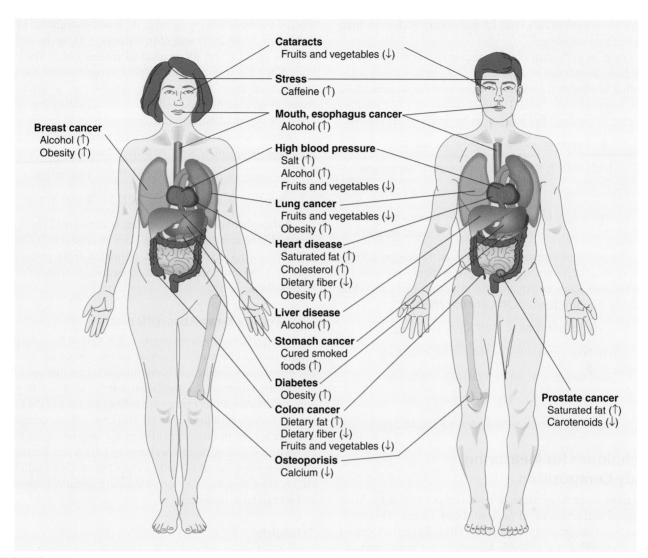

FIGURE 3-2   Possible health problems associated with poor dietary habits. (Reprinted with permission from Williams MH, ed. *Nutrition for Health, Fitness, and Sport.* 5th ed. New York: McGraw-Hill; 1999.)

A BMI score of 18.5 to 24.9 is considered ideal, whereas a BMI score less than 18.5 is considered underweight. Scores falling between 25.0 and 29.9 are considered overweight; those between 30 and 34.9, grade 1 obesity; those between 35.0 and 39.9, grade 2 obesity; and those greater than or equal to 40 represent grade 3 obesity.[52]

Body Composition Assessment

Although widely used, the BMI does not take into account the body *composition* of the individual. Use of this index supports the misconception that body weight is more important than body fatness. Many patients are concerned about losing body weight and desire to be thin, without recognizing that there is an important distinction between being *thin* and being *lean*. Although thinness is related to body weight, leanness is associated with the composition of the individual's body weight. The use of height–weight norms can lead to erroneous conclusions about one's level of body fatness and health risk. Obesity

is better defined as an excess amount of total body fat for a given body weight and is most accurately assessed through body composition analysis.

Body composition is often expressed as the relative amount of fat mass (FM) to FFM. FM is composed of both essential fat and storage fat. Essential fat represents approximately 3% of body weight in adult men and 12% of total body weight in adult women.[53] The FFM includes all body tissues, water and other fluids, muscle, bone, connective tissues, and internal organs. Although FFM and LBM are often used interchangeably, in practice LBM includes the constituents described for FFM and adds the essential fat.

To classify the level of body fatness, the relative body fat (% body fat) is obtained by dividing the FM by the total body weight. See the following equation:

$$\% \text{ body fat} = (\text{FM/body weight}) \times 100.$$

A healthy range of body fat is 12% to 18% for men and 18% to 23% for women. Most health care providers agree that men with more than 25% body fat and women with more than 30% body fat are obese.[54]

Once an individual's body composition is measured, an ideal body weight can be calculated. This can be a useful computation to educate the patient or client who has an unrealistic expectation of their "ideal" weight. *Assuming LBM remains constant,* desired or ideal weight can be computed as follows:

$$\text{fat weight} = \text{current weight} \times (\% \text{ fat}/100).$$

$$\text{lean body mass (LBM)} = \text{current weight} - \text{fat weight}.$$

$$\text{ideal weight} = \text{LBM}/[1 - (\% \text{ fat desired}/100)].$$

$$\text{desired weight loss or weight gain} = \text{present weight} - \text{ideal weight}.$$

The previous equations can be used to compute long-term or short-term goals. For example, a client weighs 68 kg, 29% fat, and wants to target an ideal body fat of 23% while retaining the same level of LBM. For this client,

$$\text{fat weight} = 68 \times (29/100) = 19.72 \text{ kg,}$$

$$\text{lean body mass (LBM)} = 68 - 19.2 = 48.8 \text{ kg,}$$

$$\text{ideal weight} = 48.8/[1 - (23/100)] = 63.38 \text{ kg,}$$

and

$$\text{desired fat loss} = 68 - 63.38 = 4.6 \text{ kg (10.2 lb).}$$

Techniques for Measuring Body Composition

The most accurate measure of body composition is by direct chemical extraction of all fat from body tissues. This technique is obviously not appropriate for clinical practice! Several indirect methods are available for measuring body composition in clinical settings. Some of the more common methods and estimated prediction errors will be described in this section. All techniques currently used to predict body density and body fat are prone to error. The "gold standard" of body composition, underwater weighing, will be described followed by common clinical techniques.

Underwater Weighing

Underwater (hydrostatic) weighing is the most widely used laboratory procedure for determining body density. The technique, often the criterion method in validation studies, is based on Archimedes' principle that "a body immersed in a fluid is acted upon by a buoyancy force in relation to the amount of fluid the body displaces." Because fat is less dense and bone and muscle mass are more dense than water, a given weight of fat will displace a larger volume of water and exhibit a greater buoyant effect than the corresponding weight of bone and muscle tissue. Body density is, therefore, equivalent to the mass (weight) of the body in air divided by the body volume. The body volume can be indirectly determined through underwater weighing. Body density (D_b) is computed as follows:

$$D_b = W_a/[((W_a - W_w)/D_w) - \text{RV} - 0.1]$$

where D_b is body density (g/mL), W_a is body weight out of the water (kg), W_w is body weight in water (kg), D_w is the density of water (g/mL), and RV is residual volume (mL). The constant of 0.1 L accounts for air volume trapped within the gastrointestinal tract. Residual lung volume can be predicted based on age, height, and gender or more accurately measured using the helium dilution or nitrogen washout techniques.

After body density is determined, percentage body fat is predicted using either Siri[55] or Brozek[56] equations:

$$\text{Siri:} \quad \% \text{ body fat} = [(4.95/D_b) - 4.50] \times 100.$$

$$\text{Brozek:} \quad \% \text{ body fat} = [(4.75/D_b) - 4.124] \times 100.$$

Although underwater weighing is considered the "gold standard," the standard error has been estimated to be 2% to 2.5%. When residual volume is estimated from prediction equations, the error of estimation of percentage of body fat can increase by up to 3%.

Dual-Energy X-ray Absorptiometry

Dual energy X-ray absorptiometry (DEXA) is an imaging procedure that can be used to quantify regional body fat, muscle, and bone mineral content. This technique is gaining popularity as a criterion method. A scintillation detector analyzes the penetration of two distinct energy peaks from a source of the high-activity isotope gadolinium-153 (^{153}Gd). Specialized computer software is used to reconstruct the image and determine body composition. Estimation errors between DEXA and densitometry have been found to be less than 2% to 4% in adults.[57] DEXA is an accepted method to measure spinal osteoporosis and related bone disorders.

Skinfolds

Assessing body composition by measuring the thickness of selected skinfold sites is probably the most commonly and widely available technique used in practice today. From the subcutaneous fat measurements made with *skinfold calipers,* percentage body fat is derived through various regression equations. Box 3-3 summarizes some of the more common standardized skinfold sites. Once the measurements are recorded, regression equations like those listed in Box 3-4 can be used to calculate body density and the Siri and Brozek equations are used to compute percentage body fat.

Because skinfold measurements are subject to intertester error, the same tester should be used for repeated measurements when possible. Intratester variability often found with inexperienced testers will also contribute to the measurement error. Therefore, it is recommended that the proficiency of skinfold technique be acquired under the direct supervision of an experienced evaluator performing several hundred assessments.

In terms of technique, it is better to take measurements when the skin is dry. The skinfold is grasped firmly by the thumb and index finger, and the caliper is placed perpendicular to the fold at approximately 1 cm (1/2 in.) below the thumb and finger. While maintaining the grasp of the skinfold, allow the caliper to be released so that the tension is exerted on the

BOX 3-3

Skinfold Sites

Abdominal fold: A vertical fold taken at a distance of 2 cm to the right of the umbilicus.

Biceps fold: A vertical fold taken (1 cm above the level used to mark the triceps) on the anterior aspect of the arm over the belly of the biceps muscle.

Chest/pectoral fold: A diagonal fold taken half of the distance between the anterior axillary line and the nipple for men and one-third of the distance between the anterior axillary line and the nipple for women.

Medial calf fold: A vertical fold at a level of the maximum circumference of the calf on the midline of the medial border.

Midaxillary fold: A vertical fold taken on the midaxillary line at the level of the xyphoid process of the sternum.

Subscapular fold: An angular fold taken at a 45-degree angle 1 to 2 cm below the inferior angle of the iliac crest taken in the anterior axillary line immediately superior to the iliac crest.

Suprailium fold: An oblique fold in line with the natural angle of the iliac crest taken in the anterior axillary line immediately superior to the iliac crest.

Thigh fold: A vertical fold on the anterior midline of the thigh, midway between the inguinal crease and the proximal border of the patella. The midpoint should be marked while the subject is seated.

Triceps fold: A vertical fold on the posterior midline of the upper right arm, halfway between the acromion and olecranon processes. The elbow should be extended and relaxed.

Data from Jackson AS, Pollock ML. Generalized equations for predicting body composition. *Brit J Nutr.* 1978;40:497-504.

Data from Jackson AS, Pollock ML, Ward A. Generalized equations for predicting body composition in women. *Med Sci Sports Exerc.* 1980;12:175-182.

BOX 3-4

Sample Regression Equations to Predict Body Density from Multiple Site Skin Skinfolds*

Males 18–61 years
$$D_b = 1.1093800 - 0.0008267 \text{ (sum of 3)} + 0.0000016$$
$$\text{(sum of 3)}^2 - 0.0002574 \text{ (age)}$$
Sum of 3 = chest, abdomen, and thigh.
(SEE = 0.0077, r = 0.91)

Male college athletes
$$D_b = 1.10647 - 0.00162 \text{ (subscapular)} - 0.00144 \text{ (abdominal)} - 0.00077 \text{ (triceps)} + 0.00071 \text{ (midaxillary)}$$
(SEE = 0.006, r = 0.84)

Females 18–55 years
$$D_b = 1.0994921 - 0.0009929 \text{ (sum of 3)} + 0.0000023$$
$$\text{(sum of 3)}^2 - 0.0001392 \text{ (age)}$$
Sum of 3 = triceps, suprailium, and thigh.
(SEE = 0.0086, r = 0.84)

Female college athletes
$$D_b = 1.096095 - 0.0006952 \text{ (sum of 4)} - 0.0000011$$
$$\text{(sum of 4)} - 0.0000714 \text{ (age)}$$
Sum of 4 = triceps, anterior suprailiac, abdomen, and thigh
(SEE = 0.0084, r = 0.85)

*SEE, standard error of estimate; r, correlation with hydrostatic weighing.

Data from Jackson AS, Pollock ML. Generalized equations for predicting body composition. *Br J Nutr.* 1978;40:497-504.

Data from Jackson AS, Pollock ML, Ward A. Generalized equations for predicting body composition in women. *Med Sci Sports Exerc.* 1980;12:175-182.

Data from Lohman TG. *Advances in Body Composition Assessment. Current Issues in Exercise Science Series.* Monograph No. 3. Champaign, IL: *Human Kinetics;* 1992.

skinfold. Wait approximately 2 seconds for a slight drop to occur resulting from initial tissue compression. Read the caliper to the nearest 0.5 mm and record. Prior to removing the caliper from the skinfold site, depress the thumb trigger to release caliper tension and tissue compression; remove the skinfold and slowly release the trigger allowing the caliper jaws to gradually come together. The tester should alternate between sites and repeat measurements. A third measurement should be taken when the first two vary by more than 1 mm. When population-specific prediction equations are appropriately selected, the predicted value of body fat for an individual usually correlates well with hydrostatic weighing ($r = 0.70$–0.90) and within $\pm 3.5\%$ of the body fat determined by the criterion method.[58,59]

The error of estimation of skinfold assessment is approximately 3%.

Bioelectrical Impedance Analysis

Another technique that holds good clinical promise is bioelectrical impedance analysis (BIA). This technique is based on the principle that the resistance to an electrical current is inversely related to body water. The richer electrolyte content of FFM has much greater conductance than does fat, allowing the establishment of a relationship between conductance and FFM. A very low-level, high-frequency current is passed through the body. Impedance is a function of resistance, the pure opposition to current flow through the body, and reactance is the opposition to current flow caused by capacitance. Because the magnitude of resistance is much greater than the reactance and resistance is a better predictor of FFM and body water, the resistance index of $(\text{height})^2/\text{resistance}$ is used in many BIA models. Both population-specific and generalized prediction equations are available to determine FFM and percentage body fat.

BIA is most accurate when the subject being tested is normally hydrated and when the temperature of the room is comfortable. Dehydrated subjects may be estimated to have less lean mass (and more fat) than if they were properly hydrated. To standardize, hydration subjects should urinate within 30 minutes of the test, consume no alcohol 48 hours prior to the test, avoid vigorous exercise within 12 hours of the test, and fast for 4 hours before the test. Excessive water intake may result in water retention, abnormally high water amounts, and a high lean mass estimation. Validation studies have yielded estimation errors comparable to skinfolds (approximately 3% body fat) when guidelines were followed to avoid alterations in hydration.

Near-infrared Interactance

The instrument consists of a small, compact, AC/DC-powered microprocessing unit and a handheld, infrared miniature flashlight-type transducer probe placed over the right biceps, halfway between the antecubital fossa and the anterior axillary fold. The NIR energy is generated at two specific wavelengths. A silicon detector located at the center of the probe measures the reemitted NIR energy. Optical density measurements are included in prediction equations for computing percentage body fat. Several manufacturer prediction equations are included for predicting body fat, FFM, and total body water in both children and adults. Studies have yielded conflicting support for this method. A trend has been that NIR overestimates body fat in lean subjects and underestimates body fat in subjects with more than 30% body fat. For these reasons, NIR cannot be considered reliable at this time.

Excess carbohydrate and fat get stored in adipose tissue as triglyceride. The body composition assessment techniques described previously are designed to measure body fat and FFM. Excessive kilocalorie intake results in increased body weight and a higher percentage of body fat. Weight-reduction programs target individuals at risk for the development of heart disease as well as individuals with manifest heart disease. **Successful weight management involves a reduction of daily caloric intake and an increase in caloric expenditure through an exercise program.** The following section describes the physiological processes involved in the use of specific fuel substrates to power specific kinds of activities.

INTRODUCTION TO ENERGY STATES

Preferential Use of Nutrients During Exercise

Normal activities of daily living place physical demands on our body that may range from sitting quietly in a chair to an all-out run to catch a bus. Activities of different intensities require different energy substrates, or a different mix of carbohydrate, fat, and protein. This section will identify three different kinds of energy states and associate these energy states with the fuel substrates that power them.

CLINICAL CORRELATE

The reader should keep in mind that an individual's degree of physical fitness determines what is "low-intensity" exercise and what is "high-intensity" exercise. A low level of activity (eg, climbing up a flight of stairs) for a healthy normal person may be a high level of activity for a sedentary obese individual or a person with chronic lung disease!

The following discussion describes exercise states relative to the healthy normal individual.

Low-Intensity Exercise

Low-intensity exercise states generally refer to most activities of daily living. These activities include walking around the house, climbing a flight of stairs, light housework, showering, and dressing, etc. These kinds of activities, *among healthy normal persons,* provoke only a mild increase in heart rate (HR) and blood pressure and do not cause undue fatigue. The metabolic energy requirements are low, generally just a few METs (eg, 3 METs), or multiples above the RMR. Oxygen is utilized by working skeletal muscle to power these low-energy activities and is matched by delivery of oxygen via the blood. As long as there is an adequate amount of energy substrates, and oxygen utilization is matched by oxygen delivery, exercise can continue for a prolonged period of time.

The predominant fuel substrate of choice for such activities is fat, in the form of free fatty acids and triglycerides.[60,61] These fatty acids are mobilized in the blood, whereas triglycerides are stored in fat vacuoles within the muscle cell. Recall the great number of hydrogen molecules attached via a single bond to the fatty acid chain: Fatty acids offer an efficient "high yield" source of hydrogens, for quick conversion to energy during low-level activities that make up a large part of our day.

Fat is stored in fat cells, called adipocytes, present in adipose tissue. The mobilization of fatty acids is augmented by glucagon, epinephrine, and norepinephrine—all of which increase as a result of exercise.

High-Intensity Exercise

High-intensity exercises of short duration occupy the other end of the energy spectrum. Running as hard and as fast as you can is a perfect example of the utilization of this system. This activity is accomplished at a very high-intensity level for a short period of time and many multiples above the RMR. Maximal running causes a dramatic increase in both HR and blood pressure. There may be shortness of breath, as the demand for oxygen by working skeletal muscle outstrips the supply, and feelings of fatigue or exhaustion. Clearly, activities of this intensity cannot be performed for very long, and there may be a prolonged recovery period while the subject "catches his or her breath."

High-intensity activities are accomplished through the utilization of circulating blood glucose and muscle glycogen. In fact, glucose is the only fuel substrate that can be used in the absence of oxygen availability.

Moderate-Intensity Exercise

The third type of exercise that humans engage in is moderate or prolonged exercise. It falls somewhere between the two extremes of low-intensity exercise and high-intensity exercise. A good example of this is the programmed exercise that we engage in when we are trying to lose weight or become physically fit. Jogging 4 miles at a comfortable pace, for instance, causes a moderate increase in MET level (eg, 7.0 METs). It places only a moderate demand on the cardiopulmonary system: For example, the HR may go up to 60% of the maximum attainable HR, and the systolic blood pressure (SBP) may go up 30 mm Hg above resting. The healthy normal subject will be breathing deeply and rapidly but will not feel short of breath. Indeed, the subject will be able to continue jogging for perhaps 30 minutes, or longer, at this level. At the end of exercise, the subject should feel comfortably fatigued, but not exhausted. **Moderate, relatively brief exercise of this kind is powered by similar amounts of glucose, muscle glycogen, cellular triglycerides, and free fatty acids.** Each skeletal muscle cell contains its own glycogen store. As exercise continues, these glycogen stores are tapped, and when these stores deplete, blood glucose is mobilized from the liver. As both glucose and glycogen deplete, fat takes over as the primary substrate. As can be seen, the relative "mix" of fuel substrates changes continually depending on what we are doing. Indeed, there is a dynamic interplay between carbohydrate and fat, as we move from varying intensities and durations of exercise (Fig. 3-3).

Carbohydrate, fat, and protein and their energy potential have been described. Significance was attached to hydrogen atoms attached with a single bond to the substrate chain, and it was noted that energy is released when these hydrogen

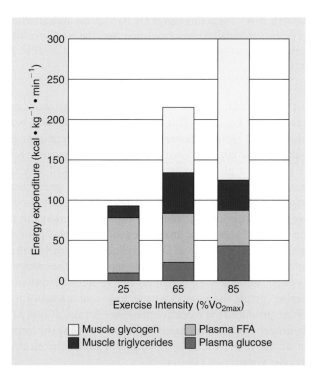

FIGURE 3-3 Change in energy substrates relative to intensity of exercise on a bicycle ergometer. Note the reliance on free fatty acids to power low-level exercise and the increased reliance on glycogen at 85% $\dot{V}O_{2peak}$. (Reproduced with permission from Romijn JA et al. Regulation of endogenous fat and carbohydrate metabolism in relation to exercise intensity and duration. *Am J Physiol.* 1993;265: E380.)

bonds are broken. Now, we will discuss how that energy is captured, transferred, and released to accomplish musculoskeletal work.

CONVERSION OF SUBSTRATES TO ENERGY

Adenosine Triphosphate: ATP

ATP Breakdown

The compound that captures and binds energy from hydrogen cleavage is adenosine triphosphate or ATP. ATP consists of an adenosine group and three phosphate groups. ATP is referred to as a high-energy phosphate compound (*phosphagen*), but compared to other high-energy phosphate compounds it occupies a middle position, somewhere between very high and very low phosphagens. **Because of its middle position, ATP can both give up and accept terminal phosphates rather easily, thus making it an ideal transporter of energy.** Energy is released when (usually) the terminal phosphate group is cleaved off; when the terminal phosphate group is reattached, energy is absorbed. When ATP loses its terminal phosphate, it becomes ADP and releases energy through the process called *hydrolysis*:

$$\text{ATPase}$$
$$\downarrow$$
$$\text{ATP} + \text{H}_2\text{O} \rightarrow \text{ADP} + \text{Pi} - 7.3 \text{ kcal/mol.}$$

This reaction does not require the presence of oxygen. It is thus an *anaerobic* process that occurs virtually all the time and under a wide variety of conditions. In addition to powering high and low exercise states, energy derived from the splitting of ATP maintains tissue BMR, provides energy to transport material across cell walls, and maintains homeostasis.

There is only a small amount of ATP stored in the body; thus, ATP must be continually resynthesized.

ATP Synthesis

There are two ways of making ATP: first, anaerobic and second, aerobic. The anaerobic reactions involve the direct transfer of energy from the substrate to ADP via phosphorylation and are termed *substrate phosphorylation*. This process occurs in the watery medium of the cell. Substrate phosphorylation produces ATP from ADP and is accomplished via another compound, phosphocreatine or PC, in the reaction

$$\text{creatine kinase} \qquad\qquad \text{creatine kinase}$$
$$\downarrow \qquad\qquad\qquad\qquad \downarrow$$
$$\text{PC} \leftrightarrow \text{P} + \text{C} + \text{energy; ADP} + \text{P} + \text{energy} \rightarrow \text{ATP.}$$

As before, breaking the bond between molecules releases energy. This released energy is used for muscular exertion, chemical work, etc. ADP is then easily reconverted back to ATP and the cycle repeats. The enzyme creatine kinase makes this reaction go very quickly. The utilization of PC as a phosphate donor for the production of ATP occurs anaerobically. PC exists in a ratio of 4:1 compared to ATP. Thus, ATP resynthesis occurs four times before this system is depleted.

The second method of making ATP occurs aerobically in the mitochondria of the cell, primarily during the later stages of glucose degradation in the citric acid (Kreb) cycle. *Oxidative phosphorylation* is the process whereby hydrogens are stripped off substrate molecules, their electrons are passed down an *electron transport chain* within the mitochondria, and energy is released, which is then packaged in the form of ATP (see Fig. 3-4). As can be seen, while water is the end product of oxidative phosphorylation, ATP is formed as a by-product.

Oxidative phosphorylation generates ATP as long as there are adequate amounts of enzymes, a supply of electrons (substrate), and oxygen. **Oxidative phosphorylation predominates during low- and moderate-intensity exercise states, when oxygen supply matches demand in the production of ATP.** The small amount of hydrogen ion present in the cytoplasm is rapidly cleared from the area by venous blood flow. However, during intense bouts of exercise, the demand for oxygen in exercising muscle outstrips the supply. The two hydrogens that "meet" oxygen and the two electrons to form water have no hydrogen receptor (see Fig. 3-4). Hydrogen ion builds up, the rate of hydrogen production exceeds the ability of the venous system to clear it, and the pH drops. This can have unpleasant consequences that take the form of cramping muscle pain, inhibition of muscle contraction, and the inability to continue exercise. We shall finish the story of excess hydrogen ion later in the discussion of glycolysis. Because glucose is the primary fuel source for chemical, electrical, and mechanical work, we shall examine the degradation of this molecule in some detail.

One final thought: Storage of ATP is minimal. However, ATP can be manufactured quickly through the aid of key enzymes in order to respond to sudden increases in activity levels.

THE METABOLIC MILL

Glucose is the primary substrate that powers physical activity and is the only fuel that can be used in high-intensity exercise. It is decomposed in two phases by way of a metabolic mill—glycolysis and the citric acid cycle. Glycolysis breaks down $C_6H_{12}O_6$ into two 3-carbon fragments to the level of pyruvic acid. The remaining energy is extracted via the citric acid cycle (Krebs or tricarboxylic acid cycle).

Glycolysis

Glycolysis occurs in the cytoplasm, or watery medium of the cell. It is thus primarily an anaerobic process and is the primary mechanism for ATP production in fast-twitch, glycolytic, or "white" muscle fibers that are resident in almost all muscle groups, especially those in the upper extremity, and the tibialis anterior, etc., where speed is a primary functional goal. Food substrates, including the many types of carbohydrates,

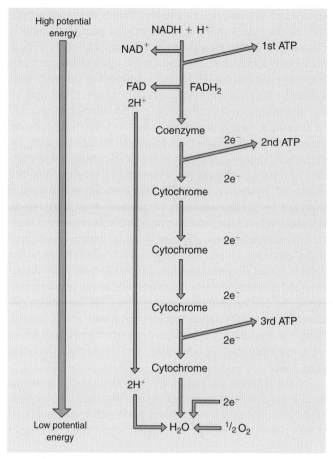

FIGURE 3-4   The production of ATP through the intramitochondrial process of oxidative phosphorylation. Note the production of metabolic water as an end product, and the production of ATP as a by-product.

must be reduced to glucose in order to enter the metabolic mill at stage I (see Fig. 3-5). This figure shows 10 chemical reactions that first reduce glucose to two 3-carbon fragments and finally degrade glucose down to 2 molecules of pyruvic acid. The process of glycolysis is essentially a downhill series of chemical reactions that break chemical bonds and release energy. Along the way, however, this released energy is used to drive uphill chemical reactions that capture this energy in the form of ATP. Evidence of anaerobic (substrate) phosphorylation is found at points C and D. Also of note is the early utilization of ATP (points A and B). This represents the *energy of activation*, initial energy that must be put into the system in order to "prime the pump." Finally, note that a total of four ATP are produced via oxidative phosphorylation, as two pairs of hydrogen electrons get passed to FAD, bypassing the formation of the first ATP, before being sent down the electron transport system (see Fig. 3-4).

By the time the glucose molecule has been reduced to pyruvic acid, a NET total of two ATP have been produced via substrate phosphorylation and four ATP have been produced via oxidative phosphorylation in skeletal muscle.[62] It should be noted that in cardiac muscle, a total of six ATP are produced via oxidative phosphorylation, as the two pairs of hydrogen

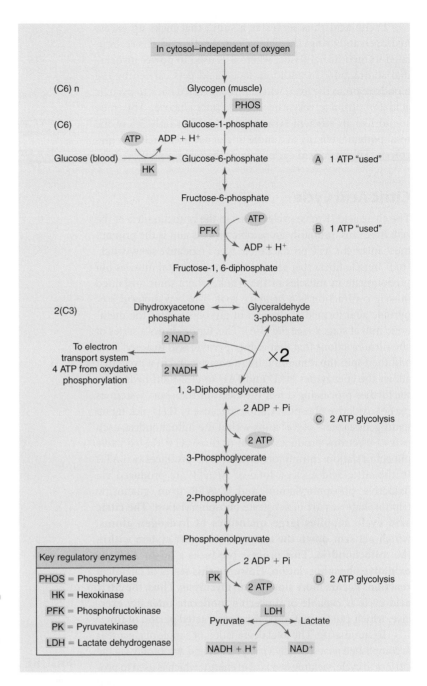

FIGURE 3-5 The degradation of the glucose molecule to the level of pyruvate in the cell cytoplasm of skeletal muscle via glycolysis. This process allows the rapid production of a small quantity of ATP via substrate phosphorylation. (Modified with permission from Foss M, Keteyian S. *Fox's: Physiological Basis for Exercise and Sport.* 6th ed. Boston, MA: WCB McGraw-Hill; 1998.)

electrons get shuttled to intermitochondrial NAD, producing three ATP per electron pair.

There are a multitude of enzymes associated with the stages of glycolysis, making the production of ATP via substrate phosphorylation relatively rapid. However, only a small amount of ATP can be generated during glycolysis. **Glycolysis is unable to make large quantities of ATP. However, the series of chemical reactions can occur very quickly. Thus, glycolysis is capable of powering high-intensity exercise but can only sustain this intensity for a short period of time.**

The formation of pyruvic acid marks the end of glycolysis. Pyruvic acid is a close cousin to lactic acid, the latter molecule having an additional two hydrogens. These two compounds play

an important role during high exercise states when oxidative phosphorylation becomes inefficient, as oxygen becomes unavailable and hydrogen ion builds up in the cytoplasm. During high-intensity exercise, local skeletal muscle pH drops, producing a crampy pain that can be very uncomfortable. A coenzyme, NAD, picks up excess hydrogen as pairs and delivers them to pyruvic acid, which then changes its name to lactic acid:

$$CH_3-\underset{\underset{}{\overset{O}{\parallel}}}{C}-\underset{\underset{}{\overset{OH}{\mid}}}{C}=O + NADH^+ + H^+ \leftrightarrow CH_3-\underset{\underset{H}{\mid}}{\overset{\overset{OH}{\mid}}{C}}-\underset{\overset{O}{\parallel}}{C}-OH$$

Pyruvic acid   Lactic acid
$C_3H_4O_3$ $C_3H_6O_3$

Lactic acid thus serves as a sump that picks up excess hydrogen and brings the pH back up. Lactic acid gets recirculated to myocardial tissue, where it is used to power myocardial contraction. In addition, lactic acid gets carried by the bloodstream to the liver, where it is converted back to pyruvic acid for ultimate resynthesis back into glucose. This may sound like an efficient system, and it is! But only 5% of the total potential energy of a mole of glucose is extracted in glycolysis. The citric acid cycle extracts the remaining 95%.

Citric Acid Cycle

The citric acid (Krebs) cycle occurs in the mitochondria of the cell. It is, thus, primarily an aerobic process and is the primary mechanism for ATP production in type I oxidative slow-twitch, "red" muscle fibers that are resident in all skeletal muscles but predominate in muscles of the trunk, where tonic sustained muscle contraction is a primary goal. The two molecules of pyruvic acid formed at the end of glycolysis enter the metabolic mill at stage I (see Fig. 3-6). This figure shows a series of chemical reactions that first reduce pyruvic acid to acetyl CoA and then spin the remaining fragments around in a cycle that allows the coenzymes NAD and FAD to cleave off hydrogens for further processing down the electron transport system as part of oxidative phosphorylation. Because NAD is picking up hydrogens as pairs of electrons within the mitochondria, each pair of electrons produces a total of three ATP via oxidative phosphorylation; intramitochondrial FAD produces two ATP. In the citric acid cycle, a total of 30 ATP are produced via oxidative phosphorylation, and 2 ATP from guanosine triphosphate as part of substrate phosphorylation. **The citric acid cycle supplies large quantities of hydrogen atoms, which get sent down the electron transport system within the mitochondria. This process produces a lot of ATP via oxidative phosphorylation. However, this series of chemical reactions occurs more slowly than glycolysis. Thus, the citric acid cycle is capable of powering moderate-intensity exercise, which can be sustained for a protracted period of time.**

To summarize: The total degradation of a mole of glucose is accomplished anaerobically via glycolysis and aerobically via the citric acid cycle, yielding 686 kcal of energy, which is used to produce a total of 36 ATP from blood glucose in skeletal muscle and 38 ATP in cardiac muscle. This remarkable process increases or decreases its production of ATP depending on the metabolic need. **The intensity of exercise, or the time rate of change of doing work, is an important signal that triggers the production of ATP. Glycolysis may predominate when the intensity of effort is high; the citric acid cycle may predominate when the metabolic demand for energy (ATP) is moderate or effort is of long duration.** Table 3-2 summarizes the relationship between energy systems and their ability to manufacture ATP.

Fat Utilization

Fat is stored in the body as triglyceride. This molecule gets mobilized, especially by slow-twitch oxidative type I, "red"

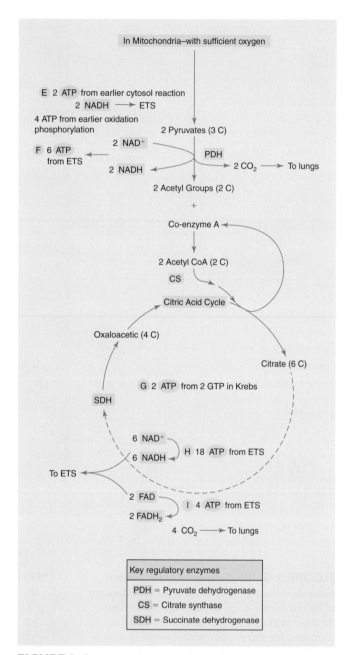

FIGURE 3-6   The degradation of pyruvate in the mitochondria of a skeletal muscle cell, producing a large quantity of ATP via oxidative phosphorylation in the citric acid cycle. (Modified with permission from Foss M, Keteyian S. *Fox's: Physiological Basis for Exercise and Sport.* 6th ed. Boston, MA: WCB McGraw-Hill; 1998.)

muscle fibers, during low levels of exercise and during prolonged exercise of moderate intensity when glycogen stores become depleted. The breakdown of triglyceride begins with the separation of the glycerol component from the three glycerides. Glycerol enters into the metabolic mill as glyceraldehyde 3-phosphate. It then becomes reduced to pyruvic acid, just like glucose, and enters the citric acid cycle for further reduction. Each of the 3 fatty acids undergoes β-oxidation in the mitochondrion, releasing hydrogen atoms that get sent down the electron transport chain, with subsequent ATP

TABLE 3-2   Summary of Interrelationship Between Energy Systems

Energy System	Substrate	O₂ Required	Speed of ATP Mobilization	Total ATP Production Per Mole of Glucose
Anaerobic: ATP-PC system	Stored phosphagens	No	Very fast	Small
Anaerobic: glycolysis	Glycogen/glucose	No	Fast	Small
Aerobic: Krebs cycle, electron transport	Glycogen/glucose, fats, proteins	Yes	Slow	Large

production. The amount of ATP produced per mole of triglyceride is enormous, compared to glucose (38 ATP):

$$glycerol:\ 19\ ATP,$$

$$3\ fatty\ acids:\ 147 \times 3 = 441\ ATP,$$

and

$$total:\ 460\ ATP$$

This makes fat a very efficient source of energy.

One final comment on the degradation of carbohydrate and fat for energy: It has been said that carbohydrates serve as a primer for fat catabolism. In order for the metabolic mill to function properly, carbohydrate (glucose) must be broken down in the presence of fat so that fat can be broken down properly. If there is no glucose present, and fat becomes the sole substrate, lipid will be broken down incompletely. This can happen in the presence of a disease, for example, diabetes or during extreme exercise states when glycogen stores have depleted. Lipid degradation under hypoglycemic conditions leads to the formation of ketone bodies that reduce the pH of body fluids and can result in a toxic condition called ketoacidosis. Diabetics and individuals on low/no-carbohydrate diets are particularly prone to this condition.

ENERGY SYSTEMS

So far, this chapter has introduced carbohydrate, fat, and protein as substrates that serve as sources for energy. We have seen how carbohydrate and fat are broken down through glycolysis and the citric acid cycle—the metabolic mill that is present in muscle cells. The energy that is released is packaged in the form of ATP. This high-energy phosphate compound is produced both aerobically and anaerobically. The manner in which it is manufactured depends in large part on the need. **These substrates and metabolic pathways will now be brought together so that the patient's response to exercise can be appreciated within the context of metabolic energy systems.**

Immediate Energy System

This energy system becomes activated when the subject moves from a resting state and first begins to exercise, as one changes steady states, and during bursts of vigorous efforts. ATP for these efforts is derived from PC present in muscle fibers. The amount of stored phosphagens is small and is generally not sufficient to power exercise for more than 40 seconds. The kinds of exercise that tend to preferentially utilize the immediate energy system include lifting a heavy package from the floor to the counter and jumping out of the way of a person trying to catch a bus! This energy system can be selectively trained by performing short bouts of maximal efforts. However, improvement is limited and may be related to genetic ability. Successful acquisition of a training effect increases intramuscular stores of ATP and PC,[63,64] and facilitates recruitment and improves the firing sequence of those motor units involved in the task.

The Short-Term Energy System

This energy system "turns on" during high-intensity, near-maximal efforts beyond the first few seconds when stored phosphagens have been reduced. Bicycling up a steep hill, or sprinting to catch a bus, preferentially activates this system. It relies on the rapid, anaerobic production of ATP through glycolysis. Glucose is the only fuel substrate that can be utilized to power this kind of exercise.

In normal subjects, shortness of breath during exercise is a symptom that is usually associated with glycolysis and the activation of the short-term energy system. At a critical exercise intensity, usually 60% to 70% of maximum exercise, hydrogen ion begins to accumulate in the blood, as the rate of lactic acid production and passage into the bloodstream exceeds the rate of removal by the liver, kidney, and other tissues. This elevation in hydrogen ion causes a reduction in blood pH. The hypothalamus responds to this relative acid state by increasing the respiratory drive, in an effort to reduce hydrogen concentration by "blowing off" carbon dioxide. This increase in minute ventilation partly compensates for the metabolic acidosis related to lactate accumulation—but only up to a point. As exercise continues, subjects ultimately hyperventilate and become short of breath as the production of lactic acid outstrips the ability of the pulmonary system to vent CO_2. On a local skeletal muscle level, shortness of breath is often accompanied by a cramping or burning sensation in these muscles, as the production of lactic acid exceeds its clearance from the area by the bloodstream.

During a graded exercise test, the power output or percent of $\dot{V}O_{2peak}$ at which ventilation departs from linearity is known as the ventilatory threshold. This ventilatory threshold is identified by an increase in the rate and depth of breathing

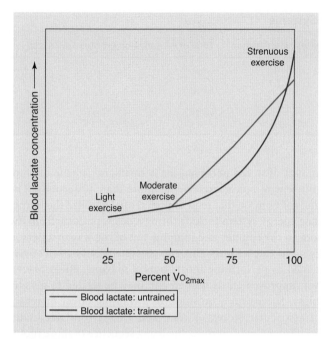

FIGURE 3-7   Onset of blood lactate accumulation (OBLA) for trained versus untrained individuals. The trained subject can perform more exercise before OBLA and can tolerate higher absolute levels.

and coincides with the onset of blood lactate accumulation (OBLA)[65] (see Fig. 3-7). Muscular fatigue at an intensity of sustained exercise greater than the OBLA is associated with the progressive accumulation of lactate in blood. However, in prolonged exercise at an intensity below OBLA, blood lactate levels reach a steady state as production is matched by clearance. In the latter instance, fatigue is usually associated with a variety of other factors, including depletion of muscular glycogen stores, dehydration, and electrolyte disturbance.

The OBLA has also been used to document the acquisition of a training effect of the short-term energy system. Training this system causes a shift in OBLA and the ventilatory threshold to higher levels of exercise, such that a glycolytically trained individual can exercise to a higher percentage of maximal $\dot{V}_{O_2}$ before lactate begins to build up. Training the short-term energy system will permit a greater tolerance to lactic acid, thus postponing the onset of fatigue (see Fig. 3-7).

The clinical decision to train the short-term energy system should be made on the basis of the age of the patient, the kinds of activities that the patient will engage in, and the presence of comorbidities, like cardiopulmonary disease. Athletes recovering from orthopedic injury who engage in soccer, basketball, or other sports requiring high-intensity efforts may be trained glycolytically. However, HR and blood pressure elevate quickly and to high levels, placing extra work on the heart. This kind of exercise can also provoke a Valsalva maneuver, which impedes blood flow back to the heart and invoke a pressor response that further compromises cardiac function.

Physical therapists should also be aware that many patients with chronic obstructive pulmonary disease fail to achieve a level of exercise that produces metabolic acidosis and thus a ventilatory threshold. This is most likely due to low exercise capacity, when the ability to attain the ventilatory threshold is precluded by the onset of shortness of breath.[66]

The Long-Term Energy System

This energy system predominates during moderate-intensity efforts. Walking or jogging at a comfortable pace preferentially activates this system. It relies on the slower, aerobic production of ATP through the citric acid cycle. **Indeed, the hallmark of the activation of the long-term energy system is the utilization of oxygen.** As long as the demand for oxygen by active skeletal muscle is matched by an adequate supply, exercise can be continued for a protracted period of time. **Activation of the long-term, or aerobic endurance, energy system tends to cause a "volume" workload on the heart, which places less stress on the heart than the higher "pressure" workload that is associated with the high-intensity, short-term energy system.**

In the way that these three energy states have been presented, it may appear that the immediate, short-term, and long-term energy systems are three discrete entities that "turn on and off" without overlap. This is not the case. Movement across exercise states and utilization of appropriate fuel substrates occur as a smooth integration of systems. All three metabolic pathways are in continuous operation; the intensity

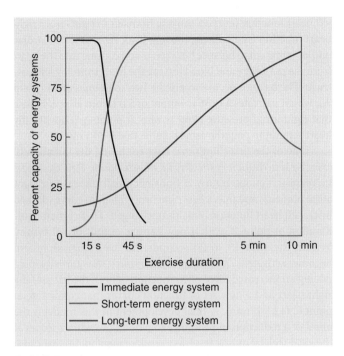

FIGURE 3-8 Utilization of three metabolic energy pathways in moving from the resting state to a moderate, prolonged level of exercise. (Modified with permission from McArdle WD, Katch FI, Katch VL. *Exercise Physiology: Energy, Nutrition, and Human Performance.* 5th ed. Philadelphia, PA: Lippincott Williams & Wilkins, 2001.)

and duration of exercise determine which system predominates[67] (see Fig. 3-8).

CARDIOVASCULAR AND PULMONARY RESPONSE TO EXERCISE

Immediate Response to Exercise: Cardiac

Exercise presents an ultimate challenge to the cardiovascular and pulmonary systems. The metabolic need for more oxygen and nutrients in working skeletal muscle during exercise initiates a long and complex series of feedforward and feedback mechanisms that occur through a dynamic interplay among somatosensory, musculoskeletal, cardiovascular and pulmonary systems. It is the amalgamation of these processes that ultimately propels the human body from point A to point B.

If metabolic need initiates the process, then cardiac output drives the process. Arterial blood carries oxygen and nutrients into metabolically active tissue, and venous blood removes metabolites and oxygen-reduced red blood cells from the area. This section will demonstrate by example what happens to these and other variables when a subject moves from rest to exercise.

Heart Rate: Revision of the Age-Related Maximum Heart Rate

During graded exercise, HR rises linearly with increasing workload. The increase in HR occurs as a result of a withdrawal in parasympathetic tone and by augmentation of sym-

pathetic neural input to the sinoatrial node. HR linearity will continue until a maximum HR (HR_{max}) is achieved, at which point exercise must stop, as cardiac output is no longer able to match metabolic need. HR_{max} decreases with age and traditionally has been calculated as 220 − age. The notion of an age-related maximum HR (ARMHR) has been universally accepted and widely used for many years. It has served as an endpoint for maximal exercise testing and has also been used as a basis for prescribing intensity of effort in rehabilitation programs. The ARMHR is constant across both gender and state of training. However, the validity of the ARMHR equation has never been established, particularly for older adults.

A recent study has sought to validate the ARMHR among healthy men and women ranging widely in age.[68] Tanaka et al. performed a meta-analysis on a total of 351 peer-reviewed research papers that met the following criteria: (1) subjects were both men and women and analyzed separately; (2) subjects were nonmedicated nonsmokers; (3) subjects were adults; and (4) maximum exercise was determined by using objective criteria. Tanaka et al. went on to perform their own research study by exposing 514 healthy men and women to maximum exercise testing. Forward stepwise multiple regression analyses demonstrated that age alone accounted for 80% of the individual variance in HR_{max}. The regression formula obtained from the research experiment was virtually identical to that of the meta-analysis. There was no significant difference in the regression equation between men and women or between sedentary and endurance-trained individuals. It was concluded that the traditional 220 − age formula overestimates true HR_{max} in young adults and underestimates true HR_{max} in persons older than 40 years. **The following formula more accurately identifies true HR_{max} among healthy adults across the life span:**

$$HR_{max} = 208 - 0.7 \times age.$$

Utilization of the new, revised formula has clinical implications. The revised formula allows older individuals to exercise to a higher HR before termination, resulting in better diagnostic validity as well as a higher level of training exercise intensity. However, it should be stressed that this formula, like 220 − age, provides only an estimate of HR_{max}. Significant variance exists at any given age. Indeed, 1 SD HR_{max} is 10 to 12 beats per minute (bpm). Finally, these results are only applicable to healthy normal adults. Individuals with overt cardiovascular disease may have a very different regression formula.

The Rate–Pressure Product

The rate–pressure product (RPP) is found by multiplying the HR and the SBP. It is usually expressed by a power of 3. Thus, for example,

$$\text{Heart rate} = 105 \text{ bpm},$$

$$\text{Systolic blood pressure} = 150 \text{ mm Hg},$$

$$\text{RPP} = 15.7 \times 10^3.$$

There is a strong linear correlation between the RPP and myocardial oxygen consumption ($M\dot{V}O_2$) during progressive, aerobic lower-extremity exercise.[69,70] The RPP has particular utility for physical therapists who treat patients with heart disease in that both the HR and SBP response to exercise are often abnormal in these patients. HR and contractility, both major determinants of $M\dot{V}O_2$, may be compromised by way of ischemia or necrosis; alterations in afterload as a function of left ventricular mechanical dysfunction can also affect $M\dot{V}O_2$. Both of these findings are captured in the measurement of the RPP. The benefit of its use in monitoring tolerance to exercise and individuating an aerobic exercise prescription is that the dynamic interplay between both HR and BP is reflected in the equation.

The cardiac response to exercise is highly individual; that is, the HR and SBP responses to exercise vary widely across individuals, especially in persons with heart disease. However, recent work by Hui and colleagues presents normative values for resting and exercise RPP among healthy normal subjects.[71] Data obtained from 1,623 subjects were used to develop a multiple regression model that recognized several factors, including age, gender, and BMI, that contribute to calculation of RPP.

The reader will recall that quantifying the amount of exercise that the physical therapist prescribes to a patient through the use of METs provides a basis for comparisons between subjects. This is not the case with the RPP, which is highly variable across patients with heart disease.

CLINICAL CORRELATE

Use of the RPP to monitor exercise benefits to the patient with heart disease because it reflects cardiac function. While comparison across patients is not possible, it can be used to monitor individual patient progress. Successful acquisition of an aerobic endurance training effect is demonstrated by a reduction of the RPP at any given submaximal workload.

Cardiac Function Curve

A *cardiac function curve* is a graphical depiction of the heart's ability to receive blood from the venous system and to pump blood out through the arterial system. Examine the cardiac function curve of a healthy normal 24-year-old individual about to begin ambulation on a treadmill[72] (Fig. 3-9). This figure isolates left heart function (curved, moving from left to right) from right heart function (more linear, moving from right to left). Cardiac output represents a balance between blood coming into the heart from the periphery and blood leaving the heart from the left ventricle. The balance occurs where the two solid lines cross (point A), which indicates a cardiac output of 5.0 L/min at rest. Notice that right atrial pressure (Pra) is zero at point A: This healthy heart is pumping out the same volume that is coming in.

One of the first things that happen during the initiation of exercise is *activation of the skeletal muscle pump*. This causes an increase in venous return, a transient small increase in right atrial pressure, and thus a new right heart function curve (dashed line). Left heart function remains unchanged. There is new equilibration at point B, with a new cardiac output of 8.0 L/min. Within the next 15 to 20 seconds, the neurological system becomes activated. *The sympathetic nervous system turns on*, producing an increased force of contraction of both the left and the right heart and a new set of function curves that equilibrate at point C (12.5 L/min). A final development in this model is the onset of a reduction in resistance to blood flow, which occurs at the local skeletal muscle level, as a result of metabolites that cause *local vasodilatation*. Final cardiac output is at 21.0 L/min, a peak exercise level that is typical for a young, healthy normal adult.

Behavioral Characteristics of Cardiac Output

Cardiac output is a function of both HR and stroke volume (see Table 3-3). This model shows HR and stroke volume data from the same individual when moving from rest to maximum exercise. Notice that the fourfold increase in cardiac output is mostly provided by an almost threefold increase in HR. Indeed, a fairly linear relationship exists between increases in HR and cardiac output for submaximal lower extremity exercise in the upright position. Stroke volume is an important, but relatively minor contributor. Stroke volume increases linearly with cardiac output in the early stages of progressive exercise. However, at approximately 40% of maximum work, stroke volume will increase at a much slower rate. Beyond 40% maximum work, the majority of further increases in exercise levels are a function of an increase in HR.

Oxygen consumption—Maintenance of the resting state requires 3.5 mL O_2/kg/min. In our 70-kg healthy 24-year-old subject, this corresponds to approximately 250 mL O_2/min in 5.0 L of blood. Measurement of $\dot{V}O_2$ at peak exercise yielded a value of 3,000 mL O_2/min—a 12-fold increase in $\dot{V}O_2$, a typical increase in a young untrained individual.

Fick equation—At this point, the reader may be wondering how a 12-fold increase in $\dot{V}O_2$ can be matched by only a 4-fold increase in cardiac output. The answer lies in the ability of working skeletal muscle to increase its *extraction* of oxygen, as represented by the Fick equation:

$$\dot{V}O_2 = \text{cardiac output} \times \text{a-}\dot{V}O_2 \text{ difference}.$$

At rest, muscle extracts approximately 25% of the available oxygen in arterial blood. The rate of oxygen removal is

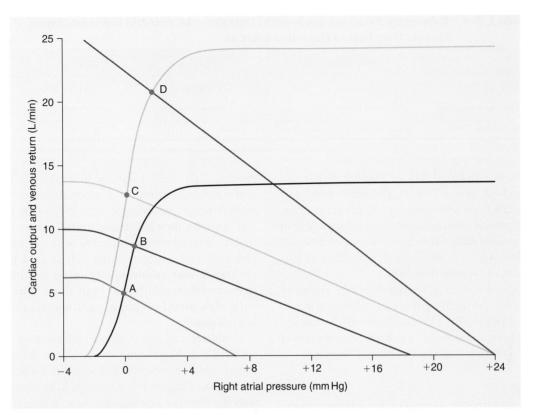

FIGURE 3-9 Cardiac function curve from a healthy untrained 24-year-old subject, representing the change in left heart and right heart function as the subject moves from the resting state to maximum exercise. Note that points A, B, C, and D represent cardiac outputs obtained during that time period. (Modified with permission from Guyton A, Jones C, Coleman T. *Circulatory Physiology: Cardiac Output and Its Regulation.* 2nd ed. Philadelphia, PA: WB Saunders; 1973.)

dependent on muscle capillarity, myoglobin content, mitochondrial number and size, and the oxidative capacity of mitochondrial units. At maximal levels of exercise, oxygen extraction can triple from a resting value of 250 mL O_2/min to 750 mL O_2/min. This phenomenon maintains tissue viability during exercise and keeps cardiac output, especially HR, from bearing the full responsibility of oxygenating tissues. Imagine the impossibility of developing HRs in excess of 600 bpm if there was a one-to-one match of cardiac output to $\dot{V}O_2$!

Immediate Response to Exercise: Pulmonary

Initiation of the exercise state provokes an increase in $\dot{V}E$ as a function of both tidal volume and frequency (see Table 3-4).

The profound increase in tidal volume is an energy-efficient way of increasing $\dot{V}E$ while keeping breathing frequency relatively low. Tidal volume increases until approximately 50% to 60% of vital capacity. Beyond this point, further increases in ventilation are primarily the result of increases in breathing frequency. Chest wall movement during exercise involves not only increased use of the diaphragm but also recruitment of the accessory muscles of ventilation.

Other Factors

Exercise provokes a massive shunting of blood away from metabolically less active tissues and toward active skeletal muscle. This is brought about by sympathetically mediated mass vasoconstriction in the renal and splanchnic circulations, skin, and inactive skeletal muscle. Vasodilatation

TABLE 3-3 Cardiac Response of a Healthy Untrained 24-Year-Old Individual When Moving from Rest to Maximum Exercise

	Cardiac Output =	Heart Rate ×	Stroke Volume
Rest	5 L/min	72 bpm	70 mL/beat
Maximum exercise	21 L/min	190 bpm	110 mL/beat
% Increase	Approximately 4×	Approximately 2.5×	Approximately 1.5×

TABLE 3-4   **Pulmonary Response of a Healthy Untrained 24-Year-Old Individual When Moving from Rest to Maximum Exercise**

	Minute Ventilation =	Frequency ×	Tidal Volume
Rest	6 L/min	12 breaths/min	0.5 L/breath
Maximum exercise	192 L/min	48 breaths/min	4.0 L/breath
% Increase	32×	4×	8×

results in an increase in blood flow to working muscle and vital organs. Indeed, blood flow to the brain and heart increases up to 25% from resting levels at maximum exercise. At rest, skeletal muscle receives only approximately 20% of total cardiac output; at maximal exercise, skeletal muscle may receive up to 80% of total cardiac output. Blood flow to kidneys may be reduced by more than 30%.

Global sympathetic stimulation, catecholamine release by the adrenal glands, and resultant shunting of blood cause an exercise-induced rise in SBP. This elevation tends to rise linearly to progressive increases in workload. Diastolic blood pressure tends to remain fairly static as exercise increases.

Gas Exchange

The process of gas exchange depends on the difference in the partial pressure of oxygen (PO_2) between lung alveoli (PAO_2) and pulmonary capillary blood (PaO_2) as well as the matching of alveolar ventilation and perfusion. During exercise, the PAO_2 rises due to an increase in alveolar ventilation. The partial pressure of oxygen of mixed venous blood is also reduced as a result of greater oxygen uptake by skeletal muscle, resulting in a greater partial pressure gradient for oxygen across the alveolar–capillary membrane. As a consequence of the overall alveolar ventilation and opening of pulmonary capillaries, matching of pulmonary ventilation to perfusion is also optimized during exercise. The saturation of hemoglobin (SaO_2) in arterial blood remains greater than 95% up to maximal exercise in healthy subjects. The oxygen content of arterial blood depends not only on the PO_2 gradient between the lung and the pulmonary capillaries but also on the oxygen-carrying capacity of blood. If hemoglobin levels are reduced (eg, anemia), the oxygen content of arterial blood will be lowered and $\dot{V}O_{2peak}$ may be reduced.

The Athletic Heart

The heart is composed of specialized contractile tissue, *myocardium*, that can respond to repetitively applied workloads in ways similar to that of skeletal muscle. The athletic heart exemplifies these adaptations to the highest degree. Like skeletal muscle, myocardium can undergo an increase in cell size, or hypertrophy. This hypertrophy is usually confined to the left ventricle, which enlarges in response to high afterload imposed by exercise. The kind of exercise that

prompts left ventricular hypertrophy (LVH) has come under recent scrutiny.[73-75] A recent review of the literature[73] related to left ventricular hypertrophy in the setting of resistance training has demonstrated only modest increases in left ventricular size, compared to the greater increases in size with endurance training.[76] **It should be noted that resistance and endurance training produces increases that are substantially less than those found in patients with high blood pressure, cardiomyopathy, or valvular heart disease.**

Athletes may also possess an *adventitious*, or extra, heart sound. The S_3 heart sound closely follows the normal S_2 heart sound, which represents closure of the aortic and pulmonic valves (see Chapter 10). Although S_3 is strongly associated with the presence of congestive heart failure in patients with heart disease, its presence in the athlete probably reflects a larger left ventricular chamber size, coupled with increased left ventricular muscle mass, and is, therefore, considered normal in this population.

Athletes may also be prone to alterations in HR and rhythm. Slow resting HRs (eg, *sinus bradycardia*) are quite common, particularly among endurance-trained athletes. This is often accompanied by a slowing of conduction through a secondary pacemaker of the heart, the atrioventricular (AV) node (ie, first-degree AV block) (see Chapter 11). Both of these findings are considered normal, as they reflect greater cardiovascular efficiency and a general shift toward vagal parasympathetic tone.

It is a tragic, though thankfully a rare event, when a young athlete dies suddenly during an athletic endeavor. These events are almost always cardiogenic and more specifically, arrhythmogenic. Lethal ventricular arrhythmias occur in the setting of preexisting structural abnormalities that are either genetically determined or acquired. The most common genetic abnormality contributing to sudden death is underlying cardiomyopathy; coronary artery disease and myocarditis are the most common of the acquired diseases. Ventricular arrhythmias that have no structural condition are not thought to be dangerous. Structural arrhythmias are life-threatening.[77] Identification of young athletic individuals judged to be at risk for sudden death is difficult. However, current best practice calls for a complete evaluation of those athletes with structural cardiac abnormalities and history of loss of consciousness (*syncope*).[78,79]

Left ventricular hypertrophy and extra heart sounds due to athletic endeavors are considered normal; these findings should not be confused with the LVH and extra heart sounds associated with chronic high blood pressure. Slow heart rates among athletes are also considered normal variants. Physical therapists should evaluate all the data and look at the total patient before making clinical decisions regarding the presence of cardiac impairment. Physical therapists should also be alert to a patient history of childhood cardiac disease and episodes of syncope and make appropriate referrals.

EXERCISE TESTING

Direct Measurement of Peak Oxygen Consumption

Most of our activities of daily living are carried out using substrates that are degraded in the presence of oxygen. Patients with cardiopulmonary disease and patients with other diseases who are deconditioned usually benefit from physical therapy interventions directed toward training the long-term (aerobic endurance) energy system. This section will describe direct and indirect measurement of $\dot{V}O_2$ during exercise as a means of both directing treatment and measuring outcome.

Traditional Modes of Exercise Testing

The measurement of $\dot{V}O_2$ is usually obtained during the application of a standardized bout of exercise, termed an exercise test or stress test. These exercise tests are typically graded from a low level to a moderate or high level. They consist of stages, each of which may last from 2 to 3 minutes. The duration of the stages and the level of exercise that each stage represents form an *exercise test protocol*. There are numerous exercise test protocols in existence, utilizing a variety of *modalities*, or ergometers. See Chapter 10 for examples of exercise test protocols and modalities.

The measurement of $\dot{V}O_2$ during a standardized exercise test allows for the comparison of results across subjects and within the same subject as a pre- and postintervention comparison.

Direct measures of $\dot{V}O_{2peak}$ are obtained through open-circuit spirometry. With the nose occluded, or while the subject wears a mask, the subject breathes through a low-resistance valve, while pulmonary ventilation and fractions of O_2 and CO_2 are measured in expired air samples. $\dot{V}O_2$ can be expressed in either absolute (L O_2/min) or weight-relative units (mL O_2/kg/min or METs). Absolute maximal aerobic power reflects the ability to perform external work. The greater the amount of the oxygen consumed at peak exercise, the more fit is the individual. When evaluating cardiorespiratory endurance, $\dot{V}O_2$ values are typically expressed relative to kilogram of body weight, as METs. Relative peak aerobic power is a better reflection of the ability to move one's body mass and is related inversely to body fatness. Classification of cardiorespiratory fitness is provided in Table 3-5.

Even in healthy individuals, many physiological variables influence and alter $\dot{V}O_{2peak}$. Higher levels of $\dot{V}O_{2peak}$ can be achieved when a larger percentage of muscle mass is involved in testing. **For example, lower extremity protocols elicit a higher $\dot{V}O_{2peak}$ than exercise tests that rely solely on upper extremity muscle mass. These values can be slightly increased when upper extremity mass is added to lower extremity mass.** Mean values for women are approximately 10% to 20% lower than those for men of comparable age and physical fitness due to the average reduction in muscle mass, higher percentage of body fat, lower hemoglobin concentration, and smaller lungs. Cross-sectional studies have shown that after the age of 25 years, $\dot{V}O_{2peak}$ declines approximately 9% per decade in sedentary individuals. It is unclear how much of this decline is due to the aging process or to reduced physical activity. $\dot{V}O_{2peak}$ is also reduced by environmental challenges such as heat stress, air pollution, or exposure to altitude.[28]

$\dot{V}O_2$ can be measured with automated measurement systems, or *metabolic carts,* which provide breath-by-breath and time-averaged data, with on-screen graphics and digital display of $\dot{V}O_2$, volume of carbon dioxide produced ($\dot{V}CO_2$), and minute ventilation. Reports may be readily generated and data may be stored for clinical and research applications. Accurate results depend on frequent calibration of the pneumotachometer and the gas analyzers using "span gases" of known concentration (see Fig. 3-10).

The ability to continue to consume oxygen at high levels of exercise is the hallmark of aerobic fitness. Knowing that glucose is the only substrate utilized during near-maximal anaerobic effort allows the examiner to assess the subject's level of physical fitness by identifying the anaerobic threshold. This can be accomplished by measuring the ratio of carbon dioxide blown off to oxygen consumed. The respiratory exchange ratio (RER) is expressed as $\dot{V}CO_2/\dot{V}O_2$ and is a ventilatory measurement obtained from the metabolic cart that reflects gas exchange between the lungs and pulmonary blood. During heavy, non–steady-state exercise, RER may exceed 1.0. This is due to the increased $\dot{V}CO_2$ released through pulmonary hyperventilation and nonmetabolic sources of CO_2 provided from lactic acid buffering in the blood.

TABLE 3-5   Cardiorespiratory Fitness

Age (y)	Maximal Oxygen Uptake (METs)				
	Low	Fair	Average	Good	High
Men					
20–29	<7.2	7.2–9.4	9.5–12.0	12.1–14.8	14.9+
30–39	<6.6	6.6–8.5	8.6–10.8	10.9–13.7	13.8+
40–49	<5.7	5.7–7.4	7.5–10.0	10.1–12.6	12.7+
50–59	<5.1	5.1–6.8	6.9–9.4	9.5–12.0	12.1+
60–69	<4.6	4.6–6.3	6.4–8.6	8.7–11.4	11.5+
Women					
20–29	<6.8	6.8–8.5	8.6–10.6	10.7–13.7	13.8+
30–39	<5.7	5.7–7.7	7.8–9.4	9.5–12.6	12.7+
40–49	<4.9	4.9–6.6	6.7–8.6	8.7–11.7	11.8+
50–59	<4.3	4.3–5.7	5.8–7.7	7.8–10.6	10.7+
60–69	<3.7	3.7–4.9	5.0–6.6	6.7–9.7	9.8+

Table 3-6 illustrates the RER and energy equivalents for various mixes of carbohydrate and fat. This table shows that RERs that fall around 0.70 indicate that fat is the predominant fuel substrate. Similarly, RERs that approach 1.0 indicate that carbohydrate is being preferentially utilized. An RER of 0.90 indicates that the subject is utilizing approximately two-third carbohydrate and one-third fat.

The utility of measuring RER using a metabolic cart becomes apparent during performance of a graded exercise test. The subject starts out at a low level of exercise: Measured RERs typically fall around 0.70, indicating utilization of free fatty acids that become catabolized in the presence of oxygen. As exercise intensity increases, the measured RER will approach 1.0, indicating more reliance on glucose as a fuel substrate, as the demand for oxygen outstrips supply and as the subject becomes more dependent on anaerobic glycolysis to continue. At peak exercise, the RER is around 1.0, indicating near-total reliance on glucose and extreme fatigue. This is because glucose is the only fuel substrate that can be used during high levels of exercise intensity. **In summary, it may be said that measurement of the RER by way of the metabolic cart allows the clinician to determine the relative mix of carbohydrate and fat at progressive levels of exercise and is an indication of which energy system is predominant. In this way, it measures the subject's level of physical fitness. Measurement of an RER value in excess of 1.0 indicates a maximal effort, whereas an RER value of less than 1.0 suggests a submaximal effort.**

The energy expenditure (kcal) associated with a given level of $\dot{V}O_2$ varies slightly with the fuel substrate being utilized and with the RER. In clinical practice and in the absence of a metabolic cart, the precise dietary mix of carbohydrate and fat is unknown. **However, if a mixed diet of carbohydrate and fat is assumed, it may be said that for every liter of oxygen consumed, 5.0 kcal of energy is liberated.**

The following example illustrates the utility of this conversion.

A 70-kg subject consumes that 4.0-oz slice of cheesecake referred to at the beginning of the chapter. Use of a bomb calorimeter has determined that the energy value of the cheesecake is 350 kcal. Recall that

$$1 \text{ MET} = 3.5 \text{ mL O}_2/\text{kg/min}$$

and

$$\text{NET} = \text{gross} - \text{resting energy expenditure.}$$

How long must the subject exercise on a treadmill at a physiological workload of 5 METs in order to expend 350 kcal of energy? The answer can be calculated as follows:

$$\text{NET} = \text{gross} - \text{resting energy expenditure,}$$

$$4 \text{ METs} = 5 \text{ METs} - 1 \text{ MET,}$$

$$4 \text{ METs} \times 3.5 \text{ mL O}_2/\text{kg/min} = 14.0 \text{ mL O}_2/\text{kg/min,}$$

$$14.0 \text{ mL O}_2/\text{kg/min} \times 70 \text{ kg} = 980 \text{ mL/min} = 0.980 \text{ L/min,}$$

$$0.980 \text{ L/min} \times 5 \text{ kcal/L} = 4.900 \text{ kcal/min,}$$

$$X \text{ min} \times 4.900 \text{ kcal/min} = 350 \text{ kcal,}$$

and

$$350 \text{ kcal}/4.900 \text{ kcal/min} = 71.4 \text{ min.}$$

TABLE 3-6   Relationship Among RER, Substrate Utilized, and Energy

Respiratory Exchange Ratio	Percentage of Carbohydrate	Percentage of Fat	Kilocalories Per Liter of Oxygen
0.71	1.1	98.9	4.690
0.85	50.7	49.3	4.862
1.00	100.0	0.0	5.047

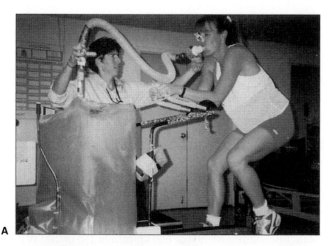

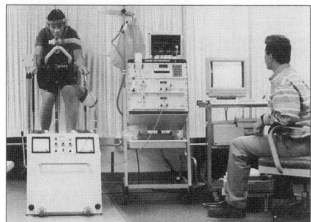

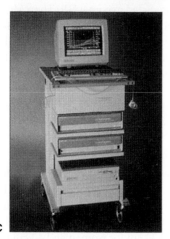

FIGURE 3-10 Common methods used to collect and sample expired gases during indirect gas analysis calorimetry. (**A**) Douglas bags, gas analyzers, and gas flow meters. (**B**) A simple, portable, time-averaged system for indirect calorimetry. (**C**) A breath-by-breath system. (Used with permission from Robergs R, Roberts S. *Exercise Physiology: Exercise Performance and Clinical Applications.* The McGraw-Hill Companies; 1997.)

CLINICAL CORRELATE

The ability to convert oxygen consumption to kilocalories has great utility for physical therapists involved in wellness and weight-reduction programs. If a subject exercised at this level on most days of the week and reduced his caloric intake by approximately 250 kcal/day, the net result would be a reduction of body weight by 1 lb/wk (1 lb = 3500 kcal).

Indirect Measurement of Peak Oxygen Consumption

Direct measurement of $\dot{V}O_{2peak}$ is complex and expensive. It is possible only if the physical therapist has access to a metabolic cart and a properly constructed laboratory. Maximal exercise testing may also pose a risk to the patient. For these reasons, it may be more feasible to subject the patient to submaximal effort and then use this information to predict maximum workload and $\dot{V}O_{2peak}$. This is possible through the use of standardized submaximal exercise testing and the use of regression equations that extrapolate the data to maximal levels. It should be noted that the numerous methods of estimating $\dot{V}O_{2peak}$ are specific to a particular protocol and ergometer. One such equation[80] is based on the length of time spent on the Bruce protocol for treadmill exercise test:

$$\dot{V}O_{2peak} (mL\ O_2/kg/min) = 14.8 - 1.379\ (time\ in\ minutes) + 0.451\ (time)^2 - 0.0.12\ (time)^3$$

It should be pointed out that use of this formula to predict $\dot{V}O_{2peak}$ carries with it a standard error of estimate (SEE) of 3.35 mL O_2/kg/min, or almost 1.0 MET. A similar formula[81] can be used to predict $\dot{V}O_{2peak}$ during the Bruce protocol while using the treadmill handrail for support, which may be appropriate for many patients with disability:

$$\dot{V}O_{2peak} (mL\ O_2/kg/min) = 2.282(time\ in\ minutes) + 8.545$$

$$SEE = 4.92\ mL\ O_2/kg/min$$

Extrapolation to peak $\dot{V}O_2$ is appropriate for individuals who are free of known cardiovascular disease, but who may be at risk for its development.

Submaximal Tests for Measuring Cardiorespiratory Fitness

Direct measurement of $\dot{V}O_{2peak}$ through the use of a metabolic cart remains the gold standard for assessment of cardiorespiratory fitness. However, direct measurement is not always possible. As such, a variety of validated exercise tests can be used to estimate $\dot{V}O_{2peak}$. These tests utilize conventional modes of exercise to obtain a submaximal HR response. An appropriate testing mode can be chosen based upon the general health status of the participant, accessibility of equipment, and consistency with the intended exercise training regime. Commonly used exercise tests include field tests, cycle ergometer tests, and step testing.

Field Tests

It should be noted that the results of these timed walking/running tests may be influenced by the subject's level of motivation and pacing ability. Because maximal effort is encouraged, greater risk may exist. Therefore, these tests may not be the test of choice for sedentary individuals at increased risk for cardiovascular or musculoskeletal complications.

The Rockport 1-Mile Fitness Walking Test—As a means of estimating cardiorespiratory fitness, the Rockport 1-Mile Fitness Walking Test has gained wide popularity. During this test, the patient/client walks 1 mile as fast as possible, preferably on a track or a level surface. HR is measured in the final minute during the final 1/4 mile. An alternative is to measure a 10-second HR immediately on completion of the 1-mile walk, but this may overestimate $\dot{V}O_{2peak}$ when compared to measurement of HR during the walk. An individual's $\dot{V}O_{2peak}$ is predicted from the regression equation:

$$\dot{V}O_{2peak} \,(\text{mL O}_2/\text{kg/min}) = 132.853 - 0.1692 \,(\text{body} \\ \text{mass in kg}) - 0.3877 \,(\text{age in years}) + 6.315 \,(\text{gender}) \\ - 3.2649 \,(\text{time in minutes}) - 0.1565 \,(\text{HR}).$$

In this equation, gender = 0 for female, 1 = male, and heart rate (HR) is taken at the end of the walk.

The 1.5-mile test—In this test, the patient/client is asked to run a 1.5-mile distance in the shortest amount of time. $\dot{V}O_{2peak}$ is estimated from the equation:

$$\dot{V}O_{2peak} \,(\text{mL O}_2/\text{kg/min}) = 3.5 + 483/\text{time in minutes}.$$

The Cooper 12-Minute Test—This test requires the patient/client to walk or run for 12 minutes on a running track, with the objective of covering the greatest distance in the allotted period of time. The distance covered is measured to the nearest 100-m interval. This test can also be performed by walking/running on a treadmill set at a 1% grade to best mimic outdoor terrain. An estimation of $\dot{V}O_{2peak}$ can be calculated by the following equation, if the participant is walking:

$$\dot{V}O_{2peak} \,(\text{mL O}_2/\text{kg/min}) = 0.1 \,(\text{speed}) + 1.8 \,(\text{speed}) \,(\text{grade}) \\ + 3.5 \,\text{mL/kg/min},$$

whereas speed is expressed in m/min and grade is expressed as a fraction. If the participant is running, the following equation can be used to estimate $\dot{V}O_{2peak}$:

$$\dot{V}O_{2peak} \,(\text{mL O}_2/\text{kg/min}) = 0.2 \,(\text{speed}) + 0.9 \,(\text{speed}) \,(\text{grade}) \\ + 3.5 \,\text{mL/kg/min}$$

Cooper reported a correlation of 0.897 between $\dot{V}O_{2max}$ and the distance covered in a 12-minute walk/run, indicating a highly significant relationship.[82] Cooper established the following normative data charts to estimate maximal $\dot{V}O_2$ and assess the patient/client's fitness level from the distance value obtained.[82]

It should be mentioned that numerous variations have been derived from the normative data charts, providing fitness levels adjusted for gender and alternate modes of exercise (ie, swimming). These charts and formulas are easily accessible on the Web from numerous sources. Caution should be exercised when the source of data is not provided with these resources.

Cycle Ergometer Tests

The Astrand–Rhyming Cycle Ergometer Test—This is a steady-state test in which the patient/client is asked to cycle at a rate of 50 rpm for 6 minutes. The suggested work rate is adjusted for gender and fitness level as follows[83]:

Men, unconditioned: 300 or 600 kg/m/min (50 or 100 W)
Men, conditioned: 600 or 900 kg/m/min (100 or 150 W)
Women, unconditioned: 300 or 450 kg/m/min (50 or 75 W)
Women, conditioned: 450 or 600 kg/m/min (75 or 100 W)

The goal is to obtain an HR value between 125 and 170 bpm. HR measurements taken at 5 and 6 minutes of work are averaged, and then compared to the Astrand–Rhyming nomogram for estimation of $\dot{V}O_{2peak}$ (see Fig. 3-11). This value must then be adjusted for age by multiplying the $\dot{V}O_{2peak}$ value by the appropriate correction factor (see Fig. 3-11).

The YMCA Cycle Ergometer Test—This submaximal test has become one of the most popular assessment tools to estimate $\dot{V}O_{2peak}$. The YMCA Cycle Ergometer Test measures the patient/client's HR at a series of work rates and adjusts the response to the subject's age-predicted maximal HR. The YMCA protocol requires the patient/client to cycle continuously for two to four 3-minute bouts, with the objective of raising the subject's steady-state HR between 110 bpm and 85% of the age-predicted maximal HR (see Fig. 3-12). HRs are taken during the last 15 to 30 seconds of the second and third minutes of each stage and must fall into the desired range for two consecutive bouts to be considered a valid predictor of $\dot{V}O_{2peak}$.

Step Tests

Step tests have been developed to estimate the subject's cardiovascular fitness based upon estimates of $\dot{V}O_{2peak}$ from direct HR response, as well as HR recovery following standardized submaximal exercise testing. Astrand and Rhyming[84] designed a step test, using a step height of 33 cm for women and 40 cm for men. The patient/client is asked to step at a rate of 22.5 steps/min, requiring oxygen uptakes of 25.8 and 29.5, respectively, for men and women. HR measurements taken at 5 and 6 minutes of work are averaged and then compared to the Astrand–Rhyming nomogram for estimation of $\dot{V}O_{2peak}$ (see Fig. 3-11).

The 3-Minute YMCA Step Test—This is a popular test designed to estimate the subject's cardiovascular fitness based upon the patient/client's HR recovery following a 3-minute bout of continuous exercise. The patient/client is asked to step at a rate of 24 steps/min, using a 30.5-cm step. Within 5 seconds from the completion of exercise, the patient is asked to sit and

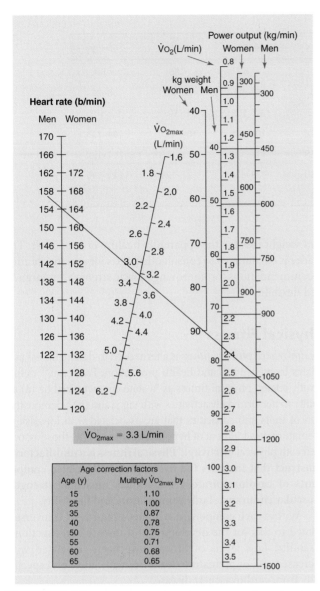

FIGURE 3-11 The Astrand–Rhyming nomogram for estimating during steady-state cycle ergometer exercise. This estimation is derived from a single submaximal effort. (Reproduced with permission from Robergs R, Roberts S. *Exercise Physiology: Exercise, Performance, and Clinical Applications.* The McGraw-Hill Companies; 1997.)

their HR is recorded for 1 minute.[85] This HR is used to obtain a qualitative rating of fitness from published normative tables (see Tables 3-7 and 3-8).

ENDURANCE TRAINING FOR THE HEALTHY INDIVIDUAL

Physical Activity

In the past 5 years, several scientific statements, consensus development conferences, and position stands have emphasized that physical inactivity is a major health problem in the United States. More than 60% of adults are not physically active on a regular basis and 25% are not active at all.[86] It is well accepted that men and women of all ages benefit from regular physical activity, and physical activity is often very beneficial in the treatment of persons with chronic disease and disabilities. People who are sedentary can improve their health, fitness, and well-being by becoming moderately active. Because vigorous physical activity can result in anginal episodes, heart attack, musculoskeletal complications, and other adverse responses in certain individuals, exercise testing and prescription are important skills for the practitioner to master.

Physical activity is a broad term used to describe all forms of large muscle movements including sports, dance, work, games, exercise, and lifestyle activities. Many health and quality-of-life benefits are derived from being physically active (Box 3-5).

In order to encourage more individuals to participate in physical activity, the Surgeon General's Report on Physical Activity and Health[86] and the American College of Sports Medicine (ACSM)[83,87] have outlined a basic recommendation for lifelong physical activity. *Every U.S. adult should accumulate 30 minutes or more of moderate-intensity physical activity on most, preferably all, days of the week.*

Strenuous physical activity is not required to achieve health benefits. Increasing evidence has shown that moderate-intensity physical activity (3–6 METs) leads to health benefits even when $\dot{V}O_{2peak}$ remains unchanged. Benefits of moderate activity may be achieved in longer sessions of moderately intense activities (ie, 40 minutes of brisk walking) or in shorter

		HR < 80	HR 80–89	HR 90–100	HR > 100
1st Stage	2nd Stage	750 kg/min (2.5 kg)[a]	600 kg/min (2.0 kg)	450 kg/min (1.5 kg)	300 kg/min (1.0 kg)
150 kg/min (0.5 kg)	3rd Stage	900 kg/min (3.0 kg)	750 kg/min (2.5 kg)	600 kg/min (2.0 kg)	450 kg/min (1.5 kg)
	4th Stage	1050 kg/min (3.5 kg)	900 kg/min (3.0 kg)	750 kg/min (2.5 kg)	600 kg/min (2.0 kg)

[a]Resistance settings shown here are appropriate for an ergometer with a flywheel of 6 m/rev.

Directions:
1. Set the first work rate at 150 kg/min (0.5 kg at 50 rpm).
2. If the HR in the third minute of the stage is:
   - less than (<) 80, set the second stage at 750 kg/min (2.5 kg at 50 rpm).
   - 80–89, set the second stage at 600 kg/min (2.0 kg at 50 rpm).
   - 90–100, set the second stage at 450 kg/min (1.5 kg at 50 rpm).
   - greater than (>) 100, set the second stage at 300 kg/min (1.0 kg at 50 rpm).
3. Set the third and fourth (if required) stages according to the work rates in the columns below the second loads.

FIGURE 3-12 YMCA cycle ergometry protocol. (Adapted from American College of Sports Medicine. *ACSM's Guidelines for Exercise Testing and Prescription.* 7th ed. Lippincott Williams & Wilkins; 2006.)

TABLE 3-7   3-Minute Step Test (Men)

	18–25 y	26–35 y	36–45 y	46–55 y	56–65 y	65+ y
Excellent	<79	<81	<83	<87	<86	<88
Good	79–89	81–89	83–96	87–97	86–97	88–96
Above average	90–99	90–99	97–103	98–105	98–103	97–103
Average	100–105	100–107	104–112	106–116	104–112	104–113
Below average	106–116	108–117	113–119	117–122	113–120	114–120
Poor	117–128	118–128	120–130	123–132	121–129	121–130
Very poor	>128	>128	>130	>132	>129	>130

sessions of more strenuous exercise (15–20 minutes of running). A moderate amount of physical activity is approximately equivalent to physical activity that uses 150 kcal/day, or 1,000 kcal/wk.[86] Physical activity may be structured (walking, running) or unstructured (washing the car, raking leaves). This report also suggests that adults who maintain a regular routine of physical activity that is of longer duration or greater intensity are likely to derive additional benefits, while excessive amounts of high-intensity exercise may increase the risk of injury or other health problems. Table 3-9 provides other examples of moderate physical activity that meet the activity recommendation.

Analogous to the USDA's Food Guide Pyramid, the Physical Activity Pyramid (PAP) has been developed to encourage a more active lifestyle. Physical therapists may use this tool to educate their patients and clients about the different types of physical activity (Fig. 3-13). As shown in this model, aerobic activities represent one way to incorporate physical activity into a healthy lifestyle. For patients or clients who are too deconditioned to meet the traditional intensities prescribed for aerobic training, a weekly activity plan incorporating activities in the base of the pyramid may result in training changes or prepare an individual to participate in a future training program. This section describes how to develop exercise prescriptions that enhance cardiorespiratory fitness and weight loss for the apparently healthy or well adult. The reader is encouraged to consult other texts for specific training recommendations for improving muscle strength, endurance, and flexibility.[28,62,83]

Physical Fitness

Health-related physical fitness is a term used to denote fitness as it relates to prevention and health promotion. Pate et al.[88] define health-related physical fitness as "a state characterized by (a) an ability to perform daily activities with vigor and (b) a demonstration of traits and capacities that are associated with low risk of premature development of hypokinetic diseases (ie, those associated with physical inactivity)." **Physical fitness is a multifactorial construct that includes the five main health-related components of cardiorespiratory endurance, muscular strength, muscular endurance, body composition, and flexibility.**

Within each component, a higher fitness level is inversely related to risk for the development of disease and functional disability. Low levels of fitness have been correlated with increased risk of premature death from all causes and specifically from cardiovascular disease.

Cardiorespiratory endurance refers to the ability to perform large-muscle, dynamic, moderate- to high-intensity exercise for prolonged periods. Performance of such exercise

TABLE 3-8   3-Minute Step Test (Women)

	18–25 y	26–35 y	36–45 y	46–55 y	56–65 y	65+ y
Excellent	<85	<88	<90	<94	<95	<90
Good	85–98	88–99	90–102	95–104	86–97	90–102
Above average	99–108	100–111	103–110	105–115	105–112	103–115
Average	109–117	112–119	111–118	116–120	113–118	116–122
Below average	118–126	120–126	119–128	121–129	119–128	123–128
Poor	127–140	127–138	129–140	130–135	129–139	129–134
Very poor	>140	>138	>140	>135	>139	>134

Canadian Public Health Association Project obtained from the following Web site: http://www.antiaging-wellness.com/Pages/Wellness/Body/Tests/step.php. Accessed July 8, 2008.

Possible Health Benefits of Physical Activity

Reduces the risk of premature death
Reduces the risk of death due to heart disease
Reduces the risk of developing hypertension
Helps reduce blood pressure in people with hypertension
Reduces the risk of developing colon cancer
Helps control body weight
Helps build and maintain healthy bones, muscles, and joints
Reduces feelings of depression and anxiety
Improves strength in older adults and reduces falls
Promotes psychological well-being and self-efficacy

Adapted from U.S. Department of Health and Human Services. *The Surgeon General's Report on Physical Activity and Health.*

depends on oxidative phosphorylation of ATP and therefore preferentially utilizes the long-term energy system. This system challenges the heart, lungs, and peripheral and pulmonary circulation to provide arterial blood to working skeletal muscle. The interrelationship between systems and steps for oxygen transport are summarized in Chapter 5, Fig. 5-7.

EXERCISE PRESCRIPTION FOR THE HEALTHY INDIVIDUAL

Principles and Assumptions of Aerobic Exercise Training

The major objective in exercise training is to produce an aerobic endurance training effect, characterized by physiological

TABLE 3-9 Examples of Moderate Amounts of Physical Activity

Activity	Time (min)
Washing and waxing car	45–60; less vigorous, more time
Washing windows or floors	45–60
Gardening	30–45
Wheeling self in wheelchair	30–40
Social dancing	30
Pushing a stroller (1.5 miles)	30
Raking leaves	30
Walking (2 miles)	30
Swimming laps	20
Bicycling 4 miles	15
Jump rope	15; more vigorous, less time

Adapted from U.S. Department of Health and Human Services. *The Surgeon General's Report on Physical Activity and Health.*

adaptations that improve performance in specific tasks. Adaptation depends on the training stimulus threshold (stimulus that elicits a response) and the ability of the organism to change. Physiological adaptation to exercise varies with the magnitude of the stimulus and the length of time over which the stimulus is applied. For example, patients who are particularly deconditioned may adapt quickly to a relatively low training stimulus, whereas an athlete may require many months to show only minimal improvement with a very high training stimulus. Additionally, training adaptations vary both *within* an individual performing different forms of exercise and *across* individuals given the same training program.

For all the reasons cited previously, an individualized exercise program is essential in order to identify a training stimulus of appropriate intensity, duration, and frequency that maximize the physiological response.

Acute Response to Aerobic Exercise

During acute aerobic exercise, the cardiorespiratory system must respond to support the energy requirements of muscle during physical exertion. The cumulative effect of adaptations in HR, stroke volume, cardiac output, blood flow, blood pressure, arteriovenous oxygen difference, and pulmonary ventilation sustain oxygen demands to the active tissues. In response to dynamic exercise, HR increases linearly with work rate and oxygen uptake. This HR response is affected by age, fitness level, intensity of the activity, blood volume, cardiac pathology, medications, body position, and environmental factors. As HR increases with higher-intensity exercise, end-diastolic volume (EDV) decreases as a result of compromised ventricular filling time. The stroke volume is the volume of blood ejected from the heart with each heart beat, and it is equal to the difference between end-diastolic volume and end-systolic volume. Thus, stroke volume initially increases with work rate, but as the cardiovascular demand increases and HR escalates, stroke volume may decrease because of decreased end-diastolic filling time. At exercise intensities up to 50% of $\dot{V}O_{2peak}$, cardiac output increases linearly with work rate due to increases in HR and stroke volume. Thereafter, increases in cardiac output depend mostly upon rising HR, although maximum values of cardiac output are affected by age, stature, fitness level, cardiovascular pathology, and body positioning during exercise. As previously discussed, there is a linear increase in SBP with increasing exercise intensity, while diastolic blood pressure may decrease slightly or remain unchanged. An SBP that fails to rise or drops in response to an exercise stimulus can signal a plateau or decrease in cardiac output and may be indicative of underlying cardiac pathology.

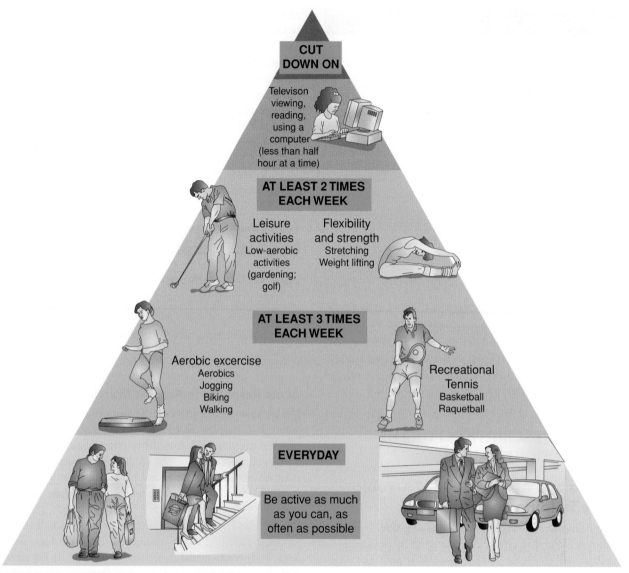

FIGURE 3-13   The Physical Activity Pyramid. (Reprinted with permission from Foss M, Keteyian S. *Fox's Physiological Basis for Exercise and Sport.* Boston, MA: McGraw-Hill; 1998.)

CLINICAL CORRELATE

While performing exercise testing on a patient/client, *exertional hypotension* is characterized by an SBP which decreases below baseline toward the end of the test stage or initially rises with exercise stimulus and then falls 20 mm Hg or more thereafter. Exercise testing/ training should be terminated immediately in subjects demonstrating exertional hypotension, as this response has been shown to correlate with myocardial ischemia, left ventricular dysfunction, and increased risk of cardiac events during follow-up.[89] See Chapter 12 for a discussion of the clinical relevance of exertional hypotension.

Pulmonary ventilation during mild- to moderate-intensity exercise increases primarily due to a rise in tidal volume, while respiratory rate response is more important to support $\dot{V}_A$ during high-intensity exercise.

Body Positioning

Posture has an effect on end-diastolic filling, which directly affects stroke volume and the overall strain placed upon the heart with steady work rate. End-diastolic volume is the highest in supine and decreases progressively as the body shifts to semi-recumbent, sitting and standing postures at rest. During exercise, end-diastolic volume remains unchanged in the supine position, while it progressively decreases in upright position, placing an increased load on the heart. Stroke volume is also highest in the supine position, resulting in a lower HR and myocardial oxygen demand at a given submaximal work rate.

Clinicians should be aware that when working with patients with cardiac pathology, initiating exercise in the supine position allows for the highest end-diastolic volume and stroke volume, thereby placing the least amount of strain on the heart. Exercising in upright positions places an increasing demand on cardiac tissues and should be monitored appropriately as the patient is progressively challenged.

Upper Extremity Versus Lower Extremity Exercise

HR, SBP, DBP, pulmonary ventilation, and $\dot{V}O_2$ are higher, while stroke volume and anaerobic threshold are lower, with upper extremity than lower extremity exercise at a steady work rate. This may reflect the dynamic involvement of smaller muscle groups, with concomitant isometric contraction and vasoconstriction of peripheral vessels in larger leg muscles during exertion. A comparison of mean RPP and estimated $\dot{M}\dot{V}O_2$ during upper extremity and lower extremity exercise is shown in Fig. 3-14. During arm exercise, $\dot{V}O_{2peak}$ generally varies between 64% and 80% of $\dot{V}O_{2peak}$ with leg exercise.[90] At high workloads, maximal HR, SBP, and RPP are similar or slightly lower with arm exercise. As such, in order to avoid an overestimation of maximal HR during upper extremity training, the prescribed target HR from lower extremity training should be reduced by approximately 10 bpm.[91]

The difference between cardiac response between arm and leg exercise has clinical relevance for the physical therapist. Recommendations regarding intensity of arm exercise training must be reduced by approximately 10 bpm to avoid overestimation of the target HR.

Low-Resistance Versus High-Resistance Training

Resistance training has been found to improve cardiorespiratory function by creating small volumes of blood that are pumped at very high pressures to the involved muscles. There is a dramatic increase in systolic and diastolic blood pressure with dynamic resistive exercise, especially during the concentric phase of the muscle contraction. For example, Mac-Dougall et al.[92] reported a mean BP of 320/250 during the double leg press. Despite speculation that this type of exercise might, therefore, increase resting blood pressure, a recent meta-analysis concluded that resistance training results in

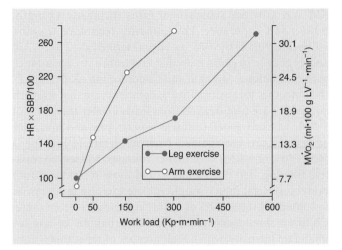

FIGURE 3-14 Mean rate–pressure product and estimated myocardial oxygen consumption ($\dot{M}\dot{V}O_2$) during arm (broken line) and leg (solid line) exercise. $\dot{M}\dot{V}O_2$ is estimated from its hemodynamic correlates, heart rate (HR) multiplied by systolic blood pressure (SBP). (Adapted with permission from Schwade J, Blomqvist CG, Shapiro W. A comparison of the response to arm and leg work in patients with ischemic heart disease. *Am Heart J.* 1977;94:203-208, and American College of Sports Medicine. *ACSM's Resource Manual for Guidelines for Exercise Testing and Prescription.* 5th ed. Philadelphia, PA: Lippincott Williams & Wilkins; 2006.)

decreases of 2% and 4% for resting systolic and diastolic pressures, respectively.[93] HR also increases substantially in response to a resistive exercise stimulus, peaking during the last few repetitions of a set. There is no difference in HR response related to the phase of muscle contraction (concentric vs eccentric). Resistance-trained individuals demonstrate resting HRs that are equal or lower than averages for the untrained. In response to resistive exercise training, maximal $\dot{V}O_2$ has been found to improve slightly with circuit training and for untrained individuals. Resistance training does little to increase $\dot{V}O_{2peak}$, although it may improve cardiovascular endurance by increasing muscle strength and endurance.[83] Lower resting HR (HR_{rest}), BP, and, consequently, RPP are positive adaptations of the cardiorespiratory system in response to resistive exercise training.

Intensity of training is often synonymous with training load (amount of weight per repetition) and most easily represented as a percentage of an athlete's repetition maximum (RM) for an exercise.[94] A true 1 repetition maximum (1-RM) indicates that after one successful repetition, the involved muscle has reached a point of fatigue whereby its force-generating capacity would fail to contract sufficiently against the imposed resistance for a second repetition. The muscle is performing at its highest intensity. Typically, exercise sets involving high resistance with low repetition to reach muscle fatigue (1–6 RM) or 90% of the RM are considered high-intensity training stimuli. High-intensity resistance training is believed to provide the most significant gains in strength and power. Moderate-intensity resistance training falls within the parameters of 6 to 12-RM or 70% to 90% of the

RM and provides submaximal gains in muscle strength, power, and endurance. Low-intensity resistance training falls below 70% of the RM, usually prescribed at 12 to 20-RM and primarily benefits muscular endurance. In accordance with the National Strength and Conditioning Association,[94] the outcomes for various load assignments are that strength and power are best derived from loads greater than 80% of 1-RM, whereas general muscle hypertrophy and muscular endurance are best gained from moderate-to-low loads (60%–80% of 1-RM) with higher volumes. Novices to resistive training, detrained athletes, and those recovering from musculoskeletal injury should initiate exercise programs at low intensity (50%–60% of 1-RM) and progress from there. Children should engage in exercise programs of low-to-moderate intensity, with a high number of repetitions, until they reach puberty.[95] It is recommended that cardiac rehabilitation patients follow a standard circuit training program using intensities of 40% to 60% of 1-RM.[96]

While 1-RM testing is the gold standard for athletes experienced in resistance training, it is not always the practical or safe means of establishing a patient/client's appropriate training workload. Novices, detrained athletes, children, sen-iors, cardiac patients, and those recovering from musculoskeletal injury are all examples of individuals who should initiate exercise programs at lower intensities (higher RM values). Estimations of 1-RM can be made from tables such as Table 3-10 to avoid the risks associated with 1-RM testing. It should be mentioned that the accuracy of these tables is controversial and should be used as a starting point to be fine-tuned by the clinician, based upon the ability and response of the client/patient.

While it is accurate to say that load assignment based upon RM is the most widely accepted means for exercise prescription in athletes, the ACSM recommends using this technique as a general guideline rather than an accurate portrayal of true intensity. They postulate that intensity can be defined as the *effort* or how difficult the training stimulus is. It has been found that the progressive increase in muscle fiber recruitment parallels increases in blood pressure, regardless of the size of the muscle mass involved.[92,97] The magnitude of the blood pressure response depends on the degree of effort (intensity), not the absolute force of contraction.[92,97] The elevation in blood pressure associated with high intensity is extreme even when recruiting a small muscle

TABLE 3-10   Estimating a 1 Repetition Maximum from a Training Load

Max Reps (RM)	1	2	3	4	5	6	7	8	9	10	12
% 1RM	100	95	93	90	87	85	83	80	77	75	67
Load (lb or kg)	10	10	9	9	9	9	8	8	8	8	7
	20	19	19	18	17	17	17	16	15	15	13
	30	29	28	27	26	26	25	24	23	23	20
	40	38	37	36	35	34	33	32	31	30	27
	50	48	47	45	44	43	42	40	39	38	34
	60	57	56	54	52	51	50	48	46	45	40
	70	67	65	63	61	60	58	56	54	53	47
	80	76	74	72	70	68	66	64	62	60	54
	90	86	84	81	78	77	75	72	69	68	60
	100	95	93	90	87	85	83	80	77	75	67
	110	105	102	99	96	94	91	88	85	83	74
	120	114	112	108	104	102	100	96	92	90	80
	130	124	121	117	113	111	108	104	100	98	87
	140	133	130	126	122	119	116	112	108	105	94
	150	143	140	135	131	128	125	120	116	113	101
	160	152	149	144	139	136	133	128	123	120	107
	170	162	158	153	148	145	141	136	131	128	114
	180	171	167	162	157	153	149	144	139	135	121
	190	181	177	171	165	162	158	152	146	143	127
	200	190	186	180	174	170	166	160	154	150	134

Data from Baechle and Earle 1989; Baechle and Earle 2000; Brzycki 1993; Chapman, Whitehead, and Binkert 1998; Epley 1985; Lombardi 1989; Mayhew, Ball, Arnold, and Bowen 1992; Morales and Sobonya 1996; and Wathen 1994. From National Strength and Conditioning Association. *Essentials of Personal Training.* Human Kinetics; 2004.

mass.[92] Therefore, the ACSM[83] recommends that individuals with hypertension, diabetes, at risk for stroke, or at other medical risk from exposure to high blood pressures should *avoid* high-intensity resistance training. They advise this population to engage in lower-intensity resistance training, by terminating lifting before fatigue. An initial goal of 12 to 13 and a final goal of 15 to 16 on the RPE scale have been recommended for submaximal training.[98–100] A target of 19 to 20 on the RPE scale is synonymous with high-intensity strength stimuli for healthy populations.[83]

CLINICAL CORRELATE

The ability to safely prescribe resistance training loads has great utility for physical therapists involved in wellness programs. While load assignment based upon RM may be used as a general guideline for healthy populations and athletes, special considerations based upon intensity must be made for populations at risk of cardiovascular insult.

Training Principles

A training stimulus must also be task specific. The *principle of specificity* tells us that the training effects derived from an exercise program are specific to the exercise performed and the muscles involved. In essence, performing specific exercises elicits specific adaptations, creating specific training effects. The concept of specificity should be used relative to the demands of the exercise, rather than to the metabolic pathway that predominates during exercise. For example, heavy resistance training is characterized by the application of high-resistance, low-repetition exercises that produce increases in strength, but with little or no change in endurance. Conversely, high-repetition, low-resistance exercises yield improvements in muscle endurance without significant changes in strength.

In order for a system to show functional improvements, it must be exposed to a high load to which it is not normally accustomed. This is referred to as the *overload principle*. Physiological adaptation occurs when exercise takes place at a level above normal. The overload principle is applicable to everyone, including the sedentary person, the athlete, persons with disabilities, and patients with cardiovascular and pulmonary disease. By progressively increasing the training variables (eg, frequency, intensity, duration), cardiovascular and/or muscular adaptations occur.

The specificity of training principle works together with the overload principle. When training for specific aerobic activities, the overload must engage the appropriate muscles required by the activity and stress central circulation. This recommendation is supported by studies that have demonstrated significant changes in aerobic capacity when the exercise used for training

is also used for testing, whereas little improvement is noted when aerobic capacity is measured by a dissimilar exercise.

The overload of specific muscle groups improves exercise performance and aerobic power by enhancing the capacity of the trained muscle to generate ATP aerobically. This aerobic improvement results from an increase in both the size and the number of mitochondria; increased capillarization of active skeletal muscles, resulting in greater regional blood flow; and a more effective distribution of cardiac output.

The *principle of reversibility* posits that detraining occurs rapidly when a person stops exercise training. Even among highly trained athletes, the beneficial effects of exercise training are transient and reversible. For example, a study demonstrated a 25% reduction in $\dot{V}O_{2max}$ in five subjects confined to bed for 20 consecutive days.[101] This reduction of nearly 1% per day was accompanied by similar reductions in maximal stroke volume, cardiac output, and the number of capillaries in the trained muscles.

Principles of Muscular Response to Training

Muscular Fitness

Muscular fitness is a term used to describe the integrated status of muscular strength and muscular endurance. Increasing muscular strength and endurance have been proven to directly impact an individual's functional ability to perform activities of daily living with less physiological stress, thereby aiding in optimizing quality of life throughout the life span. Considered a health-related fitness component, muscular fitness maintains or improves bone mass, glucose tolerance, musculotendinous integrity, FFM, and RMR. Potential consequences of declining muscular fitness include weight gain and obesity, osteoporosis, type 2 diabetes mellitus, musculotendinous injury, and the inability to carry out the activities of daily living.

Muscle strength has been defined as the maximal force a muscle can generate at a given velocity, and *muscle endurance* refers to the ability of a muscle to make repeated contractions or to resist muscular fatigue. Tests for measuring muscle strength and endurance may be placed on a continuum. Tests that allow few repetitions are used to measure strength, whereas tests involving high numbers of repetitions may be used to measure endurance. Common tests for measuring muscle strength and endurance are provided in the following section.

Muscular Strength

Muscular strength refers to the maximal force that can be generated by a specific muscle or muscle group. *Static strength* (isometric strength) can be measured using handgrip dynamometers and cable tensiometers. Measures of static strength are specific to both the muscle group and joint angle involved in testing; therefore, their utility in describing overall muscle strength is limited. Peak force development in such tests is commonly referred to as the maximum voluntary contraction. Static strength is most accurately expressed in Newtons, although kilogram is commonly used.

Dynamic strength testing is commonly tested using the 1-RM. This gold standard for dynamic strength identifies the heaviest weight that can be lifted only once using good form. Normative data are available for upper-body strength and leg strength based on a 1-RM bench press and 1-RM leg press, respectively. The 6-RM and 10-RM tests have also been used as measures of muscular fitness, but estimating a 1-RM from such tests has been problematic.

Isokinetic testing involves the assessment of maximal muscle tension throughout a range of motion set at a constant angular velocity (eg, 180 degrees/s). Equipment utilizing a dynamometer that allows control of the speed of the joint rotation (degrees/s) as well as the ability to test movement around various joints is available from several commercial sources. These devices measure peak rotational force or torque. Some of these testing methods will be discussed in Chapters 9 and 10.

Muscular Endurance

There are two types of tests designed to assess muscular endurance: one, dynamic in nature; and the other, static. Dynamic muscle tests measure the ability of a muscle group to perform repeated contractions over a period of time sufficient to cause muscular fatigue. Static muscle endurance tests assess the ability of a muscle group to maintain a specific percentage of the maximum voluntary contraction for a prolonged period of time. The abdominal muscle endurance test is an example of a dynamic test. This muscle group is tested using a curl-up (crunch) test. During this test, the individual performs slow, controlled curl-ups to lift the shoulder blades off the mat in time with a metronome at a rate of 20 curl-ups/min. A posterior pelvic tilt is maintained. The number of curl-ups completed without pausing up to 75 is compared to normative data according to age and gender. The YMCA Bench Press Test[102] provides an example of how resistance training equipment may be adapted to measure dynamic muscular endurance. In this test, standardized repetitions are performed using a 35-lb barbell for women and an 80-lb barbell for men. Subjects are scored by the number of successful repetitions they perform at a rate of 30 lifts/min. The Sorensen test is an example of a static muscular endurance test. In this test, the subject is positioned in prone on a table with the upper trunk suspended out over the end. The subject is instructed to maintain the trunk in a static posture parallel to the floor for as long as possible. The effort is timed, and the datum is compared to a normative data set. This test has been used to identify patients at risk for the development of low back pain.

Flexibility

Flexibility is the ability to move a joint through its complete range of motion. Muscle viscosity, ligament and tendon tightness, temperature, adequate warm-up, and distensibility of the joint capsule are among the many variables that affect flexibility. Maintaining flexibility of all joints facilitates movement needed to carry out activities of daily living. When an activity moves the structures of a joint beyond its shortened range of motion, tissue damage can occur.

No single test evaluates total body flexibility. Goniometers, electrogoniometers, inclinometers, tape measures, and visual estimates of range of motion can be useful in fitness screening. Flexibility of the neck, trunk, hips, and shoulders, for example, can be assessed through joint screening tests.

The sit-and-reach test has been commonly used to assess low back and hip-joint flexibility. This test is not a good measure of low back function when the distance reached is the only measure recorded. To improve this test, the administrator should examine the quality of the movement including the angle of the sacrum (90 degrees or more) and the spinal curve. One leg should be assessed at a time to evaluate symmetry. Standardized test procedures should be followed if this test is to be used. Normative data are available based on gender and age.

Essential Components of an Exercise Program

Initial screening of participants for the presence of risk factors and/or symptoms of cardiovascular, pulmonary, and metabolic disease is needed in order to maintain safety during exercise testing and training. Screening provides a mechanism for the identification of individuals who may be at risk and who should undergo a medical examination and monitored graded exercise testing prior to program initiation. Individuals who are apparently healthy (ie, low risk) and have a functional capacity of at least 8 METs may participate in unsupervised exercise programs.[83] **Supervised programs are strongly recommended for those individuals who have lower functional capacities (<8 METs) or have multiple risk factors.** Screening recommendations will be described in Chapters 9 and 10. The focus in this section will be on describing the essential components of an individualized exercise prescription.

Exercise prescriptions include the frequency, intensity, duration (time), mode(s), and progression of exercise. These five components should be utilized when prescribing exercise for individuals of all ages and fitness levels. The following recommendations are guidelines developed from the scientific evidence available on exercise training. An individualized exercise program should be based on the objective evaluation of individual responses to exercise, including measured or estimated $\dot{V}O_{2peak}$, HR, blood pressure, rating of perceived exertion, signs and symptoms of exercise intolerance, and possibly an electrocardiogram. Current guidelines do not require that a graded exercise test be completed for all individuals before beginning an exercise program. However, it is recommended that individuals older than 40 years with two or more risk factors undergo formal graded exercise testing before an exercise program is implemented.[83] As the exercise prescription is developed, an individual's goals, behavioral characteristics, and exercise preferences should be considered.

Intensity

Perhaps the most challenging component of an exercise prescription is the exercise intensity. Before setting the target intensity range, or *training window,* the goal or desired outcome must be clearly identified. A higher training window (70%–85% of HR_{max}) may be used in order to enhance cardiorespiratory endurance. Deconditioned individuals benefit from intensities as low as 40% to 49% of HR reserve (HRR) or 55% to 64% of HR_{max}.[83] A low- to moderate-intensity training window (eg, 55%–65% of HR_{max}), which is performed over a prolonged duration, appears to optimize weight reduction. Examples of these will be included in the following section that describes several methods available for determination of patient-specific exercise intensity.

The following approaches for computing exercise intensity may not be appropriate for the elderly and patients with two or more risk factors for heart disease, known cardiovascular disease, or other chronic diseases without appropriate screening and testing.

Oxygen uptake reserve ($\dot{V}o_2R$)—Because $\dot{V}o_{2peak}$ is considered the best measure of cardiorespiratory fitness, a straight percentage of measured or estimated $\dot{V}o_{2peak}$ may be used in prescribing exercise intensity. Traditionally, a training window of 60% to 80% of $\dot{V}o_{2peak}$ has been used. For example, if an individual had an estimated $\dot{V}o_{2peak}$ of 12 METs determined by a submaximal graded exercise test, the prescribed training window would be set at 7.2 to 9.6 METs.

In a 1998 position stand,[103] the ACSM recommended that exercise intensity be computed using a percentage of oxygen uptake reserve (%$\dot{V}o_2R$). The $\dot{V}o_2R$ is the difference between the $\dot{V}o_{2peak}$ and resting $\dot{V}o_2$ and it is computed by the following equation:

$$\text{Target } \dot{V}o_2 = (\text{exercise intensity}) (\dot{V}o_{2peak} - \dot{V}o_{2rest}) + \dot{V}o_{2rest}$$

In this equation, $\dot{V}o_{2rest}$ is 3.5 mL O_2/kg/min or 1.0 MET, and the exercise intensity may range from 50% to 85%, expressed as a fraction of the equation. An intensity as low as 40% may be used in very deconditioned individuals. Because $\dot{V}o_2R$ is highly correlated to the HRR, it is now considered the most accurate way to determine whether the exercise stimulus is intense enough to promote improvements in cardiorespiratory fitness.

Percent of HR_{max}—Historically, a training window of 70% to 85% of an individual's HR_{max} has been used to prescribe exercise intensity. This corresponds to 50% to 85% of $\dot{V}o_{2peak}$ and provides an adequate stimulus to improve or maintain $\dot{V}o_{2peak}$. A higher training window of 85% to 95% HR_{max} may be used for individuals with higher initial fitness levels. Ideally, HR_{max} is determined from a multistaged exercise test. As previously discussed, when HR_{max} is estimated by the formula 220 − age, significant error may be introduced. Therefore, it is recommended that the revised formula[68] be used:

$$HR_{max} = 208 - 0.7 \times \text{age}.$$

Heart rate reserve method—A second method involves the use of the HRR method, also known as the Karvonen method. The HRR is computed by subtracting the HR_{rest} from the HR_{max} to obtain HRR, then 60% and 80% of the HRR is computed and added to HR_{rest}. Sixty to eighty percent of HRR approximates 50% to 85% of $\dot{V}o_{2peak}$ in most fit individuals but more closely corresponds to 60% to 80% of $\dot{V}o_2R$.

$$\text{Target heart rate range} = HR_{rest} + ([HR_{max} - 0.50\, HR_{rest}] \times 0.50 \text{ and } 0.85)$$

Sixty percent of HRR provides an adequate stimulus for improvement of cardiorespiratory fitness in most individuals and tends to yield a higher training target HR than that obtained from the straight percentage of HR_{max}.

Rating of perceived exertion—The Borg RPE scales provide important information about how the participant feels or perceives the intensity of the work performed (see Chapter 10). Although considered a more subjective method of rating exercise intensity, the RPE is highly correlated to HR and $\dot{V}o_2$ in adult subjects across a variety of modes of exercise. This method provides a valuable alternative for self-monitoring in patients and clients who cannot palpate their own pulse. Using the original category Borg scale, a range of 12 (somewhat hard) to 16 (hard) corresponds to a training window intensity necessary for physiological adaptations to exercise training.

Intensity summary—Table 3-11 summarizes the corresponding intensities using three of the methods described. The intensity calculated for a given prescription must be developed in conjunction with the other components of exercise prescriptions (ie, duration, frequency). Time constraints and the individual's goals must also be considered. If the initial goal is weight reduction, lower-intensity exercise programs performed for a longer duration result in greater kilocalorie reduction.

TABLE 3-11   Classification of Physical Activity Intensity

Intensity	Relative Intensity		
	% HR_{max}	% HRR	RPE
Very light	<35	<20	<10
Light	35–54	20–39	10–11
Moderate	55–69	40–59	12–13
Hard	70–89	60–84	14–16
Very hard	≥90	≥85	17–19
Maximal	100	100	20

On the basis of physical activity lasting up to 60 minutes. RPE based on Borg 6–20 scale.

Data from Pollock ML, Wenger NK. Physical activity and exercise training in the elderly. A position paper from the Society of Geriatric Cardiology. *Am J Geriatr Cardiol.* 1998;7(4):45-46.

Frequency

The frequency refers to the number of times per week that an individual exercises. Because the incidence of lower-extremity injuries appears to increase with higher frequencies, the ACSM recommends an exercise frequency of 3 to 5 d/wk.[83] In most individuals, two sessions per week does not typically evoke cardiovascular changes and is more likely to maintain current levels of cardiorespiratory fitness. Deconditioned individuals, however, may improve their cardiorespiratory fitness with only two workouts per week. For individuals exercising at 60% to 80% of HRR or 70% to 85% of HR_{max}, an exercise frequency of 3 d/wk is sufficient to improve or maintain $\dot{V}O_{2peak}$. In addition, activities involving other muscle groups involved in different types of activities may occur on the off days and may consist of resistance training or recreational activities. It should be noted that lower-intensity exercise prescribed for weight loss and improved fitness goals may require 6 to 7 d/wk in order to achieve the caloric expenditure that is desired.

Duration

Duration refers to the length of time spent exercising in the training window. The optimal duration depends on the intensity, frequency, and fitness level of the individual. In general, the greater the intensity, the shorter the duration needed for adaptation and vice versa. As described previously, 20- to 30-minute durations are optimal for an intensity of approximately 70% HR_{max}. However, lower-intensity exercise may result in benefits if performed for up to 45 minutes. More frequent shorter durations (eg, completing multiple 5-minute daily bouts of exercise) may be effective in some deconditioned patients. More than 45-minute durations may increase the risk of musculoskeletal complications. Table 3-12 summarizes the dynamic interplay between intensity, frequency, and duration.

Mode

The mode refers to the exercise device or activity selected to improve cardiorespiratory fitness. The best cardiovascular training activities involve the use of large muscle groups activated in a rhythmic nature for prolonged periods. Treadmills, cycle ergometers, and rowing machines are examples of popular training modalities. Additionally, walking, jogging, swimming, and cross-country skiing exemplify outdoor activities that also improve fitness. For novice exercisers, selecting a mode that requires minimal skill and can be performed at a constant intensity with minimal interindividual variation in energy expenditure is recommended. Later, activities that require more skill may be added.

The use of multiple modalities arranged in a sequence has gained recent popularity. This "circuit training" approach is designed to engage multiple muscle groups of both the upper and lower extremities, and usually includes resistance training. The participant moves from one device to the other (eg, bike, treadmill, weight machine), as quickly as possible, typically performing 1 set of 10 repetitions on each device. The goal is to maintain an elevated HR throughout the circuit, thus evoking an aerobic endurance training effect as well as a muscle strength training effect. The efficacy of these training programs has not been well substantiated. Box 3-6 groups modalities and activities appropriate to their skill level and appropriateness.

ENVIRONMENTAL CONSIDERATIONS

A variety of environmental influences can affect the acute response and long-term adaptation of the cardiorespiratory system to exercise. The physiological stress of physical exertion

TABLE 3-12   The FIT Formula for Physical Activity— Threshold for Benefits and Target Zone for Optimal Activity Levels

	Threshold of Training	Target Zone
Frequency	Most days of the week	All, or most, days of the week
Intensity	Equivalent to normal walking	Normal to brisk walking
	Approximately 150 calories accumulated	150 to 300 calories accumulated
	500 to 1000 calories per week	500 to 2000 calories expended per week
Time (duration)	30 min or three 10-minute sessions	Approximately 30 to 60 min[a]

[a]Length of time depends on activity intensity.

BOX 3-6

Grouping of Cardiorespiratory Endurance Activities

Group 1   Activities that can be readily maintained at a constant intensity and interindividual variation in energy expenditure is relatively low. Desirable for early stages of a rehabilitation program when precise control of exercise intensity is desired.
Examples: cycling, treadmill walking.

Group 2   Activities in which the rate of energy expenditure is highly related to skill, but can provide a constant intensity for a given individual.
Examples: cross-country skiing, swimming.

Group 3   Activities where both skill and intensity of exercise are highly variable. These activities must be used cautiously and competitive factors minimized for high-risk, low-fit, and/or symptomatic individuals.
Examples: basketball, tennis, and racquetball.

Adapted from American College of Sports Medicine. *ACSM's Guidelines for Exercise Testing and Prescription.* 7th ed. Philadelphia, PA: Lippincott Williams & Wilkins; 2006.

is often complicated by environmental conditions such as extreme temperatures, altitude, and pollutants. An understanding of the interrelationships between the environment and the body at exercise is essential for the physical therapist involved in wellness programs.

Extreme Temperatures: Heat and Cold
Thermoregulation
The human body maintains a limited core temperature range of 36.1°C to 37.8°C or 97.0°F to 100.0°F under healthy conditions. Body temperature is maintained with slight deviation by the thermoregulatory center of the hypothalamus. A fine balance exists between heat gain and heat loss within the body. This balance is affected by the individual's metabolic rate, environmental conditions, and clothing. Physical exertion in extremes of heat and cold can place a heavy burden on thermoregulatory mechanisms, leading to impaired performance, temperature-related illnesses, and injury.

Heat
Energy metabolism generates the majority of internal heat gain. With exercise, there is an increase in metabolic rate, and thus an increase in the rate of internal heat generation. During locomotion 25% of metabolic energy expenditure is translated to mechanical work, while 75% is released as heat in contracting muscles.[104] *Radiation* from the sun or hot surfaces can increase heat stress through *conduction* when a hot object comes in contact with the skin, or when internally generated heat contacts adjacent tissues. Heat is also transferred by the motion of hot air or water through *convection*. The contribution of radiation and convection to overall heat gain or loss is slight, averaging 10% to 20%. See Box 3-7.

BOX 3-7

Factors Affecting Body's Mechanisms for Heat Balance and Environmental Stressors

- Air temperature and humidity
- Thermal radiation from the ground
- Metabolic heat production
- Conduction
- Convection
- Sweat evaporation
- Radiation
- Sky thermal radiation
- Respiratory evaporation
- Blood flow to the skin
- Solar radiation
- Reflected solar radiation

The complex interaction between environmental conditions and the athlete.

Data from Wilmore JK, Costill DL. *Physiology of Sport and Exercise*. 2nd ed. Human Kinetics; 1994.

During exercise, as the temperature of working muscle increases, the peripheral vascular system transports heat to central organs, raising the athlete's core temperature. In response, cardiac output increases and blood is shunted from central organs to transport heat to the skin. Water secreted onto the skin through sweat glands absorbs this heat, vaporizing the liquid. This evaporative cooling accounts for a significant amount of heat loss from the body. Despite the fact that small amounts of sweat can dissipate large amounts of heat, this mechanism usually cannot offset heat gain sufficiently to maintain core temperature.

Sweat evaporation is limited by several factors including the rate of sweat production and dehydration during prolonged activity. Sweat production is physiologically limited by the individual's state of *acclimation*, aerobic fitness level, and genetics.[105] Acclimation is a physiological adaptation that occurs with repeated exposure to heat stress during exercise. Acclimation allows an individual to produce higher volumes of sweat in a shorter period of time, while conserving sodium. This physiological adaptation results in less cardiovascular strain and a lower core temperature for a given heat stress.[106] The benefits of acclimation are evident within days of exposure, but lost upon prolonged removal of heat stress during exercise. It should be noted that 1 in 20 individuals are heat intolerant and unable to acclimate to heat stress.[107]

Sweat evaporation can also be limited by the condition of the ambient air and by clothing. The evaporative rate is dependent upon the differential between water vapor pressure on the skin and in the air. On a humid day, the water vapor pressure in the air is high, reducing the pressure gradient and decreasing evaporation rates. Air movement of 4 to 6 mph facilitates maximum evaporative cooling by convection, while lower speeds can hinder the process. Clothing can interfere with evaporation by absorbing sweat and blocking vaporization. Clothing best suited to facilitate evaporation should be a loose-fitting, lightweight fabric with an open weave, and cover the least amount of surface area. When the physiological responses to heat exposure are insufficient to balance heat gain, heat-related disorders can occur. The most common heat-related disorders encountered include heat cramps, heat syncope, dehydration, heat exhaustion, and heat stroke. See Table 3-13 for a description of the signs, symptoms, and first aid related to these disorders.

Cold
Cold stress is described as an imbalance between heat gained from metabolism and clothing, and heat loss from environmental factors through convection, radiation, evaporation, and conduction.[108] Heat is primarily lost by convection, at an increasing rate with accelerated winds or rapid motion through the air. The *windchill factor* takes this phenomenon into account, assessing the equivalent temperature for a given wind speed and thermometer reading. Individuals with low body fat and high surface area-to-mass ratios (eg, children) experience more rapid heat dissipation. Heat is

TABLE 3-13   Heat-Related Disorders, Including Symptoms, Signs, and First Aid

Disorder	Symptoms	Signs	First Aid
Heat cramps	Painful muscle cramps, especially in abdominal or fatigued muscles	Incapacitating pain in voluntary muscles	Rest in cool environment Drink salted water Massage muscles
Heat syncope	Blurred vision (gray out) Fainting (brief)	Brief fainting or near fainting Normal temperature	Lie on back in cool environment Drink water
Dehydration	No early symptoms Fatigue, weakness Dry mouth	Loss of work capacity Increased response time	Fluid and salt replacement
Heat exhaustion	Fatigue Weakness Blurred vision Dizziness, headache	High pulse rate Profuse sweating Low blood pressure Insecure gait Pale face Collapse Body temperature normal to slightly increased	Lie flat on back in cool environment Drink water Loosen clothing
Heat stroke	Chills Restlessness Irritability	Red face Euphoria Shivering Disorientation Erratic behavior Collapse Unconsciousness Convulsions Body temperature >40°C (104°F)	Immediate, aggressive, effective cooling Transport to the hospital

Data from the ACSM.

also lost through the evaporation of sweat as it soaks through clothing. Proper insulation from clothing is essential to maintain thermal balance. The physiological response to cold exposure includes peripheral vasoconstriction and contraction of inactive skeletal muscle to insulate the body, thereby conserving heat. As previously discussed, during exercise there is an increase in metabolic rate and thus an increase in the rate of internal heat generation. This metabolic heat assists in maintaining core temperature in cold environments. However, if the intensity of exercise decreases as a result of fatigue or cyclic bouts of exercise, metabolic heat declines and cold-related disorders such as hypothermia and tissue damage can ensue. See Table 3-14 for a description of the signs, symptoms, and first aid related to these disorders.

CLINICAL CORRELATE

The body is placed under considerable strain when asked to meet the thermoregulatory demands of physical exertion in extremes of heat and cold. Despite the acute and long-term physiologic adaptations to exercise in the heat, factors such as high humidity and dehydration prevent the dissipation of body heat, placing the athlete at substantial risk of heat-related illness. Exertion in cold weather should be maintained at a relatively steady workload, as sweat evaporation during cyclic bouts of exercise can lead to increased risk of hypothermia. Control of heat balance is best accomplished through prevention and management of risk factors.

High Altitude

Barometric pressure decreases at altitudes above sea level, creating a hypobaric environment with decreased partial pressure of oxygen (PO_2) in the inspired air (Table 3-15). With this decline in PO_2, there is a concomitant decrease in arterial oxygen saturation and availability of oxygen for transport to tissues throughout the body. The resulting hypoxia (oxygen deficiency) acutely triggers several compensatory mechanisms to increase oxygen availability, ultimately resulting in acclimation with prolonged exposure.

The primary physiological compensatory response with acute exposure to hypobaric conditions above 1,200 m is hyperventilation. In response to sudden hypoxia, chemoreceptors in arterial blood vessels signal the brain to increase pulmonary ventilation. Acutely, this is accomplished by increasing tidal volume, but with prolonged exposure and at very high altitudes, an increase in respiratory rate occurs as well. Hyperventilation causes high amounts of carbon dioxide to diffuse from circulating blood into the lungs for expiration. This increased carbon dioxide clearance can increase pH, causing respiratory

TABLE 3-14   Cold-Related Disorders, Including Symptoms, Signs, and First Aid

Disorder	Symptoms	Signs	First Aid
Hypothermia	Chills Fatigue or drowsiness Pain in the extremities	Euphoria Slurred speech Slow, weak pulse Shivering Collapse or unconsciousness Body core temperature ≤35°C (95°F)	Move to warm area and remove wet clothing Modest external warming Drink warm carbohydrate-containing fluids Transport to the hospital
Frostbite	Burning sensation at first Coldness, numbness, tingling	Skin color white or grayish yellow to reddish violet to black Blisters Response to touch depends on depth of freezing	Move to warm area and remove wet clothing External warming (eg, warm water) Drink warm carbohydrate-containing fluids if conscious Treat as a burn; do not rub affected area Transport to the hospital
Frost nip	Possible itching or pain	Skin turns white	Similar to that for frostbite
Trench foot	Severe pain Tingling, itching	Edema Blisters Response to touch depends on depth of cooling	Similar to that for frostbite

Data from the ACSM.

alkalosis. This physiological response further increases arterial oxygen saturation. Additionally, the cardiorespiratory system acutely responds by increasing HR to create a small increase in cardiac output. Despite these acute compensatory responses both at rest and during exercise, the overall arterial oxygen saturation remains diminished, the magnitude of which is directly dependent upon altitude and exercise intensity as depicted in Fig. 3-15. There is a steady decrease in maximal oxygen uptake of 10% per 1,000 m altitude above 1,500 m.[109] While arterial PO_2 is lessened, the PO_2 in muscle tissue remains constant, reducing the diffusion pressure gradient of oxygen into the tissue by approximately 70%. The oxygen demand for a given submaximal workload remains constant, regardless of changes in altitude. This disparity in oxygen uptake and the oxygen demand required to fuel exertion results in a higher relative exercise intensity for any given workload.[106] Because of the increased demand on the cardiorespiratory system, physical performance declines proportionately with the duration of the activity, greatly affecting the endurance athlete.[110]

TABLE 3-15   Barometric Pressure for a Standard Atmosphere and Inspired Partial Oxygen Pressure

Altitude (m)	Barometric Pressure (mm Hg)	Inspired Oxygen Pressure (mm Hg)
0	760	149
1500	627	123
2000	596	115
2500	627	107
3000	522	100

Data from the ACSM.

Over time, the human body acclimates to hypobaric conditions. The resting ventilatory rate stabilizes at 40% above sea-level values (at 3,000 m) within 3 to 4 days.[105] Pulmonary ventilation takes longer to stabilize during exercise, reaching up to 100% above sea-level norms.[105] Within the first weeks at an altitude, plasma volume progressively decreases, resulting in increased hematocrit and increased oxygen transport. Red blood cell production is augmented, increasing total blood volume and blood viscosity. This leads to reduced stroke volume and cardiac output at rest and with exercise, after

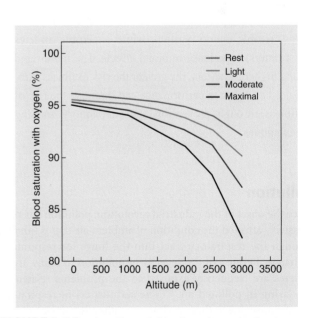

FIGURE 3-15   The effect of altitude and exercise levels on arterial oxygen saturation. Adapted from the American College of Sports Medicine. (Adapted from *ACSM's Resource Manual for Guidelines for Exercise Testing and Prescription.* 5th ed. Philadelphia, PA: Lippincott Williams & Wilkins; 2006.)

2 weeks of altitude exposure. Skeletal muscle changes include increased mitochondria, myoglobin concentration, and capillary density to improve peripheral oxygen uptake. These adaptations allow the individual to compensate for the decreased Po_2 experienced at moderate altitude after 2 to 3 weeks of exposure and are reversed after one month at seal level. For this reason, some athletes and coaches are proponents of altitude training and training in hypobaric chambers to enhance performance prior to an event.

As discussed above, the human body is placed under extreme challenge when asked to perform at high altitude and can easily fall subject to one of the several illnesses. These illnesses include acute mountain sickness, high-altitude pulmonary edema, and high-altitude cerebral edema, the symptoms of which range in severity. Mild symptoms can vary from headache, nausea, vomiting, decreased appetite, and sleep disturbances, while more serious cases experience fatigue, chest pain, dyspnea, tachycardia, and ataxia. These illnesses can best be avoided by adjusting the amount and rate of ascent, engaging in altitude training regimes, and gradually increasing the training workload. Other preventive measures include hydrating adequately, eating a high-carbohydrate diet, and taking supplemental vitamin C, E, and iron a few weeks before and after ascent.

CLINICAL CORRELATE

Unacclimated skiers, mountain climbers, cyclists, and runners who ascend to high altitudes can experience impaired physical performance and illnesses of varying severity. Endurance athletes are most significantly affected by hypobaric conditions due to their reliance on the aerobic energy system, while anaerobic athletes (sprinters) experience minimal effects. The more rapid and higher the ascent, the greater the risk of illness. Athletes can enhance performance and diminish the risk of illness through prevention and preparatory training techniques.

Pollution

Since the onset of the industrial revolution, pollution has progressively affected the condition of ambient air that is inhaled through the respiratory tract into the lungs for respiratory exchange. Because of the severity of pollution in many areas, athletes are frequently exposed to the problems related to exercising in polluted air.[106] The seriousness of respiratory compromise due to these pollutants is directly correlated with the pollutant concentration, exposure time, air temperature, humidity, and route of inspiration. The mucous membranes of the nose are an effective barrier to large particles and highly soluble gases, while allowing small particles and less soluble

gases to reach deeper airways and lung tissue. Mouth breathing during exercise provides less air filtration, allowing more pollutants to pass through the lungs to blood and ultimately body tissues. As these pollutants make their way through the body, they can reduce alveolar diffusion capacity, reduce oxygen transport capacity, and cause irritation of the airways, which may lead to bronchoconstriction.[106]

Industry and population density are directly related to pollution severity due to the emission of cardiac output, sulfur and nitrogen oxides, hydrocarbons, and particles from gas-powered equipment and automobiles. Exercising in high traffic areas can expose the athlete to high cardiac output levels, which have been found to interfere with oxygen transport and availability from hemoglobin. While no significant effect has been demonstrated on healthy individuals exercising at moderate intensities, exercise time and $\dot{V}o_{2peak}$ are inversely related to cardiac output concentration during high-intensity exercise. Cardiac patients exposed to high levels of cardiac output may be at risk of complications such as arrhythmias and early onset of angina during submaximal exercise.[106] Primary pollutants may interact with each other to magnify their effect and are compounded by temperature and humidity. The combination of high temperature and humidity can contribute to smog phenomena associated with high ozone (O_3) levels. Symptoms related to O_3 exposure include throat irritation, cough, nausea, shallow breath, headaches, and chest pain, and are predominant in asthmatic patients. In lower temperatures, pollutants emitted from increased fuel consumption for heating combined with high humidity can create fog high in sulfuric acid (acid rain) and sulfates. Sulfur oxides can irritate the upper respiratory system, causing reflex bronchoconstriction and airway impedance. Nasal mucosa can effectively remove most of sulfur oxides, when nose breathing is used. Athletes are at risk due to the common use of mouth breathing techniques as well as asthma patients with sensitive airways. Particles emitted into the air usually consist of aerosols, soot, dust, and smoke, which are associated with bronchoconstriction when inhaled. Here again, mouth breathing during exercise increases pollutant exposure.

The U.S. Environmental Protection Agency (EPA) has established national air quality standards to protect against harmful health effects and is responsible for informing and alerting the general population about air quality.[106] The EPA uses the *air quality index (AQI)* as a guideline for five primary pollutants: ground-level O_3, particulate matter, carbon monoxide, sulfur dioxide, and nitrogen dioxide. The AQI converts pollutant concentrations in the ambient air to a value rated from 0 to 500. Under the Clean Air Act, an AQI value greater than 100 indicates air pollution in an unhealthy range. Prior to engaging in outdoor activity, individuals can access local AQI ratings to prevent unsafe exercise participation by following the EPA's health advisory statement. An example of how the AQI is used to advise individuals on how to best protect themselves from pollutant exposure to O_3 is found in Box 3-8. The AQI can be easily accessed on the Web site at http://airnow.gov/index.cfm?action=airnow.currentconditions.

BOX 3-8

Air Quality Guide for Ozone

Air Quality Index	Protect Your Health
Good (0–50)	No health impacts are expected when air quality is in this range.
Moderate (51–100)	Unusually sensitive people should consider limiting prolonged exposure.
Unhealthy for sensitive groups (101–150)	The following groups should limit prolonged outdoor exertion: People with lung disease, such as asthma Children and older adults People who are active outdoors
Unhealthy (151–200)	The following groups should avoid prolonged outdoor exertion: People with lung disease, such as asthma Children and older adults People who are active outdoors Everyone else should limit prolonged outdoor exertion.
Very unhealthy (201–300)	The following groups should avoid all outdoor exertion: People with lung disease, such as asthma Children and older adults People who are active outdoors Everyone else should limit outdoor exertion.

AIRNow. Air Quality Conditions and Forecasts. http://airnow.gov/index.cfm?action= static.consumer. Accessed July 26, 2008.

CLINICAL CORRELATE

The environmental effects of pollution can affect the body's cardiorespiratory response to the physical demands of exercise. The best means for minimizing the effects of outdoor pollutants is avoidance of exposure. Limiting exercise in areas of high traffic and industry can limit cardiac output exposure, preventing undue cardiac stresses. Avoidance of exercise during conditions of high humidity with associated fog is especially important for asthmatic patients, athletes, and those with respiratory tract sensitivities. Information regarding local air pollution and current health advisories can be obtained by consulting the EPA at http://www.epa.gov.

THE EXERCISE SESSION

There are three components to the exercise session: a warm-up phase, an endurance phase, and a cool-down phase.

Warm-up Phase

The warm-up should be gradual and of sufficient intensity to increase muscle and core temperature without causing fatigue. It may consist of 5 to 10 minutes of low-intensity calisthenics and stretching, utilizing the major muscle groups, and include 5 to 10 minutes of the endurance activity performed at a low intensity and progressed to the lower limit of the training window. For example, if jogging is the endurance activity, a slow walk progressing to a brisk walk can be used to gradually increase HR.

Most of the perceived benefits of a warm-up are well documented. Benefits include gradual increases in muscle temperature and peripheral blood flow, energy metabolism (enhanced lipid catabolism and decrease in carbohydrate metabolism), and increased tissue elasticity. The warm-up has been shown to improve neuromuscular function (enhanced function of the CNS and neuromuscular recruitment of motor units), maintain acid–base balance, and reduce the oxygen deficit during more vigorous exercise. Among the unsubstantiated benefits of the warm-up is the reduced risk of musculoskeletal injuries.

Endurance Phase

The endurance phase provides the stimulus designed to develop cardiorespiratory fitness. The endurance phase maintains the HR or other marker of exercise intensity in the training window. This phase may last between 20 and 60 minutes. As previously described, the duration of this phase depends on the intensity of the exercise. For example, a duration of 20 minutes at a high intensity is generally perceived as vigorous exercise, whereas moderate-intensity programs may last 30 minutes or more. This phase may incorporate treadmill work, cycle ergometer work, recreational games or activities, resistance training, or several of the previously cited exercises. The endurance phase may consist of continuous or discontinuous (interval) activities, where periods of exercise alternate with periods of rest. A sample walking program using continuous training and a walk/jog program incorporating interval training are provided in Tables 3-16 and 3-17, respectively.

Cool-down Phase

The cool-down phase provides a gradual recovery from the endurance phase and allows elevated metabolic processes to return to baseline slowly. This phase should consist of exercise of diminishing intensity (ie, slower walking), calisthenics, or stretches, called an active cool-down. Some clinicians have advocated the inclusion of yoga, t'ai chi, and relaxation training

TABLE 3-16 **Sample Aerobic Walking Program**

Week (min)	Warm-up	Target Zone	Cool-down	Total Time
1	Walk slowly 5 min	Walk briskly 5 min	Walk slowly 5 min	15 min
2	Walk slowly 5 min	Walk briskly 7 min	Walk slowly 5 min	17 min
3	Walk slowly 5 min	Walk briskly 9 min	Walk slowly 5 min	19 min
4	Walk slowly 5 min	Walk briskly 11 min	Walk slowly 5 min	21 min
5	Walk slowly 5 min	Walk briskly 13 min	Walk slowly 5 min	23 min
6	Walk slowly 5 min	Walk briskly 15 min	Walk slowly 5 min	25 min
7	Walk slowly 5 min	Walk briskly 18 min	Walk slowly 5 min	28 min
8	Walk slowly 5 min	Walk briskly 20 min	Walk slowly 5 min	30 min
9	Walk slowly 5 min	Walk briskly 23 min	Walk slowly 5 min	33 min
10	Walk slowly 5 min	Walk briskly 26 min	Walk slowly 5 min	36 min
11	Walk slowly 5 min	Walk briskly 28 min	Walk slowly 5 min	38 min
12	Walk slowly 5 min	Walk briskly 30 min	Walk slowly 5 min	40 min

Note: This program should include at least 3 exercise sessions per week. From week 13 onward, check your pulse periodically to ensure that you are exercising within your target heart rate range. As you become more fit, walk faster to increase your heart rate toward the upper levels of your target range.

U.S. Department of Health and Human Services.

into the cool-down phase. Further evidence is needed to document the effectiveness of these approaches. Typically cool-down periods last from 5 to 10 minutes.

Active cool-down enhances venous return, prevents blood from pooling in the extremities, and permits circulatory adjustments following training. Other important benefits include prevention of postexercise hypotension and dizziness. The cool-down phase also promotes a more rapid removal of lactic acid and facilitates heat dissipation. An important benefit of cool-down in patients with heart disease is the reduced likelihood of threatening ventricular dysrhythmias and reduced sudden cardiac death.

FITNESS AND WELLNESS

In past years, the majority of fitness enthusiasts participated in traditional forms of muscular resistance training programs, aerobic activities such as jogging, and team or individual sports. Today, there exists a tremendous market geared toward attracting and retaining individuals of all fitness levels in the group class environment. These group classes are varied in difficulty, spanning a diverse range of physical demands and styles. Physical therapists involved in tailoring wellness programs have an obligation to their patients to attain a basic understanding of the components and physical demands of an exercise style prior to recommending its use. While the wide genre of classes is far too expansive to cover in this section, we will attempt to highlight the most popular fitness (aerobics and spinning) and wellness (yoga, t'ai chi, and pilates) activities.

Fitness Classes
Aerobics

Mixed-impact aerobic classes are choreographed to music approximately 130 to 150 bpm, incorporating variations of high-impact and low-impact aerobic movements to provide a full body workout. High-impact movements place greater mechanical loading stresses on the lower extremity and spine, and typically include jumping, hopping, and lunging moves. Low-impact movements, such as turns, steps, and kicks, minimize physical stresses. The benefit of mixed-impact aerobic class is that it provides both a musculoskeletal and cardiovascular challenge that can be easily modified to suit the fitness level of participants. Intensity levels can be modified by altering the speed and range of motion of the movement, altering the arm component of the move, varying the amount of traveling distance completed, and adjusting the vertical height involved.[106] A review of the literature revealed a large difference in the energy expenditure between low-impact (4–5 kcal/min) and high-impact (10–11 kcal/min) aerobic movements.[111] These mixed-impact aerobic classes can include variations such as cardio-dance and kick-boxing.

Step training is a very popular fitness class that also challenges the cardiorespiratory system, while providing a strong musculoskeletal stimulus as well. While described as a low-impact aerobic exercise program, it has been the experience of this author that intensities vary significantly based upon the instructor and fitness level of the participants. Classes are structured with a cadence averaging 120 to 130 bpm, but speeds vary. Step benches range from 4 to 12 in. in height and can easily be adjusted with risers. Novices are encouraged to initiate training at the lowest level to maintain a low-impact aerobic workout while isolating each movement with precision. Once the

TABLE 3-17 Sample Aerobic Jogging Program with Interval Training

Week	Warm-up	Target Zone Exercise	Cool-down	Total Time
1	Stretching 5 min	Walk (nonstop) 10 min	Walk slowly 3 min; stretch 2 min	20 min
2	Stretching 5 min	Walk 5 min; jog 1 min; walk 5 min; jog 1 min	Walk slowly 3 min; stretch 2 min	22 min
3	Stretching 5 min	Walk 5 min; jog 3 min; walk 5 min; jog 3 min	Walk slowly 3 min; stretch 2 min	26 min
4	Stretching 5 min	Walk 5 min; jog 4 min; walk 5 min; jog 4 min	Walk slowly 3 min; stretch 2 min	28 min
5	Stretching 5 min	Walk 4 min; jog 5 min; walk 4 min; jog 5 min	Walk slowly 3 min; stretch 2 min	28 min
6	Stretching 5 min	Walk 4 min; jog 6 min; walk 4 min; jog 6 min	Walk slowly 3 min; stretch 2 min	30 min
7	Stretching 5 min	Walk 4 min; jog 7 min; walk 4 min; jog 7 min	Walk slowly 3 min; stretch 2 min	32 min
8	Stretching 5 min	Walk 4 min; jog 8 min; walk 4 min; jog 8 min	Walk slowly 3 min; stretch 2 min	34 min
9	Stretching 5 min	Walk 4 min; jog 9 min; walk 4 min; jog 9 min	Walk slowly 3 min; stretch 2 min	36 min
10	Stretching 5 min	Walk 4 min; jog 13 min	Walk slowly 3 min; stretch 2 min	27 min
11	Stretching 5 min	Walk 4 min; jog 15 min	Walk slowly 3 min; stretch 2 min	29 min
12	Stretching 5 min	Walk 4 min; jog 17 min	Walk slowly 3 min; stretch 2 min	31 min
13	Stretching 5 min	Walk 2 min; jog slowly 2 min; jog 17 min	Walk slowly 3 min; stretch 2 min	31 min
14	Stretching 5 min	Walk 1 min; jog slowly 3 min; jog 17 minute	Walk slowly 3 min; stretch 2 min	31 min
15	Stretching 5 min	Jog slowly 3 min; jog 17 min	Walk slowly 3 min; stretch 2 min	30 min

U.S. Department of Health and Human Services.

stepping moves have been mastered, research strongly indicates that increasing bench height is the preferential method to increase aerobic intensity.[106] Way too often, overzealous steppers will incorporate high-impact bounding of the step in place of good technique. This high-impact loading poses a tremendous mechanical stress to the lower extremities, predisposing the individual to overuse injuries. Similar classes are formatted with the substitution of a BOSU balance trainer in place of the traditional step bench. The BOSU[112] is an air-filled dome with a 26-in. diameter platform, which provides a dynamic surface to challenge stepping and balancing maneuvers.

Spinning

Spinning classes have gained widespread popularity in fitness environments. Unlike other fitness and wellness activities offered in a group format, spinning is a non–weight-bearing activity that provides a challenging cardiovascular experience for the fitness enthusiast. Guided by visual imagery, cyclists are led through a virtual outdoor tour, complete with valleys, hills, straightaways, and finish lines.[113] While there is no established cadence for these aerobic classes, intensity is varied by musical tempo and commands given by the instructor. These classes appeal to cyclists of all experience levels because

students can easily control their workout intensity by adjusting their pedaling speed, wheel resistance, and body position (seated vs standing) while cycling with the group.[114]

Wellness Classes
Yoga

Developed in India more than 5,000 years ago, *yoga* is derived from a Sanskrit term meaning "to unite," as in uniting the body, mind, and spirit.[115] Yoga can be described as both a physical and psychological discipline, its complete practice consisting of an enormous body of precepts, attitudes, techniques, and spiritual values.[116] Yoga practice in Western society is predominantly focused on Hatha yoga, which encompasses many different styles. Hatha yoga forms consist of a series of *asanas* (exercises) done with specific breathing patterns and mindfulness to achieve each posture. Yoga practice is believed to produce numerous benefits including increased strength and mobility, improved posture and balance, enhanced lymphatic flow, and a relaxation response, which affects neural, cardiovascular, and respiratory systems.

The most commonly practiced forms of Hatha yoga include Iyengar, Ashtanga, Bikram, Vinyasa, and Kundalini.

Iyengar yoga is firmly based on traditional yoga doctrine, emphasizing the development of strength, stamina, flexibility, and balance, as well as concentration and meditation. It is characterized by fluid movements with great attention to detail and precise focus on body alignment. Iyengar yoga emphasizes standing postures and is known for its use of props, such as belts, blocks, blankets, and pillows to aid novices and those with physical limitations in performing asanas. Ashtanga yoga is a progressive sequence of poses performed at a rapid pace to generate intense, internal heat and profuse sweat. This heat-building process is intended to detoxify muscles and organs, improve circulation, and create a fit, strong body, with a calm mind. This athletic style of yoga is commonly referred to as "power" yoga and provides a rigorous workout for participants. Bikram, also referred to as "hot" yoga, is composed of a series of 26 poses executed in a room heated to 95°F to 100°F. Through contraction and extension of the body, these asanas are intended to address every bodily system including the digestive, respiratory, circulatory, immune, endocrine, lymphatic, skeletal, muscular, and nervous systems. Because of the heated environment, Bikram yoga challenges the cardiorespiratory system while affording the musculoskeletal system great extensibility. Vinyasa yoga is a flowing series of traditional yoga postures that is intended to warm and energize the body through an aerobic effect. The purpose of Vinyasa is to purify the body through increased circulation and sweating while improving flexibility.

Kundalini yoga is a physical and meditative style that focuses on psychospiritual growth and the body's potential for maturation to create a communication between "mind" and "body." Kundalini yoga gives special consideration to the role of the spine and endocrine system while concentrating on *chakras* (psychic centers) in the body in order to generate a spiritual power, which is known as kundalini energy. Kundalini is considered the *prana* (potential life force) lying dormant in our bodies, which can be awaked by spiritual discipline. The practice of Kundalini yoga consists of a number of bodily postures, expressive movements and utterances, breathing patterns, and concentration. The wide scope of yoga practice provides the opportunity to pursue experiences ranging from a low-intensity, relaxing state to a high-intensity athletic workout.

CLINICAL CORRELATE

When recommending yoga practice for patients in rehabilitation and wellness programs, the astute physical therapist should be aware of the physical demands associated with different forms of yoga. For instance, a healthy athlete looking for an aerobic program might best be served by the Ashtanga style, while Kundalini yoga would better suit the needs of a debilitated patient with chronic pain.

While there is limited outcome-based research on yoga as it directly applies to cardiopulmonary rehabilitation, sufficient evidence exists to support the exploration of yoga in both therapeutic and wellness environments, for patients across the lifespan. Yoga has been found to improve vital capacity of the lungs in college students,[117] while demonstrating decreased resting HR, increased $\dot{V}O_{2peak}$, and parasympathetic baroreflex sensitivity in the elderly.[118] Tandon demonstrated that yoga practice with COPD patients resulted in significantly greater gains in mean maximum work and decreased symptoms, when compared with traditional physical therapy treatment.[119] It has also been well documented that yoga has a positive impact on pulmonary and autonomic function in patients with asthma.[115] Research has demonstrated the benefit of yoga for musculoskeletal conditions, pain management, wound healing, balance, and fall prevention.

T'ai Chi

T'ai chi is an ancient martial art developed in China in the 12th century A.D. As with many alternative practices, it is considered a way of life that integrates the mind, body, and spirit. T'ai chi practice seeks to bring the forces of *yin* (negative energy) and *yang* (positive energy) into balance, allowing the individual to achieve optimal health and prevention of disease. Meditation, mental concentration, breathing, and slow, graceful movements are used to transmit *chi* (vital energy) throughout the body. While it is considered a martial art, it is important to make the distinction that t'ai chi utilizes flexibility and mental concentration over strength to beat an opponent. Movement of the trunk and limbs is coordinated with breathing and mental concentration to move chi through distinct channels in the body. The t'ai chi form includes arm raising and lowering along with weight shifts from one leg to another, steps, and rotation of the torso in combinations and sequences. These controlled, nonimpact movements displace the individual's center of gravity, making it extremely beneficial for the older population.[115]

Numerous sources have documented the effectiveness of t'ai chi exercise in improving balance and preventing falls with older individuals. T'ai chi has been found to have a measurable physiological effect on cardiorespiratory function, mental control, immune capacity, and fall prevention because of improvements in muscle strength, flexibility, and balance.[120,121] Despite the slow, rhythmic pace of moves, t'ai chi is a moderate-intensity aerobic exercise that has been shown to improve circulatory status in elderly individuals.[122,123] Lai and colleagues[124] found that elderly t'ai chi practitioners showed a significant improvement in $\dot{V}O_2$ uptake, concluding that t'ai chi could be practiced as a means for delaying the decline in cardiorespiratory function associated with aging. In a randomized trial, Yong et al. found t'ai chi exercise routines to be comparable with moderate-intensity aerobic exercise programs in reducing blood pressure in previously sedentary, hypertensive, elderly individuals.[125] It has also been demonstrated that t'ai chi exercise enhances cardiorespiratory function and improves functional outcomes following coronary artery bypass surgery.[126] Research has demonstrated improved quality of life measures for elders and debilitated populations, leading to the inclusion of t'ai chi instruction in elder care settings and cardiac rehabilitation programs.

Pilates

Pilates training, created by Joseph H. Pilates (born in Germany, 1880–1967), has become a rapidly growing trend in the United States. Originally designed to aid wounded soldiers during World War I, pilates exercises focus on core strength, flexibility, breathing, and mental concentration to execute rhythmic movements with precision and control. Introduced to the United States in 1926, pilates exercise was firmly embraced by the performing arts community for the rehabilitation and fitness training of dancers. The original system referred to as *contrology* was described by pilates as "the science and art of coordinated body–mind–spirit development through natural movements under strict supervision of the will."[127] These original works have been interpreted by many sources worldwide, including the founders of Polestar Education (a Pilates education company specializing in rehabilitation) who describe six basic principles of pilates exercise as follows: breathing; axial elongation/core control; organization of the head, neck, and shoulders; spine articulation; alignment of the extremities and spine; and movement integration.[128] The expansive series of exercise includes both mat work and techniques performed on apparatus specifically designed to accommodate all fitness levels and ages. Despite its reputation for providing a strenuous core and full body workout, the spring-based apparatus can easily be adjusted to assist extremity motion in the early stages of rehabilitation. Pilates exercise proposes to improve strength, flexibility, alignment, and circulation in enthusiasts. Workout intensity strongly relies on the expertise of the instructor and the setting (one-to-one or group session). It should be noted that careful attention should be paid to the background of the instructor, as Pilates certification programs vary significantly in their rigor. Similar to many complementary practices, pilates lacks scientific evidence to support its efficacy.

SUMMARY

This chapter on exercise physiology for the well individual has been divided into basic exercise physiology and applied physiology. The discussion of basic exercise physiology has described the strong link between fuel substrates, metabolic pathways, and exercise states. The section on applied exercise physiology has focused on measurement of body fat, maintenance of physical fitness, principles of endurance training, and exercise prescription. An understanding of both domains will lay a proper foundation on which to evaluate abnormal exercise responses in patients with cardiovascular and pulmonary disease.

In order to administer an effective treatment session, the physical therapist must make constant and ongoing comparisons between two sets of data. On the one hand, the patient's response to an exercise regimen must be compared to that same patient's physiological data acquired during the resting state. On the other hand, patient information obtained during exercise must be compared to normative data derived from healthy normal subjects in order to determine whether the response to exercise is indeed "normal." This chapter has described the normal response to exercise. Future chapters will describe abnormal responses to exercise and link those responses to disease states and treatment regimens.

Patients receive optimal care when they are neither undertreated nor overtreated. Exercise "volume" must be sufficient to provide an overload and provoke a cardiovascular and pulmonary response, but not enough to endanger the patient's health and well-being. This chapter's sections on endurance training and exercise prescription have described a well-standardized approach that can be used to develop an effective exercise prescription and produce a training effect. Clearly, however, such a standardized approach must be adjusted to fit individuals with heart and lung disease. Future chapters will provide the reader with guidelines for the application of these principles to the management of patients with cardiovascular and pulmonary impairments and functional limitations.

Heads Up!

This chapter contains a CD-ROM activity.

REFERENCES

1. Weyer C, Snitker S, Rising R, et al. Determinants of energy expenditure and fuel utilization in man: effects of body composition, age, sex, ethnicity, and glucose tolerance in 916 subjects. *Int J Obes.* 1999;23:715-722.
2. Nieman DC, Trone GA, Austin MD. A new handheld device for measuring resting metabolic rate and oxygen consumption. *J Am Diet Assoc.* 2003;103(5):588-592.
3. Goran MI. Energy expenditure and obesity. *Med Clin North Am.* 2000;84:347-362.
4. DeLorenzo A, Tagliabue A, Andrioli A, et al. Measured and predicted resting metabolic rate in Italian males and females, aged 18–59 y. *Eur J Clin Nutr.* 2001;55:208-214.
5. Taylor RW, Gold E, Manning P, Goulding A. Gender differences in body fatness content are present well before puberty. *Int J Obes Relat Metab Disord.* 1997;21:1082-1084.
6. Klausen B, Toubro S, Astrup A. Age and sex effects on energy expenditure. *Am J Clin Nutr.* 1997;65(4):895-907.
7. Muller B, Merk S, Burgi U, et al. Calculating the basal metabolic rate and severe and morbid obesity. *Schweiz Rundsch Med Prax.* 2001;90(45)1955-1963.
8. Marra M, Polito A, DeFilippo E, et al. Are the general equations to predict BMR applicable to patients with anorexia nervosa? *Eat Weight Disord.* 2002;7(1):53-59.
9. Ravussin E et al. Determination of 24-hour energy expenditure in man. *J Clin Invest.* 1986;78:1568.
10. Altman P, Dittmer D. *Metabolism.* Bethesda, MD: Federation of American Societies for Experimental Biology; 1968.
11. Bemben M et al. Age-related patterns in body composition for men aged 20–79 yr. *Med Sci Sports Exerc.* 1995;27:264.

12. Poehlman E et al. Endurance exercise in aging humans: effects on energy metabolism. *Exerc Sport Sci Rev.* 1994;22:751.

13. Wilmore J, Behnke A. An anthropometric estimation of body density and lean body weight in young men. *J Appl Physiol.* 1969;27(1):25-31.

14. Katch F, Behnke A, Katch V. Estimation of body fat from skinfolds and surface area. *Hum Biol.* 1979;51:411-424.

15. Krauss RM, Eckel RH, Howard B; American Heart Association. American Heart Association Dietary Guidelines. Revision 2000: A Statement for Health Care Professionals from the Nutrition Committee of the American Heart Association. *Stroke.* 2000;31(11):2751-2766.

16. Kirwin J et al. A moderate glycemic meal before endurance exercise can enhance performance. *J Appl Physiol.* 1998;84:53.

17. Walton P, Rhodes E. Glycaemic index and optimal performance. *Sports Med.* 1997;33:164.

18. Aro A et al. Stearic acid, trans fatty acids, and dietary fat: effects on serum and lipoprotein lipids, apolipoproteins, lipoprotein(a), and lipid transfer proteins in healthy subjects. *Am J Clin Nutr.* 1997;65:1419.

19. ASCN/AIN Task Force on Trans Fatty Acids. Position paper on trans fatty acids. *Am J Clin Nutr.* 1996;63(5):663-670.

20. Hu F et al. Dietary fat intake and the risk of coronary heart disease in women. *N Engl J Med.* 1997;337:1491.

21. Willett W, Ascherio A. Trans fatty acids: are the effects only marginal? *Am J Public Health.* 1994;84:722.

22. National Cholesterol Education Program. *Second report of the Expert Panel on the Detection, Evaluation, and Treatment of High Blood Cholesterol in Adults (Adult Treatment Panel II).* Bethesda, MD: National Institutes of Health and National Heart, Lung, and Blood Institute; 1993. NIH publication 93-3095.

23. Gaziano J et al. Moderate alcohol intake, increased levels of high density lipoprotein and its subfractions, and decreased risk of myocardial infarction. *N Engl J Med.* 1993;329:1829.

24. Burtis C, Ashold E. *Tietz Textbook of Clinical Chemistry.* 3rd ed. Philadelphia, PA: WB Saunders; 1999.

25. Kukita H, Hiwada K, Kokubu T. Serum apolipoprotein AI, AII, and B levels and their discriminative values in relatives of patients with coronary artery disease. *Atherosclerosis.* 1984;51:261-267.

26. Maciejko J, Holmes D, Kottke B, et al. Apolipoprotein AI as a marker of angiographically assessed coronary artery disease. *N Engl J Med.* 1983;309:385-389.

27. Naito H. The association of serum lipids, lipoproteins and apolipoproteins with coronary artery disease assessed by coronary arteriography. *Ann N Y Acad Sci.* 1985;454:230-238.

28. McArdle WD, Katch FI, Katch VL. *Exercise Physiology: Energy, Nutrition, and Human Performance.* Baltimore, MD: Lippincott Williams & Wilkins; 2001:188.

29. Corbin C, Lidsey R, Welk G. *Concepts of Physical Fitness: Active Lifestyles for Wellness.* 10th ed. New York: McGraw-Hill; 2000.

30. Stein R, Michielli D, Glantz M, et al. Effects of different exercise training intensities on lipoprotein cholesterol fractions in healthy middle aged men. *Am Heart J.* 1990;119:277-282.

31. American Heart Association (AHA). An eating plan for healthy Americans. 2008. http://www.heart.org/presenter. jtml?identifier-1088. Accessed March 8, 2010. cholesterol/do_plan.html. Accessed December 21, 2009.

32. Hill J, Peters J, Reed G, et al. Nutrient balance in humans: effects of diet composition. *Am J Clin Nutr.* 1991;54:10-17.

33. Golay A, Allaz A, Morel Y, et al. Similar weight loss in low and high-carbohydrate diets. *Am J Clin Nutr.* 1996;63:174-178.

34. St Jeor S, Ashley J. Dietary Strategies: issues of diet composition. In: Fletcher G, Grundy S, Hayman L, eds. *Obesity: Impact on Cardiovascular Disease.* Armonk, NY: Futura Publishing Company Inc; 1999:233-246.

35. Harats D et al. Citrus fruit supplementation reduces lipoprotein oxidation in young men ingesting a diet high in saturated fat: presumptive evidence for an interaction between vitamins C and E in vivo. *Am J Clin Nutr.* 1998;67:240.

36. Hodis H et al. Serial coronary angiographic evidence that antioxidant vitamin intake reduces progression of coronary artery disease. *JAMA.* 1995;273:1849.

37. Landry GL. Heat injuries. In: Kliegman RM, Behrman RE, Jenson HB, Stanton BF, eds. *Nelson Textbook of Pediatrics.* 18th ed. Philadelphia, PA: WB Saunders–Elsevier; 2007:chap 6.

38. Nerbrand C, Agreus L, Lenner R, et al. The influence of calcium and magnesium in drinking water and diet on cardiovascular risk factors in individuals living in hard and soft water areas with differences in cardiovascular mortality. *BMC Public Health.* 2003;3(1):21.

39. Mayo Clinic. Water: How much should you drink every day? http://www.mayoclinic.com/health/water/NU00283. Accessed December 21, 2009.

40. Mayo Clinic. Mayo Foundation for Medical Education and Research. http://www.mayoclinic.org. Accessed December 21, 2009.

41. Sacco R et al. The protective effect of moderate alcohol consumption on ischemic stroke. *JAMA.* 1999;28:913.

42. Williams PJ. Interactive effects of exercise, alcohol, and vegetarian diet on coronary artery disease risk factors in 9242 runners: the National Runners Health Study. *Am J Clin Nutr.* 1997;66:1197.

43. Pierson T. Nutrition Committee of the American Heart Association. AHA Medical Scientific Statement: Alcohol. *Circulation.* 1996;94:3023-3025.

44. Poehlman E, Melby C, Badylak S. Relation of age and physical exercise status on metabolic rate in younger and older healthy men. *J Gerontol.* 1991;46:B54-B58.

45. Goran M, Poehlman E. Total energy expenditure and energy requirements in healthy elderly persons. *Metabolism.* 1992;41:744.

46. Bray GA, Ryan DH, Harsha DW. Diet, weight loss and cardiovascular disease prevention. *Curr Treat Options Cardiovasc Med.* 2003;5(4):259-269.

47. Guerra S, Sherrill DL, Bobadilla A, et al. The relation of body mass index to asthma, chronic bronchitis, and emphysema. *Chest.* 2002;122(4):1256-1263.

48. Sinkov V, Cymet T. Osteoarthritis: understanding the pathophysiology, genetics, and treatments. *J Natl Med Assoc.* 2003;95(6):475-482.

49. Morricone L, Donati C, Hassan T, et al. Relationship of visceral fat distribution to angiographically assessed coronary artery disease: results in subjects with or without diabetes or impaired glucose tolerance. *Nutr Metab Cardiovasc Dis.* 2002;12(5):275-283.

50. Kendall DM, Sobel BE, Coulston AM, et al. The insulin resistance syndrome and coronary artery disease. *Coron Artery Dis.* 2003;14(4):335-348.

51. National Institutes of Health. Clinical Guidelines on the Identification, Evaluation, and Treatment of Overweight and Obesity in Adults. *Obes Res.* 1998;6(suppl 2):51S-209S.

52. Expert Panel. Executive summary of the clinical guidelines on the identification, evaluation, and treatment of overweight and obesity in adults. *Arch Intern Med.* 1998;158:1855-1867.

53. Behnke A, Wilmore J. *Evaluation and Regulation of Body Build and Composition.* Upper Saddle River, NJ: Prentice Hall; 1974.

54. Robergs R, Roberts S. *Estimating Body Composition. Exercise Physiology: Exercise, Performance and Clinical Applications.* St Louis, MO: Mosby; 1997.

55. Siri WE. Body composition from fluid spaces and density: analysis of methods. 1961. *Nutrition.* 1993;9(5):480-491; discussion 480, 492.

56. Brozek J, Grande F, Anderson J, et al. Densitometric analysis of body composition: revision of some quantitative assumptions. *Ann N Y Acad Sci.* 1963;110:113-140.

57. Heymsfield SB et al. Body composition of humans: comparison of two improved four component models that differ in expense, technical complexity, and radiation exposure. *Am J Clin Nutr.* 1991;52:52.

58. Heyward VH, Stolarczyk LM. *Applied Body Composition Assessment.* Champaign, IL: Human Kinetics; 1996.

59. Roche AF. Anthropometry and ultrasound. In: Roche AF, Heymsfied SB, Lohman TG, eds. *Human Body Composition.* Champaign, IL: Human Kinetics; 1996:167-198.

60. Romijn J et al. Regulation of endogenous fat and carbohydrate metabolism in relation to exercise intensity and duration. *Am J Physiol.* 1993;265:E380.

61. Wolfe R. Fat metabolism in exercise. *Adv Exp Med Biol.* 1998;441:147-156.

62. Foss M, Keteyian S. *Fox's Physiological Basis for Exercise and Sport.* 6th ed. Boston, MA: WCB McGraw-Hill; 1998.

63. Thorstenson A, Sjodin B, Karlsson J. Enzyme activities and muscle strength after "sprint training" in man. *Acta Physiol Scand.* 1975;94:313-318.

64. Karlsson J, Nordesjo L, Jorfeldt L, et al. Muscle lactate, ATP, and CP levels during exercise after physical training in man. *J Appl Physiol.* 1972;33(2):199-203.

65. Weltman A et al. Reliability and validity of a continuous incremental treadmill protocol for the determination of lactate threshold, fixed blood lactate concentrations and $\dot{V}O_{2max}$. *Int J Sports Med.* 1990;11:26.

66. Midorikawa J, Hida W, Taguchi O, et al. Lack of ventilatory threshold in patients with chronic obstructive pulmonary disease. *Respiration.* 1997;64:76-80.

67. Gastin R. Energy system interaction and relative contribution during maximal exercise. *Sports Med.* 2001;31(10):725-741.

68. Tanaka H, Monahan KD, Seals DR. Age-predicted maximal heart rate revisited. *J Am Coll Cardiol.* 2001;37:153-156.

69. Kitamura K, Jorgensen CR, Gobel FL, Taylor HL, Wang Y. Hemodynamic correlates of myocardial oxygen consumption during upright exercise. *J Appl Physiol.* 1972;32:516-522.

70. Kim KT, Choi SW, Takahashi K, Kurokawa T, Yamasaki M. Change in double product during stepwise incremental exercise. *J Physiol Anthropol Appl Human Sci.* 2003;22(3):143-147.

71. Hui S, Jackson A, Wier L. Development of normative values for resting and exercise rate pressure product. *Med Sci Sports Exerc.* 2000;32:1520-1527.

72. Guyton A, Jones C, Coleman T. *Circulatory Physiology: Cardiac Output and Its Regulation.* 2nd ed. Philadelphia, PA: WB Saunders; 1973.

73. Bloomer R. Does resistance training stimulate cardiac muscle hypertrophy? *Strength Cond J.* 2003;25(2):7-15.

74. George K, Batterham A, Jones B. Echocardiographic evidence of concentric left ventricular enlargement in female weight lifters. *Eur J Appl Physiol.* 1998;79:88-92.

75. Dickerman R, Schaller F, McConathy. Left ventricular wall thickening does occur in elite power athletes with or without anabolic steroid use. *Cardiology.* 1998;90:145-148.

76. Pelliccia A, Maron B. Outer limits of the athlete's heart, the effect of gender, and the relevance to the differential diagnosis with primary cardiac diseases. *Cardiol Clin.* 1997;15(3):381-396.

77. Link M, Homoud M, Wang P, et al. Cardiac arrhythmias in the athlete: the evolving role of electrophysiology. *Curr Sports Med Rep.* 2002;1(2):75-85.

78. Firoozi S, Sharma S, McKenna W. Risk of competitive sport in young athletes. *Heart.* 2003;89(7):710-714.

79. Seto C. Preparticipation cardiovascular screening. *Clin Sports Med.* 2003;22(1):23-35.

80. Foster C, Jackson A, Pollock M, et al. Generalized equations for predicting functional capacity from treadmill performance. *Am Heart J.* 1984;107:1229-1234.

81. McConnell T, Clark B. Prediction of maximal oxygen consumption during handrail-supported treadmill exercise. *J Cardiopulm Rehabil.* 1987;7:324-331.

82. Cooper KH. A means of assessing maximal oxygen intake. *JAMA.* 1968;203(3):135-138.

83. American College of Sports Medicine. *ACSM's Guidelines for Exercise Testing and Prescription.* 8th ed. Philadelphia, PA: Lippincott Williams & Wilkins; 2010.

84. Astrand PO, Ryhming I. A nomogram for calculation of aerobic capacity (physical fitness) from pulse rate during submaximal work. *J Appl Physiol.* 1954;7:218-221.

85. Golding LA. *YMCA Fitness Testing and Assessment Manual.* Champaign, IL: Human Kinetics; 1989.

86. U.S. Department of Health and Human Services. *Physical Activity and Public Health: a Report of the Surgeon General.* Atlanta, GA: U.S. Department of Health and Human Services, Centers for Disease Control and Prevention, National Center for Chronic Disease Prevention and Health Promotion; 1996.

87. Franklin BA, Whaley MH, Howley ET; American College of Sports Medicine. *ACSM'S Guidelines for Exercise Testing and Prescription.* 6th ed. Philadelphia, PA: Lippincott Williams & Wilkins; 2000.

88. Pate RR, Pratt M, Blair SN, et al. Physical activity and public health: a recommendation from the Centers for Disease Control and Prevention and the American College of Sports Medicine. *JAMA.* 1995;273:402-407.

89. Franklin BA. Diagnostic and functional exercise testing: test selection and interpretation. *J Cardiovasc Nurs.* 1995;10:8-29.

90. Franklin BA. Exercise testing, training and arm ergometry. *Sports Med.* 1985;2:100-119.

91. Franklin BA, Vander L, Wrisley D, et al. Aerobic requirements of arm ergometry: implications for exercise testing and training. *Phys Sportsmed.* 1983;11:81-90.

92. MacDougall JD, Tuxen D, Sale DG, et al. Arterial blood pressure response to heavy resistance exercise. *J Appl Physiol.* 1985;58:785-790.

93. Kelley GA, Kelley KS. Progressive resistance exercise and resting blood pressure: a meta-analysis of randomized controlled trials. *Hypertension.* 2000;35:838-843.

94. National Strength and Conditioning Association. *Essentials of Strength Training and Conditioning.* 2nd ed. Champaign, IL: Human Kinetics; 2000.

95. Bilcheck H. Epiphyseal injuries in young athletes. *NSCA J.* 1989;11(5):60-65.

96. Sparling P, Cantwell J. Strength training guidelines for cardiac patients. *Phys Sportsmed.* 1989;17(3):190-196.

97. MacDougall JD, McKelvie RS, Moroz DE, et al. Factors affecting blood pressure during heavy weight lifting and static contractions. *J Appl Physiol.* 1992;73:1590-1597.

98. Hass CJ, Garzarella L, de Hoyos D, et al. Single versus multiple sets in long-term recreational weightlifters. *Med Sci Sports Exerc.* 2000;32:235-242.

99. Starkey DB, Pollock ML, Ishida Y, et al. Effect of resistance training volume on strength and muscle thickness. *Med Sci Sports Exerc.* 1996;28:1311-1320.

100. Faigenbaum A, Pollock ML, Ishida Y. Prescription of resistance training for health and disease. *Med Sci Sports Exerc.* 1999;31:38-45.

101. Saltin R, Blomqvist G, Mitchell JH, et al. Response to submaximal and maximal exercise after bed rest and training. *Circulation.* 1968;38(suppl 7):1-78.

102. Goldring L, Meyers C, Sinning W, eds. *Y's Way to Physical Fitness.* 3rd ed. Champaign, IL: Human Kinetics; 1989.

103. American College of Sports Medicine Position Stand. The recommended quantity and quality of exercise for developing and maintaining cardiorespiratory and muscular fitness, and flexibility in healthy adults. *Med Sci Sports Exerc.* 1998;30(6):975-991. Review.

104. McArdle D, Katch FI, Katch VL, eds. *Exercise Physiology.* 4th ed. Philadelphia, PA: Lea & Febiger; 1996.

105. Pandolf KB, Sawka MN, Gonzalez RR, eds. *Human Performance Physiology and Environmental Medicine at Terrestrial Extremes.* Traverse City, MI: Cooper; 1988.

106. American College of Sports Medicine. *ACSM's Resource Manual for Guidelines for Exercise Testing and Prescription.* 5th ed. Baltimore, MD: Lippincott Williams & Wilkins; 2006.

107. Wyndham CH, Strydom NB, Benade JS, et al. Heat stroke risk in unacclimatized and acclimatized men of different maximum oxygen intakes working under hot humid conditions. *Chamber of Mines Research Report 12/72.* Johannesburg, South Africa: Chamber of Mines of South Africa; 1972.

108. Plog BA, ed. *Fundamentals in Industrial Hygiene.* 5th ed. Itasca, IL: National Safety Council; 2002.

109. Hegnauer AH, ed. *Biomedicine Problems of High Terrestrial Elevations.* Natick, MA: US Army Research Institute of Environmental Medicine; 1969:204-222.

110. Fulco CS. Maximal and submaximal exercise performance at altitude. *Aviat Space Environ Med.* 1998;69:793-801.

111. Williford HN, Scharff-Olson M, Blessing DL. The physiological effects of aerobic dance: a review. *Sports Med.* 1989;8:335-345.

112. Make life your playground. http://www.bosu.com/scripts/cgiip.exe/WService=BOSU/story.html. Accessed March 8, 2010.

113. Bryant CX, Wenson J, Peterson JA. Safe and enjoyable group cycling for your members. *Fit Man.* 2001;17:38-42.

114. Sherman RM. The indoor cycling revolution. *IDEA Today.* 1997;15:30-33, 35-36, 38-39.

115. Davis CM. *Complementary Therapies in Rehabilitation: Evidence for Efficacy in Therapy, Prevention, and Wellness.* 2nd ed. Thorofare, NJ: Slack Inc; 2004.

116. Feuerstein G. *The Yoga Tradition.* Prescott, AZ: Hohm Press; 1998.

117. Birkel DA, Edgren L. Hatha yoga: improved vital capacity of college students. *Altern Ther Health Med.* 2000;6(6):55-63.

118. Bowman AJ, Clayton RH, Murray A, Reed JW, Subhan MM, Ford GA. Effects of aerobic exercise training and yoga on the baroreflex in healthy elderly persons. *Eur J Clin Invest.* 1997;27(5):443-449.

119. Tandon MK. Adjunct treatment with yoga in chronic severe airways obstruction. *Thorax.* 1978;33(4):514-517.

120. Li JX, Hong Y, Chan KM. T'ai chi: physiological characteristics and beneficial effects on health. *Br J Sports Med.* 2001;35(3):148-156.

121. Hong Y, Li JX, Robinson PD. Balance control, flexibility, and cardiorespiratory fitness among older t'ai chi practitioners. *Br J Sports Med.* 2000;34(1):29-34.

122. Wang Js, Lan C, Wong MK. T'ai chi chuan training to enhance microcirculatory function in healthy elderly men. *Arch Phys Med Rehabil.* 2001;82(9):1176-1180.

123. Lai JS, Wong MK, Lan C, Chong CK, Lien IN. Cardiorespiratory responses of t'ai chi ch'uan practitioners and sedentary subjects during cycle ergometer. *J Formos Med Assoc.* 1993;92(10):894-899.

124. Lai JS, Lan C, Wong MK, Teng SH. Two-year trends in cardiorespiratory function among older t'ai chi ch'uan practitioners and sedentary subjects. *J Am Geriatric Soc.* 1995;43(11):1222-1227.

125. Young Dr, Appel LJ, Jee S, Miller ER. The effects of aerobic exercise and t'ai chi on blood pressure in older people: results of a randomized trial. *J Am Geriatr Soc.* 1999;47(3):277-284.

126. Lan C, Chen SY, Lai JS, Wong MK. The effect of t'ai chi on cardiorespiratory function in patients with coronary artery bypass surgery. *Med Sci Sports Exerc.* 1999;31(5):634-638.

127. Gallagher SP, Kryzanowska R. *The Pilates Method of Body Conditioning.* Philadelphia, PA: BainBridge Books; 1999.

128. Anderson BD. *Polestar Education Instruction Manual: Polestar Approach to Movement Principles.* Coral Gables, FL: Polestar Pilates Education, LLC; 2001.

Anatomy of the Cardiopulmonary System

Sean M. Collins* & Barbara Cocanour*

INTRODUCTION

Anatomy, from the Greek word *anatome* for dissection, is the oldest basic medical science.[1] It is the study of the structure of an organism and is primarily a morphological science (*morphology* being the study of structure without regard to function). *Function* is defined as the activity performed by any structure. To truly understand the function of the human body, whether normal or abnormal, knowledge of its structure is essential. Physical therapists examine, evaluate, and provide interventions to individuals with various cardiopul-

monary impairments. Understanding the cardiopulmonary anatomy allows comprehension of function as well as an appreciation of the relationships between body systems involved with oxygen and nutrient transport. This chapter is not intended to be an exhaustive source of cardiopulmonary anatomy, but it will describe the cardiopulmonary anatomy as it is relevant for the physical therapist. This chapter assumes a basic understanding of anatomical terms and cardiopulmonary anatomy.

The organization of this chapter is based on the functional components of the cardiopulmonary system: ventilation, respiration, and circulation. The physical therapist must understand the structures involved with ventilation, respiration, and circulation in order to examine all domains of disablement (ie, pathology, impairment, functional limitation, disability). Often pathological processes alter the anatomy, resulting in impairment of organ function. Impairment of organ function in the cardiopulmonary system impacts the vital processes in the energy transport system. The physical therapist must also understand these structures in order to effectively evaluate, treat, and recognize the various effects of medical and surgical interventions. Finally, the physical therapist must possess the anatomic language to enter into a dialogue regarding disease mechanisms, treatment rationales, and advanced therapeutic concepts. This chapter includes clinical correlates that highlight the importance of cardiopulmonary structure to function and physical therapy evaluation.

EMBRYONIC DEVELOPMENT OF THE CARDIOPULMONARY SYSTEM

This is not intended to be a full review of the embryonic development of the cardiopulmonary system. Its purpose is limited to improving the physical therapist's understanding of the structural abnormalities underlying various congenital defects, as well as the consequences of premature birth.

Development of the Heart

The heart begins development on gestational day 19 as a pair of *lateral endocardial tubes* in the cardiogenic area, in a horseshoe–shaped formation in the buccopharyngeal area that later forms the pericardial cavity (Fig. 4-1). The lateral endocardial tubes fuse to form the *primitive heart tube*, which begins beating on day 22 and circulating blood on day 24. The paired dorsal aortae form outflow tracts on the cranial end of the primitive heart tube, and three bilateral pairs of inflow tubes connect with the caudal end to form the vitelline, umbilical, and the common cardinal veins.[2]

The inflow end of the primitive heart tube subdivides into the left and right horns of the sinus venosus, the primitive atrium, the ventricle, and the bulbus cordis. The sinus venosus develops into the right atrium and a part of the coronary circulation, and the primitive atrium gives rise to the right and left auricles. An *atrioventricular sulcus* separates the primitive atrium from the primitive ventricle. The primitive ventricle later develops into the left ventricle, whereas the inferior portion of the bulbus cordis differentiates into the right ventricle and the conotruncus. The conus cordis forms from the proximal portion of the conotruncus and develops into the cardiac outflow tracts and a part of the right ventricle.[2] The distal part of the conotruncus, the truncus arteriosus, forms part of the ascending aorta and the pulmonary trunk. The most cranial segment of the heart tube, the aortic sac, gives rise to the left and right aortic arches.

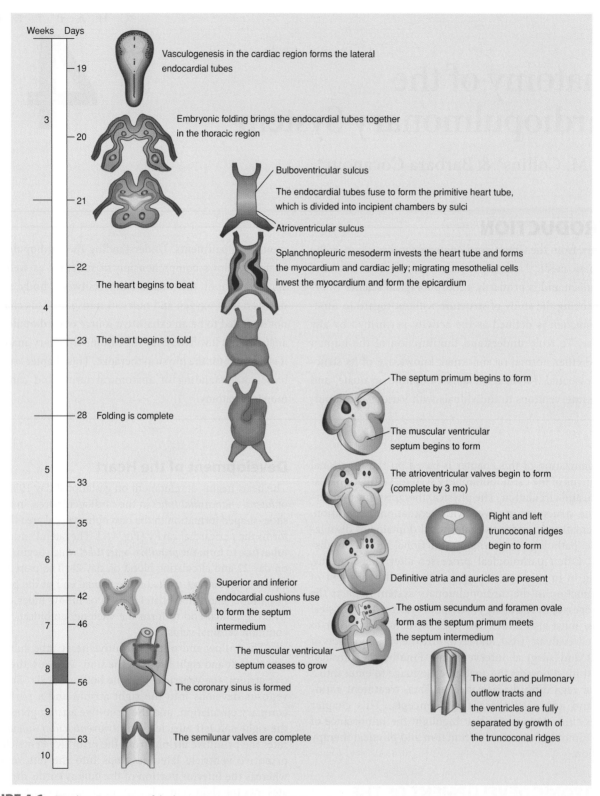

FIGURE 4-1   Timeline: Formation of the heart. (Reprinted from Larsen WJ. *Human Embryology.* Copyright 1993, with permission from Elsevier: p. 132.)

The relationship of the heart chambers is established by a series of folds and loops. The bulbus cordis is displaced ventrocaudally and to the right, the ventricle to the left, whereas the atrium and sinus venosus are displaced craniodorsally.

While the four-chambered heart is developing, the primitive vasculature is being remodeled from a bilateral symmetrical single-circuit system to asymmetrical systemic and pulmonary circuits. The heart tube is remodeled in a manner such that the blood that is returned to the two sinus horns by way of the paired vitelline, umbilical, and common cardinal veins returns to the right atrium by way of the superior and inferior venae cavae[3]. The superior vena cava develops from the right anterior cardinal vein, draining the head and the upper limbs, whereas the inferior vena cava develops from the right vitelline vein, draining the trunk and the lower limbs. The left vitelline, left cardinal, and the two umbilical veins degenerate. The left sinus horn gives rise to the coronary sinus and the oblique vein of the left atrium to drain the heart. The superior vena cava, inferior vena cava, and the coronary sinus drain into the sinus venarum—the smooth posterior wall of the right atrium. Meanwhile the pulmonary venous system is incorporated into the smooth posterior wall of the left atrium.

During the fourth week of development, the septation of the atria and division of the atrioventricular canal begin.[2] Right, left, superior, and inferior pad-like thickenings (endocardial cushions) form on the inner wall of the atrioventricular canal. The superior and inferior pads fuse forming the septum intermedium, dividing the atrioventricular canal into left and right canals. Remodeling will eventually align the left and right atrioventricular canals with the appropriate atria and ventricles.

During the remodeling, the primitive atrium is divided into left and right by the growth of the septum primum and septum secundum from the posterosuperior roof (Fig. 4-1). The opening between the descending edge of the septum primum and the atrioventricular canal is the ostium primum that allows for a right-to-left shunting of blood. The septum primum fuses with the septum intermedium, thus eliminating the ostium primum. However, before the elimination of the ostium primum, an ostium secundum develops in the superior region of the septum primum.[3] The septum secundum develops to the right of the septum primum, growing from the posterosuperior atrial roof but does not reach the septum intermedium, thus creating the foramen ovale. The foramen ovale and ostium secundum do not overlap but allow for the continual shunting of blood from right to left. At birth, the shunt is closed by the rise of left atrial pressure, pressing the septum primum against the septum secundum.

During the fourth week of development, an incomplete muscular septum develops in the ventricular area. This coordinates with the formation of the atrioventricular valves and the septation of the outflow tracts. The cardiac outflow is divided by a pair of spirally patterned longitudinal truncoconal septa.[2] The truncoconal septa arise from a pair of swellings on opposite walls of the outflow tracts (Fig. 4-1).

When these swellings fuse, they form the ascending aorta and the pulmonary trunk. The septa also grow into the ventricular area to complete the interventricular septum, dividing the area into the left and right ventricles.

As the septa are formed, the atrioventricular valves, chordae tendineae, and papillary muscles are sculpted from the surrounding myocardium between the fifth and eighth weeks of gestation. The semilunar valves develop from tubercles that appear near the inferior end of the truncus arteriosus at the level of the ventricular outflow. By the end of the eighth week, a heart with its definitive structures is functioning.

Development of the Lungs

During the third week of development, differential growth and lateral folding convert the flat embryonic disc into a tube-like structure with a midventral opening to the yolk sac.[2] The corresponding germ layers from each side fuse to form concentric layers of ectoderm (an outer layer that gives rise to integumentary structures), mesoderm (a middle layer that gives rise to muscles and related structures), and endoderm (an inner layer that gives rise to the gut structures). The endoderm region in the area of the yolk sac is the midgut, cranial to the yolk sac is the foregut, and caudal to the yolk sac is the hindgut. The formation of the tubular embryo forms an intraembryonic coelom—a cavity between two layers of mesoderm, with a layer of somatic (parietal) mesoderm next to the ectoderm, and a layer of splanchnic (visceral) mesoderm next to the endoderm.

At the cranial end of the embryo is the buccopharyngeal membrane, with the cardiogenic region cranial and lateral to the buccopharyngeal membrane, and the septum transversum (forerunner of the diaphragm and liver) cranial to the cardiogenic region. The *septum transversum* forms an incomplete separation between the thoracic (primitive pericardial) and the abdominal (peritoneal) cavities. The pericardioperitoneal canals are large openings on either side of the foregut between the thoracic and abdominal areas. The mesodermal septum transversum develops in the cervical region and later descends to its definitive region between the primitive pericardial and the peritoneal cavities taking its innervation from C3 through C5 (the spinal origin of the phrenic nerves) with it.[3] The largest part of the diaphragm, consisting of the central tendon and muscle sheets from the pleuroperitoneal membrane, takes its origin from the septum transversum.

With further development, pleuroperitoneal folds grow into the pericardioperitoneal canals to fuse with the septum transversum and the esophageal mesentery, to form separate pleural and peritoneal cavities. A peripheral rim of muscular tissue of the diaphragm originates from the surrounding mesenchyme of the body wall, whereas the crura of the diaphragm develop from the mesentery of the esophagus. The crura and the peripheral ring of muscle, lining the body wall, are innervated by the spinal nerves T7 through T12.[3]

During the fifth week, pleuropericardial folds partition the primitive pericardial cavity into the pericardial cavity and two pleural cavities. The pleuropericardial folds fuse with each other and to the mesenchyme associated with the foregut, forming a definitive pericardial sac separated from the pleural cavities. At this stage of development, the pericardioperitoneal canals connect the pleural cavities with the peritoneal cavity.

During the fourth week, the lungs develop from an outpocketing of the ventral foregut, the *lung bud*. As the lung bud expands caudally, esophagotracheal ridges form to separate the dorsal esophagus from the ventral trachea and lung bud. Communication is maintained between the esophagus and the respiratory components through the laryngeal orifice. Between days 26 and 28, the lung bud bifurcates to form two primary *bronchial buds* from the tracheal portion.[3] Around the fifth week the bronchial buds enlarge to form the right and left main bronchi. With further development, the right bronchus forms three secondary bronchi and the left forms two, the forerunners of the numbers of lobes of the lungs on the respective sides. Between weeks 6 and 16, the primordial segments undergo further divisions until the bronchopulmonary segmentation of the adult lung is completed. Further divisions will continue during postnatal life. During this process of segmentation, the developing respiratory tree is assuming a more caudal position.

STRUCTURAL ORGANIZATION OF THE CARDIOPULMONARY SYSTEM

Thoracic Cavity

The thoracic cavity (Fig. 4-2) is surrounded by the ribs and muscles of the chest wall, the diaphragm, and the root of the neck, and contains the majority of the organs involved with ventilation, respiration, and circulation. It is divided into three parts—two lateral parts, each containing a lung, and the central part called the *mediastinum* (the section containing a central band of organs including the esophagus, trachea, great vessels, and the pericardium).

STRUCTURE OF ELEMENTS INVOLVED IN VENTILATION

"Ventilation is the movement of a volume of gas into and out of the lungs."[4] The chest wall and muscles of ventilation work as a pump to produce the necessary pressure changes, whereas the lung interstitium, upper airways, trachea, bronchi, and bronchioles offer a dynamic route of passage for air during normal breathing.

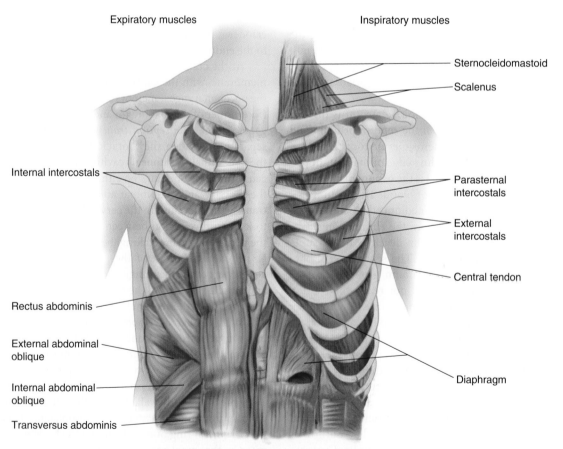

Expiratory muscles

Inspiratory muscles

Sternocleidomastoid

Scalenus

Internal intercostals

Parasternal intercostals

External intercostals

Central tendon

Rectus abdominis

External abdominal oblique

Internal abdominal oblique

Diaphragm

Transversus abdominis

FIGURE 4-2   The muscles of inspiration and expiration. Anterior view of the chest wall depicting the bony cavity formed by the ribs, vertebrae, and sternum. Muscles of expiration (**left**) and inspiration (**right**) are shown.

Thoracic Cage

The thoracic cage creates a bony framework and consists of connective tissue, fascia, muscles of the chest wall, and vascular and neural elements. The bony structure is roughly cone shaped and includes the sternum and costal cartilages anteriorly, the ribs laterally, and the vertebrae posteriorly. The thoracic cage is open superiorly where it communicates with the neck. Its inferior wall is formed by the diaphragm, which has several openings to allow communication between the thoracic and the abdominal cavities.

Sternum

The sternum consists of three parts: manubrium, body, and the xiphoid process. The superiorly located manubrium articulates with the clavicles laterally. Just beneath the clavicles, the manubrium also articulates with the first rib. The *jugular notch*, also called the *suprasternal notch,* is an indentation at the middle of the superior border of the manubrium. Inferior to the manubrium, the body consists of four separate bones that fuse after puberty and have laterally placed notches for articulation with the costal cartilages of ribs 3 through 7. A notch exists at the junction of the manubrium and the body, for articulation with the second rib. The most inferior part of the sternum, the xiphoid process, is a plate of hyaline cartilage that ossifies fully at around the age of 40.[1] The *sternal angle* is a horizontal ridge, at the level of the second rib, across the sternum where the manubrium and the body form a fibrocartilaginous joint. This joint allows "pump handle" action of the sternal body during respiration (sagittal plane motion of the superior ribs).

Ribs

There are 12 pairs of ribs that mainly form the thoracic cage. The structure of the ribs serves two important functional roles (1) to protect the thoracic organs and (2) to provide a dynamic bony lever system for ventilation. The superior seven pairs of ribs articulate with the sternum via the costal cartilages and are referred to as *true ribs.* Rib pairs 8 through 10 have indirect cartilaginous connections to the sternum and are referred to as the *false ribs.* Rib pairs 11 through 12 have their costal cartilages embedded in the lateral body wall; they do not articulate with the sternum and are referred to as the *floating ribs.* The cartilaginous attachment of rib pairs 1 through 10 to the sternum provides a strong yet flexible articulation that contributes to the respiratory "bucket handle" motion (frontal plane motion of the inferior ribs). Costal cartilages of rib pairs 7 through 10 form the costal margin—the inferior margin of the thoracic cage on the anterior body wall.

The 12 pairs of ribs articulate with the thoracic vertebrae. These vertebrae form the posterior bony framework of the thoracic cavity. The thoracic vertebrae differ from the cervical and lumbar vertebrae due to the existence of facets on their transverse processes and body that allow for their articulation with ribs 1 through 12. The facet joints of the thoracic vertebrae, which articulate with the adjacent vertebrae, are aligned almost entirely in the frontal plane and the spinous processes overlap the vertebrae inferior to their origin. The combination of these structural factors greatly limits motion available to the thoracic vertebra. The head of the ribs articulates with the vertebrae at two facet joints—one at the body of the thoracic vertebra of the same number and the other to the thoracic vertebra just superior. These are the costovertebral joints. Lateral to the neck of the rib, a tubercle articulates with the transverse process of the same number of thoracic vertebrae at the costotransverse joints. The costovertebral and costotransverse joints are synovial joints allowing movement of the ribs. The axis for the upper ribs runs almost in a frontal plane and for the lower ribs in a sagittal plane. Based on the orientation of these joint axes, the movement of the upper ribs is primarily anterior and posterior (pump handle), whereas the transverse diameter increases for the lower ribs (bucket handle).

CLINICAL CORRELATE

Based on the connection of the ribs to the thoracic vertebrae, the posture, movement, and deformities of the thoracic spine may have an impact on ventilation. With postural deformities, reductions in thoracic cage expansion and therefore decreased static lung volumes may be present. Conversely, movement of the thoracic spine can be used to facilitate either inspiration (extension of the spine) or exhalation (flexion or rotation of the spine), or to facilitate either inspiration or expiration in one lung with side bending. Flexing the trunk forward causes the diaphragm to move cranially and lengthen. In view of the possible benefit of being flexed forward for facilitating expiration (the forward lean), the question that arises is, "Can a chronically shortened diaphragm be lengthened with such simple maneuvers?" Evidence provided by Volume Reduction Surgery (VRS) and transplantation shows that the chronically shortened diaphragm cannot do so. Therefore, during an evaluation of breathing patterns, if paradoxical breathing (indicating an ineffective diaphragm) can be eliminated with a forward lean posture, it may be established that the patient does not have a shortened diaphragm and may benefit from treatments such as inspiratory muscle training or diaphragmatic muscle training.

Muscles of Ventilation

During ventilation, the muscles of the thoracic cage and of the abdomen act as "pump" muscles to move the bony thorax, thereby causing intrathoracic pressure changes that, in turn, produce airflow into the lungs (Fig. 4-2). Muscles of the larynx and pharynx (discussed later) act as "valves" that help regulate airflow and maintain airway patency. Numerous studies have been conducted on the neural control of the ventilatory muscles and their coordination in ventilatory rhythm; many are reviewed in Miller et al.[5]

Intercostals

The muscles of the thoracic cage include the 11 internal and external intercostals. These muscles connect one rib to the next. The external intercostals originate from the lower border of a superior rib and travel inferomedially to the upper border of the inferior rib. They function to elevate the ribs and increase thoracic volume. Conversely, the internal intercostals originate from the lower border of a superior rib and travel inferolaterally to the upper border of the inferior rib. They function to lower the ribs, thereby decreasing thoracic volume.

Diaphragm

The diaphragm is the primary muscle of ventilation. Structurally, the diaphragm forms a partition between the thoracic and the abdominal cavities (Fig. 4-3). It originates from the xiphoid process of the sternum, the lower six costal cartilages and their adjoining ribs, lateral and medial arcuate ligaments, and from the right and left crura attached to the anterior sur-faces of the lumbar vertebrae. The lateral and medial *arcuate ligaments* are thickenings in the thoracolumbar fascia over the quadratus lumborum and psoas major muscles, respectively. The muscle fibers of the diaphragm insert into the central tendon. There is a foramen in the central tendon to accommodate the inferior vena cava. An esophageal hiatus occurs in the right crus, whereas a median arcuate ligament that interconnects the left and right crura, forms the aortic hiatus. At rest, the diaphragm is dome shaped because of a balance between the functional residual volume of the lungs and the abdominal contents. When the diaphragm contracts, it descends over the abdominal contents and flattens, which causes the lower ribs to move outward; this decreases the intrathoracic pressure, which pulls air into the lungs. Figure 4-3 depicts the diaphragm in the transverse and sagittal planes. The diaphragm is innervated by phrenic motor neurons located in the cervical spinal cord (C3 through C5).

CLINICAL CORRELATE

In patients with chronic obstructive pulmonary disease (COPD), a greater volume of air is left in the lungs at the end of expiration (increased functional residual capacity [FRC]). Therefore, the diaphragm in such patients is of a more shortened length (flattened) as compared to normal FRC. Based on the length–tension relationship of

---

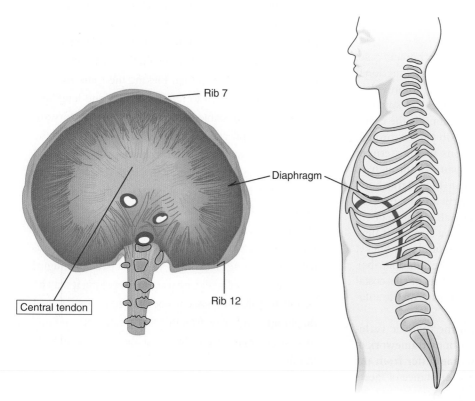

Rib 7

Diaphragm

Central tendon

Rib 12

FIGURE 4-3   Transverse and sagittal views of the diaphragm.

muscles, this shortened length results in a decreased force-generating capacity of the diaphragm. Because the diaphragm is flat, this loss of force is combined with a biomechanical alteration due to a change in the angle of pull of the diaphragm on the ribs. Despite an increased neural drive to the diaphragm, measurement of thoracoabdominal motion in COPD patients has demonstrated decreases in abdominal movement and increases in chest wall movement. This is thought to be related to the decreased mechanical capabilities of the diaphragm.[6,7] With severe airflow limitation and significant hyperinflation, static or dynamic, the separation of the ribs makes it hard to believe that the external intercostals are actually shortened. However, they are affected functionally because of the lack of remaining range of motion of the ribs at the costovertebral and costotransverse joints.

Pleurae

The pleurae are serous membranes lining the pleural region of the thoracic cavity; they consist of an outer parietal layer and an inner visceral layer. The parietal pleura lines the inner surface of the thoracic cavity, the diaphragm, the mediastinum, and the great vessels in the superior mediastinum. The visceral pleura covers the outer surface of the lungs. The space between the two pleurae (pleural cavity) is supplied with a small amount of pleural fluid that serves to hold the visceral and parietal pleurae together during ventilation, and at the same time reduces friction between the lungs and the thoracic wall. Although the layers can easily slide over each other, separation is strongly resisted. The parietal and visceral pleurae are in contact at the root of the lung. Here, during lung development, the lung bud comes into contact with the pleura. Nerves and blood vessels that communicate between the mediastinum and the lungs pass through the root enveloped in a sheet of pleura. Therefore, the lungs and the thoracic wall form a functional unit that moves together—the lungs with the thoracic wall during inspiration and the thoracic wall with the lungs during quiet expiration. In expiration and during resting ventilation, recesses exist in the pleural cavity. *Pleural recesses* are spaces between the visceral and parietal pleurae, and these recesses exist predominantly in the lower parts of the thoracic cavity. No pleural recesses exist superiorly because of the close fit between the lungs and the pleural cavity. The previously mentioned functional residual capacity is dependent on the balance of recoil forces between the lungs and the thoracic wall. The visceral pleura does not have innervation and therefore does not have sensation, whereas the parietal pleurae of the costal and peripheral diaphragm are innervated by intercostal nerves. The mediastinal and central diaphragmatic pleurae are innervated by the phrenic nerve.[8]

CLINICAL CORRELATE

Pleural effusion refers to an excess of pleural fluid in the pleural cavity; it may restrict the patient's ability to inspire and thus reduce lung volume. Other materials can invade the pleural space and cause restrictive lung dysfunction as well: There may be blood in the pleural space (*hemothorax*) or pus due to bacterial infection (*empyema*) or there may be an inflammation of the pleura, causing *pleurisy*. Pleurisy may be appreciated on lung auscultation by the presence of a *pleural friction rub*—a squeaky adventitious sound caused by the two layers of inflamed lung pleura moving against each other during ventilation.

Lungs

The lungs lie within the thoracic cavity on either side of the mediastinum. They are covered by the visceral pleura and include the conducting airways, such as the bronchi and the bronchioles that form a passageway for airflow into the lungs. The conducting airways continue to bifurcate, adding surface area with each generation, until finally they terminate into the distal airways that include the alveoli.[9] These airways are supported by a network of connective tissue known as *interstitium*. The interstitium is an elaborate system of collagen fiber bundles and proteoglycan filaments that form a fine reticular mesh which supports the functional elements of the lungs. The main role of the lungs is to provide a large surface area of contact between the air and the blood in order to accomplish gas exchange. The outer surface of the interstitium is covered by the visceral pleura. Medially, the hilum (the root of each lung) marks the entrance and exit points of bronchi, nerves, blood, and lymph vessels. The most superior aspect of each lung is called its apex. The lung surface adjacent to the ribs is called the costal surface, and the lung surface adjacent to the mediastinum is called the mediastinal surface.

Right Lung

There are three lobes in the right lung—(1) right upper (superior) lobe (RUL), (2) right middle lobe (RML), and (3) right lower (inferior) lobe (RLL) (Fig. 4-4). The RUL occupies the superior third of the right lung. Posteriorly, the RUL is adjacent to the first 3 through 5 ribs. Anteriorly, the RUL extends inferiorly as far as the fourth right rib. The right middle lobe is typically the smallest of the three lobes and appears triangular in shape in the frontal plane, being narrowest near the hilum. The RML extends inferiorly and laterally to the fifth and the sixth rib, as it passes medially. The RLL is the largest of all the three lobes, separated from the

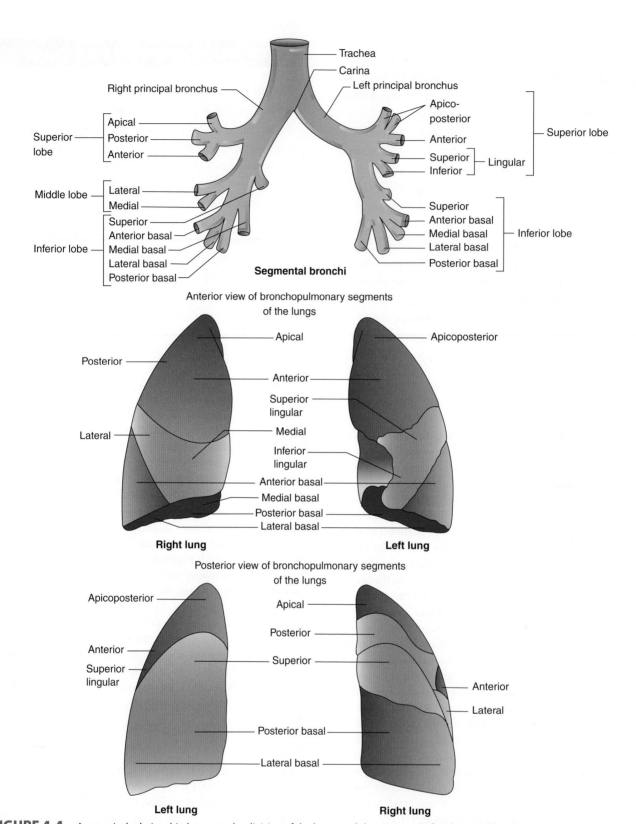

Segmental bronchi

Trachea
Carina
Right principal bronchus
Left principal bronchus

Superior lobe
— Apical
— Posterior
— Anterior

Apico-posterior
Anterior
Superior
Inferior — Lingular
— Superior lobe

Middle lobe
— Lateral
— Medial

Inferior lobe
— Superior
— Anterior basal
— Medial basal
— Lateral basal
— Posterior basal

Superior
Anterior basal
Medial basal
Lateral basal
Posterior basal
— Inferior lobe

Anterior view of bronchopulmonary segments of the lungs

Posterior
Apical
Apicoposterior
Anterior
Superior lingular
Medial
Inferior lingular
Lateral
Anterior basal
Medial basal
Posterior basal
Lateral basal

Right lung   **Left lung**

Posterior view of bronchopulmonary segments of the lungs

Apicoposterior
Apical
Anterior
Posterior
Superior lingular
Superior
Anterior
Lateral
Posterior basal
Lateral basal

Left lung   **Right lung**

FIGURE 4-4   Anatomical relationship between the division of the lungs and the airways. Refer also to Table 4-1.

TABLE 4-1   Segmental Bronchi and Associated Lung Segments

Lung and Bronchus	Lobe and Bronchus	Bronchial Divisions and Segments		
Right lung Right main bronchus	Right upper lobe and bronchus	Apical segment[1] Posterior segment[2] Anterior segment[3]		
	Right middle lobe and bronchus	Lateral segment[4] Medial segment[5]		
	Right lower lobe and bronchus	Superior segment[6] Medial basal segment[7] (not seen in lateral view)		
		Basilar trunk	Anterior segment[8] Lateral segment[9] Posterior segment[10]	
Left lung Left main bronchus	Left upper Left upper lobe and bronchus Left lower lobe and bronchus	Upper bronchi	Apico-posterior segment[1] Anterior segment[3]	
		Lower bronchi	Lingular bronchi	Superior segment[4] Inferior segment[5]
		Superior bronchus Basilar trunk	Superior segment[6] Anterior medial segment[7,8] (not seen in lateral view) Lateral segment[9] Posterior segment[10]	

others by the oblique fissure. Posteriorly, the RLL extends as far superiorly as the sixth thoracic vertebral body and extends inferiorly to the diaphragm. During full inspiration, the lower lobe can extend to as low as L2, becoming superimposed over the upper poles of the kidneys. Grossly, two fissures—horizontal and oblique—that anatomically correspond to the visceral pleural surfaces of those lobes from which they are formed separate these lobes from one another. The *horizontal fissure* separates the RUL from the RML; the *right oblique fissure* is more expansive in size than the minor fissure, separating the right upper and middle lobes from the larger right lower lobe.

Left Lung

The structure of the left lung differs slightly from that of the right lung (Fig. 4-4). The two lobes of the left lung are separated by an oblique fissure, identical to that seen on the right side, although often slightly more inferior in location. The portion of the left lung that corresponds anatomically to the right middle lobe (the lingular segment) is incorporated into the left upper lobe and extends posteriorly to the sixth rib. Posteriorly, the LLL extends as far inferiorly as the eleventh rib, and superiorly as far as the fourth rib.

AIRWAY ANATOMY

The branching nature of the bronchi contributes to the lobar structure of the lungs. This structure allows for an exponential increase in the amount of surface area for gas exchange as the bronchi continue to branch until they reach the terminal bronchioles and finally the alveoli. This branching nature also permits lung segments and lobes to function relatively inde-

pendently. Pathological processes in one lobe, such as pneumonia, will not necessarily affect other regions of the lung. It should be pointed out that considerable anatomical variation might exist between individuals. The bronchial anatomy described herein is illustrative of a typical bronchial pattern. The reader should be aware that oftentimes, two or three bronchi might arise from a common trunk rather than have separate and discrete origins. This is frequently the case for the apical and posterior segments of the upper lobe of the left lung (therefore typically combined into apicoposterior) and the anterior and medial basal segments of the lower lobe of the left lung (therefore often combined into anteromedial basal). This explains why some anatomy texts list 10 segments for the left lung and others only 8.

Conducting Airways and Lobes of the Lungs

After the bifurcation of the trachea into the main bronchi, the conducting airways pass through the hilum (the root of the lung) and continue to bifurcate. Throughout the generation of these bifurcations, the airway diameter decreases and contains less cartilage and smooth muscle (Fig. 4-4).

In the normal adult, the left main bronchus (LMB) measures approximately 4.5 cm in length and the right (RMB) measures approximately 2.5 cm in length. The shortness of the right main bronchus is due to the more proximal origin of the right upper lobe bronchus. Taken together, the two main bronchi, volumetrically, have 40% more cross-sectional area than the trachea. The left main bronchus leaves the trachea at a 135-degree angle, whereas the more superiorly located right main bronchus tends to be more vertically oriented, having a 155-degree angle of origin.

Right Upper Lobe Bronchi

Soon after its origin, the RMB gives rise to the right upper lobe bronchus, which typically is directed superiorly and slightly laterally, having an almost 90-degree angle from the RMB (Fig. 4-4). The upper lobe bronchial trunk measures approximately 1 cm in length and approximately 1 cm in diameter. The trunk then gives rise to the segmental bronchi of the RUL. A segmental bronchus supplies the apical segment of the right upper lobe and has a diameter ranging from 4 to 7 mm. Another bronchus, supplying the posterior segment, has a more horizontal course.

Finally, a third segmental bronchus supplies the anterior segment and, like the posterior segmental bronchus, has a generally horizontal course but proceeds somewhat inferiorly from its origin. The right main bronchus extends no farther inferiorly than the origin of the right upper lobe bronchus. The airway distal to the upper lobe bronchus is referred to as the bronchus intermedius (BI). The bronchus intermedius generally averages 2 cm in length and terminates at the point of origin of the right middle lobe bronchus.

Right Middle Lobe Bronchi

The middle lobe bronchial trunk measures approximately 12 mm in length and 8 mm in diameter. The origin of the middle lobe bronchus marks the point of origin of the right lower lobe bronchus. From its origin, off the anterior aspect of the BI, the right middle lobe bronchial trunk continues slightly inferiorly for a short distance before giving rise to the lateral and medial segmental bronchi. The medial segmental bronchus has a slightly more oblique course than the lateral segmental bronchus.

Right Lower Lobe Bronchi

The right superior segmental bronchus may arise at, or above, the level of the origin of the right middle lobe bronchus but more frequently arises slightly more distally. Regardless, the superior segmental bronchus is the first branch off the lower lobe bronchus and has a predominantly horizontal course. The airway distal to the superior segmental bronchus is referred to as the *basilar trunk*. The basilar segmental bronchi have a predominantly vertical orientation. The anterior, posterior, and lateral basilar segmental bronchi typically arise from a common trunk. The medial basal bronchus, oriented medially, has its origin inferior to the superior segmental bronchus.

Left Upper Lobe Bronchi

The origin of the left upper lobe bronchus occurs at a level lower than the origin of the right upper lobe bronchus. The left upper lobe bronchial trunk gives rise to the upper lobe and lingular segmental bronchi. Measuring 9 mm in length and approximately 12 mm in diameter, the left upper lobe bronchial trunk characteristically appears short but has a large diameter. The left upper lobe bronchial trunk divides into the ascending upper division (eventually giving rise to the apico-posterior and anterior segments) and the descending lower division (which then gives rise to the lingular segmental bronchi). Note that in the left upper lobe bronchus, the apical and posterior segments are combined and as such are supplied by one bronchus. The courses of apical and posterior segmental bronchi have vertically and horizontally oriented components as bronchial rami divide to supply the apicoposterior segment. The anterior segmental bronchus will have a more horizontal course similar to that seen on the right side. The lingular segmental bronchi have an oblique course. The superior lingular segmental bronchus has a more horizontal course and supplies the superior lingular segment. The superior lingular segmental bronchus is superior to the more vertically oriented inferior lingular segmental bronchus.

Left Lower Lobe Bronchi

The left superior segmental bronchus is similar to that on the right side, having a typically horizontal course and supplying the superior segment. There are only four segments in the left lower lobe, compared to five on the right. The bronchial segment that supplies the medial basal segment on the right side is not a separate entity on the left. As a result, the anterior and medial segments are combined and supplied by an anteromedial bronchus. As is the case on the right side, the basilar segmental lower lobe bronchi course predominantly vertically. Like their contralateral counterparts, lateral and posterior basal segmental bronchi may arise from a common trunk.

Upper Airways

The upper airways include the nose, pharynx, nasopharynx, oropharynx, larynx, and the trachea. These structures allow communication between the environment and the lungs. Knowledge of their structure is important for physical therapists in certain examination procedures as well as in airway clearance techniques.

Nose

The nose is supported by bone and cartilage and is covered by skin. Periosteal and perichondral membranes blend to connect the bones and cartilage to each other. The nasal cavity is a wedge-shaped passage divided vertically by a septum into right and left halves and into compartments by the nasal conchae. The nasal cavity begins with the *nares* and passes posteriorly to the nasopharynx. The lateral walls of each cavity contain prominent folds called *conchae* that project medially and inferiorly into the cavity and serve to increase the respiratory surface of the nasal mucous membrane to help warm and moisten air. The mucous membrane is formed from nasal epithelial cells; additional functions include protecting the airway from foreign substances by trapping particles in mucus and allowing for their removal by sneezing. The conchae occupy a large portion of the available space in the nasal cavity, and a small amount of inflammation can obstruct the nasal passage. The floor of the nasal cavity is formed by the palatine process of the maxilla and the horizontal part of the palatine bone. The paired nasal cavities open through the narrowed posterior apertures into the *pharynx* (Fig. 4-5).

CLINICAL CORRELATE

The nasal conchae narrow the nasal passageways, and the mucous membrane is composed of fragile cells, making suction-catheter trauma likely in the case of blind *nasotracheal suctioning*. This is why low platelet counts may be a contraindication to this form of suctioning or, at the very least, require the insertion of a *nasopharyngeal airway (nasal trumpet)*.

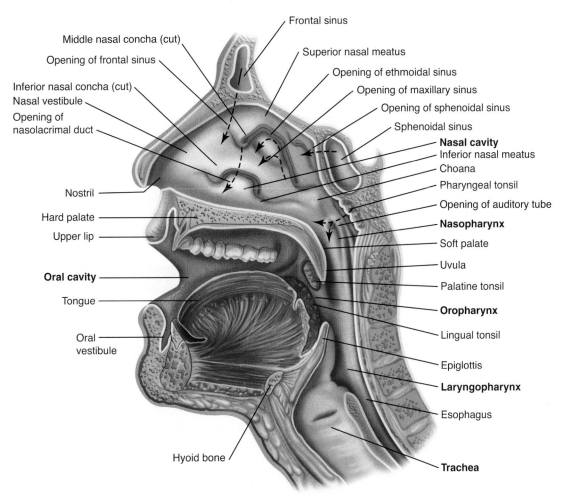

FIGURE 4-5   Sagittal view of the upper airways. (Reproduced with permission from Tintinalli JE, Kelen GD, Stapczynski JS. *Emergency Medicine: A Comprehensive Study Guide*. 6th ed. New York: McGraw-Hill; 2004:102.)

Pharynx

The pharynx is a shared structural throughway that allows the digestive system (from the mouth) and the respiratory system (from the nose) passage to their respective destinations—the esophagus and the larynx. The posterior and lateral walls of the pharynx are muscular, whereas the anterior wall consists of the opening to the nasal cavities, the soft palate, the opening to the mouth and the tongue, and finally to the posterior wall of the opening to the larynx.[1] The pharynx is surrounded by the superior, middle, and inferior constrictor muscles that run horizontally; the stylopharyngeus, which is oriented longitudinally, disappears between the superior and middle constrictors. The inferior constrictor maintains a tonic contraction until swallowing, serving as a sphincter between the esophagus and the pharynx. The pharynx normally undergoes small changes in size during normal breathing; however, structural abnormalities may impede airflow through the pharynx, particularly during sleep.

The pharynx is divided by the soft palate into the *nasopharynx* and *oropharynx*. Muscles that form the soft palate, which assist with ventilation, include the levator and tensor veli palatini, the musculus uvulae, the palatopharyngeus, and the palatoglossus. Their coordinated action regulates the route of airflow between nasal and oral pathways to meet ventilatory demands (Fig. 4-5).[10]

The roof of the nasopharynx is called the *fornix* and consists of a mucous membrane in close proximity to the basal portions of the sphenoid and occipital bones. The ostium of the auditory tube is located in the lateral wall of the pharynx and provides a structural connection to the middle ear. The soft palate forms a mobile floor of the anterior portion of the nasopharynx. The pharyngeal isthmus is posterior to the soft palate and forms the opening to the oropharynx. The isthmus can be closed by the levator veli palatini muscle pulling the soft palate backward and upward.[10] The soft palate will approximate the posterior wall to allow, for example, proper phonation of consonants, drinking under pressure, and expiration of air through the mouth and not the nose (ie, pursed-lip breathing).

The oropharynx is bordered anteriorly by the base of the tongue and extends downward posteriorly to the upward projection of the epiglottis. The epiglottis is united to the tongue by a midline and two lateral folds—the median and the lateral glossoepiglottic folds. The laryngeal part of the pharynx is continuous with the oropharynx at the level of the upper border of the epiglottis and is wide superiorly and narrows as it travels posteriorly. Distal to the cricoid cartilage of the larynx, the pharynx becomes continuous with the esophagus. At this point, the anterior wall of the pharynx is the opening to the larynx.

Larynx

The larynx (composed of nine cartilages) forms a protective connection between the pharynx and the trachea. As part of the respiratory system, the larynx protects the trachea from food and foreign bodies by acting as a valve. The larynx is also equipped with a phonating mechanism designed for voice production. Laryngeal muscles, in addition to phonation, produce large changes in the size and therefore resistance of the laryngeal opening through the vocal cords. The larynx is approximately 5 cm in length in adult males.

The nine laryngeal cartilages form joints to allow normal functioning of the laryngeal structures. The cricoarytenoid joints and the cricothyroid joints both allow movement, which approximates, tenses, relaxes, tightens, or slackens the vocal cords.

The larynx is divided into three compartments by the projecting folds of the mucous membranes of the lateral walls. The vestibule lies between the inlet and the superior folds; the ventricle, between the superior folds and the vocal cords; and the infraglottic cavity, between the vocal cords and the cricoid cartilage, where it is continuous with the trachea. Contraction of the transverse and oblique arytenoid muscles and the aryepiglottic muscles has a sphincter action and closes the laryngeal inlet as a protective mechanism during swallowing.

Trachea

The trachea begins at the level of the cricoid cartilage of the larynx, which generally is at the level of the sixth cervical vertebra. In adults, the trachea ranges from 9 to 15 cm in length and terminates as the *carina*, a ridge at the bifurcation of the trachea into the left and right main bronchi (Fig. 4-4). The trachea has a maximum transverse diameter of 16 mm, whereas sagittally the trachea is narrower, having a maximal diameter of 14 mm. The posterior wall of the trachea tends to appear slightly flattened due to posteriorly directed horse-shoe–shaped cartilages. The carina is a cartilaginous wedge at the bifurcation of the trachea into the right and left main stem bronchi. It resides approximately at the level of the fifth thoracic vertebral body and can be localized approximately at the same level as the sternal notch.

CLINICAL CORRELATE

Tracheal suctioning requires the insertion of a catheter into the upper airway, where it is passed down the trachea to the level of the carina. The carina is richly innervated by the vagus nerve. When the tip of the suction catheter comes in contact with the carina, it can provoke a strong parasympathetic response, which in turn can trigger a sudden decrease in the heart rate and produce cardiac arrhythmias. Therapists should monitor their patients carefully for the appearance of such events and provide supplemental oxygen during the procedure.

STRUCTURE OF ELEMENTS INVOLVED IN RESPIRATION (GAS EXCHANGE)

"Respiration refers primarily to the exchange of oxygen and carbon dioxide across a membrane into and out of the lungs at the cellular level."[4] In the lungs it is the close proximity of the alveoli to the capillaries of pulmonary circulation that allows the gas exchange to occur. In the tissues of the body, the capillaries form dense networks that deliver oxygen to metabolically active tissues and pick up carbon dioxide in the form of hydrogen and acids to be returned to the lungs.

Alveoli

The terminal bronchioles evolve into respiratory bronchioles that have *alveolar ducts* extending from their walls. The alveolar ducts carry in their walls strong fibers that extend to the end of the duct. The ducts are densely populated with sacs that give rise to the terminal air sacs—the *alveoli*. The portion of lung extending distal to the terminal bronchiole is called the respiratory zone or the acinus (Fig. 4-6). Whereas the distance from the terminal bronchiole to the alveoli is only approximately 5 mm, the *acinus* makes up the majority of the air volume of the lung (3,000 mL).[11] A dense network of fibers anchors the acinus to the interstitium. When the diaphragm and chest wall move, tension is transmitted through this dense network of fibers into the acinus and then to the alveolar walls. The alveolar wall consists of two thin layers of epithelial cells (*squamous and granular pneumocytes*) spread over a layer of connective tissue. Squamous pneumocytes are flat and thin, making up approximately 95% of the gas-exchange area, whereas granular pneumocytes are thick, active cells that produce surfactant. A third cell type is free floating in the alveolus and is called an *alveolar macrophage*, which engulfs and ingests foreign material in the alveoli as a protective function against disease.

CLINICAL CORRELATE

The importance of this dense interconnected fiber network becomes apparent when disease processes, such as emphysema, destroy some of the fibers, which can drastically affect both respiration (reduced surface area) and ventilation (widened and irregular airspaces) of the alveoli.

Capillaries

Capillaries are tiny blood vessels (measuring approximately 4–12 μm in diameter) composed of a single layer of flattened endothelial cells. Capillaries bring blood in close contact with tissues. In metabolically active tissues, capillaries form a dense

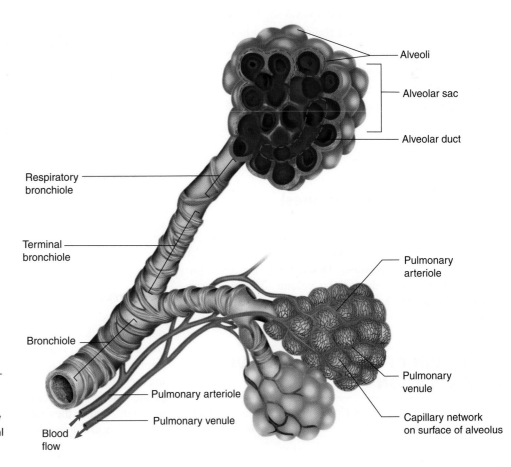

FIGURE 4-6 Terminal divisions of the bronchial tree, depicting the terminal and respiratory bronchioles leading into alveolar sacs or the acinus. Expanded view of an alveolar sac shows individual alveoli.

Alveoli

Alveolar sac

Alveolar duct

Respiratory bronchiole

Terminal bronchiole

Pulmonary arteriole

Bronchiole

Pulmonary venule

Pulmonary arteriole

Capillary network on surface of alveolus

Pulmonary venule

Blood flow

network that is fed by a number of arterioles. The density of the capillary bed is related to the functional activity of the organ—the greater the need for aerobic metabolism, the greater the density of the capillary bed. A capillary is composed of a thin layer of simple squamous cells. The capillary network is interwoven throughout the interstitium. Even though capillaries lack the elastic connective tissue component of arteries and veins they are still able to distend, thus allowing them to accommodate to the volume of blood being delivered to the lungs.

Alveolar–Capillary Membrane

It is at the alveolar–capillary interface that a common basement membrane is shared.[9] The route that oxygen must take to get from the lung to the pulmonary capillary bed begins with movement through the squamous and granular pneumocytes (alveolar epithelium) and proceeds across the basement membrane and finally across the capillary endothelium into the lumen of the capillary, where it either becomes dissolved in plasma or is picked up by the red blood cell. The alveolar–capillary membrane thickness varies throughout the lung but is approximately 0.5 to 1.0 μm.

CLINICAL CORRELATE

The thickness of the membrane may increase with fluid accumulation in the interstitium because of increased capillary hydrostatic pressure (heart failure), obstructed lymphatic flow (lung cancer), reduced osmotic pressure, or trauma. This thickening in the membrane will make diffusion of gases more difficult and will impede respiration. The thickness of the membrane may also increase by fibrotic scarring of either the alveolar cell walls or the interstitium.

Red Blood Cells (Erythrocytes)

Erythrocytes are biconcave discs with a simple structure. They do not have a nucleus and do not reproduce or carry on metabolic activities. They contain cytoplasm, protein, lipid substances, and hemoglobin. Hemoglobin accounts for approximately 33% of the cellular volume. The biconcave structure maximizes the surface available for gas exchange in the capillaries.[9]

STRUCTURE OF ELEMENTS INVOLVED IN CIRCULATION

"Circulation is the passage of blood through the heart, blood vessels, organs and tissues; it also describes the oxygen deliv-

ery system."[4] The central components of the circulatory system, all located in the mediastinum, consist of the heart, which pumps blood, and the great vessels, which transport blood to the central pulmonary and systemic circulation. The systemic circulation includes the arteries and arterioles that deliver blood to the body; the capillaries that allow oxygen, nutrient, and waste product exchange; and the veins that return blood to the heart.

Mediastinum

The mediastinum is a space that extends from the thoracic inlet superiorly to the diaphragm inferiorly, and from the sternum anteriorly to the vertebral column posteriorly. The structures contained in the mediastinum are surrounded by loose connective tissue, nerves, blood and lymph vessels and nodes, and fat. The looseness of the connective tissue, combined with the elasticity of the lungs and pleura, allows the mediastinum to accommodate movement and volume changes in the thoracic cavity related to venous return, cardiac output, ventilation, and swallowing. There may be variations in the location of the mediastinum with changes in body position and, more significantly, with changes in unilateral lung volume. The mediastinum can shift to one side with unilateral loss of lung volume, such as in the case of a pneumothorax or even atelectasis (a collapsed or airless condition of the lung).

CLINICAL CORRELATE

A mediastinal shift is a common sign that reflects lung pathology. The mediastinum shifts *toward* a pneumothorax or severe atelectasis, or *away from* a tension pneumothorax. A tension pneumothorax occurs when air leaks out of a lung through a flap of lung tissue that acts as a one-way valve, allowing air to escape into the pleural space but not allowing it to return back into the lung. Pressure and tension build up in the pleural space, pushing the mediastinum away from the pathology.

Pericardium

The pericardium, located in the middle of the mediastinum, is posterior to the sternum and to the second through sixth costal cartilages. It is a double-walled fibroserous sac that surrounds the heart and the roots of the vessels entering and leaving the heart. The fibrous outer layer fuses with the outer layer of the vessels to the sternum, forming the sternopericardial ligaments, and to the central tendon of the diaphragm, forming the pericardiophrenic ligament.

The fibrous layer is lined with the serous pericardium— the parietal layer that continues onto the heart as the visceral pericardium (the epicardium). The potential space between the parietal pericardium and the visceral pericardium is the pericardial cavity. Serous fluid fills the pericardial cavity and allows for an almost friction-free environment for cardiac function, whereas the fibrous wall provides protection from the rapid and potentially damaging overfilling of the pericardial cavity.

The phrenic nerves, which contain pain fibers, innervate the parietal pericardium; however, the visceral pericardium is insensitive to pain. The pericardium receives its blood supply through branches of the internal thoracic arteries and phrenic arteries. Venous drainage is through the azygos and pericardiophrenic veins.

CLINICAL CORRELATE

Pericardial effusion is a pathologic condition where excess fluid (hemorrhagic, inflammatory, etc) fills the pericardial cavity. This increase in pressure on the heart restricts blood flow into the right ventricle, greatly diminishing venous return and impairing cardiac output. A pericardial rub may be appreciated through cardiac auscultation, indicating inflammation of the outer thin-walled serous pericardium and the fibrous layer.

Heart

For it is the heart by whose virtue and pulse the blood is moved, perfected, made apt to nourish and is preserved from corruption and coagulation . . . . It is indeed the fountain of life, the source of all action.

WILLIAM HARVEY (1578–1697)[10]

The heart is an inverted, cone-shaped organ situated obliquely in the mediastinum. It is slightly larger than the size of a closed fist, with two-thirds of its mass extending left of the midline. The tip of the left ventricle defines the apex of the heart, whereas the base of the heart is formed by the two atria. The apex is directed downward and anteriorly, pointing inferolaterally to the left. In normal adults the apex rests at the level of the fifth intercostal space, midclavicular line in supine. The *point of maximum impulse* (PMI) is located at the apex and in some individuals may be visualized, when the left ventricle contracts and the apex of the heart moves forward, striking the chest wall. The base of the heart consists of the two atria. The base is directed upward and posteriorly and points posteromedially to the right. Finally, the heart is rotated on its long axis such that the right ventricle is an anterior structure, the left ventricle is a lateral structure positioned toward the anterior axillary line, and the wall of the interventricular septum is directed straight out away from the anterior chest.

The position of the heart in the mediastinum, as just described, implies that the heart lies on its side, with a portion of the left ventricle in direct contact with the diaphragm, and this is indeed the case. This *diaphragmatic portion* of the left ventricle is also termed as its inferior wall and is a common site of myocardial infarction.

CLINICAL CORRELATE

When the heart is hypertrophied and/or dilated, the PMI is displaced laterally because of the increase in left ventricular muscle mass. Left ventricular hypertrophy can be caused by increased systolic demands on the heart secondary to hypertension.

The great vessels enter and exit from the superiorly oriented base of the heart. The gross structure of the heart includes four chambers, four cardiac valves, and the vessels of coronary circulation. The right side of the heart pumps oxygen-poor blood from the cells of the body back to the lungs for gas exchange; the left side of the heart receives oxygen-rich blood from the lungs and pumps it through the arteries to the various parts of the body. The physical therapist must understand the normal structure of the heart in order to appreciate how the anatomy of the heart impacts physiology and pathophysiology and allows the necessary series of tightly coordinated physiological processes to occur.

Fibrous Skeleton

The cardiac skeleton is composed of fibrocartilaginous tissue, sometimes referred to as the *anulus fibrosus*, which forms a firm anchor to which the muscles and valves of the heart are attached (Fig. 4-7). The anulus fibrosus gives structure to the heart and acts as an electrical insulator between the atria and ventricles to ensure impulses move only through the AV node.[1] It consists of tough fibrous rings surrounding the atrioventricular canals and the origins of the aortic and the pulmonary trunks, which are connected by the tendon of the conus—a fibrous band. The aortic anulus and the AV anuli are connected by the left and right fibrous trigone. These fibrous rings provide not only the circular form for the canals (atrioventricular and semilunar) but also the necessary rigidity to prevent the outlets from becoming dilated from the force of blood flowing through them.

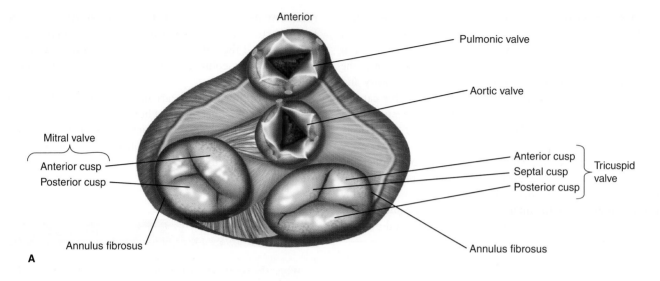

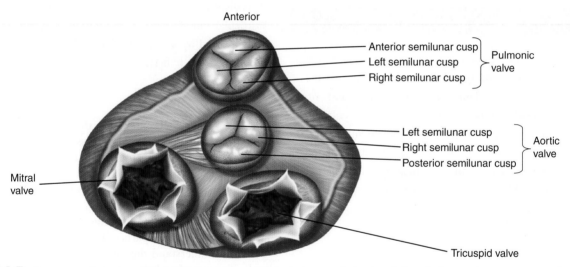

FIGURE 4-7   Transverse plane view of fibroskeleton and heart valves during systole (**top**) and diastole (**bottom**). **A:** Heart in systole: Fibroskeleton with atrioventricular and semilunar valves with atria removed. **B:** Heart in diastole: Fibroskeleton with atrioventricular and semilunar valves with atria removed.

CLINICAL CORRELATE

Cardiac arrhythmias may occur when the anulus fibrosus is damaged or diseased such as during cardiac surgery or aging. This occurs through escape of the ventricular action potential to the atria or from passage of the action potential from the atria to the ventricles by means other than the AV node and Bundle of His.

Tissue Layers

The heart wall consists of three layers. The outermost layer of the heart—the *epicardium* (visceral pericardium)—consists of epithelial cells that form a serous membrane to cover the entire heart. The innermost layer of the heart is known as the *endocardium*. It is a serous membrane that lines the inner surface of the heart, its valves, and the chordae tendineae. The endothelial cells of the endocardium are similar to and continuous with those of the tunica intima of the arteries (described in the section on circulation). The middle layer of the heart is the *myocardium*. It is responsible for the major pumping action of the ventricles due to the presence of contractile elements. The myocardial cells have an intrinsic ability to contract in the absence of stimuli (automaticity), in a rhythmic manner (rhythmicity), and to transmit nerve impulses (conductivity). The myocardium does not undergo mitotic activity and cannot replace injured cells. Therefore, in the case of cell death (due to lack of oxygen) or disease (eg, viral cardiomyopathy) the impact of loss of cells is the loss of contractile function.

Myocardial Cells

Myocardial cells are grouped into two structural categories (mechanical and conductive) representing their functional contributions. Mechanical cells have a greater capacity for mechanical shortening necessary for pump action, and conductive cells have a greater capacity for self-excitation and transmission of an action potential. Histologically the mechanical cells contain a much larger number of actin and myosin myofilaments than the conductive cells, whereas the conductive cells have more ion channels in their cell membranes.

Mechanical cells, or *myocytes,* are large cells that are joined together in series by intercalated discs forming a *syncytium* (a group of cells in which the protoplasm of one cell is continuous with that of the adjoining cells). Intercalated discs, which are cell membranes, have 1/100th the electrical resistance of the myocytes. Electrically the heart has two syncytia, the atria and the ventricles, which are separated by the fibrous skeleton. Action potentials spread rapidly through cardiac muscle, resulting in mechanical shortening, which occurs virtually simultaneously within each syncytium.[12]

Chambers of the Heart

Right Atrium

The right atrium has a thin muscular wall. It receives venous (deoxygenated) blood from the head and upper extremities via the superior vena cava, from the trunk and lower extremities via the inferior vena cava, and from the myocardium via the coronary sinus. The coronary sinus empties into the right atrium just above the tricuspid valve. The inner surfaces of the posterior and medial walls are smooth, whereas the anterior and lateral walls are composed of parallel muscle bundles known as the pectinate muscles.[11] Most of the blood flow into the right atrium occurs during inspiration when pressure drops below that in the inferior and superior venae cavae. There are no functioning valves in the adult venae cavae; thus, when the right atrial pressure rises, congestion occurs in the systemic circulation. Normal filling pressure for the right atrium ranges from 0 to 8 mm Hg and is commonly referred to as *central venous pressure* (CVP).

CLINICAL CORRELATE

Orthotopic heart transplants involve the excision of the right atrium. The donor heart is then attached to the right atrium.

Right Ventricle

The right ventricle receives blood from the right atrium through the tricuspid valve and ejects it through the pulmonic valve into the pulmonary artery where it travels to the lungs. The right ventricle is normally the most anterior cardiac chamber lying beneath the sternum. It may be divided into the body of the right ventricle (inflow region consisting of the tricuspid valve, the chordae tendineae, the papillary muscle, and a heavily trabeculated myocardium) and the infundibulum (smooth outflow region). The inflow and outflow portions of the right ventricle are separated by four muscular bands—the infundibular septum, the parietal band, the septal band, and the moderator band. The resistance of pulmonary circulation is approximately 1/10th that of the systemic circulation. Normal systolic pressure in the right ventricle ranges from 15 to 28 mm Hg and the end-diastolic pressure ranges from 0 to 8 mm Hg. The chamber is crescent shaped and has a thin myocardial wall. The right ventricle generates less than one-fourth the stroke work of the left ventricle.

Left Atrium

The left atrium receives venous (oxygenated) blood from the lungs through the right and left inferior and superior pulmonary veins. The wall of the left atrium is slightly thicker than that of the right atrium, an adaptation to the slightly higher pressures in the left atria. Normal filling pressure ranges from 4 to 12 mm Hg. Two pulmonary veins enter posterolaterally on each side and, although there are no valves, sleeves of atrial muscle extend from the atrial wall around the pulmonary veins. These may exert a sphincter-like action to reduce backflow of blood during atrial systole.[10] The auricular appendage ("dog ear") is an anteriorly directed outpocketing of the left superior aspect of the chamber, which represents the original heart tube and serves no useful function.[8]

CLINICAL CORRELATE

Certain conditions, such as mitral valve insufficiency, can result in an increase in regurgitant blood flow from the left ventricle back through the leaky mitral valve into the left atrium. This can create chronically elevated left atrial pressures that irritate the walls of the left atrium, sending it into atrial fibrillation. The left atrium, now "quivering like a bag of worms," produces no forward blood flow. Static blood is subject to clot formation, and this blood clot invariably forms in the left atrial appendage.

Left Ventricle

The left ventricle has a thick muscular wall, approximately two to three times the thickness of the right ventricular wall. It receives blood from the left atrium through the mitral valve and ejects it through the aortic valve to the systemic circulation via the aorta. Normal systolic pressure ranges from 90 to 140 mm Hg and normal end-diastolic pressure from 4 to 12 mm Hg.

The ventricular septum, a thick muscular area that becomes membranous as it nears the atrioventricular (AV) valves, separates the right and left ventricles. It contains electrical conduction tissue and provides stability to the ventricles during contraction. The left chamber is an ellipsoidal sphere with its blunt tip directed anteriorly, inferiorly, and to the left where it forms the apex of the heart. There is a funnel-shaped inflow tract formed by the mitral anulus, its leaflets, and the chordae tendineae that directs the entering blood toward the apex. The outflow tract, which is surrounded by the inferior surface of the anteromedial mitral leaflet, the septum, and the ventricular wall, sends the blood from the apex superiorly and to the right toward the aortic valve. During systole, when the mitral valve leaflets snap shut, the entire chamber is converted into an explosive outflow tract.

Valves

The valves of the heart are formed by cartilaginous cusps from the fibrous skeleton to ensure unidirectional blood flow through the heart. Figure 4-7 illustrates the valves of the heart in the transverse plane of the heart with the atria removed during both diastole and systole. The *mitral or bicuspid valve* lies between the left atrium and the left ventricle. It has two cusps that slightly overlap each other when the valve is closed. The *tricuspid valve* lies between the right atrium and the right ventricle. It has three leaflets that are thinner than those of the mitral valve. The leaflets, both of the tricuspid and bicuspid valves, are attached to strong fibrous strands called *chordae*

tendineae. These cords arise from the *papillary muscle bundles* in the inner ventricles. Two groups of papillary muscles arise from the trabeculae carneae in the left ventricle and three arise in the right ventricle. The *aortic* and *pulmonary valves* are called semilunar (ie, half-moon) valves because they have three cusps that are cuplike in nature. The AV (ie, mitral and tricuspid) valves prevent backflow of blood from the ventricles into the atria during systole. The aortic and pulmonary valves prevent backflow of blood from the aorta and pulmonary artery into the ventricles during diastole. They open and close based entirely on pressure gradient changes in the heart during the cardiac cycle.

CLINICAL CORRELATE

Abnormalities in valve structure either impede blood flow through the valve (*stenosis*) or cause retrograde blood flowback through the valve (*regurgitation*), which can produce limitations in exercise tolerance. These abnormalities can lead to a variety of *cardiac murmurs*. For a description of these heart sounds, the reader may refer to Chapter 8.

Conduction System

Figure 4-8 depicts the cardiac conduction system. The cardiac impulse arises in the sinoatrial (SA) node, which is

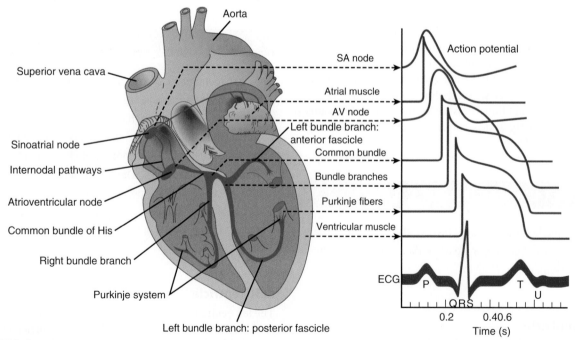

FIGURE 4-8   Anterior view of heart depicting the heart conduction system, action potentials, and ECG waveform representing a typical depolarization/repolarization cycle. (Reproduced with permission from McPhee SJ. *Pathophysiology of Disease: An Introduction to Clinical Medicine.* 6th ed. New York: McGraw-Hill; 2010:250. Redrawn with permission from Ganong WF. *Review of Medical Physiology.* 22nd ed. McGraw-Hill; 2005.)

located in the posterior wall of the right atrium near the entrance of the superior vena cava. It is known as the cardiac pacemaker because it has the fastest rate of impulse generation (ie, 60–100 bpm). Once generated, the impulse spreads via three conduction pathways—the anterior internodal tract of Bachmann, the middle internodal tract of Wenckebach, and the posterior internodal tract of Thorel—that carry the impulse to the AV node.[12] A fourth tract depolarizes the left atrium. Collectively these tracts are called the *internodal conduction pathways.*[11]

The AV node is in the floor of the right atrium near the opening of the coronary sinus. The cardiac impulse travels from the AV node to the Bundle of His, which proceeds through the fibrous skeleton and then divides into the right and left bundle branches that travel inferiorly through the interventricular septum. The left bundle branch bifurcates into anterior and posterior divisions; both bundle branches finally terminate into a network of individual Purkinje fibers that stimulate ventricular contraction.

CLINICAL CORRELATE

A normal electrocardiographic (ECG) signal relies on the structural integrity of the conduction system. Abnormalities in the conduction system will present as abnormalities in the ECG. Myocardial infarctions in the area of the interventricular septum can result in blockage of one of the bundle branches, known as a *bundle branch block.*

Innervation

The heart has its own intrinsic rate of depolarization and subsequent contraction and is not innervated in the same manner that skeletal muscle is (because there is no action potential delivered in response to neurotransmitters). Innervation of the heart allows the autonomic nervous system to influence the heart rate and contractility and therefore allows adjustment in cardiac output based on metabolic demands. The *cardiac plexus* is located anterior to the tracheal bifurcation and consists of both parasympathetic and sympathetic nerves. The parasympathetic system input to the plexus originates through the right and left vagus nerve. The sympathetic input arises from each sympathetic trunk in the neck. The superior cervical, middle cervical, and cervicothoracic ganglion give rise to the superior, middle, and inferior cervical cardiac nerves, respectively. The upper 4 through 5 thoracic ganglia feed into the thoracic cardiac nerves, which also join the cardiac plexus. Both the parasympathetic and sympathetic fibers reach the heart via two coronary plexuses, which branch off from the cardiac plexus. The nerves that branch off the coronary plexuses follow the

coronary vessels to innervate the SA node as well as other components of the conducting system and the atrial and ventricular myocardium. However, the parasympathetic innervation to the ventricular myocardium is sparse, and therefore the sympathetic nervous system has the dominant effect on myocardial contractility.

Coronary Circulation

As with lung airway anatomy, considerable anatomical variation may exist in cardiac circulatory anatomy too. The coronary arteries (CA) terminate in capillaries that supply the myocardium with blood. The *left coronary artery* (LCA) and the *right coronary artery* (RCA) arise from the sinuses of Valsalva (ie, outpouchings of the aortic wall that prevent occlusion of the coronary orifice by the open semilunar valve) just above the aortic valve.[1] The LCA has two main branches—the *left anterior descending* (LAD) and the *left circumflex* (LCX) *arteries* (Fig. 4-9). The coronary arteries course around the heart in two grooves—the atrioventricular groove and the interventricular groove, which meet at the posterior aspect of the heart, known as the crux of the heart. The AV node is located at the crux and is nourished by either the RCA or the LCA. *Right or left coronary dominance* is determined by which artery crosses the crux and supplies the AV node. Fifty percent of people are right coronary artery dominant, 10% to 15% are left coronary dominant, and 35% to 40% have mixed right and left dominance. Lesions (atheromatous plaque, embolisms) of the RCA may produce AV node disturbances. Generally, the RCA supplies the right atrium, the right ventricle, and the inferior wall of the left ventricle. The LAD artery nourishes the anterior wall of the left ventricle. The LCX artery supplies the left atrium and lateral and posterior walls of the left ventricle. In 55% of the population, the sinoatrial (SA) node is nourished by the RCA. A branch of the LCX artery supplies the SA node in the remaining 45%. The AV node is supplied by the RCA in 90%

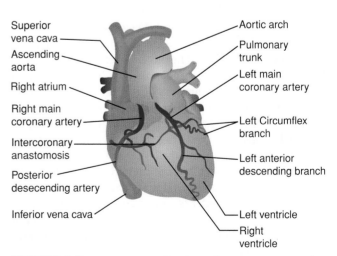

FIGURE 4-9 Anterior view of the heart depicting major vessels and coronary circulation.

of people. In the other 10%, the AV node is supplied by the LCX artery. Lesions of the LCA can interfere with ventricular pumping due to the large amount of myocardial tissue that is supplied by the LCA (Fig. 4-9).

Potential anastomoses (ie, intercoronary channels) exist between the arterial branches. These anastomoses provide collateral circulation if normal coronary vasculature becomes blocked. The heart has an extensive capillary network—approximately 3,300 capillaries/mm^2 or approximately one capillary for each muscle cell. Under conditions of pathological cardiac hypertrophy, for example, the capillary network does not enlarge to accommodate the increase in heart size. This results in lack of oxygen and nutrients to the muscle.

The coronary arteries, reviewed earlier, all travel along the epicardial surface of the heart. These coronary arteries give rise to perforating arteries that diverge at right angles from the main epicardial arteries and travel deep into the myocardium, supplying blood and oxygen to the heart muscle.

The venous system of the heart consists of the thebesian veins, the anterior cardiac veins, and the coronary sinus. The thebesian veins traverse the myocardium, draining a portion of the right atrium, right ventricle, and some of the left ventricle. The anterior cardiac veins drain a large portion of the right ventricle and empty into the right atrium. The coronary sinus and its branches drain most of the myocardium through the great, middle, and small cardiac veins, and the left vein of Marshall (Fig. 4-9).

Circulation and Lymphatics

Blood is brought into close proximity with alveolar air during pulmonary circulation, and it is during systemic circulation that this blood is delivered to the remainder of the body in order to provide oxygen and nutrients to power various metabolic processes. Lymphatic vessels will also be considered in this section because of their anatomical connections to the circulatory system and their histologic similarities with arteries and veins.

The general structure of vessels can be considered regardless of the type of vessel. Vessel wall thickness is a function that depends on the amount of pressure that the vessel must withstand. The inner layer of the vessel is termed the *intima,* which consists of a flattened layer of endothelial cells. The integrity of this layer is essential to normal blood flow and will be discussed in more detail in Chapter 6, when discussing the process of atherosclerosis. In all vessels larger than capillaries, a layer of connective tissue supports this layer of endothelial cells. The intima is surrounded by the *media,* a layer of smooth muscle and elastic tissue. Superficial to the media is a collagenous tissue called the *adventitia.* This outer layer contains the nerves and the small blood vessels that supply the wall of the vessel, and it binds the vessel loosely with connective tissue in the area that they traverse.

Arteries

When the general structure of vessels is analyzed, variation exists both between and within vessels, which can be linked to the functional demands of that vessel. Arteries, at all levels, have a more developed media than veins, and veins are more developed than lymph vessels. The well-developed media within arteries can vary in the amount of elastic versus contractile elements. The elastic elements are more dominant in the proximal arteries, in order to allow greater distension because a larger volume of blood at a higher pressure is ejected through them. This elastic tissue, after being distended, also allows for a smooth transition back to normal between heartbeats. The more distal arteries continue to branch to form the more terminal arterioles, at which point an increasing proportion of contractile elements becomes apparent. The media of smaller arteries and arterioles are almost entirely muscular. The functional benefit of this structural shift is related to the maintenance of blood pressure and to the distribution of peripheral blood flow. The presence of anastomoses is evident as arteries become arterioles and arterioles become capillary beds. *Anastomoses* are connections between arterial branches providing collateral circulation to capillary beds. Their presence is extremely variable within individuals.

CLINICAL CORRELATE

The length–tension curve for skeletal muscular contraction can be applied to the functional properties of the arteries, and the relative components of the media become more significant. Proximal arteries, such as the aorta, contain a greater proportion of elastic tissue. This increases the slope of the passive elastic component of the length–tension relationship, thereby increasing the force of the recoil after distension due to blood ejection. In the more distal arteries, especially arterioles, the media contain a greater proportion of contractile components, thereby allowing a greater proportion of movement and force of contraction by these vessels. In peripheral vascular disease (PVD), peripheral arteriosclerosis may limit contraction of the media. In the proximal arteries, atherosclerosis reduces the distension and recoil force; and in the distal arteries, it reduces the range of movement and force of contraction.

Although most arterioles empty into capillary beds, some form arteriovenous anastomoses by emptying directly into venules. These arterioles tend to have highly contractile walls and therefore assist with the regulation of local blood flow.

Veins

Capillaries terminate into venules, which also exhibit similar endothelial intima as the arterial system, but with the addition of a thin adventitia. Medium-sized veins demonstrate some media, but the media may not continue in veins as they approach the heart. Veins create anastomoses more freely than do arteries, leading to complex networks for drainage of blood from tissue. To ensure proper flow of blood toward the heart, the intima in veins is folded in upon itself, creating valves. These are often bicuspid valves, but may be unicuspid or tricuspid as well. Valves are not present in the abdominal cavity veins of the portal system. However, because of movement of the diaphragm during ventilation, the ventilatory pump assists in the necessary pressure changes for flow back to the heart.

Lymphatics

Lymphatic capillaries are similar in structure to vascular capillaries, and as such they allow certain molecules to pass freely through their walls. Lymphatic capillaries begin blindly in tissue, and the number of lymph capillaries varies depending on the body region. In the central nervous system there are no lymph vessels, whereas in the dermis of the skin, lymph capillaries form dense plexuses. Like the venous system, larger lymphatic vessels are formed by the convergence of smaller vessels and as they get larger, a media begins to appear. Lymph vessels also contain valves, similar to veins, to ensure proper one-way flow of lymph toward the heart.

As they advance toward the venous system, many lymphatics pass through *lymph nodes*. Lymph nodes are collections of lymphocytes, and their precursors are held together by connective tissue and permeated by lymphatic channels. Each lymph node receives a number of lymph vessels, and the lymph from all of these vessels circulates through the lymph channels of the node, exiting through one larger vessel. Lymph may pass through several larger vessels before entering a node, and conversely lymph may pass from one node to another before entering the venous system. All lymph passes through several nodes prior to its entrance into the venous circulation (Chapter 21).

Innervation

Motor innervation of blood vessels is carried out entirely by the sympathetic nervous system.[12] The arterioles have a particularly rich innervation for the control of local blood flow. Afferent fibers leave the blood vessels carrying sensations of pain, and in a few locations (aorta, internal carotids) afferent fibers leave the site of mechanoreceptors or chemoreceptors. Blood vessels are accompanied by nerve plexuses embedded in the adventitia. In the thoracic, abdominal, and cranial vessels, the nerve originating at the base of the vessel is likely to innervate the entire vessel. However, in the limbs a series of interlocking plexuses is fed at regular intervals by nerve branches originating from local peripheral nerves. Innervation allows the regulation of blood flow and distribution of cardiac output by changing the luminal diameter of blood vessels. **Sympathetic activity tends to vasoconstrict blood vessels, whereas local changes associated with increased metabolic rates can vasodilate vessels.**

Pulmonary Circulation

Pulmonary circulation refers to the flow of deoxygenated blood from the systemic veins into the right side of the heart and then into the lungs. Blood flows from the right ventricle through the pulmonary valve to the pulmonary trunk. The pulmonary trunk is divided into the right and left pulmonary arteries that travel to the right and left lungs, respectively. At this point the pulmonary arteries do not follow exactly the same distribution as the bronchial tree, but rather branch in a similar distribution. The pulmonary capillaries form a network in the walls of the alveolar ducts and the alveoli. The pulmonary veins grow larger and often flow between the bronchopulmonary segments draining adjacent segments, eventually leading back to the left atrium.

SUMMARY

This chapter has summarized the basic highlights of cardiopulmonary anatomy relevant to the physical therapist student about to engage in clinical practice. It provides a basis of anatomical and structural knowledge for later chapters in the text, and provides a foundation upon which to integrate knowledge of cardiovascular and pulmonary physiology, evaluation, and intervention strategies for individuals with various cardiopulmonary impairments.

REFERENCES

1. Moore KL. *Clinically Oriented Anatomy*. 3rd ed. Baltimore, MD: Lippincott Williams & Wilkins; 1992.
2. Larsen WJ. *Human Embryology*. New York: Churchill Livingston; 1993.
3. Sadler TW. *Langman's Medical Embryology*. 8th ed. Baltimore, MD: Lippincott Williams & Wilkins; 2000.
4. American Physical Therapy Association. Guide to Physical Therapist Practice. 2nd ed. *Phys Ther*. 2001 Jan;81(1):9-746.
5. Miller AD, Bianchi AL, Bishop BP. *Neural Control of the Respiratory Muscles*. Boca Raton, FL: CRC Press; 1997.
6. De Troyer A. Effect of hyperinflation on the diaphragm. *Eur Respir J*. 1997;10:708.
7. Martinez FJ, Couser JI, Celli BR. Factors influencing ventilatory muscle recruitment in patients with chronic airflow obstruction. *Am Rev Respir Dis*.1990;142: 276.

8. Stern JT. *Essentials of Gross Anatomy.* Philadelphia, PA: FA Davis Company; 1988.

9. Weibel ER. *The Pathway for Oxygen.* Cambridge, MA: Harvard University Press; 1984.

10. Hollinshead WH. *Textbook of Anatomy.* 5th ed. Hagerstown, MD: Harper and Row; 1997.

11. West JB. *Respiratory Physiology: The Essentials.* 2nd ed. Baltimore, MD: Lippincott Williams & Wilkins; 1979.

12. Guyton AC, Hall JE. *Textbook of Medical Physiology.* 9th ed. Philadelphia, PA: WB Saunders; 1998.

Physiology of the Cardiovascular and Pulmonary Systems

5

Barbara J. Morgan & Jerome A. Dempsey

CARDIOVASCULAR SYSTEM PHYSIOLOGY

The major function of the cardiovascular system is to deliver, via the blood, oxygen and nutrients to all tissues of the body and to remove from them carbon dioxide and other waste products of cellular metabolism. In this regard, the cardiovascular system is the link between external respiration (gas exchange between the atmosphere and lungs) and cellular respiration (use of oxygen for energy production by the mitochondria). Other vital functions include, transport of heat to maintain body temperature, delivery of white blood cells to sites where they defend against foreign material, and transport of hormones from the site of release to their target organs. Thus, the cardiovascular system is a key contributor to constancy of the body's internal milieu or homeostasis.

These tasks are accomplished by two interconnected yet distinct components of the cardiovascular system: the pulmonary circulation and the systemic circulation (Fig. 5-1). Each component is made up of (1) a pump (right ventricle for the pulmonary circulation, left ventricle for the systemic circulation) that provides energy to propel the blood, (2) a system of arteries and arterioles that distributes blood throughout the region each pump supplies, (3) a network of capillaries through which gases and nutrients are exchanged with the tissues supplied, and (4) a system of venules and veins that returns the distributed blood to the pump. The two components differ in the amount of the total blood volume each contains at any one point in time, the pressure of operation, thickness of vessel walls, and resistance to blood flow (Table 5-1).

Blood and Its Constituents

Blood is composed of solid components—the red and white blood cells and platelets, which are suspended in a liquid component, the plasma.[1] Plasma is an aqueous solution of gases, salts, carbohydrates, proteins, and lipids. In normal circumstances, the proportion of cells to plasma (the *hematocrit*) is approximately 45%. Normal values for the major blood constituents are shown in Table 5-2. Normal values for blood gases are shown in Table 5-3.

Red Blood Cells

The red blood cells (erythrocytes) are flexible, biconcave disks that contain hemoglobin, a protein that confers on the blood most of its oxygen-carrying capacity. Each molecule of hemoglobin can bind four molecules of oxygen. The amount of oxygen bound to hemoglobin at any point in time depends on the local partial pressure of oxygen (PO_2) (Fig. 5-2).[2] In blood perfusing the lung the high partial pressure of oxygen (100 mm Hg) allows the hemoglobin to become almost completely saturated with oxygen. In blood perfusing peripheral tissue, where the PO_2 is lower (40 mm Hg), oxygen is much less tightly bound to hemoglobin, favoring the release of oxygen to the tissues. The dissociation of oxygen from hemoglobin is facilitated by conditions of increased temperature, increased partial pressure of carbon dioxide (PCO_2), and decreased pH that exist in metabolically active tissue.

White Blood Cells

The main function of the white blood cells (leukocytes) is to protect against invasion by foreign organisms and substances. The five types of leukocytes are neutrophils, eosinophils, basophils, monocytes, and lymphocytes, all of which originate from hemopoietic tissue of the bone marrow and spleen. Many of the white blood cells responsible for the body's defense mechanisms are phagocytic; that is, they contain enzymes that are capable of digesting foreign material. T lymphocytes and B lymphocytes orchestrate the cell-mediated and humoral immune responses, respectively.

Platelets

The platelets play a major role in the body's response to hemorrhage. Platelets aggregate at the site of blood vessel injury, thereby creating a plug that can completely occlude the damaged vessel. Platelets make additional contributions to hemostasis by releasing serotonin (a vasoconstrictor chemical) and thromboplastin (a blood-clotting protein).

Plasma Proteins

The plasma proteins are responsible for a variety of important functions.[1] The clotting proteins are essential for hemostasis; others participate in the immune response; and still others transport lipid molecules, vitamins, hormones, and trace metals. Albumin, the most plentiful of the plasma proteins, is the

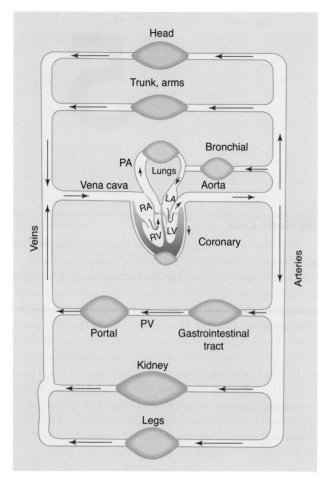

FIGURE 5-1 Schematic representation of the functional divisions of the circulatory system. Note that the pulmonary and systemic circulations are connected in series so that the blood flows through the chambers of the right heart and the lungs, then to the chambers of the left heart, and the rest of the body. RA, right atrium; RV, right ventricle; LA, left atrium; LV, left ventricle; PA, pulmonary artery; PV, portal vein. (Modified with permission from West JB, ed. *Best and Taylor's Physiological Basis of Medical Practice*. 12th ed. Baltimore, MD: Lippincott Williams & Wilkins; 1991.)

primary protein responsible for the plasma's colloid osmotic pressure (also called oncotic pressure). The colloid osmotic pressure is a major determinant of the movement of fluid across the capillary wall. Albumin and most of the other plasma proteins are manufactured in the liver.

TABLE 5-1   Comparison of the Systemic and Pulmonary Circulations

	Systemic Circulation	Pulmonary Circulation
Distribution of total blood volume (%)	80–95	5–20
Pump (ventricular) pressure (mm Hg)	120/0	25/0
Distributing artery pressure (mm Hg)	120/80	25/10
Vessel wall thickness	Thick	Thin
Resistance to blood flow	High	Low

TABLE 5-2   Normal Values for the Major Constituents of Blood

Constituent	Normal Value
Hematocrit	45%
Red blood cell count	5×10^{12} cells/L
Hemoglobin	15 g/dL
White blood cell count	5×10^{9} cells/L
Platelets	250×10^{9} cells/L
Plasma proteins	7 g/dL
Na^+	140 mEq/L
Cl^-	100 mEq/L
K^+	3.5–5 mEq/L

Heart As a Pump

The right and left ventricles function as two pumps connected in series: The right ventricle pumps blood into the lungs for the exchange of CO_2 and O_2, and the left ventricle pumps blood to all other tissues of the body (Fig. 5-1). Because of this serial arrangement, the amounts of blood pumped per unit time by the right and left ventricles are (must be) equal. An equal amount of flow can be generated at a much lower pressure in the pulmonary circulation because vascular resistance is lower than in the systemic circulation. This lower resistance is due to the shorter, wider, and more highly distensible vessels in the pulmonary circulation.

Determinants of Pump Function

How well (or poorly) the heart performs its crucial pumping role has a major impact on the health of the individual. Rhythmic, coordinated pumping of the cardiac chambers depends on the unique physical and electrical properties of the "working" myocytes that generate the energy to propel blood and the "conduction" myocytes that are responsible for the spread of electrical impulses through the heart.

In myocardial cells, as in all excitable tissues, an action potential is generated when the electrical voltage difference across the cell membrane is reduced to a threshold level.[3] The working myocytes, which have more negative resting membrane potentials, are referred to as fast-response cells because their action potentials are characterized by a rapid upstroke. The conduction cells located in the sinoatrial (SA) and atrioventricular (AV) nodes have less negative resting membrane potentials and are referred to as slow-response cells because their action potentials have gradual upstrokes (Chapter 4, Fig. 4-10). The cells of the heart's conduction system are capable of spontaneous depolarization because their resting membrane potentials are close to threshold and because their membrane potentials are inherently unstable. These electrical characteristics of conduction system cells are the basis of automaticity and rhythmicity (the ability of the heart to initiate its own beat at a regular rate)—two inherent traits of the heart.

TABLE 5-3   Blood Gas and Acid–Base Values for Healthy Subjects Under Resting Conditions

Site	O$_2$ Saturation (%)	Po$_2$ (mm Hg)	Pco$_2$ (mm Hg)	pH (Units)	[HCO$_3^-$] (mEq/Li)
Systemic arteries	97	90–95	40	7.4 (7.35–7.45)	24 (23–26)
Pulmonary artery (mixed venous)	75	40	46	7.36	28

Cardiac contraction is initiated when action potentials that arise in conduction cells spread across the working cells of the myocardium.

The myocardium, because of its multicellular structure, behaves like a syncytium. Gap junctions between adjacent cells allow cell-to-cell propagation of electrical impulses. An action potential arriving at the myocardial cell membrane depolarizes the membrane and triggers the chain of events that culminates in myocardial contraction. Calcium ion flux is the physiological basis for this excitation–contraction coupling. Depolarization of the cell membrane increases its permeability to calcium ions. In addition, the action potential is transmitted to the interior of the cell along T-tubule membranes where it mobilizes stored calcium ions from the sarcoplasmic reticulum. The resultant increase in intracellular calcium concentration initiates actin–myosin binding, cross-bridge formation, and sarcomere shortening. The magnitude of the increase in intracellular calcium concentration determines the number of cross-bridges formed and therefore the strength of the resulting contraction. During repolarization of the cell membrane, calcium is extruded from the cell and resequestered in the sarcoplasmic reticulum and, as a result, actin and myosin filaments disengage and sarcomeres lengthen.

Coordinated pumping of the upper and lower chambers— The heart functions most efficiently as a pump when atrial and ventricular contractions have the appropriate temporal relationship. That is, the ventricles discharge optimum stroke volumes only if the time delay between atrial and ventricular contraction is sufficient to allow filling of the ventricles prior to systole.

Coordinated contraction and relaxation of myocardial cells in the upper and lower chambers is ensured by the heart's conduction system, the principal components of which are the SA node, the AV node, the bundle of His and bundle branches, and the Purkinje fibers (Chapter 4, Fig. 4-10). Action potentials arising in the SA node are propagated through the atrial myocardium to the AV node—the sole route of impulse conduction from the atria to the ventricles. The relatively slow conduction velocity that is characteristic of AV nodal tissue accounts for a brief pause between atrial and ventricular contraction. From the AV node, impulses travel through the bundle of His to the bundle branches that innervate the left and right ventricles. The terminal elements in the conduction system are the Purkinje fibers. Their relatively fast conduction velocities ensure rapid spread of the wave of depolarization throughout the ventricular mass.

As mentioned earlier, the term *automaticity* refers to the inherent ability of myocardial cells to generate action potentials without depolarizing input from an external source.[3] All portions of the heart's conduction system contain automatic cells. Even though any one of them is capable of initiating a cardiac cycle, the SA node normally assumes the role of pacemaker because it has an inherent discharge rate that is faster than that of other conduction system cells. The other potential pacemakers become hyperpolarized when they are paced at rates faster than their own inherent rates—a phenomenon known as overdrive suppression. Under pathological conditions, conduction system cells outside of the SA node can assume the pacing role when SA node function is depressed, when pathways from the SA node are blocked, or when these cells become "irritable" (ie, their own rhythmicity is enhanced). In these circumstances, the cells responsible for initiating the heartbeat are referred to as ectopic pacemakers. Cardiac rhythm disturbances arise when the heart's conduction system is damaged by disease or when ectopic pacemakers usurp the pacing function.

When the coordinated pumping of the heart's chambers is compromised by rhythm disturbances, deterioration in pump

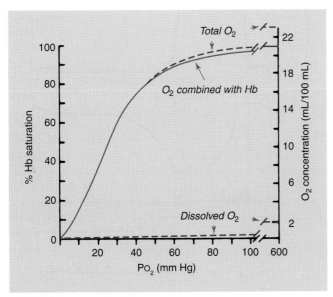

FIGURE 5-2   Relationship of Po$_2$ to O$_2$ content in plasma (dissolved O$_2$), in hemoglobin (Hbo$_2$) and in whole blood (total O$_2$ = Hbo$_2$ + dissolved O$_2$). The actual numbers for Hbo$_2$ content will depend on the hemoglobin concentration. The example above is for a normal concentration of 15 g/100 mL. This Po$_2$/% Hbo$_2$ relationship holds for conditions of normal blood pH (7.40) and temperature (37°C). (Used with permission from West JB. *Respiratory Physiology—The Essentials*. 5th ed. Baltimore, MD: Lippincott Williams & Wilkins; 1995.)

function almost always ensues. When the atria and ventricles do not contract in sequential fashion, for example, in atrial fibrillation or complete heart block (Chapter 10), loss of atrial contribution to ventricular filling leads to a decrement in ventricular pump performance. Frequent premature contractions can result in life-threatening hypotension due to inadequate ventricular filling time.

Adequacy of coronary blood supply—The heart is dependent on the coronary arteries for its own blood supply (Chapter 4, Fig. 4-11). When the coronary blood supply is inadequate to meet the myocardium's metabolic demands, for example, when the arterial lumen is narrowed by atherosclerotic plaque (Chapter 6), pump function can be compromised in several ways. The resultant ischemia has a negative effect on the contractile state of the myocardium and predisposes the heart to serious rhythm disturbances. Complete, prolonged blockage of a coronary artery (eg, in myocardial infarction) results in myocardial cell death. The necrotic cells in the affected area are eventually replaced with a firm scar; however, the noncontractile scar tissue does not contribute to the heart's pumping function. Such loss of myocardium negatively affects the contractile state of the myocardium.

Unidirectional flow of blood through the heart—Unidirectional flow of blood through the heart is ensured by two sets of valves that operate reciprocally (Chapter 4, Fig. 4-9). The atrioventricular valves (mitral and tricuspid) control blood flow from the atria to the ventricles. The semilunar valves (aortic and pulmonic) control flow out of the ventricles. These valves, which consist of thin fibrous tissue flaps, or leaflets, open and close passively in response to changes in the chamber pressure. That is, when myocardial contraction raises the pressure within a given chamber above the downstream pressure, the valve opens. When contraction ceases and pressure within the chamber drops below the downstream pressure, the valve closes. The leaflets of the atrioventricular valves are attached to papillary muscles in the ventricular walls by strong bands of fibrous tissue called chordae tendineae. The chordae are "tethers" that prevent bulging of the leaflets and the regurgitation of blood back into the atria during ventricular contraction.

Malfunctioning valves can compromise pump performance by interfering with the forward flow of blood. A valve that fails to close completely is said to be *incompetent* or *insufficient*. An incompetent valve is leaky; that is, it allows regurgitation of a portion of the stroke volume into the upstream chamber. When a *stenotic* valve fails to open fully, it forces the upstream chamber to contract more vigorously in order to discharge the stroke volume. When valvular dysfunction is present for months or years, the myocardium undergoes hypertrophy to compensate for the pressure or volume overload caused by the faulty valve, and cardiac output is maintained at relatively normal levels. In contrast, when valvular dysfunction occurs acutely, such as when a papillary muscle ruptures as a result of myocardial infarction, a life-threatening reduction in pump performance may occur.

Events of the Cardiac Cycle

The period of time between successive heartbeats is the cardiac cycle. Figure 5-3 shows the temporal relationships between the electrical and mechanical events of the cardiac cycle, the heart sounds, and changes in ventricular volume.[4] Note that Fig. 5-3 shows only left atrial, left ventricular and aortic pressures, and left ventricular volume. The relationships depicted here also exist in the right heart during the cardiac cycle; however, the operating pressures are much lower (Table 5-1).

Electrical events—The cardiac cycle is initiated when the action potentials that arise in the SA node cause *a wave of depolarization* that spreads first through the atria (Chapter 4, Fig. 4-10). The impulses are then conducted to the AV node and finally to the ventricles. The electrical fields created by summation of action potentials in myocardial cells are conducted through the electrolyte-containing fluids of the body and can be recorded from the body surface as the

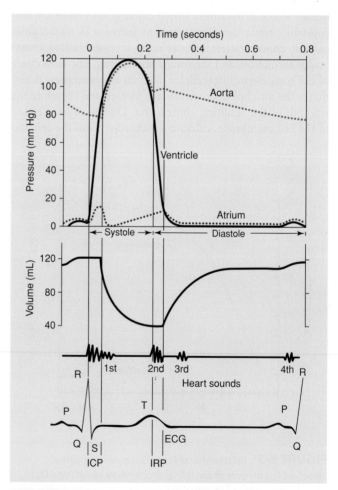

FIGURE 5-3   Mechanical and electrical events of the cardiac cycle. ICP, isovolumic contraction period; IRP, isovolumic relaxation period; ECG, electrocardiogram. (Used with permission from Smith JJ, Kampine JP. *Circulatory Physiology—The Essentials*. 3rd ed. Baltimore, MD: Lippincott Williams & Wilkins; 1998.)

electrocardiogram (ECG) (Fig. 5-3). By convention, deflections on the ECG tracing are called the P, Q, R, S, and T waves. The first positive deflection (relative to the tracing's baseline) of the cardiac cycle, the P wave, represents atrial depolarization. The first negative deflection, the Q wave, is normally small and may not always be seen. The positive deflection after the Q wave (or the second positive deflection if no Q wave is present) is the R wave. The S wave is the negative deflection after the R wave. The QRS complex represents ventricular depolarization. After a pause, the T wave follows the S wave. The T wave represents ventricular repolarization.

Ventricular systole—Close inspection of the ventricular volume tracing in Fig. 5-3 reveals that ventricular systole consists of three parts: an isovolumic contraction period (ICP), a rapid ejection period, and a slower ejection period. During the ICP, ventricular pressure rises, but there is no change in ventricular volume because the mitral and aortic valves are closed. Once the aortic valve opens, the period of rapid ejection begins. Ventricular and aortic pressures rise to a peak in this period, and approximately two-thirds of the ventricular volume is emptied into the aorta. During the subsequent slower ejection period, ventricular and aortic pressures begin to fall. When ventricular pressure falls below aortic pressure, the aortic valve closes. Closure of the aortic valve marks the beginning of the isovolumic relaxation period (IRP) during which ejection of blood ceases and ventricular pressure falls dramatically.

Note that the ventricle does not empty completely during systole. The residual volume (end-systolic volume) is roughly equal to the amount of blood ejected from the ventricle during systole. **The *ejection fraction*, that is, the percentage of the end-diastolic volume ejected during the subsequent systole, is a clinically useful index of cardiac pump function. Ejection fraction is increased in situations where force of contraction is augmented (eg, during exercise) and is reduced in situations where force of contraction is diminished (eg, cardiomyopathy, ischemic heart disease).**

Ventricular diastole—The IRP is the initial phase of ventricular diastole. When ventricular pressure falls below atrial pressure, the mitral valve opens and diastolic filling of the ventricle commences. A period of rapid filling occurs immediately after the valve opens, followed by a period of more gradual filling, called diastasis. Ventricular filling is completed when the P wave that initiates the next cardiac cycle causes atrial contraction, which leads to a further increase in ventricular volume and pressure. This atrial contribution to ventricular filling, which has been termed the *atrial kick*, is important mainly during fast heart rates, when time for ventricular filling is limited.

Regulation of Cardiac Output

The preceding sections outlined several aspects of normal physiology that enable the heart to function as an efficient pump. The end product of this pumping function, the cardiac output, must be adequate to meet metabolic needs of the tissues of the body in a wide variety of conditions that threaten homeostasis. The major determinants of cardiac output are preload, afterload, contractile state (by virtue of their influence on stroke volume), and heart rate. **Cardiac output is the product of stroke volume and heart rate. The *cardiac index*, a clinically useful indicator of pump performance in individuals of varying sizes, is calculated by dividing the cardiac output by body surface area. The normal value for cardiac index in an adult is 3 L/min/m².**

Stroke volume—Stroke volume, the amount of blood pumped with each heartbeat, is influenced both by *intrinsic factors* (ie, those determined by properties of the heart muscle itself) and by *extrinsic factors* (ie, those imposed by neural stimulation, hormones, drugs, and disease). The most important intrinsic regulator of stroke volume is myocardial cell length. Within physiological limits, the force generated by the contracting myocardium increases in direct proportion to its precontraction length (the Frank-Starling mechanism).[5] A family of curves that depict the relationship between end-diastolic volume and ventricular performance is shown in the left-hand portion of Fig. 5-4. The particular curve on which the ventricle operates at any point in time is determined by the contractile, or *inotropic*, state of the myocardium (right-hand portion of Fig. 5-4). Factors that increase contractility will cause the curve to shift up and to the left. Factors that have a negative influence on contractility will shift the curve down and to the right. The Frank-Starling mechanism is analogous to the length–tension relationship in skeletal muscle. As is the case with skeletal muscle, when the heart muscle is stretched beyond the length that is optimal for myofibrillar cross-bridge formation, force generation decreases. The dashed lines in the two lower curves illustrate this situation. The clinical concept of *preload* refers

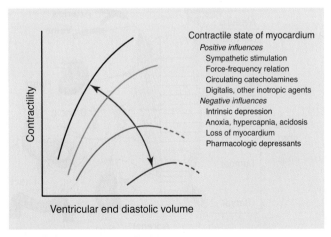

FIGURE 5-4 Determinants of myocardial contractility and ventricular performance. End diastolic volume. (Used with permission from Braunwald E, Ross J, Sonnenblick EH. *Mechanisms of Contraction of the Normal and Failing Heart*. 2nd ed. Philadelphia, PA: Lippincott Williams & Wilkins; 1976.)

to the effect of myocardial stretch prior to contraction (ie, the end-diastolic volume) on stroke volume. In patients with ventricular dysfunction due to disease, many pharmacologic treatments are aimed at optimizing ventricular performance by altering preload (Chapter 8).

Another intrinsic regulatory mechanism is the force–frequency relationship, whereby increases in the heart rate, per se, cause increases in myocardial force generation. The physiologic basis for the relationship between frequency and force is an increase in the amount of calcium ions available for excitation–contraction coupling that occurs at high heart rates.

The load against which the ventricles must pump to eject blood is referred to as *afterload*—another intrinsic regulator of pump performance.[4] Increases in afterload can have a negative effect on pump performance. For example, when pressure in the aorta is increased suddenly, the left ventricular stroke volume falls. In the healthy heart, the reduction in stroke volume is only temporary because compensatory mechanisms come into play. In patients with ventricular dysfunction, high afterload has a significant deleterious effect on cardiac output. In the clinical setting, the systemic arterial pressure provides an estimate of left ventricular afterload. Pharmacological treatment aimed at afterload reduction is a commonly used strategy for treatment of ventricular dysfunction (Chapter 8).

A chronic state of intrinsic depression can occur when myocardial cells are damaged by exposure to adverse loading conditions, toxins, and infectious processes. After myocardial infarction (Chapter 6), necrosis of cells and subsequent replacement with scar tissue can depress the contractile state, provided that sufficient numbers of cells are lost. Insufficient blood supply to myocardial tissue depresses inotropic state because of the anoxia, hypercapnia, and acidosis caused by ischemia.

Factors extrinsic to the heart also serve as important regulators of the inotropic state.[3] The neurotransmitter norepinephrine, released locally when the sympathetic nerves fire, increases inotropic state. Release of acetylcholine from the parasympathetic nerve terminals produces a negative inotropic effect, mainly in the atria. Catecholamine hormones epinephrine and norepinephrine, which are released into the blood stream by the adrenal glands, circulate to the heart and positively influence contractility. Pharmacologic agents such as digitalis, amrinone, and isoproterenol increase inotropic state, whereas barbiturates, calcium antagonists, and anesthetic agents decrease inotropic state (Chapter 8).

Heart rate—Because cardiac output is the product of heart rate and stroke volume, the heart rate contributes importantly to the heart's function as a pump. In situations when a change in cardiac output is necessary (eg, during exercise), the heart rate is regulated by neural, chemical, and intrinsic mechanisms.

Neural regulation of the heart rate is under the control of the sympathetic and parasympathetic divisions of the autonomic nervous system (Fig. 5-5).[4] Parasympathetic fibers, which travel to the heart via the vagus nerve, innervate the SA node, the AV node, and atrial muscle. When these nerve fibers are activated, they slow the heart rate and decrease the rate of conduction through the AV node. Sympathetic neurons from the thoracic cord travel to the heart in the superior, middle, and inferior cardiac nerves. They innervate the heart's conduction system as well as the atrial and ventricular muscles. When the sympathetic nerves fire, they increase heart rate and the rate of conduction through the AV node. In addition to their effects on heart rate, parasympathetic and sympathetic neural impulses regulate cardiac output by decreasing and increasing, respectively, the force of myocardial contraction.

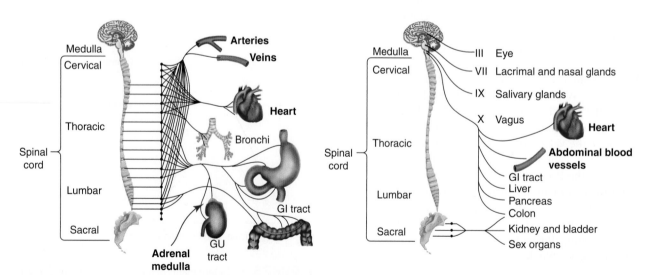

FIGURE 5-5   Sympathetic (**left**) and parasympathetic (**right**) divisions of the autonomic nervous system and the structures innervated by each division. GI, gastrointestinal; GU, genitourinary. (Modified with permission from Smith JJ, Kampine JP. *Circulatory Physiology—The Essentials*. 3rd ed. Baltimore, MD: Lippincott Williams & Wilkins; 1998.)

The most important natural chemical regulators of cardiac output are the catecholamines (norepinephrine and epinephrine) secreted by the adrenal glands. When these hormones bind to β-adrenergic receptors in the SA node and myocardial cells, they increase heart rate and the force of contraction. In the clinical setting, pharmacologic agents are used to regulate (either increase or decrease) the heart rate and force of contraction (Chapter 8).

In addition to the neural and chemical regulators of heart rate, two intrinsic factors play a small role in heart rate control. The stretch of the SA node and increased body temperature both increase heart rate. **The primary determinants of the heart's performance as a pump are preload, afterload, heart rate, and contractility.**

The Arterial Systems

Arteries comprise the distributing systems for the pulmonary and systemic circulations. Within the systemic circulation, the various vascular beds are arranged as parallel circuits (Fig. 5-1).[1] One or more large arteries supply each organ or type of tissue (eg, the kidney or skeletal muscle). These arteries divide multiple times within the organ and eventually give rise to arterioles, the primary resistance vessels in the systemic circulation. The arterioles are thick-walled, muscular vessels that regulate distribution of blood flow to the capillary beds via changes in their caliber. Arteriolar diameter is controlled by sympathetic neural activity, circulating hormones, locally produced metabolites, and local mechanical factors that influence vascular smooth muscle tone. Because of the parallel arrangement of the systemic circuits, the amount of flow through each vascular bed can be controlled separately, according to the level of tissue activity. For example, after a large meal, large amounts of blood are diverted to the gastrointestinal tract to support the process of digestion. At the same time, blood flow to nonessential (for the moment) vascular beds is reduced.

The pulmonary circulation comprises the pulmonary trunk, the right and left pulmonary arteries, and their divisions within each lung.[1] The pulmonary arteries are well supplied with sympathetic and parasympathetic nerve fibers; however, this innervation does not play an important role in regulating pulmonary vascular resistance. Instead, the vascular smooth muscle of the pulmonary bed is responsive to local chemical influences. Hypoxic vasoconstriction of the pulmonary vasculature is a local phenomenon that occurs in regions of the lung that contain oxygen-poor air. This mechanism is important in maintaining high pulmonary vascular resistance during fetal life when only a small fraction of the cardiac output circulates through the pulmonary bed. After birth, when the infant's first breath oxygenates previously hypoxic alveoli, pulmonary vascular resistance falls dramatically due to reversal of hypoxic vasoconstriction. In postnatal life, hypoxic vasoconstriction is beneficial when a portion of the lung becomes hypoxic due to bronchial obstruction. In this case, hypoxic vasoconstriction redistributes blood flow away from the hypoxic region toward adequately ventilated areas of the lung, thereby minimizing the deleterious effect of the obstruction on gas exchange. However, when the entire lung is hypoxic (eg, at high altitude or in pulmonary disease), sustained hypoxic vasoconstriction results in pulmonary hypertension and, eventually, right ventricular dysfunction.

Hemodynamics

Blood flow through the cardiovascular system is influenced both by events in the central circulation (the driving pressure generated by the pump) and by the peripheral circulation (the resistance to flow generated by the arterioles). Ohm's law, originally used to describe the factors that govern flow of electrical current, can also explain the relationships among pressure, flow, and resistance in the circulatory system.[3] The following formula shows that blood flow (F) through a vascular bed is directly proportional to the pressure gradient across the bed (ΔP) and is inversely proportional to the resistance (R) offered by the arterioles:

$$F \propto \frac{\Delta P}{R}.$$

The pressure at the inlet of any bed is roughly equal to the mean arterial pressure (one-third pulse pressure + diastolic pressure). The pressure at the outlet of the bed is equal to its venous pressure. These same principles can be applied to the circulatory system as a whole. Flow (cardiac output) is directly proportional to the pressure gradient (aortic pressure minus right atrial pressure) and inversely proportional to total peripheral resistance (the sum of the reciprocals of resistances in the individual vascular beds).

Poiseuille's law states that laminar flow through a rigid cylinder varies directly with the pressure gradient and inversely with the radius and length of the tube and the viscosity of the fluid.[3] Of course, blood flow through the cardiovascular system does not meet the criteria specified by Poiseuille; nevertheless, the following formula, based on Poiseuille's law, is useful for explaining the relationship among factors that influence vascular resistance:

$$\text{Resistance} = \frac{8nL}{\pi r^4},$$

where n = blood viscosity, L = vessel length, and r = vessel radius. Note that the radius term in this equation is raised to the fourth power. **This means that even very small changes in the radius can result in large changes in resistance.**

The term *vasoconstriction* refers to an increase in vascular resistance. Conversely, *vasodilation* refers to a decrease in resistance. Note that increases and decreases in blood flow do not always imply vasodilation and vasoconstriction. According to Ohm's law, these changes can also occur "passively" secondary to changes in perfusion pressure. **Blood flow through a vascular bed is equal to perfusion pressure divided by resistance. The primary determinant of resistance is vessel caliber.**

Regulation of Arterial Flow

The caliber of arterioles, the primary resistance vessels in the systemic circulation, is determined by the net effect of multiple, simultaneous constrictor and dilator influences. These neural, chemical, and mechanical factors are summarized in Fig. 5-6.

Arterioles throughout the body are innervated by sympathetic, noradrenergic nerve fibers.[3] When these nerves fire, norepinephrine is released from storage granules into the synaptic cleft. The released norepinephrine then binds to postsynaptic α-adrenergic receptors on vascular smooth muscle, thereby triggering vasoconstriction. Sympathetic vasoconstrictor neurons that innervate arterioles in skeletal muscle and many other vascular beds are tonically active and contribute importantly to maintaining blood pressure homeostasis. Sympathetic vasoconstrictor impulses originate from vasomotor centers in the brainstem. Reflexes arising in the peripheral sensory receptors (eg, baroreceptors and chemoreceptors) modulate the level of central sympathetic outflow in response to perturbations of homeostasis. In addition to this neural mechanism, the radius of arterioles is decreased by increases in the local concentrations of vasoconstrictor hormones (eg, angiotensin, vasopressin). Neural and humoral vasoconstrictor mechanisms both contribute importantly to the maintenance of blood pressure and blood volume (eg, during the shift from supine to upright posture).

Conversely, the radius of the resistance vessels increases and vasodilation occurs when sympathetic stimulation is withdrawn. In addition, local accumulation of vasodilator substances (eg, adenosine) plays an important role in the vasodilation that is produced by an increase in an organ's metabolic rate (eg, exercise-induced vasodilation in skeletal muscle).

The vascular endothelium plays an important role in the local regulation of vascular smooth muscle tone.[3] The endothelium participates in vasodilator responses, vasoconstrictor responses, and in vascular adaptations to long-term stimuli. It releases at least two potent vasodilator substances, nitric oxide and prostacyclin, in response to changes in chemical concentrations within the blood. This mechanism is thought to be the basis for the endothelium's role in metabolically mediated vasodilation. Vascular endothelium also mediates flow-induced vasodilation. The endothelial monolayer is in direct contact with blood flowing through the vessel lumen and therefore is subject to increased shear stress when flow increases. Nitric oxide and prostacyclin are released from the endothelium in response to an increase in shear stress. The vascular endothelium also produces locally active vasoconstrictor substances (eg, endothelin-1 and thromboxane) that participate in the regulation of arteriolar tone; however, nitric oxide seems to be the most important endothelial factor under normal conditions. In addition to its role in the regulation of vascular tone, the endothelium also plays a crucial role in preventing blood coagulation via its inhibitory effects on platelet aggregation (Chapter 6).

Myogenic contraction and relaxation are intrinsic qualities of vascular smooth muscle that contribute importantly to

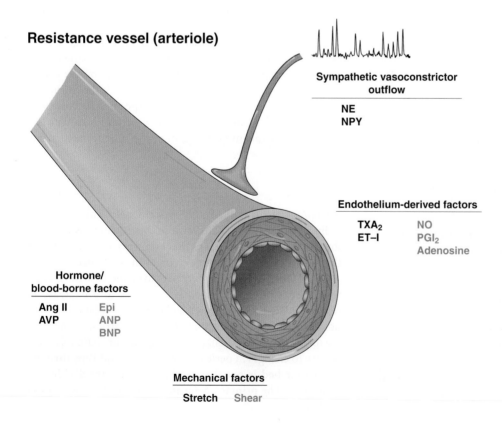

Resistance vessel (arteriole)

Sympathetic vasoconstrictor outflow

NE
NPY

Endothelium-derived factors

TXA$_2$	NO
ET–I	PGI$_2$
	Adenosine

Hormone/blood-borne factors

Ang II	Epi
AVP	ANP
	BNP

Mechanical factors

Stretch   Shear

FIGURE 5-6   Summary of the neural, chemical, and mechanical factors that determine the caliber of resistance arterioles. Constrictor influences (shown in black) are opposed by dilator influences (shown in gray). Ang II, angiotensin II; AVP, arginine vasopressin; Epi, epinephrine; ANP, atrial natriuretic peptide; BNP, brain natriuretic peptide; NE, norepinephrine; NPY, neuropeptide Y; TXA$_2$, thromboxane; ET-I, endothelin-I; NO, nitric oxide; PGI$_2$, prostacyclin.

basal tone in the arterioles. Myogenic vasoconstriction occurs in response to stretch of vascular smooth muscle; that is, when transmural pressure at the arteriolar level rises, vascular smooth muscle is stimulated to contract. When transmural pressure falls, vasodilation occurs.

Because vascular beds in the systemic circulation are arranged as parallel circuits, the resistance in each bed can be regulated separately. The resultant differential distribution of the cardiac output is essential for maintaining homeostasis under a wide range of metabolic and environmental conditions.

The Capillary Exchange System

Capillaries are narrow vessels constructed of a single layer of endothelial cells. Flow through the capillaries is continuous, nonpulsatile, and relatively slow due to the large cross-sectional area of the capillary bed. Thus, the capillary bed is well suited for exchange of gases, nutrients, and waste products between blood and tissues. These substances cross the capillary walls either by diffusion or by filtration and reabsorption, depending primarily on their lipid solubility.

Diffusion of Gases and Molecules

Lipid-soluble molecules, such as O_2 and CO_2, diffuse directly through the lipoprotein membrane of the capillary endothelium.[3] The rate of diffusion is proportional to the difference in gas partial pressures on either side of the membrane and to the area of interface, and inversely proportional to membrane thickness. The following formula illustrates the relationships between the factors that influence the rate of diffusion:

$$\text{Rate of diffusion of a gas} = \frac{A \times D \times \Delta P}{T},$$

where A = area of the sheet of tissue, D = diffusion constant (based on properties of the tissue and the gas), ΔP = pressure gradient across the sheet of tissue, and T = thickness of the tissue.

Water-soluble molecules, such as inorganic ions, proteins, and glucose, travel through pores located between the endothelial cells. The process of filtration and reabsorption aids the movement of these water-soluble substances.

Transcapillary Movement of Fluid

In addition to the exchange of gases, nutrients, and waste products, there is a constant movement of fluid across the capillary wall that is caused by the forces shown in Fig. 5-7.[4] At the arterial end of the capillary, the intravascular pressure is high (~30 mm Hg), relative to the pressure of the fluid in the interstitial space (~0 mm Hg), and is higher than the colloid osmotic pressure exerted by the plasma proteins. This pressure gradient causes the fluid to move out of the capillary into the interstitial space (filtration). At the venous end of the capillary, the intravascular pressure is still high relative to interstitial pressure, but both pressures are lower than the colloid osmotic pressure, which pulls fluid back into the capillary (reabsorption). Normally, 85% of the fluid that is filtered is reabsorbed. The remainder is drained from the area via the lymphatic system. Thus, there is no accumulation of fluid in the interstitial space. When the balance among filtration, reabsorption, and drainage is upset, edema formation occurs. Conditions that promote edema formation include venous hypertension (which limits reabsorption by raising intravascular pressure at the venous end of the capillary), blockage of lymphatic drainage vessels, decreased plasma protein concentration, and increased permeability of the capillary wall.

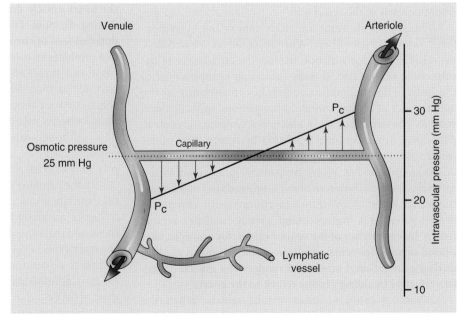

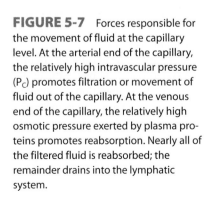

FIGURE 5-7 Forces responsible for the movement of fluid at the capillary level. At the arterial end of the capillary, the relatively high intravascular pressure (P_C) promotes filtration or movement of fluid out of the capillary. At the venous end of the capillary, the relatively high osmotic pressure exerted by plasma proteins promotes reabsorption. Nearly all of the filtered fluid is reabsorbed; the remainder drains into the lymphatic system.

The Lymphatic System

Lymphatics are tiny, extremely thin-walled vessels that are not connected in series with the arteries and veins.[4] A primary function of the lymphatic system is to return excess tissue fluid to the intravascular compartment. The lymph vessels accomplish this task by collecting fluid that has been filtered but not reabsorbed at the capillary level (Fig. 5-7) and returning it to the central circulation via a system of regional watersheds. Lymph vessels in peripheral tissue combine to form collecting ducts that are lined with smooth muscle and equipped with one-way valves that ensure unidirectional flow. As the lymph is propelled toward the central circulation, it flows through a series of successively larger vessels that merge to form the thoracic ducts that empty into the subclavian veins. On its route from peripheral tissue to the central circulation, lymph passes through at least one regional lymph node. These nodes contain filtration systems lined with phagocytic cells that engulf and neutralize bacteria and other foreign material (Chapter 22).

The Venous System

Blood is returned to the heart from the periphery through the systemic veins.[4] These veins are compliant, thin-walled vessels that contain valves to ensure one-way flow of blood. Because they are highly compliant, the veins act as reservoirs for blood; therefore, they are referred to as capacitance vessels. At any one time, approximately 60% of the total blood volume is contained within the systemic veins.

Regulation of Venous Flow and Volume

Through active and passive changes in their capacity, the veins regulate the amount of venous return to the heart. The volume of blood stored in a venous bed is dependent on the pressure gradient across the bed and the level of "tone" present in smooth muscle of the vessel wall.[6]

The splanchnic veins are richly innervated by sympathetic vasoconstrictor fibers. When these nerves are activated, the resulting venoconstriction reduces the capacitance of the splanchnic venous bed, thereby increasing venous return to the heart. This mechanism contributes importantly to the maintenance of cardiac output during postural shifts in blood volume. The cutaneous veins, also under sympathetic control, participate in temperature regulation by constricting under cold conditions and dilating in the heat. In contrast, veins in skeletal muscle do not receive sympathetic innervation. When a muscle contracts, however, blood is squeezed out of the veins contained within it. Working in concert with competent venous valves, this "muscle pump" greatly facilitates venous return. **Incompetence of the venous valves, for example, that caused by varicose veins, results in excessive venous pooling during gravitational stress and renders the muscle pump less effective in aiding venous return to the heart.**

Breathing can also affect venous return. When the diaphragm descends during inspiration, intrathoracic pressure decreases and intra-abdominal pressure rises. The gradient between the abdomen and thorax is thus increased, causing blood to flow from the inferior vena cava into the right heart. **The systemic veins act as a reservoir for blood. Through active and passive changes in their capacity, they continuously regulate central blood volume and cardiac filling pressures.**

Special Characteristics of the Regional Circulations

The factors responsible for regulation of blood flow are not the same in all organs and vascular beds. In fact, there are marked regional differences in circulatory control mechanisms. In this section, regulation of coronary, pulmonary, skeletal muscle, and cerebral blood flow will be discussed.

Coronary Blood Flow

The left and right coronary arteries and their major branches are epicardial; that is, they lie on the surface of the heart. The epicardial arteries branch to form the endocardial coronary arteries that penetrate the heart muscle at right angles. The majority of the heart's venous blood drains into the right atrium via the cardiac veins and the coronary sinus.

As blood traverses the coronary vascular bed, extraction of oxygen from it is nearly complete, even at resting levels of *myocardial oxygen consumption* ($M\dot{V}O_2$). Consequently, the oxygen content of blood in the coronary sinus is approximately one-third of that found in the venous drainage of resting skeletal muscle. **Because of this high degree of extraction, increases in $M\dot{V}O_2$ must be accommodated by increases in the rate of oxygen delivery via coronary blood flow.**

Mechanical and metabolic factors are the primary determinants of the rate of blood flow through the coronary arteries.[3] **The coronary arteries are compressed by contraction of the heart muscle during systole; therefore, they fill mainly during diastole. Diastolic pressure, then, is the primary determinant of coronary perfusion pressure.** Any condition that produces an increase in the work of the heart (eg, exercise, emotional stress) also causes an increase in the rate of coronary blood flow. Metabolic by-products of cardiac muscle contraction are thought to be responsible for this close coupling between myocardial metabolism and coronary blood flow. Although the specific chemical mediators of this response have not been identified, adenosine is thought to play an important role in metabolic vasodilation.

In the coronary circulation, unlike the peripheral circulation, the autonomic nervous system seems to have little direct influence on blood flow. Nevertheless, alterations in sympathetic and parasympathetic outflows to the heart can influence coronary blood flow indirectly because they affect heart rate and force of contraction—the two primary determinants of the myocardium's metabolic rate. The double product, an estimate of ($M\dot{V}O_2$) that is useful clinically, is calculated by multiplying heart rate by systolic blood pressure.

Autoregulation is an intrinsic regulatory characteristic of the coronary vascular bed and other beds (eg, the cerebral circulation) that have low levels of neural control. When perfusion pressure in one of these vascular beds is either increased or decreased, local resistance vessels adjust their caliber appropriately so that the impact on blood flow is minimized. Because of autoregulation, blood flow to vital organs remains relatively constant over a wide range of perfusion pressures. Although the mechanisms responsible for autoregulation are not completely understood, myogenic and flow-dependent processes are thought to be involved.

The Pulmonary Circulation

Pulmonary circulation is unique because it is the only vascular bed that receives all of the cardiac output all of the time. The pulmonary vessels—arterioles, capillaries, and venules—are highly distensible and thin walled, containing comparatively little smooth muscle.[3] The average resistance in the pulmonary vasculature is only approximately 1/10 of that in systemic circulation. The pulmonary arterioles at the entrance to the gas-exchange area of the lungs are of muscular type and they respond primarily to local hypoxia and hypercapnia. In contrast to arterioles in the systemic circulation, the pulmonary arterioles are not under significant neural (sympathetic) control.

The pulmonary microcirculation includes an extensive interdigitating capillary network, likened more to a sheet of blood rather than to individual channels. The pulmonary capillary bed has a huge surface area and yet contains only 70 to 90 mL of blood under resting conditions. This capillary blood volume can expand more than threefold with only very small changes in pressure as pulmonary blood flow increases. In pulmonary circulation, capillary hydrostatic pressure is lower than in systemic circulation (approximately 7 mm Hg vs 30 mm Hg); therefore, filtration pressure is very low. This is an important mechanism for keeping the lungs "dry." Nevertheless, there is a small outward flow of fluid ($\sim$10–20 mL/h) from the pulmonary capillaries into the interstitium of the alveolar wall and then into the perivascular and peribronchiolar spaces of the lung. The lymphatic system of the lungs transports this filtered fluid from the interstitium to the hilar lymph nodes. The flow of lymph will increase substantially if capillary hydrostatic pressure and filtration increase. This lymphatic "storm sewer" prevents accumulation of fluid in the interstitial space that can lead to alveolar flooding (pulmonary edema) and impairment in gas exchange. A common cause of pulmonary edema is increased capillary filtration pressure due to failure of the left ventricle to discharge blood. Other causes of pulmonary edema are increased capillary permeability and decreased lymphatic clearance.

Vascular resistance in pulmonary circulation—unlike systemic circulation—is not controlled to a significant extent by extrinsic neural influences; nor does the smooth muscle in pulmonary arterioles exhibit autoregulation of blood flow. Nevertheless, there is a significant amount of smooth muscle in the pulmonary arteries, arterioles, and veins. A number of factors may act locally on this smooth muscle; however, the partial pressure of oxygen (P_{O_2}) in the alveolar gas is the most important minute-by-minute regulator of local pulmonary vascular resistance. If alveolar P_{O_2} falls below approximately 65 to 70 mm Hg, for example, because of underventilation in a specific region, adjacent arterioles will constrict. Local blood flow is thereby reduced and shifted to portions of the lung with higher ventilation and higher alveolar P_{O_2}. (Note that this hypoxic vasoconstriction in the lung is the opposite of what occurs in the systemic vasculature, where local hypoxia relaxes the local resistance of vessels, thereby causing vasodilation.) Accumulation of CO_2 in underventilated lung regions will also cause localized pulmonary arteriolar vasoconstriction.

Skeletal Muscle Blood Flow

Skeletal muscle is unusual among body tissues because it can increase its resting metabolic rate by as many as 50-fold, as evidenced by increases in the arteriovenous O_2 content difference across the muscle's vascular bed. If homeostasis is to be maintained, this large increase in metabolism necessitates a proportionately large increase in blood flow. Flow and metabolic rate are well matched in skeletal muscle by a combination of neural, chemical, and mechanical regulatory factors. The relative contributions of these factors depend on the level of muscle activity. When the muscle is at rest, arterioles in skeletal muscle exhibit a relatively high level of baseline resistance that is determined by myogenic tone and tonic levels of sympathetic vasoconstrictor outflow. In contrast, during muscle contraction, chemical and mechanical vasodilatory factors become much more important and can override the vasoconstrictor effects of sympathetic nerve stimulation.[7]

Metabolic by-products of contraction would seem to be the ideally suited chemical regulators of skeletal muscle blood flow; however, the specific chemical(s) responsible for exercise vasodilation have not been identified. The difficulty arises, in part, because almost all of the substances released into the interstitial space during muscle contraction (eg, potassium, adenosine, CO_2, lactate) produce vasodilation. In addition, an exercise-induced increase in many of these vasodilator stimuli is transient, whereas vasodilation is maintained throughout the period of muscle contraction. Thus, it appears that separate mechanisms may be responsible for initiating and maintaining metabolic vasodilation.

By-products of muscle contraction may exert their relaxing effect on vascular smooth muscle, at least in part, by stimulating the release of nitric oxide from the endothelium. In addition, the endothelium contributes to exercise hyperemia via flow-mediated vasodilation.

Mechanical factors also exert local control over skeletal muscle blood flow. When a muscle contracts and shortens, blood vessels within it are compressed. Thus, blood flow to a muscle is impeded while the muscle is contracting. During rhythmic muscle activity, reductions in blood flow that occur during the contraction phase are counterbalanced by increases in flow during the relaxation phase. In contrast, during sustained (isometric) muscle contraction, blood flow to the working muscle can become severely limited.[6]

A contraction-induced increase in extravascular pressure within the skeletal muscle decreases transmural pressure in the arterioles of the muscle vascular bed. This drop in transmural pressure causes relaxation of vascular smooth muscle via a local myogenic mechanism. The resultant myogenic vasodilation is thought to contribute importantly to exercise hyperemia. Conversely, when transmural pressure across the arteriolar wall increases, for example, when intravascular pressure rises, vascular smooth muscle is stimulated to contract and myogenic vasoconstriction occurs.

Because the skeletal muscle vascular bed is so large (approximately 40% of the total body mass), it is a major contributor to total peripheral resistance and, therefore, plays a key role in blood pressure regulation.[6] The skeletal muscle bed, along with the splanchnic and renal circulations, participates importantly in baroreflex responses to orthostatic stress. Reductions in blood flow through inactive muscle, produced by reflexes arising in contracting muscle, are important for the redistribution of blood from inactive to active tissue that occurs during exercise.

Cerebral Blood Flow

The cerebrum is supplied with blood by the anterior, middle, and posterior cerebral arteries. These vessels are branches of the circle of Willis that arises from the basilar and internal carotid arteries. Venous drainage occurs via sinuses that empty into the jugular veins.[3]

The blood–brain barrier is a unique feature of the cerebral circulation. Capillaries within the central nervous system have very tight junctions between adjacent endothelial cells. This feature prevents the movement of large molecules and highly charged ions from the blood to the brain and spinal cord, and as a result, circulating hormones do not participate in the regulation of cerebral blood flow.

The cerebral vessels, unlike those in other organs, are contained within a rigid structure—the cranium. Because of this rigidity and because the brain is relatively incompressible, a balance must exist among arterial inflow, venous outflow, and extravascular fluid volume. Although regional differences in blood flow can be observed in response to evoked changes in brain activity (eg, sensory stimulation, talking, reading, problem solving), the rate of total cerebral blood flow remains remarkably constant over a large range of behavioral and environmental conditions. Maintenance of cerebral blood flow within a narrow range is advantageous to the individual because brain tissue is highly dependent on aerobic metabolism; ischemia lasting only a few minutes causes irreversible tissue damage.

Autoregulation and local chemical influences are of primary importance in the control of cerebral blood flow.

The cerebral vessels show excellent autoregulatory capacity within the arterial pressure range of approximately 60 to 160 mm Hg. Increases and decreases in arterial pressure within this range trigger local vasoconstriction and vasodilation, respectively, that maintain blood flow at the baseline level. When mean arterial pressure falls below the autoregulatory range, the resultant decrease in cerebral blood flow results in syncope. When pressure rises above this range, increased blood flow, cerebral edema, and disruption of the blood–brain barrier ensue. Both myogenic and metabolic mechanisms are thought to play an important role in autoregulation.

Even though autoregulation is a strong controller of cerebral blood flow, it can be overridden by changes in arterial P_{CO_2}. Hypercapnia causes marked cerebral vasodilation; conversely, hypocapnia causes vasoconstriction. Potassium ions, low pH, and adenosine are potent vasodilators that are thought to be responsible for the coupling of blood flow with metabolism in the cerebral circulation.

The cerebral vessels receive sympathetic nervous system innervation. Electrical stimulation of these nerves causes vasoconstriction in cerebral vessels; however, this neural mechanism does not appear to regulate cerebral blood flow under physiological conditions. In acute hypertensive episodes, sympathetic vasoconstriction may protect the brain from arterial pressure increases that exceed the autoregulatory range.

The Fetal Circulation

The heart and blood vessels begin to develop in the third to fourth week of gestation. The formation of cardiovascular structures is essentially complete by week 7, and the fetal heart begins to beat by week 12. During fetal life, the lungs are not functional gas-exchange organs; therefore, the fetus must be supplied with oxygen by the maternal cardiovascular system via the placenta. In addition, the placenta performs the absorption and excretion functions of the lungs, gastrointestinal tract, and kidneys. Because of these special requirements, the structure and function of fetal circulation differ from the postnatal circulation in several important ways.

Cardiovascular Structure and Function in the Fetus

The fetus is supplied with oxygenated blood from the placenta via the umbilical vein.[1] Approximately half of this blood is routed to the liver; the remainder flows through a bypass tract, the ductus venosus, into the inferior vena cava. There it mixes with the unoxygenated blood from the lower extremities and rejoins the stream of oxygenated blood that perfused the liver. The majority of blood from the inferior vena cava flows into the left atrium through the foramen ovale, an opening normally present only during fetal life, where it is pumped into the systemic circulation. The remainder of blood from the inferior vena cava empties into the right atrium where it mixes with deoxygenated blood from the superior vena cava. The right ventricle then pumps this blood; however, because of the high pulmonary vascular resistance that exists before birth, only a small fraction of the right ventricle's stroke volume enters the pulmonary circulation. The remainder bypasses the lungs via the ductus arteriosus, a fetal connection between the pulmonary artery and the descending aorta. The head and upper extremities are supplied with blood from the ascending aorta. A portion of blood in the descending aorta supplies the lower extremities, and the remainder is returned to the placenta via two umbilical arteries.

Oxygen delivery to the fetus is facilitated by the presence of fetal hemoglobin. This protein has a higher affinity for oxygen than does adult hemoglobin. In addition, the hemoglobin concentration in fetal blood is higher than that in adult blood. As a result of these two factors, oxygen saturation in the fetus is maintained at adult levels, even though the P_{O_2} in arterial blood is less than half of that of an adult.

Changes That Occur at Birth

At birth, several structural changes prepare the newborn for life outside the uterus. First when the umbilical cord is cut and blood flow through the umbilical veins ceases, the ductus venosus closes. The asphyxia produced by the stoppage of umbilical flow stimulates the respiratory centers in the neonate's brainstem. The resultant lung inflation and oxygenation of the alveoli causes a dramatic fall in pulmonary vascular resistance, which allows a large increase in pulmonary blood flow. The increased flow of blood from pulmonary circulation into the left atrium raises pressure in the left atrium more than that in the right atrium, thereby closing the flaplike covering of the foramen ovale. Closure of the umbilical arteries substantially increases the resistance to left ventricular outflow and aortic pressure. When the aortic pressure rises above the pulmonary artery pressure, blood flow through the ductus

arteriosus is reversed, and in 1 to 2 days the ductus closes. Persistence of fetal structures (ie, patent foramen ovale and patent ductus arteriosus) into postnatal life can result in a significant "shunt" of unoxygenated blood to the systemic circulation, thereby producing arterial hypoxemia and cyanosis in the infant.

PULMONARY SYSTEM PHYSIOLOGY

The pulmonary system's primary function is to exchange O_2 and CO_2 between tissues, blood, and environment. In this regard, the lung is the only line of defense for O_2 and CO_2 homeostasis. In addition, the pulmonary system plays an important role in maintaining the acid–base balance. The lung is solely responsible for regulating CO_2 levels; thus, it is the body's major excreter of acid. The pulmonary system contributes to temperature homeostasis via evaporative heat loss from the lungs (this is not a major thermoregulatory mechanism in humans; however, it is very important in many animals). The lung also has nonrespiratory functions. It is the only organ that always receives all of the cardiac output; therefore, it is an ideal site for filtering and metabolizing toxic substances in the blood.

Gas Transport from Atmosphere to Tissue

Fulfilling the needs of metabolizing tissues for O_2 delivery and CO_2 elimination requires a high degree of coordination among several discrete functions. The steps in gas transport can be thought of in terms of these functions (Fig. 5-8B) and by the resultant changes in the partial pressures of O_2 and CO_2 at each step (Fig. 5-8A).

Partial Pressures

O_2 and CO_2 levels in air and blood are expressed as partial pressures. The pressure exerted by each individual gas in a gas

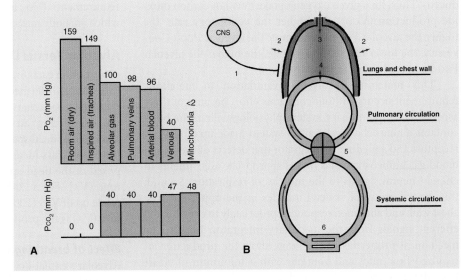

FIGURE 5-8 (**A**) Partial pressures of O_2 and CO_2 at each of the steps in their transport between ambient air and tissue. (**B**) Schematic representation of the functional links in O_2 and CO_2 transport. 1 = neural control; 2 = the pump; 3 = ventilation; 4 = pulmonary gas exchange; 5 = blood gas transport; and 6 = tissue gas exchange.

mixture is independent of the pressures of other gases; that is, each gas exerts a pressure proportional to its concentration. Thus, the partial pressure of a gas (P) equals the fractional concentration of the gas times the barometric pressure (P_B). For example, in dry atmospheric air, the O_2 concentration is 21% and the nitrogen concentration is 79%. Thus, at sea level:

$$P_{O_2} \text{ (mm Hg)} = 0.21 \times 760 \text{ mm Hg} = 160 \text{ mm Hg}$$

and

$$P_{N_2} \text{ (mm Hg)} = 0.79 \times 760 \text{ mm Hg} = 600 \text{ mm Hg.}$$

As air travels through the nasal passages and upper airways, it is warmed to 37°C and it becomes completely saturated with water vapor. At body temperature, water vapor exerts a pressure of 47 mm Hg (P_{H_2O}). In order to represent accurately the partial pressures presented to the lungs for gas exchange (ie, after warming and humidification), P_{H_2O} is first subtracted from the barometric pressure. Thus, for inspired, tracheal gases at sea level,

$$P_{O_2} = 0.21 \times (760 - 47) \text{ mm Hg} = 150 \text{ mm Hg}$$

and

$$P_{N_2} = 0.79 \times (760 - 47) \text{ mm Hg} = 563 \text{ mm Hg.}$$

Note that inspired, tracheal P_{O_2} is fixed (ie, unless supplemental O_2 is administered, an individual changes altitudes or rebreathes his or her own exhaled air). In contrast, the P_{O_2} (and P_{CO_2}) in alveolar gas and that in arterial, capillary, and venous blood are affected by many factors of health and disease. The following discussion briefly considers the determinants of P_{O_2} and P_{CO_2} at each of the four major steps in gas transport from the atmosphere to tissue mitochondria.

Steps in O_2 and CO_2 Transport

Step 1: Inspired (tracheal) to alveolar air gradient—The difference between tracheal and alveolar partial pressures is determined solely by the level of alveolar ventilation ($\dot{V}_A$) in relation to metabolic requirements (O_2 consumed or CO_2 produced). Thus, for a given oxygen uptake ($\dot{V}_{O_2}$) or carbon dioxide production ($\dot{V}_{CO_2}$) the higher the ventilatory rate, the higher the alveolar P_{O_2} and the lower the alveolar P_{CO_2}. Conversely, the lower the ventilatory rate, the higher the alveolar P_{CO_2}, and the lower the alveolar P_{O_2}.

This matching of alveolar ventilation to metabolic requirement occurs without conscious effort because of three aspects of the pulmonary system physiology. First, the body contains a neurochemical control system made up of sensory receptors and a medullary integrator that detects deviations in blood gas homeostasis and makes appropriate adjustments in efferent neural signals to the muscles of respiration. Second, this special group of skeletal muscles in the upper airways, chest wall, and abdomen respond appropriately to coordinated efferent signals from the medullary integrator. Finally, the mechanical properties of the lungs allow the production of required flow rates and volumes with a minimum of effort from the respiratory pump muscles.

Step 2: Alveolar-to-arterial P_{O_2} difference—The difference in alveolar (P_{AO_2}) and arterial (P_{aO_2}) partial pressures of oxygen is determined by the ability of the lungs to oxygenate the mixed venous blood that is returned to the lungs. This ability depends on the rate of diffusion between the alveoli and pulmonary capillaries and on the uniformity with which blood perfusing the pulmonary capillaries is matched with ventilation of the alveoli. Note that in the normal situation as shown in Fig. 5-8A, the O_2 gradient between alveolar gas and arterial blood is small (~5–10 mm Hg).

Step 3: Gas transport by the blood—The third step depends critically on the ability of hemoglobin to bind O_2 tightly at high P_{O_2} (ie, as blood leaves the lungs) and also to release O_2 readily at lower P_{O_2} (ie, as blood traverses the capillaries of active tissue). CO_2 transport from tissue back to the lung and its subsequent release is also dependent on the ability of the red blood cells to carry CO_2.

Step 4: Exchange of gases between capillary and tissue mitochondria—The final step in gas transport occurs almost entirely by diffusion. Factors governing the rate of diffusion have been discussed earlier in this chapter.

Pulmonary Ventilation and Alveolar Gases

Inspiration occurs when the respiratory muscles generate subatmospheric pressures in the pleural space and the alveoli; expiration occurs when the lungs recoil and pleural and alveolar pressures become less negative.[2] Normal values for the volume of air inhaled and exhaled under resting conditions (O_2 consumption and CO_2 production = 200–300 mL/min) by a healthy adult with a body weight of 70 kg are as follows: The volume of air inspired with each breath, or tidal volume (V_T), equals 500 mL (range = 300–800 mL), and the average breathing frequency (f_b) is 15 breaths/min (range = 10–20 breaths/min). The product of tidal volume and frequency is total minute ventilation ($\dot{V}_I$), which averages 7.5 L/min (range = 4–10 L/min). The level of $\dot{V}_I$ will change in accordance with changing tissue metabolic requirements ($\dot{V}_{O_2}$ and $\dot{V}_{CO_2}$), the primary determinants of which are body mass, diet, and level of activity.

Alveolar Versus Dead-Space Ventilation

A portion of each breath does not participate in gas exchange; this volume is termed the dead space.[2] Anatomical structures that lack gas-exchange surfaces are the pharynx, larynx, and the conducting airways. The volume of this airway (or anatomical) dead space in milliliters is approximately equal to the individual's ideal body weight in pounds. The V_T is composed of the dead-space volume (V_{DS}) plus the alveolar volume (V_A). For a 70-kg human, the average V_T (500 mL) is made up of V_{DS} (150 mL) plus V_A (350 mL). Alveolar ventilation ($\dot{V}_A$) is the product of V_A and the breathing frequency.

Effect of breathing pattern on dead-space ventilation—Alveolar ventilation depends not only on the level of $\dot{V}_I$ but also on the pattern of breathing. Because a dead-space volume accompanies each breath, a rapid, shallow breathing pattern (ie, high f_b, small V_T) provides less alveolar ventilation than the *same* $\dot{V}_I$ produced by slow, deep breathing. High breathing frequencies are commonly observed in the individual with restrictive lung disease who has stiff (noncompliant) lungs that are difficult to expand to a normal V_T. In these instances, the patient's ventilatory control system has to "make a choice," either to allow alveolar hypoventilation (with consequent CO_2 retention and hypoxemia) or to increase $\dot{V}_I$ above normal levels to achieve an adequate $\dot{V}_A$ (with consequent increase in effort and energy expenditure). Obviously, neither choice is ideal!

Other causes of increased dead-space ventilation—In addition to the dead space contained within conducting airways, a portion of $\dot{V}_I$ may be "wasted" when there is an uneven distribution of ventilation relative to perfusion throughout the lung. An extreme example of increased *dead-space ventilation* occurs when completely unperfused alveoli are ventilated (eg, when a pulmonary embolus blocks blood flow to a portion of the lung). In a less extreme example, dead-space ventilation is also increased when normally perfused alveoli are overventilated (eg, when a partially obstructed airway in one portion of the lung results in overventilation elsewhere).

In healthy individuals, the anatomical plus alveolar dead space occupies only approximately 30% of the V_T. In contrast, in patients with nonuniform structural abnormalities of the lungs, 60% to 70% of each V_T may be composed of dead-space volume. When dead-space volume is increased, the energy costs involved in providing adequate $\dot{V}_A$ can be quite high. **Dead-space ventilation may be increased (1) by increased breathing frequency because of the oxygen-poor, carbon dioxide–rich volume of gas inspired from the conducting airway or (2) by overventilation of alveoli with respect to their perfusion.**

Determinants of Alveolar P_{O_2} and P_{CO_2}

An increase in tissue metabolic activity results in increased levels of CO_2 and decreased levels of O_2 in the mixed venous blood that is returned to the lung. $\dot{V}_{O_2}$ and $\dot{V}_{CO_2}$, then, represent the metabolic load to which $\dot{V}_A$ must respond. The alveolar air can be thought of as a compartment of gas lying between the atmospheric air and the blood in the pulmonary capillaries. O_2 is constantly being removed and CO_2 is constantly being added to this reservoir by the blood flowing through the alveolar capillaries. During inspiration, alveolar P_{O_2} rises because fresh air is added to the alveolar gas. During expiration, alveolar P_{O_2} decreases and alveolar P_{CO_2} increases because fresh air is no longer being added, yet the blood flowing through the pulmonary capillaries continues to exchange gases with the alveolar air.

In addition to these within-breath variations in alveolar gas tensions, P_{AO_2} and P_{ACO_2} vary in different areas of the lung (depending on the ventilation–perfusion distribution) and they vary from breath to breath. Of practical significance are the mean values for P_{AO_2} and P_{ACO_2}, averaged throughout all alveoli and over many breaths. These mean values for P_{AO_2}

and P_{ACO_2} can be calculated using the alveolar air equation.[2] The concept underlying this equation is that the alveolar gas compartment is affected by the supply of fresh air to its $\dot{V}_A$ in relation to the amount of O_2 removed ($\dot{V}_{O_2}$) and CO_2 added ($\dot{V}_{CO_2}$). The alveolar air equation for calculating P_{ACO_2} is

$$P_{ACO_2} = \dot{V}_{CO_2}/\dot{V}_A \times K.$$

Because variations in inspired P_{O_2} must be taken into account, the alveolar air equation for O_2 is

$$P_{AO_2} = P_{IO_2} - \dot{V}_{O_2}/\dot{V}_A \times K.$$

In both equations, K is a constant (863) used to standardize gas volumes and temperatures and partial pressures.

Alveolar hyperventilation occurs when more O_2 is supplied and more CO_2 is removed than the metabolic rate requires; in this case, alveolar and arterial P_{O_2} rises and P_{CO_2} falls. *Alveolar hypoventilation* occurs when less O_2 is supplied and less CO_2 removed than the metabolic rate requires; in this case, alveolar and arterial P_{O_2} decrease and P_{CO_2} rises. Alveolar and arterial P_{CO_2} levels are almost always identical. Normally, near sea level, an alveolar and arterial P_{CO_2} of approximately 40 mm Hg (± 3 to 4 mm Hg) is maintained by adjusting ventilation appropriately for metabolic CO_2 production. **The alveolar or arterial P_{CO_2} expresses the ratio of CO_2 production ($\dot{V}_{CO_2}$) to alveolar ventilation ($\dot{V}_A$) and defines under any physiologic condition whether the individual is hypoventilating, hyperventilating, or ventilating normally.**

Mechanical Characteristics of the Lung and Chest Wall

The mechanics of the lungs and thorax play a crucial role in the physiology of breathing. For example, mechanical factors determine how much one is "willing" or "able" to ventilate, the breathing pattern, and the energy cost of breathing. In addition, mechanical factors contribute importantly to the perception of breathing effort. Moreover, lung and chest wall mechanics affect the distribution of inspiratory gas throughout the lungs, which, in turn, is a major determinant of gas exchange and arterial P_{O_2} (P_{aO_2}).

Lung Volumes and Capacities

The lung volumes that define total lung capacity (TLC) and its subdivisions are shown in Fig. 5-9.[2] The TLC and vital capacity define the maximum limits for each breath. The starting point for each breath is the functional residual capacity (FRC) or end-expiratory lung volume. The residual lung volume is the lowest possible lung volume achievable via forced expiration.

Respiratory Muscles

Inspiratory muscle contraction expands the chest cavity outward and causes pleural pressure to become more subatmospheric. This pressure change is transmitted to the interior of the lungs so that alveolar pressure also becomes subatmospheric. The pressure difference between the alveoli and the airway opening (ie, mouth and/or nose) induces airflow into

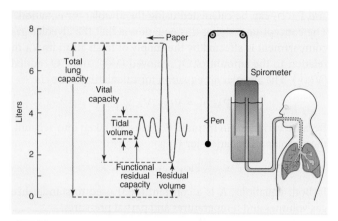

FIGURE 5-9   Normal lung volumes. In a 70-kg adult, average values are as follows: tidal volume = 0.4–0.7 L; functional residual capacity = 2.5 L (or 40%–50% of TLC); TLC = 5–7 L; residual volume = 1–2 L (or 20%–25% of TLC); vital capacity = 4–6 L. These volumes vary among healthy people according to weight, height, age, and gender. (Used with permission from West JB. *Respiratory Physiology—The Essentials.* 5th ed. Baltimore, MD: Lippincott Williams & Wilkins; 1995.)

the lungs from the atmosphere. Following activation of the inspiratory muscles, the lungs expand until their recoil (inward) force equals the opposing (outward) force of the chest wall plus that of the contracting inspiratory muscles. When these forces come into balance, inspiration ceases. Expiration occurs passively as the result of inspiratory muscle relaxation.

Two sets of respiratory muscles act in coordinated fashion to produce ventilation: (1) those of the chest wall and abdomen that cause volume and pressure changes inside the thorax and (2) those that dilate and stiffen the collapsible, extrathoracic upper airway so that it can remain patent as negative pressure is generated within the chest.

Upper Airway Muscles

The extrathoracic airway includes the larynx, pharynx, and the oral and nasal cavities (Chapter 4, Fig. 4-7). The upper airway is most susceptible to collapse at the level of the soft palate and at the base of the tongue. Neural outflow to palatal and tongue muscles is particularly important in maintaining airway patency and minimizing airway resistance during inspiration.

In the larynx, the sole abductor muscle is the posterior cricoarytenoid. This muscle is innervated by somatic fibers that originate from the nucleus ambiguus in the ventrolateral medulla and reach their destination via the recurrent laryngeal nerve. The larynx, when denervated, acts as a one-way valve that allows expiration but not inspiration. Therefore, the vocal folds must be actively abducted by the posterior cricoarytenoid during inspiration.

Oral, nasal, and pharyngeal muscles are innervated by cranial nerves VII, IX, X, and XII. These muscles act as constrictors or dilators of the upper airway and they also contribute importantly to nonrespiratory functions. Along with

the larynx, they are involved in swallowing, vocalization, coughing, and sneezing. The control of these muscles is complicated and poorly understood; however, their role in stabilizing the upper airway during inspiration is vital.

Diaphragm and Rib Cage Muscles

The diaphragm, which is innervated by the phrenic nerves arising from spinal segments C3 through C5, is a thin, dome-shaped muscle that separates the thoracic and abdominal cavities (Chapter 4, Fig. 4-5). It is a musculotendinous sheet, consisting of muscle bundles that originate from the lower ribs and insert on a flat central tendon. The diaphragm is responsible for generating most of the negative pleural and alveolar pressure during inspiration; therefore, it is the principal muscle of inspiration.

During inspiration, the dome of the diaphragm flattens as myofibrils shorten. Diaphragmatic contraction increases the cephalocaudal, anteroposterior, and lateral dimensions of the thorax, thereby increasing intrathoracic volume and decreasing intrathoracic pressure. As it contracts and descends, the diaphragm compresses the abdominal contents. This compression resists the diaphragm's descent and creates positive pressure in the abdominal compartment. As a result, the abdominal wall is pushed outward. The lower ribs remain caudal to the diaphragm, even as it descends, and positive abdominal pressure causes the lower rib cage to be displaced outward. Thus, the abdominal contents act as a fulcrum for the diaphragm.

The human rib cage consists of 12 ribs on each side that articulate with the thoracic vertebrae (Chapter 4, Figs. 4-3 and 4-4). The motion of the ribs with respect to the thoracic vertebrae is similar to the motion of a bucket's handle with respect to the bucket. Normally, each rib is tilted approximately 30 degrees below the horizontal plane. During inspiration, upward rotation of the ribs increases the cephalocaudal dimension of the thorax.

The principal inspiratory muscles of the rib cage are the external intercostals, which are so oriented that their contractions rotate the ribs ("bucket handles") upward toward the horizontal plane. The rib cage muscles are innervated by the intercostal nerves that arise from spinal segments T1 through T12. The accessory muscles of inspiration include the sternocleidomastoid and the scalene muscles, which are attached to the first two ribs and to the sternum. When the position of the head is fixed, contraction of these muscles lifts the rib cage, thereby increasing the cephalocaudal dimension of the thorax. The serratus anterior and pectoralis muscles can also function as accessory muscles of inspiration. By virtue of their attachments to the ribs and sternum, they expand the thorax in the anteroposterior plane when the position of the arms is fixed.

In normal quiet breathing, the intercostal muscles may contribute up to half of the active inspiratory volume change; the diaphragm produces the rest. The muscles of the rib cage also contribute to inspiration by preventing inward (paradoxical) movement of the chest wall. Inward movement during inspiration can be seen in the newborn, whose rib cage is very compliant. This may also occur when the rib cage loses stiffness because of activation failure of the intercostal muscles, such as in spinal cord injury or in REM (rapid eye movement) sleep. Conversely, under conditions where the diaphragm is paralyzed, the rib cage muscles must accomplish the entire work of breathing. As pleural pressure decreases in such individuals, the diaphragm is sucked up into the thorax (paradoxical motion of the diaphragm) and the abdominal wall moves in.

The diaphragm's ability to generate tension in response to motoneuron activation depends critically on its length. Tension is maximal at the diaphragm's usual ("optimal") fiber length that occurs at approximately the normal resting lung volume (ie, FRC). As the diaphragm muscle fibers are progressively shortened by increasing lung volume, the force that can be generated by the diaphragm falls, reaching zero at approximately 40% of the diaphragm's normal resting length which is achieved at TLC.

The diaphragm's function as an inspiratory muscle is also dependent on its shape. The diaphragm is normally curved, with the convexity facing cephalad and the concavity facing caudad. Its ability to convert developed tension into a pressure difference between the thoracic and the abdominal compartments depends on that curvature. Imagine what would happen if the diaphragm were a completely flat sheet of muscle separating the thorax from the abdomen. In this situation, no amount of force exerted by muscle contraction in that plane could produce a pressure difference between the diaphragm's top and bottom surfaces! A less extreme example of how the diaphragm's shape determines function is seen in patients with severe emphysema. In such individuals, lung hyperinflation creates a low, flat, shortened diaphragm that is susceptible to fatigue because it must operate at a substantial mechanical disadvantage.

In normal circumstances, the diaphragm is a highly fatigue-resistant skeletal muscle. It contains a large volume of mitochondria and high levels of oxidative enzymes. The diaphragm is rich in myoglobin and its high capillary density keeps diffusion distances for O_2 very short. In addition, the diaphragm is very sensitive to locally produced vasodilator metabolites, thereby ensuring that it has adequate levels of blood flow to meet metabolic demands during repeated contractions. Thus, this key inspiratory muscle is capable of generating high levels of force output, even over long periods of time, without fatigue. Nevertheless, the diaphragm does fatigue under certain conditions. For example, it is possible to demonstrate diaphragm fatigue when requirements for force production are very high and sustained, such as during repetitive inspiratory efforts against high resistance. Fatigue can also be demonstrated when blood flow to the diaphragm is limited in combination with high-force output, such as during very high-intensity endurance exercise.

CLINICAL CORRELATE

In the clinical setting, diaphragm fatigue occurs when the capacity for force generation is compromised, such as in neuromuscular diseases or when diaphragm length is shortened (eg, by lung hyperinflation) or in malnourished states where atrophy occurs in all skeletal muscles.

Muscles of Expiration

The most important expiratory muscles are the abdominals, which are innervated at spinal levels T6 through L1. During expiration, abdominal muscle contraction depresses the lower ribs, pulls down the anterior part of the lower chest, and compresses the abdominal contents. The resultant increase in intra-abdominal pressure forces the relaxed diaphragm upward, causing its fibers to lengthen and thereby decreasing rib cage volume. During expiration, the abdominal muscles are assisted by the internal intercostals, which depress the ribs and move them inward. Contraction of the internal intercostal muscles also stabilizes the rib cage and prevents bulging of the intercostal spaces during forceful expiratory maneuvers.

Expiratory muscles are normally inactive during quiet breathing because expiration is achieved passively via elastic recoil of the lungs. Nevertheless, the expiratory muscles are critical for performing forceful expiratory maneuvers (eg, coughing) and are readily activated during even mild exercise. In heavy exercise, when breathing frequency is increased and expiratory time greatly shortened, active expiration is crucial for maintaining end-expiratory lung volume so that the diaphragm and other inspiratory muscles can work at their optimal lengths.

Mechanics of Breathing

In order to inflate the lungs, the inspiratory muscles must perform two types of work: (1) They must overcome the tendency of the lungs to recoil inward, that is elastic work, and (2) they must overcome resistance to flow offered by the airways.[2] The following discussion of breathing mechanics will describe these processes.

Lung distensibility—In terms of its elastic properties, a lung can be likened to a balloon. While inflated, there is a tendency of the lung to recoil or collapse. In order to keep the lung inflated, a pressure difference between the alveolar pressure (P_A) and the intrapleural pressure (P_{pl}) must be maintained. This distending force is provided by the elastic properties of the chest wall (which causes a tendency to recoil outward) and by the action of the inspiratory muscles.

Compliance is the term used to describe distensibility or the ease with which the lung can be inflated. It is defined as a change in volume for a given change in pressure. In the normal range of V_T, the lung is remarkably distensible, as illustrated by the linear portion of the compliance curve of a normal lung in Chapter 9, Fig. 9-6A. However, as the lung volume approaches TLC, the lung is much stiffer (its compliance is smaller), as shown by the flatter slope of the upper portion of the compliance curve. This relationship of compliance to lung volume has substantial implications in determining how we "select" our breathing frequencies, tidal volumes, and end-expiratory lung volumes.

Compliance curves for individuals with emphysema and pulmonary fibrosis are different. With emphysema, a disease in which elastic tissue is progressively lost from the alveolar walls, compliance is high, and therefore small changes in translung pressure cause large volume changes. In contrast, in pulmonary fibrosis the lung is very "stiff"; that is, compliance is reduced and changes in translung pressure produce smaller than normal changes in volume.

Determinants of elastic characteristics of the lung—One factor responsible for the lung's elastic behavior (ie, the tendency to recoil to its resting volume after distention) is the network of elastin and collagen fibers in the alveolar walls and the surrounding blood vessels and bronchi.[2] In the geometrical arrangement of these fibers, lung tissue is like a nylon stocking in which individual fibers are difficult to stretch, whereas the entire stocking is very distensible because of its knitted construction. Changes in the structure and/or the amounts of these elastic tissues account for the loss of elastic recoil and increased lung compliance that occurs with normal aging and with emphysema.

Surface tension, created by the presence of an interface between air in the alveoli and the watery alveolar tissue, is responsible for much of the lung's elastic recoil. The strong attractive forces between molecules in the liquid phase maintain the size of the air–liquid interface at the smallest possible area. As a result, each alveolus has a spherical liquid lining layer that is pulled inward toward the center of curvature of the alveolus. Because this surface force acts like an "elastic tension," a greater pressure is required to expand the alveolus than would be necessary if the alveolar liquid lining layer were not present.

Physiological importance of surfactant—Surface tension is kept at an optimal level because of a chemical called surfactant, which is synthesized by alveolar type II cells and secreted in the alveolar lining fluid.[2] Its production is stimulated by the stretch of alveolar epithelium that occurs with a change in lung volume. If one breathes at a constant small VT for a long period of time, surfactant will not be produced and the lung will become less and less compliant, requiring more work to expand. Surprisingly, a single large inspiration that occurs periodically (eg, a sigh or a yawn) is sufficient to restore the normal surfactant layer and thereby keep compliance normal and alveoli open (surfactant also reduces the tendency for alveolar collapse [atelectasis] at low lung volumes).

In the fetal lung, surfactant production begins at between 28 and 32 weeks of gestation. In preterm infants born prior to this time, absence of surfactant results in low-compliance, difficult-to-inflate lungs and areas of atelectasis. These babies are hypoxemic and the work of breathing is greatly increased. Prior to 1980

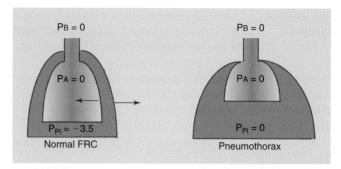

FIGURE 5-10   In a normal lung at functional residual capacity (FRC) (**left**), the tendency of the lung to recoil inward is exactly balanced by the tendency of the chest to expand outward. This causes pleural pressure (P_{pl}) to be subatmospheric. Pneumothorax (**right**) removes the lung–chest wall couple and allows the lung to collapse, the chest to spring out, and P_{pl} to go to zero. P_A, alveolar pressure; P_B, body surface (atmospheric) pressure.

this respiratory distress syndrome in the newborn was responsible for a significant fraction of infant mortality in the United States. In recent years, surfactant replacement therapy has contributed to a dramatic fall in mortality of preterm infants.

Interaction Between Lung and Chest Wall

The functional "chest wall" includes the rib cage, diaphragm, and abdominal wall. The chest wall components must work together to move the lung and to produce a breath.

Figure 5-10 (left) shows the elastic forces that act on the lung and chest wall to determine lung volume at the end of a normal expiration, defined as "relaxation volume" (or FRC). Under these static conditions, there is an equal tendency for the chest to increase in volume (spring out) as there is for the lung to decrease in volume (recoil inward). Thus, at FRC the chest wall opposes lung collapse.

The critical importance of this coupling of lung and chest wall forces is illustrated in Fig. 5-10 (right), which shows the effect of breaking the liquid seal between the parietal and visceral pleura. *Pneumothorax* occurs when the chest wall is punctured, allowing air to enter the pleural space. Under these conditions the lung shrinks down to its resting (minimal) volume while the chest wall expands to its resting (maximal) volume.

Volume-Related Changes in Recoil Pressures of Lung and Chest Wall

Transmural pressures of the lung/chest wall system vary throughout the respiratory cycle. Beginning at FRC, inspiration occurs when active muscle force is applied to the relaxed chest wall. The outward force of inspiratory muscle contraction, added to the normal recoil of the chest wall, decreases alveolar pressure so that it is negative with respect to atmospheric pressure. When the glottis is open, air flows down the pressure gradient from atmosphere to alveoli, causing an increase in lung volume. Flow continues to increase lung volume until the recoil force of the lung offsets the sum of the muscle force and recoil force of the chest wall, resulting in an alveolar pressure of zero (relative to atmospheric pressure).

Expiration is initiated when the inspiratory muscles relax and eliminate the outward muscle force, thereby allowing passive relaxation of the respiratory system back toward FRC. The positive recoil pressure of the lung then results in reduced alveolar volume and an alveolar pressure that exceeds atmospheric pressure, causing expiratory airflow. Expiration continues until lung volume is reduced to FRC, where the recoil pressures of the respiratory system are again balanced at zero.

Resistance to Airflow

Thus far, mechanical factors that influence the elastic work of breathing have been discussed. Now, the additional force that must be applied to cause air to flow into the lung (ie, the pressure required to overcome frictional resistance to airflow) will be outlined.

Poiseuille's Law has been used to describe airflow through the airway tree. Accordingly,

$$\text{Flow rate} = \frac{\Delta P}{R} = \frac{P_{ATM} - P_{ALVEOLAR}}{\text{resistance}}.$$

By rearranging this equation,

$$\text{Airway resistance (Raw)} = \frac{P_{ATM} - P_{ALVEOLAR}}{\text{airflow rate}}.$$

Airway resistance is usually expressed in centimeters of water pressure per liter per second of airflow. The factors affecting airway resistance, which are analogous to the factors affecting resistance to blood flow in the cardiovascular system, can be described by the equation:

$$\text{Raw} = \frac{8\eta l}{\pi r^4},$$

where η = viscosity of gas, l = length of the tube, and r = radius of the tube. Clearly, the radius of the airway is the major determinant of airway resistance. **Because the radius term is raised to the fourth power, even very small changes in radius greatly affect airway resistance.**

Sites of Airway Resistance

Normally, 70% to 80% of the total airway resistance is provided by the large airways (>2 mm diameter).[2] Resistance in the smaller airways is very low because flow is laminar, not turbulent, at that level. In addition, the airways distal to the terminal bronchioles branch in such a manner that the radius of successive branches remains nearly constant. The total cross-sectional area of the smallest airways exceeds that of the "parent" airway; therefore, the resistance of the distal airways is very low even though the individual radii are very small.

Factors Affecting Airway Caliber

Airways are distensible, collapsible tubes whose radii are determined by neural, chemical, and mechanical factors. Caliber of the extrathoracic upper airway is regulated mainly by tonic and phasic activation of many pairs of skeletal muscles and also by the degree of local vascular engorgement. In the intralobar airways, contraction and relaxation of bronchial smooth muscle cells regulate caliber. Bronchial smooth muscle is under autonomic nervous system control; increases in parasympathetic outflow cause bronchoconstriction, whereas sympathetic stimulation causes bronchodilation. In the clinical setting, inflammation of the airway epithelium is a major cause of increased airway resistance. The vascular engorgement and excessive secretion production that accompany inflammation can cause narrowing of the airway lumen. In addition, locally released chemical mediators (eg, histamine) can reduce airway caliber by triggering smooth muscle contraction.

Airway Resistance During Inspiration Versus Expiration

Caliber of the intrathoracic airways is also affected by a mechanical factor (ie, transmural pressure across the airway wall). When the pressure surrounding the outside of the airway (PA) is more negative than airway pressure (Paw), airway radius increases. Conversely, when PA is positive relative to Paw, airway radius decreases. These within-breath fluctuations in transmural pressure and airway radius are responsible for the characteristic shape of the flow–volume loop (Fig. 5-11).

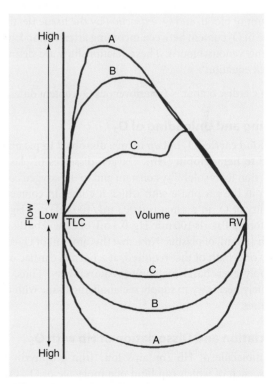

FIGURE 5-11 Flow–volume loops (inspiration down, expiration up). In curve A, maximal inspiration was followed by a maximum forced expiration. In B, both inspiration and expiration were submaximal. In C, inspiratory effort was even less than in B, and expiration was initially slow and then forced. In all three cases, the descending portions of the expiratory curves are almost superimposed on each other.

The relationship between respiratory flow rate and lung volume is represented as an X–Y plot in Fig. 5-11. Note the flow–volume relationship for inspiration has a different shape from that for expiration. Although flow rate remains relatively constant throughout a maximal inspiration to TLC, a maximal expiratory effort from TLC causes flow rate to rise rapidly to a peak and then to decline as lung volume falls over most of the remaining forced expiration. A remarkable feature of this maximal flow–volume envelope is that it is virtually impossible to penetrate it, regardless of how forcefully one exhales. Even if the individual exerts huge expiratory efforts with their accompanying increases in intrathoracic pressure, the descending portion of the flow–volume curve takes virtually the same path.

The reason for this remarkable behavior is "dynamic" compression of the airways caused by positive intrathoracic pressure. During forced expiration, the positive pressure in the pleural space acts not only on the alveoli but also on the outside of the airway walls, thereby promoting airway compression. Figure 5-11 shows that the maximum flow rate during forced expiration is effort-independent; more forceful expiratory efforts do not result in greater airflow.

Gas Transport by the Blood

O_2 consumption by tissue requires *O_2 delivery*, which is determined by the product of cardiac output and the O_2 content in each unit of blood, and *O_2 extraction* by the tissue (ie, the difference in O_2 content between incoming arterial blood and the outgoing venous blood). These relationships are defined by the Fick equation[2]:

$$\dot{V}O_2 = \text{Cardiac output} \times (\text{arteriovenous } O_2 \text{ content difference}).$$

Loading and Unloading of O_2

The blood carries O_2 in two forms: dissolved in plasma and bound to hemoglobin (Hb). Oxygen dissolves in plasma in proportion to its solubility constant and to the oxygen concentration in the gas phase with which it comes in contact. The solubility of O_2 in plasma is 0.003 mL/100 mL/mm Hg PaO_2. Therefore, if PaO_2 is 100 mm Hg, 0.3 mL of O_2 will be dissolved in each 100 mL of plasma. Note that this amount of O_2 content is only one-sixth of that required, at a normal cardiac output, to supply even basal metabolic requirements. Thus, Hb is absolutely necessary to supply metabolizing tissue with the O_2 it requires.

Association and Dissociation of Hb with O_2

Each molecule of Hb contains four iron-porphyrin heme groups, each of which can bind one molecule of O_2. Oxygen binding to Hb is proportional to the PO_2 of the blood; however, because of interaction among heme groups within each hemoglobin molecule, the binding is not linear. As each O_2 molecule binds to Hb, it increases the affinity of the remaining heme sites for additional O_2 molecules. The relationship between binding of oxygen and PO_2 is shown in Fig. 5-2, where it is assumed that the pH is 7.4 and the temperature is 37°C.[2]

The upper portion of the curve represents arterial blood after it leaves the lung. Usually, the lower, steeper part of the curve represents systemic tissue capillary blood or venous blood. Note that at PO_2 above approximately 80 mm Hg, the saturation changes little; however, at PO_2 below approximately 50 mm Hg, the saturation drops more steeply.

Memorization of a few key points on the curve provides the clinician with immediate insight into how seriously systemic O_2 transport is threatened by varying levels of arterial hypoxemia. The points to remember are

- the normal values for mixed venous blood (75% saturation and 40 mm Hg PO_2);
- the normal values for arterial blood (97% saturation and 90–95 mm Hg PO_2);
- the "shoulder" of the curve where saturation (and content) begin to fall precipitously (90% saturation and 55–65 mm Hg PO_2).

Calculation of O_2 Content of Whole Blood

Oxygen content of whole blood can be calculated if the PaO_2 and the Hb concentration are known.

- First, determine the oxygen-carrying capacity (HbCC) of fully saturated Hb, which varies directly with the Hb concentration:

$$\text{HbCC} = \text{Hb (g/100 mL)} \times 1.39 \text{ mL } O_2/\text{g Hb}.$$

Note that 1.39 mL O_2/g Hb is a fixed value for all normal hemoglobin. In normal circumstances (15 g Hb):

$$\text{HbCC} = 15 \times 1.39 = 20.9 \text{ mL } O_2/100 \text{ mL}.$$

- Second, determine the percentage of HbO_2 saturation, given the PaO_2. The HbO_2 dissociation curve (Fig. 5-2) must be consulted to obtain this value. HbO_2 content can then be calculated according to the following formula:

$$\text{HbO}_2 \text{ content} = \text{HbCC} \times \% \text{ HbO}_2 \text{ saturation}.$$

For normal arterial blood, at $PaO_2 = 90$ mm Hg,

$$\text{HbO}_2 \text{ content} = 20.9 \times 97\% = 20.2 \text{ mL } O_2/100 \text{ mL}.$$

- Third, to calculate the whole blood O_2 content, the amount of O_2 dissolved in plasma must be added to the HbO_2 content. The plasma O_2 content is the product of PaO_2 and the solubility constant (0.003 mL O_2/100 mL/mm Hg). Thus, in normal circumstances,

$$\text{plasma } O_2 \text{ content} = 90 \text{ mm Hg} \times 0.003$$
$$= 0.27 \text{ mL } O_2/100 \text{ mL}.$$

The whole blood O_2 content can then be calculated as follows:

$$\text{whole blood } O_2 \text{ content} = (\text{HbCC} \times \% \text{ HbO}_2 \text{ saturation})$$
$$+ (\text{plasma } O_2 \text{ content}).$$

So, for the normal example in arterial blood,

$$\text{whole blood } O_2 \text{ content} = (20.9 \times 97) + (0.27)$$
$$= 20.5 \text{ mL } O_2/100 \text{ mL}.$$

Shape of the HbO_2 Dissociation Curve

The sigmoid shape of the HbO_2 dissociation curve has many physiological advantages—all geared toward delivery of O_2 in sufficient amounts to maximize the capillary to tissue diffusion gradient and thereby ensure tissue oxygenation.[2] For example, in Fig. 5-2, contrast the loss of O_2 content along the flatter versus the steeper portions of the dissociation curve. Along the upper part of the curve, lung function must fail substantially (ie, PaO_2 must fall more than 30 mm Hg) before O_2 saturation, O_2 content, and therefore systemic O_2 transport are significantly reduced. In contrast, at the steeper portion of the curve, Hb binds O_2 less tightly, which means that as the Hb loses O_2 by diffusion to the metabolizing tissue from beginning to end of the tissue capillary, the PO_2 falls much less (than on the flatter portion of the curve).

Unloading O_2 at the tissue occurs at a rate demanded by tissue mitochondria. This unloading of O_2 from Hb occurs in the arterioles and capillaries. Passive diffusion of O_2 is the primary process by which O_2 moves from blood to tissue. In skeletal muscle, myoglobin may facilitate the diffusion process.

Position of the HbO_2 Dissociation Curve

The following conditions shift the HbO_2 dissociation curve to the right: increased temperature, carbon dioxide concentration, and hydrogen ion concentration (decreased pH). Changes in these variables in the opposite direction shift the curve to the left.[2]

Shifts in the HbO_2 dissociation curve can facilitate or impede oxygen delivery to tissue, especially during periods of increased metabolic activity. For example, exercising muscle generates heat, CO_2, and acidic metabolites, all shifting the HbO_2 dissociation curve to the right. Thus, in normal circumstances during exercise, Hb unloads O_2 at the muscle at higher capillary PO_2 than it does when the dissociation curve is not right-shifted. As a result, the gradient for O_2 diffusion from blood to tissue is increased and O_2 delivery is improved.

Leftward shifts in the HbO_2 dissociation curve also occur. For example, humans hyperventilate at high altitudes, causing pH to increase. Also, fetal hemoglobin has an increased O_2 affinity at any given PO_2. Leftward shifts are beneficial under these conditions of O_2 deficiency.

Carriage of CO_2

Resting metabolism results in the production of approximately 200 mL CO_2/min in a 70-kg adult. It is important for the body to dispose of this promptly because CO_2 combines spontaneously with the water in plasma to produce carbonic acid. Thus, the resting $\dot{V}CO_2$ would produce approximately 13 mol of H^+ in a 24-hour period, which is an enormous acid load. Therefore, CO_2 must be continuously removed from the body via the lungs.

CO_2 is transported to the lungs by the venous blood in three forms: dissolved in plasma, bound to plasma proteins and hemoglobin, and as bicarbonate (HCO_3^-).[2] The first two forms each account for only approximately 5% to 10% of the total CO_2 carried, whereas the third form accounts for approximately 90% of all CO_2 carried in the blood.

The first step in CO_2 transport is the spontaneous hydration of CO_2 to carbonic acid (H_2CO_3) by the reaction:

$$CO_2 + H_2O \leftrightarrow H_2CO_3 \leftrightarrow HCO_3^- + H^+.$$

This reaction occurs mainly within red blood cells, where it is catalyzed by carbonic anhydrase. The second step in this process, the ionic dissociation of carbonic acid to H^+ and HCO_3^- is rapid, not requiring a catalyst. As concentrations of the ions rise, HCO_3^- diffuses out of the red cell but H^+ cannot do this because the cell membrane is relatively impermeable to cations. Thus, in order to maintain electrical neutrality, Cl^- ions diffuse into the cell from the plasma. Some of the hydrogen ions are removed from the solution by combining chemically with the large amount of hemoglobin present within the red cell and to a lesser extent with the plasma proteins. This "buffering" effect of Hb contributes importantly to pH regulation, especially in venous blood where the deoxygenated Hb has a greater ability to buffer H^+ than does oxygenated Hb.

These reactions occur within the circulation of metabolizing tissue and account for the addition of CO_2 to venous blood. When the venous blood returns to the lung, the entire process is reversed. CO_2 diffuses from red cells through plasma and into alveolar gas where the CO_2 concentration is lower. There is a net shift of bicarbonate into the red cell, which is converted to CO_2 and a net shift of chloride out.

Pulmonary Gas Exchange

Arterial hypoxemia, (ie, a reduction in PaO_2 below normal) can be caused by alveolar hypoventilation (which reduces PaO_2) or by widening the difference between alveolar and arterial PO_2. In humans, the alveolar to arterial PO_2 difference is governed primarily by the uniformity of ventilation ($\dot{V}$) to perfusion ($\dot{Q}$) distribution ($\dot{V}/\dot{Q}$) ratio.[2] Alveolar to capillary diffusion disequilibrium may also play a small role in special circumstances.

Distribution of Ventilation and Perfusion: Ventilation Distribution

Interregional factors are the most important determinants of ventilation distribution in healthy individuals. In a normal, upright lung, inspired ventilation is distributed more toward the lung bases than toward the lung apex.[2] This occurs because alveoli at the top of the lung are more expanded than those at the bottom, mainly because the weight of the lung below pulls down on them and distends them. Because the lung is less stiff at low lung volumes, the less distended lower regions of the lung are easier to expand (and therefore, to ventilate) than the more distended regions in the upper portions of the lung. Thus, because of gravity, approximately two times as much inspired ventilation is delivered to the bottom versus the top regions of the upright lung. In contrast, intraregional nonuniformities in ventilation distribution are the major cause of $\dot{V}/\dot{Q}$ mismatch and arterial hypoxemia in individuals with lung disease. These nonuniformities are caused by variations in resistance and compliance in different regions of the lung. Thus, a unit with narrowed airways and increased resistance will take longer to fill with air during inspiration. Even at normal breathing frequencies, inspiratory time (T_I) may not be sufficient for every terminal respiratory unit to achieve the same volume expansion during inspiration. **Nonuniformity of ventilation distribution can result from alterations in local distensibility or resistance to airflow. The magnitude of the nonuniformity in these expanding units during inspiration will depend on the breathing frequency, that is, the time available for filling.**

Distribution of Ventilation and Perfusion: Perfusion Distribution

Blood flow distribution in the upright lung is (like inspired ventilation) directed primarily to the lung bases, which receive five times more flow than the apices. Blood flow distribution in the low-resistance pulmonary circulation is primarily under passive (ie, nonneural) control; thus, this interregional effect is purely due to gravity.[2] Given that the pulmonary artery pressure is relatively low (15 mm Hg), there is an insufficient pressure head to push blood up to the top of the upright lung throughout the entire cardiac cycle. Therefore, blood flow at the apices will be reduced (with respect to the bases), especially during diastole.

When cardiac output increases during exercise, the pulmonary circulation accommodates the increased blood flow by recruiting and distending capillaries, and as a result there is a substantial reduction in pulmonary vascular resistance. Thus, interregional blood flow during exercise is much more evenly distributed among lung regions than it is at rest.

Even in the healthy lung, not all maldistribution of perfusion is due to gravity. A likely source of within-region perfusion nonuniformity is simply the random structural differences in the diameter, length, and branching angles of the vessels. In disease states, structural heterogeneity of vessel and airway caliber is the major cause of $\dot{V}/\dot{Q}$ maldistribution.

Hypoxia-induced pulmonary vasoconstriction is a local mechanism that provides an extremely effective and "low cost" means of causing a more uniform distribution of perfusion to ventilation, thereby preventing arterial hypoxemia. Hypoxic vasoconstriction is most effective when the involved area of the lung is relatively small (ie, <20% of total lung mass). In such circumstances, blood flow can be redistributed without large effects on pulmonary vascular resistance. In contrast, if all or a majority of the lung is made hypoxic (eg, global alveolar hypoventilation, high altitudes), the resultant widespread vasoconstriction will cause pulmonary vascular resistance to rise markedly. If global hypoxia is sustained, hypertrophy of the pulmonary artery smooth muscle and chronic pulmonary hypertension will occur. Under conditions of chronic, global hypoxia, hypoxic vasoconstriction is of little or no help in maintaining alveolar to arterial O_2 exchange because *all* areas of the lung are hypoxic; that is, there are no well-oxygenated areas available for perfusion.

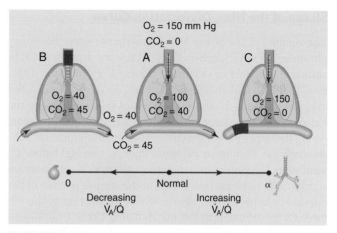

FIGURE 5-12   Effect of altering the ventilation-perfusion ratio on P_{O_2} and P_{CO_2} in a lung unit. Note that mixed venous blood has a $P_{CO_2} = 45$ and a $P_{O_2} = 40$ mm Hg in all three units.

Importance of $\dot{V}/\dot{Q}$ Ratio

Figure 5-12 demonstrates how altering the $\dot{V}/\dot{Q}$ ratio of a lung unit affects its gas exchange.[2] Three lung units (A, B, and C) are shown, all with inspired tracheal $P_{O_2} = 150$ mm Hg and $P_{CO_2} = 0$ mm Hg. The mixed venous blood entering each of the units has a $P_{O_2} = 40$ mm Hg and $P_{CO_2} = 45$ mm Hg. Lung unit A has a normal $\dot{V}/\dot{Q}$ of nearly 1.0. In this unit, $P_{A_{O_2}}$ is determined by the balance between addition of O_2 by ventilation and its removal by blood flow. $P_{A_{CO_2}}$ is determined in an analogous manner. In lung unit B, $\dot{V}/\dot{Q}$ is reduced by blocking its ventilation while leaving its blood flow intact. It is clear that the $P_{A_{O_2}}$ in the unit will fall and $P_{A_{CO_2}}$ will rise so that eventually the P_{O_2} and P_{CO_2} in the alveolar gas and end-capillary blood are the same as that of mixed venous blood. In lung unit C, $\dot{V}/\dot{Q}$ is increased by obstructing its blood flow. Now the alveolar O_2 rises and CO_2 falls, eventually reaching the composition of tracheal inspired gas.

Effect of $\dot{V}/\dot{Q}$ Inequality on Gas Exchange

The reason the lung with uneven $\dot{V}/\dot{Q}$ has difficulty oxygenating arterial blood is illustrated for the upright lung in Fig. 5-13.[2] Here, $P_{A_{O_2}}$ at the apex is 40 mm Hg greater than at the base. At the same time, the major share of blood flow leaving the lung comes from the lower areas where $P_{A_{O_2}}$ is the lowest. This combination of greatest flow and lowest P_{O_2} has the effect of depressing the P_{O_2} in the mixed arterial blood outflow. In contrast, the expired alveolar gas comes more uniformly from the apex and base because the between-region differences in ventilation are much less than those for blood flow. The result is that the mean alveolar P_{O_2} is approximately 101 mm Hg and the arterial blood P_{O_2} is 97 mm Hg; the 4 mm Hg difference between alveolar and arterial O_2 is due to $\dot{V}/\dot{Q}$ nonuniformities.

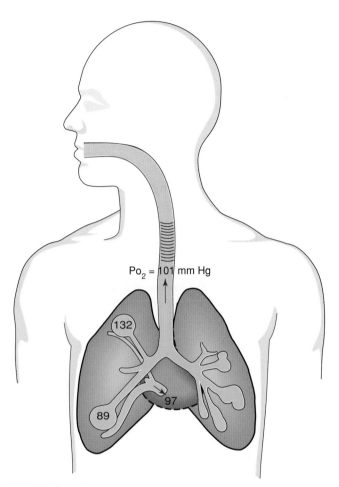

FIGURE 5-13 Depression of Pa_{O_2} by ventilation–perfusion inequality. In this diagram of the upright lung, only two groups of alveoli at the apex and base are shown. The relative sizes of the airways and blood vessels indicate their relative ventilations and blood flows. Because most of the blood comes from the poorly oxygenated base, depression of the Pa_{O_2} is inevitable.

In the figure: $P_{O_2} = 101$ mm Hg, with values 132, 97, and 89 shown.

Another reason for mean Pa_{O_2} to be less than mean P_{AO_2} is that not all of the mixed venous blood is exposed to alveolar gas for oxygenation. One to two percent of the total cardiac output bypasses the alveolar capillaries and directly enters the left ventricle, some via the bronchial airway circulation and some via the intracardiac thebesian veins. This small amount of "anatomical shunt" of blood with mixed venous O_2 composition also reduces the Pa_{O_2} and widens the alveolar to arterial P_{O_2} difference to approximately 10 mm Hg.

In disease states, $\dot{V}/\dot{Q}$ maldistribution can have devastating effects on arterial blood gases. Wasted ventilation occurs clinically when a large blood clot (pulmonary embolism) obstructs a pulmonary artery. Immediately after the occlusion, all perfusion is diverted to the unaffected lung, but half of the ventilation still goes to the affected lung. Clearly, the ventilation to the affected lung is wasted because it is ineffective in oxygenating any of the mixed venous blood. This wasted ventilation greatly increases the alveolar dead-space ventilation.

In addition, the overall efficiency of lung ventilation is decreased, because more than half the power used in breathing moves air that serves no useful purpose.

Shunt refers to a communication between two parts of the cardiovascular system that allows passage of blood from the venous to the arterial circulation without participating in gas exchange. Shunt occurs in the lung when there is a substantial and selective airway obstruction (eg, aspiration of a foreign body into a main stem bronchus or airway disease causing obstruction of a specific area of the lung). In this circumstance, a significant fraction of the pulmonary blood flow does not participate in gas exchange. The effect on Pa_{O_2} is substantial.

Alveolar–Capillary Diffusion

Fick's law states that the rate of transfer of a gas through a sheet of tissue is proportional to the tissue area and to the difference in gas partial pressure between the two sides, and inversely proportional to the tissue thickness. The large area of the blood–gas barrier in the lung (50–100 m^2) and its thinness ($<1/2$ μm) make it an ideal surface for diffusion.

The blood entering the pulmonary capillary normally has a P_{O_2} of approximately 40 mm Hg (ie, that of mixed venous blood). Across the blood–gas barrier, less than a micrometer away, is the alveolar gas with its P_{O_2} of 100 mm Hg. Oxygen moves down this large pressure gradient, and P_{O_2} in the blood rises so rapidly that it very nearly reaches equilibrium with P_{AO_2} in the time it takes for a red cell to traverse one-third of the capillary length. Thus, in normal circumstances, the difference in P_{O_2} between alveolar gas and end-capillary blood is immeasurably small (ie, a mere fraction of a millimeter of mercury).

The average transit time of a red cell through the pulmonary capillary bed, as through any vascular bed, is determined by the ratio of the size of the capillary bed (ie, the "sink," divided by the rate of blood flow into the capillary bed):

$$\text{Mean transit time} = \frac{\text{pulmonary capillary blood volume}}{\text{blood flow}}.$$

The pulmonary capillary blood volume consists of the "sheet" of blood contained in the alveolar walls and exposed to alveolar gas. It averages 80 mL in the resting human. Pulmonary blood flow consists of the entire cardiac output; therefore,

$$\text{Mean transit time (at rest)} = \frac{80 \text{ mL}}{5,000 \text{ mL/min}} = \frac{80 \text{ mL}}{83 \text{ mL/s}}$$
$$= 0.9 \text{ seconds.}$$

This is clearly sufficient time for equilibration of mixed venous and alveolar P_{O_2}. During heavy exercise, however, blood flow increases to approximately four times the resting level. If the pulmonary capillary bed were *not* capable of expanding as pulmonary blood flow increased, then

$$\text{Mean transit time (exercise)} = \frac{80 \text{ mL}}{20,000 \text{ mL/min}}$$
$$= 0.24 \text{ seconds.}$$

This might not be sufficient time to reach full equilibrium of mixed venous and alveolar P_{O_2}. In normal circumstances, however, this failure to equilibrate does *not* occur because the low-resistance pulmonary vasculature is capable of expanding its capillary blood volume during exercise to its maximum morphologic capacity (200–250 mL, or three times the resting value) by recruiting more capillaries. So,

$$\text{Mean transit time} = \frac{210 \text{ mL}}{20,000 \text{ mL/min}} = \frac{210 \text{ mL}}{333 \text{ mL/s}}$$
$$= 0.6 \text{ seconds.}$$

Thus, during exercise, marked reductions in transit time are prevented, and sufficient time is provided for diffusion equilibrium.

Neurochemical Regulation of Breathing

A complex control system is responsible for regulating ventilation so that (1) alveolar gases are precisely regulated to meet tissue needs for O_2 and CO_2; (2) ventilatory movements are integrated with other body movements, such as speech, coughing, chewing and swallowing, and posture and locomotion; and (3) the energy required to provide the needed ventilation is not excessive. A related critical need is that ventilation must remain, as much as possible, an *involuntary* act of which we are unaware. A schematic of the respiratory control system and its components is shown in Fig. 5-14.[8]

Central Integration and Rhythm Generation

Contraction of the respiratory muscles produces the tidal flow of gas within the pulmonary system. Rhythmic phrenic nerve activity emerging from the central nervous system (CNS) is the source of diaphragmatic electrical activity. Without input from the CNS, normal ventilation ceases. Note that this occurs in marked contrast to the cardiovascular system, where the heart can contract and pump blood, even when isolated from the CNS.

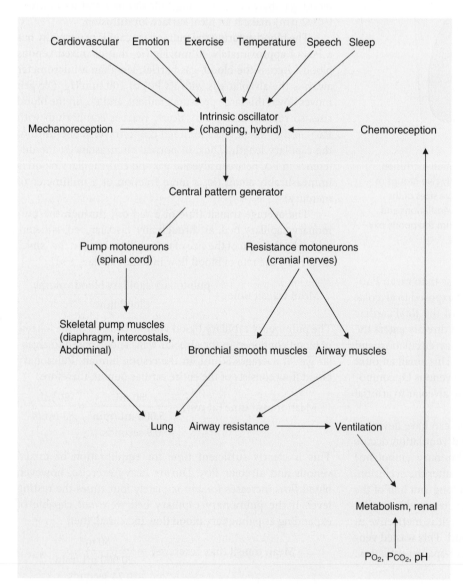

FIGURE 5-14 Schematic representation of major components of the ventilatory control system: the central oscillator and pattern generator, the sensory inputs, and the distribution of respiratory motor output to the thoracic pump muscles and the airways.

Location of Respiratory Neurons

The breathing controller is located in the pons and medulla, portions of the brain that are continuous with the spinal cord. These regions of the brainstem also contain the cardiovascular (vasomotor) centers, and it is at this level that cranial nerves IX through XII, which contain most of the sensory information about breathing, enter the CNS.

Groups of neurons in the dorsal and ventral portions of the medulla show activity that is synchronous with inspiration and expiration. The inherent rhythm of these neurons activates the bulbospinal, premotor neurons in the medulla that integrate the basic rhythm with other inputs from sensory and higher centers. The premotor neurons, in turn, relay the neural signals to α-motoneurons in the spinal cord, resulting in rhythmic breathing. The external inputs to the medullary respiratory controller from the pons and peripheral sensors influence the speed of the respiratory cycle (ie, breathing frequency) and the strength of the respiratory muscle output (tidal volume).

Descending Pathways to Respiratory Muscles

The main "pump" muscles of respiration—the diaphragm, intercostals, and abdominal muscles—are rhythmically activated by spinal α-motoneurons. In humans, phrenic motoneurons occupy a column lying in the third through fifth cervical segments. The α-motoneurons that innervate the internal and external intercostals occupy motor columns that extend the entire length of the thoracic spinal cord. The abdominal muscles, which have an expiratory function, have α-motoneurons occupying the lower thoracic and upper lumbar spinal cord segments.

The pharyngeal and laryngeal "respiratory" muscles are activated by the motoneurons of cranial nerves IX through XII. Activity in these nerves precedes phrenic activity; thus, its function is to prepare (ie, dilate and stiffen) the upper airway prior to each inspiration.

Neural pathways that exert voluntary control over breathing are important for speaking, singing, and breath-holding. These corticospinal pathways bypass, in a large part, the medullary respiratory network.

Afferent Inputs

Sensory inputs to the medullary integrator neurons are essential for generating a breath that is large enough to affect pulmonary gas exchange. These inputs act primarily as feedback regulators.

Chemoreceptors—Mammals have two types of chemoreceptors: One set peripherally located and affected by arterial blood composition and the other in the medulla, bathed by the brain interstitial fluid.[8]

The *carotid bodies*, located bilaterally at the bifurcations of the common carotid arteries, sense changes in Po_2, Pco_2, and pH of the arterial blood. Sensory information is carried from the carotid chemoreceptors to the brainstem medullary neurons via cranial nerve IX. This mechanism augments res-

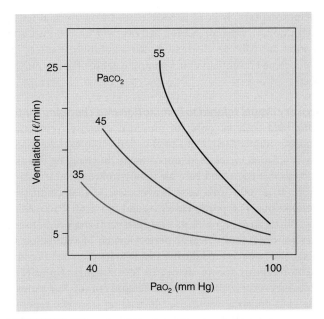

FIGURE 5-15 Effects of hypoxia on minute ventilation. As Pao_2 is reduced (by gradually reducing inspired Po_2), ventilation increases in a hyperbolic fashion and this effect of hypoxia is enhanced by increasing $Paco_2$. Thus, in the lowest response curve arterial, Pco_2 is maintained at 35 mm Hg and at the highest curve at 55 mm Hg (by adding CO_2 to inspired gas as the Po_2 is reduced).

piratory muscle activity in response to hypoxia-induced carotid chemoreceptor stimulation (Fig. 5-15). Note that the ventilatory response to hypoxia is curvilinear; at normal $Paco_2$ the response becomes quite brisk at 60 mm Hg Pao_2. This Pao_2 corresponds to the "shoulder" of the HbO_2 dissociation curve, below which O_2 saturation drops severely and tissue hypoxia probably occurs. Note also that decreased Po_2 and increased Pco_2 both stimulate ventilation via the carotid body and that, when applied together (ie, "asphyxia"), they have a multiplicative effect on ventilatory output. The carotid chemoreceptors also respond briskly to other perturbations, especially metabolism-induced changes in pH (ie, acidosis or alkalosis).

Although the *medullary chemoreceptors* have not yet been isolated anatomically, they are believed to lie on the ventrolateral surface of the medulla. The medullary chemoreceptors are very sensitive to changes in the pH of brain interstitial fluid, especially when the pH change is caused by an increase or a decrease in Pco_2. Note that the chemical environment of the medullary chemoreceptors has a closely regulated ionic composition. This regulation is due, in part, to the selective permeability of the cerebral blood vessels (ie, the blood–brain barrier). Because of the blood–brain barrier, metabolic acids and bases in the plasma enter the brain interstitial fluid very slowly. In contrast, CO_2 crosses readily and alters the pH of the interstitial fluid very quickly and substantially (it is a poorly buffered fluid because of its low protein content).

The ventilatory response to increased CO_2 in the arterial blood and the brain is due to stimulation of both the peripheral carotid chemoreceptors and the central medullary chemoreceptors. If P_{CO_2} is reduced to below normal levels (hypocapnia), chemoreceptor activity will be reduced and ventilation will be decreased. This inhibitory effect of hypocapnia on ventilation is a common cause of apnea during sleep.

Sensory inputs related to locomotion and changing metabolic rate—At the onset of muscular exercise, ventilation increases immediately. With each increment in exercise intensity, ventilation increases in proportion to the changing $\dot{V}_{O_2}$ and $\dot{V}_{CO_2}$ so that Pa_{CO_2} and Pa_{O_2} are tightly controlled near resting levels. It is only with very heavy exercise that ventilation increases out of proportion to $\dot{V}_{CO_2}$, and as a result, Pa_{CO_2} falls.[9]

What can account for this very fast ventilatory response at exercise onset and the near-perfect match of ventilation to metabolic rate required during steady-state exercise? Because chemoreceptors see no change or "error signal" (in arterial P_{CO_2}, P_{O_2}, or pH), these chemical factors cannot play a major role in stimulating ventilation. Instead, at least two types of stimuli and receptors are probably involved.

Neurons located in the motor areas of the higher CNS perform the dual roles of (1) initiating movement by means of neural impulses reaching the spinal cord via corticospinal tracts and (2) simultaneously stimulating medullary respiratory neurons via direct corticomedullary pathways. This means that stimulating breathing during exercise is considered a *feedforward* mechanism because ventilation is increased without knowledge of feedback from the periphery.

Receptors in limb skeletal muscles are responsive to tension, stretch, and metabolic stimuli such as changes in pH and potassium. These receptors are activated by muscle contraction and, in turn, exert a positive *feedback* influence on the ventilatory response via afferent pathways in the spinal cord. This influence explains at least a portion of the increase in ventilation during muscular exercise.

Metabolic rate (CO_2 production, in particular) influences breathing so that $\dot{V}_A$ tracks changes in tissue CO_2 production. As a result, the average Pa_{CO_2} is tightly regulated within narrow limits. For example, increased carbohydrate ingestion (which increases $\dot{V}_{CO_2}$ and the respiratory exchange ratio), changes in body mass, hypo- and hyperthyroidism, and renal dialysis all alter the amount of tissue CO_2 production and all also cause corresponding changes in $\dot{V}_A$. The exact nature of the stimulus and location of receptor sites responsible for this coupling of $\dot{V}_A$ to $\dot{V}_{CO_2}$ in the resting subject remain unknown.

Mechanical feedback—Whereas most of the sensors mentioned previously are concerned with providing adequate $\dot{V}_A$, receptors in the chest wall and lung are concerned with "how" we take individual breaths, that is, with the optimization of the mechanical work. As discussed previously, mechanical impedances offered by the lung and airways must be overcome by the respiratory muscles in order to produce volume expansion of the lungs and gas flow through the airways. To keep respiratory muscle work to a minimum, receptors in the muscles are sensitive to their own rate and magnitude of tension develop-

ment and relay this activity to the medulla via the spinal cord or phrenic nerve afferents.[10] Receptors in the lung and airways also sense the rate and magnitude of lung stretch. This input, which is relayed to the medulla via the vagus nerves, has substantial effects on the breathing pattern.

The pulmonary stretch receptors affect breathing pattern—During inspiration, vagal afferent fibers from the pulmonary stretch receptors (PSRs) fire in proportion to lung volume, thereby inhibiting medullary inspiratory neurons, so that expiration can begin. Thus, vagal feedback is an important inhibitory "off-switch" to determine breathing pattern; however, it is not the only mechanism available to terminate inspiration. Pontine neurons also signal medullary neurons to make the switch from inspiration to expiration.

In adult humans, PSRs seem to be less sensitive than those in other mammals; that is, the lung volume at which PSRs exert their inhibitory effect is much higher. Thus, PSRs play little role during normal tidal ventilation in the human at rest, but become important during exercise to ensure that V_T is constrained to the linear and more compliant part of the pressure–volume relationship for the respiratory system.

Many other types of lung mechanoreceptors, present in the airways and lung parenchyma, affect a wide variety of respiratory responses. Other receptors served by the vagus nerves include the *irritant receptors* that are stimulated by inhaled chemicals and particulates and by changes in bronchiolar smooth muscle tone. Stimulation of these receptors elicits cough and bronchoconstriction. They also respond to airway narrowing or closure and, accordingly, they are responsible for the augmented inspirations or "sighs" which we take periodically to maintain patent airways. In addition, *J-receptors* located in the lung parenchyma have afferent fibers that travel in the vagus nerves. These fibers elicit tachypnea (rapid, shallow breathing) when stimulated by increased interstitial fluid pressure (eg, in pulmonary edema).

Chest wall proprioceptors play an important role in "load compensation." Like all skeletal muscles, the respiratory muscles of the chest wall develop forces that depend on their starting length (preload) and their afterload. Preload varies with body posture and afterload is a function of the magnitude of lung and chest wall expansion and the resistance to airflow. Receptors in the chest wall reflexively modify motor nerve discharge to the respiratory muscles in such a manner that ventilation changes are minimized, despite varying preloads and afterloads.

Phrenic afferents—When the diaphragm is overworked to the point of showing signs of fatigue, end products of metabolism such as lactic acid and hydrogen and potassium ions begin to accumulate in the muscle's interstitial space. These metabolites activate muscle receptors with small, unmyelinated phrenic afferents, and as a result, phrenic efferent activity is inhibited. As a result, the diaphragm no longer works at the same high level and further fatigue is avoided.

Distribution of efferent outputs—As mentioned previously, many different respiratory muscles are important to taking a breath. By distributing motor output to the various muscles, the medullary controller coordinates their actions very precisely.

Inspiration is accomplished primarily by phrenic activation and diaphragmatic contraction, but intercostal muscles also play a major role, especially if the level of ventilation is increased. Thus, the "load" is shared and the diaphragm is spared. Activation of intercostal muscles also helps (along with the rib cage) to stiffen the chest wall. This allows the diaphragm to contract and create a negative pleural presence without inward movement of the thoracic wall. In some pathological conditions (eg, obstructive lung disease), the diaphragm is shortened and flattened because of hyperinflation and therefore must work from a mechanical disadvantage. In these cases, accessory muscles of respiration, such as the scalenes and sternocleidomastoids, assist with inspiration by lifting the rib cage.

The greatest and most variable site of resistance to airflow is the upper extrathoracic airway. The calibers of the pharynx and larynx are controlled by abductor muscles innervated by hypoglossal motor nerves that originate from the medulla in close proximity to the respiratory controller neurons. This arrangement means that just prior to the activation of the chest wall inspiratory muscles, the airway is stiffened and the orifice diameter increased. Like the chest wall, these respiratory muscles of the upper airway are under both feedforward and feedback control. For example, during exercise the pharyngeal and laryngeal orifices are fully abducted during both inspiration and expiration, beginning with the first augmented breath (probably a feedforward mechanism). If upper airway narrowing occurs during sleep, increased negative pressure in the airway triggers a reflex activation of upper airway dilator muscles, so that further collapse is prevented (a feedback mechanism).

Conscious Perception of Breathing Effort: Dyspnea

Muscle spindle afferents originating in the chest wall and vagal afferents from the lung, project to the cerebellum and cerebral cortex, as well as to the medulla. Furthermore, medullary inspiratory and expiratory neurons also project to the higher CNS. It is likely that such connections form the anatomical pathways by which feedback from respiratory movements and loads and even chemoreceptor stimuli are perceived consciously.

In normal circumstances, sensory inputs to the brain from the pulmonary system do not enter the individual's awareness, even when VT and force production increase substantially (eg, during moderate exercise). In contrast, an unpleasant perception of breathing, dyspnea, seems to arise when either the drive to breathe is excessive or a mechanical impediment to ventilation exists. Increased drive occurs when the medullary respiratory neurons are bombarded with feedback inputs from chemoreceptors or from feedforward inputs from the motor cortex. Mechanical impediments to breathing occur with airway obstruction or restriction of lung volume. **Dyspnea is most likely to occur when there is a discrepancy between the neural drive to breathe and the level of ventilation achieved.[11]**

Control of Breathing in the Newborn

The transition from placental gas exchange during intrauterine life to air breathing brings with it multiple, rapid changes in the newborn's pulmonary system.[12] Consider, for example, that functional alveoli multiply at a rate of approximately 200 per minute over the first year of life, that thousands of neural synapses turn over each day in the CNS, and that the PaO_2 almost doubles within the first few breaths of postnatal life. Thus, all feedback and feedforward systems in the ventilatory control system are affected by birth and maturation, in addition to concomitant changes in the mechanical characteristics of the lung and chest wall. The following events are known to occur with maturation in the infant.

- The carotid bodies appear to be more vital for maintaining adequate ventilation in the newborn, as shown by the marked apneas and significant mortality caused by carotid body denervation at birth. Carotid sinus nerve activity has been shown to be significant in the fetal animal and the carotid body response to hypoxia increases over the first few weeks of life.

- Mechanoreceptor feedback from lung stretch and upper airway narrowing are much stronger in newborn than adult humans. Brief apneas and periodicities in breathing pattern are common in the first weeks of life, as are frequent augmented inspirations (or sighs)—the latter serving to homogenize the distribution of ventilation and to increase surfactant production during the transition to air breathing. Brief apneas are accompanied by profound brachycardia in the newborn, signifying a powerful diving reflex.

- The infant's ribs are cartilaginous and extend at near right angles (rather than obliquely as in the adult) from the vertebral column, thereby providing a more circular ribcage shape. The area of apposition of the diaphragm on the ribs is also very small and the diaphragm is relatively flat. Thus, the rib cage expands slightly on inspiration and the diaphragm is mechanically disadvantaged.

- The relative compliances of the rib cage and lungs in the newborn means that passive FRC is reduced to approximately 10% of TLC (rather than 50% as in the adult). Accordingly, in order to preserve an adequate end-expiratory lung volume (and oxygen reservoir), the infant "actively" regulates an end-expiratory lung volume by showing a strong continued postinspiratory activity of the diaphragm during early expiration, along with a strong adduction of the upper airway. Both these mechanisms oppose the normal elastic recoil of the lungs, prolong expiration, and maintain a high end-expiratory lung volume.

- Body temperature is highly labile and more subject to environmental temperature in the newborn, and the infant quickly changes tissue heat production as environmental temperature changes. With hypoxia, the newborn also reduces the metabolic rate in order to preserve ATP production in the face of a reduced O_2 supply. This hypometabolic response probably explains the infant's ventilatory response to hypoxia, which consists of a brisk initial hyperventilation, followed quickly by ventilatory depression.

- An infant spends more than twice as much time in REM (rapid eye movement) sleep as does an adult, and this is believed to be important to the neuronal maturation of the central nervous system. It also means that most skeletal muscles, including the intercostal muscles, are atonic much of the time and when this atonicity is added to the already highly compliant cartilaginous rib cage structure, the rib cage will (paradoxically) be sucked in with each diaphragmatic inspiration. Thus, in REM sleep, for any given V_T the infant must augment the amount of diaphragmatic effort.

Despite the maturation required of most key mechanical and neural characteristics of the ventilatory control system, full-term and even the great majority of preterm infants survive and thrive while this maturation is taking place (ie, during the first 1–2 years of life). Rarely does the control system fail, as it apparently does in sudden infant death syndrome (SIDS). Some scientists have attributed this breakdown to an immature, unstable ventilatory control system that allows apneas to worsen and persist, upper airways to obstruct, and arousal mechanisms to fail. On the other hand, not all evidence supports this apnea hypothesis of SIDS. Clearly, the pathogenesis of this extremely difficult-to-study malady must be multifactorial.

SUMMARY

In this chapter we have reviewed the basic concepts of cardiovascular and pulmonary physiology for the entry-level physical therapy practitioner. To provide a framework for understanding the pathophysiology of these two systems, we have emphasized the regulatory mechanisms responsible for maintenance of tissue homeostasis. Knowledge of how pathology affects function in patients with cardiovascular and pulmonary disease is a basic, essential component of patient–client management.

Heads Up!

This chapter contains a CD-ROM activity.

REFERENCES

1. West JB, ed. *Best and Taylor's Physiological Basis of Medical Practice.* 12th ed. Baltimore, MD: Lippincott Williams & Wilkins; 1991.
2. West JB. *Respiratory Physiology—The Essentials.* 5th ed. Baltimore, MD: Lippincott Williams & Wilkins, 1995.
3. Berne RM, Levy MN. *Cardiovascular Physiology.* 7th ed. St Louis, MO: Mosby; 1997.
4. Smith JJ, Kampine JP. *Circulatory Physiology—The Essentials.* 3rd ed. Baltimore, MD: Lippincott Williams & Wilkins; 1998.
5. Braunwald E, Ross J, Sonnenblick EH. *Mechanisms of Contraction of the Normal and Failing Heart.* 2nd ed. Boston, MA: Little, Brown; 1976.
6. Rowell LB. *Human Cardiovascular Control.* New York: Oxford University Press; 1993.
7. Rowell LB, Shepherd JT, eds: *Handbook of Physiology: Exercise: Regulation and Integration of Multiple Systems.* New York: Oxford University Press for the American Physiological Society; 1996.
8. Feldman JL, Smith JC. Neural control of respiratory pattern in mammals: an overview. In: Dempsey JA, Pack AI, eds. *Regulation of Breathing.* New York: Marcel Dekker; 1995:39-69.
9. Dempsey JA, Forster HV, Ainsworth DM. Regulation of hyperpnea, hyperventilation, and respiratory muscle recruitment during exercise. In: Dempsey JA, Pack AI, eds. *Regulation of Breathing.* New York: Marcel Dekker; 1995:1065-1134.
10. Jammes Y, Speck DF. Respiratory control by diaphragmatic and respiratory muscle afferents. In: Dempsey JA, Pack AI, eds. *Regulation of Breathing.* New York: Marcel Dekker; 1995:543-582.
11. Shea SA, Banzett RB, Lansing RW. Respiratory sensations and their role in the control of breathing. In: Dempsey JA, Pack AI, eds. *Regulation of Breathing.* New York: Marcel Dekker; 1995: 923-957.
12. England SJ, Miller MJ, Martin RJ. Unique issues in neonatal respiratory control. In: Dempsey JA, Pack AI, eds. *Regulation of Breathing.* New York: Marcel Dekker; 1995:797-827.

6

Cardiovascular Pathophysiology

Sandra L. Cassady & Lawrence P. Cahalin

INTRODUCTION

Despite the increased emphasis on health promotion and prevention, advances in technology, and the development of evidence-based treatment regimens, coronary atherosclerotic heart disease (ASHD) remains the leading cause of cardiovascular death and disability in the United States.[1–3] All physical therapists, regardless of area of specialization or practice setting, treat patients with cardiovascular disease. Common symptoms of cardiovascular disease include dyspnea, chest pain, claudication, palpitations, syncope, and fatigue. None of these symptoms, however, are specific to a given system or cardiovascular disorder. By understanding the pathophysiology and clinical manifestations of common cardiovascular diseases, physical therapists are more likely to deliver safe interventions. The onset or change in symptoms detected during an examination may indicate the development or progression of a serious and potentially life-threatening disease.

This chapter presents the pathophysiology and clinical manifestations of most common cardiovascular diseases found in the adult. Medical care and therapeutic interventions are presented elsewhere in this text. Before discussing specific diseases, several important facts necessary to understand common pathologies of the cardiovascular system are presented. These facts provide a very brief introduction and rationale for the material presented in the remainder of the chapter.

OVERVIEW OF MAJOR CARDIOVASCULAR DISEASES

1. ***More than half of all deaths in industrialized countries are due to cardiovascular diseases.*** More than 50% of all adults in the United States and in other industrialized countries die of atherosclerosis and other major manifestations of this disease.[4,5] Most of the related morbidity in this country can be accounted for by atherosclerosis of the coronary arteries, the cerebral blood vessels, and the aorta and its main branches. Hypertension, an important complication of atherosclerosis, contributes to the severity of the disease and aggravates its symptoms. Accounting for approximately 10% of all cases of heart disease,[6] hypertension may occur independent of atherosclerosis or precede it. Clotting disturbances complicate atherosclerosis. Thrombosis of atherosclerotic coronary arteries is the main cause of myocardial infarction (MI).[7–9] Thrombi may occur without preexisting atherosclerosis and are common in the venous system.

2. ***Abnormal cardiac development during fetal life is a significant cause of disease in newborns.*** Within the first 2 months after conception, the heart develops through several complex embryologic processes (see Chapter 4). The true incidence of cardiovascular malformations is difficult to determine accurately. It has been estimated that approximately 0.8% of livebirths are complicated by a cardiovascular malformation.[10] Although many infants born with cardiac defects have anomalies that are not life-threatening and heal on their own, almost one-third (2.6 per 1,000 livebirths)[11] have disease severe enough to result in a cardiac catherization, cardiac surgery, or death in the first year of life. Ventricular septal defects represent the most common congenital cardiac malformation in infants and children.[5] In adults, the incidence of this defect and others is much lower due to spontaneous or surgical closure during infancy and death before adulthood. Further information about congenital cardiac abnormalities is found in Chapter 21.

3. ***Cardiac function is dependent on a constant supply of oxygen and nutrients.*** Reduction of the lumen secondary to narrowing or occlusion of the arteries affects blood supply to the myocardium and causes ischemia. Current theories for the pathogenesis of atherosclerosis will be presented. Other mechanisms (ie, vasospasm) will also be described in this chapter. Either sudden occlusion of arterial blood flow (MI) or chronic ischemia may lead to cardiac pump dysfunction or failure. Patients with ischemia may present with bouts of angina pectoris. Angina pectoris

is one of the many causes of chest pain that physical therapists must be able to differentiate from other forms of chest discomfort.

4. ***Although regulated by hormones and biogenic amines, arterial blood pressure is dependent on both the action of the heart and elastic and contractile properties of the arteries and arterioles.*** Blood flow depends on pressure gradients generated by the action of the heart and the peripheral resistance of arteries and arterioles. Smooth muscle cells in the arteries and arterioles contract under the influence of adrenergic nerves, which release the catecholamines epinephrine and norepinephrine. These catecholamines are also produced by adrenal medullary cells and released into the circulation. Epinephrine and norepinephrine affect both the heart and the blood vessels. Blood pressure is also regulated by the hormones renin, angiotensin, and aldosterone. Abnormalities in the regulation of blood pressure may result in hypertension or hypotension. Both are commonly found in patients with cardiovascular disease.

5. ***Heart failure is a clinical syndrome, or a group of signs and symptoms, that results from abnormalities in the function of the heart.*** Heart (cardiac) failure is recognized as a pathophysiological state in which the heart is unable to pump blood at a rate commensurate with the requirements of metabolizing tissues. This results in elevated filling pressures due to loss of myocardial contractility.[10] More than 6 million patients suffer from heart failure in the United States.[12] This growth is not only due to the aging population but also due to the decrease in mortality from other cardiovascular diseases.

6. ***The heart is susceptible to blood-borne pathogens.*** A variety of inflammatory processes may be responsible for coronary artery abnormalities. Some of these mimic atherosclerotic disease and may predispose the individual to true atherosclerosis. Recent developments in our understanding of the inflammatory mechanisms and their direct and indirect effects on vascular wall cells have led to the consideration that chronic bacterial and viral infections may be potential initiating factors.[13] *Chlamydia pneumoniae,*[14,15] *Helicobacter pylori,*[16] and cytomegalovirus[17] are among the prominent potential infectious causes of atherosclerosis. Although there are several examples of positive associations between pathogens and disease, at present there is insufficient evidence[18] to designate infection as a causal risk factor for coronary heart disease.

7. Bacteria and other pathogens found in blood-producing septicemia may invade the endothelium of blood vessels and the endocardium of the heart. Because the endocardium is in direct contact with blood, bacterial endocarditis is a common infectious lesion of the heart.[19] With the exception of immunosuppressed persons, intramural bacterial abscesses of the myocardium and bacterial pericarditis are uncommon. Patients with preexisting lesions, as in congenital heart disease, valve deformities, or mural thrombi, are predisposed to cardiac infections. Blood clots provide a very suitable growth medium for bacteria. Clots within the ventricles and those attached to the valves often become infected. Emboli may result from infected thrombi, and embolization of peripheral arteries may result in infectious arteritis. Venous infections (eg, thrombophlebitis) are usually related to preexistent thrombosis.

8. ***Systemic metabolic diseases often affect the heart and the blood vessels.*** Diabetes mellitus is a very strong risk factor for the development of coronary artery disease (CAD) and stroke.[20,21] Eighty percent of all deaths among patients with diabetes are due to atherosclerosis. Among all hospitalizations for diabetic complications, more than 75% are due to atherosclerosis.[5] Caused by an absolute or relative deficiency of insulin or a resistance of tissues to insulin, this systemic disorder of intermediary metabolism primarily affects small blood vessels (microangiopathy). In all groups of patients, diabetes accelerates the natural course of atherosclerosis and involves a greater number of coronary vessels with more diffuse atherosclerotic lesions.[22–25]

9. ***Inflammatory and destructive cardiac lesions may result from immune complexes and immunoglobulins in the blood that may be deposited in the heart and blood vessels.*** Immunoglobulins are found in normal blood and have no adverse influences on the heart and blood vessels. However, when circulating immunoglobulins are complexed with antigen into immune complexes, they become pathogenic and cause vasculitis or endocarditis. Hypersensitivity reactions that elicit formation of antibodies to the body's own tissues can damage the heart and blood vessels, as in rheumatic fever. Both fatal and nonfatal acute MIs and sudden coronary death may occur early in the course of autoimmune disorders. For example, patients with fatal systemic lupus erythematosus (SLE), who receive treatment with glucocorticoids for more than 2 years, demonstrate a high incidence of coronary atherosclerosis at the time of autopsy.[26–28] Accelerated atherosclerosis is increasingly recognized as a leading cause of morbidity and mortality, especially among young women with systemic lupus erythematosus who receive long-term glucocorticoid administration.[26,27]

10. ***Malignant tumors of the cardiovascular system are rare.*** Primary tumors of the heart are less common (incidence of 0.002%–0.3%)[29–35] than metastatic tumors of the heart.[36] Benign tumors occur more frequently than malignant ones,[37] and many tumors are curable by surgery. The most common cardiac tumor is the myxoma. Malignant tumors of the heart and blood vessels are classified as sarcomas and hemangiosarcomas, respectively. Small benign vascular tumors, hemangiomas, are very common and are of limited clinical significance.[38,39]

11. ***Within each form of cardiovascular disease, the level of impairment and limitation on activity may vary within and between patients.*** As a means of quantifying the activity limitations imposed by symptoms, the classification

BOX 6-1

The Functional Classification of Heart Disease: New York Heart Association Classification System

Class I   No limitation of physical activity. Ordinary physical activity does not cause undue fatigue, dyspnea, or anginal pain.

Class II   Slight limitation of physical activity. Ordinary physical activity results in symptoms.

Class III   Marked limitation of physical activity. Comfortable at rest but less than ordinary activity causes symptoms.

Class IV   Unable to engage in any physical activity with out discomfort. Symptoms may be present even at rest.

BOX 6-2

Characteristics and Lifestyles Associated with Increased Risk of Future Coronary Artery Disease

Personal Characteristics (Nonmodifiable)
Male gender
Age
Family history of CAD or other atherosclerotic vascular disease before age 55 in men, before age 65 in women
Personal history of CAD or other atherosclerotic vascular disease (eg, cerebrovascular or occlusive peripheral vascular disease)

Biochemical or Physiologic Characteristics (Modifiable)
Blood lipid abnormalities
    Elevated blood total cholesterol
    Elevated LDL cholesterol or VLDL cholesterol
    Low HDL cholesterol
Elevated blood triglycerides
Hyperglycemia/diabetes mellitus
Obesity
Hypertension

Lifestyles (Modifiable)
Tobacco smoking
Diet high in saturated fat, cholesterol, and calories
Excess alcohol consumption
Physical inactivity

LDL, low-density lipoprotein; HDL, high-density lipoprotein; CHD, coronary heart disease; VLDL, very low-density lipoprotein.

Adapted from Kasper EK, Agema WR, Hutchins GM, et al. The causes of dilated cardiomyopathy: a clinicopathologic review of 673 patients. *J Am Coll Cardiol.* 1994; 23:586.

system of the New York Heart Association (NYHA)[40] displayed in Box 6-1 is commonly used. Physical therapists are trained to address the needs of their patients and clients across all delivery settings, and they are encouraged to incorporate the principles of the disablement model as outlined in the *Guide to Physical Therapist Practice.*[41] This resource *guides* therapists through the essential elements of patient/client management. Classifications such as that of the NYHA help facilitate communication among professionals about the functional limitations resulting from their active pathologies.

CARDIAC DISEASE

Atherosclerotic Heart Disease (Coronary Artery Disease)

As stated previously, coronary atherosclerotic heart disease is the most common cause of cardiovascular disability and death in the United States. Men are more often affected than women by an overall ratio of 4:1. Before age 40 this ratio is 8:1, but beyond age 70 it is 1:1. In men, the peak incidence of the clinical manifestations is in the fifth decade of life compared to the sixth decade for women.[3]

Atherosclerotic heart disease (ASHD), also known as coronary artery disease (CAD), is a progressive disease process characterized by irregularly distributed lipid deposits in the intimal layer of medium and large coronary arteries. Although the mechanisms of atherogenesis are still under investigation, epidemiological studies have identified several risk factors associated with an increased likelihood of developing premature CAD. Risk factors classified as modifiable characteristics, nonmodifiable characteristics, and lifestyle preferences are shown in Box 6-2. Alterable risk factors are the focus of interventional risk-factor reduction studies and cardiac rehabilitation. Blood homocysteine levels and hypoestrogene-

mia in women are two important risk factors under investigation. Several retrospective studies have identified mild-to-moderate increases in homocysteine, an amino acid, as a strong and independent risk factor for CAD, stroke, and peripheral vascular disease.[42–45] However, some prospective studies[46–48] have failed to show this association. In these patients, elevated plasma homocysteine appears to be more closely linked to thrombus-mediated coronary events (ie, MI) than to coronary atherosclerosis seen on angiography.[49] Elevated homocysteine is also linked to venous thrombosis. The exact mechanisms remain unclear but may include endothelial toxicity, accelerated oxidation of cholesterol, an impairment of endothelial-derived relaxing factor, and a reduction in flow-mediated arterial vasodilation.[50–53] As previously mentioned, chronic infections may also be involved and remain under investigation as causal risk factors for atherosclerosis.[13]

Recent research has also focused on abnormalities of lipid metabolism. Risk *increases* progressively with higher levels of low-density lipoprotein (LDL) cholesterol and *declines* with higher levels of high-density lipoprotein (HDL) cholesterol.

The ratio of LDL to HDL cholesterol provides a composite marker of risk. Ratios below 3:1 indicate lower risk, whereas ratios above 5:1 indicate a higher risk.[54] There is further evidence that other abnormalities of lipid metabolism may also play a role in the pathogenesis of CAD. Patterns associated with increased atherosclerosis include elevated levels of apolipoprotein (A) and small, dense LDL lipoprotein particles. These lipoproteins and their accompanying lipids appear more likely to pass into the vessel wall and may be more difficult to clear. Although elevated triglyceride levels often occur in association with other lipid abnormalities, accumulating evidence suggests that hypertriglyceridemia is an independent risk factor for CAD.[54–57] A more thorough review of the epidemiological evidence for the risk factors associated with cardiovascular disease can be found in Chapter 15.

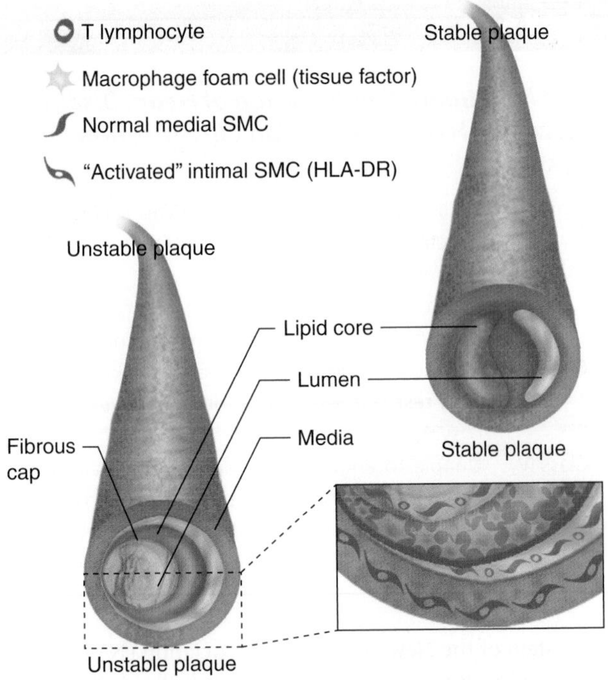
T lymphocyte
Macrophage foam cell (tissue factor)
Normal medial SMC
"Activated" intimal SMC (HLA-DR)
Stable plaque
Unstable plaque
Lipid core
Lumen
Media
Fibrous cap
Stable plaque
Unstable plaque

FIGURE 6-1 Characteristics of "stable" and "vulnerable" coronary atherosclerotic lesions. Initially, vulnerable plaques grow outward. The vulnerable plaque has a substantial lipid core and thin fibrous cap separating the thrombogenic macrophages from the blood. At sites of lesion disruption, smooth muscle cells (SMC) are activated and detected by the presence of human leukocyte antigen-DR (HLA-DR). The stable plaque has a relatively thick fibrous cap protecting the lipid core from contact with the blood. Stable plaques often cause luminal narrowing.

The Atherosclerotic Lesion

Our knowledge of the pathophysiology of atherosclerosis and the clinical presentations of CAD continue to accumulate rapidly. **Abnormal lipid metabolism and/or the excessive intake of cholesterol and saturated fats, especially when superimposed on genetic predisposition, initiate the atherosclerotic process and development of atherosclerotic plaque.**[5,10]

Atherosclerotic plaque consists of accumulated intracellular and extracellular lipids, connective tissue, smooth muscle cells, and glycosaminoglycans (eg, several sulfates and hyaluronic acid). The earliest detectable lesion of atherosclerosis is the *fatty streak*. The fatty streak consists of lipid-laden *foam cells,* which are macrophages that have migrated as monocytes from the circulation into the subendothelial layer of the intima. Later, the fatty streak evolves into fibrous plaque that is made up of intimal smooth muscle cells surrounded by connective tissue and intracellular and extracellular lipids.

Pathogenic Mechanisms of Plaque Formation

Although the exact mechanism of plaque formation remains under study, many hypotheses have been developed. The most pervasive include the lipid hypothesis and the chronic endothelial injury hypothesis. Both are described in the following sections.

The lipid hypothesis—The lipid hypothesis states that elevation in plasma LDL levels results in penetration of LDL into the arterial wall, leading to lipid accumulation in smooth muscle cells and in macrophages (foam cells) (see Fig. 6-1). LDL also augments smooth muscle cell hyperplasia and migration of cells into the subintimal and intimal regions in response to growth factors. LDL is modified or oxidized in this environment and is rendered more atherogenic. Small, dense LDL cholesterol particles are also susceptible to modification and oxidation. The modified or oxidized LDL is chemotactic to monocytes, which promotes their migration into the intima, their early appearance in the fatty streak, and their transformation and retention in the subintimal compartment as macrophages. Scavenger receptors on the surface of macrophages facilitate the entry of oxidized LDL into these cells, transforming them into lipid-laden macrophages and foam cells. Oxidized LDL is also cytotoxic to endothelial cells and may be responsible for their dysfunction or loss from the more advanced lesion.[58–60]

An atherosclerosis model has been studied in monkeys fed a cholesterol-rich diet.[61,62] This study demonstrated that within 1 to 2 weeks of inducing hypercholesterolemia, monocytes attached to the surface of the arterial endothelium through the induction of specific receptors, migrated into the subendothelium, and accumulated lipid in macrophages (ie, foam cells). Proliferating smooth muscle cells also accumulate lipid. As the fatty streak and fibrous plaque enlarge and bulge into the lumen, the subendothelium becomes exposed to the blood at sites of endothelial retraction or tear, and platelet aggregates and mural thrombi form. It is postulated that the release of growth factors from the aggregated platelets may increase smooth muscle proliferation in the intima. The organization and incorporation of the thrombus into the atherosclerotic plaque may contribute to its growth.[63]

The chronic endothelial injury hypothesis—The chronic endothelial injury hypothesis states that, through various mechanisms, endothelial injury produces loss of endothelium, adhesion of platelets to subendothelium, aggregation of platelets, chemotaxis of monocytes and T-cell lymphocytes,

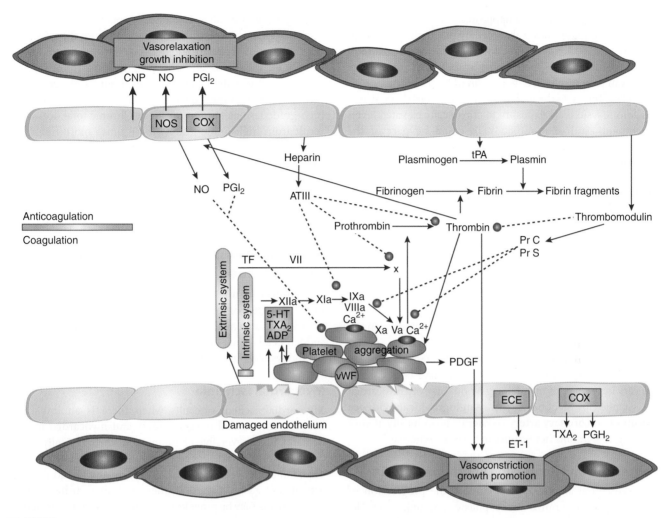

FIGURE 6-2 The complex interaction of the endothelium, platelet aggregation, and coagulation. Vasorelaxation: nitric oxide (NO), nitric oxide synthase (NOS), C-type natriuretic peptide (CNP), prostaglandin I_2 (PGI$_2$), cyclooxygenase (COX). Anticoagulation: antithrombin (ATIII), tissue plasminogen factor (tPA), protein C, protein S (Pr C, Pr S), Coagulation: tissue factor (TF), von Willebrand factor (vWF). Platelet aggregation: serotonin (5-HT), adenosine diphosphate (ADP). Vasoconstriction and growth promotion: platelet-derived growth factor (PDGF), endothelin-converting enzyme (ECE), enthothelin-1 (ET-1), prostaglandin H_2, thromboxane A_2 (TXA$_2$). (Reproduced with permission from Volta SD. *Cardiology*. Berkshire, UK: McGraw-Hill; © 1999.)

and release of platelet-derived and monocyte-derived growth factors. This induces migration of smooth muscle cells from the media into the intima, where they replicate, synthesize connective tissue and proteoglycans, and form a fibrous plaque (see Fig. 6-2). Other cells (eg, macrophages, endothelial cells, arterial smooth muscle cells) also produce growth factors that can contribute to smooth muscle hyperplasia and extracellular matrix production.[5]

Modified LDL is cytotoxic to cultured endothelial cells and may induce endothelial injury, attract monocytes and macrophages, and stimulate smooth muscle growth. Modified LDL also inhibits the mobility of macrophages, so that once they transform into foam cells in the subendothelial space they may become trapped. In addition, regenerating endothelial cells (after injury) are functionally impaired and increase the absorbed LDL from plasma.

The atherosclerotic plaque may grow slowly and over several decades may result in severe arterial stenosis or may progress to total arterial occlusion. With time, the plaque becomes *calcified*. Some plaques are stable, but others, especially those rich in lipids and inflammatory cells (eg, macrophages) and covered by a thin fibrous cap, may undergo spontaneous fissure or rupture, exposing the plaque contents to flowing blood (see Fig. 6-2). These plaques are believed to be unstable or vulnerable and are more closely associated with the onset of an acute ischemic event.[5] The ruptured plaque stimulates thrombosis; the thrombus may (1) embolize, (2) rapidly occlude the lumen to precipitate myocardial ischemia or infarction, or (3) gradually become incorporated into the plaque, contributing to its stepwise growth.

The two hypotheses just described are closely linked and not mutually exclusive. The lipid hypothesis suggests that remnants of triglyceride-rich lipoproteins or modified LDL of hyperlipidemic subjects are absorbed by macrophages to form the early atherosclerotic lesion and that chronic exposure of endothelium to these lipoproteins leads to cell injury. Cell necrosis in turn results in a deposition of lipid in the extracellular space. Injury to the endothelium and progression of atherosclerotic lesions by exposure to chronically elevated levels of remnants and/or modified LDL could be part of the sequence leading to the formation of occlusive plaques and to their clinical sequelae.[64,65]

As previously introduced, recent studies[13,66,67] have validated an old theory that atherosclerosis progresses as the result of an inflammatory response in the vessel wall. The process may be initiated or worsened by an infectious agent as diverse as cytomegalovirus, *C. pneumoniae*, and *H. pylori*. A high circulating level of the nonspecific inflammatory marker, *C-reactive protein*, has been correlated with a higher rate of ischemic events.

Coronary Anastomosis (Collaterals)

Larger caliber collaterals develop below adjacent arteries on the epicardial surface. These are believed to be preexisting smaller arteries altered by flow-induced pressure differentials between different coronary beds. Functionally, these have been considered very important for maintaining blood supply to myocardial cells supplied by stenotic vessels.[5] **Angiographical evidence indicates that coronary artery collaterals form locally at sites of high-grade lesions in response to chronic ischemia.**[5]

Progression and Regression of Atherosclerosis

With sequential angiographical studies, the progression of atherosclerosis is known to be phasic and unpredictable.

High-grade lesions do not necessarily appear where low-grade lesions were once found. New lesions of more than 50% can occur between repeated angiograms. Sites of future lesions cannot be identified and the progression cannot be predicted.[68-71] Individual plaques may progress at accelerated rates unrelated to their degree of stenosis. We do know that high-grade lesions tend to progress. Chronic total occlusions result from high-grade lesions three times more frequently than in cases of less severe lesions but frequently do not result in infarction because of collateral development.[72] Stenotic *regression* can also be demonstrated angiographically in some but not all cases after either aggressive pharmacologic treatment with statins or very low-fat diets.

Manifestations of Atherosclerotic Heart Disease

The clinical manifestations of ASHD typically evolve after many decades of progressive atherosclerosis and include myocardial ischemia, infarction, congestive heart failure, and sudden death. Each of the possible manifestations and related pathophysiology are presented.

Myocardial Ischemia

Myocardial ischemia results when there is an imbalance between myocardial oxygen supply and myocardial oxygen demand. It is a reversible phenomenon, which typically comes on with exertion and goes away with rest. The factors affecting the balance between myocardial oxygen supply and demand are illustrated in Fig. 6-3. Increased myocardial oxygen requirements may be provoked by a number of factors including

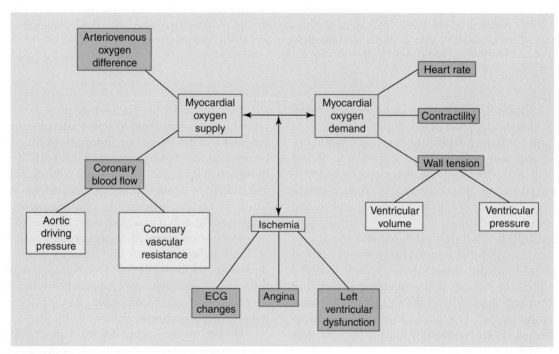

FIGURE 6-3   Factors influencing myocardial oxygen supply and demand.

exercise, mental stress, or even spontaneous fluctuations in heart rate and blood pressure. Decreased oxygen supply may result from a reduction in coronary blood flow. (The reader may recall the already-high extraction of oxygen from blood flowing through myocardial tissue, with the resultant dependence on coronary blood flow to meet myocardial demand. See Chapters 3 and 5.) Decreased blood flow may be due to decreased aortic driving pressure or increased coronary vascular resistance, which may be due to coronary vasospasm, platelet aggregation, or partial thrombosis.

It is a commonly held belief that coronary artery occlusion greater than 70% produces myocardial ischemia, which in turn provokes the symptoms that bring the patient to the doctor's office. The patient at this stage of atherosclerotic progression is comfortable at rest but will complain of chest pressure during mild-to-moderate exercise, which is relieved by rest. The diagnosis of ischemic heart disease is usually made on the basis of a formal exercise stress test.

Coronary atherosclerosis and coronary arterial spasm both reduce coronary blood flow and thus reduce myocardial oxygen supply. When this happens, myocardial ischemia and irritability occur, which may produce arrhythmias, impaired myocardial contractility (systolic dysfunction), and impaired myocardial relaxation (diastolic dysfunction). This diastolic dysfunction prolongs systole and reduces ventricular filling time. Ventricular compliance decreases and the ventricular end-diastolic pressure rises, causing aortic driving pressure to be further reduced. Myocardial ischemia often manifests itself on an electrocardiogram (ECG) as ST-segment displacement (see Chapter 11).

The threshold for myocardial ischemia can be either predictable or unpredictable. Abnormal endothelial function appears to play a role in the unpredictable, fluctuating threshold for ischemia. The majority of studies suggest that endothelium-dependent vasodilator mechanisms predominate in nondiseased epicardial coronary arteries. During interventions that normally induce increases in myocardial oxygen consumption and blood flow (eg, exercise, stress, induced tachycardia), epicardial vascular dilation occurs. This dilation is at least partially endothelial dependent. However, the presence of even nonocclusive, early atherosclerosis appears to *impair* the release of endothelium-relived relaxing factor (nitrous oxide), attenuating this vasodilator mechanism, which results in prevailing, unopposed vasoconstriction. Moderate vasoconstriction in an area of minimal occlusion may be of little hemodynamic consequence; however, the same degree of vasoconstriction in an area of greater occlusion may markedly decrease blood flow and induce ischemia.[73–75]

Stable angina—The classical symptom of myocardial ischemia is *angina pectoris*. This discomfort is described as pressure, heaviness, or tightness that may be located in the middle of the chest (substernal); over the heart (precordial); or in the shoulder, arm, throat, or jaw. Angina may be precipitated by exertion, stress, emotions, and heavy meals. Stable angina usually lasts for several minutes and is usually relieved by rest and/or nitroglycerin. The patient is pain free at rest.

Anginal pain arises within the myocardium and is thought to stimulate free nerve endings in or near small coronary vessels. Impulses travel in afferent unmyelinated or small myelinated cardiac sympathetic nerves through the upper thoracic ganglia to dorsal horn cells and through the spinothalamic tract of the thalamus to the cortex.[5,76] The cerebral cortex integrates and modifies these impulses. This modulation may contribute to the variability in the perception of angina across patients. Psychosocial and cultural factors may also influence the perception of pain at the cortical level.

Unstable angina—The term *unstable angina* is usually used to denote either a change in the anginal pattern or angina at rest. Unstable angina may occur with less exertion than previously described, may last longer, or become less responsive to medication. Angiography has shown that a high proportion of patients with unstable angina have complex coronary stenoses characterized by plaque rupture, ulceration, or hemorrhage with subsequent thrombus formation. This inherently unstable situation may progress to complete occlusion and infarction, or may heal, with reendothelialization and return to a stable though possibly more severe pattern of ischemia. New-onset angina is sometimes considered unstable, but if it presents in response to exertion and responds to rest and medication, it does not carry the same poor prognosis.

Prinzmetal (variant) angina—*Prinzmetal angina,* also called atypical or variant angina, is an unusual type of cardiac pain due to myocardial ischemia that occurs almost exclusively at rest. Prinzmetal and colleagues[77] hypothesized that variant angina was the result of transient increases in vasomotor tone or *vasospasm.* Vasospasm causes a transient, abrupt, marked decrease in the diameter of the coronary artery that results in myocardial ischemia. In such cases, no preceding increases in myocardial oxygen demand occur. Vasospasm can occur in both normal and diseased coronary arteries. Often the decrease in the diameter can be reversed by nitroglycerin.[10] Variant angina is usually not associated with physical exertion or emotional stress and is associated with ST-segment elevation, rather than with depression on ECG.[78] This form of angina is often severe and characteristically occurs in the early morning, awakening patients from sleep. It tends to involve the right coronary artery and is likely to be associated with arrhythmias or conduction defects.[5] Prinzmetal angina may be associated with acute MIs and severe cardiac arrhythmias, including ventricular tachycardia and fibrillation (see Fig. 6-4).[79]

Asymptomatic (silent) myocardial ischemia—Many individuals have some episodes of "silent" ischemia (ischemia without symptoms); some patients have only silent ischemia. Asymptomatic ischemic episodes may be present in patients with any of the aforementioned ischemic coronary syndromes or after an MI. Some patients never complain of chest pain with episodes of ischemia; others *inconsistently* report chest pain

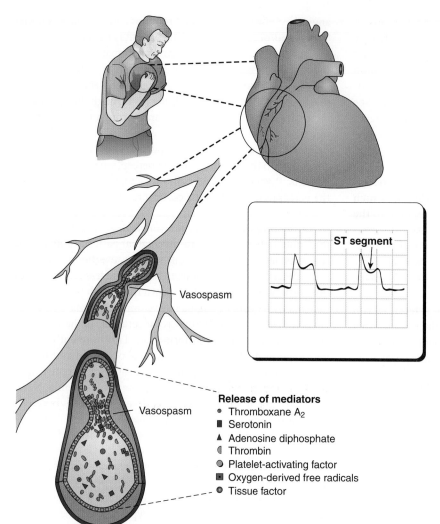

FIGURE 6-4   Clinical presentation, electrocardiographic, chemical, and arterial changes associated with coronary artery spasm. Note the ST-segment elevation above baseline.

with episodes of ischemia. The true prevalence of silent ischemia is undetermined, but it is believed to be high. Important factors include age, the presence and extent of CAD, and other disease processes that include peripheral neuropathy as a component (eg, diabetes mellitus, alcoholic neuropathy).

Some clinicians have attempted to explain silent ischemia as angina that is less noxious than reported angina. The correlation between ECG evidence of ischemia and the report of anginal pain in patients with chronic stable angina is only fair.[80,81] Therefore, the most likely explanation is neurologic. Neuropathy with defective sensory efferent nerves occurs commonly in persons with diabetes. The variable expression of ischemic pain may be explained by modification of pain stimuli in the central nervous system. Patients with diabetes have a relatively high incidence of painless MIs and definite silent ischemic episodes as documented by ambulatory ECG recordings and exercise testing.[82–85]

Anginal equivalents—These include dyspnea, fatigue, light-headedness, and belching brought on by exercise or stress and relieved by rest or nitroglycerin. We have said that some patients with diabetes may not complain of chest discomfort due to impaired peripheral sensation (eg, silent ischemia).

Alterations in neural processing can, by extension, also give rise to anginal equivalents. Ischemic episodes in this group can present as a fullness in the throat and jaw, a desire to cough, or dyspnea. Elderly patients and patients with peripheral neuropathies may also present with anginal equivalents.

The rich variety of radiation patterns associated with angina pectoris is determined by the levels of the spinal cord, which share sensory inputs with somatic structures (eg, gut) and the heart. The precise mechanisms causing angina and anginal equivalents are yet to be defined.

Myocardial Infarction

Pathogenesis—MI results from prolonged myocardial ischemia and is precipitated in most cases by an occlusive coronary thrombus at the site of a preexisting atherosclerotic plaque. Less frequently,[3,65,86] infarction may result from prolonged vasospasm, inadequate myocardial blood flow (eg, hypotension), or excessive metabolic demand. Very rarely, MI may be caused by embolic occlusion, aortitis, vasculitis, or coronary artery dissection. Cocaine[87] and other similar types of drugs can induce coronary artery vasoconstriction and may lead to myocardial ischemia as well as to infarction.

Regardless of the etiology, an MI results in the complete interruption of blood supply to an area of myocardium, almost always in the left ventricle, and more rarely in the right ventricle. Cells die and tissues become necrotic in an area referred to as the *zone of infarction*. Within 18 to 24 hours after MI, an inflammatory response occurs in response to necrosis. Leukocytes aid in the removal of dead cells, and fibroblasts form a connective tissue scar within the area of infarction. Visible necrosis is present in 2 to 4 days. During this time, proteolytic enzymes remove debris while catecholamines, lipolysis, and glycogenolysis elevate plasma glucose and increase free fatty acids to assist depleted myocardium recovery from an anaerobic state. By 4 to 10 days the debris is cleared and a collagen matrix is laid down. Between 10 and 14 days, weak, fibrotic scar tissue with beginning revascularization is present. This area remains vulnerable to stress. **Usually, the formation of fibrous scar tissue is complete within 6 to 8 weeks.**[88,89] Inelastic scar tissue replaces the necrotic tissue and the region is unable to contract and relax like healthy myocardial tissue. When a *transmural MI* occurs with full-thickness necrosis, wall motion may be reduced (hypokinetic), abnormal (dyskinetic), or absent (akinetic). When necrosis is limited to the innermost layer of the heart (ie, *subendocardial MI*), wall motion will usually appear to be normal.

CLINICAL CORRELATE

The completed scar is tough, usually thick, and fibrous and serves to protect the heart from further damage. Current best practice calls for the implementation of low-level exercises designed to maintain function and prevent the deleterious effects of prolonged inactivity during this initial 6- to 8-week period.

Adjacent to the zone of infarction is a less seriously damaged area of injury called the *zone of hypoxic injury*. This zone is able to return to normal, but may become necrotic if blood flow is not restored. With adequate collateral circulation, this area may regain function within 2 to 3 weeks. Immediately surrounding the zone of injury is another reversible zone known as the *zone of ischemia* (see Fig. 6-5).

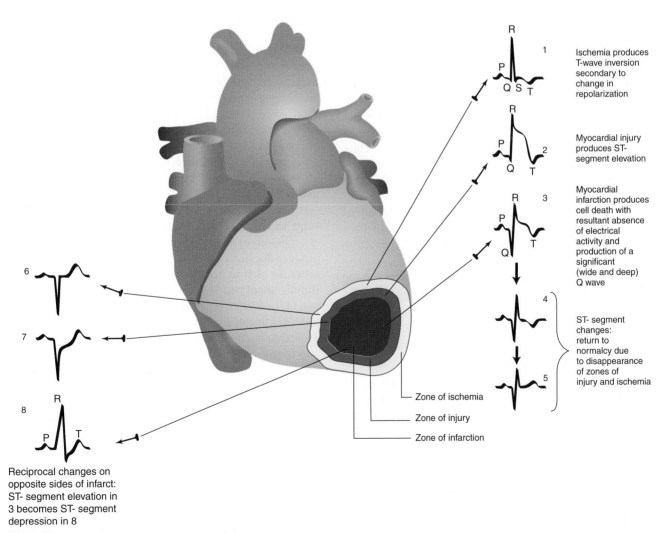

1 Ischemia produces T-wave inversion secondary to change in repolarization

2 Myocardial injury produces ST-segment elevation

3 Myocardial infarction produces cell death with resultant absence of electrical activity and production of a significant (wide and deep) Q wave

4 ST-segment changes: return to normalcy due to disappearance of zones of injury and ischemia

5

Zone of ischemia
Zone of injury
Zone of infarction

Reciprocal changes on opposite sides of infarct: ST-segment elevation in 3 becomes ST-segment depression in 8

FIGURE 6-5 ECG changes associated with the three zones of infarction.

The location and extent of infarction depend on the anatomic distribution of the occluded vessel, the presence of additional stenotic lesions, and the adequacy of collateral circulation. Occlusion in the anterior descending branch of the left coronary artery results in infarction of the anterior left ventricle and the interventricular septum. Occlusion of the left circumflex artery produces anterolateral or posterolateral infarction. Right coronary thrombosis leads to infarction of the posteroinferior portion of the left ventricle and may involve the right ventricular myocardium and interventricular septum. The arteries supplying the atrioventricular node and the sinus node more commonly arise from the right coronary; thus, atrioventricular blocks at the nodal level and sinus node dysfunction occur more frequently during inferior infarctions. A general rule is that the more proximal the lesion, the greater the extent of the infarct. Individual variation in coronary anatomy and the presence of collateral vessels can make it difficult to locate the precise site of the lesion responsible for infarction. The gold standard for identification of the blockage and infarct site remains that of coronary angiography rather than that of ECG. The necrotic, ischemic, and injured myocardial tissue cause characteristic ECG changes as the myocardium heals. These changes are described in the following sections.

As mentioned previously, MIs are classified as either *transmural* (full-thickness) or *subendocardial* (partial-thickness) infarctions. Transmural MIs are characterized by electrocardiographic evolution of ST-segment elevation with significant Q waves. Subendocardial MIs are characterized by ST-T wave changes but without the development of significant Q waves (see Chapter 11). On pathologic examination, however, most infarctions involve the subendocardium initially, and some transmural extension is common even in the absence of Q waves. Thus, some cardiologists prefer the classification of Q wave or non–Q-wave infarction. The non–Q-wave infarction generally results from incomplete occlusion or spontaneous lysis of the thrombus and signifies the presence of additional jeopardized myocardium; non–Q-wave infarctions are associated with a higher incidence of reinfarction and recurrent ischemia.[90,91]

CLINICAL CORRELATE

Because of this high incidence of reinfarction, patients with subendocardial MIs are considered less stable than those with transmural MIs. Indeed, many of these patients will be referred to surgery for surgical management. For this reason, physical therapy interventions tend to be more conservative than those directed toward patients with full-thickness MIs.

The size and anatomic location of the infarction strongly influence the acute course, the early complications, and the long-term prognosis. Hemodynamic stability is related to the extent of necrosis. In small infarctions, cardiac function may be normal, whereas with more extensive damage, early heart failure and cardiogenic shock[92] may appear. Prevention of infarct extension by reducing both the zones of injury and ischemia is a major goal of early intensive care unit management.

Diagnosis of an MI relies upon the presentation of classical symptoms, elevation of specific enzymes, and an acute injury pattern on ECG with evolutionary ECG changes over time.[93–95] Because of the multiple neural innervation levels, pain presentation with MI may vary (see CD-ROM). It has been estimated that up to 25% of MIs occur without any symptoms.[96] These silent MIs present a challenge to the clinician who must utilize other monitoring techniques and instruct patients about symptom recognition and provide activity guidelines. These alternative methods of therapeutic intervention are described in Chapter 10.

Diagnosis and laboratory findings—Diagnosis of an acute MI requires that at least two of the following three elements be present: (1) a history of ischemic-type chest discomfort, (2) evolutionary changes on serially obtained ECG tracings, and (3) a rise and fall in serum cardiac enzymes.[97] With respect to these three elements, there is considerable variation in presentation.

Clinical presentation of myocardial infarction—The most notable symptom of an MI is the sudden sensation or onset of chest discomfort that is often described as "crushing chest pain or pressure," which occasionally radiates to the arms, neck, throat, and back. This pain is usually constant, lasts for 30 minutes or more, and may be associated with pallor and shortness of breath. The pain of MI is qualitatively different from the pain of angina. The former is usually more severe and prolonged and unrelieved by rest. Patients who are prescribed nitroglycerin are instructed to report to the hospital if their angina is unrelieved after three doses, because of the likelihood of an evolving MI.

The chest pain of an MI is accompanied by a dramatic surge in sympathetic nervous system activity. The release of catecholamines results in sympathetic stimulation, which may produce diaphoresis and peripheral vasoconstriction that may cause the skin to become cool and clammy to touch. Reflex stimulation of vomiting centers may cause nausea and vomiting. In the first 24 hours, fever may develop and persist for up to a week because of the inflammatory responses within the myocardium. If cardiac output is compromised, the patient may complain of lightheadedness due to a reduction in blood pressure. The patient experiencing an acute MI may also be in denial and not seek care for several days following the event. It should be noted that patient denial of symptoms will result in the delay of medical care. This delay does not only affect diagnosis and treatment—it can also have tragic consequences. Indeed, the sooner the patient presents to the hospital, the better the chances of survival. "Time is muscle" is a phrase that can save a patient's life!

Electrocardiography—Electrocardiographic changes are almost always present in patients experiencing acute infarctions. A normal tracing obtained during an MI is rare. The

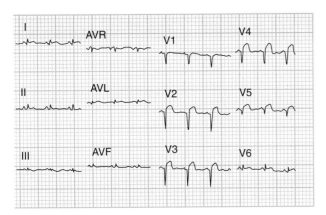

FIGURE 6-6 Twelve-lead electrocardiogram showing an acute anterolateral wall myocardial infarction. Note the ST-segment elevations in V2–V6, coupled with deep Q waves in V1–V5, representing areas of myocardial injury and necrosis, respectively.

extent of the electrocardiographic abnormalities provides only a rough estimate of the magnitude of infarction. The earliest signs are usually peaked or "hyperacute" T waves, followed by ST-segment elevation, Q-wave development, and finally T-wave inversion. This sequence of events may develop over a few hours or over several days. The evolution of new Q waves (>30 ms in duration and one-third the height of the R wave) is diagnostic for transmural MI. Q waves do not develop in 30% to 50% of acute infarctions, representing subendocardial MI. If these patients have a typical clinical presentation (ie, elevated cardiac enzymes and ST-segment changes, usually depression or T-wave inversion lasting at least 48 hours), they are classified as having non–Q-wave infarctions.[93,94] Some of these changes are shown in acute and subacute tracings for an anterior and lateral wall infarction (Fig. 6-6). Further discussion of electrocardiography can be found in Chapter 11.

Cardiac enzymes—As myocytes become necrotic, the integrity of the sarcolemmal membrane is compromised and serum cardiac markers diffuse into the cardiac interstitium. These markers eventually reach the microvasculature and lymphatics in the region of the infarct.[98] Intracellular location, molecular weight, local blood and lymphatic flow, and the rate of elimination from the blood are all factors that determine the rate of appearance of the markers.[99–101] Markers currently monitored include creatine kinase (CK), myoglobin, and the cardiac-specific troponins (troponin T, and troponin I). Lactic dehydrogenase (LDH) and serum glutamic–oxaloacetic transaminase (SGOT) are also enzymes that are frequently used to rule in an MI.

CK is released when cells die. Three isoenzymes of CK have been identified by electrophoresis: The MM band is specific to skeletal muscle death, the BB band is specific to brain cell death, and the MB band is specific to myocardial cell death. Rapid assays are now available for CK-MB isoforms. A ratio of CK-MB2/CK-MB1 greater than 2.5 has a sensitivity for the presence of myocardial cell necrosis of 46.4% at 4 hours and 91.5% at 6 hours.[62] **Serum CK levels exceed the normal range within 4 to 8 hours after the onset of an acute MI and returns to normal within 2 to 3 days.[10] Peak CK occurs on average at approximately 24 hours.** Although the elevation of CK is considered a sensitive detector of an acute infarction, false positives are found in many patients including those with muscle disease, diabetes mellitus, skeletal muscle trauma, pulmonary embolism, and alcohol intoxication.[99,101,102]

Myoglobin is a protein released into circulation from injured myocardial cells and can be detected within a few hours after the onset of infarction. Peak levels of myoglobin are reached within 1 to 4 hours. Myoglobin is excreted into the urine. Its measurement has been suggested as a useful index of successful reperfusion.[103] Patients presenting with ST-segment elevation less than 6 hours from symptoms and a diagnosis of MI are at increased risk of mortality when myoglobin is elevated.

The cardiac troponins are the newest markers. The troponin complex consists of three subunits that regulate the calcium-mediated contractile processes of striated muscle. Troponin C binds Ca^{2+}; troponin I binds to actin and inhibits actin–myosin interactions; and troponin T binds to tropomyosin. Troponin T and troponin I are highly cardiac selective and are released into the blood during an MI. These regulatory proteins rise within 4 to 6 hours of the onset of cell necrosis and remain elevated for several days after the infarction.[10]

CLINICAL CORRELATE

Because of the rapid elevation and decline in CK-MB assays, patients who are in denial and who delay presentation to the emergency room may show normal CK-MB values. However, troponin levels remain elevated for a longer period of time and may "salvage" a diagnosis (see Fig. 6-7).

Treatments and complications—Management of patients with MI can be divided into medical and surgical interventions. Medical interventions include the use of pharmacological agents aimed at reducing myocardial oxygen demand (eg, β-blockade, calcium channel blockade), increasing myocardial oxygen supply (eg, coronary artery vasodilators), and improving/maintaining myocardial function (eg, digitalis glycosides). These medical interventions are covered in some detail in Chapter 8. Current surgical interventions for patients with MI include thrombolysis, intra-aortic balloon pump, angioplasty, and stent placement[104–106] (see Table 6-1).

Some of the surgical interventions in Table 6-1 deserve comment. Drugs that have the potential to dissolve ("lyse") a thrombus within a coronary artery are called *thrombolytic agents* and are introduced surgically by way of a catheter whose tip is placed in the coronary artery at the site of the blockage. Thrombolytic agents such as streptokinase and tissue plasminogen activator (tPA) are then administered, usually within a few hours of an acute MI in hope of dissolving a

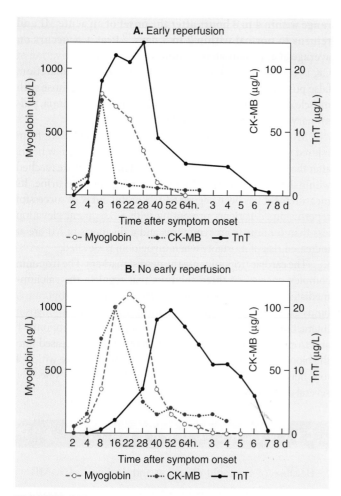

A. Early reperfusion

--o-- Myoglobin   --•-- CK-MB   --•-- TnT

B. No early reperfusion

--o-- Myoglobin   --•-- CK-MB   --•-- TnT

FIGURE 6-7 Evolution of three major serum markers (CK-MB, myoglobin, and troponin T) after myocardial infarctions in patients in whom (**A**) reperfusion with thrombolytics was successful and (**B**) not achieved. (Reprinted with permissions of Chapelle JP. *Diagnosticum.* 1993;93(1):8-15).

thrombus and improving blood flow to areas of myocardium in the zones of injury and ischemia.

Coronary artery stents were first introduced into clinical practice in the mid-1980s. These are cylindrical wire-mesh devices that are placed at the site of vascular occlusion via balloon angioplasty. Stents are now used in 80% of all percutaneous cardiac interventions.[107] However, their propensity to restenosis has led to the recent development in drug-eluting "coated stents." These devices are coated with antiproliferative substances, most notably rapamycin. Early results show extremely low restenosis rates averaging between 0% and 9% after 6 and 12 months,[107] respectively.

The use of intracoronary radiation therapy (brachytherapy) is a relatively recent addition to management options of patients with MI and/or residual ischemia. It was developed to address the relatively high rate of restenosis in patients following stent placement.[108–110] This technique involves the use of radiation delivered either via a stent or a catheter-based system. It is believed that this radiation inhibits smooth muscle cell mitosis and proliferation of adventitial myofibroblasts.[111]

The use of enhanced external counterpulsation (EECP) devices demonstrates early promise in the treatment of ischemia.[112–116] It is a noninvasive outpatient series of treatment sessions that consists of total 35 hours, divided into one or two 60-minute treatment sessions 5 days a week. A series of pneumatic compressive cuffs is wrapped around the calves and thighs. Inflation of the cuffs is synchronized with the cardiac cycle such that inflation occurs during diastole and deflation occurs during systole (see Table 6-1). The benefits of enhanced external counterpulsation have been shown to last up to 5 years following initial treatment.

With all these interventions, it is important to remember that early recognition and prompt intervention provide the most options and increased chance of salvaging injured myocardium.

Even when treatment is initiated promptly, a variety of complications can occur following an MI (Box 6-3). Approximately 10% of patients experience a recurrent infarction in the first 10 to 14 days.[3] Infarct extension is at least twice as common in non–Q-wave infarcts when compared to Q-wave infarcts. The recurrent infarct may be relatively silent or associated with prolonged or intermittent chest pain. Abnormalities of rhythm and conduction are common. Myocardial dysfunction is proportionate to the extent of necrosis. A large MI will destroy a large portion of myocardium and likely result in extensive myocardial dysfunction. Extensive myocardial dysfunction is likely to produce acute heart failure, hypotension, and possibly shock, all of which are indicative of a poor prognosis after an acute MI.[95]

Heart Failure

In this chapter, heart failure is presented as one of the possible manifestations of ASHD. Further information about heart failure can be found in Chapter 18. Heart failure exists when the

TABLE 6-1 Current Treatment of Myocardial Infarction

Intervention	Description	Outcome
Early initiation of emergency services	CPR, defibrillation, aspirin, nitroglycerin, oxygen, etc	Cardiovascular stabilization, maintaining myocardial oxygen supply, decreasing myocardial oxygen demand
Intracoronary thrombolysis	Administration of clot-dissolving drugs (eg, streptokinase, tPA)	Salvage of jeopardized myocardium
Intra-aortic balloon pump (IABP)	Placement of balloon-tipped catheter in aorta distal to the aortic arch	Increases ejection of blood from left ventricle during systole; improves coronary artery perfusion during diastole
Percutaneous transluminal coronary angioplasty (PTCA)	Inflation of balloon-tipped catheter in coronary artery at the site of occlusion	Restoration of myocardial blood flow via plaque compression
PTCA with stent placement	Placement of a cylindrical wire mesh at the site of occlusion in coronary artery	Restoration and maintenance of myocardial perfusion via plaque compression
Intracoronary radiation therapy (brachytherapy)	Local ionizing g- or b-radiation is delivered to the site of coronary stenosis	Reduction of restenosis via plaque irradiation
Coronary artery bypass graft (CABG)	Use of select veins or arteries obtained from the patient, which bypasses atherosclerotic lesions	Restoration of myocardial blood flow via revascularization
Left ventricular assist devices (LVAD)	Mechanical device that surrounds the ventricles and assists in ventricular ejection	Improves stroke volume and cardiac output, used as either bridge to transplantation or destination therapy
Cardiac transplantation	Replacement of heart from a suitable donor	Improves cardiac performance
Enhanced external counterpulsation (EECP)	Pneumatic cuffs applied to the lower extremities that alternately inflate and deflate	Increases collateral blood flow to ischemic areas of the myocardium

heart is unable to pump sufficient cardiac output to meet the body's metabolic demands. Clinically, *heart failure* is defined as a syndrome with a variety of interrelated pathophysiologic phenomena, of which impaired ventricular function is the most important. This results in a reduction of exercise capacity and other characteristic clinical manifestations.[64] Many of the signs and symptoms are related to systolic dysfunction.

Systolic function of the heart is determined by four major determinants: (1) the end-diastolic volume and the resultant fiber length of the ventricles prior to onset of the contraction (*preload*), (2) the impedance to left ventricular ejection (*afterload*), (3) the contractile state of the myocardium (*contractility*), and (4) the rate of contraction, or heart rate (*chronotropy*).[3]

Heart function may be impaired as a result of alterations in any of these four determinants. The most common problem is depression of myocardial contractility, caused either by a loss of functional muscle due to infarction or by processes diffusely affecting the myocardium. The heart may fail as a pump because of excessive preload (eg, valvular regurgitation) or when afterload is excessively elevated, as occurs in severe hypertension. Pump function may also be inadequate when the heart rate is too slow or too rapid. The normal heart is capable of handling considerable variation in preload, afterload, and heart rate; however, the diseased heart often has limited reserve for handling such challenges.

Cardiac pump function may be normal or even supranormal at rest, but inadequate when metabolic demands or requirements for blood flow are in excess. This situation is termed high-output heart failure. Hyperthyroidism, beriberi, severe anemia, arteriovenous shunting, osteitis deformans (Paget disease), and sepsis may result in high-output heart failure.[117]

Cardiac failure may also occur as a result of isolated or predominant *diastolic dysfunction* of the heart. In these cases, filling of the left or right ventricle is impaired because of excessive hypertrophy or changes in the composition of the myocardium. Contractility may be preserved; however, diastolic pressures are elevated and cardiac output may be reduced.[10,118]

A number of cardiac and systemic adaptations occur when the heart fails. If the stroke volume of either ventricle is reduced by depressed contractility or excessive afterload, end-diastolic volume and pressure in that chamber will rise. This increases end-diastolic myocardial fiber length, resulting in a greater systolic shortening in the normal heart; but in the failing heart, Starling's law is less applicable. If the condition is chronic, *ventricular dilatation* will occur. Although this may restore resting cardiac output, the resulting chronic elevation of diastolic pressures will be transmitted back up to the atria and to the pulmonary and systemic venous circulation. Ultimately, increased pulmonary capillary pressure may lead to transudation of fluid, with resulting *pulmonary or systemic edema*. Reduced cardiac output will also activate several neural and humoral systems. Increased activity of the sympathetic nervous system will stimulate myocardial contractility, heart rate, and venous tone. This change results in a rise in central blood volume, which serves to further elevate preload. Although these adaptations are designed to increase cardiac output, tachycardia and increased contractility may result and cause ischemia in patients with underlying CAD. The rise in preload may worsen pulmonary congestion. Sympathetic nervous system activation also increases *peripheral vascular resistance*. Because peripheral vascular resistance is also a major determinant of left ventricular afterload, excessive sympathetic activity may further depress cardiac function. Lower cardiac output causes a reduction in renal blood flow and glomerular filtration rate, which leads to sodium and fluid retention. The renin–angiotensin–aldosterone system is also activated, leading to further increases in peripheral vascular resistance and left ventricular afterload as well as sodium and fluid retention. Heart failure is also associated with increased circulating levels of arginine vasopressin, a vasoconstrictor and inhibitor of water excretion.[118,119]

Myocardial failure is characterized by two hemodynamic alterations. The first is a reduction in the ability to increase cardiac output in response to increased demands imposed by activity or exercise (*cardiac reserve*). The second major abnormality is the elevation of ventricular diastolic pressure. This is considered a result of compensatory processes.

Heart failure may be left sided or right sided, or involve both sides of the heart (biventricular failure). Patients with *left heart failure* have symptoms of low cardiac output and elevated pulmonary and venous pressures. In *right-sided heart failure,* signs of fluid retention predominate. Many patients exhibit signs and symptoms of both right- and left-sided failure. Left ventricular failure is the most common cause of right-sided failure. The pathophysiology and manifestations for left- and right-sided heart failure are listed in Table 6-2.

Left ventricular failure (congestive heart failure)—Intrinsic myocardial disease (eg, ASHD, cardiomyopathy), excessive workload on the heart (eg, hypertension, valvular disease, congenital defects), and cardiac arrhythmias or iatrogenic damage (eg, drug toxicity, irradiation) can result in the development of left ventricular failure. Systolic ventricular dysfunction results in a reduced stroke volume and increased end-diastolic volume with a resultant drop in the ejection fraction (stroke volume/end-diastolic volume). Increased left ventricular end-diastolic volume (LVEDV) decreases left ventricular compliance and causes the left atrial volume to expand, which results in left atrial dilatation. The elevated end-diastolic volume will produce higher end-diastolic pressure, which will be reflected back to the left atria, and pulmonary vessels and their pressures will be elevated. If pulmonary pressures rise high enough to cause transudation of intravascular fluid from the pulmonary capillaries (and if the rate of transudation exceeds the rate of lymphatic drainage), then dyspnea and possibly pulmonary edema will develop. In addition, the diastolic dysfunction or delayed

TABLE 6-2   Clinical Manifestations of Heart Failure

Left Ventricular Failure	Right Ventricular Failure
Progressive dyspnea (on exertion first)	Dependent edema
Dyspnea and orthopnea	Hepatomegaly
Paroxysmal nocturnal dyspnea	Ascites
Fatigue, weakness	Fatigue
Pulmonary rales	Anorexia, nausea, bloating
S_3 heart gallop	Right-sided S_3 or S_4
Enlarged heart	Accentuated P2
Possible functional mitral and tricuspid regurgitation RV lift of sternum	Murmurs with pulmonary or tricuspid valve insufficiency

S/S of pulmonary edema
  Marked dyspnea
  Pallor
  Cyanosis
  Diaphoresis
  Tachypnea
  Anxiety
  Agitation
	Jugular venous distension
	Weight gain
	Right upper quadrant (liver) pain
	Jaundice
	Cyanosis (nail beds)
	Decreased urine output

Cerebral hypoxia
  Irritability
  Restlessness
  Confusion
  Impaired memory
  Sleep disturbances	

ventricular relaxation resulting from left ventricular hypertrophy causes an even greater left ventricular end-diastolic pressure (LVEDP). Elevated LVEDP inhibits diastolic coronary blood flow to the endocardium and thus increases the risk of subendocardial ischemia. Finally, marked left ventricular dilatation can stretch the mitral valve annulus, resulting in functional mitral regurgitation.

Left heart failure may cause a reduction in physical exercise capacity. Systolic dysfunction may result in a marked decrease in stroke volume and ejection fraction, producing an elevated end-diastolic pressure, which causes blood to be reflected backward into the lung fields. The lungs become soggy and difficult to move, resulting in premature exercise-induced shortness of breath. Redistribution of blood flow due to reduced cardiac output during exercise will also cause a reduction of blood flow to the kidneys and skin initially and later to the brain, gut, and skeletal muscle. However, during exercise, peripheral arteriovenous oxygen extraction will increase, which may compensate for reduced blood flow.

Right ventricular failure—Elevated pulmonary artery pressures caused by left ventricular failure, mitral valve regurgitation, or chronic or acute pulmonary disease can result in an increased pressure load on the right ventricle, with resultant right ventricular dilatation. Right ventricular hypertrophy may or may not develop, depending on the acuteness and severity of the pressure load. If the pressure rises acutely (eg, massive pulmonary embolism or acute mitral regurgitation), there will be right ventricular dilatation and failure without right ventricular hypertrophy. If pulmonary hypertension is a chronic problem (eg, COPD), the right ventricle will undergo hypertrophy in response to chronically increased right ventricular afterload.

Prolonged pulmonary hypertension causes irreversible anatomic changes in the walls of the small pulmonary arteries so that the hypertension becomes chronic, with resultant right ventricular dilatation and right ventricular hypertrophy. Hypoxia, hypercapnia, and/or acidosis cause further pulmonary vasoconstriction, resulting in an even greater degree of pulmonary hypertension. The workload on the right ventricle is subsequently increased. Eventually the right ventricular end-diastolic pressure increases, which will be reflected back to the right atrium and the venous system with resultant jugular venous distension, liver engorgement, ascites, and peripheral edema. Also, right ventricular hypertrophy reduces right ventricular compliance that may interfere with right ventricular filling and further reduce cardiac output. If there is a reduction in blood flow to the pulmonary vascular bed, or an increase in cardiac output, heart rate, or blood volume, then pulmonary hypertension will worsen, producing increased signs and symptoms of right ventricular failure. The manifestations of left- and right-sided heart failure are summarized in Table 6-2.

When possible, the treatment of heart failure targets the underlying cause (eg, ischemia, hypertension, valvular disease, arrhythmias).[120,121] Pharmacologic therapy includes a wide variety of agents that attempt to improve contractility, reduce preload, promote vasodilation, impede the stimulation of the sympathetic nervous system, or relieve hypoxia. See Chapter 8. Nonpharmacologic, surgical, and therapeutic interventions for the management of heart failure are presented in Chapter 18.

Sudden Death

Sudden death is characterized by a loss of consciousness and absence of an arterial pulse without prior circulatory collapse. It is the result of a fatal cardiac arrhythmia, which is typically due to CAD in the middle-aged and elderly adult. In as many as 25% of patients, sudden death may be the first clinical manifestation of coronary disease.[122] Sudden death is a multifactorial problem and is more likely to occur in patients with prior infarct and moderate to severe left ventricular dysfunction. Ischemic heart disease is most often the underlying cause, but cardiomyopathy, valvular heart disease, electrophysiologic abnormalities, and idiopathic ventricular fibrillation may also cause sudden death. Triggering factors include physical or mental stress, ionic or metabolic disorders, an acceleration of sinus rhythm, or the appearance of a supraventricular arrhythmia. Other factors are the arrhythmogenic effect of certain drugs and the interaction of electri-

cal instability with ischemia and/or left ventricular dysfunction due to multiple causes.[64] Approximately 20% of patients with acute MI die before reaching a hospital.[3] Most of these deaths are caused by ventricular fibrillation. Transient ischemia is rarely the cause of sudden death. Most patients who die suddenly have a vulnerable myocardium. The risk of sudden death in postinfarction patients is strongly related to the presence of electrical instability and its interaction with left ventricular dysfunction and residual ischemia. Patients at high risk of sudden death are those with a history of malignant ventricular arrhythmias (sustained ventricular tachycardia or out-of-hospital arrest), heart disease with markers of a vulnerable myocardium for malignant ventricular arrhythmias (depressed contractility, ischemia, electrical instability), and severe bradyarrhythmias.[64]

VALVULAR HEART DISEASE

Cardiovascular problems secondary to impaired valves may be caused by congenital deformities, infection, or disease (eg, coronary thrombosis or rheumatic fever). Any of the valves within the heart may become stenotic, insufficient, or prolapsed (Fig. 6-8).

Stenosis is a narrowing or constriction that prevents the valve from fully opening. Scars and abnormal deposits on the valve leaflets are often the cause. Valvular stenosis obstructs blood flow, and the chamber behind the narrowed valve must contract more forcefully in order to sustain cardiac output. *Insufficiency* refers to regurgitation or a leakage of blood back into the heart chamber through a valve whose leaflets fail to close completely. As a result of the leaky valve, the chamber behind (retrograde to) the valve initially dilates, and then ultimately hypertrophies, in response to the increased volume of work. Severe degrees of incompetence are possible in the absence of symptoms. *Prolapse* of the mitral valve occurs as enlarged leaflets bulge backward into the left atrium.

The mitral and tricuspid valves have larger cross-sectional areas than the semilunar valves and are subject to less mechanical force during valve opening and closure. Higher pressures generated during systole lead to greater valve dysfunction on the left side of the heart than on the right side, and often more than one valve is involved.[10,123] Valvular dysfunction increases the work of the heart, requiring the chamber to pump harder to force blood through a stenosed valve or to maintain adequate flow if blood is seeping back. Patients with valvular disease are often asymptomatic for many years, or may present with easy fatigue. However, abnormal valve structure results in turbulent blood flow, which increases the hemodynamic stress on these structures and leads to progressive damage and dysfunction. **Compensatory mechanisms including ventricular hypertrophy, chamber dilation, and peripheral processes can help maintain the overall performance of the heart for many years, even when there is malfunction of more than one valve. Eventually, these compensatory**

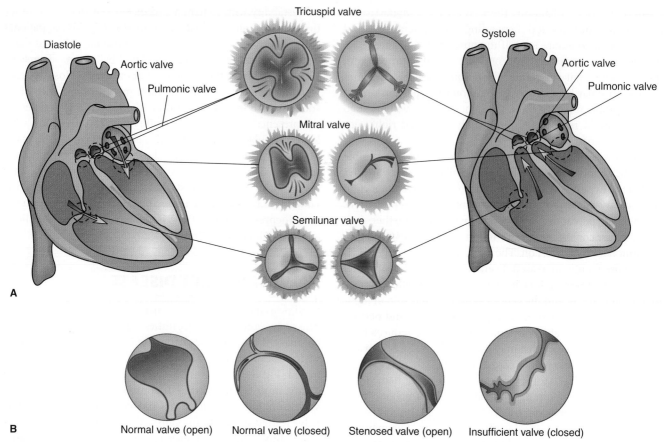

FIGURE 6-8   Valves of the heart. (**A**) The pulmonic, aortic, mitral, and tricuspid valves are shown here as they appear during diastole (ventricular filling) and systole (ventricular contraction). (**B**) Normal position of the valve leaflets, or cusps, when the valve is open and closed; fully open position of stenosed valve; closed regurgitant valve showing abnormal opening for blood and flow back into the heart chamber. (Reprinted from Goodman CC, Boissonnault WG. *Pathology: Implications for the Physical Therapist.* Philadelphia, PA: WB Saunders; Copyright 1998, with permission from Elsevier.)

mechanisms fail or the stenosis or insufficiency progresses. Patients may become exhausted and symptoms of heart failure may develop (eg, breathlessness, dyspnea). The etiology,[124] pathophysiology, and clinical manifestations[125,126] of common valvular abnormalities are described in Table 6-3. Medical and therapeutic interventions including valvuloplasty and valve replacement are described elsewhere in this chapter and in related references.

CARDIOMYOPATHIES

The cardiomyopathies consist of a diverse group of diseases involving a primary disorder of the myocardial cells with resultant myocardial dysfunction. Current classification is based on the presentation, pathophysiology, and type of abnormal myocardial structure and function. Dilated cardiomyopathies, hypertrophic cardiomyopathies, and restrictive cardiomyopathies represent the three main categories.[127] The pathophysiology and common signs and symptoms for each group of cardiomyopathies are found in Table 6-4. A brief description of each group follows.

Primary Dilated Cardiomyopathy

Dilated cardiomyopathies are characterized by an increased cardiac mass, dilatation of all four cardiac chambers with little or no wall thickening and systolic dysfunction.[128] Patients with dilated cardiomyopathies often present with dyspnea as well as with the other signs and symptoms of heart failure. In some patients, the presenting event is a symptomatic ventricular arrhythmia (ie, palpitations). Dilated cardiomyopathy may be idiopathic or may result from infectious and noninfectious inflammatory processes; toxins such as alcohol and drugs; pregnancy; a variety of metabolic disorders including endocrine, nutritional, altered metabolism, and myocardial ischemia; or hereditary diseases such as glycogen storage diseases and muscular dystrophies.[129] Chronic alcohol abuse and myocarditis are also frequent causes of dilated cardiomyopathy.

Dilated cardiomyopathy results in a decreased stroke volume, which is compensated at rest by an increase in heart rate. These patients have an impaired ability to increase cardiac output during exercise, which results in an increase in LVEDP and reduced exercise tolerance. The patient's cardiac reserve

TABLE 6-3 Etiology, Pathophysiology, and Clinical Manifestations of Valvular Heart Disease

Abnormality	Etiology	Pathophysiology	Clinical Manifestations
Aortic stenosis	Congenital, inflammatory valvulitis, senile calcification, rheumatic fever, severe atherosclerosis	Restricted opening of the aortic valve causes increased pressure load on LV, increased LV systolic pressure, and LV hypertrophy. Reduced compliance leads to increased LV filling pressure, greater dependence of LV filling on atrial contraction, and increased risk of subendocardial ischemia. Cardiac output fails to rise on exertion but is usually normal at rest. When prolonged, aortic stenosis leads to LV systolic dysfunction, LV dilatation, and increased pressure in lungs and right heart.	Dyspnea on exertion Angina pectoris Lightheadedness, syncope on exertion Systolic ejection murmur Sudden death
Aortic insufficiency/ aortic regurgitation	Congenital, rheumatic fever, infective endocarditis, arthritis, lupus, aortic root disease	Incomplete closure of the aortic valve causes regurgitation of blood to the LV during diastole. If aortic insufficiency is chronic, it leads to LV dilatation and compensatory LV hypertrophy. If severe, acute aortic insufficiency, increase in total stroke volume, and increased LV end-diastolic volume and pressure occur. Significant LV hypertrophy, LV compliance decreases producing a greater dependence of adequate LV filling on atrial systole.	Asymptomatic for decades then patient presents with dyspnea on exertion Systolic ejection murmur Usually less angina pectoris, lightheadedness, and syncope on exertion Signs and symptoms of LV failure if acute; may have diastolic decrescendo murmur at sternal borders
Mitral stenosis	Rheumatic fever, congenital	Restricted opening of the mitral value produces a pressure and volume load on the LA leading to LA dilatation and increased LA pressure. This produces increased pressure in the pulmonary vessels and increased workload on RV culminating in RV hypertrophy. Pulmonary edema may result from increased LA pressure. Pulmonary hypertension may result and lead to possible RV failure. Adequate LV filling is dependent on atrial systole.	Often asymptomatic for 20–25 y and then a gradual increase in the following symptoms over a 5-y period: dyspnea, fatigue, chest pain, chronic bronchitis, orthopnea, hemoptysis, palpitations, and a loud S_1 (diastolic rumble) unless there is severe calcification
Mitral regurgitation	LV dilatation, calcification, rheumatic fever, infective endocarditis, papillary muscle dysfunction, chordal rupture, mitral valve prolapse	Regurgitation of blood from the LV into the LA during early systole produces an increased volume load and LA and decreased impedance to LV emptying. If acute, small LA cannot handle regurgitant flow producing higher LA pressure, pulmonary HTN, and acute pulmonary edema. If chronic, the dilated LA absorbs the regurgitant flow in most patients producing normal or only slightly increased A and pulmonary pressures at rest. If LA dilatation is inadequate, LA and pulmonary pressures increase.	If acute, signs and symptoms of LV failure; loud high-pitched murmur is transmitted to axilla, S_3 is common If chronic, usually asymptomatic for decades or life if mild regurgitation is present; once LV fails, patient has signs and symptoms of chronic weakness, fatigue, lightheadedness, dizziness and those listed under mitral stenosis
Mitral valve prolapse	Heredity, congenital, acquired	Usually normal hemodynamics. Possible mitral regurgitation due to ballooning of the MV leaflets into the LA during systole.	Atypical chest pain Fatigue Palpitations Dyspnea Late systolic crescendo murmur

(continued)

TABLE 6-3   Etiology, Pathophysiology, and Clinical Manifestations of Valvular Heart Disease *(Continued)*

Abnormality	Etiology	Pathophysiology	Clinical Manifestations
Pulmonary stenosis	Congenital, rheumatic fever	Restricted opening of the PV causes increased pressure load on RV, RV hypertrophy, and dilatation. Decreased compliance results in an elevated RV end-diastolic pressure, increased RA and systemic venous pressures, and dependence of adequate RV filling on atrial systole. Once RV systolic dysfunction develops, cardiac output decreases and RV failure results.	Dyspnea on exertion Fatigue, weakness Possible cyanosis Signs and symptoms of RV failure Pulsations in throat Possible angina or syncope on exertion Growth delayed in children Harsh systolic ejection murmur S_4 may be present
Pulmonary regurgitation	Dilatation of pulmonary valve due to pulmonary hypertension or pulmonary artery, endocarditis, congenital, other	Regurgitation of blood from the PA to the RV during diastole produces an increased volume load on the RV. RV failure worsens if pulmonary HTN coexists.	Signs and symptoms of pulmonary hypertension and/or RV failure Diastolic ejection murmur
Tricuspid stenosis	Rheumatic fever, congenital, carcinoid	Restricted opening of the TV causes atrial fibrillation producing a further increase in RA and systemic venous pressures. Cardiac output decreases at rest and fails to rise during exercise. If TS and MS coexist, RV flow decreases and the severity of pulmonary HTN decreases.	Dyspnea Signs and symptoms of decreased cardiac output Prominent pulsations in neck Jugular venous distention Ascites Peripheral edema Diastolic murmur
Tricuspid regurgitation	Secondary to pulmonary HTN, congenital, rheumatic fever	TR implies and aggravates severe RV failure. Systolic regurgitation into RA causes an increased volume load on RA, RA dilatation, and increased RA pressure with reflection to the venous system. If afib, RA volume, and pressure increase, RA dilatation increases and TR increases.	Similar to tricuspid stenosis Signs and symptoms of biventricular failure if caused by left heart dysfunction Atrial fibrillation common on ECG Holosystolic murmur at lower sternal border

LV, left ventricle; RV, right ventricle; LA, left atrium; RA, right atrium; HTN, hypertension; ECG, electrocardiogram; PV, pulmonic valve; TV, tricuspid valve; TR, tricuspid regurgitation; TS, tricuspid stenosis; MS, mitral stenosis; MV, mitral valve; afib, atrial fibrillation.

Adapted from Reader GS. Identification and treatment of complications of myocardial infarction. *Mayo Clin Proc.* 1995;70:880.

depends on preservation of right ventricular function and systemic vasodilator reserve during exercise. Eventually, the patient develops left ventricular failure and right ventricular failure. Oxygen desaturation occurs, which results in an increased arteriovenous oxygen difference. Increased left ventricular filling pressure increases the risk of subendocardial ischemia. Without clinical heart failure, the prognosis of dilated cardiomyopathy is good but usually worsens. The natural history resembles that of other causes of heart failure once heart failure becomes manifest.

Hypertrophic Cardiomyopathy

Hypertrophic cardiomyopathy is characterized by a considerable increase in cardiac mass (hypertrophy), which may be symmetrical or asymmetrical, without cavity dilatation, accompanied by normal or increased systolic function.[130] In addition, there may be a left ventricular outflow obstruction,

known as hypertrophic obstructive cardiomyopathy and formerly referred to as idiopathic hypertrophic subaortic stenosis (IHSS). In IHSS, impaired systolic anterior motion of the mitral valve apparatus can bring the leaflet into contact with the interventricular septum and cause outflow tract obstruction. In hypertrophic cardiomyopathy, left ventricular hypertrophy results in diastolic dysfunction due to abnormal left ventricular relaxation and distensibility, which leads to decreased left ventricular compliance and increased left ventricular filling pressures. Decreased left ventricular compliance causes an increased dependence on left ventricular filling from atrial systole. Hyperdynamic left ventricular function produces rapid ejection. Myocardial ischemia is common and may result from impaired vasodilator reserve, increased oxygen demands, especially if hypertrophic obstructive cardiomyopathy develops. Increased filling pressures cause subendocardial ischemia.

TABLE 6-4 Classifications of the Cardiomyopathies

	Dilated	Hypertrophic	Restrictive
Common causes	Idiopathic, alcoholic, myocarditis, postpartum, doxorubicin, endocrinopathies, genetic diseases	Hereditary syndrome, possibly chronic hypertension	Amyloidosis, postradiation, post–open-heart surgery, diabetes, endomyocardial fibrosis
Ventricular volume	↑		
End diastolic	↑↑		
End systolic	↑		
Ventricular mass	↓	↑↑↑	↑
Mass/volume ratio		↑↑	↑
Systolic function			
Ejection fraction	↓-↓↓	↑	
Myocardial shortening	↓-↓↓	↑	
Wall stress			
Diastolic function			
Chamber stiffness	↑	↑↑	↑↑
Filling pressure	↑↑	↑	↑
Symptoms	Left or biventricular failure, fatigue, weakness	Dyspnea, fatigue, angina, syncope, or presyncope	Dyspnea, fatigue, RV failure
Findings on physical examination	Cardiomegaly, S₃, elevated JVP, rales	Sustained PMI, S₄, variable systolic murmur, bisferiens carotid pulse	Elevated JVP, Kussmaul sign
Chest X-ray	Enlarged heart, pulmonary congestion	Mild cardiomegaly	Mild-to-moderate cardiomegaly
Echocardiogram, nuclear studies	LV dilation and dysfunction	LVH, asymmetrical septal hypertrophy, small LV size, normal or supranormal function, systolicanterior mitral motion, diastolic dysfunction	Small or normal LV size, normal or mildly reduced LV function
Electrocardiogram	ST-T changes, conduction abnormalities, ventricular ectopy	LVH, exaggerated septal Q waves	ST-T wave changes, conduction abnormalities, low voltage
Cardiac catheterization	LV dilation and dysfunction, high diastolic pressures, low cardiac output	Small, hypercontractile LV dynamic outflow gradient, diastolic dysfunction	High diastolic pressures, normal or mildly reduced LV function

JVP, jugular venous pressure; PMI, point of maximal impulse.

Restrictive Cardiomyopathy

Restrictive cardiomyopathy is characterized by a restriction of ventricular filling caused by endocardial or myocardial disease or both. The ventricular walls lose compliance and become excessively rigid. In the presence of endocardial or myocardial disease, decreased left ventricular compliance causes a reduction in ventricular filling. This creates a back pressure that leads to atrial enlargement and increased atrial pressures, which are reflected back to filling vessels. Distortion of the ventricular cavity and involvement of the papillary muscles and chordae tendineae can cause mitral and/or tricuspid regurgitation.[131] Partial obliteration of the fibrous tissue and thrombus results in reduced stroke volume and often compensatory tachycardia. Eventually systolic function becomes impaired. If there is left ventricular involvement, pulmonary hypertension is common.

OTHER CARDIAC DISORDERS

Acute Myocarditis

Inflammation of the myocardial wall most frequently results from streptococcal infection leading to rheumatic fever or viral infections, such as coxsackie B virus, but can also be caused by other bacterial, rickettsial, fungal, or parasitic infections as well as by immunologic reactions, pharmacologic agents, toxins, and some systemic diseases. Myocarditis can be an acute or chronic process, may involve a limited area of myocardium, or may be diffuse. Many patients have nonspecific cardiovascular complaints, including fatigue, dyspnea, palpitations, and precordial discomfort.[132]

Infectious myocarditis often follows an upper respiratory infection. The patient may present with chest pain or signs of heart failure. Myocarditis is often accompanied by pericarditis.

Pericarditis

Acute inflammation of the pericardium may be either infectious in origin or caused by a wide variety of systemic diseases. Viral infections represent the most common cause of acute pericarditis. Other causes include bacterial infections, uremia, acute MI, and pericardiotomy associated with cardiac surgery, tuberculosis, malignancy, and trauma. Systemic diseases, which may lead to pericarditis, include autoimmune disorders (ie, connective tissue diseases), other inflammatory disorders (eg, sarcoidosis, amyloidosis, inflammatory bowel disease), drug toxicity, chest irradiation, and hypothyroidism. Pericarditis presents with a wide range of signs and symptoms as it progresses from a simple inflammatory response with no cardiovascular compromise to pulmonary effusions and cardiac tamponade, which may limit ventricular filling, stroke volume, and cardiac output.[133]

Initially, patients with pericarditis may present without signs or symptoms. When present, symptoms of acute pericarditis include chest pain, dyspnea, a higher resting heart rate, and an elevated temperature. Over time, the chest pain associated with pericarditis may mimic that of an MI. Position, breathing, and movement rarely affect the pain associated with an MI. The pain associated with pericarditis may be relieved with leaning forward, kneeling on all fours, or sitting upright.

Pericardial Effusion

Pericardial effusion may develop during pericarditis. The speed with which the fluid accumulates within the pericardial sac determines the physiological significance of the effusion. Because the pericardium stretches, a large effusion (>1000 mL) that develops slowly may produce no hemodynamic effects and the patient may remain asymptomatic. However, smaller effusions that appear rapidly can cause *tamponade*. Cardiac tamponade is characterized by elevated intrapericardial pressure (>15 mm Hg), which restricts venous return and ventricular filling.[134,135] As a result, stroke volume and pulse pressure fall and the heart rate and venous pressure rise. If left untreated, tamponade may result in shock and death.

Pericardial effusions may be painful, most commonly as the result of an acute inflammatory process, or painless as is often the case with uremic or neoplastic effusion. Dyspnea and cough are common. A *pericardial friction rub* may be present with large effusions. Tachycardia, tachypnea, and a narrow pulse pressure with a relatively preserved systolic blood pressure are characteristic of cardiac tamponade. Pulsus paradoxus (more than 10 mm Hg decline in systolic pressure

during inspiration) is the classic finding. Central venous pressure is elevated in patients with pericardial effusion. Edema and ascites may also be present. When tamponade is present, urgent pericardiocentesis is required. Although significant improvements in cardiac hemodynamics may be noted when a small amount of fluid is removed from the pericardium, continued drainage with a catheter is often required.

Rheumatic Heart Disease

Rheumatic fever is a systemic immune process that may result subsequent to a hemolytic streptococcal infection of the pharynx, for example, "strep throat," and leads to infection of the endocardium, usually the mitral valve leaflets. Acute rheumatic fever most commonly affects children 5 to 15 years of age, whereas chronic rheumatic heart disease may develop in older patients, especially those with more severe carditis. The mitral valve is attacked in 75% to 80% of the cases, the aortic valve is affected in 30% of the cases, and the tricuspid and pulmonary valves are affected in less than 5% of the cases.[3,136] Often more than one valve is affected. There appear to be two different clinical groups. One group shows evidence of significant valvular disease with a higher percentage of death within the first 5 years after onset. The other group has relatively mild valve disease that slowly develops progressive dysfunction due to gradual wear and tear on the valve caused by turbulent flow through its defective structures. The pathophysiology and clinical manifestations of rheumatic heart disease are incorporated into Table 6-3.

Infective Endocarditis

Bacterial or fungal infection of the heart valves causes vegetations to form along the cusps, which may interfere with proper opening and closing. Any abnormality of either a heart valve or the blood flow through a heart valve increases the risk of infective endocarditis. The degree of risk varies substantially according to the specific abnormality. The development of infective endocarditis is associated with situations where infective organisms may be introduced directly into the bloodstream (eg, dental, urinary, or intestinal procedures; intravenous drug abuse; central venous catheter placement). The clinical manifestations of infective endocarditis are highly variable and depend on the involvement of other organ systems because of embolization of valvular vegetation fragments, bacterial seeding of distant foci, or the development of immune complex–associated disease. Generally, there are symptoms suggestive of a flulike illness and possibly the clinical manifestations of specific valvular lesions and/or congestive heart failure.

Intracardiac infection can result in perforation of valve leaflets; rupture of the chordae tendineae, intraventricular septum, or papillary muscle; valve ring abscesses; occlusion of a valve orifice; coronary emboli; burrowing abscesses of the myocardium; and purulent pericardial effusions. Treatment is directed toward the specific infective organism with high serum levels of an effective antibiotic. Surgical intervention (eg, valve replacement or resection) is indicated if medical treatment is unsuccessful or for an unusual pathogen, myocardial abscess formation, refractory heart failure, serious embolic complications, or refractory prosthetic valve disease. Antibiotic prophylaxis is indicated for all patients with congenital or acquired valvular dysfunction, prosthetic heart valves, obstructive hypertrophic cardiomyopathy, a number of other congenital cardiac defects or shunt repairs, and for patients with previous endocarditis. Antibiotics are recommended before all dental, respiratory, and surgical procedures.

VASCULAR DISEASE

Atherosclerosis is a systemic disease that affects all major arteries. It represents the most common form of arterial wall disease. Clinical manifestations result most often from the narrowing and occlusion of a limited number of arteries, usually at the bifurcation of larger arteries. Additionally, with a reduction in elastin and collagen, the arterial wall weakens and may result in aneurysmal dilation. It is beyond the scope of this chapter to present every form of vascular disease. Common forms of arterial vascular disease include hypertension, aneurysms, and peripheral arterial occlusive disease.

This section begins with a description of hypertension. Although a disorder of vascular system, hypertension is a risk factor of coronary heart disease. If untreated, hypertension may result in many of the common cardiac disorders presented earlier in this chapter. Hypertension is also a risk factor for peripheral arterial occlusive disease, which is briefly discussed following a review of the common diseases found in the aorta and in other large vessels. For a description of the less common forms of vascular disease (ie, vasculitis, thromboangiitis obliterans, syphilitic aortitis, fibrodysplasia of visceral arteries, and radiation arteritis) the reader may refer to other comprehensive references.[3,64] This section ends with a description of metabolic syndrome, an increasing problem for adults, children, and adolescents.

Hypertension

Definition and Classification

Systemic hypertension is defined as a persistent elevation in systolic blood pressure above 140 mm Hg and/or diastolic pressure above 90 mm Hg measured on at least two separate occasions at least 2 weeks apart. An estimated 50 million Americans have elevated arterial blood pressure; of these, 68% are aware of their diagnosis, 53% are receiving treatment, and 27% are under control by the 140/90 threshold.[137] Table 6-5 provides the current (2003) classification for blood pressure measurements. Morbidity and mortality increase as both systolic and diastolic blood pressure rise. Therefore, both systolic hypertension and diastolic hypertension are clinically significant. When systolic and diastolic pressures fall into different categories, the higher category should be selected to classify the individual's blood pressure. Isolated systolic hypertension

TABLE 6-5 Classification of Blood Pressure Measurements in Adults

Classification	Systolic HTN (mm Hg)	Diastolic HTN (mm Hg)
Normal	<120	<80
Prehypertension	120–139	80–89
Hypertension		
Stage 1	140–159	90–99
Stage 2	≥160	≥100

Reproduced from National Heart, Lung, and Blood Institute, U.S. Department of Health and Human Services. The Seventh Report of the Joint National Committee on Preventions, Detection, Education, and Treatment of High Blood Pressure (JNCVI). *Medscape Cardiol.* 2003;7(1). http://www.medscape.com/viewarticle/455849. Accessed July 1, 2003. NIH Publication 04-5230.

refers to the case where systolic blood pressure is 140 mm Hg or more and diastolic blood pressure is less than 90 mm Hg (see Table 6-5).

When hypertension is the result of an unidentifiable cause, it is called *primary* or *essential hypertension*. In approximately 95% of the cases, no cause can be established.[3] Essential hypertension[123] is relatively uncommon before the age of 20 and usually presents between the ages of 25 and 55. When hypertension results from an identifiable cause such as renal insufficiency, renal artery stenosis, or coarctation of the aorta, it is referred to as *secondary hypertension*.

The fact that hypertension and its sequela appear to "run in families" was observed in sibling pair studies, twin studies, and family studies and has led to some inaccurate assumptions that hypertension was inherited as a simple, autosomal dominant trait. In the 1950s, a research team showed that primary hypertension was a complex genetic condition where 5 to 20 or more genes were involved. Further research has demonstrated that some unusual forms of inherited hypertension are indeed inherited as a simple monogenic trait.[138]

Blood pressure is a function of two main determinants: (1) the amount of blood flow (cardiac output) and (2) the peripheral vascular resistance. The pathogenesis of primary hypertension involves a series of feedback loops and interrelated regulatory systems. Disturbances within any of these systems can increase blood pressure. In the past 10 years, the vascular endothelium has been identified as a major blood pressure regulatory organ. Endothelial cells produce potent vasodilator substances. The most important may be the endothelial-derived relaxing factor nitric oxide. Other substances secreted by the endothelium are the vasodilator prostaglandins. The endothelium also produces potent vasoconstrictors, such as endothelin, which is the most potent constrictor known and may contribute to increased peripheral vascular resistance in advanced hypertension. Through these substances, the endothelium responds to sheer stress and a variety of circulating factors; modulates underlying vascular smooth muscle cell tone; and facilitates growth, differentiation, and angiogenesis.

Changes in blood pressure are sensed by *baroreceptors* located primarily in the aortic arch and the carotid sinus. These receptors relay information to the central nervous system via the vagus and glossopharyngeal nerves. When blood pressure is low, sympathetic output produces vasoconstriction and a reflex increase in heart rate. When blood pressure is high, sympathetic tone should be reduced and the heart rate should reflexively decrease through parasympathetically mediated mechanisms. However, in patients with primary or secondary hypertension, these baroreceptor mechanisms are altered or reset and their sensitivity to a given pressure level is decreased.

Hypertension is an important risk factor for heart disease. Over time, elevated blood pressure causes an increased pressure load on the left ventricle, which responds by developing compensatory left ventricular hypertrophy in order to maintain forward flow. Over time, however, diastolic dysfunction develops while normal left ventricular systolic function is maintained. The left ventricular hypertrophy and the resultant prolonged relaxation time produce a stiffer and less compliant left ventricle, causing a higher LVEDP at any volume. This in turn increases the load on the left atrium, which slows ventricular filling rate and reduces the passive filling volume. The stiffer left ventricle becomes more dependent on active atrial contraction for adequate filling. If there is inadequate filling volume, stroke volume will decrease and symptoms of inadequate cardiac output and pulmonary congestion may develop. Higher filling pressures exert pressure on the left ventricular wall. This inhibits coronary blood flow and increases the risk of subendocardial ischemia, as the demand for oxygen exceeds the supply.

As hypertension becomes more severe and more prolonged, systolic dysfunction develops. With the progression of left ventricular hypertrophy, the metabolic demand of the hypertrophied left ventricle will exceed the supply of blood to the heart muscle, causing myocardial ischemia. As a result, stroke volume will fall, causing a further elevation in left ventricular end-diastolic volume and LVEDP. The rise in end-diastolic pressure will be reflected back to the left atrium and pulmonary vessels. If the pulmonary pressures rise high enough to cause transudation of intravascular fluid from the capillaries, pulmonary edema will result. This systolic dysfunction will initially manifest itself as reduced left ventricular functional reserve during exercise. Later, the signs and symptoms of systolic dysfunction may develop even at rest.

The longer the hypertension is present, the greater the tendency of resistance vessels to adapt to the elevated blood pressure by way of media hypertrophy and increased wall-to-lumen ratio (vessel remodeling), which makes the vessels even more susceptible to vasoconstrictors. Thus, the original mechanism (ie, primary or secondary) eventually becomes less relevant, because the altered vascular structures themselves serve to perpetuate the condition. Renal blood flow declines and renal vascular resistance rises. Consequently, the sodium-excreting capacity of the kidneys further declines, making the hypertension more volume dependent over time. Compliance of large vessels, including the aorta, declines, produces a stiffer arterial wall, and impairs the ability of the arterial wall to contribute to pulsatile blood flow (Windkessel effect). This creates more work for the heart and leads to further increases in systolic blood pressure.[138]

Patient Presentation

The patient with hypertension, known as the "silent killer," is generally asymptomatic. Untreated or poorly managed hypertension results in multiple complications including cerebral vascular accidents, congestive heart failure, ASHD, renal failure or nephrosclerosis, simple or dissecting aortic aneurysms, peripheral vascular disease, and retinopathy. Pharmacologic therapy is addressed in Chapter 8 and incorporates many groups of cardiovascular drugs including β-blockers, diuretics, α-adrenergic blockers, central acting α-adrenergic agonists, angiotensin-converting enzyme (ACE) inhibitors, and calcium channel blockers. Nonpharmacologic treatment includes weight reduction, alcohol moderation, sodium restriction, relaxation training, and exercise training. Although nonpharmacologic interventions may not eliminate the need for antihypertensive medications, they often permit lower dosages with fewer side effects.

Aneurysms

An *aneurysm* is a localized dilatation of the wall of a blood vessel, usually caused by atherosclerosis and hypertension, or less frequently by trauma, infection, or a congenital weakness in the vessel wall. Aneurysms are common in the aorta but can occur in any peripheral vessel.[5,10] They are common in the popliteal arteries of the elderly. The sign of an aneurysm is a pulsating swelling that produces a blowing murmur on auscultation. An aneurysm may rupture, causing hemorrhage, or thrombi may form in the dilated pouch and give rise to emboli that may obstruct smaller vessels.

Aortic Aneurysm

More than 90% of abdominal atherosclerotic aneurysms originate below the renal arteries and many are located at the bifurcation of the aorta.[3] The infrarenal aorta is normally 2 cm in diameter; an aneurysm at this site is diagnosed when the diameter exceeds 4 cm. Aneurysms are typically asymptomatic and usually are discovered on routine physical examination in men over 50 years of age. Severe back or abdominal pain indicates rupture. Aortic aneurysms are not necessarily associated with atherosclerotic occlusive disease.

Patients may be asymptomatic or symptomatic. In those who are symptomatic, chronic midabdominal and/or low back pain may be present. Symptoms often occur as a result of an inflammatory process. Peripheral emboli may occur, and symptomatic arterial insufficiency may result. A ruptured aortic aneurysm typically results in death before the patient can be hospitalized or before the patient reaches the operating room. Patients with bleeding confined to the retroperitoneal area may have severe pain in the abdomen, flank, or back and a pulsating abdominal mass. Abdominal ultrasonography is the preferred diagnostic study. Surgical excision and grafting is the treatment of choice for most aneurysms of the infrarenal abdominal aorta. The complication rate following repair is 5% to 10% and includes MI, bleeding, respiratory insufficiency, limb ischemia, ischemic colitis, renal insufficiency, and stroke.[139,140]

Aneurysms of the Thoracic Aorta

Thoracic aneurysms are most commonly due to atherosclerosis. Other causes of thoracic aneurysms include Marfan syndrome, cystic medial necrosis, and vasculitis. Traumatic aneurysms may result from rapid deceleration accidents and may occur at the ligamentum arteriosis just beyond the left subclavian artery. Most thoracic aneurysms are asymptomatic. Manifestations depend on the size and position of the aneurysm and its rate of growth. When symptomatic, substernal, back or neck pain may occur. Pressure on the trachea, esophagus, left recurrent laryngeal nerve, and the superior vena cava may result in dyspnea, stridor, dysphagia, hoarseness, and edema in the cervical and upper extremities and jugular venous distention.

Thoracic aneurysms are most commonly detected by imaging techniques (ie, CT scan and MRI). Aortography may be used to confirm the diagnosis and delineate the location and extent of the aneurysm. In total, less than 10% of aortic aneurysms are thoracic.[3]

Aortic Dissection

Aortic dissection is the most common aortic catastrophe requiring admission to the hospital. It originates at the site of an intimal tear and then propagates distally. More than 95% of the intimal tears occur either in the ascending aorta just distal to the aortic valve or just distal to the left subclavian artery.[141] The initial intimal tear probably results from the constant torque applied to the ascending and proximal descending aorta occurring at these two points associated with the pulsatile blood flow from the heart, usually under hypertensive conditions.[142] Dissection occurs on rare occasions in an aorta without an apparent intimal tear. Invariably, these aortas show histological abnormalities of the media. Proximal dissections occur more often in aortas[143] with abnormalities of the smooth muscle, elastic tissue, or collagen. Distal dissections occur more commonly in patients with hypertension. When undiagnosed and untreated, aortic dissection is a lethal disease. Death is usually due to rupture of the aorta into the pericardial sac or pleural space or to acute aortic regurgitation with left ventricular failure.[5]

Aortic dissection is most commonly confused with MI and other causes of chest pain. It may simulate numerous neurologic lesions and various abdominal conditions related to renal–visceral ischemia. Aggressive medical measures are taken to lower hypertension when aortic dissection is present using a fast-acting antihypertensive agent with continuous blood pressure monitoring. Emergent surgical repair is necessary for patients with tears in the ascending aorta just distal to

the aortic valve. Tears distal to the left subclavian artery may be managed successfully with aggressive drug therapy unless the patient has severe pain, aortic rupture, ischemia, or a progression of the dissection. Without treatment, the mortality rate of aortic dissection at 3 months exceeds 90%.[3]

Popliteal and Femoral Aneurysms (Peripheral Artery Aneurysms)

Popliteal aneurysms account for approximately 85% of all peripheral artery aneurysms.[3] Peripheral aneurysms occur almost exclusively in men, and about half are symptomatic at the time of diagnosis. Symptoms result from thrombosis, peripheral embolization, or compression of adjacent structures with resultant venous thrombosis or neuropathy. Ultrasound is used to diagnose and measure the diameter of the aneurysm. Arteriography is needed to define the anatomy of the outflow arteries in preparation for the operative repair. A reversed saphenous vein bypass graft with proximal and distal ligation is generally used.

A femoral aneurysm manifests itself as a pulsatile mass on one or both sides of the thigh. Potential complications are the same as described for popliteal aneurysms. Complications occur less frequently, and asymptomatic aneurysms are typically not repaired. Pseduoaneurysms often develop at distal anastomotic sites from previous aortic surgery and may require repair.[144]

Peripheral Arterial Occlusive Disease

Occlusive disease of the aorta and the iliac arteries begins most frequently just proximal to or just distal to the bifurcation of the aorta. Atherosclerotic changes occur in the media and intima, often with perivascular inflammation and calcified plaques in the media. Progression involves the complete occlusion of one or both common iliac arteries and then the abdominal aorta up to the segment just below the renal vessels. Although a generalized disease, occlusion tends to be segmental in distribution, and when the involvement is in the aorto–iliac vessels there may be minimal atherosclerosis in the more distal external iliac and femoral arteries. Patients with localized occlusion beyond the aortic bifurcation are good candidates for angioplasty, atherectomy, and stenting.

The classic symptom of peripheral arterial occlusive disease is *intermittent claudication*. This condition is initially manifested as cramp-like pains in the calves during walking and is relieved by rest.[145,146] Patients with multisegmental disease usually have more symptoms and are at greater risk of losing a limb. Abrupt worsening of claudication may be associated with plaque rupture (crescendo claudication) as with myocardial ischemia.

Clinical Findings

As indicated previously, patients with occlusive arterial disease present with pain or weakness in the lower extremities, which is brought on by walking, and relieved after a few minutes of rest. It is almost always present in the calf muscles and often in the thighs and buttocks as well. Resting pain is infrequent but a serious symptom when present. Resting pain usually presents as a nocturnal pain located in the region of the heads of the metatarsal bones of the feet. It is relieved by placing the legs in the dependent position such as hanging them over the side of the bed.

Metabolic Syndrome

Definition and Categorization

Metabolic syndrome has been loosely described as a constellation of metabolic risk factors that is strongly associated with type 2 diabetes and the promotion of atherosclerotic cardiovascular disease.[147] In 2001, the National Cholesterol Education Program (NCEP)—Adult Treatment Panel III (ATP III) proposed that metabolic syndrome be based on several common clinical measures including waist circumference, triglycerides, HDL-C, blood pressure, and fasting glucose level.[147] Abnormalities in any three of the above five measures result in a diagnosis of metabolic syndrome.[147] The presence of an abnormality in the above five measures is defined in Table 6-6 by using the categorical cut points for each of the five areas.

The threshold cut points listed in Table 6-6 identify levels that have been observed to confer greater risk of type 2 diabetes and atherosclerotic cardiovascular disease.[147] The individual and interrelated methods by which each of the five factors contributes to the development of these diseases is shown in Fig. 6-9.[148,149] As shown in Fig. 6-9, the major components of metabolic syndrome and subsequent effects on the development of diabetes and atherosclerotic cardiovascular disease include the presence of vascular abnormalities, oxidative stress, visceral fat, inflammation, adipocytokines, and cor-

tisol.[147,148] The separate and interrelated characteristics of these factors promote the development of diabetes and atherosclerotic cardiovascular disease, which are both interrelated (and overlapping as shown in Fig. 6-9). In fact, prospective population studies reveal that presence of metabolic syndrome is associated with a twofold increase in atherosclerotic cardiovascular events and a fivefold increase in the risk of developing diabetes in persons without established type 2 diabetes.[147,148]

TABLE 6-6   Diagnostic Criteria for Metabolic Syndrome

Measure	Categorical Cut Points
Elevated waist circumference	≥102 cm (≥40 in.) in men ≥88 cm (≥35 in.) in women
Elevated triglycerides	≥150 mg/dL (1.7 mmol/L) Or Drug treatment for elevated triglycerides
Reduced HDL-C	<40 mg/dL (1.03 mmol/L) in men <50 mg/dL (1.3 mmol/L) in women Or Drug treatment for reduced HDL-C
Elevated blood pressure	≥130 mm Hg systolic blood pressure Or ≥85 mm Hg diastolic blood pressure Or Drug treatment for hypertension
Elevated fasting glucose	≥100 mg/dL Or Drug treatment for elevated glucose

Reproduced with permission from Diagnosis and management of the metabolic syndrome: an American Heart Association/National Heart, Lung, and Blood Institute scientific statement: executive summary. *Circulation.* 2005;112;285-290.

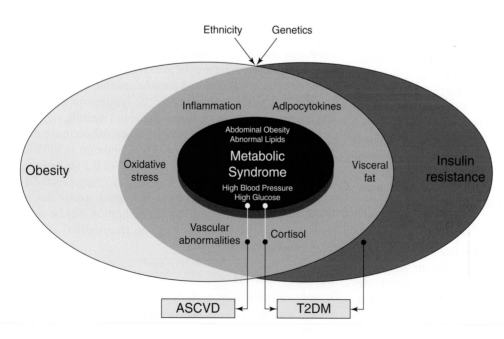

FIGURE 6-9 Schematic of the components of metabolic syndrome. (Reprinted with permission from Steinberger J, Daniels SR, Eckel RH, et al. Progress and challenges in metabolic syndrome in children and adolescents: a scientific statement from the American Heart Association Atherosclerosis, Hypertension, and Obesity in the Young Committee of the Council on Cardiovascular Disease in the Young; Council on Cardiovascular Nursing; and Council on Nutrition, Physical Activity, and Metabolism. *Circulation.* 2009;119:628-647.)

Also, as shown in Fig. 6-9, ethnic and genetic factors are also related to metabolic syndrome, which highlights the importance of examining the presence of metabolic syndrome in children and adolescents.[147,148] White, black, and Hispanic individuals (both adults and children), as opposed to Asian individuals, have been observed to have greater propensity for metabolic syndrome, but with different predisposing factors. For example, black children and adults have lower total cholesterol and triglyceride levels and higher HDL-C levels than white children, but black and Hispanic children are more insulin resistant than white children.[147,148] Although ethnic differences are poorly understood, they are important to consider in the examination and management of persons with metabolic syndrome.[147,148]

The clinical management of metabolic syndrome has centered on reducing the risk factors identified in Table 6-6 and in Fig. 6-9.[147,148] Thus, the management of metabolic syndrome involves both lifestyle treatment and appropriate pharmacologic therapy for metabolic risk factors. Lifestyle recommendations include weight maintenance/reduction, increased physical activity, and a healthy diet (reduction of saturated fat, trans fat, and cholesterol). Optimal pharmacologic therapy for metabolic syndrome risk factors may include lipid-lowering drugs, antihypertensive drugs, aspirin therapy, and drug therapy to control elevated plasma glucose for individuals with diabetes. Currently, drug therapy to reduce plasma glucose or insulin resistance is not recommended for individuals with impaired fasting glucose.[147,148]

SUMMARY

This chapter reviewed the pathophysiology of the common forms of cardiovascular disease including CAD, heart failure, valve disease, and cardiomyopathies. Special emphasis was placed on the pathogenesis of atherosclerosis, the most common cause of CAD. The discussion of peripheral vascular disorders focused on hypertension, aneurysms, and arterial occlusive disease. Finally, the chapter ended with a description of metabolic syndrome. The interested reader may seek additional information in other excellent, comprehensive cardiology references.[5,10]

Heads Up!

This chapter contains a CD-ROM activity.

REFERENCES

1. Deedwania PC, Amsterdam EA, Vagelos RH. Evidence-based, cost-effective risk stratification in management after myocardial infarction. *Arch Intern Med.* 1997;157:273.
2. Gillum RF. Trends in acute myocardial infarction and coronary heart disease death in the United States. *J Am Coll Cardiol.* 1994;23:1273.
3. Tierney LM, McPhee S, Papadakis MA. *Current Medical Diagnosis and Treatment 1999.* 38th ed. Stamford, CT: Appleton & Lange; 1999:358.
4. Damjaniv I. *Pathology for the Health Related Sciences.* Philadelphia, PA: WB Saunders; 1996:155-156.
5. Fuster V, Alexander RW, O'Rourke RA. *Hurst's the Heart.* 10th ed. New York: McGraw-Hill; 2001.
6. Srikanththan VS, Dunn FG. Hypertension in coronary artery disease. *Med Clin North Am.* 1997;81:1141.
7. Zhou J, Chew M, Ravn HB, Falk E. Plaque pathology and coronary thrombosis in the pathogenesis of acute coronary syndromes. *Scand J Clin Lab Invest Suppl.* 1999;230:3-11.
8. Shah PK. Plaque disruption and thrombosis: potential role of inflammation and infection. *Cardiol Rev.* 2000;8(1):31-39.
9. Noll G. Pathogenesis of atherosclerosis: a possible relation to infection. *Atherosclerosis.* 1998;140(suppl 1):S3-S9.
10. Braunwald E, Zipes DP, Libby P. *Heart Disease: A Textbook of Cardiovascular Medicine.* 6th ed. Philadelphia, PA: WB Saunders; 2001.
11. Hoffman J. Congenital heart disease. *Pediatr Clin North Am.* 1990;37:45.
12. Alexander RW, Schlant RC, Fuster V, et al. *Hurst's The Heart, Arteries and Veins Companion Handbook.* 9th ed. New York: McGraw-Hill; 1999.
13. Danesh J, Collins R, Peto R. Chronic infections and coronary heart disease: is there a link? *Lancet.* 1997;350:430-436.
14. Muhlestein JB, Hammond EH, Carlquist JF, et al. Increased incidence of *Chlamydia* species within the coronary arteries of patients with symptomatic atherosclerosis versus other forms of cardiovascular disease. *J Am Coll Cardiol.* 1996;27:1555-1561.
15. Maass M, Bartels C, Engel PM, et al. Endovascular presence of viable *Chlamydia pneumoniae* is a common phenomenon in coronary artery disease. *J Am Coll Cardiol.* 1998;31:827-832.
16. Pasceri V, Cammarota G, Patti G, et al. Association of virulent *Helicobacter pylori* strains with ischemic heart disease. *Circulation.* 1998;97:1675-1679.
17. Hendrix MG, Salimans MM, van Boven CP, Bruggeman CA. High prevalence of latently present cytomegalovirus in arterial walls of patients suffering grade III atherosclerosis. *Am J Pathol.* 1979;96:673-706.
18. O'Donnell CJ, Levy D. Weighing the evidence for infection as a risk factor for coronary heart disease. *Curr Cardiol Rep.* 2000;2(4):280-287.
19. Shively BK. Infective endocarditis. *Curr Treat Options Cardiovasc Med.* 2001;3(1):25-35.
20. Schwartz CJ, Valente AJ, Sprague EA, et al. Pathogenesis of the artherosclerotic lesion: implications for diabetes mellitus. *Diabetes Care.* 1992;15:1156-1167.
21. Stamler J, Vaccaro O, Neaton JD, Wentworth D. Diabetes, other risk factors and 12-year cardiovascular mortality for men screened in the multiple risk factor intervention trial. *Diabetes Care.* 1993;16:434-444.
22. Kawate R, Yamakido M, Nishimoto Y, et al. Diabetes mellitus and its vascular complications in Japanese migrants on the island of Hawaii. *Diabetes Care.* 1979;2:161-170.
23. Head J, Fuller JH. International variations in mortality among diabetic patients: the WHO Multinational Study of Vascular Disease in Diabetics. *Diabetologia.* 1990;33:447-481.
24. Vigorita VJ, Morre GW, Hutchens GM. Absence of correlation between coronary arterial atherosclerosis and severity or duration of diabetes mellitus of adult onset. *Am J Cardiol.* 1980;46:535-542.

25. Waller BF, Palambo PJ, Lie JT, Roberts WC. Status of the coronary arteries at necropsy in diabetes mellitus after age 30 years: analysis of 229 diabetic patients with and without evidence of coronary heart disease and comparison to 183 control subjects. *Am J Med*. 1980;69:498-506.

26. Roberts WC, High ST. The heart in systemic lupus erythematosus. *Curr Probl Cardiol*. 1999;24:1-56.

27. Sturfelt G, Eskilsson J, Nived O, et al. Cardiovascular disease in systemic disease in systemic lupus erythematosus: a study from a defined population. *Medicine* (*Baltimore*). 1992;71:216-223.

28. Petri M, Spence D, Bone LR, Hochberg MC. Coronary risk factors in the Johns Hopkins Lupus Cohort: prevalence by patients, and preventive practices. *Medicine* (*Baltimore*) 1992;71:291-302.

29. Allard MF, Taylor GP, Wilson JE, McManus BM. Primary cardiac tumors. In: Goldhaber SZ, Braunwald E, eds. *Cardiopulmonary Diseases and Cardiac Tumors: Atlas of Heart Diseases*. Vol 3. Philadelphia, PA: Mosby; 1995:15.1-15.2.

30. Reynan K. Frequency of primary tumors of the heart. *Am J Cardiol*. 1996;77:107.

31. Lam KYL, Dickens P, Chan ACL. Tumors of the heart. *Arch Pathol Lab Med*. 1993;117:1027.

32. Tazelaar HD, Locke TJ, McGregir CGA. Pathology of surgically excised primary cardiac tumors. *Mayo Clin Proc*. 1992;67:957.

33. Salcedo EE, Cohen GL, White RD, Davison MB. Cardiac tumors: diagnosis and treatment. *Curr Probl Cardiol*. 1992;17:73.

34. Pollia JA, Gogol LJ. Some notes on malignancies of the heart. *Am J Cancer*. 1996;27:329-333.

35. Burke A, Virmani R. *Tumors of the Heart and Great Vessels. Atlas of Tumor Pathology*. 3rd series. Washington, DC: Armed Forces Institute of Pathology; 1995.

36. Hanson EC. Cardiac tumors: a current perspective. *NY State Med*. 1992;92:41.

37. Allard MF, Taylor GP, Wilson JE, McManus BM. Primary cardiac tumors. In: Golhaber S, Braunwald E, eds. *Atlas of Heart Diseases*. Philadelphia, PA: Mosby; 1995:15.1-15.22.

38. Paysk KA, Argenta LC, Erickson RP. Familial vascular malformations: report of 25 members of one family. *Clin Genet*. 1984;26:221.

39. Walter JW, Blei F, Anderson JL, et al. Genetic mapping of a novel familial form of infantile hemangioma. *Am J Med Genet*. 1999;82:77-83.

40. Criteria Committee of the New York Heart Association. *Nomenclature Criteria for Diagnosis of Diseases of the Heart and Great Vessels*. 9th ed. Boston, MA: Little, Brown and Company; 1994:253-256.

41. American Physical Therapy Association. Guide to Physical Therapist Practice. 2nd ed. *Phys Ther*. 2001 Jan;81(1):9-746.

42. Boushey CF, Beresford SA, Omenn GS, Motulsky AG. A quantitative assessment of plasma homocysteine as a risk factor for vascular disease: probable benefits of increasing folic acid intakes. *JAMA*. 1995;274:1049-1057.

43. Robinson K, Arheart K, Refsum H, et al. Low circulating folate and vitamin B_6 concentrations: risk factors for stroke, peripheral vascular disease, and coronary artery disease. *Circulation*. 1998;97(5):437-443.

44. Refsum H, Ueland PM, Nygard O, Vollset SE. Homosysteine and cardiovascular disease. *Annu Rev Med*. 1998;49:31-62.

45. Malinow MR, Bostom AG, Krauss RM. Homocyst(e)ine, diet, and cardiovascular diseases: a statement for healthcare professionals from the Nutrition Committee, American Heart Association. *Circulation*. 1999;99:178-182.

46. Stampfer MJ, Malinow MR, Willett WC, et al. A prospective study of plasma homocyst(e)ine and risk of myocardial infarction in US physicians. *JAMA*. 1992;268:877-881.

47. Arnesen E, Refsum H, Bonaa KH, et al. Serum total homocysteine and coronary heart disease. *Int J Epidemiol*. 1995;24: 704-709.

48. Ridker PM, Manson JE, Buring JE, et al. Homocysteine and risk of cardiovascular disease among postmenopausal women. *JAMA*. 1999;281:1817-1821.

49. Nygard O, Nordrehaug JE, Refsum H, et al. Plasma homocysteine levels and mortality in patients with coronary artery disease. *N Engl J Med*. 1997;337:230-236.

50. Welch GN, Loscalzo J. Homocysteine and atherothrombosis. *N Engl J Med*. 1998;338:1042-1050.

51. Tsai JC, Perrella MA, Yoshizumi M, et al. Promotion of vascular smooth muscle cell growth by homocysteine: a link to atherosclerosis. *Proc Natl Acad Sci U S A*. 1994;91:6369-6373.

52. Stamler JS, Osborne JA, Jaraki O, et al. Adverse vascular effects of homocysteine are modulated by endothelium-derived relaxing factor and related oxides of nitrogen. *J Clin Invest*. 1993;91:308-318.

53. Chambers JC, McGregor A, Jean-Marie J, et al. Acute hyperhomocysteinaemia and endothelial dysfunction. *Lancet*. 1998;351:36-37.

54. Steinberf D. Oxidative modifications of LDL and atherogenesis. *Circulation*. 1997;95:1062.

55. O'Keefe JE, Lavie CJ, McCallister BD. Insights into the pathogenesis and prevention of coronary artery disease. *Mayo Clin Proc*. 1995;70:69.

56. American College of Physicians. Guidelines for using serum cholesterol, high-density, lipoprotein cholesterol, and triglyceride levels as screening test for preventing coronary heart disease in adults. *Ann Intern Med*. 1996;124:515.

57. Abrams J, Vela BS, Coultas DB. Coronary risk factors and their modifications. *Curr Probl Cardiol*. 1995;20:535.

58. Vasankari T, Ahotupa M, Toikka J, et al. Oxidized LDL and thickness of carotid intima media are associated with coronary atherosclerosis in middle-aged men. *Atherosclerosis*. 2001;155(2):403-412.

59. Keaney JF. Atherosclerosis: from lesion formation to plaque activation and endothelial dysfunction. *Mol Aspects Med*. 2000;21(4-5):99-166.

60. Craig WY, Rawstron MR, Rundell CA, et al. Relationship between lipoprotein- and oxidation-related undergoing coronary artery bypass graft surgery. *Arterioscler Thromb Vasc Biol*. 1999;19(6):1512-1517.

61. Kritchevsky D. Atherosclerosis: aortic lipid changes induced by diets suggest diffuse disease with focal severity in primates that model human atheromas. *Nutrition*. 1998;14(1):17-22.

62. Wissler RW, Vesselinovitch D, Hughes R, et al. Arterial lesions and blood lipids in rhesus monkeys fed human diets. *Exp Mol Pathol*. 1983;38(1):117-136.

63. Worthey SG, Osende JI, Helft G, et al. Coronary artery disease: pathogenesis and acute coronary syndromes. *Mt Sinai J Med*. 2001;68(3):167-181.

64. Cheitlin MD, Skilow M, McIllroy MB. *Clinical Cardiology*. Los Altos, CA: Lange Medical Publications; 1993:147.

65. Mittleman MA. Triggering of acute myocardial infarction by heavy physical exertion. *N Engl J Med*. 1993;329:1677-1683.

66. George J, Harats D, Gilburd B, Shoenfeld Y. Emerging cross-regulatory roles of immunity and autoimmunity in atherosclerosis. *Immunol Res*. 1996;15(4):315-322.

67. Zhou X, Caligiuri G, Hamsten A, Lefvert AK, Hansson GK. LDL immunization induces T-cell-dependent antibody formation and protection against atherosclerosis. *Arterioscler Thromb Vasc Biol*. 2001;21(1):108-114.

68. Moise A, Lesperance J, Theroux P, et al. Clinical and angiographic predictors of new total occlusion in coronary artery disease: analysis of 313 non-operated patients. *Am J Cardiol*. 1984;54:1176-1181.

69. Ambrose JA, Tannenbaum MA, Alexopoulos D, et al. Angiographic progression of coronary artery disease and the development of myocardial infarction. *J Am Coll Cardiol*. 1988;12:56-62.

70. Little WC, Constantinescu M, Applegate RJ. Can coronary angiography predict the site of a subsequent myocardial infarction in patients with mild-to-moderate artery disease? *Circulation*. 1988;78:1157-1166.

71. Giroud D, Li JM, Urban P, et al. Relation of the site of acute myocardial infarction to the most severe coronary arterial stenosis at prior angiography. *Am J Cardiol*. 1992;69:729-732.

72. Petursson KK, Jonmundsson EH, Brekkan A, Hardarson T. Angiographic predictors of new coronary occlusions. *Am Heart J*. 1995;129:515-520.

73. Bortone AS, Hess OM, Eberli FR. Abnormal coronary vasomotion during exercise in patients with normal coronary arteries and reduced coronary flow reserve. *Circulation*. 1991;83:26-37.

74. Yeung AC, Vekshtein VI, Krantz DS, et al. The effect of atherosclerosis on the vasomotor response of coronary arteries to mental stress. *N Engl J Med*. 1991;325:1551-1556.

75. Nabel EG, Ganz P, Gordon JB, et al. Paradoxical narrowing of atherosclerotic coronary arteries induced by increases in heart rate. *Circulation*. 1990;81:850-859.

76. Rosen SD, Paulesu E, Frith CD, et al. Central nervous pathways mediating angina pectoris. *Lancet*. 1994;344:147-150.

77. Prinzemetal M, Kennamer R, Merliss R, et al. Angina pectoris. I. A variant form of angina pectoris: preliminary report. *Am J Med*. 1959;27:375.

78. Chevalier P, Dacosta A, Defaye P, et al. Arrhythmic cardiac arrest due to isolated coronary artery spasm: long-term outcome of seven resuscitated patients. *J Am Coll Cardiol*. 1998;31:57.

79. Cohen M. Variant angina pectoris. In: Fuster V, Ross R, Topol EJ, eds. *Atherosclerosis and Coronary Artery Disease*. Philadelphia, PA: Lippincott-Raven; 1996:1367-1376.

80. Mongiardo R, Finocchiaro ML, Beltrame J, et al. Low incidence of serotonin-induced occlusive coronary artery spasm in patients with recent myocardial infarction. *Am J Cardiol*. 1996;78:84.

81. Pristipino C, Beltrame JF, Finocchiaro ML, et al. Major racial differences in coronary constrictor response between Japanese and Caucasians with recent myocardial infarction. *Circulation*. 2000;101:1102.

82. Versaci F, Tomai F, Nudi F, et al. Differences of regional coronary flow reserve assessed by adenosine thallium-201 scintigraphy early and six months after successful percutaneous transluminal coronary angioplasty or stent implantation. *Am J Cardiol*. 1996;78:1097.

83. Kern MJ, Puri S, Bach RG, et al. Abnormal coronary flow velocity reserve after coronary artery stenting in patients: role of relative coronary reserve to assess potential mechanisms. *Circulation*. 1999;100:2491.

84. Kosa I, Blasini R, Schneider-Eicke J, et al. Early recovery of coronary flow reserve after stent implantation as assessed by positron emission tomography. *J Am Coll Cardiol*. 1999;34:1036.

85. Gregorini L, Marco J, Kozakova M, et al. Alpha-adrenergic blockade improves recovery of myocardial perfusion and function after coronary stenting in patients with acute myocardial infarction. *Circulation*. 1999;99:482.

86. Davis MJ. The pathology of coronary atherosclerosis. In: Schlant RC, Alexander RW, eds. *Hurst's the Heart, Arteries and Veins*. Vol 2. 8th ed. New York: McGraw-Hill; 1994.

87. Hollander JE, Hoffman RS, Burstein JL. Cocaine-associated myocardial infarction: mortality and complication. *Arch Intern Med*. 1995;155:1081.

88. Haak SW, Richardson SJ, Davey SS. Alterations in cardiovascular function. In: McCance KL, Huether SE, eds. *Pathophysiology: The Biological Basis for Disease in Adults and Children*. 2nd ed. St. Louis, MO: Mosby Year Book; 1994.

89. McCance KL, Huether SE, eds. *Pathophysiology: The Biological Basis for Disease in Adults and Children*. 2nd ed. St Louis, MO: Mosby Year Book; 1994.

90. Reeder GS, Gersh BJ. Modern management of acute myocardial infarction. *Curr Probl Cardiol*. 1996;21:585.

91. Ryan TJ, Anderson JL, Antman EM, et al. ACC/AHA guidelines for the management of patients with acute myocardial infarction. A report of the American College of Cardiology/American Heart Association Task Force on Practice Guidelines. *J Am Coll Cardiol*. 1996;28:1328.

92. Barry WL, Sarenbock IJ. Cardiogenic shock: therapy and prevention. *Clin Cardiol*. 1998;21:72.

93. Hathaway WR, Peterson ED, Wagner GS, et al. Prognostic significance of the initial electrocardiogram in patients with acute myocardial infarction. *JAMA*. 1998;279:387.

94. Cannon CP, McCabe CH, Stone PH, et al. The electrocardiogram predicts one year outcomes of patients with unstable angina and non-Q-wave MI: results of the TIMI III Registry Ancillary Study. *J Am Coll Cardiol*. 1997;30;1333.

95. Reader GS. Identification and treatment of complications of myocardial infarction. *Mayo Clin Proc*. 1995;70:880.

96. Goodman CC, Boissonnault WG. *Pathology: Implications for the Physical Therapist*. Philadelphia, PA: WB Saunders; 1998.

97. Tunstall-Pedoe H, Kuulasmaa K, Amouyel P, et al. Myocardial infarction and coronary deaths in the World Health Organization MONICA project. *Circulation*. 1994;90(1):583-612.

98. Adams J III, Abendschein D, Jaffe A. Biochemical markers of myocardial injury. Is MB creatine kinase the choice for the 1990s? *Circulation*. 1993;88:750-763.

99. Antman EM, Grudzien C, Sacks DB. Evaluation of a rapid bedside assay for detection of serum cardiac troponin T. *JAMA*. 1995;273:1279-1282.

100. Ellis AK. Serum protein measurements and the diagnosis of acute myocardial infarction. *Circulation*. 1991;83:1107-1109.

101. Mair J, Dienstl F, Pluschendorf B. Cardiac troponin T in the diagnosis of myocardial injury. *Crit Rev Clin Lab Sci*. 1992;29:31-57.

102. Zimmerman J, Fromm R, Meyer D, et al. Diagnostic marker cooperative study for the diagnosis of myocardial infarction. *Circulation*. 1999;99:1671-1677.

103. Apple FS. Creatine kinase isoforms and myoglobin: early detection of myocardial infarction and reperfusion. *Coron Artery Dis*. 1999;10:75-79.

104. Soloman AJ, Gersh BJ. Management of chronic stable angina, medical therapy, PTCA, and CABG. *Ann Intern Med*. 1998;128:216.

105. Bell G et al. Stenting for ischemic heart disease. *Prog Cardiovasc Dis*. 1997;40:159.

106. Bittl JA. Advances in coronary angioplasty. *N Engl J Med*. 1996;335:1290.

107. Amann FW. Coronary stents. *Ther Umsch*. 2003;60(4):179-182.

108. Verin PY, deBruyne B, Baumgart D, et al. The dose-finding study group: endoluminal beta-radiation therapy for the prevention of coronary artery restenosis after balloon angioplasty. The Dose Finding Study Group. *N Engl J Med*. 2001;344(4):243-249.

109. Frishman WH, Chiu R, Landzberg BR, et al. Medical therapies for the prevention of restenosis after percutaneous coronary interventions. *Curr Probl Cardiol*. 1998;23(10):534-635.

110. Leon MB, Teirstein PS, Moses JW, et al. Localized intracoronary gamma-radiation therapy to inhibit the recurrence of restenosis after stenting. *N Engl J Med*. 2001;344(4):250-256.

111. Minnesota Department of Health, Health Technology Advisory Committee. *Executive Summary, June 2001. Intracoronary Brachytherapy*. http://www.health.state.mn.us/htac/brachydr.htm. Accessed December 14, 2009.

112. Linnemeier G. Enhanced external counterpulsation—a therapeutic option for patients with chronic cardiovascular problems. *J Cardiovasc Manag*. 2002;13(6):20-25.

113. Soran O, Kennard ED, Kelsey SF, Holubkov R, Strobeck J, Feldman AM. Enhanced external counterpulsation as treatment for chronic angina in patients with left ventricular dysfunction: a report from the International EECP Patient Registry (IEPR). *Congest Heart Fail*. 2002;8(6):297-302.

114. Michaels AD, Accad M, Ports TA, Grossman W. Left ventricular systolic unloading and augmentation of intracoronary pressure and Doppler flow during enhanced external counterpulsation. *Circulation*. 2002;106(10):1237-1242.

115. Holmes DR Jr. Treatment options for angina pectoris and the future role of enhanced external counterpulsation. *Clin Cardiol*. 2002;25(12)(suppl 2):II22-II25.

116. Beller GA. A review of enhanced external counterpulsation clinical trials. *Clin Cardiol*. 2002;25(12)(suppl 2):II6-II10.

117. Massie BM, Shah NB. Evolving trends in the epidemiology of heart failure. *Am Heart J*. 1997;133:703.

118. Dauterman KW. Heart failure with preserved systolic function. *Am Heart J*. 1998;135:S310.

119. Poole-Wilson PA. Chronic heart failure: definition, epidemiology, pathophysiology, clinical manifestations and investigations. In: Julion DG, Camm AJ, Fox KM, Hall RJC, Poole-Wilson PA, eds. *Diseases of the Heart*. 2nd ed. London, UK: WB Saunders; 1996;467-481.

120. ACC/AHA guidelines for the management of heart failure. *J Am Coll Cardiol*. 1995;26:1396.

121. Cohn JN. The management of heart failure. *N Engl J Med*. 1996;335:490.

122. Burke AP, Farb A, Malcom GT, et al. Coronary risk factors and plaque morphology in men with coronary disease who die suddenly. *N Engl J Med*. 1997;336:1276.

123. Watchie J. *Cardiopulmonary Physical Therapy: A Clinical Manual*. Philadelphia, PA: WB Saunders; 1995.

124. Rose AG. Etiology of valvular heart disease. *Curr Opin Cardiol*. 1996;11:98.

125. Carabello BA. Valvular heart disease. *N Engl J Med*. 1997;337:32.

126. Connolly HM. Valvular heart disease. *N Engl J Med*. 1997;337:1775.

127. Richardson P, McKenna W, Bristow M, et al. Report of the 1995 World Health Organization/International Society and Federation of Cardiology Task Force on the definition and classification of cardiomyopathies. *Circulation*. 1996;93:841.

128. Kasper EK, Agema WR, Hutchins GM, et al. The causes of dilated cardiomyopathy: a clinicopathologic review of 673 patients. *J Am Coll Cardiol*. 1994;23:586.

129. Dec GW, Fuster V. Idiopathic dilated cardiomyopathy. *N Engl J Med*. 1994;331:1564.

130. Maron BJ. Hypertrophic cardiomyopathy. *Lancet*. 1997;350:127.

131. Kushwaha SS, Fallon JT, Fuster V. Restrictive cardiomyopathy. *N Engl J Med*. 1997;336:267.

132. Pisani B, Taylor DO, Mason JW. Inflammatory myocardial diseases and cardiomyopathies. *Am J Med*. 1997;102:459.

133. Hoit BD. Pericardial heart disease. *Curr Probl Cardiol*. 1997;222:353.

134. Ball JB, Morrison WL. Cardiac tamponade. *Postgrad Med J*. 1997;73:141.

135. Fowler NO. Constrictive pericarditis: its history and current status. *Clin Cardiol*. 1995;18:341.

136. Stollerman GH. Rheumatic fever. *Lancet*. 1997;349:935.

137. He J, Welton TK. Epidemiology and prevention of hypertension. *Med Clin North Am*. 1997;81:1077.

138. Vota SA. *Cardiology*. Berkshire, UK: McGraw-Hill; 1999.

139. Patel MI, Hardman DT, Fisher CM, et al. Current views on the pathogenesis of abdominal aortic aneurysm. *J Am Coll Surg*. 1995;181(4):371-382.

140. Van der Vliet JA, Boll AP. Abdominal aortic aneurysm. *Lancet*. 1997;349(9055):863-866.

141. Braverman AC. Aortic dissection. *Curr Opin Cardiol*. 1997;12(4):389-390.

142. Hagan PG, Nienaber CA, Isselbacher EM, et al. International Registry of Acute Aortic Dissection (IRAD)—new insights into an old disease. *JAMA*. 2000;283:897.

143. Pretre R, Von Segesser LK. Aortic dissection. *Lancet*. 1997;349(9063)1461-1464.

144. Dawson I, Sie RB, Van Bockel JH. Atherosclerotic popliteal aneurysm. *Br J Surg*. 1997;84(3):293-299.

145. Allen RC, Smith RB. Diseases of the peripheral arteries and veins. In: Schlant RC, Alexander RW, eds. *Hurst's The Heart*. 8th ed. New York: McGraw-Hill; 1995.

146. Regensteiner JG, Hiatt WR. Exercise rehabilitation for patients with peripheral arterial disease. In: Holloszy JO, ed. *Exercise and Sports Sciences Reviews*. Vol 23. Baltimore, MD: Williams & Wilkins; 1995.

147. Grundy SM, Cleeman JI, Daniels SR, et al. Diagnosis and management of the metabolic syndrome: an American Heart Association/National Heart, Lung, and Blood Institute scientific statement: executive summary. *Circulation*. 2005;112:285-290.

148. Steinberger J, Daniels SR, Eckel RH, et al. Progress and challenges in metabolic syndrome in children and adolescents: a scientific statement from the American Heart Association Atherosclerosis, Hypertension, and Obesity in the Young Committee of the Council on Cardiovascular Disease in the Young; Council on Cardiovascular Nursing; and Council on Nutrition, Physical Activity, and Metabolism. *Circulation*. 2009;119:628-647.

149. Adams JE, Bodor GS, Davila-Roman VG, et al. Cardiac troponin I: a marker with high specificity for cardiac injury. *Circulation*. 1993;88:101-106.

Pulmonary Pathology

Chris L. Wells

INTRODUCTION

The goal of this chapter is to provide a review of pulmonary diseases and disorders that impact pulmonary function. The pulmonary system is responsible for the delivery of oxygen and the release of carbon dioxide, which is vital for normal cellular function. The lungs also assist the renal system in the regulation and maintenance of acid–base balance. When lung function becomes impaired, multiple systems may be affected. Consequently, it is important that physical therapists have an understanding of lung pathologies and their clinical presentation to perform a thorough evaluation, properly monitor the patient, and design an appropriate treatment plan.

This chapter is divided into sections that are based on common pathological impairments and clinical presentations. The first group of pathologies has been classified as chronic obstructive pulmonary diseases (COPD). The second section involves diseases that cause a pulmonary restrictive breathing pattern. Other smaller categories include infections, diseases that disrupt the pulmonary vascular system, and diseases that have pleural involvement. Separate chapters (Chapters 13 and 14) will address neuromuscular and musculoskeletal disorders that affect pulmonary functioning.

CHRONIC OBSTRUCTIVE PULMONARY DISEASES

Chronic obstructive pulmonary disease (COPD) is a generic term that refers to lung diseases that result in air trapping in the lungs, causing hyperinflation of the lungs, and a barrel-chest deformity. The American Thoracic Society and European Respiratory Society recently updated the definition of COPD, which commonly refers to emphysema and chronic bronchitis as "a **preventable and treatable** disease state characterized by airflow limitation that is not fully reversible. The airflow limitation is usually progressive and associated with an abnormal inflammatory response of the lungs to noxious particles/gases, **primarily caused by cigarette smoking. Although COPD affects the lungs it also produces systemic consequences**" (The text in bold has been added to this new definition in 2004).[1,2] This classification of pulmonary disease can be further subdivided based on the presentation of chronic production of purulent sputum. Nonseptic obstructive diseases typically do not clinically present with chronic and consistent sputum production.

Nonseptic obstructive disease includes diagnoses such as emphysema, α_1-antitrypsin deficiency (α_1-ATD), and asthma. Patients with a nonseptic disease may produce a small quantity of sputum, but it is not as significant as it is in diseases like cystic fibrosis (CF), chronic bronchitis, and bronchiectasis, which are classified as *septic obstructive pulmonary diseases.* These diseases are clinically associated with large volumes of sputum production, colonization of bacteria and fungus, and chronic infections. This division may assist the physical therapist in anticipating where bronchial hygiene techniques will be a primary focus of intervention.

Nonseptic Obstructive Airway Diseases

As a classification of pulmonary disease, COPD is the fourth leading cause of death in the United States, afflicting 16 million Americans with 20% of the population affected with some type of COPD. By 2010, it is estimated that COPD will be the third biggest cause of mortality within the world. Acute exacerbations of COPD account for $16 million spent annually in doctor visits. Forty thousand people die from COPD annually.[3] This group of diseases is characterized by an increase in lung compliance with larger lung volumes and air trapping due to premature closure of the airways. The destruction of the lung architecture leads to hypoxia and hypercapnia (see Fig. 7-1).

These diseases are classified under COPD because the patients' presentations have similar characteristics (see Table 7-1). These patients present with hyperinflation, a barrel chest, and excessive use of accessory respiratory muscles. The pulmonary function test (PFT) demonstrates an increase in total lung capacity (TLC), inspiratory reserve capacity (IRC), and residual volume (RV) and a decrease in forced vital capacity (FVC),

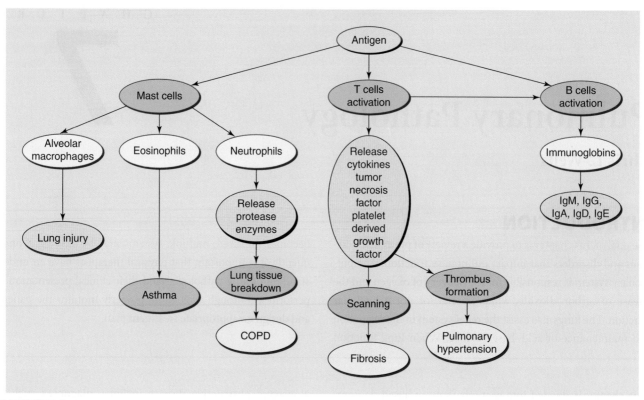

FIGURE 7-1　This diagram summarizes the general immune response that leads to various pulmonary diseases through destruction of lung tissue. This may lead to hypoxia and hypercapnia.

forced expiratory volume in 1 second (FEV_1), diffusion capacity of carbon monoxide (DLCO), and an FEV_1/FVC ratio (see Fig. 7-2 and Table 7-2).[4] Blood gases typically show hypoxia with or without hypercapnia. In the case of septic obstructive disease, like CF or bronchiectasis, the patient will have a chronic pro-ductive cough with excessive sputum production. Finally, from the adverse effects of treatment and a decrease in activity, many of these patients will also have muscle weakness, both type 1 and type 2 muscle fiber atrophy, osteopenia, or osteoporosis and may develop right-sided heart failure.

TABLE 7-1　Clinical Summary

	Nonseptic COPD	Septic COPD	Pulmonary Fibrosis	Pulmonary Hypertension
Lung compliance	↑	↑	↓	↓
Dyspnea	↑	↑	↑	↑
Cough	Variable	Productive	Dry, ↑ exertion	If present, nonproductive and weak
X-ray	Hyperinflation ↓ Diaphragm	Hyperinflation ↓ Diaphragm	↓ Volume Honeycombing	↑ Vascular markings
Hypoxemia	+	+	+	+ If HTN is severe
Hypercapnia	+	+	+ At end stage	
Auscultation	↓ Breath sounds	Rales, wheezes	Rales	=, Rales
Breathing pattern	Prolonged expiration	Prolonged expiration	Rapid rate, shallow	=, Increase rate
FVC	↓	↓	↓	=, ↓
FEV_1	↓	↓	↓	=, ↓
FEV_1/FVC	↓	↓	=	=, ↓
DLCO	↓	↓	↓↓	↓
TLC	↑	↑	↓	=
RV	↑	↑	↓	=

TABLE 7-2 Classification of Lung Disease by Pulmonary Function Test

PFT	Normal (%)	Mild (%)	Moderate (%)	Severe (%)
Obstructive				
FVC	80–120	65–80	50–65	<50
FEV$_1$	80–120	65–80	50–65	<50
FEF$_{25\%–75\%}$	80–120	60–80	40–60	<40
FEV$_1$/FVC	>80	70–80	50–70	<50
RV/TLC	<0.3	0.3–0.45	0.45–0.6	>0.6
Restrictive				
FVC	80–120	65–80	50–65	<50
FEV$_1$	80–120	65–80	50–65	<50
FEV$_1$/FVC	>80	>80	>80	>80
RV/TLC	<0.3	<0.3	<0.3	<0.3
TLC	>80	65–80	50–65	<50

Modified with permission from Vedantam R, Crawford A. The role of preoperative pulmonary function tests in patients with adolescent idiopathic scoliosis undergoing posterior spinal fusion. *Spine.* 1997;22(23):2731-2734.

Asthma (*ICD-9-CM* Code: 493)

Asthma is a chronic disease characterized by reversible obstruction to airflow within the lungs. Between asthmatic episodes lung function is relatively normal, and only exposure to a stimulant results in airway hyperreactivity and airway obstruction.[5–7] It is estimated that there are 15 million people who suffer from asthma within the United States,[8] and the World Health Organization reports an estimated 300 million with asthma worldwide.[9] Asthma is the most common chronic disease in children with an incidence rate of 5.9% annually. There has been a 160% increase in asthma cases in children younger than 4 years since the 1980s.[8] The increased incidence of asthma has been associated with increased exposure to

TABLE 7-3 Risk Factors of Asthma

Childhood asthma	Occupational exposures
Family history	Environmental exposures
Atopy	Second smoke
Maternal smoking	Gender

Modified from Sears M. Evolution of asthma through childhood. *Clin Exp Allergy.* 1998;28(suppl 5):82-89.

nitric oxide, ozone, secondhand smoke, and indoor pollutants.[10] It has been theorized that most cases of atopic or allergy-associated asthma is related to indoor exposure to irritants such as tobacco smoke, carbon monoxide, and nitric oxide from poorly vented heating systems, pesticides, dust mites, mold, rodents, cockroaches, and animal dander.[8] There is a higher rate of asthma in females.[6] Occupational exposure, which is related to the duration and intensity of exposure, is a factor for discussing adult-onset asthma. Asthma accounts for more than 10.4 million doctor appointments annually and more than $23 million is spent on medical management and on the loss of work time related to exacerbation of occupational asthma.[8] Table 7-3 lists the most common risk factors associated with asthma.

Thirty-four percent of children who develop asthma present with wheezing before the age of 3 years. The incidence rate in children younger than 3 years is 11.3%, whereas 15% present for medical evaluation between 3 and 6 years of age.[11] Eighty percent of all asthmatic cases have an onset before the age of 5 years with 50% to 70% of these children reporting diminishing or absent symptoms in late adolescence or adulthood.[7] Approximately 10% will continue to

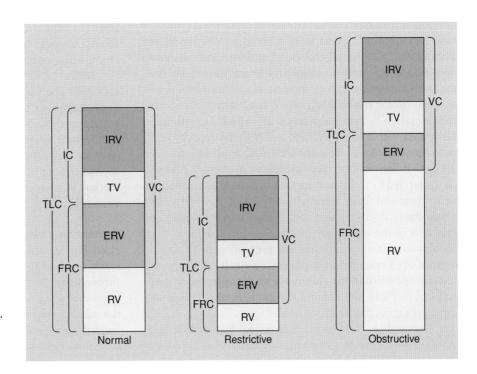

FIGURE 7-2 Pulmonary function tests.
(Reprinted with permission from Ali J, Summer W, Levitzky M. *Pulmonary Pathophysiology.* New York: McGraw-Hill; 1999.)

TABLE 7-4   Classification of Asthma

	Symptoms	Peak Expiratory Flow	FEV$_1$
Mild	Twice a week, nocturnal twice per month, exacerbation with exertion	20%–30% predicted	70%–90% predicted
Moderate	Once a day	Wide variations >30%	60%–80% predicted
Severe	Significant intolerance to exertion	>30% predicted	<60% predicted

Modified from Beck K. Control of airway function during and after exercise in asthmatics. *Med Sci Sports Exerc.* 1999;31(suppl 1):S4-S11 and Kemp J. Comprehensive asthma management: guidelines for clinicians. *J Asthma.* 1998;35(8):601-620.

have symptoms, but these symptoms will be controllable, whereas 30% of children will remain symptomatic, with 17% of these children being classified as having severe asthma.[12] Therefore, approximately 35% to 40% of children will be limited by lung disease in their activities and play. The most widely recognized phenotype of childhood asthma is atopic asthma. Atopic asthma is an allergy-associated form of asthma that accounts for 85% of all school-age asthma cases. It is associated with wheezing, cough, and shortness of breath, and the child may present with other atopic diseases such as eczema and hay fever.[13] It has been suggested that children are most susceptible to atopic asthma due to the maturation process of lymphocytes as the immune system is developing along with the maturation and development of the lung and airway tissue.[14]

Asthma affects people across the lifespan—The majority of asthmatic children have a family history of asthma, particularly on their mother's side. Maternal smoking compounds the risk of childhood asthma.[11] There is a twofold increase in the risk of asthma development in the first year of life and a fourfold increase if the mother smokes and has allergies in the prenatal period.[7] There is a 40% to 50% risk of a child developing asthma if one of the parents or the child's primary caregiver smokes.[10] There is an increase in obesity-related asthma with 6.6% of all childhood asthma cases related to obesity. Obesity-related asthma is characterized by low-grade inflammation with an increase in cytokines and tumor necrosis factor α (TNF-α), which may upregulate airway inflammation.[15] The persistence of childhood asthma is associated with a low FEV$_1$ and a FEV$_1$/vital capacity (VC) ratio less than 0.8 L, frequent asthmatic episodes, the need for anti-inflammatory medications, and *atopy*.[11] Atopy is characterized by an immediate skin hypersensitivity reaction with wheal and flare.[7] Approximately 3% of the elderly have a past medical history that includes asthma. It is estimated that 25% of the elderly are undiagnosed with asthma, even though the classic symptoms are present, and it takes an average of .5 years before a diagnosis is made. Only approximately one-third of the elderly are under appropriate medical care.[16] Table 7-4 includes the guidelines for classifying asthma as mild, moderate, or severe.

The etiology is unknown, but several factors have been associated with the development of asthma. It has been theo-rized that children are most susceptible to the development of asthma because there is less epithelial cell differentiation leading to more fragile airways. The exposure to allergens and, particularly, respiratory viral infections lead to an increase in the proliferation and migration of endothelial cells, recruitment of perivascular supporting cells, an increase in fibroblastic cells, and less normal epithelial cells. The consequence is the development of a hyperactive respiratory immune response.[9,14,17] Maternal smoking has been linked to the increased exacerbation of existing asthma in children. These children also have a higher incidence of infections that may contribute to the development of asthma. Early infections, particularly infections due to the respiratory syncytial virus (RSV) and ureaplasma urealyticum, are associated with asthma.[7,14,18] There also appears to be a genetic link. Chromosomes 5, 11, and 14 appear to contribute to the inflammatory process of asthma.[12,19]

The stimulants that cause asthmatic episodes are similar whether the patient is a child or an adult. Stimulants may include air pollutants, pollen associated with allergies, respiratory infections, exertion, and medications. Children are more at risk because of allergies, whereas the elderly are more susceptible to pollutants and medications. Medications that have been linked to asthma include nonsteroidal anti-inflammatory drugs (NSAIDS), aspirin, nonselective β-blockers, and angiotensin-converting enzyme (ACE) inhibitors.[16]

Airways are characterized by the infiltration of inflammatory cells. There is evidence of remodeling in composition and organization of the walls of the airways. Smooth muscle hyperplasia and hypertrophy are present as well as increased proliferation of epithelial cells. There is hyperplasia of the goblet cells and hypertrophy of vascular tissue and finally, an increased accumulation of myofibroblast cells.[9] The inflammation is associated with the increase in mast cells and eosinophils.[20]

Asthma may also be exacerbated by exercise—It is theorized that *exercise-induced asthma* (EIA) is due to loss of water and heat from the lower respiratory system. Breathing through the mouth during exercise bypasses the nasal passages that warm and humidify the inspired air. By bypassing the nasal passages, there is a resultant loss of heat and water from the mucosa and the lower airways, and the lower airways have to compensate. It is postulated that the loss of heat causes hyperemia, vascular engorgement, and bronchial edema, which reduce the lumen size of the bronchioles.[21] The severity of EIA is determined by minute ventilation during exercise, temperature, humidity of air, and baseline airway reactivity.[21]

Whether antigens, allergies, or exercises stimulate the asthmatic episode, the result is the onset of an inflammatory process (see Fig. 7-1). There is a release of T cells that causes a cell-mediated immune response of particularly CD4 helper/inducer cells. The activation of T cells stimulates the release of antibodies from the humoral-mediated immune system. The elevation of immunoglobin E (IgE) antibodies is associated with asthma-activated mast cells and eosinophils, which in turn help to further promote this inflammatory process by releasing other proinflammatory mediators.[7,12,19] This inflammatory process is associated with bronchoconstriction and airway obstruction.[16]

Asthma is associated with an increase in airway resistance. It is theorized that the drying of the airways, in the presence of EIA, stimulates the inflammatory process and leads to *bronchoconstriction* and an increase in airway resistance.[22] The resistance is related to contraction of the smooth muscle of the bronchioles. There is edema and cellular infiltration of the airways that also contribute to airway obstruction.[23]

The classic symptoms of asthma are wheezing, dyspnea, chest pain, facial distress, and usually a nonproductive cough[18] (see Fig. 7-3). Airways may become obstructed with viscous, tenacious mucus during acute exacerbation that leads to further hyperinflation. These symptoms are more severe in children than in adults. There is an increased risk of an asthmatic attack in children because of the natural lower lung compliance and less compliance with medication.[18] Symptoms in adults may also include paroxysmal nocturnal dyspnea, morning chest pain, and increased symptoms with exposure to cold.[16] In the case of a severe asthma attack that is refractory to bronchodilators, called *status asthmaticus*, the patient may present with decreased breath sounds, cyanosis, exhaustion, hypercapnia, and pending respiratory failure.[24] **It is important to note that EIA symptoms related to bronchoconstriction may present 6 to 8 hours after cessation of submaximal aerobic exercise or immediately after short intense bouts of exercise**.[22,21]

The guidelines for diagnosis vary and are based on the age of the patient. In infants, the diagnosis of asthma is made based on at least three episodes of wheezing observed by a physician.[18] In children, asthma is diagnosed by a history of intermittent episodes of wheezing, coughing, shortness of breath, and chest tightness. These symptoms are worse at night or in the early morning hours. An allergen, pollutant, or exercise may be identified as stimulant.[18] In older children and adults, an improvement in FEV_1 by 15% or more after use of a bronchodilator and sustained improvement in symptoms and lung function with corticosteroids are also consistent with the diagnosis of asthma.[16,18] Finally, the diagnosis of EIA requires the documentation of a 15% decrease in the peak expiratory flow recording following exercise.[21]

The first intervention for asthma is *prevention*. Smoking cessation, as well as minimizing the exposure to secondhand smoke, is important for any woman who is pregnant. It is also important to receive an annual flu shot and avoid stimulants that precipitate an asthmatic episode.[21] The use of high-efficiency particulate air vacuums, mattress covers, and methods to improve heating and home ventilation systems may be effective in reducing the incidence of asthmatic episodes or atopic asthma.[8]

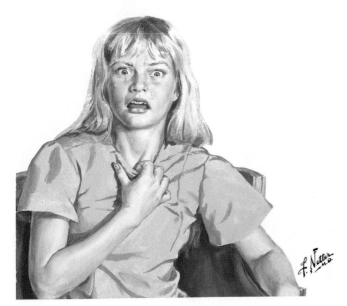

FIGURE 7-3 Patient in an acute asthmatic attack. Note the shortness of breath, anxiety, and general increase in sympathetic discharge. (Image from www.netterimages.com. Reused with permission of Elsevier, Inc. All rights reserved.)

CLINICAL CORRELATE

EIA exacerbation can be minimized through medication and by performing a warm-up approximately 45 to 60 minutes before the exercise program. This warm-up exercise period should consist of 30-second exercise bouts with 2-minute rest periods. This reduces the severity of signs and symptoms of EIA.[21]

The goal of treatment is to minimize exacerbation[25]— The use of short- and long-acting *bronchodilators* is the main defense in controlling asthma.[21] There are several types of bronchodilators that can be prescribed, and it is important that the patient and the therapist understand the proper use of the medication (refer to Table 7-5). β-Adrenergic agonists can be used to increase smooth muscle relaxation that results in bronchodilation and inhibits the release of mediators. Cromolyn, a

TABLE 7-5   Common Medications Used for Asthma and Other COPD

Drug (Inhalation)	Onset (min)	Peak (h)	Duration (h)	Action
Albuterol (Ventolin, Proventil)	5–15	1–1.5	3–6	β_2-Selective bronchodilators
Bitolterol (Tornalate)	3–4	0.5–1	5–8	β_2-Selective bronchodilators
Pirbuterol (Maxair)	<5	0.5–1	5	β_2-Selective bronchodilators
Terbutaline (Brethaire)	15–30	1–2	3–6	Nonselective bronchodilators
Atrovent (w/albuterol, Combivent)	15	1–2	3–4	Prevents bronchoconstriction (anticholinergic)
Salmeterol (Servent)	10–20	3	12	β_2-Bronchodilators

Modified from Kemp J. Comprehensive asthma management: guidelines for clinicians. *J Asthma*. 1998;35(8):601-620 and Cypcar D, Lemanske R. Asthma and exercise. *Chest*. 1994;15(2):351-365.

corticosteroid, is also effective as a prophylactic but not as a rescue drug.[21] More recently, there are other medications being trialled for management of asthma when more traditional methods are not sufficient. These include the use of leukotriene modifiers that block the proinflammatory mediators that promote smooth muscle contraction, vascular leakage, mucus secretion, and airway hyperactivity. IgE inhibitors such as malizurals and other medications like etanercept that block TNF-α are also under investigation. Finally, immunosuppressive medications, methotrexate, and cyclosporine are also being used for the chronic severe cases of asthma.[20]

Establishment of a routine exercise program is also important in the treatment of asthma. Fifty percent of children with asthma are severely deconditioned, but the level of deconditioning cannot be predicted by the history of asthma.[5] People with asthma have a positive response to exercise with improved minute ventilation and oxygen consumption and decrease in blood lactate.[21]

Wheezing and breathlessness are poor predictors for asthma.[16] Asthma that persists into adulthood can be associated with irreversible obstructive disease that may increase the incidence of deaths related to end-stage obstructive disease and increases the risk of pneumonia. *Severe asthma* is defined as asthmatic symptoms that persist despite maximized medical therapy with one or more exacerbation annually. There is a predominance of neutrophil cells associated with airway inflammation and there is a 30% to 50% loss in expiratory airflow, which appears to be associated with a fixed loss of the elastic recoil of the lung that is not associated with emphysema.[26,27]

Emphysema (*ICD-9-CM* Code: 492)

Emphysema is the second most prevalent disease within the category of COPD, with only asthma having a higher incidence. Emphysema is characterized by abnormal, irreversible enlargement of the airways distal to the terminal bronchioles, leading to decrease in driving pressure and intraluminal pressure, which leads to the impairment in expiratory airflow and maintenance of airway patency during inspiration[28,29] (see Figs. 7-4 and 7-5). This may result in destruction of the acini, which are the functional units of the lungs for gas exchange. Each acinus is composed of one to three respiratory bronchioles and the alveolar ducts and sacs.

Emphysema can be classified as *centriacinar, panacinar,* or *paraseptal,* based on the location of the anatomical disruption. See Fig. 7-6 for the illustrations of different types of emphysema. The key structure in the classification of emphysema is the *respiratory bronchiole.* Centriacinar or centrilobular emphysema involves the enlargement and destruction of the first- and second-order respiratory bronchioles, and the alveoli remain intact. Centriacinar emphysema is most commonly associated with smoking. In contrast, the enlargement and

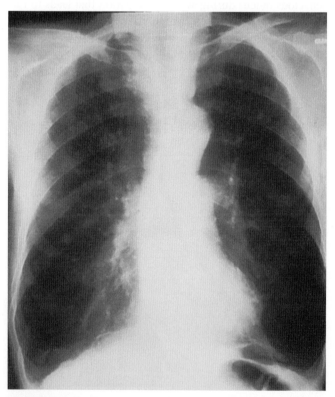

FIGURE 7-4   Emphysema. Notice the hyperinflation of the lungs on this P-A (posterior-anterior) X-ray with flattening of the diaphragm and elongation of the cardiac silhouette. (Courtesy of Dana Gryzbicki, MD, University of Pittsburgh, PA.)

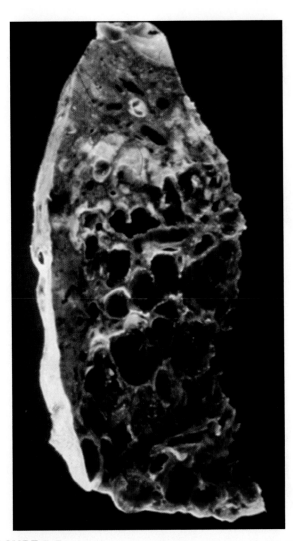

FIGURE 7-5 Emphysema. This disease results in the destruction of bronchioles and parenchymal tissue, which leads to the loss of elastic recoil properties of the lung. This results in the dilatation of airways, which leads to air trapping and hyperinflation. (Courtesy of Dana Gryzbicki, MD, University of Pittsburgh, PA.)

of FEV_1 function occurs more than twice as fast as the aging process and declines by 25% for each pack year of smoking.[28,31] It is associated with a very insidious onset, which occurs over 30 to 40 years.

Cigarette smoking is associated with an increase in cellular apoptosis, early and excessive cell death. There is an increased accumulation of apoptotic cells and slow cell removal with macrophage dysfunction. There is also an increase in TNF-α and a decrease in surfactant protein. These changes lead to alteration of alveolar and small airway function, inflammatory and proteolytic activity, and changes in the endothelium and epithelium cells. The consequences of destruction of the alveolar wall, decrease in surface area, loss of functioning pulmonary capillary bed, and loss of the parenchyma lead to air trapping and ventilation–perfusion ($\dot{V}/\dot{Q}$) mismatch.[3,32]

The etiology of emphysema is based on the protease–antiprotease hypothesis in which there is an imbalance between protease, which causes tissue breakdown, and antiprotease enzymes. This imbalance leads to the loss of lung parenchyma and elastic recoil, which the small airways depend on return to their resting states during exhalation. The elastic property of the parenchyma also provides a normal level of airway resistance during inspiration. This loss of parenchyma tissue results in the loss of *radial traction* on the airways. The end result is dilation of airways, premature airway closure and air trapping, and an increase in RV.[28,29,33]

The nicotine in cigarette smoke attracts neutrophils, activates alveolar macrophages, and inactivates the protective nature of antiprotease.[34] The alveolar macrophages and neutrophils contain protease enzymes, which are capable of destroying the elastic property of the lung tissue, thus producing emphysema.[28] The cigarette smoke also causes a proliferation of endothelial cells, smooth muscle cells, platelet aggregation, and destruction of pulmonary capillaries. The impairment to the small blood vessels within the pulmonary system may lead to the decrease in DLCO and the development of secondary hypertension.[3,31,32]

As a consequence of intrinsic pulmonary damage, hyperinflation of the lungs occurs, which eventually leads to the compensatory changes of the chest wall. This disruption of normal chest wall mechanics leads to dysfunction of the inspiratory muscles, particularly of the diaphragm. The dysfunction of the diaphragm is an important cause of respiratory failure in patients with emphysema. Hyperinflation causes shortening of inspiratory muscles and flattening of the diaphragm with the loss of sarcomeres. The end result is a loss of diaphragmatic excursion and subsequent decline in the mechanical effectiveness of the diaphragm, and other respiratory muscles needed to support the increased demand of ventilation.[35]

The most common complaint of patients with emphysema is *dyspnea on exertion* (DOE). The result of a physical examination reveals the following findings: diminished breath sounds and wheezing, which are typically associated with exertion, and a prolonged expiratory phase.[36] The patient will

destruction of the entire acinus are the defining characteristics of panacinar emphysema, where there is a more even distribution of destruction and dilatation of the entire acinus.[30] Paraseptal emphysema involves the periphery of the secondary lobule along the septum. Paraseptal emphysema is not typically associated with the progression of end-stage COPD but can be associated with an increased risk of pneumothorax (PTX).[28]

Cigarette smoking has been linked to the development of centriacinar emphysema; however, a small proportion of smokers will develop panacinar emphysema. Approximately 10% to 15% of patients with a significant history of smoking will develop clinically significant obstructive disease. A large proportion of the small particles in cigarette smoke are distributed to the first- and second-order bronchioles. Many of the particles are removed through a well-developed lymphatic system of the lower lobes; however, the particles that are also deposited in the upper lobes are revoked at a slower removal rate due to the smaller size of its lymphatic system.[28] The loss

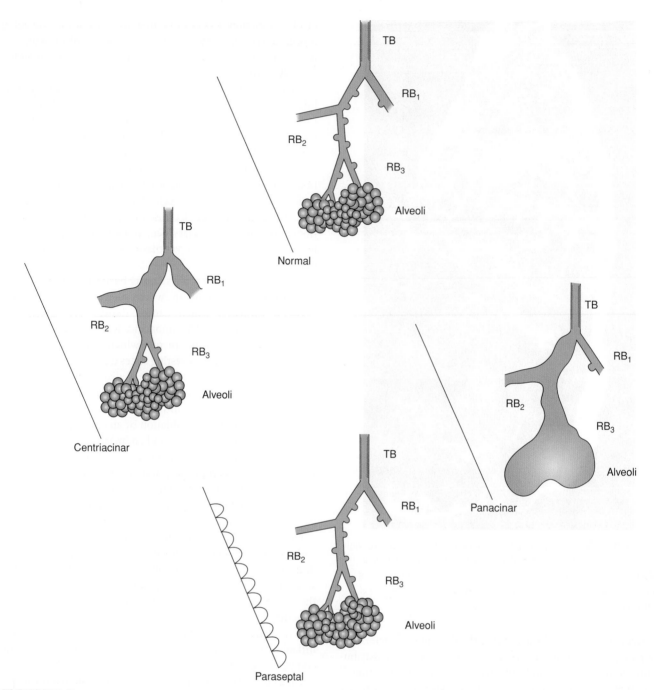

FIGURE 7-6   Types of emphysema. (Modified with permission from Gurney JW. Pathophysiology of obstructive airways disease. *Radiol Clin North Am.* 1998; 36(1):15-27.)

present with an enlarged anterior–posterior dimension of the chest wall, called a *barrel chest,* with an increase in rib angle. The accessory muscles are commonly hypertrophied from overuse. There is hyperresonance sound upon mediate percussion, which is consistent with the hyperinflation of the lungs. The presence of a chronic cough and sputum production will vary and depend on the infectious history of the patient. As the disease advances, many patients become *cachectic,* or emaciated, and begin to show signs of right-sided heart failure due to secondary pulmonary hypertension. The classic signs and symptoms of right-sided heart failure include

peripheral pitted edema, weight gain, jugular vein distension, diminished appetite, right upper quadrant discomfort, and ventricular gallop, S_3 heart sound (see Fig. 7-7). Emphysema is considered as a systemic disease with the increase of the inflammatory process. Patients with emphysema commonly suffer from osteoporosis, skeletal muscle disease, depression, and an increase in incidence of cardiovascular disease.[29,37] Beyond the physical examination, PFT results are consistent with other obstructive airway diseases, which include a decline in FVC, FEV_1, and FEV_1/FVC ratio that indicates small airway disease. There is an increase in TLC and RV.[38]

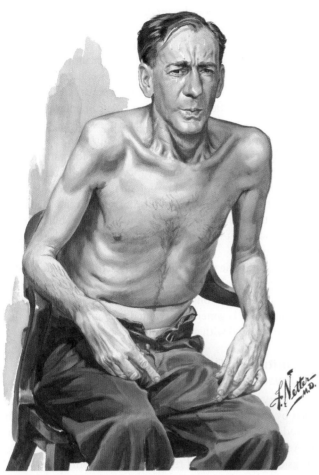

FIGURE 7-7 Patient with a diagnosis of emphysema. Note the generalized muscle wasting, shortness of breath with pursed-lip breathing, and use of accessory muscles with a forward-leaning posture. (Image from www.netterimages.com. Reused with permission of Elsevier, Inc. All rights reserved.)

TABLE 7-6 Indications for Supplemental Oxygen

Recommended Indications

$Pao_2 \leq 55$ mm Hg or $Sao_2 \leq 89\%$ at rest

$Pao_2 \leq 55$ mm Hg or $Sao_2 \leq 89\%$ with exercise

$Pao_2 \leq 55$ mm Hg or $Sao_2 \leq 89\%$ during sleep

Evidence of pulmonary hypertension or cor pulmonale, mental or psychological impairment, polycythemia, and a Pao_2 of 56–59 mm Hg or an $Sao_2 \leq 90\%$ at any time

Medicare Criteria for Reimbursable Oxygen Supplementation[a]

$Pao_2 \leq 55$ mm Hg or $Sao_2 \leq 88\%$

Pao_2 of 56 to 59 mm Hg or $Sao_2 \leq 89\%$ if there is evidence of cor pulmonale, polycythemia, or congestive heart failure, hematocrit $> 56\%$)

Drop in $Pao_2 > 10$ mm Hg or $Sao_2 > 5\%$ with signs and symptoms of hypoxia

[a]Medicare requires recertification and retesting in 60 to 90 days if $Pao_2 > 55$ mm Hg, or $Sao_2 > 88\%$ when oxygen was prescribed; recertification in all patients required after 1 year.

Modified from Dasgupta A, Maurer J. Late stage emphysema: when medical therapy fails. *Cleve Clin J Med.* 1999;65(7):415-424 and Heath J, Mongia R. Chronic bronchitis: primary care management. *Am Fam Physician.* 1998;57(10):2365-2372, 2376-2378.

The chest X-ray reveals hyperinflation with a flattened diaphragm, decreased vascular markings, and possible enlargement of the right side of the heart. Because of the destruction of the gas-exchange areas of the lungs, there is also a mismatch between ventilation and perfusion ($\dot{V}/\dot{Q}$) that is demonstrated on a $\dot{V}/\dot{Q}$ scan.[36]

Patients who present with the classic presentation of emphysema will have arterial blood gas analysis that typically reveals hypoxia and normal-to-slight hypocapnia. These patients present with tachypnea, labored breathing, and a normal-to-low body mass index (BMI). Some patients with emphysema will present with signs more associated with chronic bronchitis including hypoxemia, hypercapnia, signs of right-sided heart failure, copious secretions, and an above-normal BMI.[3] **Caution must be taken in this basic medical description because many patients with emphysema will present with a mixture of clinical features**.

Smoking cessation is instrumental in the care of patients with emphysema because it leads to a slower decline in FEV_1

when compared to the patients who continue to smoke.[39] Smoking cessation has been the only treatment that has shown to slow the alterations in the natural progression of emphysema with patients with mild disease.[29] In addition, there are several other treatment options. Pharmacology interventions include short-acting and long-acting β_2-agonists that cause bronchodilation of the airways. Anticholinergic drugs can be used, but are not usually the first line of medications. These medications, such as Atrovent, block bronchoconstriction. Refer to Table 7-5 for a summary of medications used in treating emphysema. Xanthine derivatives (eg, theophylline) also produce bronchodilation, accelerate mucociliary transport, and limit the inflammatory response. Corticosteroids are common agents used for their anti-inflammatory effects. It is also important that the patients receive the preventive vaccinations against influenza and pneumococcus.[20]

Long-term oxygen therapy helps correct hypoxemia and minimizes secondary pulmonary hypertension. The threshold for oxygen prescription include a Pao_2 less than 55 mm Hg, an oxygen saturation less than 88%, evidence of cor pulmonale, or a hemocrit greater than 56% (Table 7-6).[39] Oxygen therapy has been shown to reduce the level of dyspnea, decrease maximal voluntary ventilation and polycythemia by correcting hypoxemia, decrease pulmonary hypertension, improve quality and quantity of sleep, and decrease nocturnal arrhythmias. **Supplemental oxygen can also improve cognitive function and exercise tolerance.** The use of BiPAP ventilation, which is a form of mechanical ventilation, provides airway pressure on both inspiration and expiration to decrease the work of breathing and prevent early airway closure. This minimizes air trapping and has also been found to reduce the retention of carbon dioxide.

CLINICAL CORRELATE

Pulmonary rehabilitation has become a widely accepted intervention in the care of patients with emphysema but is still not covered by many insurance plans, although research supports its positive effects of increasing maximal exercise tolerance, oxygen uptake, and exercise endurance. There is also an improvement of the perceived level of dyspnea and a decrease in muscle fatigue. There is an improvement in quality of life, including the improvement in self-worth, well-being, and an increased sense of self-control.[39] Pulmonary rehabilitation should include general muscle strengthening with emphasis on the upper body; aerobic conditioning; and education about smoking cessation, nutrition, vaccinations, proper use of medications and supplemental oxygen, and the disease process.

Bullectomy is a common surgical intervention for a patient with emphysema with significant bullae disease. A *bulla* is a large air space greater than 1 cm in diameter, which is the result of destruction of the parenchyma. A bulla no longer participates in gas exchange or diffusion. A bulla may also cause compression of adjacent functional lung tissue, which further impairs diffusion. Bullae are associated with a 15% to 20% incidence of PTX. A bullectomy is indicated when there is a significant level of dyspnea, clear presence of bullae that compress viable tissue, and when there is a high incidence of PTX. A bullectomy results in the reduction of pulmonary vascular and airway resistance, a reduction of functional residual capacity (FRC), and less air trapping. If enough diseased tissue is removed, the diaphragm may return to a more normal position that will improve muscle contraction.[39,40]

Volume reduction is the surgical resection of approximately 20% of dysfunctional lung tissue, thus reducing the hyperinflated state (see Figs. 7-8 and 7-9). The most common complication is air leaking in which there is a disruption of subatmospheric pressure within the thorax.[39] From the outcomes of the NIH *National Emphysema Treatment Trial* (NETT) study, it has been determined that the patients with the best outcome have primarily upper lobe disease and have a decrease in exercise capacity, less than 25 W for women and less than 40 W for men.[40]

Lung transplantation is a viable option for patients with end-stage disease who have maximized medical intervention. Patients with emphysema are potential candidates for either single- or double-lung procedures. Transplantation has the potential to significantly improve quality of life, but there are still questions as to whether transplantation extends the life of the recipient.[39,40]

In general, the prognosis of emphysema varies depending on the degree of obstruction, the presence of hypercapnia, the recurrence of infections, and the development of right-sided heart failure. It is generally accepted that an FEV_1 of less than 25% is associated with a 50% mortality rate in 2 years.[39]

α_1-Antitrypsin Deficiency (Genetically Acquired Emphysema) (*ICD-9-CM* Code: 493.8)

α_1-Antitrypsin is an enzyme that is predominantly synthesized by the liver parenchymal cells and counterbalances the degradation of tissue caused by protease, a proteolytic enzyme. α_1-Antitrypsin primarily inhibits neutrophil elastase, which works to break down and remove bacteria from the airways.[41] The normal level of α_1-AT is 104 to 276 mg/dL. At an α_1-AT level below 50 mg/dL, the genetic disorder α_1-ATD should be suspected.[42] Genetic emphysema or α_1-ATD commonly presents as panacinar disease.[42,43] The degree of deficiency is associated with the severity of the disease.

α_1-ATD is the most common autosomal recessive genetic cause of liver disease in children[43,44] and only second to CF in genetic pulmonary disease.[44] Beyond the second decade of

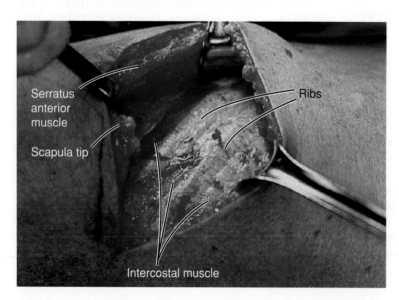

FIGURE 7-8 Surgical entrance into the chest wall via *thoracotomy* as a precursor to volume reduction surgery. The ribs and intercostal muscles are identified. The ribs are counted to ascertain the proper level for entering the chest cavity. (Courtesy of Peter Fergen, MD, University of Pittsburgh, PA.)

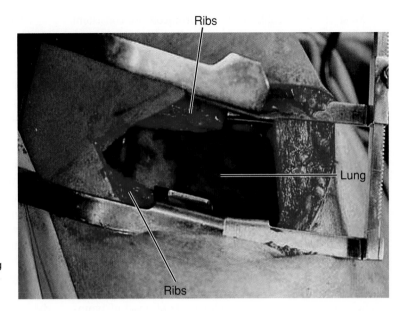

Ribs

Lung

Ribs

FIGURE 7-9 Volume reduction surgery. Rib-spreading retractors increase the exposure of the chest cavity. (Courtesy of Peter Fergen, MD, University of Pittsburgh, PA.)

life, α_1-ATD is primarily associated with lung disease.[45] It is estimated that 1.29 million patients suffer from α_1-ATD in the United States and another 1.1 million worldwide, which causes end-stage obstructive lung disease.[44–46] There is an estimated 25 million carriers of α_1-ATD worldwide. The prevalence is 1 in 1,500 people of European descent.[41]

α_1-ATD can be divided into four categories based on variation in *allele.* An allele is one or more alternative forms of a gene on a chromosome. There have been more than 100 alleles identified with 34 associated with functional deficiency in the circulating α_1-AT.[41] Allele M involves a variation that carries little to no risk of disease, because the α_1-AT level is sufficient enough not to cause cellular damage.[42] The deficient variants that most commonly lead to liver or lung disease are allele S, allele Z, and allele null (0). Allele Z is the most common variant that is characterized by a normal level of α_1-AT synthesis, but the secretion is only 15% of predicted levels. Allele Z accounts for 95% of severe α_1-ATD. Allele S and allele 0 with the null variants are characterized by little α_1-AT production, accounting for the most severe expression of the disease. The Z allele and null variants most predictably lead to premature lung disease.[42,43]

The onset of symptoms associated with pulmonary dysfunction typically begins in the 30s with the diagnosis of α_1-ATD occurring between 40 and 50 years of age.[42,45] **It is estimated that up to 13% of patients with emphysema actually have α_1-ATD.** Only approximately 10% of α_1-ATD cases are actually diagnosed correctly. Most are initially diagnosed with asthma or nongenetic emphysema.[43] A correct diagnosis takes 7.2 years on an average, and it is not uncommon that the patient is seen by 6 to 10 physicians before a correct diagnosis is made.[45] Diagnosis prior to 20 years of age is typically related to liver dysfunction.[44]

Smoking has been associated with the acceleration of lung disease in the presence of α_1-ATD. It has been estimated that cigarette smoking accelerates the progression of the lung disease by 19 years.[45] Patients with α_1-ATD or a family history of α_1-ATD should not smoke! The tobacco smoke increases the level of oxidant exposure, alveolar macrophages, and neutrophils in the airways, along with other inflammatory cells. Cigarette smoke also inactivates α_1-AT and leads to neutrophil protease being unopposed, thus causing the degradation of proteins within the lungs.[43] An elastase–antielastase hypothesis has been proposed to explain the destructive changes that occur because of this deficiency. Neutrophil protease is capable of cleaving many of the proteins from connective tissue within the lung. Without the appropriate level of α_1-AT, neutrophil protease is unopposed, which leads to an imbalance, with degradation occurring at a faster rate than repair and remodeling.[43]

The primary significance of α_1-ATD is the premature development of emphysema, occurring in the third or fourth decade of life. Shortness of breath is typically the first symptom that causes the patient to present for medical intervention.[43] Patients also report a chronic cough in 37% of all cases, sputum production (38%), wheezes (44%), and hyperreactive airways (20%).[45] Many patients may present with weight loss, cor pulmonale, and polycythemia as the disease progresses to end stage.[47] For up to 20% of patients, the clinical presentation of pulmonary impairment will also have liver disease, and up to 70% of patients will have abnormal liver enzymes.[42]

Upon examination of α_1-ATD, the diagnostic testing shows similar findings to smoke-related emphysema. The results of PFTs demonstrate an obstructive pattern with a decline in FVC, FEV_1, and FEV_1/FVC ratio. DLCO is also diminished. There is an increase in TLC and RV. Radiological studies show the classic signs of hyperinflation and a decrease in vascular markings particularly of the lower lobes. Smoking-related emphysema shows more upper lobe or uniform disease throughout the lungs.[42,44,47] High-resolution CT scan is the gold standard for diagnosis. When a patient younger than 50 years presents with signs and symptoms of emphysema or asthma with impairment more excessive than expected, blood testing should be conducted to test the serum α_1-AT level.[43]

Most of the available treatment protocols are consistent with the treatments for emphysema such as bronchodilators, aerosolized or systemic corticosteroids, cessation of smoking, and preventive vaccinations. Pulmonary rehabilitation and supplemental oxygen therapy also are effective in the management of α_1-ATD. It has been recommended that if the plasma level of α_1-AT is less than 11 μmol/L, the patient should be given augmentation therapy (Prolastin, Aralast, and Zemaira), with the goal to increase α_1-AT above 15 μmol/L (80 mg/dL), which appears to protect the lungs and slow down the decline of PFTs.[41,42] Work is also being done to develop gene therapy for the treatment of α_1-ATD. The most common surgical intervention for end-stage lung disease due to α_1-ATD is lung transplantation. The clinical trials for lung volume reduction have shown that it is an ineffective procedure because of the primary presence of lower lobe disease. However, the effectiveness of this procedure is still in question.[42]

The prognosis of α_1-ATD depends on the type of variant or allele, history of cigarette smoking, age of onset of symptoms, and the development of infectious bronchiectasis. Rapid decline in PFTs is associated with a worse prognosis.[42] Sixty-two percent of patients with α_1-ATD will die from respiratory failure, whereas 13% will die from end-stage liver disease.[45,47]

Chronic Bronchitis (*ICD-9-CM* Code: 491)

Chronic bronchitis is a clinical diagnosis that consists of a persistent cough that produces sputum for more than 3 months per year for at least two consecutive years in the absence of another definable medical cause. It is associated with obstruction of the airways and mucus plugging.[1,23] It is estimated that 15 million people suffer from chronic bronchitis in the United States.[48] **Cigarette smoking is the most important risk factor in the development of chronic bronchitis.**[49]

Smoking causes inflammation throughout the lung tissue with an increase in macrophages and T lymphocytes found within the airways. This inflammation is associated with airway remodeling, hypertrophy of submucosal glands, enlargement of smooth muscle cells, fibrosis of airway walls, and goblet cell hyperplasia.[50] Polymorphonuclear neutrophils are suspected to be the primary cause of the chronic airway inflammation.[51] The increased activity of macrophages and neutrophils leads to the release of various enzymes such as interleukin 8, TNF-α, and elastase, which leads to further inflammation and airway destruction.[52] The inflammation within the airways is correlated with alveolar wall destruction and rupture of the attachment between the outer airways and the alveoli. The end result is the loss of the elastic recoil within the lung tissue, which leads to airway obstruction and hyperinflation of the lungs.[34]

Approximately 15% of smokers will develop emphysema or chronic bronchitis. In the smokers who go on to develop chronic bronchitis, the exposure to nicotine causes an inflammatory response, as discussed previously, which stimulates mucus secretion, and disruption of the architecture of the airways and capillary system.[34,53]

There are other risk factors that have been identified in the development of chronic bronchitis. Age and the degree of airway obstruction along with the degree of hypoxia and hypercapnia are associated with chronic bronchitis. Aging is associated with a decline in B cells and T cells and a decrease in responsiveness to protect the airway. There is also a decrease in ciliary function and in the presence of chronic bronchitis, there is a further decline in CD4 and CD8 cells. This imbalance increases airway destruction and mucus production and retention.[52] There is a greater risk of chronic bronchitis if the patient requires systemic steroids for medical management. At times of exacerbation, the patient may develop acute respiratory failure with secretion retention and severe abnormal blood gases requiring mechanical ventilation.[54]

Chronic bronchitis can be divided into subsets based on the degree of pulmonary dysfunction and sputum production. Acute tracheobronchitis is not associated with any pulmonary dysfunction but is typically associated with an acute viral infection. With simple chronic bronchitis, there is a mild-to-moderate decline in FEV_1 and an increase in sputum production. Complicated chronic bronchitis pertains to a patient who is of advanced age, has an FEV_1 of less than 50% of predicted, and has repeated exacerbations, poor nutrition, and comorbidities. Exacerbations that are associated with an increase in purulent secretions are likely from a bacteria infection such as streptococcus or *Haemophilus influenzae*. Finally, with chronic bronchitis, infection is distinct from the other subsets in that the patient has constant sputum production throughout the year.[54]

Upon inspection of the lung tissue in the presence of chronic bronchitis, there is hypertrophy and increased density of the secretory cells down the tracheobronchial tree. Along with airway obstruction from the loss of elastic recoil, there is inflammation of the respiratory bronchioles, hypertrophy of the smooth muscle at the level of the small noncartilaginous airways, and mucus plugging that further narrows or occludes the small airways.[24,49] The end result is a retention of mucus in the airways that lead to further airway obstruction and creates a vicious cycle of further pulmonary infections and destruction.[54]

These patients commonly present with an increase in shortness of breath and a productive cough during the acute exacerbation. There is an increase in sputum production and purulence along with a positive culture that confirms an infection. *H. influenzae* is the most common source of infection. A wheeze may be present upon auscultation. The physical examination and testing will reveal a barrel chest; decline in the FVC, FEV_1, and FEV_1/FVC ratio; decrease in DLCO; and commonly, hypercapnia and hypoxemia. The patients may also report anorexia associated with dyspnea while eating[24,49] (see Fig. 7-10).

The standard of care includes antibiotic treatment in the presence of an acute infection and short-acting β-agonists, long-acting bronchodilators, and inhaled corticosteroids. Frequently, these patients may be on chronic inhaled or

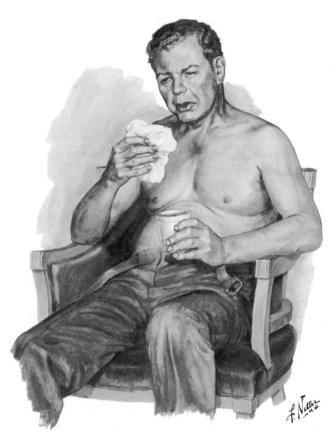

FIGURE 7-10   Patient with a diagnosis of chronic bronchitis. Note the cyanosis, use of accessory muscles, and sputum production. (Image from www.netterimages.com. Reused with permission of Elsevier, Inc. All rights reserved.)

intravenous antibiotics on a monthly basis to control infections. Smoking cessation is the most effective way to decrease mortality. The patients may also be taking expectorants and mucolytics to assist in management of sputum. Patients are encouraged to be well-hydrated. Bronchodilators may be used to manage bronchospasms. As this disease progresses, supplemental oxygen may be required to correct hypoxemia, and some form of pulmonary hygiene may need to be incorporated into the patient's daily routine. Pulmonary rehabilitation is becoming recognized as a key component in the medical treatment plan. Finally, some pulmonologists are administrating an antiprotease, such as prolastin, to counteract the destruction of elastase caused by the chronic inflammatory process.[49,55]

The prognosis of chronic bronchitis is dependent on age, smoking, and the degree of airway obstruction. The 10-year mortality rate is 60% in smokers, whereas it is only 15% in nonsmokers. If the FEV_1 is less than 1 L, the median survival rate is 4 years. Patients who spend at least 50% of the day in bed are four times more likely to die than patients who are mobilized early and frequently.[49,54]

Bronchiolitis Obliterans (*ICD-9-CM* Code: 496)

Bronchiolitis obliterans (OB) is an acute inflammatory injury usually characterized by a diffuse destruction of the bronchioles.

There are multiple causes of OB in the adult population including an infectious process, toxic fume exposure, collagen vascular disease, chronic bronchitis, and lung transplantation. Most recently it has been recognized as the exposure to diacetyl, an additive used in artificial butter flavoring for popcorn, has been linked to OB.[56] In pediatric patients, OB is primarily a complication of severe lower airway infection.[57,58]

The characteristics of OB may vary based on the underlying disease. In the presence of OB with organizing pneumonia (BOOP), an infection, there is fibroblastic proliferation in the small airways and mild chronic inflammatory infiltrates consistent with increased composition of alveolar macrophages in the alveoli.[59] Polyp formation within the bronchioles consisting of granulation tissue can extend into the terminal bronchioles, which can partially or completely obstruct the airway. These polyps form at the site of epithelial injury. The proliferative form of OB is characterized by inflammation and infiltration of mesenchymal cells, which are composed of fibroblasts, myofibroblasts, and other extracellular substances, that leads to fibrosis and airway destruction.[60] The proliferative form of OB has three principal processes that include an acute inflammatory phase with reversible fibrosis. In the first form, the basement membrane is intact, which allows for recovery. The second is described as an acute to subacute inflammatory presence with irreversible bronchiole fibrosis, and the most severe pattern is the chronic inflammatory picture with irreversible fibrosis. This third pattern is mostly associated with complications from transplantation and graft-versus-host disease.[60] With obstructive pulmonary disease like emphysema and asthma, injury of the bronchioles is associated with mucus plugging, inflammatory infiltration, smooth muscle hypertrophy, goblet cell hyperplasia, and bronchial gland hypertrophy. This leads to narrowing of the airways that compounds the loss of elastic recoil and results in further airway obstruction.[59]

Constrictive OB is an uncommon idiopathic form of OB. The usual site of injury with constrictive OB is isolated to the bronchioles with preservation of distal airways. It is characterized by mural fibrosis, resulting in reduction in the lumen size of the bronchioles. Compared to nonconstrictive idiopathic OB, there is luminal narrowing due to scarring rather than smooth muscle hypertrophy.[59,60]

Recently, the most common cause of OB is associated with lung transplantation and is associated with the loss of graft function. It is speculated that OB is the result of chronic rejection. The hallmark sign is submucosal bronchiolar fibrosis preceded by bronchiolar inflammation resulting in epithelial necrosis through a process of lymphohistiocytic-mediated cytotoxicity that targets the respiratory bronchioles. The end process is the deposition of collagen and airway obliteration also referred to as vanishing airway disease. Transplanted OB is associated with frequency and severity of acute cellular rejection, ischemic and reperfusion injury, cytomegalovirus (CMV), and other bacterial or fungal respiratory infections. The incidence of OB associated with transplantation has been reported as high as 80% in recipients after 5 years with an onset of 16 to 20 months.[58,61] More than 50% of recipients who survive beyond 3 months will develop OB.[62] OB in transplant recipients can be classified as active or inactive, based on the presence or absence of lymphocytic infiltration, respectively.[63] There are three typical patterns that OB can follow: a rapid and relentless decrease in FEV_1 with death within 1 year of diagnosis, an insidious onset with a slow decline in FEV_1, and finally, a rapid decrease in FEV_1 onset followed by a stabilization over a prolonged period of time.[61]

In children and infants, OB is the primary cause of obstructive pulmonary disease. The primary site of injury involves the inflammation of the peripheral, small airways. The onset is typically the result of a viral infection, adenovirus, RSV, parainfluenza, influenza, and rhinovirus. Thirty-four percent of children who require mechanical ventilatory support as part of the medical therapy for severe respiratory infection will go on to develop OB as opposed to only 3% in cases where children did not require mechanical ventilation.[57] Hyperactivity of the airways may develop as a result of this chronic inflammatory process.[24,59]

In general, there is a pronounced degree of fibroproliferative activity in the bronchioles that leads to or adds to further airway obstruction. There is the presence of derangement of epithelial function, local necrosis, fibropurulent exudate, and deposition of collagen.[57,60] The damage is typically confined to the cartilaginous airways, with sparing of the respiratory bronchioles, alveolar ducts, pulmonary alveoli, and interstitium. In larger airways, there may be signs of bronchiectasis, mucus plugs, and chronic inflammatory infiltrates by lymphocytes, macrophages, and plasma cells.[59,63]

Frequently, there is an insidious onset with progressive dyspnea with exertion, often associated with a cough in the development of OB. Upon auscultation, wheezing and crackles are present when OB presents with an obstructive pattern. In the stage where there is an increase in sputum production, there may be the presence of low-pitched wheezing or rhonchi. Patients commonly complain of dyspnea, a low-grade fever, and a persistent cough.[63] In children, the signs and symptoms will include hypoventilation and hypercapnia, intercostal retractions, tachypnea, grunting, expiratory wheezes, crackles, hyperinflation, and atelectasis.[57,59] On examination of lung function, there is a decrease in FVC and FEV_1 as well as an increase in RV[57,61]; in the presence of small airway involvement, there will also be a reduction of the FEV_1/FVC ratio. A chest X-ray will illustrate hyperinflation and patchy atelectasis, and a high-resolution CT scan will reveal mosaic perfusion, vascular attenuation, and central bronchiectasis.[57,58]

Medical management begins with prevention, primarily to decrease the incidence of exposure to toxic gases, minerals, and organic particulates.[60] Therapy also includes the use of supplemental oxygen, antiviral medications, and corticosteroids to suppress the inflammatory process. Bronchodilators may be used for the management of bronchospasm. For transplant recipients, prevention and early treatments of acute rejection and viral infection are the best medical approaches to preserve the function of the donor lung.[63]

Mortality is generally low for OB and is predominantly associated with the underlying pathology that is responsible for the inflammatory process. Death due to OB in children is approximately 1%.[59] In the transplant population, the mortality rate has been reported as high as 56% with more than 60% of the deaths related to a respiratory infection.

Lymphangioleiomyomatosis (*ICD-9-CM* Code: 496)

Lymphangioleiomyomatosis (LAM) is a rare disease that affects women in their reproductive years. It is a multisystem disease that is characterized by nonneoplastic proliferation of atypical smooth muscle cells in the parenchyma and lymphatic system. It is also associated with the development of renal angiomyolipomas in approximately 50% of the cases.[64,65]

The etiology of LAM is unknown, but there may be a genetic link because LAM is present in the autosomal genetic disorder *tuberous sclerosis complex* on chromosome 16. Typically, the onset of LAM is in the early to mid-30s and has an incidence of 1 per 1 million.[66] The pulmonary system is the primary site of dysfunction.[64] There are two patterns of LAM: tumor sclerosis gene LAM, which is also associated with central nervous system involvement including seizures and cognitive impairments, and sporadic LAM, which does not have any neurological involvement.[67]

Upon examination of the lung tissue, there is diffuse formation of cysts that leads to degradation of supportive elastic fibers by an imbalance between α_1-AT and elastase. There is a proliferation of immature smooth muscle cells (LAM cells) within the walls of the airways, which leads to the destruction of alveoli and obstruction of the small airways.[64-66]

This disease is frequently misdiagnosed as asthma, COPD, pulmonary fibrosis, tuberculosis (TB) infection, or sarcoidosis. On an average, there is a 4-year delay between the onset of symptoms and the diagnosis, unless the patient experiences a spontaneous PTX; then the average time to obtain a correct diagnosis is slightly more than 2 years.[67] The chest X-ray demonstrates nonspecific changes with preserved or increased lung volumes, hyperinflation, diffuse reticular opacities, pleural effusions, and a PTX. High-resonance CT scan is the best tool for diagnosis because it is very sensitive in detecting cystic formation and honeycombing without fibrosis and dilatation of the thoracic duct. There may also be the dilatation of the thoracic duct. The results of PFTs may show an obstructive, restrictive, or mixed pattern.[65] The majority of cases demonstrate an obstructive volume pattern. Approximately 35% of patients will have normal a PFT until late into the disease[67]; however, a reduction of DLCO is seen in most cases regardless of the pattern.[65,66]

The most common presenting signs and symptoms are DOE and PTX. The patient may also present with a nonproductive cough, hemoptysis, chylous pleural effusion, wheezing, chest pain, abdominal pain, and ascites, if associated with dilatation and cysts involving the lymphatic system of pelvis and abdomen. Symptoms may worsen with the use of oral contraceptives.[64,66] Signs and symptoms of right-sided heart failure may be documented in association with pulmonary hypertension.[65,67]

Treatment includes counseling the patient to avoid pregnancy because the hormonal changes worsen the disease. The patient should also be encouraged to avoid labor-intensive jobs because of the risk of PTX. Corticosteroids and cytotoxin are typically not effective in alleviating signs and symptoms. It has been suggested that the use of progesterone and tamoxifen may stabilize the disease progression.[66] More recently, antiestrogen and luteinizing hormone are being used to manipulate the endocrine system as well as oophorectomy, which appears to slow the progression of the disease.[68]

Death is usually due to respiratory failure. Mortality rates are variable and are greatly influenced by the degree of small airway obstruction and impairments in DLCO. On an average, there is a 50% to 80% survival rate at 8 to 10 years after the onset of symptoms.[64,66] Patients whose primary complaint is dyspnea have a significantly higher mortality rate as opposed to those suffering from PTX; 10-year survival rates are 47% and 89%, respectively.[67]

Septic Obstructive Airway Diseases

This group of diseases is also under the umbrella term of COPD, but these diseases are classified as septic diseases because of the presence of purulent sputum production and a high incidence of pulmonary infections. The hallmark clinical feature is a productive cough with excessive secretion production. The PFT findings are similar with a decrease in expiratory effort despite an increase in TLC. Many of these patients develop hypercapnia, which leads to pulmonary hypertension and cor pulmonale.

Cystic Fibrosis (*ICD-9-CM* Code: 277)

CF is the most common autosomal recessively inherited disorder in Caucasians.[69] Within the lungs, this genetic defect leads to excessive production of thick, dehydrated, hyperviscous mucus and impairment of the mucociliary blanket.[70,71] The incidence is 1 in 3,000 births in the United States and Europe. Chronic bouts of inflammation and infection lead to the breakdown of protein in the lungs. Obstructions of small airways develop from mucus plugs and destruction of the cartilaginous support of the airways. The end result is bronchiectasis, which is a permanent dilatation of the bronchi that is characterized by inflamed airways, which are full of purulent sputum[23] (see Figs. 7-11 and 7-12).

CF is the result of mutation of the gene, CF transmembrane regulator (CFTR), which is associated with the failure of chloride secretion that results in dehydration of endobronchial secretions and cripples the mucociliary function as well as disrupts the function of the pancreas and reproductive system. This leads to an increased attraction to bacteria because of the decreased ability to contain and remove bacteria. CFTR is also associated with the transportation of bicarbonate and sodium and has been linked to the differentiation of osteoblastic cells.[72,73]

Ninety percent of people who are diagnosed with CF will also have pancreatic insufficiency.[69] Recently, it has been recognized that early diagnosis and treatment is important to the aggressive nutritional support that aids in the management of musculoskeletal and pulmonary health.[74] Through infancy and childhood, patients with CF will suffer from nasal polyps; failure to thrive syndrome; chronic or recurrent pneumonia; and a chronic cough, pancreatitis, and gastroesophageal reflux disease (GERD).[69]

The diagnostic findings are similar in patients with other obstructive lung diseases. A chest X-ray typically demonstrates hyperinflation and flattening of the diaphragm. High-resolution CT scans are more sensitive than conventional

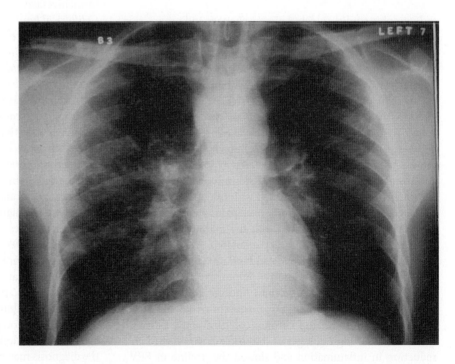

FIGURE 7-11 Cystic fibrosis. Notice the hyperinflation of the lung, the fibrotic changes throughout the lung fields, particularly the upper lobes, and decreased aeration. (Courtesy of Joseph Pilewshi, MD, University of Pittsburgh, PA.)

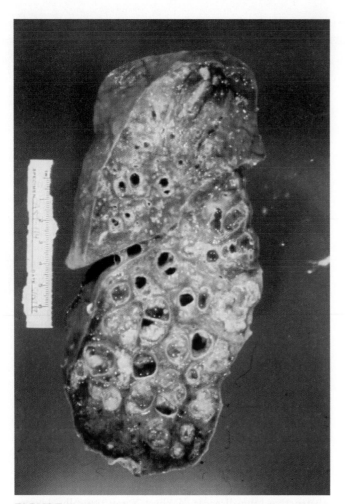

FIGURE 7-12   Cystic fibrosis. This gross pathology slide clearly illustrates destruction of the parenchymal tissue and the large cyst formation. (Courtesy of Dana Gryzbicki, MD, University of Pittsburgh, PA.).

radiographic studies to detect airway changes and progression of bronchiectasis; there is a strong correlation between CT scan findings and PFTs.[72] PFTs reveal an obstructive pattern and a decline in DLCO as the disease progresses. Abnormal arterial blood gases will be consistent with hypoxia and hypercapnia with advancement of the disease.

Most patients will present with a chronic productive cough, dyspnea with accessory muscle use, inspiratory crackles and wheezing, and clubbing of the nail beds.[69,75] Patients also present with weight loss, decreased activity tolerance, pancreatic insufficiency, hemoptysis, and sputum production. This clinical picture may be complicated with osteoporosis, muscle wasting, diabetes mellitus, chronic back pain, and developmental delays.[24,76] CF is associated with the following complications: massive hemoptysis and spontaneous PTX, which are associated with chronic infection and inflammation.[77]

Treatment primarily addresses pulmonary care and management of pancreatic insufficiency. Antibiotic and antifungal medications have become the mainstay in managing active infection and minimizing chronic colonization.[78] Research has shown that high dosages of ibuprofen have resulted in a reduction in inflammation and slowed the decline in FEV$_1$.

Clinically, the risk to renal and gastrointestinal system is too high, and most physicians will not prescribe the use of ibuprofen. Also, low-dose levels have also been linked to the increase of neutrophil migration into the lungs. Other pharmaceutical interventions are being directed at the primary CFTR defect or the direct consequences of its mutation.[79] Sputum retention is managed by a variety of airway and pulmonary hygiene techniques.[76,80] Additionally, the primary surgical intervention for CF is a double-lung transplantation. Therapy should also include management of osteoporosis and proper nutritional support. Finally, a well-rounded exercise program should be prescribed that addresses aerobic and endurance training, muscle strengthening, spine and osteoporosis care, and energy conservation as the disease progresses. See Chapter 17 for more information on the disease and treatment of CF.

The prognosis is dependent on the aggressiveness of the genetic expression of the disease as well as on the quality of the medical care. Certainly the lifespan of patients with CF has improved with advances in antibiotics, management of pancreatic insufficiency, hypoxia, and hypercapnia. The median life expectancy has increased over the years to 38 years of age.[72] Eighty percent of people with CF will succumb to respiratory failure; others will die from complications of right-sided heart failure, severe hemoptysis, and spontaneous PTX.[81,82]

Bronchiectasis (*ICD-9-CM* Code: 494)

Bronchiectasis is the permanent dilatation of the bronchi from the destruction of the muscular and elastic properties of the lung. It is characterized by thickening of the bronchial walls, impairment of the mucociliary blanket, hypersecretion of purulent sputum, and bacterial colonization.[23,83,84] Indeed, purulent overproduction of secretions is the hallmark of this pulmonary disease.[85] There is a classification system for bronchiectasis that describes the distortion of the bronchi. *Cylindrical bronchiectasis* is associated with relatively uniform dilatation, whereas *varicose bronchiectasis* is characterized by local constrictions superimposed on cylindrical bronchiectasis. Finally, *saccular or cystic bronchiectasis* is associated with more severe disease and leads to the formation of bullae.[84]

Bronchiectasis is usually associated with other underlying pulmonary diseases, but there are rare cases of idiopathic bronchiectasis that accounts for approximately 30% of the cases.[86] Bronchiectasis is typically associated with CF, primary ciliary dyskinesia, and connective tissue disorders, such as rheumatoid arthritis (RA), lupus, α_1-ATD, emphysema, and recurrent pulmonary infections.[84]

There is a higher prevalence of bronchiectasis in underdeveloped countries because of the lack of antibiotics. There is an increased number of patients being treated for bronchiectasis because people are living longer due to medical advances with various pulmonary diseases.[87] It has been suggested that there may be a genetic predisposition, as well as environmental factors, that contributes to the development of bronchiectasis.[84] The onset of bronchiectasis is commonly seen in the middle aged or in the elderly, but in the cases of congenital lung disease, the diagnosis may be made in childhood or early adulthood.[85]

There are two key factors that account for the development of bronchiectasis: the presence of intense and chronic inflammation and an inadequate defense mechanism to minimize the effects of infection resulting in tissue damage. These are the foundations for bronchial dilatation, inflammation, and weakening of the bronchial walls, which account for the impairment of the mucociliary escalator. Pooling of secretions creates an environment for bacterial colonization and infection. The increased levels of macrophages contribute to the influx of neutrophils. This increase in neutrophils stimulates phagocytosis; the production of reactive oxygen mediators; the release of proinflammatory mediators such as interleukin-1, interleukin-8, tumor necrosis factor; and the release of protease that causes irreversible loss of the elastin layer and causes the destruction of the smooth muscle and cartilaginous support of airways.[85] There is a dysfunction of natural killer cells and the consequences of this cellular response leads to the increase in oxidative stress that causes further tissue damage. A *vicious circle hypothesis* has been proposed to describe the cycle of infection and chronic immune response, both of which cause lung tissue damage.[88]

The clinical presentation of bronchiectasis is associated with persistent production of large volumes of secretions, frequent hemoptysis, and recurrent infections. Secretions collect within the bronchioles in dependent positions.[85] Crackles, high- and low-pitched rhonchi, and pleural rubs may be heard on auscultation. The patient may also present with fever, fatigue, dyspnea, finger clubbing, and a chronic productive cough with foul-smelling sputum, which may have a bloody tinge to it.[84,85] The remaining part of the physical examination is consistent with the underlying disease process. When the underlying disease is an obstructive process such as emphysema or CF, there will be a barrel chest and an obstructive pattern on the PFT. Bronchiectic changes can be seen on X-ray in the presence of a restrictive disease process but, typically, are not associated with overproduction of sputum.[84]

The diagnosis is primarily made upon clinical history and physical examination. The chest X-ray is relatively nonspecific, but usually illustrates hyperinflation with focal areas of atelectasis. A high-resolution CT scan is the gold standard for diagnosis, which documents dilatation of bronchi with or without bronchial wall thickening.[84]

The principal treatment for bronchiectasis involves the management of the underlying disease, which commonly includes the use of antibiotics, corticosteroids, and bronchodilators. Nutritional support, supplemental oxygen, airway clearance, and rehabilitation are also key components in the management of a patient with bronchiectasis. Surgical resection of the lung tissue that is the source of repeated infections or hemoptysis and lung transplantation may be an effective treatment plan to minimize recurrent exacerbations and further loss of lung function.[85,87]

The prognosis is dependent on the underlying disease and its severity, the quality and responsiveness to medical treatment, and the age of the patient. The majority of patients will succumb to respiratory failure or right-sided heart failure related to pulmonary hypertension.[87,88]

PULMONARY VASCULAR DISEASES

Pulmonary Embolism (*ICD-9-CM* Code: 415.1)

More than 600,000 patients suffer a pulmonary embolism (PE) annually in the United States.[89] *PE* is closely linked to the presence of deep vein thrombus (DVT), blood clots, or a thrombus in the peripheral venous system, and it is the third leading cardiovascular cause of death, accounting for 200,000 deaths annually in the United States and Europe.[90,91] Refer to Table 7-7 for risk factors associated with PE.[92] The prevalence of suffering a PE is 28% and 74% with moderate and strong risk factors, respectively.[90] A medical history that includes PE as a potential risk of another PE may be a fatal event.[93] Typically, embolic events arise from the upper legs and pelvis. Air, fat, and amniotic fluid are also sources of embolisms.[94] Small emboli may have little compromise to a healthy individual but may cause severe respiratory failure in an elderly individual with a reduced reserve of the cardiopulmonary system.[94]

PE accounts for 3% of deaths related to patients who had undergone surgical intervention, and a PE is found in 24% of surgical cases in an autopsy series. In one study of approximately 1,000 autopsies, a PE was reported as the primary cause of death in 26% of the cases; and in another 35%, PE was a primary contributor of death.[95] Untreated PE accounts for 30% of hospital mortality, whereas, if treated, the mortality rate is reduced to 2%.[85,96] Only one-third of patients diagnosed with a venous thromboembolism (VTE), which include a PE or DVT, are symptomatic and, if left untreated, can raise the mortality rate to as high as 25%.[96,97] The formation of a thromboembolus is associated with three pathological features. *Stasis*, which typically occurs with immobility or bed rest, is due to a decrease in muscle contraction, lower cardiac output, and

TABLE 7-7 Risk Factors Associated with Pulmonary Embolism

[a]Previous DVT or PE	[b]Congestive heart failure
[a]Orthopedic surgery on lower extremity (hip fracture, total knee arthroplasty, total hip arthroplasty)	[b]Acute myocardial infarction
[a]Oral contraceptives	[b]Cerebrovascular accident
[a]Major trauma	
[a]Spinal cord injury[a]	Older than 40 years Immobilization or bed rest Obesity Lupus

[a]Strong risk factors.

[b]Moderate risk factors.

Data from Wood M, Spiro S. Pulmonary embolism: clinical features and management. *Hosp Med.* 2000;61(1):46-50, Alexander P, Giangola G. Deep vein thrombosis and pulmonary embolism: diagnosis, prophylaxis, and treatment. *Ann Vasc Surg.* 1999; 13(3):318-327, and Philbrick JT, Shumate R, Siadaty MS, Becker DM. Air travel and venous thromboembolism: a systemic review. *Soc Gen Intern Med.* 2007;22:107-114.

subsequent venodilation. There is usually the presence of *endothelial injury* that activates the inflammatory process, platelet aggregation, and the formation of the thrombus typically in the area of the venous valves. Finally, *hypercoagulability* may be related to the immobility.[95]

It is difficult to initially diagnose a PE in the elderly because the signs and symptoms are often vague and typically mimic the signs and symptoms of other comorbidities.[90] The most pronounced clinical presentation of a PE includes an unexplained rapid onset of dyspnea (87% of all cases) and pleuritic chest pain (52%). Hemoptysis (44%) indicates pulmonary hemorrhage or infarction, cough (20%), leg pain and edema (37%), and syncope (14%). Tachycardia is present in 25% of all cases as well as tachypnea (65%), decreased breath sounds and abnormal lung sounds with rales (55%), and abnormal heart sounds (15%). Pleuritic chest pain, dyspnea, and tachypnea are present in 97% of all diagnosed cases of PE.[89]

During the process of evaluation, it is important to develop a differential diagnostic list as you proceed with testing to begin to formulate a clinical diagnosis. The differential diagnoses may include the following conditions: acute myocardial infarction, asthma, PTX, congestive heart failure, acute pulmonary edema, pleurisy, pericarditis, musculoskeletal trauma to the chest wall, sepsis, tamponade, and aortic dissection.[94]

Upon physical examination, the findings will vary based upon the size of the embolism. There may be a low-grade fever, cyanosis, tachycardia, jugular venous distension, tachypnea, and hypotension. Upon auscultation, there may be a pleural rub and a split of the S_2 heart sound heard over the pulmonic valve. One-third of cases are associated with the presence of a pleural effusion. Ninety percent of all cases are associated with DVT, but what is alarming is that the DVT is only clinically present in 10% of all PE cases.[89] The degree of respiratory compromise is dependent on the size of PE and on the preexisting cardiopulmonary reserves.

The clinical diagnosis is nonspecific, with false-negative physical examination findings in 50% of patients, and 50% confirmed false-positive findings in patients who present with symptoms related to conditions other than DVT.[95] The Homan Test is very nonspecific and lacks sensitivity in the diagnosis of a DVT. Examination of the arterial blood gases usually reveals hypoxia, hypocapnia, and a high alveolar–arterial gradient.[45] An echocardiogram may be suggestive of right heart strain or ischemia, and the ECG may demonstrate a T-wave inversion in one or more precordial leads.[93] Examination of the cardiac biomarkers may reveal an elevation in troponin, which indicated myocardial microinfarctions and release of brain-type natriuretic peptide from the myocytes because of increased workload and stress of the right ventricle.[98]

The usual first step when a PE is suspected is to obtain a $\dot{V}/\dot{Q}$ scan,[85] although the results may be inconclusive. Pulmonary angiography is the definitive study to evaluate the pulmonary artery system and assess the presence of a PE.[93] The helical CT scan has largely replaced the use of $\dot{V}/\dot{Q}$ scan for rapid diagnosis.[90] It is also important to determine the *source* of the PE. A contrast and compression venogram is the definitive study for DVT but is invasive and carries risks.[93] Most recently, *color flow duplex imaging* has become an acceptable and sensitive tool for the detection of DVT.[95]

The key to quality medical care is the identification of patients who are at high risk and the implementation of effective prophylactic treatment. In one multicenter study, it was reported that only 32% of patients at high risk for DVT actually received some form of prophylactic intervention.[95] Prophylaxis includes early mobilization and the use of graduated compression stockings, or compression stockings. Intermittent pneumatic compression stockings are used to provide a peripheral pump to enhance venous return and reduce venous stasis. Many patients are prescribed anticoagulants for the prevention and treatment of DVT formation. An *inferior vena cava filter* is the treatment of choice for patients who have a history of recurrent PEs, proximal DVT, or acute PE and who cannot be administered anticoagulation medications. The use of a filter is suggested for patients who have suffered multiple trauma and cancer.[99] In patients who cannot take anticoagulants, an *inferior vena cava filter* may be placed to decrease the risk of a PE occurring from a lower extremity or pelvic thrombus.

Acute management for a PE includes the use of thrombolytic therapy, which is most effective if used within the first 48 hours, and surgical intervention. Alteplase and recombinant tissue plasminogen activator are most effective and used with 92% response rate. There is a 13% incident of major hemorrhage complications and 1.8% incidence of intracranial or fatal hemorrhage. Pulmonary embolectomy has become an effective intervention for a massive PE, with a 5% to 10% mortality rate with an increase in death rate as the pulmonary vascular resistance increases.[91,98]

The prognosis of patients suffering from PE is dependent on the size of the embolism, its impact on the cardiopulmonary system, primarily acute failure of the right ventricle because of rapid rise in pulmonary vascular resistance, and the promptness of medical care. It is estimated that PE has a 35% mortality rate.[91]

Pulmonary Hypertension (*ICD-9-CM* Code: 417)

The normal mean pressure within the pulmonary arterial system is less than 15 mm Hg. *Pulmonary hypertension* can be defined as a mean pulmonary arterial pressure (PAP) greater than 25 mm Hg at rest and greater than 30 mm Hg during exercise, and pulmonary capillary wedge pressure, which is the pressure to assess the delivery of blood to the left atria and left heart function, is of 15 mm Hg or less. More recently, it has become evident that the definition of pulmonary hypertension should also include an elevation in

TABLE 7-8 Classification for Pulmonary Hypertension[a]

Group I: Pulmonary arterial hypertension (PAH)
  Idiopathic PAH (primary)
  Familial PAH

PAH associated with
  Collagen vascular disease
  Congenital systemic to pulmonary shunts
  Portal hypertension
  HIV infections
  Drugs and toxins
  Other diseases: glycogen storage disease, Gaucher disease, etc.
  PAH associated with significant venous or capillary involvement
  Pulmonary venoocclusive disease
  Pulmonary capillary hemangiomatosis

Group II: Pulmonary venous hypertension
  Left-sided atrial or ventricular heart disease
  Left-sided valvular disease

Group III: Pulmonary hypertension associated with lung diseases and/or hypoxemia
  COPD
  Interstitial lung disease
  Sleep disordered breathing
  Alveolar hypoventilation disorders
  Chronic exposure to high altitudes

Group IV: Pulmonary hypertension due to chronic thrombotic and or embolic disease
  Thromboembolic obstruction of proximal pulmonary arteries
  Thromboembolic obstruction of distal pulmonary arteries
  Nonthrombotic pulmonary embolism (tumor, parasites, foreign material)

Group V: Miscellaneous
  Sarcoidosis
  Histiocytosis X
  Lymphangiomatosis

Compression of pulmonary vessels

[a]Third World Conference on Pulmonary Hypertension.

Data from Simonneau G, Galei N, Rubin LJ, et al. Clinical classification of pulmonary hypertension. *J Am Coll Cardiol.* 2004;43:5S-12S.

pulmonary vascular resistance.[100,101] In the past, pulmonary hypertension was classified as primary, or idiopathic, and secondary, which was associated with a contributing disease or disorder. Recently, there has been a new classification of pulmonary hypertension put forth that clusters the clinical presentation by similarities in pathology, clinical presentation, and therapy options.[102] See Table 7-8 to review the new classification of pulmonary hypertension.[103]

Pulmonary arterial hypertension (PAH) is defined as elevated PAP with normal left atrial and/or ventricular pressure. The pathology stems from abnormal vascular proliferation and remodeling of the small pulmonary arteries and arterioles. These changes lead to progressive elevation in pulmonary vascular resistance and eventually, right-sided heart failure. PAH includes such pathologies as idiopathic and familial, which accounts for approximately 6% of all cases and is associated with a mutation of bone morphogenetic protein receptor II genes.[101,102] This category also includes connective tissue

disorders such as scleroderma, congenital systemic to pulmonary shunts, HIV, thyroid diseases, and portal pulmonary hypertension.

Idiopathic pulmonary hypertension (iPAH), formally referred to as primary pulmonary hypertension, is a rare disease that predominantly affects women in their mid-30s; however, children may also be affected. The annual incidence of iPAH is one to two cases per million. iPAH is associated with systemic increases in the inflammatory process leading to muscle dysfunction and osteoporosis.[104] The diagnosis of iPAH involves the elimination of any known cause for the hypertension and has a survival rate of 2.8 years after diagnosis.[100,105]

Most patients present with nonspecific symptoms and diagnosis may be delayed for an average of 2 to 3 years for iPAH. Delayed diagnoses of pulmonary hypertension may also occur for patients with other causes, but the delay occurs at a low incidence. Shortness of breath is typically the first symptom and is usually attributed to physical deconditioning by the patient as well as by the physician (see Table 7-1). Other symptoms include chest pain from right ventricular ischemia, near syncope or syncope, fatigue, and peripheral edema. These symptoms intensify as the pressure rises and is related to right-sided heart failure. A decrease in quality and volume of voice as well as a weak, ineffective cough is caused by the enlarged pulmonary artery compressing the left recurrent laryngeal nerve.[104,106,107]

PAH also presents from the sequelae of a congenital heart defect, which is referred to as Eisenmenger syndrome.[108] Hypertension related to a congenital heart defect is underestimated by at least 10% and is typically the result of the blood shunted from the left side of the heart to the right, therefore inducing high volume and pressure through the pulmonary system resulting in hypertension.[109] There is a decrease in Eisenmenger syndrome associated with many types of congenital heart defects due to improved detection and medical care; however, there is a rise in Eisenmenger syndrome in children with more complex congenital heart defects because children are surviving longer despite these defects.[105]

Pulmonary hypertension can also be associated with intrinsic lung disease. With intrinsic lung disease there is a disruption of the capillary beds and a destruction of the gas-exchange area of the parenchymal tissue that leads to hypoxia and vasoconstriction, which can cause hypertension.[110]

Despite the underlying cause of pulmonary hypertension, there are three conditions that contribute to the development of hypertension. These include *vasoconstriction, remodeling of the vascular wall,* and the *dysfunction of platelets.* Vasoconstriction is associated with endothelial dysfunction, overproduction of endothelin-1, and a reduction in vasodilatation enzymes such as nitric oxide and prostacyclin. Vascular remodeling is the key factor and involves the presence and proliferation of smooth muscle cells in the small pulmonary arteries of the respiratory acini. There is endothelial cell proliferation that contributes to the remodeling and formation of plexiform lesions that are characteristic of pulmonary hypertension. Platelet dysfunction leads to thrombosis formation and contributes to further increases in vascular resistance and hypertension.[111]

Physical examination typically reveals abnormal heart sounds including S_4, or atrial gallop, and a split S_2 due to the asynchronous closure of the semilunar valves. As the disease progresses, an S_3, or ventricular gallop, can also be heard and is indicative of advanced right-sided heart failure. The point of maximal impulse will be shifted to the left, indicative of right ventricular hypertrophy. The electrocardiogram is consistent with right ventricular hypertrophy and includes changes in the T wave. As the disease progresses, there will be overt signs of right-sided heart failure, jugular vein distension, hepatic congestion, peripheral edema, ascites, and systemic hypotension in most cases.[111]

The gold standard for diagnosing and documenting the severity of pulmonary hypertension is *heart catheterization*. This diagnostic procedure can determine whether there is a congenital or acquired intracardiac shunt or any abnormalities of the valves. It can also rule out myocardial dysfunction through biopsy and can measure pressures within the heart and cardiac output. PFTs may show a mild restrictive pattern in cases of severe hypertension and a decrease in DLCO. Echocardiograms can be used to monitor the progression of the disease and the effectiveness of treatment. Pulmonary angiography is the gold standard for determining the pulmonary arterial anatomy and assists in the diagnosis of thromboembolic disease. $\dot{V}/\dot{Q}$ scans and CT scans are also used to rule out thromboembolic disease. Finally, desaturation during the 6-minute walk test is associated with lower survival rates.[102,111] There is no cure for iPAH or many of the other causes of pulmonary hypertension, but many medical advances have improved quality of life and prolonged survival. These medical interventions may also be applied to the treatment of PAH. The antihypertensive benefits of calcium channel blockers are effective in the early stages of iPAH. Today there are three major pharmacological options. The most common is oral or continuous intravenous prostacyclin, such as Flolan or treprostinil. Prostacyclin is a group of potent vasodilators that, when infused into the pulmonary arterial system, improve hemodynamics. In many cases, there is an immediate reduction in PAP, whereas in others, there may be no or minimal immediate response but with long-term use, there is an improvement in symptoms. The dosage of prostacyclin is limited by complaints of jaw pain and joint pain, particularly in the foot and ankles. Nitric oxide–derived medications, such as sildenafil, are effective vasodilators. Endothelin-antagonist medications, bosentan, sitaxsentan, and phosphodiesterase 5 inhibitors, and sildenafil, inhibit the release of endothelin and improve the effects of brain natriuretic peptide and nitric oxide to reduce pulmonary pressures. The most common positive effects of these drugs include the improvement in exercise tolerance and a decrease in symptoms experienced at rest and with exertion. Supplemental oxygen may be helpful in patients who have hypoxemia either at rest or with activity. The use of anticoagu-

lants and diuretics is common to prevent and minimize further thrombus formation and for the management of heart failure, respectively.[100,112]

Beyond the advances in medical treatment, the options of surgical intervention have also improved significantly. There have been improvements in the surgical correction for multiple congenital defects. Lung transplantation is the most common surgical intervention for iPAH and for many patients with PAH. More recently other surgical procedures including pulmonary thromboendarterectomy for thromboembolic disease and atrial septostomy are being conducted to decrease pulmonary hypertension. In children with congenital heart defects, the success of surgical intervention depends on the age at the time of the surgery, the degree of heart failure, and the reversibility of the endothelial damage.[105,108]

The prognosis for iPAH is very poor despite advances in care with a mean survival time of 2.8 years. The National Institute of Health reports a 1-year survival in 64% of the patients and a 3-year survival in 48% of the patients. The prognosis of the patients with PAH depends on the progression of the underlying disease including the progression of PAH and how responsive the patient is to intervention and management.[104,105]

Pulmonary Edema (*ICD-9-CM* Code: 518.8)

Pulmonary edema is defined as failure of the microvascular endothelium that leads to an abnormal accumulation of fluid in the extravascular components of the lungs.[113,114] Pulmonary edema is the result of a breakdown of the capillary endothelium and the alveolar epithelium barriers that protect the respiratory system.[53] Along with these barriers, the lymphatic system is impaired and is unable to eliminate excess fluid from the pulmonary system.[113,114]

Pulmonary edema can be classified based on the pathological changes that lead to the edema. *Hydrostatic pulmonary edema* is due to an imbalance between the intravascular and extravascular space that allows fluid to move into the interstitial space and eventually into the alveoli. Hydrostatic edema is mostly associated with postoperative fluid overload, near drowning, and PE.[113,115] Pulmonary edema with diffuse alveolar disease (DAD) is associated with acute lung injury (ALI) and acute respiratory distress syndrome (ARDS), and actually involves damage to the endothelial cells.[113-115] Please refer to the section on ARDS for more specific information. Pulmonary edema without DAD is primarily associated with drug-induced reactions that may be related to hypoxia and acidosis. This edema typically occurs with reversible cellular damage with rapid recovery.[113,115] Finally, mixed pulmonary edema is associated with severe head injury. Fifty percent of the patients will experience pulmonary edema that is most likely related to an increase in microvascular pressure that causes arterial hypertension and vasoconstriction.[113,115] Mixed edema is also seen in high-altitude illness with hypoxic-induced vasoconstriction and reperfusion injury after following lung transplantation and pneumonectomy.[116]

There are several factors that may predispose the patient to developing pulmonary edema. The function of the cardiac, renal, and hepatic systems contributes to the homeostasis of the body fluid and blood volume. Body weight, age, vascular tone, and fluid overload related to surgery also contribute to pulmonary edema.[117] Postoperative pulmonary edema has an incidence of 8% and accounts for 12% of the deaths in patients during the postoperative period.[117]

Damage to the endothelial lining is a key factor in the development of pulmonary edema because the endothelial cells regulate permeability, modulate vascular tone and $\dot{V}/\dot{Q}$ matching, and interact with blood-borne cells. Injury to the endothelial cells leads to an excessive inflammatory response with the release in interleukin-8, leading to increased vascular leaking and further endothelial damage. Platelet aggregation and a subsequent clot increase oxidative stress. Finally, the angiotensin-converting enzymes impairment is associated with more severe lung injury and lower survival.[114,118]

The clinical presentation of pulmonary edema does not depend on the underlying cause. The patient could present with acute or subacute onset of dyspnea, tachypnea, restlessness, crackles, and eventual peripheral cyanosis with hypoxemia.[115] When a significant amount of the gas-exchange area is impaired, the patient will succumb to respiratory distress and possibly to respiratory failure, which would require mechanical ventilatory support. The clinical presentation is the primary focus for the diagnosis of pulmonary edema.

It is important to diagnose the underlying cause of the edema because this determines prognosis and helps to identify a treatment. Diuretics will be used to minimize fluid but fluid status needs to be monitored carefully to prevent a decline in cardiac function. Medications are used to support cardiac function and blood pressure and to treat or prevent infection. Corticosteroids are used to minimize the inflammatory response in the care of patients with pulmonary edema.

PLEURAL DISEASES AND DISORDERS

Pneumothorax (*ICD-9-CM* Code: 512)

PTX is defined as the presence of air in the pleural cavity between the parietal and visceral pleura. PTX can be classified as primary, secondary, iatrogenic, traumatic, or tension. Primary PTX typically has a spontaneous occurrence particularly in young, tall, thin men with no underlying lung disease. Secondary PTX is associated with underlying disease, with COPD being the most common.[119-121] In both primary and secondary spontaneous PTX, it appears that blebs and bullae play roles in the pathogenesis. There is an imbalance between protease and antiprotease enzymes and an increase in the number of neutrophils and macrophages that result in the development of bullae. These bullae and blebs can rupture under increased pressure, as with a cough or Valsalva maneuver, causing air to leak into the pleural space.[119]

Iatrogenic PTX is due to a complication from a diagnostic or treatment procedure. The introduction of a central line into the subclavian vein is the most common procedure associated with PTX. *Traumatic* PTX is caused by the entry of air through the chest wall or from a laceration of the lung because of the penetrating wound of a gunshot or from a nonpenetrating wound of a rib fracture. The pleural space can become filled with air or blood (hemothorax) or both.[119,120]

Finally, *tension PTX* may be a potentially life-threatening situation and is associated with many etiologies. In this case, air enters the pleural space, but cannot escape. The increasing pressure will cause a progressive collapse of the lung and will eventually displace the mediastinum to the contralateral side (see Fig. 7-13). This can compromise venous return and subsequently decrease cardiac output.

Signs and symptoms will vary based on the size of the PTX and any other underlying pulmonary dysfunction. If the

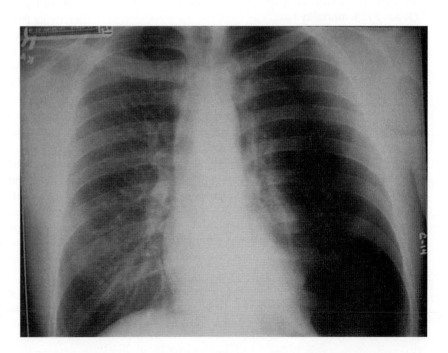

FIGURE 7-13 Left lung tension pneumothorax. When the right and left lung fields are compared, you can appreciate a loss of the lung markings of the left lung, the subtle outline of the compressed lung, and a shift of the mediastinum to the right. (Courtesy of Dana Gryzbicki, MD, University of Pittsburgh, PA.)

PTX is small and there is no underlying pulmonary disease, the patient may be asymptomatic. The most common symptom is acute dyspnea and pleuritic chest pain. The chest pain may be initially described as sharp and later as a steady ache. Symptoms may resolve within 24 hours even though the PTX has not resolved. Patients with underlying pulmonary disease will be symptomatic with even a small loss of lung function. As more lung tissue is involved, the symptoms will escalate. Breath sounds will be absent or diminished, there will be a hyperresonant sound upon mediate percussion, and a decrease in tactile fremitus.

A chest X-ray at peak inspiration and peak expiration is recommended to establish the diagnosis and determine the size of the PTX.[56] Large PTX is defined as a 2 cm or greater distance between the chest wall and rim of the lung. PFTs will demonstrate a decrease in VC and an increase in the alveolar–arterial gradient causing varying degrees of hypoxemia. In severe cases, the patient may become hemodynamically unstable with tachycardia, hypotension, cyanosis, and cardiovascular and/or pulmonary arrest.[119,121]

If the PTX has affected less than 15% of the lung, it can be treated conservatively with an estimated resolution of 1.8% daily. When a patient is symptomatic, it typically means that the PTX is larger than 15% of lung tissue. The lung can be reexpanded with placement of a needle or a chest tube to aspirate the air or blood from the pleural space.[120] A more aggressive treatment approach is *chemical pleurodesis,* the placement of a chemical, talc, or tetracycline into the pleural space to adhere visceral pleura to parietal pleura. The chemical causes an inflammatory response with resultant fibrosis and scarring.[119,120] Finally, through a thoracotomy, the bullae can be resected.[119–121]

The prognosis is related to the size of the PTX, to the presence of an underlying pulmonary disease, and to the extent of the trauma. There is approximately a 32% recurrence rate within the first 2 years after the initial PTX, and, in general, PTX has a 15% mortality rate.[23]

Pleural Effusion (*ICD-9-CM* Code: 518)

Pleural effusion is an excessive collection of fluid between the parietal and visceral pleurae. Pleural effusions can be classified into two types: transudate and exudate. Transudate effusion is generally noninfectious and typically results from mechanical factors influenced by the rate of formation or reabsorption of pleural fluid. Transudate effusions are the results of an increased pulmonary capillary pressure such as in congestive heart failure, a decrease in lymphatic drainage as in thoracic surgery, a decrease in osmotic pressure resultant from renal disease, or an increase in intrapleural pressure from atelectasis. Exudative pleural effusion is generally the result of an infectious process with the most common cause being pneumonia.[122–124]

In children, the most common causes of effusion are parapneumonia; however, 40% to 50% of all pneumonia cases having documented effusions also have a congenital heart disease.[122,124,125] A small number of childhood pleural effusions are associated with malignancy and liver failure.[126]

The development of pleural effusion can be separated into phases. The first phase is the *exudative phase* in which the fluid is free flowing and contains a predominance of neutrophils, elevated proteins, and a normal level of glucose. The effusion may be the result of fluid overload, an alteration in the permeability of the pleura, or an inflammatory process. Parapneumonia, in which the infection involves the visceral pleura, may initiate an outpouring of fluid into the pleural space.[127] The second phase is the *fibrinopurulent stage* with continued influx of inflammatory cells and proteins. The increased permeability of the pleura will permit bacteria to enter the pleural cavity when the effusion is associated with pneumonia and fibrin will begin to deposit over the visceral and parietal pleurae. The final stage is the *organization stage* with the development of an *empyema.* In this stage, the fluid becomes more viscous, the inflammatory process progresses, bacteria multiply, and there is a deposition of fibrin and subsequent formation of *a pleural peel.* This infected pleura, or peel, can cause restriction of ventilation.[125,128]

The most common symptom is dyspnea, cough, and pleuritic chest pain. The severity of the distress depends on the size of the effusion, the rate of fluid collection, and the condition of pulmonary function. Dyspnea is the consequence of the restrictive lung defect from the compression of the effusion, $\dot{V}/\dot{Q}$ mismatch, and the decrease in cardiac output. The cough is dry and nonproductive and is the consequence of inflammation and compression of the bronchial walls. If the cough is productive, the clinician should suspect pneumonia, and if hemoptysis is present, it is more likely related to PE or cancer.[123] If there is pleuritic pain, it is usually an initial symptom and worsens with deep inspiration or in the supine position, but it can suggest an inflammation or infiltration of the parietal pleura or the presence of a PE.[123,124] If the pain is constant, the underlying pathology may be cancer. Pain on palpation of the chest wall may be an indication of an empyema or metastatic cancer.[127] The most common symptoms in children are chest or abdominal pain and vomiting. If children have pneumonia along with effusion, they may also present with cough, fever, and dyspnea.[126]

Results of physical examination are associated with the size of the effusion and may reveal a decrease in chest expansion, dullness on percussion, and diminished breath sounds over the effusion. A zone of bronchial breathing may be heard upon auscultation at the upper border of the effusion.[124] A pleural rub may be appreciated in the early stages of the effusion.[126] If the effusion is large, the fluid can compress the lung and displace the mediastinum to the contralateral side. There can be a decrease in chest wall expansion and mild hypoxemia, which can be corrected with supplemental oxygen.[123,124]

Chest X-ray will be positive for the presence of a fluid collection and distortion of the dome of the diaphragm if at least 300 mL of fluid is in the space. A CT scan or ultrasound is more sensitive for the diagnosis, particularly if there is a small effusion. The effusion can also cause a mismatch between V̇/Q̇ because the fluid is compressing the lung tissue. Needle aspiration of the fluid can also be performed for diagnostic purposes.[124]

If the effusion is small and the patient is asymptomatic, the patient is typically monitored closely. If the patient is symptomatic, the fluid can be drained either by *thoracentesis* or by placement of a pigtail catheter or chest tube. The primary focus for the treatment of pleural effusion, once the symptoms have been alleviated, is to treat the underlying process. The use of fibrinolytic therapy such as urokinase or streptokinase can also be used to decrease the viscosity of the effusion to allow for drainage with the goal to avoid the need for surgical intervention.[125] The prognosis is dependent on the underlying disease.[124]

PULMONARY INFECTION

Empyema (*ICD-9-CM* Code: 510)

Empyema is the presence of pus in the pleural space. The pus is highly viscous with an opaque whitish yellow color and consists of fibrin, cellular debris, and dead and live bacteria.[129] An empyema can develop if a pleural effusion is not treated or is not responsive to treatment, the effusion progresses into the organization phase, and the fluid is contaminated with bacteria.

Approximately 40% of bacterial pneumonias will develop pleural effusion and approximately 15% of these cases will go on to develop empyema. There is an increased risk of empyema for children diagnosed with bacterial pneumonia.[122] Empyema can also be caused by contamination of the pleura during a surgical procedure, with trauma, or with aspiration pneumonia.[124]

If the patient does not quickly respond to the treatment for a pleural effusion, further diagnostic testing should be conducted to evaluate for the presence of an empyema, particularly if this slow recovery is associated with a persistent fever, weight loss, malaise, and an elevation of white blood cells.[124]

The empyema should be drained and antibiotics should be prescribed. If a simple aspiration is unsuccessful, use of fibrinolytic medications can improve the ability to drain infection. An open thoracotomy or open drainage with rib resection for debridement of the empyema and infusion of an antibiotic can also be completed to treat an empyema.[124,125] The mortality rate associated with an empyema can range between 20% and 75%, particularly in the elderly and children and in patients who are severely debilitated.[122,130]

Pneumonia (*ICD-9-CM* Codes: 482.2, 483, 484, 486)

Pneumonia is defined as an acute inflammation of the lungs, which usually occurs when the normal defense mechanisms of the respiratory system fail to keep the lower respiratory tract sterile, causing the small bronchioles and alveoli to become plugged with fibrotic exudate. The cellular response gives rise

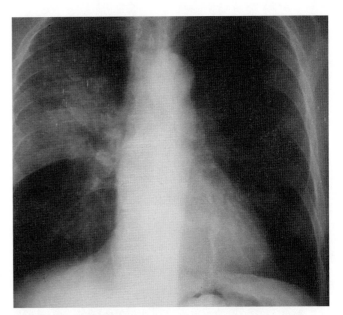

FIGURE 7-14   Right middle lobe (RML) pneumonia. This chest X-ray illustrates the consolidation of the RML with minimal involvement of right upper lobe (RUL), which is consistent with pneumonia. (Courtesy of Dana Gryzbicki, MD, University of Pittsburgh, PA.)

to the appearance of consolidation on chest X-ray. There are many etiologies that underlie the infection including bacterial, viral, and fungal sources (see Figs. 7-14 and 7-15).[23,131]

Various reference points can be used to classify pneumonia for medical intervention and research. One common classification system uses the infectious agent, such as *bacterial, viral, or fungal pneumonia*. The infections can also be classified according to the incidence of the infectious agent for a particular population or region of the country, such as typical versus atypical pneumonia.

Another classification system is based on the environment in which the patient becomes infected with the agent that produces the pneumonia. This system allows health care professionals to identify specific interventions to minimize, prevent, and treat the common characteristics of the environmental setting. *Community-acquired pneumonia* (CAP) is an infection that occurs while the patient is living out in the community or the infection manifests itself within the first 72 hours of a hospitalization. CAP accounts for 1.7 million hospital admissions at the cost of $9 million annually and is the sixth leading cause of death in the United States.[132] The incidence of CAP is 34 out of 1,000 cases for patients older than 75 years with up to 40% requiring hospitalization and 10% requiring admission into an intensive care unit with a 5% to 10% mortality rate.[133] *Hospital-acquired pneumonia* (HAP) is the second leading cause of *nosocomial infections*, only exceeded by urinary tract infections, and is defined as an acute infection that is neither present nor incubated at the time of hospital admission up to 48 hours postadmission. The source of the infection is introduced to the patient within the hospital and accounts for 5 to 10 cases per 1,000 hospital admissions annually. Approximately 25% to 50% of *hospital-acquired*

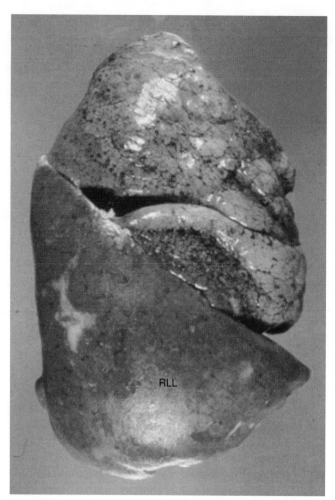

RLL

FIGURE 7-15   Pneumonia. The examination of this lung reveals infiltration and consolidation of the right lower lobe (RLL) with relatively normal lung tissue in the superior lobes. (Courtesy of Dana Gryzbicki, MD, University of Pittsburgh, PA.)

pneumonia is associated with mechanical ventilation (ventilator-associated pneumonia [VAP]).[134,135] More recently a third large category, *nursing home–acquired pneumonia,* has been included in this environmental classification system because of the increasing number of people who are living in nursing care facilities and the higher incidence of pneumonia within this group. Nursing home–acquired pneumonia has an annual incidence rate of 32 cases per 1,000.[136]

Many risk factors have been identified that are associated with the development of pneumonia. These risk factors can be divided into medical and environmental conditions and respiratory function. A medical condition includes such factors as age; the integrity of the immune system; the presence of acute or residual effects of head, neck, or chest trauma; and surgery. The environmental situation takes into account the increased risk of pulmonary infection due to admission into a hospital and particularly into an intensive care unit, placement or use of tracheal or gastric devices, and exposure of other individuals. Finally, respiratory function risk factors include the increased infection rate associated with the use of mechanical ventilation and the need for aerosolized breathing treatments.[132,137]

Risk factors that have been associated with nosocomial infections include surgery and the depressive effects of the anesthesia, smoking within 8 weeks of admission, age, number and severity of comorbidities, recent hospital admissions, wound care or infusion care including hemodialysis, immuno-suppressive medications, and the presence of atelectasis from immobility and aspiration.[136,138] Age is a key factor because the elderly demonstrate a decrease in the function of the mucociliary cells, a decrease in lung compliance with a lower FEV_1 and VC, as well as a decrease in muscle mass and an increase in comorbidities. [138,139]

The most common pathogens found in sputum identified in pneumonia are streptococcus, pneumococcus, *H. influenzae, Pseudomonas aeruginosa, Acinetobacter, Staphylococcus aureus,* and anaerobes obtained from aspiration. Less common sources of infections include legionella, aspergillus and candida fungal infections, CMV, RSV, and protozoan-like *Pneumocystis carinii,* most commonly seen in immunocompromised patients from HIV infections, transplant recipients, and the very ill.[130,140] There has been a rise in the incidence of multiple-resistant *S. aureus* that accounts for up to 50% of VAP with an associated mortality rate reported between 25% and 76%.[141]

The infection actually occurs because an agent, bacterial, viral or fungal, has reached the lower respiratory track where it has multiplied to a point the mucociliary blanket or macrophages cannot cleanse the system. An inflammatory process will be activated along with the immune response, causing localized edema and collateral cellular damage from toxins released by the pathogen, reactive oxidative enzymes, and lysosomal enzymes released by neutrophils and macrophages. The moist, warm environment of the lung is a breeding ground for growth of the pathogen and a vicious cycle between the immune response and the infection. The result is the consolidation of the lung tissue impairing the lungs' ability to perform proper gas exchange. This infection can also spread to other segments of the lungs as well as to the pleural space and pericardium.[142]

When pneumonia in patients with HIV is examined, the infection appears to be related to the CD4 count. If the CD4 count is above 200/μL, the pneumonia is more likely to be caused by more typical agents such as streptococcus pneumococcal, *H. influenzae,* and *S. aureus.* If the CD4 count is less than 200/μL, patients with HIV are more likely to become infected with disseminated mycobacterium TB, fungal, CMV, and pneumocystis pneumonia (PCP).[143,144]

Aspiration has been clearly identified as a common contributing factor to the development of pneumonia. There is an increased risk of aspiration for the patient who has nasal or oral gastric tubes, an endotracheal tube, head and neck trauma, and a depressed mental status.[141] Aspiration is also associated with malnutrition, tube feeding, contracture of cervical extensors, and use of CNS depressant medications.[140] Other events have been linked to aspiration including dysphagia due to loss of dentition and poor hygiene, decreased saliva production, and weakening of muscles of mastication. Aging is associated with a delay in the neural processing to perform the proper swallowing sequence and a decrease in sensation of the oral cavity. Finally, there is an increased incidence of aspiration in the presence of some diseases such as Parkinson disease, cerebral vascular accident, GERD, connective tissue disorders, and Alzheimer disease.[145]

There are three clinical presentations for aspiration. The first syndrome occurs if the aspiration causes *airway obstruction.* If the obstruction is in the large bronchus, it will produce stridor and dysphonia. If the obstruction is more distal, a high-pitched wheeze is likely to be present. Clinically, the patient may present with fever, hemoptysis, and pleuritic chest pain. There will also be a decrease in breath sounds to the obstructed area. The second aspiration syndrome is a *chemical pneumonitis,* which is typically associated with gastric content aspiration but can also be caused by aspiration of bile, medications, and alcohol. These patients will present with dyspnea, high-pitched wheezing, cyanosis, and hypoxemia. If extensive lung tissue is involved, the presentation will include cough, pulmonary congestion, and shock. There may also be crackles upon auscultation along with dyspnea and respiratory distress. The last aspiration syndrome is *pleuropulmonary infection,* which includes acute pneumonitis, necrotizing pneumonia, lung abscess, empyema, and infectious pneumonia. These patients present with fever, productive cough, crackles and/or low-pitched wheezes, and an increase in fremitus and dullness on percussion over the area of consolidation.[133,145]

The typical clinical presentation for pneumonia includes fever and a productive cough with sputum production that is usually yellowish green or rust colored. There is also an elevation in the WBC count and a positive sputum culture identifying the infectious agent in most cases.[135] The patient may report an increased level of fatigue and weight loss. If a substantial amount of lung tissue is involved, the patient may also present with dyspnea, tachycardia and tachypnea, and hypoxemia with desaturation upon exertion. Unfortunately, the elderly present with atypical signs. The health care professional should be monitoring for unexplained changes in mental status and functional impairments including an increase in falls, anorexia, incontinence, low-to-normal WBC count, tachypnea, and tachycardia.[133,140] The health care professional should also be concerned with aspiration pneumonia if the patient presents with drooling, poor oral motor control, poor phonation quality, and choking. The patient may also complain of dry mouth, difficulty in chewing, hoarseness, and throat discomfort.[145]

The diagnosis for pneumonia is made based on a positive X-ray showing infiltration or consolidation of the infected segment for at least 48 hours and at least two clinical signs and symptoms of dyspnea, fever, productive cough, leukocytosis, or leukopenia. The accuracy of diagnosis is dependent upon the analysis of the sputum.[146] The severity of the infection can be graded by the use of the CURB 65 (confusion, urea nitrogen, respiratory rate, blood pressure, 65 years of age and older) scoring system. This is a scale graded from 0 to 5 with a point given for each of the positive response to the categories: confusion, increased respiratory rate, low blood pressure (<90/<60), urea levels greater than 7 mmol/L, and 65 years of age or older. A score of 3 or higher is associated with an increase in mortality.[133]

The primary focus of intervention should first begin with prevention. Annual flu vaccination is an important preventative measure. Facilities should properly clean all respiratory equipment and engage in good hand-washing techniques. If aspiration is a concern, the patient should be positioned in a semirecumbent position and should avoid overfeeding. Good dental hygiene will decrease the colonization of bacteria in the upper airway.

CLINICAL CORRELATE

Early mobilization that encourages an increase in tidal volume and secretion mobilization is critical.[135,140] In patients who cannot be mobilized, the facility should implement chest physical therapy, a bed-positioning schedule, and use of incentive spirometers. Many of these preventive techniques can also be implemented in the home.

Once the diagnosis of pneumonia has been made, treatment should include administration of the proper pharmacological therapy. Typically for bacterial infections, the patient is placed on a wide-spectrum antibiotic. If the signs and symptoms do not resolve or become recurrent, a sputum culture should be done. These results will allow the physician to prescribe a more precise and effective antibiotic. Treatment should also include early mobilization and chest physical therapy as mentioned earlier.[140]

There are several factors that have been identified as prognostic indicators. They include age greater than 65 years, inability to protect the airway, a respiratory rate greater than 30 breaths/min, fever, X-ray showing more than one lobe involvement, and the need for mechanical ventilation. The clinical outcome is also negatively affected by the presence of comorbidities such as COPD, chronic renal failure, diabetes mellitus, chronic heart failure, malnutrition, recent splenectomy, and diminished mental status.[132,147]

Pneumonia is the sixth leading cause of death.[132] CAP mortality is 1% to 2% for mild pneumonia, 5% to 10% for patients who require hospitalization, 30% in the elderly, and 20% to 50% in cases of severe pneumonia. In community dwellers who are ambulatory, the mortality rate is 5% whereas it is 37% for patients in an ICU.[130] In the cases of nursing home–acquired pneumonia, mortality rates are as high as 48% for patients who are dependent in activities of daily living (ADL) and are nonambulatory.[140] Thirty-two percent of all nursing home residents who survive the pneumonia will die within the next 24 months because of associated functional impairments and severity of the comorbidities.[136]

Mycobacterium Tuberculosis (*ICD-9-CM* Code: 486)

According to the World Health Organization, it is estimated that one-third of the world's population is infected with TB and 1.8 million deaths annually are TB related. Globally, there are 8.3 million new cases of TB diagnosed every year. These data support that more individuals are being diagnosed with TB at the same death rate in the past decade.[148] Ninety-five percent of individuals with a new diagnosis and 98% of all deaths are related to TB and HIV coinfection.[149] In the United States, 15 million people are infected with TB. There has been a rise in TB since the early 1980s because of the HIV/AIDS epidemic. *TB is a social disease that disproportionately affects the under-privileged who are malnourished, homeless, substance abusers, and people who live in underdeveloped countries or who are institutionalized in extended care facilities and prisons.*[148,150,151]

Mycobacterium TB is primarily an infection in which the lung is the primary site of incubation (see Figs. 7-16 and 7-17). This mycobacterium is an immobile organism that thrives in warm, well-oxygenated tissues. **The mode of transmission is the inhalation of small, dry droplet nuclei that becomes airborne from the cough or sneeze of an infected person.** To become infected, the person needs to be exposed to an actively infected person for an extended period of time, to a person who is infected with laryngeal TB, or to a person who has extensive pulmonary disease. The particles need to reach the alveoli to replicate. The lung is usually the site of the primary infection. The risk of infection is dependent on the concentration of organism in the air particles, the length of exposure time to the infected person, and the host's immune system.[151]

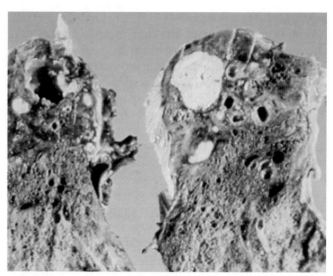

FIGURE 7-17   TB. In the RUL there is a large granuloma. A necrotic cavitation is present in the LUL. (Courtesy of Dana Gryzbicki, MD, University of Pittsburgh, PA.)

The incubation period is 2 to 12 weeks. At approximately 6 to 8 weeks, the TB skin test, purified protein derivative (PPD), will be positive because the count of the organism is high enough to cause an immune response to the invasion. Diagnosis by a sputum smear is difficult owing to the difficulty in obtaining sufficient sample. Diagnosis is made by an increase in interferon gamma, early-secreted antigen, and culture filtrate protein 10 (CFP-10). Diagnosis in children is very difficult with nonspecific signs and symptoms of failure to thrive, persistent fever, and malaise.[148]

The infection can spread via the blood and lymphatic system to other organs such as the kidneys, bones, and brain. The immune system will surmount an attack against the organism and will surround the TB to form a granuloma.[151] Healing will cause fibrosis and calcification of the granulomas. If the patient is immunocompromised, the TB will not be contained within the lungs and can cause a disseminated disease.[149,151]

Reactivation or secondary infection can occur from an encapsulated lesion containing virulent TB. The secondary infection usually occurs at a time when the immune system is in a compromised state due to an illness or to aging. **The site of reactivation is usually the upper lobes of the lungs or an extrapulmonary site.**[151]

During the primary infection, most patients are asymptomatic. If the patient presents with signs and symptoms, they are typically similar to the clinical presentation of pneumonia, such as an unproductive cough and a fever. If the pleura is involved, the patient may also experience dyspnea and pleuritic pain. Crackles may be present in the area of infection along with bronchial breath sounds if there is consolidation. X-ray will be abnormal with fluffy shadows of the upper lobes, atelectasis, enlarged lymph nodes, and cavitations, mainly in the upper lobes. There is also scarring of the lungs with a loss of tissue function.[148]

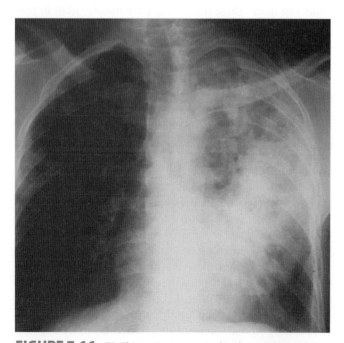

FIGURE 7-16   TB. This patient presented with a primary pulmonary infection of TB. The chest X-ray illustrates unilateral, patchy parenchymal infiltrates with pleural effusion. (Courtesy of Dana Gryzbicki, MD, University of Pittsburgh, PA.)

The secondary infection is associated with a cough, which becomes increasingly productive as the disease progresses, accompanied by night sweats, weight loss, low-grade fever, and sometimes pleuritic pain. There will be subtle inspiratory crackles, a decrease in tactile fremitus, and adventitious breath sounds over areas of pleural thickening and cavitation.[151] The signs and symptoms of extrapulmonary disease are dependent on the tissue infected. Mycobacterium osteomyelitis of the upper thoracic spine is associated with chronic hypercapnic respiratory insufficiency or failure.[152]

The first line of defense is prevention of the transmission of this disease. Universal precautions should be used around anyone who has a cough. One should avoid overcrowded housing as in homeless shelters and prisons. Finally, people should be vaccinated and screened for TB exposure. If the purified protein derivative test is positive, the person should undergo at least 6 months of treatment to minimize the risk of a secondary infection. During the primary infection, respiratory isolation is important to minimize the spread of the disease. Patients are usually given rifampin and isoniazid (INH) for 6 months to suppress the infection followed by another 2 months of pyrazinamide and ethambutol administration. Further medical or surgical intervention will depend on the site and severity of the extrapulmonary infections.[148,151]

The mortality rate in patients who go untreated is as high as 80%, and a median time period to death is 2.5 years. In the HIV population, mortality exceeds 80%.[151] Respiratory failure associated with acute hypoxia may require mechanical ventilation and is associated with a mortality of 70%.[152]

Meconium Aspiration (*ICD-9-CM* Code: 770.1; Practice Pattern 5B, 6G)

Meconium aspiration syndrome (MAS) is one of the primary causes of neonatal respiratory distress that frequently leads to respiratory failure and death.[153] Meconium is the green viscous fluid that consists of fetal gastrointestinal secretions, cellular debris, mucus, blood, and other waste products. This material appears in the 10th to 16th week of gestation. In approximately 12% of deliveries, the meconium is passed in the later weeks of the pregnancy and contaminates the amniotic fluid.[153,154] Over the past decade there has been a significant decrease in the incidence of MAS due to early detection, amniotransfusion, and caesarean deliveries.[155] Approximately one-third of these infants will require mechanical ventilation. It is estimated that 1.5% of all infants will suffer from MAS, and mortality rates vary based on gestational time of MAS with the mortality rate as high as 30% in the second trimester and 22% in the third trimester.[155] The reader may refer to Chapter 21 for a more detailed description of this disease.

RESTRICTIVE PULMONARY DISEASES (PULMONARY FIBROSIS)

This next group of pathologies has more than 200 different diseases. Pulmonary fibrosis has been linked to immune disorders, occupational exposures, genetic and hormonal abnormalities, and a complication of lung injury. These diseases are classified together because they have similar clinical features such as a shallow, rapid breathing pattern due to a loss in the compliance of the lungs and the chest wall. One of the most pronounced features is significant hypoxemia with rapid desaturation on exertion. Many patients develop pulmonary hypertension and cor pulmonale (Table 7-1). The PFTs consistently show decreased levels in FVC and FEV_1 with the FEV_1/FVC within normal limits. There is a significant reduction in VC and TLC and the DLCO is usually quite diminished (Fig. 7-2 and Table 7-2).

Idiopathic Pulmonary Fibrosis (*ICD-9-CM* Code: 518)

Idiopathic pulmonary fibrosis (IPF) is a type of interstitial pulmonary fibrosis, which encompasses a large heterogeneous group of diseases that involves an inflammatory to fibrotic process of the parenchyma. IPF is also referred to as cryptogenic fibrosis alveolitis and includes such pneumonias as nonspecific, desquamative, cryptogenic, and lymphocytic interstitial.[156] The onset of IPF occurs in mid- to late life, and the prevalence is approximately 14 to 15 per 1,000 in the general population. There is a slightly higher incidence in men and there appears to be no racial differences. The cause is unknown, but much work has been done to develop a classification system of IPF that is based on pathological findings and clinical presentation. In general, usual interstitial pneumonia (UIP) is characterized by patchy, nonuniform, and variable destruction of interstitial tissue (see Figs. 7-18 and 7-19) and accounts for 60% of the cases of IPF. There is also a minimal

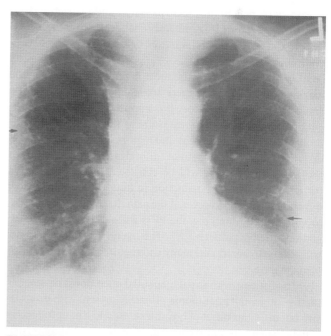

FIGURE 7-18 Interstitial pulmonary fibrosis. Note the relatively small lung volumes with the diffuse infiltrates, mostly apparent in the lower lobes. (Courtesy of Dana Gryzbicki, MD, University of Pittsburgh, PA.)

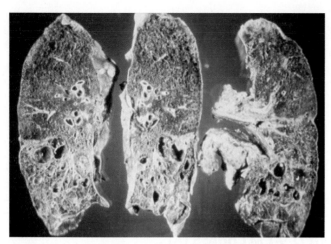

FIGURE 7-19   Interstitial pulmonary fibrosis. The progression of this inflammatory and fibrotic process leads to large cyst formation, which is referred to as *honeycombing*. This destructive process typically predominates in the lower lobes. (Courtesy of Dana Gryzbicki, MD, University of Pittsburgh, PA.)

inflammatory component to this disease with collagen deposition that thickens the alveolar septum.[157] Desquamative interstitial pneumonia (DIP) is another form of IPF that presents with little fibrosis but a significant inflammatory response with an accumulation of alveolar macrophages within the alveolar spaces and interstitium.

The initial injury appears to damage the alveolar and epithelial cells. It has been suggested that the immune response to some unknown stimulant is what starts a cascade of events. There also appears to be an autosomal dominant genetic link for some patients with the prevalence of familial IPF being 5.9 per million.[158] The damage causes inflammatory cells to release cytokines, tumor necrosis factor, and platelet-derived growth factor. These inflammatory chemicals result in smooth muscle and fibroblast proliferation, degradation of the alveoli, and collagen deposition.[159]

Open lung biopsy is the most definitive method for the diagnosis of IPF because there are many diseases that have a similar clinical presentation. It is important to rule out occupational or environmental exposure as the cause for the pulmonary fibrosis. Chest X-ray and high-resonance CT scan will document bilateral interstitial infiltrates typically starting in the upper lobes. PFTs will be consistent with a restrictive pattern that includes a reduction in lung volumes and a low diffusing capacity. However, if the patient has a significant history of cigarette smoking, the PFTs will show both restrictive and obstructive patterns.[160,161] The majority of these patients will also be hypoxic, and many will require high levels of supplemental oxygen.[162]

The patients with usual interstitial pneumonia or desquamative interstitial pneumonia primarily present with progressive but insidious onset of breathlessness and a nonproductive cough. Patients may also complain of systemic symptoms such as low-grade fever, malaise, arthralgias, weight loss, and clubbing of the fingers and toenails.[160,161,163] These patients usually desaturate quickly, even when attempting to complete activi-

ties of daily living. Severe desaturation may also be associated with light-headedness, dizziness, and arrhythmias. Exertion is commonly associated with pleuritic chest pain as the patient struggles to increase tidal volume and the respiratory pattern is shallow and rapid. Along with the interstitial fibrosis, up to 84% of these patients will also develop pulmonary hypertension. The hypertension is multifactorial as it relates to chronic hypoxia leading to vascular remodeling, vascular obstruction and destruction associated with the inflammatory and fibrotic processes, and also heart dysfunction. These patients may present with chest pressure, arrhythmias, dizziness upon exertion, and signs and symptoms of right-sided heart failure.[164]

Treatment is very limited in its effectiveness in stopping the progression of this disease, although there are new drugs currently under clinical trials, such as growth factor β and endothielin-1, which have been shown to interfere with the adverse effects of the immune response.[156] High levels of systemic corticosteroids are commonly used as the first line of intervention. Cyclophosphamide impairs the function of neutrophils that eventually decreases fibroblastic and collagen proliferation. Azathioprine and cyclosporine suppress the production and maturation of T and B cells involved in the immune response.[165] More recently, patients with moderate-to-severe pulmonary hypertension may be administered Flolan or UT15. These medications are very potent vasodilators that may be effective in lowering the level of hypertension and making the patient less symptomatic.

The prognosis is dependent on the rate of progression of the disease. Death is usually the result of respiratory failure or heart failure in the presence of pulmonary hypertension. The mean survival of IPF is 5 to 6 years but will vary based on the aggressiveness and type of IPF, duration of symptoms, presence of pulmonary hypertension, and responsiveness to therapy.[156]

Acute Respiratory Distress Syndrome (*ICD-9-CM* Code: 769)

ARDS has more recently been referred to as ALI to reflect the cellular status. The ALI results in pulmonary infiltrates, severe refractory oxygenation, and fibrin deposition leading to lung stiffness and a subsequent decrease in compliance. It has been suggested that ALI/ARDS is the most severe form of pulmonary edema in which diffuse alveolar involvement contributes to further injury.[118] A diagnosis of ALI/ARDS is made when the ratio of the partial pressure of oxygen (Pa_{O_2}) and the fraction of oxygen inhaled (Fi_{O_2}) (Pa_{O_2}/Fi_{O_2}) is less than 200 mm Hg and when all cardiac sources for pulmonary edema have been ruled out. A low value of 200 mm Hg represents severe lung injury (normal Pa_{O_2}/Fi_{O_2} is 380–486 mm Hg).

The development of ARDS can be the result of direct injury to the lung tissue as with a blunt chest trauma or as a result of an indirect injury that is associated with systemic inflammation and elevations in inflammatory mediators such as in sepsis and mechanical VAP, which can precipitate further lung injury.[118,166] The causes of ALI/ARDS are multiple, but the development of ARDS is associated with damage to the alveolar epithelial cells and the disruption of the pulmonary vascular endothelium.[114,118] Barotrauma, volutrauma, and oxygen toxicity caused by the use of mechanical ventilator to compensate for respiratory dysfunction or failure can also lead to further inflammation and cellular damage.[167]

There are several factors that predispose an individual to ARDS, which can include, but are not limited to, pneumonia, aspiration, lung contusion, fat emboli, near drowning, inhalation injury, sepsis, severe trauma, and blood product transfusion.[168] It has been estimated that the incidence of ARDS is 75 per 100,000. Despite advancements in medicine, the incidence has not really declined in the last 30 years.[168] Forty-two percent of patients diagnosed with ARDS will be associated with a complication of sepsis, whereas orthopedic trauma accounts for 11% of the cases. Twenty-two percent of trauma cases that are complicated with ARDS will involve a lung contusion. Finally, 50% of aspiration cases will progress to ARDS, with 85% of the cases showing signs of ARDS within 72 hours.[169]

ARDS is characterized as a heterogeneous disorder that changes over time. There are three stages in the process of ARDS. The first stage is an *exudate phase,* which is characterized by pulmonary edema, hemorrhage, and hyaline membrane formation. Clinically, there is a rapid onset of respiratory failure that is refractory to supplemental oxygen.[167] Damage to the type I alveolar epithelial cells leads to an increased risk of infection, alveolar remodeling, alveolar edema, and a decrease in antioxidative function. Damage to the type II cells impairs the ability of the epithelium to transport fluid that accumulates and causes additional and persistent edema. The dysfunction of type II cells also causes the reduction of surfactant, which increases airway resistance and pressure to ventilate, and is associated with the increased risk of bacterial infection and colonization.[118] The inflammatory mediators, such as tumor necrosis factor α and interleukin-1 and interleukin-6, lead to an increased vascular permeability and thrombus formation.[114] The second phase involves *cellular proliferation* with the elevation of neutrophils and other inflammatory cells. The influx of neutrophils, whose duration and severity of the level of neutrophils is a predictor of mortality, leads to intrafibrin deposition and pulmonary vascular thrombi.[118] This phase is characterized by DAD, which is associated with cellular necrosis, epithelial hyperplasia, and further inflammation that leads to destruction of the delicate structures of the lung. The third phase is *fibroproliferation,* which is the result of chronic inflammation whereby injured lung tissue is replaced with fibrotic tissue.[168] The inflammatory response leads to a reduction in protein C and antithrombinase, and an increase in plasminogen activator inhibitor and angiotensin II, which leads to vascular remodeling and thrombi.[114,166] If the remodeling and destruction of the pulmonary vascular bed are significant, the patient will also develop pulmonary hypertension and will present clinically with right-sided heart failure.[167,168]

The initial clinical presentation is characterized by acute respiratory failure that typically requires mechanical ventilatory support. Upon examination, diffuse crackles can be observed, along with pink frothy secretions, a sign of alveolar edema. This respiratory failure is associated with difficulty in ventilating the patient and is refractory to supplemental oxygen.[168]

Once the patient has been weaned from the mechanical ventilator, a restrictive breathing pattern is common for the first 12 months. Some patients will have a complete recovery, whereas others will continue to demonstrate a mild-to-moderate restrictive breathing process with a decrease in TLC, VC, and low diffusion capacity. The recovery is associated with the degree of lung injury, inflammatory response, particularly level and duration of increased neutrophil levels, and vascular remodeling.[114] Patients with significant residual deficits will present with DOE, hypoxemia, functional impairments, hypertrophy of accessory respiratory muscles, and a shallow, rapid breathing pattern. The duration on the ventilator and severity of illness are associated with a higher level of pulmonary impairment as well as mild-to-moderate decline in quality of life.[115,168]

The diagnosis of ALI/ARDS is based on the clinical presentation of respiratory failure with severe hypoxia and a decrease in lung compliance. The chest X-ray will illustrate a patchy, diffuse airspace disease. The CT scan is consistent with diffuse damage due to injury and edema, which compresses uninvolved tissue that further impairs the respiratory system.[115,170] In patients with residual pulmonary dysfunction, the PFTs will show a restrictive process with a decline in lung volumes.

There is a delicate art involved in the treatment of patients with pulmonary edema and ALI/ARDS. High ventilation pressures and high oxygen concentration need to be avoided because these factors can actually contribute to further cellular injury. **The common approach to mechanical ventilator support is to use a low tidal volume to minimize barotrauma and a low percentage of oxygen to avoid tissue damage from oxygen toxicity. The ventilator is usually set with a high positive end-expiratory pressure (PEEP) to keep airways open and allow for easier ventilation.**[167] The newer mechanical ventilators have two modes of ventilation, which are beginning to be recognized as valuable components in the treatment of ARDS. BiVent ventilation or airway pressure release ventilation (APRV) is combining high and low positive end-expiratory pressure levels over two separate time intervals with the goal to recruit alveoli and improve gas exchange with a decreased exposure to high airway pressure.[171] The other mode of ventilation is pressure-regulated volume control (PRVC) mode of ventilation in which the ventilator adjusts pressure to deliver a prescribed tidal volume under the lowest pressure.

There are many other treatments used in the management of ARDS. Treatment also includes management of fluid balance to minimize pulmonary edema and still maintain cardiac output. The administration of surfactant replacement therapy is undergoing clinical trials in adults. Nitric oxide gas mixture is used to promote bronchodilation to reduce the positive

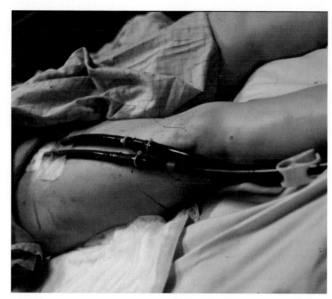

FIGURE 7-20   Extracorporeal membranous oxygenator. This patient is being supported on ECMO because of cardiopulmonary failure. The cannulas are connected to the femoral artery and vein. (Courtesy of Chris L. Wells, University of Pittsburgh, PA.)

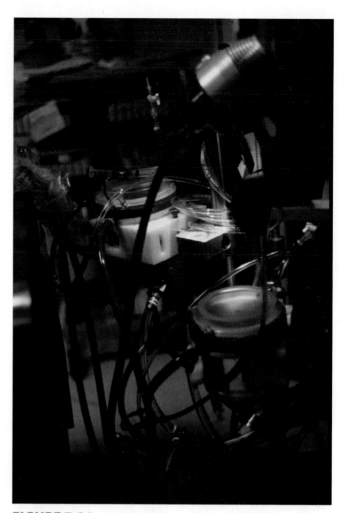

FIGURE 7-21   ECMO. This device is used to oxygenate the blood outside the body (white canisters) and then pump the blood back into the patient's body (pump is in the right upper corner). The patient is in critical condition and cannot be supported by mechanical ventilation alone. (Courtesy of Chris L. Wells, University of Pittsburgh, PA.)

pressure required to ventilate the lungs, thus reducing risk of barotrauma.[166] Antibiotics and systemic corticosteroids are used to minimize infection and inflammation, respectively.[168] In extreme cases an extracorporeal membranous oxygenator (ECMO) may be used to completely support the respiratory system and allow the lungs to rest (see Figs. 7-20 and 7-21). Finally, it is suggested to try positioning the patient in prone. Prone positioning seems to improve oxygenation in approximately 50% of cases. The reason for this improvement is unclear, but it may be related to a reduction in pleural pressure, more uniform ventilation, decreased atelectasis, or reduced abdominal pressure on the thoracic cavity. In addition, lying prone appears to promote postural drainage and promote the redistribution of perfusion.[170]

There is a 40% to 60% mortality rate associated with ARDS.[168] Mortality is highly associated with sepsis, especially when there is a high concentration of neutrophilic activity.[118] These deaths are primarily associated with respiratory failure among the elderly. This fact should support early detection and aggressive medical management of respiratory infections in elderly patients. This is different in the younger patient, whose death is primarily due to multisystem organ failure, including right-sided heart failure due to pulmonary hypertension.[114,169]

Bronchopulmonary Dysplasia (*ICD-9-CM* Code: 769)

Bronchopulmonary dysplasia (BPD) is a chronic, restrictive pulmonary disorder that is a consequence of unresolved or abnormally repaired lung disease. BPD is most prevalent in premature infants who are exposed to high concentrations of supplemental oxygen and positive-pressure mechanical ventilation in order to compensate for immature lungs.[172] The reader may refer to Chapter 21 for a more detailed description of this disease.

Hypersensitivity Pneumonitis (*ICD-9-CM* Codes: 503, 505)

Hypersensitivity pneumonitis (HP), or external allergic alveolitis, is an immunologically mediated disease that is typically associated with sensitivity from repeated exposure or large dosage exposure to an antigen. Further exposure results in an inflammatory response that involves the distal airways and alveoli.[173-175] There are numerous agents that can be the impetus for HP including organic material such as agents from moldy hay or grains; fungi from water reservoirs; and bird serum, feathers, and excreta. HP can also be caused from exposure of mining dust and pharmacological products such as gold, amiodarone, and minocycline.[173,175-177] Acute HP is a nonprogressive and intermittent inflammatory response to the exposure of an antigen. There is spontaneous improvement in the individual's condition once the person is removed from the antigen. The onset of symptoms usually occurs 4 to 8 hours after exposure and there is a resolution of signs and symptoms within a month of onset.[173,175,176] Subacute HP is more common than acute HP and it is caused by intermittent or continuous exposure to the antigen with symptoms presenting within weeks to months after exposure. Chronic HP is from persistent and recurrent exposure to low levels of the antigen, which can be divided into two cases. The first case is where the individual is suffering recurrent acute bouts of acute HP triggered by repeated exposures and the second case involves the individual who has low dosage exposures that progress in an insidious manner without any history of acute symptoms. The presentation and progression of this disease are dependent on the exposure dosage and duration as well as the individual's genetic susceptibility.[173]

Host factors are important for the pathogenesis of this disease process, because many individuals are exposed to the same materials and do not develop HP. It is unclear exactly what are these host factors that allow for the induction of the inflammatory process, but hypersensitivity testing is generally negative for the antigen. In the acute phase, there is infiltration of macrophages, lymphocytes, and neutrophils into the alveolar spaces and small vessel vasculitis. In the subacute stage, the histological changes are consistent with three findings: interstitial inflammatory cell infiltrates, poorly formed non-necrotizing granuloma formation, and cellular bronchiolitis with destruction and intra-alveolar fibrosis.[173] If the disease progresses into the chronic phase, the granulomas will disappear and be replaced by peribronchial fibrosis, smooth muscle hyperplasia, and fibrotic formation predominantly in the respiratory bronchioles.[175]

Four to eight hours after exposure, the individual will present with fever, chills, cough, dyspnea, and inspiratory crackles. In the acute phase there will be an increase in leukocytes and neutrophils in the bronchoalveolar fluid. In severe cases, hypoxemia may also be present and there will be infiltrates seen on the chest X-ray, which can be mistaken for a viral pneumonia.[175,178] A low-level, long-term exposure is characteristic of the exposure history of individuals that progress to the chronic phase. There is extensive fibrosis and a honeycombing pattern on radiologic studies as well as severe hypoxia.[178] Along with the classic symptoms presented in the acute and subacute phases, these individuals also present with malaise, weight loss, and significant fatigue and weakness. Hypoxemia is commonly present from diffuse infiltrates, hilar lymphadenopathy, and pleural effusion as can be seen on a chest X-ray.[89,162,178] There will be a decrease in lung volumes on pulmonary function studies and a low DLCO, which is consistent with a restrictive lung pattern.

Part of the diagnosis of HP is the elimination of other granulomatous diseases such as sarcoidosis, viral pneumonia, aspergillus infection, and other collagen vascular diseases. The ratio of the CD4 (T-helper cells, which assist the B-cell response and interact with macrophages to strengthen the immune system) to the CD8 count (T-suppressor cells which assist in the body's defense) may also assist in the diagnosis, in that elevation of CD8 cells and a decrease in the CD4/CD8 ratio are associated with an increase in cytokines that modulate inflammation and granuloma formation.[175]

An increase in the CD4/CD8 ratio is associated with lymphocytic infiltration.[173,174]

The first line of treatment is the prevention of HP with removal of the antigen when possible or the use of individual protective equipment to minimize exposure to harmful materials. With the presentation of HP, exposure to the antigen should be eliminated. The patient is typically treated with a high dose of corticosteroids followed by a slow taper.

Prognosis is dependent on the responsiveness to corticosteroids in the acute and subacute phases. If the inflammatory process persists, even despite aggressive treatment, the prognosis is poor. The progression of the fibroblastic activity destroys the small airways and alveoli and leads to refractory hypoxemia and progressive respiratory failure.[174] Prognosis is also associated with the presence of pulmonary hypertension with higher mortality rates with up to 80% mortality at 5 years of onset of symptoms.[162]

Occupational Diseases (*ICD-9-CM* Codes: 502, 503)

There is a subset of pulmonary interstitial disorders that result from the inhalation of inorganic dusts (pneumoconioses), organic particles (hypersensitivity pneumoconioses), and industrial gases, fumes, and smoke. These occupational lung diseases are associated with a chronic inflammatory process that leads to scarring and pulmonary fibrosis.[179]

Pneumoconioses involve the permanent deposition of inorganic material (coal, asbestos, silica, beryllium, etc) within the pulmonary system. Pneumoconiosis is also referred to as allergic alveolitis and is considered an immunologically mediated disease.[173] These diseases are typically associated with occupations such as miners, pipe fitters, welders, cutters, stonecutters, and fabric mill and quarry workers.[180,181] This section focuses on asbestos and silica exposure, but the different exposures tend to be clinically similar.

Recently, attention has been focused on reports of pulmonary disease related to work in microwave popcorn production. A cluster of people who work in the butter-flavoring room or the packing room have been diagnosed with fixed OB (fixed meaning unresponsive to bronchodilators). They have a history of inhalation exposure to diacetyl, which is a volatile butter-flavoring chemical. The reader is referred to the section on OB for a more detailed clinical presentation.[56]

Asbestos is a generic term for a group of naturally occurring complex crystalline mineral fibers that are ideal for a variety of construction purposes because of their tensile strength.[181] Small particles from these fibers can deposit in the distal airways depending upon the size of these particles and pressure gradient within the lung.[182] This deposition is associated with a high incidence of pulmonary carcinomas. Mesothelioma is a highly aggressive tumor associated with asbestos exposure. It has a high mortality rate due to the late diagnosis and resistance to treatment.[183] Other fibers have a high concentration of iron and are associated with scarring and pulmonary fibrosis. Finally, the most common fiber type, which is used commercially for building material, is frequently associated with pleural disease.[182,183]

The clinical presentation of asbestosis depends upon the type, length, and concentration of the fibers inhaled and the immunological response. For example, crocidolite asbestos fibers are associated with more fibrogenic changes and mesotheliomas due to greater cytotoxicity, cell proliferation and inflammation, and the production of reactive oxygen molecules.[184–186] In many cases, the pulmonary fibrosis and malignancies are associated with a history of 20-plus years of exposure.[187] The incidence of pleural disease and fibrosis varies, but it is reported that the parenchyma is involved in up to 82% of cases. Isolated fibrosis is diagnosed in approximately 15% cases. Pleural disease is found in 48% and presents as either effusion, fibrotic plaque, or malignant mesothelioma.[187,188]

Silica is a group of naturally occurring minerals with quartz being the most common form used in construction. Silicosis is associated with progressive fibrotic pneumoconiosis and formation of nodules (see Fig. 7-22).[180] Although the environmental control of exposure has improved over the last

two decades, the incidence of lung disease associated with silica is still on the rise. The increase in the documented onset of pneumoconiosis is due to the long latency period between the time of exposure and the actual onset of disease. The latency between exposure and disease can extend for 20 to 40 years, and it has been estimated that the incidence will not peak until 2030. The risk factors involved in the development of pulmonary disease include the duration and intensity of the exposure to the inorganic material and to the size and water solubility of the particles.[189,190]

Regardless of the fine particles that are inhaled, these inorganic particles trigger the accumulation of alveolar macrophages and inflammation that extends into the terminal respiratory bronchioles and adjacent alveolar interstitium. The release and activation of macrophages cause the release of inflammatory mediators such as cytokines, tumor necrosis, tumor growth factor, platelet-derived growth factor, and fibroblasts. This histological response amplifies cellular injury, fibroblastic proliferations, and collagen deposition.[191] Toxic oxygen and nitrogen species are released and further lead to cell mutation and death. Neutrophils and lymphocytes are also released and this immune response can be characterized by the loss of alveolar type I and type II cells, an increase in WBCs, fibroblast proliferation, and collagen accumulation. Damage to type I cells is regarded as an early sign of fibrosis followed by hyperplasia and hypertrophy of type II epithelial cells.[180] Type II alveolar cells, which produce surfactant, play a role in the repair of the injured alveolar epithelium and determine the extent of the lung disease. This cascade of events leads to the alteration of biological function of lipids, damage and mutation of cellular DNA and RNA resulting in cellular dysfunction, fibrosis, and malignant transformation.[182,189]

Pneumoconiosis is associated with radical oxygen and nitrogen species, which are linked to cellular mutation, RNA, and DNA alterations and apoptosis. The damage to the DNA leads to neoplastic transformation and apoptosis. Apoptosis, the disposal of cellular debris, is the major pathway responsible for alveolar type II cell hyperplasia in acute lung. Normally, there exists a balance between apoptosis and cell proliferation. When proliferation exceeds apoptosis, it leads to the triggering of the inflammatory process or malignant cell formation. If the apoptosis rate exceeds proliferation, there is epithelial dysfunction and lung injury. Apoptosis and tumor growth are stimulated by the presence of the reactive oxygen molecules.[182,188]

Pneumoconiosis is classified in two forms: acute and classic. Acute pneumoconiosis is associated with a high concentration exposure leading to severe alveolitis. Neutrophils and eosinophils infiltrate the alveolar spaces and cause small vessel vasculitis.[173] Acute alveolitis clinically presents with progressive respiratory failure, bilateral pulmonary consolidation, and a high incidence of deaths related to respiratory failure or right-sided heart failure.[190] The classic form has a more insidious clinical presentation with pulmonary nodules, collagen deposition, and macrophage infiltrates. The classic form can be divided into simple and complicated subtypes.

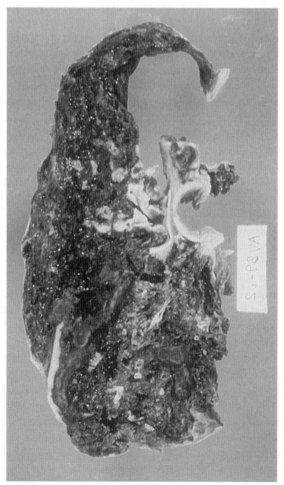

FIGURE 7-22   Silicosis. This disease is associated with deposits of foreign material that causes inflammation, progressive scarring, and destruction of the lung. (Courtesy of Dana Gryzbicki, MD, University of Pittsburgh, PA.)

In the simple form, the radiological findings show multiple nodules with well-defined borders. The nodules are less than 10 mm in diameter. The complicated form is associated with massive fibrosis, nodules are greater than 1 cm in diameter, and have irregular margins and calcifications.[189,190]

Regardless of the various causes of pneumoconioses, the patient presents with a similar clinical picture of a slowly progressive respiratory and functional decline, with exertional dyspnea, a dry nonproductive cough, and cyanosis. The disease can progress regardless of any further exposure. There is usually the presence of expiratory wheezing, bilateral inspiratory crackles in the lower lung fields, and clubbing of the nail beds. In the advanced stages of the disease, the patient may develop cor pulmonale typically due to pulmonary hypertension.[180]

The radiological findings by chest X-ray reveal *a ground-glass appearance*, and as the disease progresses, honeycombing will develop throughout the lungs. With asbestosis, the abnormality is first documented in the lower lung fields, but with silicosis most of the pathology is first seen in the upper lobes and posterior lung fields.[189,190] Plaque formation may occur in the parietal or visceral pleura. **Pleural disease is the hallmark of asbestosis and is used to help differentiate asbestosis from other fibrotic pathologies.**[187] There may also be signs of pleura-based masses that may resemble cancerous tumors.[180,181] Occasionally, there will be calcification of the hilar nodes with silicosis.[191]

In the simple form of pneumoconiosis, typically, lung function is preserved, but in the complicated form, there is a restrictive pattern with a reduction in lung volumes, especially VC and TLC; a decrease in DLCO; and a decrease in pulmonary compliance with a normal FEV_1/FVC ratio. The earliest physiological abnormalities include a reduction in VC, DLCO, and desaturation with exertion. If FEV_1 is <75% of the age- and gender-matched predictive value, it is usually associated with a history of smoking. Occasionally, in the presence of silicosis, there will initially be a normal PFT result that can progress into an obstructive airflow pattern or a milder restrictive pattern.[181,191]

The best defense against pneumoconioses is prevention. The exposure to inorganic dust should be avoided by using a proper respiratory filter device if the exposure risk is high and the ventilation in the work area is poor. Prevention should also include proper protective clothing and employee education. Employees should be encouraged to undergo annual physical check ups that include chest X-rays and spirometry. Once the diagnosis has been made, medical management should include the use of corticosteroids to minimize the inflammatory response. Monitoring the progression of the disease should be done through radiological studies, PFTs, and exercise testing. With the progression of the disease, medical care may include the use of supplemental oxygen and prostacyclin drugs for right-sided heart failure due to pulmonary hypertension; chemotherapy, radiation and surgical resection for cancer; and ventilatory support for respiratory failure. In the presence of isolated pulmonary fibrosis, lung transplantation should be considered on a case-by-case basis.[181,191]

With the insidious onset of the clinical signs and symptoms and the long latency between exposure and pathology, many clients are diagnosed with advanced disease and therefore, prognosis is poor. Twenty percent of the deaths from asbestos exposure are due to pulmonary fibrosis. Deaths related to cancer account for 39% and malignant mesothelioma accounts for 9% of the deaths associated with asbestos exposure. Compared to age-matched smokers, clients with a history of smoking and asbestos exposure have a 4.5-fold increased risk of developing bronchogenic carcinoma.[181]

IMMUNOLOGICAL DISEASES

This is a group of diseases that are suspected to have been mediated by an immune response, which activates an inflammatory process. RA is a systemic disease that is characterized by persistent inflammation of the synovial joints with hyperplasia of the synovium resulting in destruction of the joint.[192] RA can be associated with pleural disease, OB, chronic pulmonary infections, and interstitial pulmonary fibrosis.[23,192,193] The etiology of *systemic lupus erythematosus* (SLE) is unknown, but it has been suggested that there is a genetic, environmental, and hormonal influence that leads to a variety of pulmonary diseases and dysfunctions. Besides the pulmonary diseases mentioned earlier, lupus is also associated with pulmonary hypertension, alveolar hemorrhage, and respiratory muscle weakness.[194,195] Scleroderma; *c*alcinosis, Raynaud phenomenon, *e*sophageal dysfunction, *s*clerodactyly *t*elangiectasia (CREST); and mixed connective tissue disease (MCTD) are three diseases that are associated with dysfunction of collagen tissue throughout the body.[196–198] Pulmonary involvement typically presents with pulmonary fibrosis and/or hypertension.[23,196] Finally, Sjögren syndrome is a chronic autoimmune inflammatory disease that is usually associated with another immune disease like RA.[199] This disease is characterized by dryness of the airways with mucus retention and pulmonary fibrosis.[200]

This group of diseases has similar pulmonary manifestations based on the presenting pulmonary disease. Many patients will present with a chronic cough that worsens with exertion, dyspnea, Raynaud syndrome, pulmonary crackles, fever, and signs of right-sided heart failure.[192,193] PFTs typically document a restrictive breathing pattern with low DLCO, hypoxia, and cyanosis.[192,194,201,202]

Treatment and prognosis are also dependent on the clinical signs and symptoms, aggressiveness of the disease, and the specific underlying immunological disease. Functional impairment and dysfunction are primarily linked to hypoxia due to fibrosis, right-sided heart failure from pulmonary hypertension, and pulmonary infections with mortality rates exceeding 50%, 2 years after presentation of pulmonary involvement.[145,194,201,203] Please refer to Chapter 13 for more specific details about these diseases, their clinical presentation, and management.

Drug Toxicity (*ICD-9-CM* Code: 518.82)

Many of the medications that are prescribed to treat systemic autoimmune diseases and oncological disorders can lead to pulmonary toxicity. The most common pulmonary complications include bronchospasm, OB, interstitial pneumonitis, pulmonary edema, and lupus.[111]

Pulmonary interstitial pneumonitis and fibrosis are associated with methotrexate, gold, and NSAIDS.[204] The patient usually presents with DOE and a nonproductive cough. The symptoms may have an acute onset with a clinical presentation that is similar to HP. However, symptoms may also have a gradual presentation like pulmonary fibrosis.[23] Acute reaction is associated with fever and cough. The clinician may also observe tachypnea and cyanosis. The chronic reaction is associated with inspiratory crackles, hypoxemia, and infiltrates can be seen on X-ray. PFTs illustrate a restrictive pattern in the chronic process with a decline in FVC, IRC, and TLC.[204]

Pulmonary edema is associated with the overuse of salicylates, narcotics, and chemotherapeutic agents. This edema is noncardiac in origin and patients usually present with chest tightness, coughing, wheezing, dyspnea, and respiratory depression and distress. The symptoms may present 24 to 48 hours after drug administration.[204]

A patient can present with pulmonary hemorrhage if the patient is taking anticoagulants or has been given thrombolytic therapy. Hemorrhage may also be a complication of cocaine abuse. The patient may present with crackles, dyspnea, a bloody productive cough, and respiratory distress.[23]

The presence of bronchospasm is common in the presence of NSAIDS, salicylates, and β-blocker administration. It is theorized that the drug causes an imbalance between bronchodilation and bronchoconstriction by inhibiting the production of prostaglandin, which is a potent bronchodilator. The patient may present clinically with wheezing, dyspnea, and a cough.[23,204]

With the use of gold and penicillamine for RA, the patient can potentially develop OB, which is characterized by the inflammation of the small airways. If the drug is not discontinued, OB will progress to destruction of the bronchioles and an obstructive breathing pattern with dyspnea at rest and on exertion, and hyperinflation of the lungs will be seen.[23,204]

SLE may be induced from the side effects of penicillamine, gold, procainamide, and phenylbutazone. The most common clinical feature is pleural effusion.[23,204] The degree of symptoms and signs will depend on size of the effusion. With a small effusion, the patient may be asymptomatic, whereas a large effusion may cause dyspnea, tachypnea, oxygen desaturation, and pain on inspiration.

The primary treatment in any of these pulmonary complications, first and foremost, is to monitor the patient for signs and symptoms of the above diseases, once the drug has been administered, and to educate the patient on self-examination for signs and symptoms. It is important to take a thorough history including examining the patient's medications when the patient presents with pulmonary symptoms with no history of disease. Once the signs and symptoms have been evaluated and a diagnosis of drug-induced pulmonary dysfunction has been made, the medications should be discontinued. Further medication intervention should be provided to support the respiratory system and to treat the clinical presentation. This intervention may include bronchodilators, corticosteroids, and supplemental oxygen.

PULMONARY ONCOLOGY (*ICD-9-CM* CODE: 239.9)

Lung cancer is the leading cause of cancer-related deaths in the United States, only surpassed by cardiac disease.[205] The rate of diagnosis and mortality has not declined over the past decade despite advances in diagnostic procedures and treatment. In 2007, 213,380 new cases of lung cancer were diagnosed and accounted for 160,390 deaths.[206]

Lung cancer has also been linked to occupational exposures of asbestos, arsenic, beryllium, cadmium, radon, and silica, just to name a few; but 80% to 90% of all lung cancer cases can be attributed to smoking.[207,208] A genetic propensity has been identified in 71% of the cases of patients diagnosed with lung cancer before the age of 50 years. This is compounded by a history of smoking. In patients who are older than 70 years, smoking alone has been linked to 72% of these cancer cases.[209] There has been a decline in lung cancer in men, which is associated with a decline in smoking, but smoking is on the rise in women, particularly young women, with lung cancer diagnosis also on the rise.[210] Smoking accounts for more cases of cancer in men, with a higher incidence in black men, but the rise in cancer in women is associated not only with the increase in smoking behavior, but also with a family history, a genetic link, of lung cancer that is a dominant factor in incidence and deaths.[209]

Smoking behavior is an important information to obtain during the interview process. It is vital to determine the number of cigarettes smoked per day, years of smoking, frequency of breaths per cigarette, and the depth of inhalation. All these factors contribute to risk of developing lung cancer.[211]

There have been several risk factors linked to lung caner. Passive or secondhand smoke exposure needs to be investigated during the interview because **patients who do not smoke themselves, but have a spouse who smokes, have a 20% higher death rate from lung cancer than those who live with nonsmokers.**[207] Approximately 12,200 people die annually from lung cancer that is not linked directly to a personal history of smoking. Of those cases, as many as 8,400 deaths are attributed to passive exposure to tobacco smoke.[212] Besides tobacco smoke, radiation exposure to the chest, asbestos, radon, chromium, arsenic, air, and air pollutants have also been identified as risk factors.[213,214]

There are several components in tobacco that are carcinogenic, such as polyaromatic hydrocarbons, and *N*-nitroso compounds from the nicotine and nicotine-like tobacco compounds. There are reactive metabolites from the smoke that

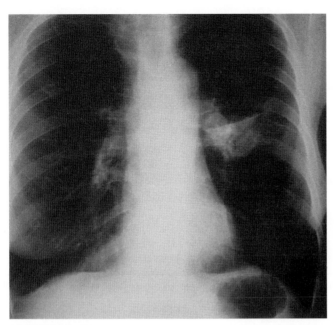

FIGURE 7-23 Lung cancer. On this chest X-ray, notice the irregular, mass located in the left upper lobe (LUL) that has been diagnosed as an adenocarcinoma. (Courtesy of Dana Gryzbicki, MD, University of Pittsburgh, PA.)

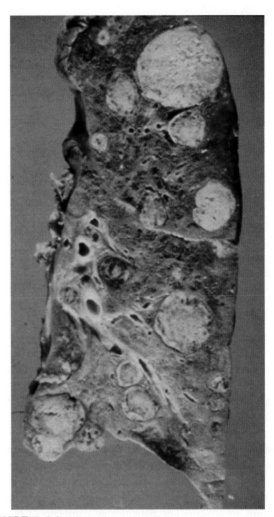

FIGURE 7-24 Metastatic cancer. This gross specimen clearly illustrated multiple tumor formation throughout this lung. (Courtesy of Dana Gryzbicki, MD, University of Pittsburgh, PA.)

bind to the DNA and damage the cell's genetic composition. As the cell repairs itself, the mutation is incorporated into the DNA sequence. If this process occurs in cells that naturally undergo mitosis frequently, like the epithelium of the bronchi, the mutation is replicated rapidly.[209] The carcinogenetic process is a complex series of events driven by the accumulation of DNA changes. These DNA changes or mutations occur in three stages: initiation, promotion, and progression. The initiation is the phase where there is an actual genetic change due to exposure causing injury. This is followed by the promotion phase in which there may be further mutations and reproduction of the changes. Finally, the progression of the mutations determines the aggressiveness of the tumor growth and determines the characteristics of malignancy.[209]

Lung carcinomas are divided into *small-cell* and *non–small-cell* cancers (see Figs. 7-23 and 7-24). Small-cell carcinoma is diagnosed if the tumor cells are smaller than the diameter of the mature lymphocytes.[215] Small-cell lung cancer accounts for 15% of all new diagnoses and 25% of lung cancer deaths annually.[210] Ninety-five percent of small-cell lung cancer cases are linked to smoking, and 70% of patients with small-cell cancers are metastatic at the time of diagnosis and are generally considered inoperable.[216] There are two distinct types of small-cell lung cancer: small-cell carcinoma or oat-cells cancer and combined small cell. Staging is classified as *limited*, which means tumors are involving one lung, tissue between lung and nearby lymph nodes; *extensive* disease where the cancer has spread outside the lungs; *recurrent* disease of the thorax or metastatic lesions to the bone and 15% will have lesions within the brain. Frequently, small-cell carcinomas are classified as limited or extensive.[214]

Non–small-cell lung cancer is the leading cause of cancer deaths worldwide. These carcinomas include squamous cell, adenocarcinoma, and large cell cancer. Non–small-cell cancer comprises approximately 80% to 85% of the newly diagnosed cases with primary lung cancer annually.[217] The high death rate is due to advanced stage of non–small-cell cancer when the diagnosis is made. Approximately 40% of patients with newly diagnosed non–small-cell cancer have a local, advanced, and inoperable cancer.[218,219] Non–small-cell lung cancer encompasses squamous cell, large cell, or adrenocarcinoma, which is the most common of non–small-cell lung cancer.[214]

Non–small-cell cancers are staged based on the tumor node malignancy (TNM) system (see Tables 7-9 and 7-10).[220,221] T indicates site and size of tumor, N is related to lymph node involvement, and M indicates the presence or absence of malignancy.[222] Staging is the evaluation of the tumor for classification, which is used for prognosis, and medical or surgical intervention. This method to stage the cancer is still evolving particularly with the use of computer tomography and other pathological procedures.[223]

TABLE 7-9   TNM Classification for Cancer

Tis	Carcinoma in situ
T1	Tumor is ≤ 3 cm, surrounded by parenchyma or visceral pleura and no evidence of invasion
T2	Tumor is > 3 cm, involves the main bronchus, invades visceral pleura, or presents with atelectasis or pneumonia
T3	Tumor of any size that has invaded chest wall, diaphragm, mediastinal pleura, pericardium, or main bronchus, but <2 cm distal to carina. Without involvement of carina, no atelectasis or obstructive pneumonitis of the entire lung
T4	Tumor of any size that directly invades structures of mediastinum. There is also malignant pleural or pericardial effusion
N0	No regional lymph node metastasis
N1	Metastasis to ipsilateral peribronchial and/or hilar and intrapulmonary nodes
N2	Metastasis to ipsilateral mediastinal and/or subcarinal nodes
N3	Metastasis to contralateral mediastinal and/or hilar involvement of scalene or supraclavicular nodes
M0	No distant metastasis
M1	Distant metastasis present

Modified from National Cancer Institute. U.S. National Institutes of Health. http://www.cancer.gov and Mountain C. Revisions in the international system for staging lung cancer. *Chest*. 1997;111:1710-1717.

Approximately 5% of patients with lung cancer are asymptomatic at the time of diagnosis with the finding occurring during some medical screening for another medical procedure. The majority of patients will present with symptoms related to the primary impairment of lung function or symptoms related to dysfunction of distant sites due to metastases. **The most common symptoms related to pulmonary involvement include dyspnea, persistent nonproductive cough, and hemoptysis. Some patients will complain of a dull aching chest pain.**[210,214] If the lesion obstructs a main airway, then the patient may present with dyspnea, postobstructive atelectasis, pneumonia, wheezing, or stridor. The patient may complain of pleuritic chest pain if there is involvement of the chest wall or pleura. The patient may present with signs or symptoms that are related to tissue dysfunction from metastasis such as headaches or seizures with CNS metastasis or jaundice with liver metastatic cancer. Finally, the performance of a thorough interview may reveal unexplained weight loss, night sweats, a decrease in activity, fatigue, anorexia, and pain that cannot be attributed to musculoskeletal or neuromuscular dysfunction.[210,214]

An important part of the diagnostic process is determination of the tumor type. There are certain characteristics that are associated with benign and malignant tumor cells. The presence of fat or a calcification pattern on CT scan and stability of tumor growth over a 2-year period are characteristics of a benign tumor. The border of a benign tumor is typically smooth and well-defined. Benign tumors are also more likely to occur in patients who are younger than 35 years with no smoking history and no occupational exposure to carcinogenic substances.[220] Common indicators of malignancy include spiculated or non–smooth edges of the tumor. There is an absence of a calcification pattern and the tumor typically doubles in size within 400 days. The rate of tumor growth is a poorer prognostic indicator than the size of the tumor at the time of diagnosis.[224] Tumors that are greater than 3 cm have a greater tendency of being malignant. Finally, the patients diagnosed with a malignant tumor usually have a history of smoking or occupational exposure and are around 65 years of age.[220]

There are various tests to assist in the diagnosis and staging of lung cancer. A chest X-ray is not sensitive enough to detect small nodules until they are greater than 1 cm in diameter.[220] CT or MRI can be used to detect calcification and fat composition of the tumor that may be used for the diagnosis of malignant versus benign tumor.[208] Bronchoscopy is the procedure of choice to obtain a biopsy when the lesion is centrally located.[220] Transthoracic needle biopsy through the chest wall, or needle biopsy, can be obtained via bronchoscopy, or video-assisted thoracotomy, which is the most effective procedure for evaluation of peripheral parenchymal lung tissue.[208,220] The thoracic surgeon may also choose to perform endoscopic ultrasonography with fine-needle aspiration to obtain enough tissue for both diagnosis and staging.[220] If a pleural effusion is present, a thoracentesis can be performed to examine the cellular makeup of a pleural effusion, which is also helpful for diagnostic purposes.[220]

TABLE 7-10   Revised Stage Grouping

0	TisN0M0
I-a	T1N0M0
I-b	T2N0M0
II-a	T1N1M0
II-b	T2N1M0, T3N0M0
III-a	T1–3N2M0, T3N1M0
III-b	T4N0–2M0, T1–4N3M0
IV	Any T, any N, M1

Modified from National Cancer Institute. U.S. National Institutes of Health. http://www.cancer.gov and Mountain C. Revisions in the international system for staging lung cancer. *Chest*. 1997;111:1710-1717.

Lung cancer can be primary, with the lung as the initial site of the carcinoma, or secondary, meaning the cancer has spread or metastasized from another site other than the lungs. *Metastasis* requires a complex series of events to occur including cell growth, vascularization of the tumor, and transportation of the cancerous cells to other systems. The malignant cells must adhere to a distant site and there must be a presence of various cytokines and other tumor and host factors to promote the survival and growth of these new cells in distant sites.[225]

The most common sites of metastasis from the lungs are the brain (10%), bone (7%), liver (5%), and adrenal gland (3%).[216,222] Metastasis from malignant lung cancer to the brain can present with signs and symptoms of headaches, hemiplegia, seizures, and behavioral changes. Metastasis to the skeletal system can present with complaints of dull, deep pain, muscle weakness, and pathological fractures. If the cancer invades the spinal cord, the patient may become paraplegic and have bowel and bladder dysfunction.[220,225]

Metastatic cancer to the lungs is typically from the primary sites: colorectum, breast, kidney, thyroid, or skin. The patients are usually asymptomatic until the advanced stages. If the cancer is adrenocarcinoma, non–small-cell cancer, with lymphatic involvement leading to breast, stomach, colon, prostate, or pancreas cancers, the patient usually presents with progressive dyspnea.[225]

The options for treatment have expanded significantly in the past decade and aggressive research continues to develop new interventions. Treatment decisions are dependent on the patient's goals, staging of the tumor and extent of the disease, adverse effects of the treatment, respiratory function, operative risk, and the size of tumor growth.[217,225,226]

Surgical intervention is dependent on many factors including preoperative and predicted postoperative pulmonary function. Postoperative pulmonary function (PPO) can be quantified by assuming that each segment of the lung contributes to 5.2% of total lung function. Prior to surgical intervention, the surgeon must determine the effects of the resection on pulmonary function. Each segment can result in approximately a 5% decline in preoperative FEV_1. Postoperative pulmonary complications can be expected if there is a preoperative decrease in FVC and FEV_1, presence of hypercapnia, and a low $\dot{V}O_2$ capacity. If the FEV_1 is less than 80% of the predicted value, a postoperative predicted value for FEV_1 multiplied by the DLCO should be calculated. If this calculation is less than 30%, the patient would be considered a nonoperative candidate.[227] Also, the patient would be nonoperative if an exercise test revealed a $\dot{V}O_2$ of less than 10 mL/kg/min. Surgery is the treatment of choice for non–small-cell cancer stages 0 through IIIA. Surgical intervention is commonly offered in conjunction with chemotherapy and/or radiation.[214] The preoperative assessment is more complex when the patient has an underlying airway obstructive disease like emphysema. In cases where the patient has emphysema, the surgical resection may actually improve pulmonary function because the resection may decompress viable tissue to assist in ventilation and diffusion.[218]

Besides surgical intervention, the other leading treatment intervention includes the use of *chemotherapy* or *radiation therapy (XRT)* for the surgical and the nonsurgical candidates. Small-cell lung cancer has traditionally been treated with a combination of at least three chemotherapy drugs. The most common agents include cyclophosphamide, vincristine, cisplatin, etoposide, doxorubicin, methotrexate, and lomustine. Etoposide plus cisplatin in conjunction with XRT has shown to be an effective intervention for the limited stage of small-cell cancer.[210] Seventy percent to ninety percent of the patients with small-cell cancer will initially respond to chemotherapy but more suffer recurrence and death within 2 years.[210] The median survival for limited and extensive small-cell cancer is 14 to 16 months and 6 to 8 months, respectively, after intervention.[23,216]

Intervention for non–small-cell lung cancer depends upon the stage of the disease. Besides the surgical intervention, XRT is recommended in most cases. There are multiple clinical chemotherapy trials that are being studied in non–small-cell cancers of various stages. With the advances in treatment, there has been an increase in survival rates with a mean survival of 36 months and the 5-year survival of 29% for stage III cancer.[226] Platinum-based chemotherapy followed by docetaxel appears to be the chemotherapy of choice but docetaxel is associated with high incidence of central nervous system or pulmonary toxicity.[226] Carboplatin and paclitaxel along with traditional radiation have been effective in the management of locally advanced tumors.[228] The combination of cisplatin and radiation improves survival by improving the local control of tumor growth.[219]

Survival depends on the staging of the tumor at the time of diagnosis. It is generally viewed that stages I and II tumors are surgically resectable and carry a higher survival rate than stages III and IV tumors, which are not resectable. If the tumor involves the mediastinal nodes, the 5-year survival rate is only 10%, whereas it is 50% with nonmediastinal involvement in stage I or II.[218] Appropriately there is a 25% 5-year survival rate for stage III lung cancers.[210,214,226] The mortality rate is higher in smokers and increases as the number of cigarettes smoked per day increases. There is also a higher mortality rate in male over female smokers.[207]

MECHANICAL PULMONARY DISORDERS (*ICD-9-CM* CODE: 518.83)

This group of extrapulmonary disorders can impair the pulmonary system since these disorders can lead to hypoxemia and pulmonary hypertension. They can also lead to a restrictive breathing pattern that may eventually lead to functional impairments and ultimately, high levels of morbidity and mortality.

Obstructive Sleep Apnea Syndrome

Obstructive sleep apnea syndrome (OSAS) is defined as recurrent episodes of apnea or the temporary cessation of ventilation during sleep. The obstruction is commonly due to occlusion of the upper airway. Obstructive sleep apnea is commonly associated with obesity, nasal obstruction, facial bony abnormalities such as retrognathia or micrognathia, hypertrophy of the uvula, and enlargement of the adenoids/tonsils. This syndrome affects approximately 4% of adults and 9% of children but is on the rise due to the elevating incidence in obesity in both groups in the United States.[228,229] There is also an increased risk of developing OSAS in patients with a history of smoking.[23,230]

The hallmark signs of OSAS are *snoring* and *daytime somnolence*. Sleep apnea is associated with fragmented sleep, repeated arousal, intermittent hypoxemia, hypercapnia, and nocturnal hypertension. Apneic periods occurring more than 30 times/min is classified as severe sleep apnea and is associated with desaturation and a decrease in FEV_1/VC ratio and a forced expiratory flow at 25% and 75% of vital capacity FEF of 25% to 75%.[230] A long-term consequence of sleep apnea includes daytime or chronic pulmonary hypertension in 42% of OSAS cases, which contributes to the increase in cardiovascular and cerebral morbidity.[228,231]

In children, sleep apnea is associated with sinus disease, which may be related to elevated airway resistance due to an inflamed upper airway. This may be caused by the higher incidence of bronchial hyperreactivity in children. Sleep apnea may also trigger nocturnal asthmatic exacerbations. Obesity in children increases the risk of sleep apnea threefold.[124]

Pregnancy

Pregnancy is associated with several temporary cardiopulmonary changes that support the fetal development. There is a 50% increase in cardiac output and oxygen consumption to support the increased work of breathing by the end of the gestational period. There is a drop in pulmonary vascular resistance, which is likely due to dilation and expansion of the pulmonary arterioles and capillaries.[232]

As the fetus grows, there are chest wall changes that occur early and progress throughout the pregnancy. There is an increase in the transverse diameter and in the circumference of the mother's chest. Although the thorax expands, there is a decrease in chest wall compliance, which accounts for the increased work of breathing. The level of the diaphragm raises approximately 4 cm and diaphragm excursion increases. The elevated level of progesterone, which acts as a respiratory stimulant, leads to hyperventilation and chronic respiratory alkalosis.[232]

Clinically, dyspnea is the most common respiratory complaint during pregnancy. Approximately 50% of pregnant women complain about dyspnea at 20 weeks of gestation. By 31 weeks, this complaint rate increases to 75%. Women also commonly report fatigue and lower extremity edema. Upon auscultation, there is a decrease in breath sounds in the lower lung fields that is consistent with bibasilar atelectasis. Lung volumes are also altered during the pregnancy. Tidal volume increases as much as 40%, which accounts for the increased

minute ventilation. VC remains unchanged, but inspiratory capacity increases slightly, which is consistent with the increase in diaphragmatic excursion. Expiratory reserve volume decreases by a mean of 15%, RV decreases by 20%, and functional reserve capacity decreases by 20% at the end of gestation. Finally, FEV_1 remains stable. When the relationship between $\dot{V}/\dot{Q}$ is examined there is a mismatch that can be three times higher than the 2% to 5% found in nonpregnant women. This mismatch is associated with an alteration in the distribution of ventilation.[232]

Obesity (*ICD-9-CM* Code: 278.0; Practice Pattern 6A)

Obesity has reached epidemic proportions in adults and children in the United States. Obesity is associated with several comorbidities including cardiovascular disease and diabetes. Severe obesity can also lead to pulmonary impairments, as it is associated with obstructive sleep apnea, obesity hypoventilation, atelectasis, and respiratory failure.[233]

In cases of mild-to-moderate obesity, it is uncommon to see deficits in VC and TLC, but severe or morbid obesity is likely to have decreased lung volumes. There is an inverse relationship between VC and torso circumference. It has been suggested that the distribution of fat is an important factor is determining pulmonary impairment. A decrease in FEV_1 and TLC is associated with the weight distribution, primarily in the upper body. There is a decrease in chest wall compliance and diaphragmatic excursion. With substantial weight loss there is a normalization of lung volumes.[234]

Obesity hypoventilation syndrome (OHS) may develop in the most markedly obese individuals. This syndrome is associated with chronic hypercapnia. There are several factors that may contribute to the development of hypoventilation, including a decrease in chest wall compliance and an increase in work of breathing. It also appears that these individuals have a blunted respiratory drive with a diminished sensitivity to carbon dioxide. It has been suggested that OSAS may contribute to the development of obesity hypoventilation syndrome. The clinician should be alerted if the patient reports fragmented sleep and morning headaches that resolve when awakening.[235]

Diaphragmatic Hernia (*ICD-9-CM* Code: 553.3)

Congenital diaphragmatic hernia (CDH) may occur through a defect in various areas of the diaphragm. The congenital defect allows herniation of abdominal contents into the thoracic cavity. The most common sites for hernia ion are posterolateral, anterior, and adjacent to the esophagus. The posterolateral defect or herniation through the foramen of Bochdalek is the most common form of CDH. CDH is associated with a high mortality because approximately 40% of the infants with CDH also have other congenital or acquired defects that may be fatal. It also has a high morbidity, associated with the development of BPD, neurological deficits, and GERD. CDH occurs in approximately one infant per 2,000 births with 80% of the hernias involving the left diaphragm. The lungs of these infants are typically underdeveloped, which may be caused by the disruption of lung development during a critical growth period.[236]

Clinical presentation ranges from being asymptomatic to signs of pulmonary dysfunction due to entrapment of bowel in the thoracic cavity. In the newborn, the most common signs and symptoms are associated with respiratory insufficiency or failure occurring within minutes to hours after birth. Within the first 24 hours the infant's respiratory function may deteriorate with the development of pulmonary hypertension, which can lead to a shunting of blood through the foramen ovale causing cyanosis. Upon examination, there will be absent breath sounds on the affected side. Chest X-ray may reveal the displacement of bowel or other visceral organs into the thoracic cavity.[236]

Medical management initially focuses on achieving hemodynamic stability. This is typically accomplished with high-frequency oscillation or intratracheal mechanical ventilation. The use of surfactant and liquid ventilation shows some promise in managing these patients during the acute critical phase. In critical cases, an extracorporeal membrane oxygenator may be utilized to rest the lungs. These invasive interventions are associated with some serious complications including intracranial bleeding and sepsis. Surgical repair of the diaphragm is warranted ideally when the infant is medically stable, which is usually after the first 24 hours.[236]

SUMMARY

This chapter has described most of the pulmonary disease processes that the physical therapist may encounter. After the physical therapist completes the examination, he or she should classify the patient into the most appropriate practice pattern. The selection of the practice pattern will be based on the documented findings of impairments, functional limitations, and disability. **It is important that the physical therapist remembers that not every impairment leads to a limitation, but there are impairments underlying every functional limitation.** This is also true for disabilities; there may be impairments or limitations, but these deficits do not necessarily lead to the perception of a disability by the patient. A patient may be classified into more than one practice pattern based on the severity of the pathology, or the patient may require reclassification into another practice pattern based on the progression of the disease or disorder or the effects of intervention. The process of selecting a practice pattern must be based on a priority system, which is the integration of the evaluation findings and the patient's goals for rehabilitation. For most of the patients with a primary lung disease, the focus of treatment will center on the pulmonary impairment. Under these conditions, the physical therapist will use the cardiopulmonary Practice Patterns A, C, G, and H, which address impairments in ventilation, respiration, and a decline in aerobic capacity with or without airway clearance dysfunction. In the presence of respiratory failure, Pattern I or J may be the most appropriate selection. In some patients, the focus of physical therapy may be to address musculoskeletal problems, such as muscle weakness, osteoporosis, and arthralgias. If the primary physical therapy focus is nonpulmonary, the therapist may best select a musculoskeletal practice pattern that is included in A, B, C, or H.[237] The goal of utilizing the *Guide to Physical Therapist Practice* is to complete a thorough evaluation, identify the disabilities and functional limitations, and select the most appropriate practice pattern based on the findings.

REFERENCES

1. Grossman R. Guidelines for the treatment of acute exacerbations of chronic bronchitis. *Chest.* 1997;112(suppl 6):310S-313S.
2. Celli BR, MacNee W. Standards for the diagnosis and treatment of patients with COPD: a summary of the ATS/ERS position paper. *Eur Respir J.* 2004;23:932-946.
3. Banning M. Chronic obstructive pulmonary disease: clinical signs and infections. *Br J Nurs.* 2006;15(16):874-880.
4. Vedantam R, Crawford A. The role of preoperative pulmonary function tests in patients with adolescent idiopathic scoliosis undergoing posterior spinal fusion. *Spine.* 1997;22(23): 2731-2734.
5. Clark C, Cochrane L. Physical activity and asthma. *Curr Opin Pulm Med.* 1999;5:68-75.
6. Hartert T, Peebles RS. Epidemiology of asthma: the year in review. *Curr Opin Pulm Med.* 2000;6:4-9.
7. Weiss S. Environmental risk factors in childhood asthma. *Clin Exp Allergy.* 1998;28(suppl 5):29-34.
8. Wu F, Takaro TK. Childhood asthma and environmental interventions. *Environ Health Prospect.* 2007;115:971-975.
9. Warner SM, Knight DA. Airway modeling and remodeling in the pathogenesis or asthma. *Curr Opin Allergy Clin Immunol.* 2008;8(1):44-48.
10. Eggleston PA. The environment and asthma in US inner cities. *Chest.* 2007;132(suppl 5):782S-788S.
11. Sears M. Evolution of asthma through childhood. *Clin Exp Allergy.* 1998;28(suppl 5):82-89.
12. Cullinan P, Newman Taylor A. Aetiology of occupational asthma. *Clin Exp Allergy.* 1997;27(suppl 1):41-46.
13. Townshend J, Hails S, McKean M. Diagnosis of asthma in children. *Br Med J.* 2007;335(7612):198-202.
14. Holt PG, Sly PD. Prevention of allergic respiratory disease in infants: current aspects and future perspectives. *Curr Opin Allergy Clin Immunol.* 2007;7(6):547-555.
15. Story RE. Asthma and obesity in children. *Curr Opin Pediatr.* 2007;19(6):680-684.
16. Dow L. Asthma in older people. *Clin Exp Allergy.* 1998;28 (suppl 5):195-202.
17. Walters EH, Soltani A, Reid DW, Ward C. Vascular remodeling in asthma. *Curr Opin Allergy Clin Immunol.* 2008;8(1):39-43.
18. Grimfeld A, Just J. Clinical characteristics of childhood asthma. *Clin Exp Allergy.* 1998;28(suppl 5):67-70.
19. Kim H, Tsai P, Oh C. The genetics of asthma. *Curr Opin Pulm Med.* 1998;4:46-48.
20. Hanania NA. Targeting airway inflammation in asthma: current and future therapies. *Chest.* 2008;133(4):989-998.
21. Cypcar D, Lemanske R. Asthma and exercise. *Chest.* 1994;15 (2):351-365.

22. Beck K. Control of airway function during and after exercise in asthmatics. *Med Sci Sports Exerc.* 1999;31(suppl 1):S4-S11.

23. Fishman A. *Pulmonary Diseases and Disorders: Companion Handbook.* 2nd ed. New York: McGraw-Hill; 1994.

24. Ali J, Summer W, Levitzky M. *Pulmonary Pathophysiology.* New York: McGraw-Hill; 1999.

25. Kemp J. Comprehensive asthma management: guidelines for clinicians. *J Asthma.* 1998;35(8):601-620.

26. Reddy RC. Severe asthma: approach and management. *Postgrad Med J.* 2008;84(989):115-120.

27. Gelb AF, Zamel N, Kristnan A. Physiological similarities and differences between asthma and chronic obstructive pulmonary disease. *Curr Opin Pulm Med.* 2008;14(1):24-30.

28. Gurney J. Pathophysiology of obstructive airways disease. *Radiol Clin North Am.* 1998;36(1):15-27.

29. Rennard SI. Chronic obstructive pulmonary disease: linking outcomes and pathology of disease modification. *Proc Am Thorac Soc.* 2006;3:276-280.

30. MacNee W. Pathogenesis of chronic obstructive of pulmonary disease. *Proc Am Thorac Soc.* 2005;2:258-266.

31. O'Byrne P, Postma D. The many faces of airway inflammation. *Am J Resp Crit Care Med.* 1999;159:S41-S66.

32. Hensen PM, Vandivier W, Douglas IS. Cell death, remodeling and repair in chronic obstructive pulmonary disease? *Proc Am Thorac Soc.* 2006;3:713-717.

33. Churg A, Coslo M, Wright JL. Mechanism of cigarette smoke induced COPD: an insight from animal model. *Am J Physiol Lung Cell Mol Physiol.* 2008;294:L612-L631.

34. Cosio M, Guerassimov A. Chronic obstructive pulmonary disease: inflammation of small airways and lung parenchyma. *Am J Resp Crit Care Med.* 1999;160(5, pt 2):S21-S25.

35. Poole D, Sexton W, Farkas G, et al. Diaphragm structure and function in health and disease. *Med Sci Sports Exerc.* 1997;29(6):738-754.

36. Martinez F. Diagnosing chronic obstructive pulmonary disease. *Postgrad Med.* 1998;103(4):112-125.

37. Agusti A. Effects of chronic obstructive pulmonary disease: what we know and what we don't know (but should). *Proc Am Thorac Soc.* 2007;4:522-525.

38. Martinez F. Diagnosing chronic obstructive pulmonary disease: the importance of differentiating asthma, emphysema, and chronic bronchitis. *Postgrad Med.* 1998;103(4):112-117, 121-122, 125.

39. Dasgupta A, Maurer J. Late stage emphysema: when medical therapy fails. *Cleve Clin J Med.* 1999;65(7):415-424.

40. Bennditt JO. Surgical options for patients with COPD: sorting out the choices. *Respir Care.* 2006;51(2):173-182.

41. Sandhaus RA. α-1 Antitrypsin deficiency. 6: new and emerging treatments for α-1 antitrypsin deficiency. *Thorax.* 2004;59:904-909.

42. Richmond RJ, Zellner KM. α-1 Antitrypsin deficiency. *Dimens Crit Care Nurs.* 2005;24(6):255-260.

43. Schwaiblmair M, Vogelmeier C. Alpha 1 antitrypsin: hope on the horizon for emphysema suffers? *Drugs Aging.* 1998;12(6):429-437.

44. Hogarth DK, Rachelefsky G. Screening and familial testing of patients for α-1 antitrypsin deficiency. *Chest.* 2008;133:981-988.

45. Stoller J. Clinical features and natural history of severe alpha 1 antitrypsin deficiency. *Chest.* 1997;111:123S-128S.

46. Luisetti M. Seersholm N. α-1 Antitrypsin deficiency. 1: epidemiology of α-1 antitrypsin deficiency. *Thorax.* 2004;59:164-169.

47. Mahadeva R, Lomas D. Genetics and respiratory disease. 2: alpha 1 antitrypsin deficiency, cirrhosis and emphysema. *Thorax.* 1998;53(6):501-505.

48. Boucher RC. Relationship of airway epithelial ion transport to chronic bronchitis. *Proc Am Thorac Soc.* 2004;1:66-70.

49. Heath J, Mongia R. Chronic bronchitis: primary care management. *Am Fam Physician.* 1998;57(10):2365-2372, 2376-2378.

50. Guddo F, Vignola AM, Saetta M, et al. Upregulation of basic fibroblast growth factor in smokers with chronic bronchitis. *Eur Respir J.* 2006;27:L957-L963.

51. Kim JS, Okamoto K, Rubin BK. Pulmonary function is negatively correlated with sputum inflammatory markers and cough clearability in subjects with cystic fibrosis but not those with chronic bronchitis. *Chest.* 2006;129:1148-1154.

52. Hayes D, Meyer KC. Acute exacerbations of chronic bronchitis in elderly patients: pathogenesis, diagnosis and management. *Drugs Aging.* 2007;24(7):555-572.

53. Saetta M. Airway inflammation in chronic obstructive pulmonary disease. *Am J Respir Crit Care Med.* 1999;160(5, pt 2):S17-S20.

54. Wilson R, Wilson C. Defining subsets of patients with chronic bronchitis. *Chest.* 1997;112(suppl 6):303S-309S.

55. Jones K, Robbins R. Alternative therapies for chronic bronchitis. *Am J Med Sci.* 1999;318(2):96-98.

56. Kanwal R. Bronchiolitis obliterans in workers exposed to flavoring chemicals. *Curr Opin Pulm Med.* 2008;14:141-146.

57. Moonnumakal SP, Fan LL. Bronchiolitis obliterans in children. *Curr Opin Pediatr.* 2008;20:272-278.

58. Kreiss K. Flavoring-related bronchiolitis obliterans. *Curr Opin Allergy Clin Immunol.* 2007;7:162-167.

59. Colby T. Bronchiolitis: pathologic considerations. *Am J Clin Pathol.* 1997;109:101-109.

60. Cordier JF. Challenges in pulmonary fibrosis: bronchiolocentric fibrosis. *Thorax.* 2007;62:638-649.

61. Chan A, Allen R. Bronchiolitis obliterans: an update. *Curr Opin Pulm Med.* 2004;10:133-141.

62. Boehler A, Kesten S, Weder W, et al. Bronchiolitis obliterans after lung transplantation. *Chest.* 1998;114(5):1412-1421.

63. Kelly K, Hertz M. Obliterative bronchitis. *Clin Chest Med.* 1997;18(2):319-333.

64. Johnson S. Lymphangioleiomyomatosis: clinical features, management and basic mechanisms. *Thorax.* 1999;54(3):254-264.

65. Niku S, Stark P, Levin DL, Friedman PJ. Lymphangioleiomyomatosis: clinical, pathologic, and radiologic manifestations. *J Thorac Imaging.* 2005;20:98-102.

66. Sullivan E. Lymphangioleiomyomatosis: a review. *Chest.* 1998;114(6):1689-1703.

67. McCormack FX. Lymphangioleiomyomatosis: a clinical update. *Chest.* 2008;133:507-516.

68. Alalawi R, Whelan T, Bajwa RS, Hodges TN. Lung transplantation and interstitial lung disease. *Curr Opin Pulm Med.* 2005;11:461-466.

69. Rosenstein B. What is a cystic fibrosis diagnosis? *Clin Chest Med.* 1998;19(3):423-441.

70. Dinwiddie R. Pathogenesis of lung disease in cystic fibrosis. *Respiration.* 2000;67:3-8.

71. Rowe SM, Clancy JP. Advances in cystic fibrosis therapies. *Curr Opin Pulm Med.* 2006;18:604-613.

72. Elizur A, Cannon CL, Ferkol TW. Airway inflammation in cystic fibrosis. *Chest.* 2008;133:489-495.

73. Boyle MP. Update on maintaining bone health in cystic fibrosis. *Curr Opin Pediatr Med.* 2006;12:453-458.

74. Kalnins D, Durie PR, Pencharz P. Nutritional management of cystic fibrosis patients. *Curr Opin Clin Nutr Metab Care.* 2007;10: 348-354.

75. Parasa R, Maffulli N. Musculoskeletal involvement in cystic fibrosis. *Bull Hosp Joint Dis.* 1999;58(1):37-43.

76. Prasad S, Main E. Finding evidence to support airway clearance techniques in cystic fibrosis. *Disabil Rehabil.* 1998;20(6/7):235-246.

77. Ferkol T, Rosenfeld M, Milla CE. Cystic fibrosis pulmonary exacerbations. *J Pediatr.* 2006;148:259-264.

78. Rubin B. Emerging therapies for cystic fibrosis lung disease. *Chest.* 1999;115:1120-1126.

79. Ratjen F. New pulmonary therapies for cystic fibrosis. *Curr Opin Pediatr.* 2007;13:541-546.

80. Langenderfer B. Alternatives to percussion and postural drainage. *J Cardiopulm Rehabil.* 1998;18:283-289.

81. Rosenstein B, Cutting G. The diagnosis of cystic fibrosis: a consensus statement. *J Pediatr.* 1998;132(4):589-595.

82. Stenbit A, Flume PA. Pulmonary complications in adult patients with cystic fibrosis. *Am J Med Sci.* 2008;355(1):55-59.

83. Ilowite J, Spiegler P, Chawla S. Bronchiectasis: new findings in the pathogenesis and treatment of this disease. *Curr Opin Infect Dis.* 2008;21:163-167.

84. Hansell D. Bronchiectasis. *Radiol Clin North Am.* 1998;36(1): 107-125.

85. Mysliwiee V, Pina J. Bronchiectasis: the "other" obstructive lung disease. *Postgrad Med.* 1999;106(1):123-131.

86. Spencer DA. From hemp seed and porcupine quill to HRCT: advances in the diagnosis and epidemiology of bronchiectasis. *Arch Dis Child.* 2005;90:712-714.

87. Chang AB, Bilton D. Exacerbation in cystic fibrosis: 4. Non-cystic fibrosis bronchiectasis. *Thorax.* 2008;63:269-276.

88. Fushillo S, De Felice A, Balzano G. Mucosal inflammation in idiopathic brnochiectasis: cellular and molecular mechanisms. *Eur Respir J.* 2008;31:396-406.

89. Porcel JM, Light RW. Pleural effusions due to pulmonary embolism. *Curr Opin Pulm Med.* 2008;14:337-342.

90. Bounameaux H, Perrier A. Diagnosis of pulmonary embolism: in transition. *Curr Opin Hematol.* 2006;13:344-350.

91. Konstantinides SV. Acute pulmonary embolism revisited. *Heart.* 2008;94:795-802.

92. Philbrick JT, Shumate R, Siadaty MS, Becker DM. Air travel and venous thromboembolism: a systemic review. *Soc Gen Intern Med.* 2007;22:107-114.

93. Tia N, Atwal A, Hamilton G. Modern management of pulmonary embolism. *Br J Surg.* 1999;86:853-868.

94. Wood M, Spiro S. Pulmonary embolism: clinical features and management. *Hosp Med.* 2000;61(1):46-50.

95. Alexander P, Giangola G. Deep vein thrombosis and pulmonary embolism: diagnosis, prophylaxis, and treatment. *Ann Vasc Surg.* 1999;13(3):318-327.

96. Segal JB, Streiff MB, Hoffman LV, Thornton K, Bass EB. Management of venous thromboembolism: a systemic review for a practice guideline. *Ann Intern Med.* 2007;146:211-222.

97. McRae SJ, Ginsberg JS. Update in the diagnosis of deep vein thrombosis and pulmonary embolism. *Curr Opin Anaesthesiol.* 2006;19:44-51.

98. Perrot M, Granton J. Pulmonary hypertension after pulmonary embolism: an underrecognized condition. *Can Med Assoc J.* 2006;174:1706-1707.

99. Young T, Tang H, Aukes J, Hughes R. Vena caval filters for the prevention of pulmonary embolism. *Cochrane Database Syst Rev.* 2007;4:1-18.

100. Archer SL, Michelakis ED. An evidence based approach to the management of pulmonary arterial hypertension. *Curr Opin Cardiol.* 2006;21:385-392.

101. Fox DJ, Khattar RS. Pulmonary arterial hypertension: classification, diagnosis, and contemporary management. *Postgrad Med J.* 2006;82:717-722.

102. Highland KB. Pulmonary arterial hypertension. *Am J Med Sci.* 2008;335(1):40-45.

103. Simonneau G, Galei N, Rubin LJ, et al. Clinical classification of pulmonary hypertension. *J Am Coll Cardiol.* 2004;43:5S-12S.

104. Desai SA, Channick RN. Exercise in patients with pulmonary arterial hypertension. *J Cardiopulm Rehabil Prev.* 2008;28:12-16.

105. Diller GP, Gatzoulis MA. Pulmonary vascular disease in adults with congenital heart disease. *Circulation.* 2007;115:1039-1050.

106. Rubin L. Current concepts: primary pulmonary hypertension. *New Engl J Med.* 1997;336(2):111-117.

107. Gaine S, Rubin L. Primary pulmonary hypertension. *Lancet.* 1998;353(9129):719-725.

108. Barst R. Recent advances in the treatment of pediatric pulmonary artery hypertension. *Pediatr Clin North Am.* 1999;46(2):331-345.

109. Auger W, Channick R, Kerr K, et al. Evaluation of patients with suspected chronic thromboembolic pulmonary hypertension. *Semin Thorac Cardiovasc Surg.* 1999;11(2):179-190.

110. Rabinovitch M. Pulmonary hypertension: pathophysiology as a basis for clinical decision making. *J Heart Lung Transplant.* 1999;18(11):1041-1053.

111. Minai OA, Budev MM. Diagnostic strategies for suspected pulmonary arterial hypertension: a primer for the internist. *Cleve Clin J Med.* 2007;74(10):736-747.

112. Traiger GL. Pulmonary arterial hypertension. *Crit Care Nurs Q.* 2007;30(1):20-41.

113. Gluecker T, Capasso P, Schnyder P, et al. Clinical and radiologic features of pulmonary edema. *Radiographics.* 1999;19:1507-1531.

114. Maniatis NA, Orfanos SE. The endothelium in acute lung injury/acute respiratory distress syndrome. *Curr Opin Crit Care.* 2008;14:22-30.

115. Ketai L, Godwin D. A new view of pulmonary edema and acute respiratory distress syndrome. *J Thorac Imaging.* 1998;13: 147-171.

116. Clarke C. Acute mountain sickness: medical problems associated with acute and subacute exposure to hypobaric hypoxia. *Postgrad Med J.* 2006;82:748-753.

117. Zwischenberger J, Alpand S, Bidani A. Early complication: respiratory failure. *Chest Surg Clin North Am.* 1999;9(3):543-559.

118. Gropper MA, Wiener-Kronish J. The epithelium in acute lung injury/acute respiratory distress syndrome. *Curr Opin Crit Care.* 2008;14:11-15.

119. Sahn S, Heffner J. Spontaneous pneumothorax. *New Engl J Med.* 2000;342(12):868-875.

120. Schramel F, Postmus P, Vanderschueren R. Current aspects of spontaneous pneumothorax. *Eur Resp J.* 1997;10:1372-1379.

121. Currie GP, Alluri R, Christie GL, Legge JS. Pneumothorax: an update. *Postgrad Med J.* 2007; 83:461-465.

122. Beers SL, Abramo TJ. Pleural effusions. *Pediatr Emerg Care.* 2007;23(5):330-339.

123. Rolston D, Diaz-Guzman E, Budev MM. Accuracy of the physical examination in evaluating pleural effusion. *Cleve Clin J Med.* 2008;75(4):297-304.

124. Parfrey H, Chilvers E. Pleural disease: diagnosis and management. *Practitioner.* 1999;243:412-423.

125. Cameron RJ, Davies HRHR. Intra-pleural fibrinolytic therapy versus conservation management in the treatment of adult parapneumonic effusions and empyema. *Cochrane Database Syst Rev.* 2008;2:1-48.

126. Givan D, Eigen H. Common pleural effusions in children. *Clin Chest Med.* 1998;19(2):363-371.

127. Colice G, Rubins J. Practical management of pleural effusions: when and how should fluid accumulations be drained? *Postgrad Med.* 1999;105(7):67-78.

128. Anthony V, Mohammed K. Pathophysiology of pleural space infections. *Semin Respir Infect.* 1999;14(1):9-17.

129. Strange C, Sahn S. The definitions and epidemiology of pleural space infection. *Semin Respir Infect.* 1999;14(1):3-8.

130. Heffner J. Infection of the pleural space. *Clin Chest Med.* 1999; 20(3):607-618.

131. Scott JAG, Brooks A, Peiris JSM, Holtzman D, Mullholland EK. Pneumonia research to reduce childhood mortality in the developing world. *J Clin Invest.* 2008;118(4):1291-1301.

132. Talwar A, Lee H, Fein A. Community acquired pneumonia: what is relevant and what is not? *Curr Opin Pulm Med.* 2007; 13:177-185.

133. Hoarse Z, Lim S. Pneumonia: update on diagnosis and management. *Br Med J.* 2006;323:1077-1080.

134. McNabb B, Isakow W. Probiotics for the prevention of nosocomial pneumonia: current evidence and opinions. *Curr Opin Pulm Med.* 2008;14:168-175.

135. Kharana P, Litaker D. The dilemma of nosocomial pneumonia: what primary care physicians should know. *Cleve Clin J Med.* 2000;67(1):25-41.

136. Ewing S. Community-acquired pneumonia: definition, epidemiology, and outcome. *Semin Respir Infect.* 1999;14(2): 94-102.

137. Croce M. Postoperative pneumonia. *Am Surg.* 2000;66:133-138.

138. Jackson WL, Shorr AF. Update in ventilator associated pneumonia. *Curr Opin Anaesthesiol.* 2006;19:117-121.

139. Feldman C. Pneumonia in the elderly. *Clin Chest Med.* 1999;3: 563-574.

140. Medina-Walpole A, Katz P. Nursing home-acquired pneumonia. *J Am Geriatr Soc.* 1999;47:1005-1015.

141. Bratzler DW, Nsa W, Houck PM. Performance measures for pneumonia: are they valuable, and are process measures adequate? *Curr Opin Infect Dis.* 2007;20:182-189.

142. Tsai KS, Grayson MH. Pulmonary defense mechanisms against pneumonia and sepsis. *Curr Opin Pulm Med.* 2008;14:260-265.

143. Barry S, Lipman M, Johnson M, et al. Respiratory infections in immunocompromised patients. *Curr Opin Pulm Med.* 1999;5: 168-173.

144. Wallace J. HIV and the lung. *Curr Opin Pulm Med.* 1998;4: 135-141.

145. Lee-Chiong T. Pulmonary aspiration. *Compr Ther.* 1997;23(6): 371-377.

146. Soto GJ. Diagnostic strategies for nosocomial pneumonia. *Curr Opin Pulm Med.* 2007;13:186-191.

147. Boersma W. Assessment of severity of community-acquired pneumonia. *Semin Respir Infect.* 1999;14(2):103-114.

148. Campbell IA, Bah-Sow O. Pulmonary tuberculosis: diagnosis and treatment. *Br Med J.* 2006;332:1194-1197.

149. Furin JJ, Johnson JL. Recent advances in the diagnosis and management of tuberculosis. *Curr Opin Pulm Med.* 2005;11:189-194.

150. Hirsch C, Johnson J, Ellner J. Pulmonary tuberculosis. *Curr Opin Pulm Med.* 1999;5:143-150.

151. ATS, CDC, IDS. Diagnostic standards and classification of tuberculosis in adults and children. *Am J Respir Crit Care Med.* 2000;161:1376-1395.

152. Shneerson JM. Respiratory failure in tuberculosis; a modern perspective. *Clin Med J Royal Coll Physicians.* 2004;4(1):72-76.

153. Srinivasan H, Vidyasagar D. Meconium aspiration syndrome: current concepts and management. *Compr Ther.* 1999;25(2): 82-89.

154. Klingner M, Kruse J. Meconium aspiration syndrome: pathophysiology and prevention. *J Am Board Fam Pract.* 1999;12: 450-466.

155. Ahanya SN, Lakshmanan J, Morgan BLG, Ross MG. Meconium passage in utero: mechanisms, consequences, and management. *Obstet Gynecol Surv.* 2004;60(1):45-57.

156. Afshar K, Sharma OP. Interstitial lung disease: trials and tribulations. *Curr Opin Pulm Med.* 2008;14:427-433.

157. Dempsey OJ, Kerr KM, Gomersall L, et al. Interstitial pulmonary fibrosis: an update. *Q J Med.* 2006;99:643-654.

158. Allam JS, Limper AH. Idiopathic pulmonary fibrosis: is it a familiar disease? *Curr Opin Pulm Med.* 2006;12:312-317.

159. Patel NM, Lederer DJ, Borczuk AC, et al. Pulmonary hypertension in idiopathic pulmonary fibrosis. *Chest.* 2007;132:998-1006.

160. Nicod L. Recognition and treatment of idiopathic pulmonary fibrosis. *Drugs.* 1998;55(4):55-62.

161. Ryu J, Colby T, Hartman T. Idiopathic pulmonary fibrosis: current concepts. *Mayo Clin Proc.* 1998;73(11):1085-1101.

162. Myers JL, Tazelaar HD. Challenges in pulmonary fibrosis: problematic granulomatous lung disease. *Thorax.* 2008;63; 78-84.

163. Katzenstein A, Myers J. Idiopathic pulmonary fibrosis: clinical relevance of pathologic classification. *Am J Respir Crit Care Med.* 1998;157(4, pt 1):1301-1315.

164. Ryu JH, Krowka MJ, Pellikka PA, et al. Pulmonary hypertension in patients with interstitial lung diseases. *Mayo Clin Proc.* 2007; 82(3):342-350.

165. Egan J. Pharmacologic therapy of idiopathic pulmonary fibrosis. *J Heart Lung Transplant.* 1998;17(11):1039-1044.

166. Schultz MJ, Haitsma JJ, Zhang H, Slutsky AS. Pulmonary coagulopathy as a new target in therapeutic students of acute lung injusry: a review. *Crit Care Med.* 2006;34:871-877.

167. ATS, ERS, ESICM, et al. International consensus conferences in intensive care medicine. *Am J Respir Crit Care Med.* 1999; 160:2118-2124.

168. Ware L, Matthay M. The acute respiratory distress syndrome. *N Engl J Med.* 2000;342(18):1334-1346.

169. Hudson L, Steinberg K. Epidemiology of acute lung injury and ARDS. *Chest.* 1999;116:74S-82S.

170. Wyncoll D, Evans T. Acute respiratory distress syndrome. *Lancet.* 1999;354:497-501.

171. Frawley PM, Habashi NM. Airway pressure regulated ventilation and pediatrics: theory and practice. *Crit Care Nurs Clin North Am.* 2004;16(3):337-348.

172. Farrell P, Fiascone J. Bronchopulmonary dysplasia in the 1990s: a review for the pediatrician. *Curr Probl Pediatr.* 1997;27(4): 129-163.

173. Takemura T, Askahi T, Ohtani Y, et al. Pathology of hypersensitivity pneumonitis. *Curr Opin Pulm Med.* 2008;14:440-454.

174. Daroowala F, Raghu G. Hypersensitivity pneumonitis. *Compr Ther.* 1997;23(4):244-248.

175. Ando M, Suga M, Kohrogi H. A new look at hypersensitivity pneumonitis. *Curr Opin Pulm Med.* 1999;5:299-304.

176. Selman M, Vargas M. Airway involvement in hypersensitivity pneumonitis. *Curr Opin Pulm Med.* 1998;4:9-15.

177. Craig T. Update on hypersensitivity pneumonitis. *Compr Ther.* 1996;22(9):559-564.

178. Salvaggio J. Extrinsic allergic alveolitis (hypersensitivity pneumonitis): past, present and future. *Clin Exp Allergy.* 1997;27 (suppl 1):18-25.

179. Erdogdu G, Hasirci V. An overview of the role of mineral solubility in silicosis and asbestosis. *Environ Res.* 1998;78(1):38-42.

180. Mossman B, Churg A. Mechanisms in the pathogenesis of asbestos and silicosis. *Am J Respir Crit Care Med.* 1998;157 (5, pt 1):1666-1680.

181. Kamp D, Weitzman S. Asbestos: clinical spectrum and pathogenic mechanisms. *Proc Soc Exp Biol Med.* 1997;214(1):12-26.

182. Miserocchi G, Sancini G, Mantegazza F, et al. Translocation pathways for inhaled asbestos fiber. *Environ Health.* 2008;7(4): 1-8.

183. Schneider J, Hoffman H, Dienemann H, et al. Diagnostic and prognostic value of soluble mesothelin-related proteins in patients with malignant pleural mesothelioma in comparison with benign asbestosis and lung cancer. *J Thorac Oncol.* 2008;3:1317-1324.

184. Robledo R, Mossman B. Cellular and molecular mechanisms of asbestos induced fibrosis. *J Cell Physiol.* 1999;180(2):158-166.

185. Rudd R. New developments in asbestos related pleural disease. *Thorax.* 1996;51(2):210-216.

186. Nishimura S, Broaddus V. Asbestos induced pleural disease. *Clin Chest Med.* 1998;19(2):311-329.

187. Murlidhar V, Kanhere V. Asbestosis composite mill at Mumbai: a prevalence study. *Environ Health.* 2005;4(24):1-7.

188. Kamp D, Weitzman S. Molecular basis of asbestos induced lung injury. *Thorax.* 1999;54(7):638-652.

189. Huaux F. New developments in the understanding of immunology in silicosis. *Curr Opin Allergy Clin Immunol.* 2007;7:163-173.

190. Chong S, Lee KS, Chung MJ, et al. Pneumoconiosis: comparison of imaging and pathological findings. *Radiographics.* 2006; 26:59-77.

191. Steenland K, Goldsmith D. Silica exposure and autoimmune disease. *Am J Ind Med.* 1995;28(5):603-608.

192. Anaya J, Diethelm L, Ortiz L, et al. Pulmonary involvement in rheumatoid arthritis. *Semin Arthritis Rheum.* 1995;24(4):242-254.

193. Tanoue L. Pulmonary manifestations of rheumatoid arthritis. *Clin Chest Med.* 1998;19(4):667-683.

194. Murin S, Weidemann H, Matthay R. Pulmonary manifestations of systemic lupus erythematosus. *Clin Chest Med.* 1998;19(4): 641-665.

195. Godfrey T, Khamashta M, Hughes G. Therapeutic advances in systemic lupus erythematosus. *Curr Opin Rheumatol.* 1998; 10(5):435-441.

196. Minai O, Dweik R, Arroliga A. Manifestations of scleroderma pulmonary disease. *Clin Chest Med.* 1998;19(4):713-727.

197. Silman A. Epidemiology of scleroderma. *Ann Rheum Dis.* 1991;50:846-853.

198. Steen V. Clinical manifestations of systemic sclerosis. *Semin Cutan Med Surg.* 1998;17(1):48-54.

199. Cain H, Noble P, Matthay R. Pulmonary manifestations of Sjogren's Syndrome. *Clin Chest Med.* 1998;19(4):687-697.

200. Tavoni A, Cirigliano C, Frigelli S, et al. Shrinking lung in primary Sjogren's syndrome. *Arthritis Rheum.* 1999;42(10):2249-2250.

201. Wiedemann H, Matthay R. Pulmonary manifestations of the collagen vascular disease. *Clin Chest Med.* 1989;10(4):677-715.

202. Corley D, Winterbauer R. Collagen vascular disease. *Semin Respir Infect.* 1995;10(2):78-85.

203. Bulpitt K, Clements P, Lachenbruch P, et al. Early undifferentiated connective tissue disease: III. Outcome and prognostic indicators in early scleroderma (systemic sclerosis). *Ann Intern Med.* 1993;118:602-609.

204. Libby D, White D. Pulmonary toxicity of drugs used to treat systemic autoimmune disease. *Clin Chest Med.* 1998;19(4): 809-821.

205. Bradbury PA, Shepherd FA. Immunotherapy for lung cancer. *J Thorac Oncol.* 2008;3(suppl 2):S164-S170.

206. Gomez M, Silvestri GA. Lung cancer screening. *Am J Med Sci.* 2008;335(1):46-50.

207. Osann K. Epidemiology of lung cancer. *Curr Opin Pulm Med.* 1998;4:198-204.

208. McLoud T, Swenson S. Lung carcinoma. *Clin Chest Med.* 1999; 20(4):697-714.

209. Christini D. Smoking and the molecular epidemiology of lung cancer. *Clin Chest Med.* 2000;21(1):87-93.

210. Sher T, Dy GK, Adjei AA. Small cell lung cancer. *Mayo Clin Proc.* 2008;83(3):355-367.

211. Lillington G. Neoplasms of the lung. *Curr Opin Pulm Med.* 1999;5:185-188.

212. Leonard C, Sachs D. Environmental tobacco smoke and lung cancer incidence. *Curr Opin Pulm Med.* 1999;5:189-193.

213. Smith RA, Cokkinides V, Brawley OW. Cancer screening in the United States, 2009. *CA Cancer J Clin.* 2009;59:27-41.

214. National Cancer Institute. U.S. National Institutes of Health. http://www.cancer.gov.

215. Franklin W. Diagnosis of lung cancer: pathology of invasive and preinvasive neoplasia. *Chest.* 2000;117:80S-89S.

216. Adjei A. Management of small cell cancer of the lung. *Curr Opin Pulm Med.* 2000;6:384-390.

217. Bunn PA, Thatcher N. Introduction. *Oncologist.* 2008;13 (suppl 1):1-4.

218. Leonard C, Whyte R, Lillington G. Primary non–small-cell lung cancer: determining the suitability of the patient and tumor for resection. *Curr Opin Pulm Med.* 2000;6:391-395.

219. Johnson D. Locally advanced, unresectable non–small cell lung cancer. *Chest.* 2000;117:123S-126S.

220. Hyer J, Silvestri G. Diagnosis and staging of lung cancer. *Clin Chest Med.* 2000;21(1):95-108.

221. Mountain C. Revisions in the international system for staging lung cancer. *Chest.* 1997;111:1710-1717.

222. Deslauriers J, Gregoire J. Clinical and surgical staging of non–small-cell lung cancer. *Chest.* 2000;117:96S-103S.

223. Jacobs PCA, Mali W, Grobbee DE, van der Graaf Y. Prevalence of incidental findings in computed tomographic screening of the chest. *J Comput Assist Tomogr.* 2008;32:214-221.

224. Hillerdal G. Indolent lung cancers: time for a paradigm shift. *J Thorac Oncol.* 2008;3:208-211.

225. Yoneda K, Louie S, Shelton D. Approach to pulmonary metastases. *Curr Opin Pulm Med.* 2000;6:356-363.

226. Govindan R, Bogart J, Vokes EE. Locally advanced non–small cell lung cancer: the past, present and future. *J Thorac Oncol.* 2008;3:917-928.

227. Brunelli A, Salati M. Preoperative evaluation of lung cancer: predicting the impact of surgery on physiology and quality of life. *Curr Opin Pulm Med.* 2008;14:275-281.

228. Belani C. Combined modality therapy for unresectable stage III non–small-cell lung cancer. *Chest*. 2000;117:127S-132S.

229. Redline S, Tishler P, Schluchter M, et al. Risk factors for sleep-disordered breathing in children: associations with obesity, race, and respiratory problems. *Am J Respir Crit Care Med*. 1999;159:1527-1532.

230. Zerha-Lancner F, Lofaso F, Coste A, et al. Pulmonary function in obese snorers with or without sleep apnea syndrome. *Am J Respir Crit Care Med*. 1997;156:522-527.

231. Kay J. Hypoxia, obstructive sleep apnea syndrome, and pulmonary hypertension. *Hum Pathol*. 1997;28(3):261-263.

232. O'Day M. Cardiopulmonary physiological adaptation of pregnancy. *Semin Perinatol*. 1997;21(4):268-275.

233. Sue D. Obesity and pulmonary function: more or less? *Chest*. 1997;111(4):891-898.

234. Chen Y, Rennie D, Cormier Y, Dosman J. Waist circumference is associated with pulmonary function in normal-weight, overweight, and obese subjects. *Am J Clin Nutr*. 2007;85: 35-39.

235. Klein S, Burke L, Bray G, Blair S, Allison D. Clinical implications of obesity with specific focus on cardiovascular disease. *Circulation*. 2004;110:2952-2967.

236. Langer J. Congenital diaphragmatic hernia. *Chest Surg Clin North Am*. 1998;8(2):295-311.

237. American Physical Therapy Association. Guide to Physical Therapist Practice. *Phys Ther*. 1997;77(11):1231-1619.

Medications

Charles D. Ciccone

INTRODUCTION

Medications play an integral role in the treatment of patients with cardiovascular and pulmonary disorders. Drugs can be used to prevent or treat various pathologies and impairments in the heart, lungs, and circulation, and thereby reduce the functional limitations and disability associated with cardiopulmonary disease. Medications can likewise have a synergistic effect with physical therapy interventions. Drugs, for example, that improve cardiac pumping ability, may enable patients to participate more effectively in interventions that improve aerobic capacity and endurance. All medications likewise produce side effects that can have a direct impact on physical therapy interventions. For instance, drugs that lower blood pressure (antihypertensives) may produce dizziness and incoordination if they cause excessive hypotension. It, therefore, makes sense that physical therapists have a basic understanding of the common cardiovascular and pulmonary medications and how these medications can affect patients receiving physical therapy.

In this chapter, pharmacologic agents are grouped according to the preferred practice patterns listed in Chapter 6 of the *Guide to Physical Therapist Practice,* 2nd edition (revised).[1] For each preferred practice pattern, medications that specifically address cardiovascular or pulmonary problems will be discussed as they relate to that practice pattern. It is, of course, not possible to describe all medications that might be related to each pattern. For example, medications used to control infection, treat cancer, and so forth, may help improve the patient's overall health, thereby helping the patient participate in aerobic conditioning, respiratory exercises, and other activities that will ultimately lead to better cardiovascular and pulmonary function. This chapter, however, will focus only on the medications that directly affect the heart, circulation, or lungs and describe how these medications relate to the physical therapy interventions described in the preferred practice patterns. This chapter will likewise present an overview of these medications, their side effects, and the potential impact of these medications on patients receiving physical therapy. For more information about specific drugs, the reader is also encouraged to consult one of the resources listed at the end of this chapter.[2–4]

MEDICATIONS RELATED TO PREFERRED PRACTICE PATTERN A: PRIMARY PREVENTION/RISK REDUCTION FOR CARDIOVASCULAR/PULMONARY DISORDERS

Many medications are designed to control specific aspects of cardiovascular function so that the risk of cardiac and related diseases is reduced. Controlling blood pressure, for example, can reduce the risk of myocardial infarction, cerebrovascular accident, kidney disease, and so forth. In some cases, drug therapy can be initiated to prevent the first episode of a cardiovascular incident (primary prevention), or drug therapy can be used to prevent the reoccurrence of a specific problem (secondary prevention). Four primary pharmacological strategies that can be used to reduce cardiovascular risks include controlling high blood pressure (antihypertensives), decreasing plasma lipids (antihyperlipidemia drugs), treatment of overactive blood clotting (anticlotting agents), and cessation of cigarette smoking. These drug categories are described here.

Antihypertensive Medications

Controlling high blood pressure (hypertension) is perhaps one of the most important ways to reduce the risk of cardiovascular disease. *Hypertension,* defined as a sustained and reproducible increase in blood pressure, typically leads to a number of problems including heart disease, stroke, and renal failure.[5] The exact cause of hypertension is often unclear in the majority of people with high blood pressure. Many people become hypertensive because of the combined influence of several physiological and lifestyle factors such as increased body weight, poor diet, cigarette smoking, lack of stress management, physical inactivity, and so forth. Although resolution of these factors may successfully reduce blood pressure, drug therapy remains the most common way to control hypertension.

Antihypertensive drugs are organized into several major categories, and these categories are listed in Table 8-1. Each major category exerts an effect at a specific organ or tissue as indicated in Fig. 8-1. Details about the antihypertensive effects and potential problems of these drugs are presented here.

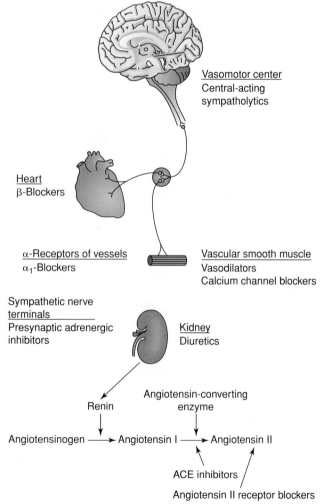

FIGURE 8-1   Sites of action of the major antihypertensive drug categories.

Diuretics

Diuretics act on the kidneys to increase the excretion of sodium and water.[6] The loss of sodium and water will reduce the total amount of fluid in the vascular system, thereby reducing blood pressure by decreasing excess fluid within the peripheral vasculature. Diuretics also reduce cardiac workload by decreasing the amount of fluid the heart must pump, and this effect is helpful in decreasing hypertensive heart disease and in treating certain forms of heart failure.

Many diuretics are currently available, and these drugs are classified according to their chemistry or mechanism and site of action (see Table 8-1). Specifically, thiazide diuretics are chemically similar to one another, loop diuretics are so named because they act on the loop of Henle in the nephron, and potassium-sparing diuretics increase the excretion of sodium and water without a concomitant increase in potassium excretion. Selection of a specific diuretic is based on the needs of each patient, with factors such as the patient's medical condition, age, and use of other medications influencing the choice of each diuretic.

Diuretics are remarkably safe when taken as directed. Problems may occur, however, if the patient overdoses and excretes too much water and electrolytes (sodium and potassium) from the body.[7,8] Patients may become confused, dizzy, and unreasonably fatigued because the fluid and electrolyte balance in the body is disturbed. Potassium supplementation is frequently provided to patients on diuretic therapy in order to maintain potassium levels and thus prevent undue fatigue. Patients may likewise experience similar problems if they take the correct diuretic dosage but severely restrict their fluid intake. Consequently, physical therapists should watch for any change in the patient's behavior or physical ability that might indicate a problem in diuretic use.

Sympatholytic Agents

As indicated earlier, hypertension typically results from the interaction of several physiological and lifestyle factors. These factors, however, seem to conspire and exert their effect on the cardiovascular system by activating the sympathetic nervous system.[9] This idea makes sense when one considers that increased sympathetic activity will invariably increase blood pressure by stimulating cardiac output and increasing peripheral vascular resistance. Sympatholytic drugs are so named because they act at various sites in the sympathetic nervous system and attempt to break up or produce a "lytic" effect on sympathetic drive to the heart and vasculature. The primary sympatholytic drug strategies are described here.

β-Blockers—β-Blockers decrease sympathetic stimulation of the heart and decrease cardiac output with a subsequent decrease in blood pressure.[10] Specifically, these drugs occupy the type 1 beta-adrenergic (β_1) receptor located on the heart and thereby prevent other chemicals such as the catecholamines (epinephrine and norepinephrine) from stimulating these receptors. Through their ability to occupy or "block" β_1-receptors, β-blockers reduce cardiac stimulation and help normalize blood pressure. These drugs are useful under other conditions

TABLE 8-1 Antihypertensive Medications

Category	Generic Name	Trade Name(s)	Category	Generic Name	Trade Name(s)
Diuretics			**Vasodilators**		
Thiazides	Chlorothiazide	Diuril, others	Nitrates	Nitroglycerin	Nitrostat, others
	Chlorthalidone	Thalitone		Isosorbide dinitrate	Isordil, others
	Hydrochlorothiazide	Microzide, others		Isosorbide	Monoket, others
	Hydroflumethiazide	Saluron		mononitrate	
	Methyclothiazide	Enduron	Other direct-acting	Diazoxide	Proglycem
	Metolazone	Zaroxolyn	vasodilators	Hydralazine	Generic
	Polythiazide	Renese		Minoxidil	Generic
Loop diuretics	Bumetanide	Bumex		Sodium nitroprusside	Nitropress
	Ethacrynic acid	Edecrin			
	Furosemide	Lasix, others	**Drugs affecting the renin–angiotensin system**		
	Torsemide	Demadex	Angiotensin-converting	Benazepril	Lotensin
Potassium-sparing	Amiloride	Generic	enzyme (ACE) inhibitors	Captopril	Capoten
diuretics	Spironolactone	Aldactone		Enalapril	Vasotec
	Triamterene	Dyrenium		Fosinopril	Monopril
				Lisinopril	Prinivil, Zestril
Sympatholytics				Moexipril	Univasc
β-Blockers	Acebutolol	Sectral		Quinapril	Accupril
(cardioselective)	Atenolol	Tenormin		Ramipril	Altace
	Betaxolol	Kerlone		Trandolapril	Mavik
	Bisoprolol	Zebeta	Angiotensin II receptor	Candesartan	Atacand
	Esmolol	Brevibloc	blockers	Eprosartan	Teveten
	Metoprolol	Lopressor, Toprol		Irbesartan	Avapro
β-Blockers	Carvedilol	Coreg		Losartan	Cozaar
(nonselective)	Labetalol	Trandate		Olmesartan	Benicar
	Nadolol	Corgard		Telmisartan	Micardis
	Penbutolol	Levatol		Valsartan	Diovan
	Pindolol	Visken			
	Propranolol	Inderal	**Calcium channel blockers**		
	Sotalol	Betapace, Sorine	Dihydropyridine agents	Amlodipine	Norvasc
α-Blockers	Doxazosin	Cardura		Felodipine	Plendil
	Prazosin	Minipress		Isradipine	DynaCirc
	Terazosin	Hytrin		Nicardipine	Cardene
Presynaptic adrenergic	Reserpine	Serpalan, others		Nifedipine	Adalat, Procardia, others
inhibitors				Nimodipine	Nimotop
Central-acting agents	Clonidine	Catapres, others		Nisoldipine	Sular
	Guanabenz	Generic	Others	Diltiazem	Cardizem, Dilacor, others
	Guanfacine	Tenex		Verapamil	Calan, Verelan, others
	Methyldopa	Generic			

marked by excessive sympathetic cardiac stimulation, and β-blockers are also indicated in certain types of angina pectoris, cardiac arrhythmias, heart failure, and in helping the heart recover function after a myocardial infarction.[11]

Some commonly used β-blockers are listed in Table 8-1. Although all these drugs have the ability to block β_1-receptors in the heart, specific β-blockers have additional properties that may make them more or less suitable for use in individual patients. Certain agents, for example, are known as cardioselective because they are fairly specific for β_1-receptors located in the heart (see Table 8-1). Other β-blockers are nonselective because they affect cardiac β_1-receptors as well as β_2-receptors located on bronchiole smooth muscle and other tissues. Various other properties and side effects of each drug are also taken into account when selecting a specific drug for each patient.

Although β-blockers are generally tolerated well by most patients, these drugs can cause certain side effects that impact physical therapy interventions. By virtue of their ability to reduce cardiac stimulation, these drugs may reduce heart rate during exercise. β-Blockers, for example, should reduce maximal heart rate by approximately 20 to 30 beats per minute (bpm). This effect could potentially limit maximal exercise capacity, but this effect is probably not substantial at the submaximal exercise workloads that are typically used in physical therapy interventions. Certain patients may, in fact, be able to exercise more effectively at submaximal workloads because β-blockers help control other symptoms (angina, arrhythmias) that limit exercise in these patients.

Bronchoconstriction may also occur in certain patients if they have some type of bronchoconstrictive lung disease (asthma, chronic obstructive pulmonary disease [COPD]) and they are also taking a nonselective β-blocker that affects the lungs as well as the heart. This situation is typically resolved by switching the patient to a β_1-specific (cardioselective) drug that also does not affect β_2-receptors on the lungs. As with many antihypertensives, β-blockers may cause orthostatic hypotension, which is characterized as an excessive fall in blood pressure when the patient sits or stands up too rapidly.

Older individuals may not tolerate β-blockers as well as younger individuals because these drugs tend to cause confusion, depression, and other behavioral changes in the elderly.

Finally, there is some controversy about how β-blockers can be used most effectively in treating hypertension.[12] Although these drugs have often been used in the initial stages of treatment, recent studies suggest that these drugs might not be the best method for treating early, uncomplicated hypertension. It likewise appears that other agents such as diuretics (as already discussed) and ACE inhibitors (see later) might be a better first choice for treating hypertension because these drugs might prevent cardiac events (stroke, coronary artery disease) more effectively than β-blockers.[11,13] Future research should help clarify how β-blockers and other drugs can be used most effectively in the treatment of high blood pressure.

Other sympatholytics—In addition to β-blockers, several other drug strategies are available that decrease sympathetic activity at other locations within the sympathetic nervous system (see Table 8-1). α-Blockers, for example, bind to the α_1-adrenergic receptor located on vascular smooth muscle and prevent catecholamines from reaching these α_1-receptors and causing vasoconstriction.[14] Decreased vasoconstriction will reduce peripheral vascular resistance with a concomitant decrease in blood pressure. Another strategy for reducing peripheral vascular resistance is to decrease the release of norepinephrine from the presynaptic sympathetic nerve terminals that normally supply vascular smooth muscle. These drugs, known as presynaptic adrenergic inhibitors, will lower vascular resistance and decrease blood pressure because the sympathetic neurons cannot release as much neurotransmitter on the vascular smooth muscle. Finally, a small group of drugs is classified as centrally acting sympatholytics because they directly affect sympathetic nervous system activity in the brain stem. Specifically, these drugs either stimulate α_2-adrenergic receptors or stimulate specific imidazoline receptors located in the vasomotor area located in the pons and medulla.[15] By acting on these brainstem receptors, these drugs reduce sympathetic discharge to the heart and peripheral vasculature, and this effect should reduce blood pressure and produce an antihypertensive effect.

Sympatholytics, which were described previously, are listed in Table 8-1. These drugs share some side effects including a tendency for hypotension and orthostatic hypotension. That is, these drugs may be too effective in reducing sympathetic activity, and patients may have abnormally low blood pressure at rest or when moving suddenly to a sitting or standing position. Another problem commonly associated with these sympatholytics is reflex tachycardia. Drugs such as the α-blockers and presynaptic adrenergic inhibitors typically cause a substantial decrease in peripheral vascular resistance thereby producing a beneficial antihypertensive effect. The body, however, will sense this reduction in blood pressure and use various mechanisms including the baroreceptor reflex to increase heart rate (reflex tachycardia) to bring blood pressure

back to the original hypertensive levels. Hence, reflex tachycardia is a misguided attempt on the part of the body to maintain blood pressure at high levels, even though this increased blood pressure is not normal. Clearly, reflex tachycardia is an indication that the normal control of blood pressure has been disrupted and the mechanisms that regulate blood pressure have been reset to maintain blood pressure at higher levels in people who are hypertensive.

Nonetheless, reflex tachycardia can often be controlled nicely by combining a β-blocker with the sympatholytic agent that caused this problem. In addition to controlling reflex tachycardia, the combination of a β-blocker and α-blocker or presynaptic adrenergic inhibitor often provides synergistic antihypertensive effects by reducing sympathetic drive to the heart and peripheral vasculature, respectively.

Vasodilators

Certain sympatholytics (α-blockers, presynaptic adrenergic inhibitors) and other drugs (ACE inhibitors, calcium channel blockers; see later) cause vasodilation. There is, however, a select group of drugs classified specifically as *vasodilators* because these drugs have a direct effect on the vascular endothelium or vascular smooth muscle. Organic nitrates such as nitroglycerin, for example, are converted to nitric oxide within the vascular wall, where they inhibit smooth muscle contraction and allow the vessel to dilate. Other agents such as hydralazine and minoxidil increase the intracellular production of cyclic adenosine monophosphate (cAMP), which serves as a chemical messenger that causes vascular relaxation and vasodilation. Vasodilators are quite effective in reducing peripheral vascular resistance, and they are often called on to help control more severe or resistant forms of hypertension.[16,17]

Vasodilators can cause several side effects that are related to their ability to decrease peripheral vascular resistance. Reflex tachycardia can occur for the same reasons stated earlier; that is, a sudden or profound fall in peripheral vascular resistance will activate the baroreflex and cause an increase in heart rate in an attempt to return blood pressure to the original, albeit hypertensive, levels. Orthostatic hypotension and dizziness may also occur, because the peripheral vasculature is maintained in a relaxed and dilated state and is less able to cope with changes in posture. Patients may complain of headaches because of vasodilation in meningeal vessels, and peripheral edema (swollen ankles and so forth) may occur because vasodilation increases the pressure gradient that forces fluid out of the capillaries and into the extravascular (interstitial) space.

Drugs Affecting the Renin–Angiotensin System

The renin–angiotensin system (see Fig. 8-2) helps maintain blood pressure and regulate vascular perfusion throughout the body.[18,19] If, for example, blood pressure suddenly decreases and remains at hypotensive levels for more than a few seconds, the kidneys sense this change and release an enzyme called renin. Renin converts angiotensinogen (a small protein) into angiotensin I. Angiotensin I is inactive until it contacts an enzyme known as ACE. The ACE is located in the lungs and

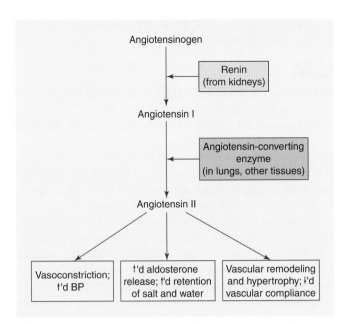

FIGURE 8-2 The renin–angiotensin system and effects of angiotensin II. Angiotensin-converting enzyme inhibitors interrupt this system by blocking the conversion of angiotensin I to angiotensin II, and angiotensin II receptor blockers prevent angiotensin II from stimulating vascular tissues.

other tissues, and this enzyme converts angiotensin I into a very powerful vasoconstrictor, angiotensin II. By increasing vascular resistance, angiotensin II elevates blood pressure back to reasonable levels, thus averting hypotensive problems including shock. Angiotensin II also stimulates the release of aldosterone, and aldosterone helps maintain vascular fluid volume by increasing renal sodium and water reabsorption.

The renin–angiotensin system is, therefore, a normal physiologic process that helps maintain blood pressure. Many people with hypertension, however, have elevated renin levels, even though blood pressure is already too high. The normal function of the renin–angiotensin system has obviously been disturbed in these individuals, resulting in production of a powerful vasoconstrictor (angiotensin II) that leads to additional increases in blood pressure that perpetuate hypertension in these people. In addition to producing vasoconstriction, prolonged increases in angiotensin II also stimulate hypertrophy and remodeling of the vasculature (see Fig. 8-2) so that the vascular wall becomes less compliant and begins to encroach on the lumen and reduce blood flow through the vessel. These changes, both the acute vasoconstriction and the more chronic and permanent effects on vascular wall hypertrophy, are devastating to cardiovascular function because they produce dramatic increases in blood pressure and workload on the heart. Drugs that help reduce activity in the renin–angiotensin system are therefore critical in decreasing the risks associated with elevated renin activity.

A primary strategy for reducing activity in the renin–angiotensin system is to administer drugs known as ACE inhibitors.[20] By inhibiting the enzyme that converts angiotensin I to angiotensin II, these drugs reduce the vasoconstriction and

vascular hypertrophy associated with angiotensin II. ACE inhibitors are, therefore, helpful in controlling high blood pressure, especially in individuals who have increased activity in the renin–angiotensin system. These drugs are also beneficial in certain forms of heart failure because they reduce the stress and workload on the myocardium that is caused by increased production of angiotensin II.

Table 8-1 lists some common ACE inhibitors. As indicated in the table, ACE inhibitors are usually identified by generic names that end with a "-pril" suffix (captopril, enalapril, and so forth). Regarding side effects, these drugs are relatively safe and well tolerated in most individuals. Some people may experience an allergic reaction, but this reaction is usually not severe. Other people may develop some annoying side effects, including nausea, dizziness, and a dry, persistent cough.

ACE inhibitors were the first drug strategy developed for reducing activity in the renin–angiotensin system. More recently, a second option has become available, where drugs can be administered that bind to and occupy the angiotensin II receptor located on cardiovascular tissues, thereby preventing angiotensin II from reaching these tissues and causing vasoconstriction and other detrimental effects. These newer drugs, known as angiotensin II receptor blockers, can also be used to control cardiovascular damage associated with increased production of angiotensin II. Angiotensin II receptor blockers appear to be at least as effective as ACE inhibitors, but the angiotensin II receptor blockers tend to have fewer side effects and they do not produce the dry cough commonly associated with ACE inhibitors. Hence, several angiotensin II receptor blockers, such as losartan and eprosartan, are currently available (see Table 8-1), and these drugs offer an alternative for people who cannot tolerate the more traditional ACE inhibitors. Likewise, recent studies suggest that some patients with kidney disease might benefit from a combination of an angiotensin II receptor blocker and an ACE inhibitor.[21] Methods for controlling the renin–angiotensin system in hypertension and other forms of cardiovascular disease continue to be investigated, and future research will clarify how ACE inhibitors and angiotensin II receptor blockers can be used most effectively in clinical situations.

Calcium Channel Blockers

Calcium channel blockers decrease the entry of calcium into cardiovascular tissues.[22] As is the case with all contractile tissues, calcium ions are the key intracellular mediators that influence the interaction between thick (myosin) and thin (actin) contractile filaments within these tissues. In vascular smooth muscle, an increase in intracellular calcium typically results in a stronger interaction between these contractile filaments, thereby increasing the strength of smooth muscle contraction and the amount of vasoconstriction in the vessel. Calcium channel blockers restrict the entry of calcium ions into vascular tissues by inhibiting the opening of specific protein channels located on the smooth muscle cell membrane. These drugs, therefore, reduce the strength of vascular smooth muscle contraction and help reduce high blood pressure by promoting vasodilation in the peripheral vasculature.[22] Calcium is also important in regulating cardiac rhythm, and some calcium channel blockers can be used to control certain types of arrhythmias that are caused by abnormal calcium stimulation within the heart (see later).

Calcium channel blockers are listed in Table 8-1. These agents can be subclassified according to their chemical structure, with several drugs being grouped together as dihydropyridine agents because they share a common chemical background. Because of their vasodilating properties, these drugs may cause dizziness, orthostatic hypotension, and peripheral edema (swollen ankles), and so forth. Because of their effects on calcium entry in the heart, these drugs may also affect cardiac rhythm and may increase the risk of arrhythmia in certain patients. There was likewise concern that some calcium channel blockers such as the short-acting form of nifedipine may actually increase the risk of heart attack in older individuals, and that these drugs might exacerbate certain problems such as kidney disease and diabetes mellitus.[23,24] Nonetheless, calcium channel blockers are a mainstay in the treatment of hypertension and other cardiovascular diseases, and careful use of these drugs can produce beneficial effects with minimal risk in many patients.

Control of Hyperlipidemia

A significant risk factor in cardiovascular disease is the unfavorable accumulation of cholesterol and other lipids in the bloodstream.[25] Elevated plasma lipids (hyperlipidemia) and certain lipid–protein complexes such as the low-density lipoproteins (LDL) are associated with an increased risk of cardiovascular disease. Hyperlipidemia causes accumulation of fatty deposits within the arterial walls, thus leading to atherosclerosis and various other cardiovascular pathologies (thrombosis, infarction, and so forth). Proper diet and exercise are critical in improving the plasma lipid profile in people with lipid disorders. In addition, several drug strategies are available that can help control the quantity and type of lipids

present in the bloodstream. These strategies are listed in Table 8-2, and they are discussed briefly here.

Statins

The term *statin* describes a group of drugs that inhibit a key enzyme responsible for cholesterol biosynthesis.[26,27] Specifically, these drugs inhibit the 3-hydroxy-3-methylglutaryl coenzyme A (HMG-CoA) reductase that catalyzes one of the early steps in cholesterol synthesis in the liver and other cells. Statins are, therefore, also known as HMG-CoA reductase inhibitors, and these drugs can directly inhibit hepatic cholesterol production and reduce total cholesterol levels in the bloodstream. Statins also decrease plasma LDL cholesterol levels by increasing the production of receptors on liver cells that degrade LDLs, and they inhibit the production of LDL precursors such as very low-density lipoproteins (VLDLs), thus further decreasing plasma LDL cholesterol levels. These drugs may produce other favorable changes in the plasma lipid profile including decreased triglyceride levels and increased high-density lipoprotein (HDL) levels, although the exact reasons for these effects are not clear.[27] Statins may likewise have direct beneficial effects on the vascular endothelium, and they can help reduce atherosclerotic plaque formation, presumably by inhibiting specific enzymes and metabolic pathways that lead to atherosclerosis within the vascular wall.[28] These drugs, therefore, produce multiple beneficial effects on lipid and vascular function, and statins have become one of the primary methods for controlling hyperlipidemia in patients at risk for cardiovascular disease.

Statins consist of atorvastatin (Lipitor), rosuvastatin (Crestor), simvastatin (Zocor), and several similar drugs (see Table 8-2). These drugs are typically used in people who have not been successful in controlling plasma lipid levels by using just diet and exercise interventions, or in any individuals who are at high risk for developing coronary artery disease.[26,29] Administration of statins may substantially decrease the risk of

TABLE 8-2   Drugs Used to Control Hyperlipidemia

Category	Drugs	Primary Effect(s) on Plasma Lipids
Statins	Atorvastatin (Lipitor) Fluvastatin (Lescol) Lovastatin (Mevacor, others) Pravastatin (Pravachol) Rosuvastatin (Crestor) Simvastatin (Zocor)	Reduce total cholesterol and LDL cholesterol levels; may also produce a modest decrease in triglycerides and a slight increase in HDL levels
Fibric acids	Clofibrate (generic) Fenofibrate (TriCor, Triglide, others) Gemfibrozil (Lopid)	Decrease triglyceride levels; gemfibrozil may also decrease VLDL levels and increase HDL concentrations
Bile acid sequestrants	Cholestyramine (Questran, others) Colesevelam (Welchol) Colestipol (Colestid)	Reduce total cholesterol and LDL concentrations by adhering to bile acids in GI tract (liver uses excess cholesterol to synthesize more bile)
Others	Niacin (Niacor, Niaspan, others) Ezetimibe (Zetia)	Decreases total cholesterol and triglyceride concentrations Reduces total cholesterol by inhibiting cholesterol absorption from GI tract

LDL, low-density lipoproteins; HDL, high-density lipoproteins; VLDL, very low-density lipoproteins.

heart attack, and the magnitude of this benefit seems to be related directly to the extent that cholesterol and other lipid abnormalities can be reduced.[26] The most common side effects associated with these drugs are gastrointestinal problems, such as stomach pain, nausea, diarrhea, gas, and heartburn.

Although less common, some patients may also experience muscle pain, cramps, and severe weakness and fatigue.[30,31] These symptoms may indicate myositis that can lead to severe breakdown and destruction of skeletal muscle (rhabdomyolysis). Statin-induced rhabdomyolysis is a serious problem that can cause renal failure as the kidneys try to excrete myoglobin and other muscle constituents that have been released into the bloodstream during muscle breakdown. In addition to statin-induced myopathy, peripheral neuropathies may occur in some patients.[30] Physical therapists should therefore be alert for any unexplained increase in muscle pain and weakness or neuropathic symptoms (numbness, tingling) in patients receiving statin drugs. Therapists should alert the medical staff so that drug therapy can be changed before these neuromuscular problems become severe or life-threatening.

Other Antihyperlipidemia Drugs

Other drugs used to treat hyperlipidemia include fibric acids such as clofibrate and gemfibrozil (Lopid) (Table 8-2). These drugs can decrease total plasma triglyceride and VLDL levels, probably by increasing the activity of the lipoprotein lipase enzyme that metabolizes triglycerides in the liver and other tissues.[32] Several agents including cholestyramine (Questran) act as bile acid sequestrants, meaning that these drugs gather up and retain bile acids in the GI tract. This action increases the elimination of bile acids from the body, thereby forcing the liver to divert cholesterol to form more bile acids and decreasing the amount of cholesterol available for causing lipid disorders.[33] Niacin (nicotinic acid, Niacor, Niaspan, others) can also be used to reduce plasma LDL levels because this drug inhibits VLDL synthesis, thus decreasing the production of the primary LDL precursor.[34] Finally, agents such as ezetimibe (Zetia) inhibit the absorption of cholesterol from the GI tract, thereby limiting the total amount of cholesterol available from dietary sources.[35]

These antihyperlipidemia drugs are associated with various side effects. In particular, many of these drugs cause gastrointestinal problems including nausea, stomach pain, gas, and diarrhea. Other side effects may occur depending on the particular agent, therapeutic dosage, and length of time the drugs are administered. Nonetheless, these agents can be used alone or combined with one another or statin drugs to improve the plasma lipid profile of people with hyperlipidemia. Proper drug management used in conjunction with diet and exercise will hopefully reduce the risk of cardiovascular disease in people with lipid disorders.

Treatment of Overactive Blood Clotting

Adequate blood clotting or hemostasis is essential for maintaining normal cardiovascular function. If the blood clots too rapidly, a thrombus can form in the arterial or venous system and disrupt or block blood flow through the occluded vessel.[36] This occlusion can be especially harmful if it occurs in the coronary artery or carotid artery because it leads to myocardial or cerebral infarction, respectively. There is likewise the risk that a piece of the thrombus can break off and form an embolism that subsequently lodges elsewhere in the vascular system. For example, a thrombus that forms in the large veins in the legs can dislodge and travel to the lungs where it creates a pulmonary embolism.

Consequently, drugs are often administered to reduce the risk of various clotting problems in people with evidence of excessive blood clotting.[36] These drugs typically work by affecting one or more of the clotting factors illustrated in Fig. 8-3. These drugs are likewise categorized as anticoagulant, antithrombotic, and thrombolytic agents depending on how they affect the clotting activity. The three drug categories are summarized in Table 8-3, and they are addressed here.

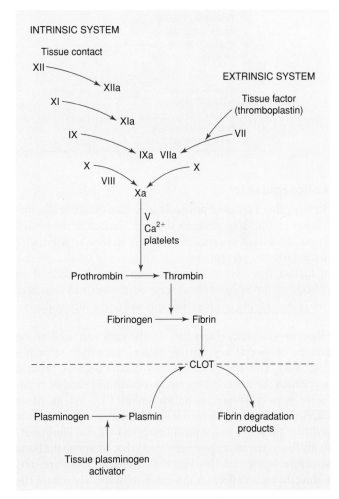

FIGURE 8-3 Mechanism of blood coagulation. Factors involved in clot formation are shown above the dashed line; factors involved in clot breakdown are shown below the dashed line. See text for details about how specific drugs can modify these clotting mechanisms. (Ciccone CD. *Pharmacology in Rehabilitation*. 4th ed. Philadelphia, PA: FA Davis; 2007:348, with permission.)

TABLE 8-3   Drugs Used to Treat Overactive Clotting

Drug Category	Primary Effect and Indication

Anticoagulants
  Heparins
    Unfractionated heparin (generic)
    Low-molecular-weight heparins
      Dalteparin (Fragmin)
      Enoxaparin (Lovenox)
      Tinzaparin (Innohep)
  Oral anticoagulants
    Warfarin (Coumadin, Jantoven)
  Direct thrombin inhibitors
    Argatroban (generic)
    Bivalirudin (Angiomax)
    Lepirudin (Refludan)
  Factor Xa inhibitor
    Fondaparinux (Arixtra)
	Inhibit synthesis and function of clotting factors; used primarily to prevent and treat venous thromboembolism

Antithrombotics
  Aspirin
  Other platelet aggregation inhibitors
    Clopidogrel (Plavix)
    Ticlopidine (Ticlid)
    Abciximab (ReoPro)
    Eptifibatide (Integrilin)
    Tirofiban (Aggrastat)
	Inhibit platelet aggregation and platelet-induced clotting; used primarily to prevent arterial thrombus formation

Thrombolytics
  Alteplase (Activase)
  Reteplase (Retavase)
  Streptokinase (Streptase)
  Tenecteplase (TNKase)
  Urokinase (Kinlytic)
	Facilitate clot dissolution; used to reopen occluded vessels in arterial and venous thrombosis

Anticoagulants

Anticoagulants are used primarily to reduce excessive clot formation in the large veins in the legs (venous thrombosis). These drugs act on specific clotting factors to normalize hemostasis and prevent venous thrombosis or reduce the risk of further thrombosis in people who have already had an episode of thromboembolic disease. Anticoagulants consist of two primary types of drugs: heparin and oral anticoagulants.

Heparin—Heparin enters the bloodstream and inhibits the activity of several key clotting factors, including thrombin (Fig. 8-3). This inhibition actually occurs because heparin accelerates the reaction between thrombin and another circulating protein known as antithrombin III.[37] As its name implies, antithrombin III binds to thrombin and decreases the ability of thrombin to convert fibrinogen to fibrin. Fibrin normally forms the sticky protein strands that comprise the basic structure of the clot (see Fig. 8-3). Heparin, therefore, acts indirectly via an effect on thrombin to ultimately reduce the formation of one of the components that creates a clot (fibrin), thereby reducing the risk of thrombosis.

The anticoagulant effects of heparin occur rapidly; that is, this drug begins to affect thrombin, fibrin, and so forth, as soon as it enters the bloodstream. Unfortunately, heparin is absorbed poorly from the upper gastrointestinal tract, and this drug must, therefore, be administered by parenteral (nonoral)

routes. The traditional form of heparin, known as unfractionated heparin, is typically administered by repeated intravenous infusion. More recently, a subtype of heparin has been extracted from the unfractionated form of this drug. These newer forms are known as low-molecular-weight heparins (LMWHs) to distinguish them chemically from the more general or unfractionated forms of heparin.[38] Some common LMWHs include enoxaparin (Lovenox), dalteparin (Fragmin), and similar drugs with generic names that end with the "-parin" suffix. LMWHs also offer some distinct advantages over the unfractionated forms, including the ability to administer the LMWHs by subcutaneous injection, much in the same way that insulin is administered to treat diabetes mellitus. Other advantages of LMWHs over unfractionated heparin include a more predictable response, fewer side effects, and less need to perform laboratory monitoring of clotting time.[38,39]

Heparin treatment is, therefore, helpful in the initial treatment of venous thrombosis because of its rapid effects. The emergence of the LMWHs has also substantially improved the convenience and safety of these drugs in helping control venous thromboembolic disease. The development of LMWHs has also expanded the use of this form of anticoagulant therapy, and LMWHs are now being considered for the treatment of other forms of thrombosis including acute myocardial infarction and ischemic stroke.[40,41] Still, heparin therapy, including use of LMWHs, is associated with some potentially serious side effects including an increased risk of bleeding in various tissues throughout the body. In certain patients, heparin and LMWHs can also activate the immune system to form antibodies that cause increased platelet aggregation (thrombocytopenia) that results in a paradoxical *increase* in blood coagulation. This condition, known commonly as heparin-induced thrombocytopenia (HIT), can be severe and life-threatening because of widespread platelet-induced clotting in various blood vessels.[42]

Oral anticoagulants—This group of *anticoagulants* consists of warfarin (Coumadin), dicumarol, and similar agents (Table 8-3). These drugs act on the liver to inhibit the production of certain clotting factors. Specifically, these drugs inhibit the regeneration of vitamin K in the liver.[43,44] Vitamin K normally helps to catalyze the hepatic production of certain clotting factors (eg, clotting factors VII, IX, and X; see Fig. 8-3). By limiting the amount of vitamin K that is available in the liver, oral anticoagulants (also known as vitamin K antagonists) delay the production of these clotting factors, thereby decreasing the ability of the blood to clot.

As their name implies, these drugs can be administered orally. There is, however, a time lag of 3 to 5 days before these drugs exert their therapeutic effects and reduce hemostasis to normal levels.[43] This time lag occurs because these drugs gradually reduce the hepatic production of clotting factors while the body metabolizes the clotting factors that are already in the bloodstream. Several days are needed to reach a balance between reduced clotting factor production in the liver and the appearance of lower and more reasonable amounts of these clotting factors in the circulation.

Hence, oral anticoagulants are often used sequentially with heparin. At the onset of a thrombosis, heparin therapy is initiated to cause a rapid effect and normalization of clotting time. Traditional treatment protocols then called for a change from heparin to oral anticoagulants within 2 to 3 days, with heparin being discontinued after 4 to 5 days.[45] This sequence allowed the rapid effects of heparin to overlap with the more gradual effects of the oral anticoagulants. With the advent of LMWHs, however, some patients are now remaining on the LMWH heparin for much longer periods (12 days or more) before being switched to oral anticoagulants such as warfarin. Regardless of when the patient is switched to the oral anticoagulant, many patients must remain on the oral anticoagulant for several weeks to several months depending on the specific needs of each patient.[45]

As is the case with all anticlotting drugs, the primary problem associated with oral anticoagulants is the increased risk of bleeding and hemorrhage in various tissues and organs.[43] This risk is obviously increased if patients are taking these drugs in high doses for extended periods of time. Overdose can likewise cause serious or even fatal bleeding. Physical therapists should, therefore, be aware of any symptoms or discomfort that might indicate hemorrhage in patients taking these drugs. A patient, for example, with sudden or unexplained joint pain may be experiencing intrajoint hemorrhage. Therapists should alert the medical staff about any increase in symptoms that might be associated with increased hemorrhage in patients taking oral anticoagulants or any anticlotting drug.

Other anticoagulants—Several other strategies have been developed to prevent excessive clotting that leads to venous thrombosis (see Table 8-3).[46] These strategies include drugs that directly inhibit thrombin activity, such as lepirudin (Refludan), bivalirudin (Angiomax), and argatroban. Drugs have also been developed that inhibit other specific clotting factors, including fondaparinux (Arixtra), which inhibits the active form of clotting factor 10 (factor Xa). Efforts continue to develop other agents that can serve as alternatives to traditional anticoagulants such as heparin and warfarin.

Antithrombotics

Antithrombotics are characterized by their ability to decrease platelet activity and reduce clots formed by platelet aggregation.[36,47] These platelet-induced clots often occur in arteries including the coronary arteries and carotid arteries. Antithrombotic drugs are, therefore, useful in preventing myocardial infarction, ischemic stroke, and other problems associated with arterial thrombus formation. These drugs essentially work by inhibiting the ability of specific endogenous chemicals to stimulate platelets (see Fig. 8-3), thereby preventing abnormal platelet activation. The primary antithrombotic strategies are described here.

Aspirin—*Aspirin* is well known for its analgesic, anti-inflammatory, and antifever effects. Over the past several years, the realization that aspirin can also produce therapeutic antithrombotic effects has led to some exciting and innovative treatment for myocardial infarction.[48] Aspirin exerts all of its therapeutic effects by inhibiting the production of prostaglandins. Specifically, aspirin inhibits the cyclooxygenase enzyme that is responsible for producing prostaglandins in various cells throughout the body. Prostaglandins are small lipid compounds that help regulate cell activity during normal function and when cells are injured or diseased. Certain prostaglandins, known as thromboxanes, are particularly important in regulating platelet activity. Thromboxanes that are produced by the cyclooxygenase enzyme cause platelets to change their shape and begin to stick together (aggregate) at the site where a clot is forming. By inhibiting the production of thromboxanes, aspirin can reduce this platelet activity and prevent excessive or abnormal platelet-induced clotting (Fig. 8-4).[49]

Aspirin can, therefore, be considered an "antiplatelet" drug that is useful in preventing heart attacks. Aspirin can also be used to help prevent other platelet-induced thrombi, including certain forms of ischemic stroke.[47] Use of aspirin in stroke remains somewhat controversial, however, and aspirin must be used very cautiously in treating stroke because of the risk of increased intracranial bleeding. Aspirin can likewise be used to help prevent deep vein thrombosis, to prevent occlusion

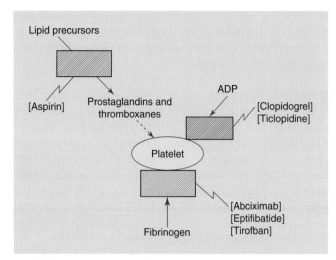

FIGURE 8-4   Effects of antithrombotic agents on platelet activation. Platelets are normally activated by endogenous chemicals such as the thromboxanes, adenosine diphosphate (ADP), and fibrinogen. Specific drugs (indicated in brackets) limit the production or block the effects of these chemicals on the platelet, thereby reducing platelet-induced clotting.

of arterial grafts (including coronary bypass surgery), and to decrease the risk of thrombogenesis following valve replacement and similar cardiac procedures.

What is also remarkable is that substantial antithrombotic effects can be achieved using very low doses of aspirin. Many antithrombotic regimens use aspirin doses of 1 adult aspirin tablet (325 mg) or even 1 pediatric tablet (81 mg) per day.[50,51] At these doses, the side effects commonly associated with aspirin, including gastric irritation and liver/kidney toxicity, are minimal. As indicated earlier, all drugs that reduce clotting may increase the risk of hemorrhage, and the risk of intracranial hemorrhage and other types of bleeding must be considered in each patient receiving aspirin therapy. Nonetheless, aspirin therapy has become a well-accepted method for preventing an initial episode of myocardial infarction, and aspirin is often an essential part of the treatment of secondary prevention in people who have already had a heart attack or certain people with ischemic stroke.

Other antithrombotic agents—Although aspirin is commonly used to decrease platelet-induced clotting, this drug is only a weak inhibitor of platelet activity. Hence, other strategies have been explored to provide more powerful antiplatelet effects. One alternative is to use drugs that block the effects of adenosine diphosphate (ADP) on the platelet[52] (Fig. 8-4). Like thromboxanes, ADP also stimulates platelet activity and causes the platelet to aggregate and form a thrombus. Certain drugs such as clopidogrel (Plavix) and ticlopidine (Ticlid) occupy and block the ADP receptor located on the platelet, thereby preventing ADP from activating the platelet and causing aggregation and thrombogenesis. Another option is to use drugs known as glycoprotein (GP) IIb/IIIa inhibitors.[53] These drugs inhibit the effects of other platelet-stimulating sub-

stances such as fibrinogen (Fig. 8-4). Fibrinogen normally activates the platelet by binding to the GP IIb/IIIa receptor, but drugs such as abciximab (ReoPro), eptifibatide (Integrilin), and tirofiban (Aggrastat) block this receptor and prevent fibrinogen from increasing platelet aggregation.

These newer antiplatelet drugs, therefore, offer some alternatives to aspirin therapy. Once again, the primary problem associated with these drugs is the increased risk of hemorrhage, especially with the GP IIb/IIIa inhibitors. The ADP inhibitors seem to be safer in terms of less chance of bleeding, but clopidogrel can cause pain in the chest and elsewhere throughout the body, and ticlopidine may cause skin rashes and gastrointestinal disturbances.

Thrombolytics

Drugs such as the anticoagulants (heparin, Coumadin) and antithrombotics (aspirin, others) can help normalize blood clotting and prevent further thrombogenesis. These drugs, however, do not appreciably affect clots that have already formed. A third category of drugs known as thrombolytics is so named because they activate clot breakdown (thrombolysis) and reestablish blood flow through the occluded vessel.[54] If administered in a timely manner, thrombolytics can reopen the vessel, restore blood flow to the tissue supplied by that vessel, and prevent tissue death.

Commonly used thrombolytics include streptokinase (Streptase), urokinase (Kinlytic), and several similar agents (Table 8-3). Although these drugs differ from one another in their exact mechanism of action, they all increase the conversion of plasminogen to plasmin in the bloodstream.[55] Plasmin (also known as fibrinolysin) is the activated form of the enzyme that initiates fibrin degradation and clot breakdown (Fig. 8-3). Thrombolytic drugs, therefore, stimulate the body's endogenous mechanism for destroying clots and help maintain blood flow through any vessels that have become occluded by a thrombus.

Thrombolytic drugs have been used primarily to reopen occluded coronary vessels in people who are in the process of developing a myocardial infarction.[56] When administered intravenously, these drugs activate plasmin throughout the systemic circulation. Plasmin travels throughout the systemic circulation until it arrives at the occluded coronary vessel and lyses the thrombus, thereby restoring blood flow to the myocardium and salvaging the function of the cardiac tissue. Although thrombolytic drugs can provide benefits if administered up to 12 hours after the onset of symptoms, optimal effects are realized if these drugs are administered as soon as possible after coronary thrombosis.[57]

Thrombolytic agents, therefore, represent one of the most important advances in the treatment of acute myocardial infarction, and proper use of these drugs has helped to increase the survival and outcome of many people who would have otherwise succumbed to a heart attack. These drugs may also provide benefits in other types of acute infarction including severe deep venous thrombosis and pulmonary embolism. Thrombolytics may likewise be considered as an option in treating ischemic stroke.[58] By lysing cerebral thrombi, these drugs have the potential to restore blood flow to the brain and attenuate the damage that occurs in ischemic stroke. Thrombolytics must, however, be used very cautiously in treating stroke because of the increased risk of intracranial bleeding, and these drugs should be administered only after diagnostic tests (eg, computerd tomography) have conclusively ruled out the possibility of cerebral hemorrhage. There is likewise a much smaller window of opportunity for administering these drugs during ischemic stroke, and they must typically be administered within 3 hours to decrease neurological deficits and improve outcomes in people with ischemic stroke.[58]

The primary drawback of thrombolytic therapy is the increased risk of bleeding and hemorrhage.[59] These drugs activate clot breakdown throughout the systemic circulation in a rather nonselective manner. As a result, the ability to generate and sustain beneficial clots in the vasculature can also be impaired leading to hemorrhage in the brain, abdominal cavity, joints, and so forth. This chance of hemorrhage is increased in certain high-risk patients, including older individuals, people with severe or untreated hypertension, and people with a history of hemorrhagic stroke or other bleeding disorders. Thrombolytic drugs should, therefore, be used cautiously in situations where the benefit of restoring blood flow through an occluded vessel far outweighs the risk of hemorrhage elsewhere in the vascular system.

Smoking Cessation Drugs

Cigarette smoking is one of the primary risk factors for developing cardiovascular disease and pulmonary problems such as emphysema and lung cancer. Strategies to quit smoking are, therefore, an essential component in the prevention and risk reduction for cardiopulmonary disorders. Three primary drug strategies addressed here are nicotine replacement therapy, bupropion, and varenicline.

Nicotine Replacement Therapy

The primary pharmacological intervention used to help people quit smoking is *nicotine replacement*.[60] Cigarettes are essentially a method for delivering nicotine, and smokers typically become hooked on cigarettes because of nicotine's strong addictive potential. Alternative methods for delivering nicotine have therefore been developed. Nicotine can be administered via patches, gum, tablets/lozenges, inhalers, or nasal sprays.[60] Nicotine patches have received a great deal of publicity, because this method of administration is convenient and provides a slow, steady influx of nicotine to help diminish the craving for this drug. A series of patches can also be used as part of a plan to wean the person from nicotine, with the dose of nicotine in these patches being progressively diminished over the course of several weeks.

Nicotine replacement therapies can increase the likelihood that a person can successfully quit smoking by approximately 50% to 75%.[60] The success of nicotine replacement therapy can also be enhanced when combined with other nonpharmacological interventions including social support and counseling that provides strategies to resist or avoid the cues that initiate the desire for a cigarette.[60]

Problems associated with nicotine patches or gum include nausea and mild headache. Because nicotine stimulates catecholamine release, nicotine replacement may be contraindicated in people with certain types of cardiovascular disease including severe angina pectoris, life-threatening arrhythmias, recent myocardial infarction, or recent cerebrovascular accident. Nicotine patches may likewise cause skin irritation and may be contraindicated in people with sensitive skin or dermatological disease.

Bupropion

Bupropion (Zyban) is another pharmacological strategy used to help people quit smoking.[61] This drug was developed originally as an antidepressant but is also marketed as a method for smoking cessation. Exactly how bupropion helps people quit smoking is not clear, but this drug may decrease nicotine cravings by potentiating the effects of dopamine and norepinephrine in the brain.[62] Bupropion acts on specific CNS synapses in the limbic system that release dopamine and norepinephrine. This drug inhibits the reuptake of these neurotransmitters after they are released from the presynaptic terminal, thus potentiating their effects on the postsynaptic neuron. Nicotine and other addictive substances may mediate some of their effects through increased dopamine release in the limbic system, and bupropion may, therefore, help substitute for the nicotine effects by increasing dopamine influence in the brain. By also increasing norepinephrine influence in the brain, bupropion may help diminish the severity of nicotine withdrawal.[62]

When used as an antismoking agent, bupropion is typically administered at a dose of 300 mg/d for 7 to 12 weeks. This dosage regimen is generally well tolerated, with the most common side effects being insomnia and dry mouth, although seizures can occur in rare cases.[61] As is the case with nicotine replacement therapy, the success of bupropion is enhanced when this drug is combined with nonpharmacological interventions such as counseling and social support. Still, bupropion is only partially successful in long-term smoking cessation, with only 23% of people using this drug remaining cigarette-free 1 year after quitting smoking.[63] The success rate of people who took bupropion, however, was approximately twice that of people who took a placebo.[63] The rather poor success rates of bupropion and other interventions such as nicotine replacement therapy underscore a basic fact: Nicotine is highly addictive, and it is often very difficult to quit smoking after developing a habit for cigarettes.

Varenicline

Varenicline (Chantix) is a relatively new non-nicotine drug developed to help people quit smoking. This drug binds to nicotine receptors in the brain, thereby preventing nicotine from stimulating these receptors.[64] This drug, however, is classified as a nicotine receptor *partial agonist*, which means that it blocks the receptor from nicotine supplied by cigarettes while still providing some stimulation of the receptor. Low-level stimulation of the nicotine receptor will hopefully reduce nicotine cravings and prevent the smoker from going into withdrawal.[64] This drug can, therefore, be substituted for cigarettes and then slowly withdrawn as other interventions (counseling and support) are implemented.

Varenicline can increase the success rate of quitting cigarettes when compared to a placebo or other pharmacological interventions such as bupropion.[65] Some possible side effects include headache, drowsiness, GI problems (nausea, gas, constipation), and disturbed sleeping. This drug, however, is generally tolerated well by most people at the dosages used to quit smoking.[65] Varenicline is, therefore, an alternative treatment for patients who cannot tolerate other pharmacological treatments (nicotine replacement, bupropion), or when other interventions have not been successful in maintaining abstinence from cigarettes.

MEDICATIONS RELATED TO PREFERRED PRACTICE PATTERN B: IMPAIRED AEROBIC CAPACITY/ENDURANCE ASSOCIATED WITH DECONDITIONING

Many medications can help increase endurance and reduce deconditioning by treating systemic disorders. Pharmacologic treatment of conditions such as cancer, acquired immune deficiency syndrome (AIDS), and various musculoskeletal and neuromuscular disorders can enable patients to participate in endurance conditioning and other activities that help maintain and improve function and overall health. It is, however, beyond the scope of this chapter to discuss all of the medications that are directly used to treat these noncardiopulmonary conditions. There are likewise several groups of medications that are used to directly treat cardiopulmonary disorders, thereby helping improve endurance and aerobic capacity. These medications are described in other sections of this chapter that are related more closely to the preferred practice patterns used to treat specific cardiovascular and pulmonary problems (cardiovascular pump dysfunction, airway clearance dysfunction, and so forth). Hence, please refer to the other sections of this chapter for cardiopulmonary medications that have more direct effects on the cardiovascular and respiratory systems, and can, therefore, have a secondary effect on improving endurance and aerobic capacity in various systemic disorders.

There are, nonetheless, some systemic disorders that are associated closely with the cardiopulmonary systems and where the drug treatment of these disorders is directly implicated in maintaining proper cardiovascular and respiratory function. Two of these disorders, diabetes mellitus and obesity, are addressed here.

Diabetes Mellitus

Diabetes mellitus is a disease caused by inadequate insulin production (type 1 diabetes) or decreased tissue sensitivity to insulin (type 2 diabetes).[66] Problems related to decreased production or effects of insulin include an impaired ability to store glucose in muscle and other tissues as well as alterations in the ability to store lipids and synthesize proteins. Defects in glucose storage can result in acute problems such as hypoglycemia because the body is not able to draw upon glucose reserves in muscle and other tissues. Likewise, blood glucose levels often increase dramatically following a meal (postprandial hyperglycemia), and prolonged, repeated exposure of blood vessels to elevated blood glucose levels can lead to pathological changes in the blood vessel wall (angiopathy) that ultimately causes narrowing and occlusion of the vessel. Angiopathy subsequently leads to many of the chronic sequelae associated with poorly controlled diabetes, including cardiovascular pathology (hypertension, myocardial infarction, cerebrovascular accident) and other problems such as poor wound healing, neuropathy, nephropathy, and retinopathy.

Fortunately, drug therapy used in combination with proper diet and exercise can help maintain normal blood glucose levels and therefore prevent the complications seen with uncontrolled diabetes mellitus. The drugs commonly used to control blood glucose levels in people with diabetes are summarized in Table 8-4, and these drugs are briefly discussed here.

Insulin

Insulin replacement is the cornerstone of drug treatment for type 1 diabetes, with the dosage and type of insulin determined according to the specific needs of each patient.[67] *Insulin* is a polypeptide and is typically administered by parental methods such as subcutaneous injection. In addition to regular insulin (insulin that is identical to human insulin), biosynthetic techniques have been used to modify the insulin molecule to either increase or decrease the rate of insulin absorption. People can, therefore, use these insulin analogues to achieve optimal glycemic control as needed throughout the day or night.[68] Some alternative ways to administer insulin have also been explored, including insulin pumps, transcutaneous insulin administration, or administration via other routes (nasal sprays, intrapulmonary inhalation, and so forth). It is beyond the scope of this chapter to describe these innovative methods for insulin delivery, and more information can be found in other sources.[69,70]

Oral Antidiabetic Agents

The primary form of drug treatment in type 2 diabetes consists of drugs that can be administered orally and help maintain normal blood glucose levels, that is, *oral antidiabetic agents* (see Table 8-4).[71] These drugs work by various methods summarized in Table 8-4. In some patients, a single agent may be successful in managing blood glucose levels, but specific combinations may also be used to provide optimal glycemic control. For example, a drug that increases insulin release from the pancreas (eg, a sulfonylurea) might be combined with a drug that decreases hepatic glucose production and increases insulin sensitivity (metformin) and possibly a third agent that decreases glucose absorption from the gastrointestinal tract (acarbose). Insulin therapy can also be included in this drug regimen, especially in patients with severe or poorly

TABLE 8-4 Drugs Used to Treat Diabetes Mellitus

Type of Insulin	Effects (h)			Common Examples[a]	
	Onset	Peak	Duration	Human	Animal
Rapid acting					
Regular insulin	0.5–1	2–4	5–7	Humulin R, Novolin R	Regular Iletin II
Aspart	0.25	0.6–0.8	3–5	NovoLog	—
Lispro	<0.5	0.5–1.5	2–5	Humalog	—
Glulisine	—	0.5–1.5	1–2.5	Apidra	—
Intermediate acting					
Isophane insulin	3–4	6–12	18–28	Humulin N, Novolin N	NPH insulin, NPH purified insulin, NPH Iletin II
Insulin zinc	1–3	8–12	18–28	Humulin L, Novolin L	Lente insulin, Lente insulin II
Long acting					
Glargine	2–5	5–24	18–24	Lantus	—
Extended insulin zinc	4–6	18–24	36	Humulin U	—

Oral Antidiabetic Agents	Mechanism of Action and Effects	Primary Adverse Effects
Classification and examples[b]		

Sulfonylureas
  Acetohexamide (Dymelor)
  Chlorpropamide (Diabinese)
  Glimepiride (Amaryl)
  Glipizide (Glucotrol)
  Glyburide (DiaBeta, Micronase)
  Tolazamide (Tolinase)
  Tolbutamide (Orinase)
	Increase insulin secretion from pancreatic beta cells; increased insulin release helps reduce blood glucose by increasing glucose storage in muscle and by inhibiting hepatic glucose production	Hypoglycemia is the most common and potentially serious side effect of the sulfonylureas; other bothersome effects (GI disturbances headache, etc) may also occur depending on the specific agent

Biguanides Metformin (Glucophage)	Act directly on the liver to decrease hepatic glucose production; also increase sensitivity of peripheral tissues (muscle) to insulin	Gastrointestinal disturbances; lactic acidosis may also occur in rare cases, but this effect could be severe or fatal

α-Glucosidase inhibitors
  Acarbose (Precose)
  Miglitol (Glyset)
	Inhibit sugar breakdown in the intestines and delay glucose absorption from the GI tract	Gastrointestinal disturbances

Thiazolidinediones
  Pioglitazone (Actos)
  Rosiglitazone (Avandia)
	Similar to the biguanides (metformin)	Headache, dizziness, fatigue/weakness, back pain; rare but potentially severe cases of hepatic toxicity may also occur

Benzoic acid derivatives
  Repaglinide (Prandin)
  Nateglinide (Starlix)
	Similar to the sulfonylureas	Hypoglycemia, bronchitis, upper respiratory tract infections, joint pain and back pain, GI disturbances, headache

[a]Examples are trade names of insulin preparations derived from recombinant or biosynthetic techniques (human insulin) or purified pork insulin (animal sources).

[b]Examples include generic names with trade names listed in parentheses.

Reprinted from Ciccone CD. *Pharmacology in Rehabilitation.* 4th ed. Philadelphia, PA: FA Davis; 2007:484 and 487, with permission.

controlled type 2 diabetes.[72] Specific drug combinations must be selected based on the individual needs of each patient, but the use of several agents may ultimately provide the best treatment by controlling different aspects of glucose metabolism in people with type 2 diabetes.

The primary adverse effect associated with all antidiabetic medications (insulin, oral antidiabetics) is hypoglycemia.[73] If these drugs are too effective in lowering blood glucose, patients may become irritable, confused, or diaphoretic, have increased heart rate, or exhibit other signs typical of hypoglycemia. Acute episodes of hypoglycemia can usually be resolved by administering some source of glucose, such as fruit juice or glucose tablets. Repeated episodes of hypoglycemia may require an adjustment in drug dosage or a change in the type of drug being administered.

Obesity

Obesity increases the risk for developing many pathological conditions including hypertension, diabetes mellitus, and myocardial infarction.[74] Successful treatment of obesity typically requires a combination of several interventions including diet, exercise, counseling, and so forth.[74] The use of drugs to manage obesity is often controversial because of the potential for drug abuse and adverse effects of these drugs. Nonetheless, judicious use of antiobesity drugs can be a valuable part of a comprehensive treatment plan for people who are obese but have been unable to lose weight through nonpharmacological interventions (diet and exercise).[74] Drugs used to treat obesity are listed in Table 8-5, and the rationale for using these drugs is addressed here.

TABLE 8-5   Drugs Used to Treat Obesity

Category and Examples[a]	Primary Effects

Sympathomimetic appetite suppressants
  Benzphetamine (Didrex)
  Diethylpropion (Tenuate)
  Methamphetamine (Desoxyn)
  Phendimetrazine (Bontril, others)
  Phentermine (Adipex-P)
	May decrease appetite with a subsequent reduction in caloric intake by increasing the influence of norepinephrine and dopamine in the lateral hypothalamic feeding center

Lipase inhibitors Orlistat (Alli, Xenical)	Reduces fat absorption into the body by inhibiting fat breakdown in the gastrointestinal tract
Serotonin–norepinephrine reuptake inhibitors Sibutramine (Meridia)	May suppress appetite by increasing the effects of serotonin and norepinephrine in the brain

[a]Examples are the generic name with common trade names shown in parentheses.

Sympathomimetic Appetite Suppressants

Many common appetite suppressants have amphetamine-like properties and generally increase sympathetic nervous system (sympathomimetic) effects in the body. When used as appetite suppressants, these agents are thought to increase the effects of norepinephrine and possibly dopamine at specific synapses located in the lateral hypothalamic feeding center.[75,76] Although the details are not clear, increased release or effects of these neurotransmitters in the hypothalamus decrease hunger sensations and increase feelings of satiety. Consequently most, if not all, of the weight loss that occurs with these drugs is due to decreased food intake rather than other effects such as increased tissue metabolism or thermogenesis.

Common appetite suppressants are listed in Table 8-5. Although these agents can be used as part of a comprehensive weight loss program, their use as appetite suppressants is often questionable because of their strong potential for adverse effects and abuse. In particular, these drugs are notorious for producing CNS excitation and cardiovascular stimulation.[77] That is, these agents increase sympathetic nervous activity via their influence on sympathetic transmitters such as norepinephrine. These sympathomimetic effects can be quite severe, and cardiovascular problems such as hypertension and cardiac arrhythmias may occur, especially in people with preexisting cardiovascular disease. Tolerance to these agents also develops within a few weeks after initiating treatment, and dosages often need to be increased to maintain their therapeutic effects.[77] Considering these limitations, appetite suppressants may be helpful in short-term management to get the patient's weight under control, but these drugs can hopefully be discontinued in favor of more long-term solutions such as diet and exercise.

Other Antiobesity Drugs

Several other drugs can be used to help treat obesity (Table 8-5). *Orlistat* (Xenical) is a lipase inhibitor that acts within the gastrointestinal tract to limit the breakdown and subsequent absorption of dietary fat.[78] This effect helps reduce body weight because less dietary fat is absorbed and stored within the body. Orlistat may, however, cause a number of gastrointestinal problems including abdominal pain, flatulence, and fecal incontinence.[79] *Sibutramine* (Meridia) is another form of appetite suppressant, but this drug differs from the typical suppressants described earlier because sibutramine increases the effects of serotonin and norepinephrine in the CNS.[79] The benefit of increased serotonin activity may be especially helpful in providing feelings of satiety and therefore reduced food intake. Side effects associated with sibutramine include increased blood pressure, insomnia, dizziness, dry mouth, and nausea.

In recognition of the benefits of increasing serotonin activity to help control appetite, several other strategies have been used to increase CNS serotonergic activity. One strategy combined fenfluramine, a serotonin-enhancing drug, with phentermine, an amphetamine-like appetite suppressant.[80] This combination, known commonly as fen/phen, caused severe cardiopulmonary problems including pulmonary vasoconstriction and cardiac valve damage.[80] Consequently, fenfluramine and a related drug, dexfenfluramine, were removed from the market.

It is also recognized that certain endogenous neuropeptides are critical in regulating appetite and energy metabolism. Central neuropeptides such as neuropeptide Y, agouti-related peptide, orexins, and the melanocortins appear to regulate hypothalamic function, while peripheral neuropeptides such as cholecystokinin, leptin, and ghrelin may provide feedback control of CNS appetite mechanisms.[81] Research is currently under way to develop drugs that might influence these neuropeptides, and thereby help control appetite. Although this research has not yet produced any commercially successful products, drugs that help suppress appetite by influencing these central and peripheral neuropeptides might soon be forthcoming.[82]

Drug treatment for obesity, therefore, remains somewhat questionable at the present time. There is little doubt that antiobesity interventions should center on a lifelong program of diet and exercise.[83] The drugs addressed here may help complement such a program, but all the currently available antiobesity drugs produce side effects, and there is no guarantee that weight loss will be maintained if the drug is discontinued and poor eating habits are resumed. Perhaps new antiobesity drugs will be developed in the future that are safer and more effective, but the best way to prevent and treat obesity at the present time remains centered around nonpharmacological methods.

MEDICATIONS RELATED TO PREFERRED PRACTICE PATTERN C: IMPAIRED VENTILATION, RESPIRATION/GAS EXCHANGE, AND AEROBIC CAPACITY/ENDURANCE ASSOCIATED WITH AIRWAY CLEARANCE DYSFUNCTION

Airway clearance dysfunction can be treated pharmacologically in several different ways (Table 8-6). Certain medications can be used to decrease irritation and control excessive airway secretions in fairly minor and transient situations such as seasonal allergies and common upper respiratory tract infections. Some of these same medications can likewise be used to facilitate airway clearance in more chronic and potentially serious conditions such as asthma, chronic bronchitis, and emphysema. Specific medications that relax bronchiole smooth muscle (bronchodilators) or decrease airway inflammation are also essential in helping maintain airway function in many forms of pulmonary disease. These pharmacological strategies for treating problems related to airway clearance are addressed in this section.

TABLE 8-6   Respiratory Medications

Drug Category	Common Examples[a]
Drugs used to control airway irritation and secretion	
Antitussives	Benzonatate (Tessalon)
	Codeine (contained in many cough/cold products)
	Dextromethorphan (contained in many cough/cold products)
	Hydrocodone (contained in many cough/cold products)
Antihistamines	Brompheniramine (Veltane, others)
	Cetirizine (Zyrtec)
	Chlorpheniramine (Chlor-Trimeton, others)
	Clemastine (Tavist)
	Diphenhydramine (Benadryl, others)
	Desloratidine (Clarinex)
	Loratadine (Claritin)
Decongestants	Epinephrine (Primatene, other cough/cold products)
	Oxymetazolone (Afrin, Neo-Synephrine, many others)
	Phenylephrine (Vicks Sinex, others)
	Pseudoephedrine (Afrinol, Sudafed, others)
	Tetrahydrozoline (Tyzine)
Mucolytics	Acetylcysteine (Mucomyst, others)
	Dornase alfa (recombinant human deoxyribonuclease I, Pulmozyme)
Expectorants	Guaifenesin (Mucinex, contained in other cough/cold products)
Bronchodilators	
β-Adrenergic agonists	Albuterol (Accuneb, Proventil, others)
	Epinephrine (EpiPen, others)
	Formoterol (Foradil, others)
	Isoproterenol (Isuprel)
	Metaproterenol (Alupent)
	Salmeterol (Serevent)
	Terbutaline (generic)
Xanthine derivatives	Aminophylline (generic)
	Theophylline (Theochron, Theolair, many others)
Anticholinergic agents	Ipratropium (Atrovent, others)
	Tiotropium (Spiriva)
Anti-inflammatory agents	
Glucocorticoids[b]	Beclomethasone (BeconaseAQ, QVAR Oral Inhaler)
	Budesonide (Pulmicort, others)
	Flunisolide (AeroBid, others)
	Fluticasone (Cutivate, Flovent, others)
	Mometasone (Asmanex, Nasonex, others)
	Triamcinolone (Azmacort)
Leukotriene modifiers	Zileuton (Zyflo)
	Montelukast (Singulair)
	Zafirlukast (Accolate)
Cromones	Cromolyn (Intal, Nasalcrom, other trade names)
	Nedocromil (Alocril, Tilade)

[a]Some categories may contain additional agents; only the most commonly used medications are listed here.

[b]Only glucocorticoids that are administered routinely by inhalation are listed here. Other glucocorticoids can be administered systemically in acute or severe conditions.

Drugs Used to Control Respiratory Tract Irritation and Secretion

Antitussives and Antihistamines

Antitussives, known commonly as cough medicines, and antihistamines are among the most commonly used medications worldwide. Antitussives often consist of agents that are classified chemically and functionally as opioids. Although opioids are often used as analgesics, these drugs can also act as antitussives because they suppress the sensitivity of the cough reflex at the brainstem.[84] Irritation of afferent pathways from the airways is normally integrated at the brainstem level, and the cough reflex is initiated from the brainstem through efferent pathways to the respiratory muscles. By suppressing this brainstem integration, airway irritants are less able to stimulate the cough reflex. Hence, certain opioids are typically used as antitussives (see Table 8-6), and these agents are found in many prescription and over-the-counter (OTC) preparations.

The primary problem associated with opioids is the chance for developing addiction. Fortunately, most of the opioids used to treat coughing have a relatively small chance for causing addiction compared with the more powerful opioids used to treat pain (eg, morphine, meperidine, and so forth). Still, excessive and prolonged use of opioid antitussives can produce some degree of tolerance (the need for more drug to achieve therapeutic effects) and dependence (the onset of withdrawal when the drug is stopped), and these drugs should, therefore, be used only for the occasional treatment of coughing.

Antihistamines are so named because these drugs occupy and block the type 1 histamine receptors (H_1 receptor) located on respiratory and other tissues. Histamine is typically released from airway mast cells, following some allergic or infectious challenge, and histamine irritates the upper airway tissues leading to coughing and other symptoms (sneezing, itching in the eyes and nose). By blocking the H_1 receptors, antihistamines prevent histamine from reaching the respiratory tissues, thus reducing the coughing and sneezing that is commonly associated with seasonal allergies, upper respiratory tract infections, and so forth. Antihistamines are, therefore, used alone or in combination with other medications (decongestants, antitussives, and so forth) to treat a wide variety of respiratory tract problems associated with increased histamine release.[85]

Antihistamines, unfortunately, are often associated with sedation, dizziness, and psychomotor slowing. These symptoms occur if the antihistamine crosses the blood–brain barrier and affects areas within the brain that control the level of alertness, including the reticular activating system. Several antihistamines, however, have been developed that do not cross the blood–brain barrier and thus do not cause significant sedation and other CNS-related side effects. These nonsedating antihistamines include loratadine (Claritin), desloratadine (Clarinex), and cetirizine (Zyrtec) (Table 8-6), and these agents are a useful option if sedation must be avoided during antihistamine administration.

As indicated, antitussive and antihistamine medications are often used for the treatment of transient or occasional coughing and other symptoms associated with relatively minor respiratory infections (common cold), seasonal allergies, and similar conditions.[85] A vast array of antitussive products are available directly to consumers, and patients receiving physical therapy may take these OTC products to decrease coughing associated with colds, hay fever, and so forth. There is concern, however, that many of the OTC cough suppressants do not work and that use of these agents is no more effective than placebo in reducing coughing.[85] Hence, some experts have questioned whether OTC cough preparations are justified, especially considering that these preparations might still pose risks to certain populations such as children.[86,87]

On the other hand, prescription agents may help control coughing in patients with more chronic and serious conditions, including asthma and COPD. Hence, physical therapists will often encounter patients who take antitussives for the treatment of coughing associated with more serious problems. There is concern, however, that indiscriminate use of antitussive medications may be counterproductive because these drugs may impair the ability of a "productive" cough to raise secretions and clear harmful substances from the airway. Coughing is the primary defense mechanism used by the lungs to maintain airway patency. To suppress this mechanism may, in some cases, do more harm than good because mucus and other harmful substances will accumulate in the airway. Consequently, antitussives still play an important role in treating patients with persistent and annoying coughs, but these drugs are being used more carefully, especially in people who have a productive cough that is helping to keep the airways open.

Decongestants

Nasal congestion typically occurs because the vasculature within the nasal mucosa dilates in response to some allergen or viral stimulus.[88] Vasodilation within the mucosa causes feelings of congestion and "stuffy head" as well as an increase in discharge from dilated capillaries that creates the familiar "runny nose" associated with allergies, symptoms of the common cold, and so forth. To decrease these symptoms, decongestant medications cause vasoconstriction in the nasal vasculature, thus reducing the swollen nasal membranes and nasal discharge.

Decongestants are classified as α-receptor agonists because they mediate their vasoconstrictive effects by stimulating α_1-receptors located on nasal arterioles and β_2-receptors located on venous smooth muscle.[89] Some α-receptor agonists that are commonly used as decongestants are listed in Table 8-6. Decongestant products can also be administered in several ways, including orally (as tablets, in syrups, and so forth), or by nasal sprays. The effects and side effects of these products are influenced largely by the method of administration and the dosing frequency. A decongestant, for example, will produce relatively specific effects on the nasal vasculature with few side effects if correct amounts of the drug are administered directly to the nasal mucosa via a nasal spray. Overuse and abuse of nasal sprays or oral forms of decongestant medications will produce more side effects because excessive amounts of the drug reach the systemic circulation and affect adrenergic receptors on other tissues, including the CNS, heart, and peripheral vasculature.

Side effects associated with decongestants include headache, nausea, and nervousness. More serious problems will occur if these drugs stimulate cardiac β_1-receptors or cause widespread stimulation of α_1-receptors in the systemic circulation. The effects on the heart and peripheral vasculature can lead to palpitations, arrhythmias, and increased blood pressure, especially if the patient has some preexisting cardiovascular problems. As indicated earlier, the likelihood of these problems is increased if large doses of the decongestant are administered indiscriminately. Patients may also become dependent on decongestants if high dosages are administered for prolonged periods. This dependence is probably caused by excessive stimulation of adrenergic receptors located in the CNS.

Hence, decongestant medications are used to control discharge associated with fairly minor and transient irritation in the nasal mucosa.[90] These drugs are available in many OTC medications and can be easily obtained by consumers. Decongestants are, however, relatively powerful drugs that can produce serious side effects if they are misused. Physical therapists should be aware that inappropriate use can lead to cardiovascular problems, and therapists should monitor heart rate and blood pressure in patients who may be developing cardiovascular problems from the misuse or abuse of these medications.

Mucolytics and Expectorants

Mucolytic medications break up mucus in the airways, thereby enabling the patient to cough up respiratory secretions more easily.[91] Mucolytics such as acetylcysteine (Mucomyst) degrade disulfide bonds within mucus secretions, thus making the mucus less viscous and more fluid. Another type of mucolytic is dornase alfa (Pulmozyme), which is a deoxyribonuclease enzyme that breaks up DNA in respiratory secretions. Under conditions such as cystic fibrosis, DNA is released from various inflammatory cells as these cells degenerate in the airway lumen. The accumulation of this DNA contributes to the viscosity of respiratory secretions and increases the likelihood that these secretions will clog the airway and cause infection and atelectasis. Dornase alfa catalyzes the breakdown of this DNA, thereby making the respiratory secretions less viscous and more amenable to being coughed up and cleared from the airway.

Mucolytics can, therefore, be helpful in various conditions where there is a chance that respiratory secretions may accumulate in the airways. These conditions range from fairly minor respiratory tract secretions to chronic conditions such as cystic fibrosis and COPD. These medications are also tolerated fairly well, although excessive use can cause nausea and vomiting, and irritation of the mouth and throat may occur

when these drugs are administered by inhalation in high doses for prolonged periods. These drugs are nonetheless helpful during physical therapy interventions that increase discharge and clearance of sputum. Airway clearance techniques will be more productive and easier to perform if the mucus in the respiratory tract is less viscous and easier to cough up.

Expectorant medications are also used to facilitate mucus secretion and clearance. Expectorants increase the secretion of a thin, watery sputum in the upper respiratory tract. By increasing the volume while also decreasing the viscosity of respiratory secretions, these drugs may enable the patient to cough up these secretions more easily. The most common expectorant currently used is guaifenesin, which is typically indicated in treating relatively acute and transient upper respiratory tract problems (infections, bronchitis, and so forth). This drug is available in several prescription forms, and it is also included in many OTC products. Guaifenesin is tolerated fairly well, with no major side effects that would jeopardize the therapeutic use of this medication or have a direct impact on the patient's response to physical therapy. There is some concern, however, about whether or not this medication is actually effective in treating respiratory disorders. Despite the widespread use of guaifenesin, there is a little evidence that this drug actually improves airway clearance and increases pulmonary function. Nonetheless, guaifenesin continues to be administered, often in combination with other agents (mucolytics, antitussives), to treat various pulmonary disorders that cause congestion and accumulation of sputum in the airways.

Bronchodilators

Bronchodilators relax airway smooth muscle and increase or maintain the size of the airway lumen. These drugs can be helpful in diseases associated with bronchospasm, including asthma and COPD. The most common bronchodilators are classified as β-adrenergic agonists, xanthine derivatives, or anticholinergic agents (Table 8-6), and these agents are described here.

β-Adrenergic Agonists

β-Adrenergic agonists cause bronchodilation via the mechanism illustrated in Fig. 8-5. These drugs bind to and activate the β_2-receptors located on airway smooth muscle cells. Stimulation of these receptors inhibits respiratory smooth muscle contraction, thus causing relaxation and bronchodilation. This effect is actually mediated by the production of an intracellular chemical known as cAMP (see Fig. 8-5). By activating the β_2-receptor located on the smooth muscle cell membrane, these drugs increase activity of the adenyl cyclase enzyme located on the inner surface of the cell membrane. This enzyme catalyzes the conversion of adenosine triphosphate (ATP) to cAMP within the cell. Increased intracellular cAMP causes activation of other enzymes within the cell (protein kinases) that ultimately cause inhibition of airway smooth muscle contraction. The action of cAMP in this situation is a

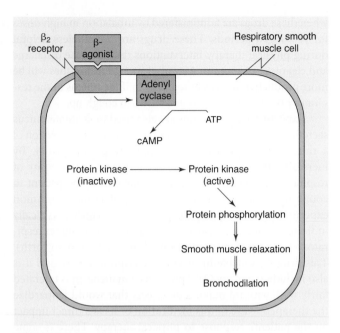

FIGURE 8-5   Mechanism of action of β-agonists on respiratory smooth muscle. β-Agonists facilitate bronchodilation by stimulating adenyl cyclase activity, which in turn increases intracellular cAMP production. cAMP activates protein kinase, which appears to add an inhibitory phosphate group to contractile proteins, thus causing muscle relaxation and bronchodilation. (Ciccone CD. *Pharmacology in Rehabilitation.* 4th ed. Philadelphia, PA: FA Davis; 2007:374, with permission.)

classic example of an intracellular second messenger system. The drug acts as an extracellular "first messenger" that binds to a surface receptor, then initiates the production of an intracellular "second messenger" (cAMP) that relays the message within the cell, and ultimately changes cell function in some way.

β-Adrenergic agonists that are used clinically as bronchodilators can be classified according to their selectivity for β-receptors. Certain agents such as albuterol and terbutaline (see Table 8-6) are fairly selective for β_2-receptors located on respiratory tissues, whereas other agents such as isoproterenol and metaproterenol are not as selective and also stimulate β_1-receptors located on the heart and other tissues. Some agents such as epinephrine may even stimulate α-receptors located on the peripheral vasculature (α_1-receptors) or in the central nervous system (α_2-receptors). A drug that is more selective for β_2-receptors will have the obvious advantage of causing relatively fewer side effects because this drug predominately affects respiratory tissues with minimal effects on the heart, peripheral vasculature, and so forth.

β-Adrenergic bronchodilators can also be classified as either short acting or long acting depending on how long they can sustain their bronchodilating effects with each dose.[92] Long-acting agents are typically more convenient because they do not have to be administered as often, and they may produce a somewhat more stable and predictable response. Finally, β-adrenergic drugs are typically administered orally or by inhalation. By inhaling these drugs through a nebulizer or

metered-dose inhaler, the drug is applied more directly to the respiratory tissues, thus minimizing absorption into the systemic circulation and reducing the chance of side effects on other tissues. Inhalation, however, may not be effective in distributing the drug to the more distal parts of the airway, especially, if the airway is already constricted to some degree. In this case, oral administration may be advantageous because the drug will be absorbed into the bloodstream where it can then be distributed to all aspects of the airway via the pulmonary circulation.

Side effects associated with β-adrenergic agonists are related to drug selectivity and the dose and route of administration. A β_2-selective drug that is administered in limited amounts by inhalation will be relatively free from serious side effects. Overuse of this type of drug, however, can cause irritation of the mouth and upper respiratory tract, which can actually increase the risk of a bronchoconstrictive attack.[93] If high doses of a nonselective β-agonist reach the systemic circulation, this drug may cause stimulation of the heart that leads to cardiac palpitations and arrhythmias. High levels of a nonselective agent in the bloodstream can also cause stimulation of adrenergic receptors in the CNS, resulting in nervousness, irritability, and insomnia.

β-Adrenergic agonists can, therefore, be used safely and effectively as bronchodilators, but overuse should be avoided because of potential toxicity to the lungs and other organs. Proper use of these drugs can allow physical therapists to capitalize on their bronchodilating properties during airway clearance techniques and respiratory exercises. That is, it will be easier for patients to raise secretions and participate in respiratory muscle training if the airways are fairly open and dilated. Therapists should, however, also be alert for any signs of overuse, including cardiac abnormalities (increased pulse rate, arrhythmias) or signs of agitation, anxiety, and so forth.

Xanthine Derivatives

Theophylline and similar drugs (see Table 8-6) are classified chemically as xanthine derivatives because these drugs are structurally similar to other xanthines such as caffeine. For simplicity, theophylline will be used to represent this drug category and illustrate the therapeutic and adverse effects associated with the xanthines. Theophylline is a powerful bronchodilator that appears to relax airway smooth muscle through a combination of several effects.[94] This drug may, for example, inhibit the breakdown of cAMP, thus allowing intracellular cAMP to remain at higher levels and mediate smooth muscle relaxation for longer periods. Theophylline may also cause bronchodilation by inhibiting calcium release within airway smooth muscle cells and by blocking the ability of adenosine to stimulate airway smooth muscle contraction. This drug also appears to have anti-inflammatory effects, and theophylline may mediate some of its bronchodilating effects by controlling airway inflammation (inflammation as a causative factor in bronchospasm is discussed in the next section). Theophylline is, therefore, a fairly complex drug that often helps control bronchoconstriction in asthma, COPD, and other conditions that cause airway constriction.

Theophylline is typically administered orally, although this drug can also be injected intravenously in acute or severe bronchoconstrictive episodes. As indicated earlier, theophylline is structurally and chemically similar to caffeine, and the major problems associated with theophylline are the caffeine-like effects of this drug. Symptoms such as nervousness, trembling, insomnia, nausea, and tachycardia can occur even when plasma drug levels are in the therapeutic range. As plasma levels approach toxic levels, excessive CNS and cardiac stimulation can cause seizures and potentially severe cardiac arrhythmias. Theophylline toxicity is, therefore, a serious concern when this drug is used in fairly high doses.[94] Physical therapists should acknowledge that this drug can produce beneficial effects by helping to maintain airway patency, but therapists should also be alert for any behavioral or cardiac signs (severe nervousness, tremors, arrhythmias, and so forth) that may indicate theophylline toxicity.

Anticholinergic Agents

Anticholinergic drugs are so named because they decrease acetylcholine (cholinergic) activity at various sites in the body. One such site is the lungs, where acetylcholine normally stimulates bronchiole smooth muscle contraction and causes constriction of the airway. By inhibiting this effect, anticholinergic agents help facilitate bronchodilation.[95] Use of these drugs, however, is limited because they tend to inhibit acetylcholine activity on many tissues throughout the body rather than exert anticholinergic effects on only the lungs. By inhibiting acetylcholine activity in other tissues, these drugs cause an array of side effects including dry mouth, constipation, tachycardia, confusion, and blurred vision. Nonetheless, the anticholinergic drugs ipratropium (Atrovent) and tiotropium (Spiriva) can produce fairly localized effects on the lungs, especially when these drugs are administered by inhalation. Consequently, these anticholinergic agents may be used alone or in combination with other bronchodilators such as the β_2 agonists (addressed earlier) to prevent bronchospasm in patients with COPD or asthma.[96]

Treatment of Airway Inflammation

Inflammation within the airway may be the underlying factor that initiates the airway constriction associated with asthma, bronchitis, and other forms of bronchospastic disease.[97] Although the cause of this inflammation may not be clear, the presence of chronic inflammation appears to sensitize the airway and bring about a hyperreactive bronchoconstrictive response. If this inflammation is reduced, many of the problems related to increased airway reactivity (bronchospasm, coughing, and accumulation of secretions) can likewise be controlled or eliminated. Three primary strategies for treating airway inflammation are glucocorticoids, leukotriene modifiers, and cromones (see Table 8-6), and these strategies are described here.

Glucocorticoids

Glucocorticoids are anti-inflammatory steroids that include drugs such as prednisone, cortisone, and agents with similar chemical structures and pharmacological effects. These agents, known also as corticosteroids, are effective in treating inflammation in various tissues because they affect specific regulatory genes within key inflammatory cells such as lymphocytes, eosinophils, neutrophils, and mast cells.[98] Within these cells, glucocorticoids increase the expression of genes that ultimately produce anti-inflammatory proteins (eg, lipocortins), and they decrease the expression of genes that code for inflammatory mediators such as tumor necrosis factor α, interferon-γ, and certain interleukins. Because of their effect at the genomic level, glucocorticoids can inhibit virtually all steps of the inflammatory response.

Glucocorticoids can, therefore, be used to treat inflammation in respiratory and other tissues, but these drugs can also produce several serious side effects. When high doses are administered systemically for prolonged periods, glucocorticoids can cause breakdown (catabolism) of muscle, tendon, bone, skin, and other tissues. Glucocorticoids can potentially cause many other side effects including hypertension, gastric ulcers, exacerbation of diabetes mellitus, glaucoma, and suppression of normal production of cortisol (the body's endogenous glucocorticoid) from the cortex of the adrenal gland (adrenocortical suppression).[99,100] Hence, the benefit of using these drugs to control inflammation must always be balanced against the potential risk of side effects.

With regard to treating bronchoconstrictive diseases, glucocorticoids have long been successful in reducing the inflammation that underlies these diseases and thereby reducing the incidence of bronchospasm. In the past, however, these drugs needed to be administered systemically, usually as oral preparations or by injection during severe attacks. Systemic administration increased the risk of catabolic and other side effects because the drug reached virtually all tissues in the body, rather than just the respiratory tissues.[100] A major breakthrough occurred when glucocorticoids were synthesized in an aerosol format and thus could be administered by inhalation. That is, the chemistry of certain compounds was modified so that these drugs retained their anti-inflammatory effects but were soluble enough to be packaged in aerosol forms, including metered-dose inhalers.

Several glucocorticoids are now available in forms that can be administered by inhalation (see Table 8-6). This type of administration offers the obvious advantage of applying the drug more directly to the inflamed respiratory tissues, with minimal absorption into the systemic circulation. There is, of course, the danger that some of the drug will be absorbed into the pulmonary circulation and eventually be distributed systemically, thus increasing the risk of systemic side effects. This danger seems minimal, however, if the total amount of glucocorticoid inhaled each day is kept below a certain level. Beclomethasone, for example, seems to produce relatively few systemic side effects if less than 1,000 μg is administered by inhalation each day.

Consequently, the development of inhaled forms of glucocorticoids has revolutionized the treatment of asthma and other bronchoconstrictive diseases.[101] These drugs are now incorporated into the treatment regimen much sooner because they do not pose as great a risk as the oral (systemic) forms of treatment. Use of glucocorticoids earlier in the course of the disease may also help delay disease progression and reduce the need for subsequent medications and medical treatment. Physical therapists should realize that the inhaled forms of these drugs can now serve as the cornerstone for treating asthma and other conditions. Therapists should, however, also be aware that these drugs can still cause substantial problems if they are overused or if the patient must revert to systemic administration in severe cases of asthma or COPD.

Leukotriene Modifiers

Leukotrienes are lipid compounds that are produced within cells lining the respiratory mucosa. These compounds are similar in structure and function to prostaglandins. Like the prostaglandins, leukotrienes tend to augment the inflammatory response, and leukotrienes seem to be especially prevalent in mediating inflammation and other effects (edema, increased mucus secretion) in asthma and in similar conditions associated with airway hyperreactivity.[102] It follows that drugs that help control the biosynthesis and effects of leukotrienes will be useful in reducing airway inflammation and preventing bronchospastic attacks.

One way to modify leukotriene effects is to inhibit the enzyme that synthesizes these compounds.[103] Leukotrienes are produced from arachidonic acid by the lipoxygenase enzyme, and several drugs have been developed that selectively inhibit this enzyme. An agent that is currently available is zileuton (Zyflo), with the likelihood that other lipoxygenase inhibitors will be in the market soon. A second option for controlling leukotriene effects is to administer drugs that occupy and block the leukotriene receptor located on respiratory cells.[104] These leukotriene receptor blockers prevent leukotrienes from activating these receptors, thus reducing their ability to inflame the airways and cause bronchoconstriction. Leukotriene receptor blockers that are currently available include montelukast (Singulair) and zafirlukast (Accolate) (Table 8-6).

Agents that modify leukotriene production or effects are tolerated fairly well. Some fairly minor problems such as headache and nausea may occur, and some patients may need to be monitored periodically to guard against more serious problems such as liver toxicity. Nonetheless, the emergence of leukotriene modifiers has been a significant advancement in treating airway inflammation because these drugs may help reduce the need for anti-inflammatory steroids in conditions such as asthma. Development of additional drugs that affect leukotrienes should provide more options for nonsteroidal management of respiratory diseases that have an inflammatory and bronchospastic component.

Cromones

Cromolyn (Intal, Nasalcrom, other trade names) and nedocromil (Alocril, Tilade) help prevent inflammation in the airway by inhibiting the release of inflammatory mediators from cells in the respiratory mucosa. Although the exact cellular mechanism is not known, these drugs stabilize mast cells and possibly other cells (eosinophils, macrophages, neutrophils, and so forth) and thereby decrease the release of histamine, leukotrienes, and other inflammatory chemicals from these cells. These cells, therefore, cannot fully participate in the chemical response that is needed to provoke irritation and inflammation in the airway.

Cromolyn and nedocromil can be administered by inhalation or nasal spray to treat relatively transient conditions such as seasonal allergies. These drugs can likewise be used alone or in combination with other agents (anti-inflammatory steroids, bronchodilators) to decrease inflammation and prevent bronchospasm in more chronic conditions including asthma.[105] When administered in the appropriate inhaled dose, these drugs are remarkably free of serious side effects. One important limitation, however, is that these drugs must be administered prior to exposure to the allergen or irritant that causes inflammation in the airway. That is, cromolyn and nedocromil must be present to stabilize mast cells and other inflammatory cells before these cells become stimulated and release histamine, leukotrienes, and so forth. These drugs can prevent an allergic or bronchospastic attack, but they cannot stop an attack that is already in progress. When used to control chronic conditions, these drugs must, therefore, be taken continuously to provide a prophylactic effect and control airway inflammation. Still, these agents afford one more option in the treatment of airway inflammation and bronchospasm, and physical therapists may see these drugs used as part of the comprehensive treatment of asthma, COPD, and similar respiratory conditions.

MEDICATIONS RELATED TO PREFERRED PRACTICE PATTERN D: IMPAIRED AEROBIC CAPACITY/ENDURANCE ASSOCIATED WITH CARDIOVASCULAR PUMP DYSFUNCTION OR FAILURE

Discussed in this section are drugs that help to treat cardiovascular pump dysfunction associated with myocardial ischemia (antianginal medications) and altered cardiac rhythm (antiarrhythmic medications) and cardiovascular pump failure. Other medications can, of course, help improve myocardial function indirectly by treating other cardiovascular problems such as high blood pressure, increased plasma lipids. These medications are addressed in other sections of this chapter.

Drugs Used to Treat Cardiovascular Pump Dysfunction

Angina Pectoris

Angina pectoris is chest pain that typically occurs when the supply of oxygen to the heart is inadequate to meet myocardial

TABLE 8-7 Organic Nitrates

Dosage Form	Onset of Action	Duration of Action
Nitroglycerin		
Oral	20–45 min	4–6 h
Buccal (extended release)	2–3 min	3–5 h
Sublingual/lingual	1–3 min	30–60 min
Ointment	30 min	4–8 h
Transdermal patches	Within 30 min	8–24 h
Isosorbide dinitrate		
Oral	15–40 min	4–6 h
Oral (extended release)	30 min	12 h
Chewable	2–5 min	1–2 h
Sublingual	2–5 min	1–2 h
Isosorbide mononitrate		
Oral	30–60 min	6–8 h
Amyl nitrate		
Inhaled	30 s	3–5 min

Reprinted from Ciccone CD. *Pharmacology in Rehabilitation.* 4th ed. Philadelphia, PA: FA Davis; 2007:308, with permission.

oxygen demands. An imbalance between myocardial oxygen supply and demand can occur for several reasons, and angina pectoris is subclassified according to the factors that precipitate an anginal attack. Drug therapy is likewise focused on resolving the precipitating factors and on helping to restore the normal balance between myocardial oxygen supply and utilization. The primary drug therapies used to relieve symptoms of angina pectoris are described here.

Organic nitrates—Organic nitrates include nitroglycerin, isosorbide dinitrate, isosorbide mononitrate, and amyl nitrate (see Table 8-7). These drugs act primarily as vasodilators in the peripheral vasculature.[106] That is, nitroglycerin and other nitrates are converted to nitric oxide within the vasculature, thereby relaxing vascular smooth muscle, which leads to vasodilation. These drugs also cause some degree of vasodilation in the coronary arteries and can increase blood flow to the myocardium. Their primary benefits in treating angina pectoris, however, are related to their ability to cause vasodilation in the systemic circulation, including the peripheral venous and arterial systems. This systemic vasodilation decreases the amount of blood returning to the heart (cardiac preload) and decreases the pressure that the heart must pump against (cardiac afterload). By decreasing cardiac preload and afterload, nitrates reduce the workload on the myocardium, which helps reduce angina by decreasing myocardial oxygen demand. By normalizing cardiac workload and oxygen demand, nitrates may also produce other beneficial effects including improved myocardial contractility and decreased risk of cardiac arrhythmias.

Although several different types of organic nitrates can be used to treat angina, nitroglycerin is the most common. Nitroglycerin can be administered by placing a tablet under the patient's tongue (sublingually) at the onset of an angina attack. Sublingual administration allows rapid absorption into the circulation via the venous drainage from the oral mucosa. More importantly, sublingual administration allows the drug to be introduced into the systemic circulation before passing through the liver. If a nitroglycerin tablet is swallowed, it will be absorbed from the upper gastrointestinal tract where it then passes directly to the liver via the hepatic portal vein. This so-called "first-pass effect" results in more than 99% of the active form of nitroglycerin being metabolized and inactivated before the drug reaches the systemic circulation. Hence, sublingual administration avoids this first-pass inactivation and allows more active nitroglycerin to reach the peripheral circulation where it can exert beneficial effects.

Another option for administering nitrates is to use a nitroglycerin patch. Small adhesive patches that are impregnated with this drug can be adhered to various sites on the surface of the skin. The drug is then slowly absorbed through the skin and into the systemic circulation. Transdermal nitroglycerin patches offer several advantages including a convenient method for administering the drug and a better chance for preventing the onset of an angina attack compared to sublingual pills that are typically taken after an attack has already started. Nitroglycerin patches also avoid the first-pass effect because they can be applied to any site on the skin, and the drug will be absorbed into the subcutaneous venous drainage at that site and reach the systemic circulation before reaching the liver.

The side effects most commonly associated with nitroglycerin and other nitrates are related to their vasodilating effects.[107] Problems with dizziness, hypotension, and orthostatic hypotension may occur because these drugs cause blood to pool in the peripheral circulation. These problems may be especially common when a patient takes a sublingual tablet and gets a sudden absorption of nitroglycerin into the systemic circulation. Patients may complain of headaches because nitrates dilate the meningeal vessels. Finally, nitrates may lose their effectiveness because the body becomes tolerant to the drug when it is administered continuously via patches.[107] Fortunately, this form of drug tolerance is rapidly reversed when the drug is discontinued for even a few hours. Consequently, patches are often applied in a 24-hour cycle where the patch is applied for 12 to 14 hours and then removed for the other 10 to 12 hours. This cycle avoids the development of drug tolerance while still allowing adequate control of angina symptoms.

Other drugs used to treat angina—Other strategies for decreasing angina symptoms include β-blockers and calcium channel blockers.[108] As discussed earlier, β-blockers decrease heart rate and myocardial contraction force because they block the effects of catecholamines (epinephrine and norepinephrine) on the heart. These drugs are, therefore, helpful in reducing angina symptoms because they reduce myocardial oxygen demand. In contrast, calcium channel blockers are effective in reducing angina symptoms primarily because they increase myocardial oxygen supply. By limiting the entry of calcium into coronary vascular smooth muscle, these drugs maintain coronary artery vasodilation and prevent coronary vasospasm. Calcium channel blockers are, therefore, especially useful in the type of angina known as Prinzmetal ischemia, which occurs because of increased reactivity and vasospasm in the coronary arteries.[109]

Side effects and other details about β-blockers and calcium channel blockers have been discussed earlier in this chapter. These drugs are often used in various combinations with organic nitrates to provide optimal management of angina symptoms in each patient.[108] A patient, for example, with classic or stable angina might take a β-blocker orally every day, with sublingual nitroglycerin being used at the onset of an angina attack. Patients with more severe or unstable forms of angina may require a more aggressive regimen that also incorporates calcium channel blockers along with oral β-blockers and oral or transdermal nitroglycerin.

Cardiac Arrhythmias

Cardiac arrhythmias can be characterized as any disturbance in cardiac excitability that results in a heart rate that is too fast, too slow, or simply irregular.[110] The causes and classification of specific arrhythmias are fairly complex and well beyond the scope of this chapter.[110] Drug treatment of arrhythmias is likewise a detailed and difficult topic that involves a number of potentially useful agents. Nonetheless, this topic can be simplified somewhat by classifying the commonly used antiarrhythmic agents into four categories.[110] These categories are listed in Table 8-8 and they are described briefly here.

Sodium channel blockers—Drugs in this category control myocardial excitability by stabilizing the opening and closing of sodium channels located on heart cell membranes. These drugs are helpful in treating a variety of arrhythmias because they tend to normalize the function of cardiac sodium channels; that is, these drugs can decrease the activity of sodium channels that are firing too rapidly or increase the activity of channels that are firing too slowly. This category of antiarrhythmics is further subdivided according to exactly how these drugs influence cardiac excitability (see Table 8-8).

β-Blockers—As discussed earlier in this chapter, β-blockers bind to β₁-receptors on the heart and prevent excessive stimulation by sympathetic catecholamines (epinephrine, norepinephrine). This effect helps normalize cardiac sympathetic activity and is helpful in controlling arrhythmias associated with increased sympathetic excitation of the myocardium.

Drugs that prolong repolarization—These drugs stabilize heart rate by delaying repolarization and prolonging the refractory period of cardiac action potentials. This effect lengthens the time between successive heart beats (diastole) and is especially helpful in treating certain types of tachycardia.

Calcium channel blockers—By inhibiting calcium entry into cardiac pacemaker cells, these drugs stabilize myocardial excitability and help reestablish the normal generation of cardiac rhythm in the sinoatrial node. Calcium channel blockers also decrease the conduction of electrical impulses throughout the heart by limiting the entry of calcium into cardiac muscle cells.

TABLE 8-8   Classification of Antiarrhythmic Drugs

Generic Name	Trade Name(s)
Class I: Sodium channel blockers	
Subclass A	
Disopyramide	Norpace
Procainamide	Promine, Pronestyl, Procan
Quinidine	Cardioquin, Quinidex, others
Subclass B	
Lidocaine	Xylocaine
Mexiletine	Mexitil
Moricizine[a]	Ethmozine
Subclass C	
Flecainide	Tambocor
Propafenone	Rythmol
Class II: β-Blockers	
Acebutolol	Sectral
Atenolol	Tenormin
Esmolol	Brevibloc
Metoprolol	Lopressor
Nadolol	Corgard
Propranolol	Inderal
Sotalol	Betapace
Timolol	Blocadren
Class III: Drugs that prolong repolarization	
Amiodarone[b]	Cordarone
Bretylium	Bretylol
Dofetilide	Tikosyn
Ibutilide	Corvert
Class IV: Calcium channel blockers	
Diltiazem	Cardizem, Dilacor
Verapamil	Calan, Isoptin, Verelan

[a]Also has some class IC properties.

[b]Also has some properties from the other three drug classes.

Reprinted from Ciccone CD. *Pharmacology in Rehabilitation*. 4th ed. Philadelphia, PA: FA Davis; 2007:325, with permission.

Consequently, a large number of drugs are available that can be used to treat cardiac arrhythmias, and selection of a specific agent obviously depends on the type of arrhythmia and other medical and physiological factors in each patient. There are likewise variable side effects associated with individual antiarrhythmic drugs depending on the category and chemical features of each drug. The primary problem, however, is that these agents may be "proarrhythmic," meaning that they can increase the chance of cardiac arrhythmias.[111] In an attempt to resolve one type of arrhythmia, these drugs may inadvertently alter cardiac excitability so that a different type of arrhythmia emerges. Consequently, physical therapists should occasionally monitor a patient's pulse or look for other symptoms (severe fatigue, diaphoresis, and so forth) that may indicate the presence of these proarrhythmic effects, especially when patients are exercising.

Drugs Used to Treat Cardiovascular Pump Failure

Cardiovascular pump failure occurs when the heart is unable to adequately supply oxygen to the tissues throughout the body.[112] This problem, described more simply as heart failure,

TABLE 8-9 Drugs Used to Treat Heart Failure

Drug Category	Rationale for Use	Examples
Drugs that increase myocardial contractility (positive inotropic agents)		
Digitalis glycosides	Increase myocardial contraction force by increasing intracellular calcium in heart tissues; may also normalize autonomic control of heart by increasing cardiac parasympathetic activity and decreasing cardiac sympathetic activity	Digoxin (Lanoxin)
Phosphodiesterase inhibitors	Prolong activity of cyclic adenosine monophosphate (cAMP) in cardiac cells, which results in increased intracellular calcium concentrations and stronger myocardial contraction	Inamrinone (generic) Milrinone (Primacor)
Other positive inotropic agents	Generally increase myocardial contraction force by selective stimulation of cardiac β_1-receptors	Dobutamine (generic) Dopamine (generic)
Drugs that decrease cardiac workload		
Diuretics	Increase excretion of excess sodium and water to reduce the volume of fluid the heart must pump	See Table 8-1
Vasodilators	Decrease cardiac preload and afterload by vasodilating the venous and arterial systems, respectively	See Table 8-1
Renin–angiotensin system inhibitors	Prevent angiotensin II–induced vasoconstriction and vascular hypertrophy	See Table 8-1
β-Adrenergic blockers	Normalize sympathetic influence on the heart; prevent damage from excessive sympathetic stimulation	See Table 8-1

is often a progressive decline in myocardial function that produces several characteristic symptoms including shortness of breath, poor exercise tolerance, tachycardia, and edema in the lungs and peripheral tissues. Drug treatment of heart failure consists of two primary strategies: to increase myocardial pumping ability and to decrease the workload on the failing heart (Table 8-9). Drugs used to achieve these strategies are described here.

Drugs That Increase Myocardial Pumping Ability

Digitalis—Digitalis is the term commonly used to represent a group of drugs known as the cardiac glycosides. This group includes agents such as digoxin and digitoxin, and these drugs have been used extensively in the treatment of heart failure.[113] Digitalis exerts a positive inotropic effect on the heart, meaning that this drug increases myocardial contraction force.[114] Digitalis exerts some of its positive inotropic effect by increasing the amount of calcium inside heart muscle cells. This increase in intracellular calcium results in a greater interaction between actin and myosin filaments, which results in increased contractile force. Digitalis also exerts beneficial electrophysiological effects on the heart, including an increase in cardiac parasympathetic activity (by stimulating the vagus nerve) and a decrease in cardiac sympathetic activity.[114] These electrophysiological effects contribute to digitalis's positive inotropic properties because they prevent tachycardia and allow the heart to fill more completely during diastole and pump more effectively during systole.

Digitalis can, therefore, be helpful in increasing myocardial contraction force and improving the symptoms of heart failure. There is concern, however, that digitalis does not produce any long-term benefits and that the use of this drug does not really improve the survival of people with heart failure. More importantly, digitalis is notorious for having a small

margin of error between the amount of drug that causes therapeutic effects and the amount that causes toxicity.[115] A relatively small increase in blood levels beyond the therapeutic range can result in digitalis toxicity. Digitalis toxicity is characterized by several symptoms including loss of appetite, fatigue, confusion, depression, and blurred vision. By altering calcium concentration in certain areas of the heart, digitalis can also disturb cardiac rhythm and cause severe arrhythmias such as ventricular tachycardia and ventricular fibrillation. Digitalis must, therefore, be used carefully, and patients experiencing any untoward effects should be quickly evaluated for possible digitalis toxicity.

Other positive inotropic agents—Because of the limitations and potential problems associated with digitalis, other drugs that selectively increase myocardial contraction force have been developed (Table 8-9).[116] These drugs, however, have not proven to be substantially better than digitalis in improving outcomes in people with heart failure. Many of these other positive inotropes must also be given by parenteral (nonoral) routes and are typically administered by continuous intravenous infusion to treat acute or severe heart failure.

Other positive inotropic agents include inamrinone and milrinone (Primacor).[117] These drugs are classified as phosphodiesterase inhibitors because they inhibit the phosphodiesterase enzyme that degrades cAMP in cardiac cells. By inhibiting cAMP degradation, these drugs increase intracellular cAMP levels, which leads to increased intracellular calcium and a stronger muscle contraction. Another option for increasing myocardial contraction force is to use dobutamine (Dobutrex).[117] This drug selectively stimulates cardiac β_1-receptors, which results in a stronger cardiac contraction. Finally, dopamine can be used to increase myocardial contraction force because this drug stimulates β_1-receptors on the heart.[117] At the appropriate dosage, dopamine also stimulates vascular dopamine receptors, which causes vasodilation in the peripheral vasculature and kidneys. Dopamine's vasodilating effects contribute to this drug's benefits in severe, acute heart failure because peripheral vasodilation helps decrease the workload on the failing heart, and dilation of the kidneys helps preserve renal function and allows the excretion of excess sodium and water.

Drugs That Decrease Cardiac Workload

Heart failure tends to become progressively worse because changes occur in the cardiovascular system, which increase myocardial workload. These changes, mediated primarily by increased sympathetic nervous system activity and increased activity in the renin–angiotensin systems, create a vicious cycle where increased cardiac workload causes additional damage to the heart, which further diminishes cardiac pumping ability, perpetuates increased sympathetic and renin–angiotensin activity, adds to the stress and workload on the myocardium, and so forth.[118] It is, therefore, essential to try to stop this vicious cycle by administering drugs that decrease cardiac workload and spare the heart from additional damage.

Several drugs already discussed in this chapter can be used to decrease cardiac workload in people with heart failure (Table 8-9). These drugs include the diuretics, vasodilators, renin–angiotensin system inhibitors, and β-blockers.[118] Diuretics help excrete excess fluid and electrolytes in the vascular system, thereby reducing the volume of fluid that needs to be pumped by the failing heart. Vasodilators decrease cardiac workload by reducing the pressure in the arterial system (cardiac afterload) and by allowing more blood to pool in the peripheral venous system, thereby reducing the volume of blood returning to the heart (cardiac preload). By reducing the acute and chronic vasoconstriction produced by angiotensin II, drugs that inhibit the renin–angiotensin system (ACE inhibitors, angiotensin II blockers) can substantially reduce detrimental effects on the heart and vascular systems. Finally, β-blockers reduce the excitatory effects of the sympathetic nervous system on the heart, and these drugs help prevent further damage caused by excessive sympathetic stimulation.

Side effects and other details about these drugs were discussed earlier in this chapter. Drugs that decrease cardiac workload can be combined with digitalis and other positive inotropic drugs to provide optimal treatment for people with various forms of heart failure. In fact, drugs such as the renin–angiotensin inhibitors and β-blockers are now considered essential for the treatment of heart failure because these drugs may actually decrease morbidity and increase life expectancy in people with heart failure.[119] Hence, drug treatment of heart failure has improved substantially over the past few years, and we may see additional benefits as more is learned about how various drugs can be combined to effectively treat this disease.

MEDICATIONS RELATED TO PREFERRED PRACTICE PATTERN E: IMPAIRED VENTILATION AND RESPIRATION/GAS EXCHANGE ASSOCIATED WITH VENTILATORY PUMP DYSFUNCTION OR FAILURE

Drugs Used to Treat Ventilatory Pump Dysfunction

Several pharmacological strategies already discussed in this chapter can be used to indirectly treat ventilatory pump dysfunction. For example, bronchodilators, mucolytics, and other drugs that facilitate airway clearance can help improve airway patency, thereby reducing the workload on the ventilatory musculature. There are likewise many pharmacological strategies that can improve the patient's general health in various musculoskeletal, neuromuscular, and other disorders, thereby enabling the patient to perform general aerobic conditioning exercises and specific exercises that improve the strength and endurance in the respiratory muscles. There are not, however, any medications that specifically increase respiratory muscle strength or endurance. Hence, pharmacological treatment of ventilatory pump dysfunction typically focuses on resolving other pathologies and impairments that will ultimately help the patient increase ventilation and improve gas exchange.

Nonetheless, administration of supplemental oxygen is a strategy that is commonly used to help alleviate the sequelae of ventilatory pump dysfunction.[120] A brief overview of the therapeutic use of oxygen follows.

Oxygen

Oxygen is typically administered to correct the hypoxia that often accompanies poor ventilation and impaired gas exchange that is secondary to a number of respiratory problems. By inhaling supplemental oxygen, arterial oxygen levels can be sustained so that oxygen delivery to peripheral tissues remains adequate to meet the metabolic demands of these tissues. This strategy, of course, will not provide a permanent solution to respiratory dysfunction. Oxygen can, nonetheless, help alleviate the hypoxia that often accompanies ventilatory pump dysfunction in acute situations. Long-term oxygen therapy is likewise generally felt to improve exercise tolerance, decrease morbidity, and improve quality of life in people with chronic conditions such as COPD.[121]

Supplemental oxygen can be administered via nasal cannulae, oxygen mask, oxygen tent/hood, or directly into an endotracheal tube.[120] Other parameters such as the oxygen dose (liters per minute), hours per day of oxygen administration, supply system (canister of compressed gas, liquid oxygen reservoir), and the dosage required during exercise must all be considered on the basis of the needs of each patient. Despite the obvious benefit of preventing hypoxia, great care must be taken to avoid administering too much oxygen and subjecting the patient to oxygen toxicity. Oxygen toxicity occurs because of the increased production of various reactive oxygen species or oxygen "free radicals."[120] These highly reactive oxygen species cause damage to many cellular components including membrane lipids, cellular proteins, and DNA. As a result, cell death often occurs with subsequent loss of tissue and organ function. In particular, the respiratory tissues may be especially prone to excessive doses of supplemental oxygen, which can lead to airway inflammation, increased alveolar permeability, and pulmonary edema that can lead to death.[120] Hence, oxygen administration is a two-edged sword; therapeutic doses can be helpful in preventing hypoxia, but excessive administration may ultimately cause severe damage to many tissues, including the pulmonary system.

Drugs Used to Treat Ventilatory Pump Failure

Medications related to this condition are designed to treat the problem that is potentiating respiratory failure. For pulmonary conditions such as asthma and COPD, medications already described in this chapter can be used in higher doses and in greater numbers (combining several synergistic drugs) to thwart respiratory failure. An aggressive drug regimen can hopefully prevent respiratory failure so that the patient can resume treatment of the underlying condition at lower (maintenance) drug doses, whereas other interventions including physical therapy are used to prevent subsequent episodes of respiratory failure. However, even pharmacological therapy can fail, in which case the patient must be placed in mechanical ventilation.

MEDICATIONS RELATED TO PREFERRED PRACTICE PATTERN F: IMPAIRED VENTILATION AND RESPIRATION/GAS EXCHANGE ASSOCIATED WITH RESPIRATORY FAILURE

The following medications are not designed to directly improve ventilation, but rather to improve patients' tolerance to mechanical ventilation. Although the *Guide* does not associate assistive ventilatory support with Practice Pattern 6F, many patients with respiratory failure may ultimately require this intervention. Three primary pharmacological interventions include antianxiety/sedative drugs, analgesics, and neuromuscular blockers. Examples of these drugs are listed in Box 8-1, and the use of these agents in patients receiving mechanical ventilation is addressed here.

Antianxiety and Sedative Agents

Antianxiety agents are often administered to patients receiving mechanical ventilation, especially when these patients are being treated in the intensive care unit (ICU).[122] Patients in the

---

BOX 8-1

Medications Commonly Used As Adjuncts to Mechanical Ventilation

Antianxiety agents and sedatives
Benzodiazepines*
    Lorazepam (Ativan)
    Midazolam (generic)
Others
    Propofol (Diprivan)
    Haloperidol (Haldol)

Analgesics
Morphine (Kadian, Duramorph, others)

Neuromuscular blockers
Atracurium (Tacrium)
Pancuronium (generic)
Rocuronium (Zemuron)
Succinylcholine (Anectine, Quelicin)
Vecuronium (generic)

*All benzodiazepines have antianxiety effects; selection of a specific agent in patients with mechanical ventilation is based on the individual needs of each patient.

ICU are subjected to a bright, noisy, and potentially intimidating environment. Use of an antianxiety agent can help keep the person calm and relaxed and also decrease the apprehension that typically occurs when the patient is intubated and mechanically ventilated.[122]

The most common antianxiety agents are the benzodiazepines (see Box 8-1). These drugs increase the effects of γ-aminobutyric acid (GABA), which is an inhibitory neurotransmitter found throughout the CNS. Increased CNS inhibition produces an antianxiety effect and may likewise cause some degree of sedation and muscle relaxation, which can also be beneficial in helping the patient tolerate mechanical ventilation in the ICU. Hence, benzodiazepines such as lorazepam (Ativan) and midazolam are commonly used to provide a calming effect and maintain adequate relaxation in patients who are being mechanically ventilated.[123] Sedation is the most common side effect associated with benzodiazepine agents. This effect is not usually a problem, however, and as indicated, sedation may be somewhat beneficial when these drugs are administered for relatively short periods of time to patients who are acutely ill and receiving mechanical ventilation in the ICU.

In addition to the benzodiazepines, other drugs can be used to induce sedative effects (Box 8-1). In particular, propofol (Diprivan) is a sedative–hypnotic that is often used as an adjunct during general anesthesia, but can also be used to help provide sedation to people who are being ventilated in the ICU.[122] Certain antipsychotics such as haloperidol (Haldol) may also provide sedation, especially in patients who are agitated.[124] The exact choice of an antianxiety or sedative agent depends on the particular needs of the patient undergoing mechanical ventilation.

Analgesics

Analgesics are also administered frequently to patients who are being mechanically ventilated.[124] These drugs help alleviate pain that accompanies trauma, surgery, and so forth, and may also help the patient tolerate the discomfort and apprehension associated with intubation and ventilation. Opioids such as morphine are the most common type of analgesics used in these situations (see Box 8-1).[124] These drugs inhibit CNS synapses that mediate painful sensations and reduce the patient's awareness and perception of all painful stimuli.[125] Opioid analgesics also cause sedation, but this side effect often complements their analgesic effects during short-term use in patients who are mechanically ventilated.

Neuromuscular Blockers

Drugs that eliminate skeletal muscle contraction may need to be administered to some patients undergoing mechanical ventilation.[126] These drugs, known as neuromuscular blockers (see Box 8-1), bind to the postsynaptic receptor at the skeletal neuromuscular junction and negate the excitatory effects of acetylcholine on skeletal muscle. This effect causes skeletal muscle paralysis throughout the body so that the patient remains immobile and does not thrash about. The thoracic wall likewise remains relaxed and compliant, thus allowing the ventilator to control chest inflation and deflation without resistance from the patient's respiratory and thoracoabdominal musculature.

The use of neuromuscular blockers in patients receiving mechanical ventilation is understandably a rather extreme and potentially dangerous intervention. These drugs are, therefore, used as a last resort when other drugs (antianxiety agents, analgesics) are not able to adequately control agitation. The primary problem associated with neuromuscular blockers is that prolonged muscular weakness sometimes occurs after these drugs are discontinued. Neuromuscular blockers, or possibly the combination of neuromuscular blockers with anti-inflammatory steroids (prednisone, cortisone, other glucocorticoids), may precipitate a syndrome of severe muscle weakness in certain patients who receive mechanical ventilation during an acute illness. This syndrome is identified by several different names, including acute steroid myopathy, critical illness polyneuromyopathy, prolonged neurogenic weakness, and the floppy person syndrome. Muscle weakness associated with this syndrome occurs because of direct muscle pathology (myopathy), abnormalities at the neuromuscular junction, nerve pathology (neuropathy), or a combination of muscle and nerve pathology (polyneuromyopathies).[127] The type and extent of this muscle weakness vary from patient to patient, but weakness can often be quite severe and last for several months after these drugs are discontinued and the patient is removed from ventilation.

Hence, a syndrome of acute, severe muscle weakness may emerge in certain patients who receive mechanical ventilation during an acute illness, especially if drugs such as the neuromuscular blockers and glucocorticoids are administered. Neuromuscular blockers, either used alone or in combination with glucocorticoids, are often considered a risk factor in the development of neuromuscular pathology in people who are acutely ill and receiving mechanical ventilation.[128] There are, however, cases where severe muscle weakness developed in patients who were mechanically ventilated but were not exposed to either neuromuscular blockers or glucocorticoids. Consequently, the exact cause of these neuromuscular problems is not known, and the development of severe muscle weakness following mechanical ventilation remains a serious and poorly understood phenomenon. Future research into the exact factors that increase the risk of this problem will hopefully lend insight into how these neuromuscular pathologies can be avoided.

Drugs Used to Treat Acute Respiratory Failure and Acute Respiratory Distress Syndrome

There are several supportive measures that can be used in cases of acute respiratory failure in adults or acute respiratory distress syndrome (ARDS). ARDS typically occurs following some recent insult such as trauma, pneumonia, sepsis, or drug overdose.[129] Patients typically exhibit bilateral infiltrates on chest radiograph, high ventilatory inflation pressures, and a high requirement for supplemental oxygen.[129] Interventions used during ARDS are targeted at providing cardiopulmonary support and preventing organ failure or infection secondary to poor oxygenation and perfusion.

With regard to pulmonary medications, three primary strategies are typically used to maintain adequate gas exchange and tissue oxygenation. These strategies are surfactant therapy, nitric oxide, and anti-inflammatory steroids. Surfactant is an oily substance produced by cells within the alveoli that helps reduce surface tension and prevent alveolar collapse. Nitric oxide relaxes vascular smooth muscle with subsequent vasodilation of the pulmonary vasculature, and this effect helps improve gas exchange, especially in areas of the lung that are underperfused. Anti-inflammatory steroids (glucocorticoids, see Table 8-6) help prevent airway inflammation and bronchoconstriction, thus maintaining airway patency and ventilation. Additional details about the use of these strategies and side effects of these drugs can be found in the next section of this chapter.

MEDICATIONS RELATED TO PREFERRED PRACTICE PATTERN G: IMPAIRED VENTILATION, RESPIRATION/GAS EXCHANGE, AND AEROBIC CAPACITY/ ENDURANCE ASSOCIATED WITH RESPIRATORY FAILURE IN THE NEONATE

Respiratory failure in neonates can be caused by myriad problems including prematurity, infection (pneumonia), postsurgical complications, congenital anomalies, and so forth. There have likewise been many advances in pharmacological and nonpharmacological treatment of neonatal respiratory problems, including innovative ways to control acid–base balance, fluid–electrolyte levels, and mechanical ventilation. Although it is not possible to review all of these treatment approaches, there are a few pharmacological strategies that have emerged as being especially important in the treatment of neonatal respiratory distress syndrome. Addressed here are three such strategies: surfactant replacement therapy, nitric oxide administration, and glucocorticoid therapy.

Surfactant Replacement Therapy

Respiratory problems often arise in neonates because of inadequate production of surfactant. Surfactant is a mixture of phospholipids, neutral lipids, and proteins that is normally synthesized by alveolar pneumocytes. Surfactant decreases surface tension within the alveolus, thus allowing the alveolus to expand during inspiration. Without sufficient surfactant, the alveoli will collapse rendering gas exchange impossible. Neonates may not produce enough surfactant because they are born prematurely, or because surfactant is inactivated by other problems (pneumonia, meconium aspiration, and so forth).[130] Insufficient surfactant production, known also as hyaline membrane disease, can lead to respiratory distress syndrome and acute respiratory failure simply because the neonate cannot inflate his or her lungs.

Hence, the development of methods to supplement inadequate surfactant production is arguably the most important advancement in treating neonatal respiratory distress syndrome. Various types of surfactant that can be used therapeutically are listed in Table 8-10. Administration of surfactant has proven to reduce the morbidity and mortality associated with acute respiratory distress in the newborn, and early surfactant replacement may reduce the risk of the child developing subsequent chronic lung disease.[130] Surfactant can be obtained from one of the three sources: human surfactant (extracted from human amniotic fluid), animal surfactant (harvested from cow or pig lungs), or artificial surfactant (synthetic mixtures of lipids and phospholipids) (see Table 8-10).[131] Although the natural forms (human or animal) were originally thought to be safer and more effective than synthetic agents, recent studies suggest that the newer synthetic surfactants may provide equivalent results in terms of improved lung function and lower mortality.[132] Efforts continue to produce a safe, effective, and relatively inexpensive method for providing surfactant replacement to neonates with ARDS.

Surfactant is typically administered to neonates via an endotracheal tube by using repeated bolus doses of the drug in aerosol form. The optimal dose and number of treatments will vary depending on the type of surfactant and the needs of each infant.[129] Surfactant replacement may cause some side effects as the drug is being administered, including airway obstruction, bradycardia, and oxygen desaturation.[129] There is likewise a slight risk of more serious complications including pulmonary hemorrhage, intracranial hemorrhage, and an increased chance of maintaining a patent ductus arteriosus.[129] Nonetheless, surfactant replacement therapy is the most common and effective pharmacological method for resolving neonatal respiratory distress syndrome, and this intervention is typically the cornerstone of treatment for preventing respiratory failure in infants.

Nitric Oxide

Nitric oxide causes vascular smooth muscle relaxation with subsequent vasodilation of vascular beds. Vascular endothelial cells, including the cells that line the pulmonary vessels, normally produce this substance. With regard to neonates, nitric oxide may play a critical role in dilating the pulmonary vessels and supplying blood to areas of the lungs that are beginning to be ventilated as the infant begins to breathe.[133] Endogenous production of nitric oxide, therefore, helps facilitate gas exchange by promoting a match between vascular perfusion and alveolar ventilation (the so-called ventilation–perfusion ratio).[134] In neonatal respiratory distress syndrome, certain

TABLE 8-10 **Source and Composition of Surfactants**

Type of Surfactant	Source	Components
Human surfactant	Amniotic fluid	Surfactant lipids; surfactant proteins A, B, C, and D
Animal surfactants		
Infasurf	Calf lung lavage	Surfactant lipids; surfactant proteins B and C
Alveofact	Cow lung lavage	Surfactant lipids; surfactant proteins B and C
Curosurf	Pig lung extract purified by chromatography	Lung phospholipids; surfactant proteins B and C
Surfactant-TA (Surfacten)	Cow lung extract plus synthetic lipids	Lung lipids plus dipalmitoyl phosphatidylcholine (DPPC), tripalmitin, palmitic acid
Survanta	Cow lung extract plus synthetic lipids	Lung lipids plus DPPC, tripalmitin, palmitic acid, surfactant proteins B and C
Artificial surfactants		
Artificial lung-expanding compound (ALEC) (Pumactant)	Synthetic	DPPC, unsaturated phosphatidylglycerol
Colfosceril palmitate (Exosurf)	Synthetic	DPPC, hexadecanol, tyloxapol

Modified from DiPiro JT, Talbert RL, Yee GC, et al., eds. *Pharmacotherapy: A Pathophysiologic Approach.* 5th ed. The McGraw-Hill Companies Inc; 2002. Used with permission.

areas of the pulmonary vascular bed may not adequately dilate because the infant is premature or because of other problems (infection, meconium aspiration, hypothermia, and so forth). Inadequate vasodilation increases pulmonary arterial pressure, leading to a syndrome of persistent pulmonary hypertension in the newborn (PPHN).[133] Inhalation of nitric oxide will dilate the pulmonary vasculature and supply blood to areas of the lung that are being ventilated. This effect will help reduce pulmonary hypertension and improve gas exchange by normalizing the ventilation–perfusion ratio.

Nitric oxide is typically administered to neonates by inhalation in doses ranging from 5 to 80 parts per million.[129] This treatment generally decreases the symptoms of neonatal respiratory distress syndrome and improves arterial oxygenation because of better ventilation–perfusion ratios throughout the lung.[135] Nitric oxide may also produce optimal benefits if combined with other pharmacologic interventions such as surfactant replacement therapy.

Short-term inhalation of nitric oxide is tolerated fairly well, although this substance can irritate the respiratory tissues, inhibit platelet aggregation, inactivate surfactant, and cause severe acute pulmonary edema in some infants.[136] When administered to term or near-term infants, or preterm infants who are not severely ill, nitric oxide may improve the chance of survival and decrease the chance that the child will develop chronic lung disease.[137,138] On the other hand, nitric oxide inhalation may not be effective in severely ill, premature babies and may increase the risk of other problems such as intraventricular hemorrhage in this population.[137] Nitric oxide therapy, therefore, continues to be an option for treating certain cases of neonatal respiratory distress syndrome, and future studies should help clarify how this intervention can be used most effectively with minimal risk to the infant.

Glucocorticoids

As indicated earlier in this chapter, glucocorticoids are anti-inflammatory steroids that play a key role in controlling airway inflammation in diseases such as asthma and COPD (see Table 8-6). These drugs may also help prevent and treat respiratory distress syndrome in neonates. When administered to the mother before the infant is born (antenatally), glucocorticoids cross the placenta and facilitate lung maturation in the infant. This treatment can, therefore, be used when premature birth is imminent and help improve respiratory function after the baby is born.[139] Glucocorticoids can likewise be administered directly to the neonate (postnatally) to treat inflammation and reduce the risk of the infant developing chronic respiratory problems.[140]

The use of glucocorticoids is always associated with some potentially severe side effects. Administration to neonates can increase the risk of gastrointestinal bleeding, hyperglycemia, and hypertension.[141] There is also a concern that antenatal and postnatal glucocorticoid administration could impair growth and development of the lungs, brain, and other tissues in the neonate.[139,142] One study investigated the chance of developmen-

tal problems and failed to see any detrimental effects of a single antenatal glucocorticoid dose on individuals who ultimately reached adulthood (mean age 31 years).[143] Another study found that premature infants receiving a specific postnatal glucocorticoid regimen (4.75 mg/kg dexamethasone over 2 weeks) did not experience any adverse effects on growth or neurodevelopment when the children reached 3 years of age.[144] These findings, however, cannot rule out the possibility that problems may occur if multiple or higher doses are given antenatally or postnatally. Despite these concerns, glucocorticoids remain, along with surfactant therapy and other pharmacological and nonpharmacological interventions, an important option for reducing the incidence of neonatal respiratory distress syndrome and preventing chronic respiratory problems as the child matures.

MEDICATIONS RELATED TO PREFERRED PRACTICE PATTERN H: IMPAIRED CIRCULATION AND ANTHROPOMETRIC DIMENSIONS ASSOCIATED WITH LYMPHATIC SYSTEM DISORDERS

General Treatment Strategies for Lymphedema

The lymphatic system drains excess fluid and macromolecules (proteins, other cells) from the interstitial spaces throughout the body and returns these substances to the vascular system via the thoracic duct. Any disruption in this drainage system results in accumulation of excess fluid in the affected region, a condition known commonly as lymphedema. Because the affected body part is often the patient's arm or leg, physical therapists play a critical role in helping to reduce the swelling and improving function in the affected extremity.

Lymphedema is typically classified as either primary or secondary depending on the causative factors.[145] Primary lymphedema occurs because of some inherent defect in the development or function of the lymphatic vessels, such as congenital malformation of the lymphatics or fibrosis of lymph nodes. Secondary lymphedema is associated with a specific insult to the lymphatics such as surgical removal of lymph nodes, infection, trauma. Regardless of the initiating factor, lymphedema often results in substantial disability because of pain, decreased movement, impaired circulation, and increased risk of infection in the affected limb(s).

Treatment of lymphatic system disorders typically focuses on physical methods (massage, exercise, compressive dressings or garments) to reduce the accumulation of fluid in the affected arm or leg.[146] This fact is especially true in chronic lymphedema associated with removal or damage to the lymph nodes following treatment for breast cancer and other malignancies. Operative treatment for lymphedema is also an option in selected cases where a specific blockage of the lymphatics can be removed surgically.

Drug therapy may also play a role in resolving specific lymphatic disorders. Infection in the lymphatic system, for example, can impair lymph drainage, and the use of appropriate anti-infectious agents is often useful in treating this form of lymphedema. This fact is especially true for filarial infections, where small parasitic worms (filariae) invade the lymphatics and restrict lymph flow resulting in severe lymphedema known commonly as elephantiasis.[147] Specific anti-infectious agents such as ivermectin, diethylcarbazine, and albendazole destroy these parasitic worms, and these drugs can often be very effective in resolving this type of lymphedema.

Other anti-infectious agents can be used to treat infection in limbs with chronic lymphedema.[145] The accumulation of lymph, a fluid rich in proteins, in a limb with poor circulation creates a milieu for the growth of bacteria and other microorganisms. Hence, an appropriate anti-infectious drug can help resolve these infections and reduce the pain and swelling in the affected limb.

In addition, anti-inflammatory agents such as glucocorticoids (prednisone, others) can be used to treat cellulitis and other inflammatory responses associated with lymphedema. Pain medications may also be useful for the short-term management of pain and tenderness in affected extremities. These medications do not directly resolve edema, but can help reduce pain and inflammation so that the patient can participate in exercises and other interventions that help reduce swelling.

Hence, several drug strategies are available to treat the causative factor in certain lymphatic disorders (eg, infection), and to help treat other problems associated with lymphedema. There is, however, considerable controversy about whether any drugs can reduce the accumulation of lymph in either primary or secondary lymphedema. Several drug strategies have been proposed to actually reduce the swelling associated with lymphatic system disorders, and these strategies are addressed briefly in the next section.

Specific Drugs That May Decrease Lymphedema

Diuretics

As discussed earlier in this chapter, diuretics increase the renal excretion of sodium and water and thereby, remove excess fluid from the body. These drugs would seem like a logical choice to reduce the accumulation of fluid in a lymphedematous arm or leg. Diuretics, however, are often not effective in the long-term management of lymphedema because they can reduce the fluid content in the affected limb, but do not remove the proteins and other cells that create an osmotic force to draw fluid into the interstitial space.[148,149] In other words, any loss of fluid from the interstitial space will quickly be replaced because the proteins and other osmotically active substances are still present to pull fluid out of the capillaries and cells and maintain the lymphedema.

Hence, diuretics fail to resolve the underlying factors that cause lymph to accumulate in the tissues, and the affected limb does not really undergo a substantial reduction in size or volume. Long-term use of diuretics is, therefore, not typically helpful in chronic lymphedema, and their use is often discouraged because of the risk of disturbing the body's fluid and electrolyte balance.[149]

Benzopyrone Derivatives

Benzopyrones are a group of compounds that include coumarin and flavonoid drugs.[150,151] These compounds are believed to stimulate macrophage function and thereby increase the breakdown and removal of proteins and other waste products in lymphedema. By helping remove these osmotically active substances, these drugs would reduce the tendency for fluid to accumulate in the interstitial space and thereby reduce lymphedema.

There is, however, conflicting evidence about the effectiveness of coumarin and other benzopyrones in treating lymphedema.[152,153] Although some studies suggest beneficial effects, other studies have failed to determine conclusively that these drugs are useful in reducing limb volume and improving function in people with lymphedema.[152] Hence, coumarin is used in certain countries (eg, parts of Europe), but this drug is not approved for treating lymphedema in the United States. It is not clear if additional research will establish a more definitive role for this drug in treating lymphedema.

Selenium

Selenium is a trace element in the body that can also act as an antioxidant and free-radical scavenger. This effect purportedly helps reduce free-radical damage thereby decreasing the inflammation and tissue damage that can increase lymphedema after surgery or following radiation treatments.[154] The actual effects of this treatment remain unclear, and additional studies are needed to verify that selenium can actually reduce the severity and improve outcomes in people with lymphedema.[155]

Several drug strategies have, therefore, been advocated for reducing lymphedema. None of these strategies have been overwhelmingly successful, however. At the present time, drug therapy plays a secondary role in the treatment of lymphedema, with physical interventions (massage, exercise, and compression) being a much more accepted method for reducing chronic lymphedema.

SUMMARY

This chapter described medications that are commonly used to help prevent or treat cardiopulmonary disease. These medications were grouped according to how they relate to the preferred cardiopulmonary practice patterns listed in the *Guide to Physical Therapist Practice*. Medications often promote improvements in function that are synergistic with the interventions and anticipated goals listed in the practice patterns. These medications, however, also produce side effects that can have a negative impact on the patient and on the patient's response to physical therapy. By understanding the therapeutic and adverse effects of these medications, physical therapists will hopefully be able to capitalize on the beneficial effects while being aware of the potential side effects of these drugs.

REFERENCES

1. American Physical Therapy Association. *Guide to Physical Therapist Practice*. 2nd rev ed. Alexandria, VA: American Physical Therapy Association; 2003.

2. Brunton LL, ed. *The Pharmacological Basis of Therapeutics*. 11th ed. New York: McGraw-Hill; 2006.

3. Ciccone CD. *Pharmacology in Rehabilitation*. 4th ed. Philadelphia, PA: FA Davis; 2007.

4. DiPiro JT, Talbert RL, Yee GC, et al., eds. *Pharmacotherapy: A Pathophysiologic Approach*. 5th ed. New York: McGraw-Hill; 2002.

5. Higgins B, Williams B; Guideline Development Group. Pharmacological management of hypertension. *Clin Med*. 2007;7:612.

6. Wang DJ, Gottlieb SS. Diuretics: still the mainstay of treatment. *Crit Care Med*. 2008;36(suppl):S89.

7. Khan NA, Campbell NR. Thiazide diuretics in the management of hypertension. *Can J Clin Pharmacol*. 2004;11:41.

8. Papadopoulos DP, Papademetriou V. Metabolic side effects and cardiovascular events of diuretics: should a diuretic remain the first choice therapy in hypertension treatment? The case of yes. *Clin Exp Hypertens*. 2007;29:503.

9. Del Colle S, Morello F, Rabbia F, et al. Antihypertensive drugs and the sympathetic nervous system. *J Cardiovasc Pharmacol*. 2007;50:487.

10. Prichard BN, Cruickshank JM, Graham BR. Beta-adrenergic blocking drugs in the treatment of hypertension. *Blood Press*. 2001;10:366.

11. Bangalore S, Messerli FH, Kostis JB, Pepine CJ. Cardiovascular protection using beta-blockers: a critical review of the evidence. *J Am Coll Cardiol*. 2007;50:563.

12. Bangalore S, Kamalakkannan G, Messerli FH. Beta-blockers: no longer an option for uncomplicated hypertension. *Curr Cardiol Rep*. 2007;9:441.

13. Wiysonge CS, Bradley H, Mayosi BM, et al. Beta-blockers for hypertension. *Cochrane Database Syst Rev*. 2007;CD002003.

14. Zusman RM. The role of alpha 1-blockers in combination therapy for hypertension. *Int J Clin Pract*. 2000;54:36.

15. Sica DA. Centrally acting antihypertensive agents: an update. *J Clin Hypertens*. 2007;9:399.

16. Sica DA. Minoxidil: an underused vasodilator for resistant or severe hypertension. *J Clin Hypertens*. 2004;6:283.

17. Toto RD. Treatment of hypertension in chronic kidney disease. *Semin Nephrol*. 2005;25:435.

18. Atlas SA. The renin–angiotensin aldosterone system: pathophysiological role and pharmacologic inhibition. *J Manag Care Pharm*. 2007;13(suppl B):9.

19. Schmieder RE. Renin inhibitors: optimal strategy for renal protection. *Curr Hypertens Rep*. 2007;9:415.

20. White WB. Angiotensin-converting enzyme inhibitors in the treatment of hypertension: an update. *J Clin Hypertens*. 2007;9:876.

21. Linas SL. Are two better than one? Angiotensin-converting enzyme inhibitors plus angiotensin receptor blockers for reducing blood pressure and proteinuria in kidney disease. *Clin J Am Soc Nephrol*. 2008;3(suppl 1):S17-S23. Review.

22. Triggle DJ. Calcium channel antagonists: clinical uses—past, present and future. *Biochem Pharmacol*. 2007;74:1.

23. Liebson PR. Calcium channel blockers in the spectrum of antihypertensive agents. *Expert Opin Pharmacother*. 2006;7:2385.

24. Opie LH, Yusuf S, Kübler W. Current status of safety and efficacy of calcium channel blockers in cardiovascular diseases: a critical analysis based on 100 studies. *Prog Cardiovasc Dis*. 2000;43:171.

25. Bertolotti M, Maurantonio M, Gabbi C, et al. Review article: hyperlipidaemia and cardiovascular risk. *Aliment Pharmacol Ther*. 2005;22(suppl 2):28-30.

26. Green ML. Management of dyslipidemias in the age of statins. *Prim Care*. 2003;30:641.

27. Sviridov D, Nestel P, Watts G. Statins and metabolism of high density lipoprotein. *Cardiovasc Hematol Agents Med Chem*. 2007;5:215.

28. Selwyn AP. Antiatherosclerotic effects of statins: LDL versus non-LDL effects. *Curr Atheroscler Rep*. 2007;9:281.

29. Garg A, Simha V. Update on dyslipidemia. *J Clin Endocrinol Metab*. 2007;92:1581.

30. Ahn SC. Neuromuscular complications of statins. *Phys Med Rehabil Clin N Am*. 2008;19:47.

31. Harper CR, Jacobson TA. The broad spectrum of statin myopathy: from myalgia to rhabdomyolysis. *Curr Opin Lipidol*. 2007;18:401.

32. Després JP, Lemieux I, Robins SJ. Role of fibric acid derivatives in the management of risk factors for coronary heart disease. *Drugs*. 2004;64:2177.

33. Insull W Jr. Clinical utility of bile acid sequestrants in the treatment of dyslipidemia: a scientific review. *South Med J*. 2006;99:257.

34. Drexel H. Nicotinic acid in the treatment of hyperlipidaemia. *Fundam Clin Pharmacol*. 2007;21(suppl 2):5.

35. Bays HE, Neff D, Tomassini JE, Tershakovec AM. Ezetimibe: cholesterol lowering and beyond. *Expert Rev Cardiovasc Ther*. 2008;6:447.

36. Chakrabarti R, Das SK. Advances in antithrombotic agents. *Cardiovasc Hematol Agents Med Chem*. 2007;5:175.

37. Li W, Johnson DJ, Esmon CT, Huntington JA. Structure of the antithrombin–thrombin–heparin ternary complex reveals the antithrombotic mechanism of heparin. *Nat Struct Mol Biol*. 2004;11:857.

38. McRae SJ, Eikelboom JW. Latest medical treatment strategies for venous thromboembolism. *Expert Opin Pharmacother*. 2007;8:1221.

39. Hull RD, Pineo GF. Heparin and low-molecular-weight heparin therapy for venous thromboembolism: will unfractionated heparin survive? *Semin Thromb Hemost*. 2004;30(suppl 1):11-23.

40. De Luca G, Marino P. Adjunctive benefits from low-molecular-weight heparins as compared to unfractionated heparin among patients with ST-segment elevation myocardial infarction treated with thrombolysis. A meta-analysis of the randomized trials. *Am Heart J*. 2007;154:1085.

41. Sandercock P, Counsell C, Stobbs SL. Low-molecular-weight heparins or heparinoids versus standard unfractionated heparin for acute ischaemic stroke. *Cochrane Database Syst Rev*. 2005;CD000119.

42. Castelli R, Cassinerio E, Cappellini MD, et al. Heparin induced thrombocytopenia: pathogenetic, clinical, diagnostic and therapeutic aspects. *Cardiovasc Hematol Disord Drug Targets*. 2007;7:153.

43. Ansell J, Hirsh J, Poller L, et al. The pharmacology and management of the vitamin K antagonists: the Seventh ACCP Conference on Antithrombotic and Thrombolytic Therapy. *Chest*. 2004;126(suppl):204S.

44. Lemos Silva R, Carvalho de Sousa J, Calisto C, et al. Oral anti-coagulant therapy. Fundamentals, clinical practice and recommendations. *Rev Port Cardiol.* 2007;26:769.

45. Huisman MV, Bounameaux H. Treating patients with venous thromboembolism: initial strategies and long-term secondary prevention. *Semin Vasc Med.* 2005;5:276.

46. Majerus PW, Tollefsen DM. Blood coagulation and anticoagulant, thrombolytic, and antiplatelet drugs. In: Brunton LL, ed. *The Pharmacological Basis of Therapeutics.* 11th ed. New York: McGraw-Hill; 2006:1467-1488.

47. Diener HC. Antiplatelet agents and randomized trials. *Rev Neurol Dis.* 2007;4:177.

48. Patrono C, Rocca B. Aspirin: promise and resistance in the new millennium. *Arterioscler Thromb Vasc Biol.* 2008;28:s25.

49. Behan MW, Storey RF. Antiplatelet therapy in cardiovascular disease. *Postgrad Med J.* 2004;80:155.

50. Campbell CL, Smyth S, Montalescot G, Steinhubl SR. Aspirin dose for the prevention of cardiovascular disease: a systematic review. *JAMA.* 2007;297:2018.

51. Kong DF. Aspirin in cardiovascular disorders. What is the optimum dose? *Am J Cardiovasc Drugs.* 2004;4:151.

52. Savi P, Herbert JM. Clopidogrel and ticlopidine: P2Y12 adenosine diphosphate-receptor antagonists for the prevention of atherothrombosis. *Semin Thromb Hemost.* 2005;31:174.

53. Tricoci P, Peterson ED. The evolving role of glycoprotein IIb/IIIa inhibitor therapy in contemporary care of acute coronary syndrome patients. *J Interv Cardiol.* 2006;19:449.

54. Kiernan TJ, Gersh BJ. Thrombolysis in acute myocardial infarction: current status. *Med Clin North Am.* 2007;91:617.

55. Perler B. Thrombolytic therapies: the current state of affairs. *J Endovasc Ther.* 2005;12:224.

56. Hilleman DE, Tsikouris JP, Seals AA, Marmur JD. Fibrinolytic agents for the management of ST-segment elevation myocardial infarction. *Pharmacotherapy.* 2007;27:1558.

57. McNamara RL, Herrin J, Wang Y, et al. Impact of delay in door-to-needle time on mortality in patients with ST-segment elevation myocardial infarction. *Am J Cardiol.* 2007;100:1227.

58. Wardlaw JM, Zoppo G, Yamaguchi T, Berge E. Thrombolysis for acute ischaemic stroke. *Cochrane Database Syst Rev.* 2003;CD000213.

59. Fitchett D. The impact of bleeding in patients with acute coronary syndromes: how to optimize the benefits of treatment and minimize the risk. *Can J Cardiol.* 2007;23:663.

60. Stead LF, Perera R, Bullen C, et al. Nicotine replacement therapy for smoking cessation. *Cochrane Database Syst Rev.* 2008;CD000146.

61. Richmond R, Zwar N. Review of bupropion for smoking cessation. *Drug Alcohol Rev.* 2003;22:203.

62. Dwoskin LP, Rauhut AS, King-Pospisil KA, Bardo MT. Review of the pharmacology and clinical profile of bupropion, an antidepressant and tobacco use cessation agent. *CNS Drug Rev.* 2006;12:178.

63. Holm KJ, Spencer CM. Bupropion: a review of its use in the management of smoking cessation. *Drugs.* 2000;59:1007.

64. Glover ED, Rath JM. Varenicline: progress in smoking cessation treatment. *Expert Opin Pharmacother.* 2007;8:1757.

65. Potts LA, Garwood CL. Varenicline: the newest agent for smoking cessation. *Am J Health Syst Pharm.* 2007;64:1381.

66. Salsali A, Nathan M. A review of types 1 and 2 diabetes mellitus and their treatment with insulin. *Am J Ther.* 2006;13:349.

67. Bhatia E, Aggarwal A. Insulin therapy for patients with type 1 diabetes. *J Assoc Physicians India.* 2007;55(suppl):29.

68. Phillips LK, Phillips PJ. Innovative insulins—where do analogues fit? *Aust Fam Physician.* 2006;35:969.

69. Khafagy el-S, Morishita M, Onuki Y, Takayama K. Current challenges in non–invasive insulin delivery systems: a comparative review. *Adv Drug Deliv Rev.* 2007;59:1521.

70. Lassmann-Vague V, Raccah D. Alternatives routes of insulin delivery. *Diabetes Metab.* 2006;32(pt 2):513.

71. Krentz AJ, Bailey CJ. Oral antidiabetic agents: current role in type 2 diabetes mellitus. *Drugs.* 2005;65:385.

72. Nelson SE, Palumbo PJ. Addition of insulin to oral therapy in patients with type 2 diabetes. *Am J Med Sci.* 2006;331:257.

73. Frier BM. How hypoglycaemia can affect the life of a person with diabetes. *Diabetes Metab Res Rev.* 2008;24:87.

74. Karam JG, El-Sayegh S, Nessim F, et al. Medical management of obesity: an update. *Minerva Endocrinol.* 2007;32:185.

75. Bray GA. Drug insight: appetite suppressants. *Nat Clin Pract Gastroenterol Hepatol.* 2005;2:89.

76. Halford JC, Cooper GD, Dovey TM. The pharmacology of human appetite expression. *Curr Drug Targets.* 2004;5:221.

77. Fernstrom JD, Choi S. The development of tolerance to drugs that suppress food intake. *Pharmacol Ther.* 2008;117:105.

78. Drew BS, Dixon AF, Dixon JB. Obesity management: update on orlistat. *Vasc Health Risk Manag.* 2007;3:817.

79. Padwal RS, Majumdar SR. Drug treatments for obesity: orlistat, sibutramine, and rimonabant. *Lancet.* 2007;369:71.

80. Wellman PJ, Maher TJ. Synergistic interactions between fenfluramine and phentermine. *Int J Obes Relat Metab Disord.* 1999;23:723.

81. Arora S, Anubhuti. Role of neuropeptides in appetite regulation and obesity—a review. *Neuropeptides.* 2006;40:375.

82. King PJ. The hypothalamus and obesity. *Curr Drug Targets.* 2005;6:225.

83. Sharma M. Behavioural interventions for preventing and treating obesity in adults. *Obes Rev.* 2007;8:441.

84. Chung KF. Drugs to suppress cough. *Expert Opin Investig Drugs.* 2005;14:19.

85. Smith SM, Schroeder K, Fahey T. Over-the-counter medications for acute cough in children and adults in ambulatory settings. *Cochrane Database Syst Rev.* 2008;CD001831.

86. Kelley LK, Allen PJ. Managing acute cough in children: evidence-based guidelines. *Pediatr Nurs.* 2007;33:515.

87. Schroeder K, Fahey T. Should we advise parents to administer over the counter cough medicines for acute cough? Systematic review of randomised controlled trials. *Arch Dis Child.* 2002;86:170.

88. Miyahara S, Miyahara N, Lucas JJ, et al. Contribution of allergen-specific and nonspecific nasal responses to early-phase and late-phase nasal responses. *J Allergy Clin Immunol.* 2008;121:718.

89. Corboz MR, Rivelli MA, Mingo GG, et al. Mechanism of decongestant activity of alpha(2)-adrenoceptor agonists. *Pulm Pharmacol Ther.* 2008;21:449.

90. Taverner D, Latte J. Nasal decongestants for the common cold. *Cochrane Database Syst Rev.* 2007;CD001953.

91. Rogers DF. Mucoactive agents for airway mucus hypersecretory diseases. *Respir Care.* 2007;52:1176.

92. Ingenito EP. Medical therapy for chronic obstructive pulmonary disease in 2007. *Semin Thorac Cardiovasc Surg.* 2007;19:142.

93. Cockcroft DW. Clinical concerns with inhaled beta2-agonists: adult asthma. *Clin Rev Allergy Immunol.* 2006;31:197.

94. Barnes PJ. Theophylline in chronic obstructive pulmonary disease: new horizons. *Proc Am Thorac Soc.* 2005;2:334.

95. Restrepo RD. Use of inhaled anticholinergic agents in obstructive airway disease. *Respir Care.* 2007;52:833.

96. Gross NJ. Anticholinergic agents in asthma and COPD. *Eur J Pharmacol.* 2006;533:36.

97. Barnes PJ. Immunology of asthma and chronic obstructive pulmonary disease. *Nat Rev Immunol.* 2008;8:183.

98. Adcock IM, Caramori G, Ito K. New insights into the molecular mechanisms of corticosteroids actions. *Curr Drug Targets.* 2006;7:649.

99. Gulliver T, Morton R, Eid N. Inhaled corticosteroids in children with asthma: pharmacologic determinants of safety and efficacy and other clinical considerations. *Paediatr Drugs.* 2007;9:185.

100. Irwin RS, Richardson ND. Side effects with inhaled corticosteroids: the physician's perception. *Chest.* 2006;130(suppl):41S.

101. Phua GC, Macintyre NR. Inhaled corticosteroids in obstructive airway disease. *Respir Care.* 2007;52:852.

102. Ogawa Y, Calhoun WJ. The role of leukotrienes in airway inflammation. *J Allergy Clin Immunol.* 2006;118:789.

103. Berger W, De Chandt MT, Cairns CB. Zileuton: clinical implications of 5-lipoxygenase inhibition in severe airway disease. *Int J Clin Pract.* 2007;61:663.

104. Riccioni G, Bucciarelli T, Mancini B, et al. Antileukotriene drugs: clinical application, effectiveness and safety. *Curr Med Chem.* 2007;14:1966.

105. Sridhar AV, McKean M. Nedocromil sodium for chronic asthma in children. *Cochrane Database Syst Rev.* 2006;CD004108.

106. Smulyan H. Nitrates, arterial function, wave reflections and coronary heart disease. *Adv Cardiol.* 2007;44:302.

107. Thadani U, Rodgers T. Side effects of using nitrates to treat angina. *Expert Opin Drug Saf.* 2006;5:667.

108. Bhatt AB, Stone PH. Current strategies for the prevention of angina in patients with stable coronary artery disease. *Curr Opin Cardiol.* 2006;21:492.

109. Van Spall HG, Overgaard CB, Abramson BL. Coronary vasospasm: a case report and review of the literature. *Can J Cardiol.* 2005;21:953.

110. Bauman JL, Schoen MD. Arrhythmias. In: DiPiro JT, Talbert RL, Yee GC, et al., eds. *Pharmacotherapy: A Pathophysiologic Approach.* 5th ed. New York: McGraw-Hill;2002:273-303.

111. Roden DM, Anderson ME. Proarrhythmia. *Handb Exp Pharmacol.* 2006;171:73.

112. Fukuta H, Little WC. The cardiac cycle and the physiologic basis of left ventricular contraction, ejection, relaxation, and filling. *Heart Fail Clin.* 2008;4:1.

113. Morris SA, Hatcher HF, Reddy DK. Digoxin therapy for heart failure: an update. *Am Fam Physician.* 2006;74:613.

114. Johnson JA, Parker RB, Patterson JH. Heart failure. In: DiPiro JT, Talbert RL, Yee GC, et al., eds. *Pharmacotherapy: A Pathophysiologic Approach.* 5th ed. New York: McGraw-Hill;2002: 185-218.

115. Bauman JL, Didomenico RJ, Galanter WL. Mechanisms, manifestations, and management of digoxin toxicity in the modern era. *Am J Cardiovasc Drugs.* 2006;6:77.

116. Petersen JW, Felker GM. Inotropes in the management of acute heart failure. *Crit Care Med.* 2008;36(suppl):S106.

117. Parissis JT, Farmakis D, Nieminen M. Classical inotropes and new cardiac enhancers. *Heart Fail Rev.* 2007;12:149.

118. Hamad E, Mather PJ, Srinivasan S, et al. Pharmacologic therapy of chronic heart failure. *Am J Cardiovasc Drugs.* 2007;7:235.

119. Jneid H, Moukarbel GV, Dawson B, et al. Combining neuroendocrine inhibitors in heart failure: reflections on safety and efficacy. *Am J Med.* 2007;120:1090.

120. Simon BA, Moody EJ, Johns RA. Therapeutic gases: oxygen, carbon dioxide, nitric oxide, and helium. In: Brunton LL, ed. *The Pharmacological Basis of Therapeutics.* 11th ed. New York: McGraw-Hill; 2006:387-399.

121. Ambrosino N, Di Giorgio M, Di Paco A. The patients with severe chronic obstructive pulmonary disease and chronic respiratory insufficiency. *Monaldi Arch Chest Dis.* 2007;67:148.

122. Kress JP, Hall JB. Sedation in the mechanically ventilated patient. *Crit Care Med.* 2006;34:2541.

123. Olkkola KT, Ahonen J. Midazolam and other benzodiazepines. *Handb Exp Pharmacol.* 2008;182:335.

124. Wong C, Burry L, Molino-Carmona S, et al. Analgesic and sedative pharmacology in the intensive care unit. *Dynamics.* 2004;15:23.

125. Zöllner C, Stein C. Opioids. *Handb Exp Pharmacol.* 2007;177:31.

126. Vilela H, Ferreira D. Analgesia, sedation and neuromuscular blockade in mechanically ventilated cardiac intensive care unit patients. Part III—neuromuscular blockade. *Rev Port Cardiol.* 2006;25:341.

127. Goodman BP, Boon AJ. Critical illness neuromyopathy. *Phys Med Rehabil Clin N Am.* 2008;19:97.

128. Stevens RD, Dowdy DW, Michaels RK, et al. Neuromuscular dysfunction acquired in critical illness: a systematic review. *Intensive Care Med.* 2007;33:1876.

129. Gal P, Shaffer CL. Acute respiratory distress syndrome. In: DiPiro JT, Talbert RL, Yee GC, et al., eds. *Pharmacotherapy: A Pathophysiologic Approach.* 5th ed. New York: McGraw-Hill; 2002:531-548.

130. Engle WA; American Academy of Pediatrics Committee on Fetus and Newborn. Surfactant-replacement therapy for respiratory distress in the preterm and term neonate. *Pediatrics.* 2008;121:419.

131. Walther FJ, Waring AJ, Sherman MA, et al. Hydrophobic surfactant proteins and their analogues. *Neonatology.* 2007;91:303.

132. Pfister RH, Soll RF, Wiswell T. Protein containing synthetic surfactant versus animal derived surfactant extract for the prevention and treatment of respiratory distress syndrome. *Cochrane Database Syst Rev.* 2007;CD006069.

133. Abman SH. Recent advances in the pathogenesis and treatment of persistent pulmonary hypertension of the newborn. *Neonatology.* 2007;91:283.

134. Dahlem P, van Aalderen WM, Bos AP. Pediatric acute lung injury. *Paediatr Respir Rev.* 2007;8:348.

135. Bloch KD, Ichinose F, Roberts JD Jr, Zapol WM. Inhaled NO as a therapeutic agent. *Cardiovasc Res.* 2007;75:339.

136. Gnanaratnem J, Finer NN. Neonatal acute respiratory failure. *Curr Opin Pediatr.* 2000;12:227.

137. Barrington KJ, Finer NN. Inhaled nitric oxide for respiratory failure in preterm infants. *Cochrane Database Syst Rev.* 2007;CD000509.

138. Finer NN, Barrington KJ. Nitric oxide for respiratory failure in infants born at or near term. *Cochrane Database Syst Rev.* 2006;CD000399.

139. Crowther CA, Harding JE. Repeat doses of prenatal corticosteroids for women at risk of preterm birth for preventing neonatal respiratory disease. *Cochrane Database Syst Rev.* 2007;CD003935.

140. Shah SS, Ohlsson A, Halliday H, Shah VS. Inhaled versus systemic corticosteroids for the treatment of chronic lung disease in ventilated very low birth weight preterm infants. *Cochrane Database Syst Rev.* 2007;CD002057.

141. Halliday HL. Clinical trials of postnatal corticosteroids: inhaled and systemic. *Biol Neonate.* 1999;76(suppl 1):29.

142. Cavalieri RL, Cohen WR. Antenatal steroid therapy: have we undervalued the risks? *J Matern Fetal Neonatal Med.* 2006;19:265.

143. Dalziel SR, Lim VK, Lambert A, et al. Antenatal exposure to betamethasone: psychological functioning and health related quality of life 31 years after inclusion in randomised controlled trial. *BMJ.* 2005;331:665.

144. Romagnoli C, Zecca E, Luciano R, et al. A three year follow up of preterm infants after moderately early treatment with dexamethasone. *Arch Dis Child Fetal Neonatal Ed.* 2002;87:F55.

145. Zuther JE. *Lymphedema Management.* New York: Thieme Medical Publishers; 2005.

146. Warren AG, Brorson H, Borud LJ, Slavin SA. Lymphedema: a comprehensive review. *Ann Plast Surg.* 2007;59:464.

147. Nutman TB. Lymphatic filariasis: new insights and prospects for control. *Curr Opin Infect Dis.* 2001;14:539.

148. Kligman L, Wong RK, Johnston M, Laetsch NS. The treatment of lymphedema related to breast cancer: a systematic review and evidence summary. *Support Care Cancer.* 2004;12:421.

149. Mortimer PS. Therapy approaches for lymphedema. *Angiology.* 1997;48:87.

150. Badger C, Preston N, Seers K, Mortimer P. Benzo-pyrones for reducing and controlling lymphoedema of the limbs. *Cochrane Database Syst Rev.* 2004;CD003140.

151. Boursier V. Lymphedema: which drug therapy? *Rev Med Interne.* 2002;23(suppl 3):421s.

152. Burgos A, Alcaide A, Alcoba C, et al. Comparative study of the clinical efficacy of two different coumarin dosages in the management of arm lymphedema after treatment for breast cancer. *Lymphology.* 1999;32:3.

153. Loprinzi CL, Kugler JW, Sloan JA, et al. Lack of effect of coumarin in women with lymphedema after treatment for breast cancer. *N Engl J Med.* 1999;340:346.

154. Bruns F, Micke O, Bremer M. Current status of selenium and other treatments for secondary lymphedema. *J Support Oncol.* 2003;1:121.

155. Dennert G, Horneber M. Selenium for alleviating the side effects of chemotherapy, radiotherapy and surgery in cancer patients. *Cochrane Database Syst Rev.* 2006;CD005037.

C H A P T E R

9

Pulmonary Evaluation

Lawrence P. Cahalin

INTRODUCTION

Examination of the pulmonary system requires optimal use of auditory, observational, tactile, auscultatory, and medical information. A significant part of this chapter will focus on the actual physical therapy examination process. Perturbation of initial examination findings with auditory, positional, or tactile maneuvers may yield information that could (1) direct further examination techniques, (2) direct treatment techniques, and (3) provide important prognostic information. The following section will review each of the examination techniques

and the application of specific maneuvers that may help to direct and predict the effects of these techniques. A review of medical information and the specific tests and measures providing the most clinically useful information will also be presented.[1-5] Much of this information and the approach used to examine a patient with pulmonary disease are outlined in Box 9-1. This information can be documented in the initial patient note presented in Appendix 1 of this chapter.

PHYSICAL THERAPY EXAMINATIONS

Medical Information and Risk Factor Analysis

The past medical history is an important part of the systems review of all patients. This is particularly true of patients with known or suspected pulmonary disease. A number of previous medical problems may predispose a person to pulmonary disorders. Examples of such previous medical problems are shown in Box 9-2 and include recurrent pulmonary infections, cardiac disease (eg, heart failure), and neuromuscular disorders.[6-8]

The primary and secondary risk factors for pulmonary diseases are also listed in Box 9-2 and include environmental and self-imposed risks. Of all risks, a history of smoking is the greatest key to unlocking the likelihood and severity of pulmonary disease. A smoking history is typically reported in pack years (the number of packs of cigarettes per day multiplied by the number of years smoked). A smoking history of greater than 70 pack years appears to be associated with a

greater likelihood of developing emphysema.[9] Smoking less than 70 pack years is associated with less of a risk of developing lung disease, but not smoking at all is associated with far less risk of developing lung disease. Secondhand smoke is also associated with a greater risk of emphysema and other pulmonary disorders.[10-12]

Listening to a patient's past history and primary complaints is critical in the examination process. In fact, a good history can provide important information that can be very useful in diagnosing a variety of pulmonary disorders. Badgett et al. found that a previous diagnosis of chronic obstructive pulmonary disease (COPD) and smoking for 70 or more pack years yielded a diagnosis of COPD with a sensitivity of 40% and a specificity of 100%.[9] The only physical examination findings that significantly improved the sensitivity were diminished breath sounds and peak flow. Adding these two variables increased the sensitivity of diagnosing COPD to 77% and slightly decreased the specificity to 95%.[9] Overall, diminished breath sounds were the best sign of moderate COPD. The

---

BOX 9-1

A Suggested Examination Approach to the Patient Designed to Determine the Disablement of Pulmonary Disorders and Direct and Predict Physical Therapy: a Patient Case Example

1. **Why are you here today?***
2. **Have you been diagnosed with a pulmonary disorder in the past?**
3. **Have you had any special tests to examine your lungs like pulmonary function tests?**
4. **Do you experience shortness of breath at rest, only with activity/exercise, or both at rest and with activity/exercise?**
5. If you become short of breath during activity or exercise, could you please **describe the type of activity or exercise that produces your shortness of breath?**
6. Can you **describe your shortness of breath?** Can you help me understand your shortness of breath by pointing to your level of shortness of breath using this 10-point scale or by marking this Visual Analog Scale?
7. Can I **place this finger probe on your index finger to obtain an oxygen saturation measurement?**
8. Can I **listen to your lungs with my stethoscope?**
9. Could I **place one of my hands on your stomach and one hand on your upper chest to determine how you breathe?**
10. Could I **place my hands on the lowermost ribs on each side of your chest to determine how you breathe?**
11. Could I **place my hands on your back to determine how you breathe?**
12. Could I **wrap my tape measure around your chest at several different sites to determine how you breathe?**
13. Now that I understand some very basic information about the manner in which you breathe, could you please **breathe in the manner I instruct you via sounds I make, pressure from my hands, methods I show to you, or different body positions?** I will occasionally place my hands on your chest and wrap my tape measure around your chest to determine how you breathe during these simple tests, and I will ask you to identify your level of shortness of breath using the 10-point scale or Visual Analog Scale—Is this OK with you?
14. Could I **measure the strength of your breathing muscles** by having you place this mouthpiece in your mouth and breathe in and out as deeply and as forcefully as you are able to do?
15. I would like you to **now perform the activity or exercise that produces your shortness of breath**—Could you please do this now?
16. Thank you for giving me the chance to examine you today. I will call your physician to get some more information about you such as the **pulmonary function tests that you said were performed last week as well as the arterial blood gas results, chest X-ray, and exercise test results.** In the meantime, I would like you to practice breathing in the manner that we discovered that helped you feel less short of breath and produced the best chest wall motion that I felt with my hands and measured with the tape measure. I will see you next week for further examinations and treatments.

*The information given in bold identifies important examination procedures for patients with pulmonary disorders.

---

importance of good listening as the beginning part of the auditory examination cannot be overstated. **Listening to a patient's past history, habits, and complaints (and attempting to quantify these variables) are instrumental in understanding the absence or presence of disease, severity of disease, treatment choice, treatment effects, and quality of life.** A patient's appearance can also provide information about the presence and severity of pulmonary disease.

Patient Appearance

The appearance of a patient can suggest the presence and severity of several pulmonary disorders such as emphysema, chronic bronchitis, or restrictive lung disease such as spinal cord injury. In fact, appearance, historically, has been a method to categorize patients with COPD. Patients with spinal cord injury often lack adequate abdominal muscle support, which results in a characteristic posture described as a "pot-belly" appearance. These examples are just a few of the many characteristics that can be observed in a patient's appearance (Table 9-1). Other signs of pulmonary disease are also presented in Table 9-1.

Dyspnea—Methods to Evaluate Shortness of Breath

One of the major complaints of patients with pulmonary disorders is shortness of breath. The purpose of this section is to present the different methods that may be used to evaluate shortness of breath. A variety of different methods to evaluate dyspnea are available and are shown in Table 9-2.[13-15] The strengths and weaknesses of each of the methods to measure dyspnea are also presented in Table 9-2. The most common method to evaluate dyspnea is likely the Borg-modified dyspnea scale of 0 to 10, which is anchored with descriptive terms that describe the sensation and amount of dyspnea a patient is experiencing. The original Borg rating of perceived exertion is occasionally used to evaluate dyspnea and overall systemic exertion at rest or during exercise. Both the original and the modified dyspnea scales and their descriptive terms are provided in Table 9-3. Other scales such as the Mahler dyspnea scale are available, but often their clinical utility is diminished because of the time and effort needed to administer them to patients.[16] Other important aspects of the auditory examination will be presented in the following section.

BOX 9-2

Risk Factors for Pulmonary Disorders

Previous medical problems predisposing a person to pulmonary disorders

1. Recurrent pulmonary infections
2. Heart failure
3. Neuromuscular disorders (eg, cerebrovascular accident (CVA), Guillain–Barré syndrome, muscular dystrophy)
4. Musculoskeletal disorders (eg, scoliosis, ankylosing spondylitis, pectus excavatum)
5. Integumentary disorders (eg, marked burns to thorax, scleroderma)
6. Past oncologic disorder treated with chemotherapy or radiation therapy
7. Obesity
8. Premature birth

Primary and secondary risk factors for pulmonary diseases
Obstructive lung disease

1. Smoking
2. Occupational exposure to irritants or allergens (eg, asbestos, chemicals)
3. Residing in locations with high levels of air pollution
4. Premature birth—bronchopulmonary dysplasia
5. Emphysema
6. α_1-Antitrypsin deficiency
7. Asthma
8. Bronchitis
9. Bronchiectasis
10. Cystic fibrosis

Restrictive lung disease

1. Occupational exposure to irritants or allergens (eg, asbestos, chemicals)
2. Cardiovascular disorders (eg, pulmonary edema from heart failure, pulmonary emboli)
3. Neuromuscular disorders (eg, spinal cord injury [SCI], CVA, Guillain–Barré syndrome, muscular dystrophy)
4. Musculoskeletal disorders (eg, scoliosis, ankylosing spondylitis, pectus excavatum)
5. Integumentary disorders (eg, marked burns to thorax, scleroderma)
6. Immunologic disorders (eg, Wegener granulomatosis, Goodpasture syndrome)
7. Past oncologic disorder treated with chemotherapy or radiation therapy
8. Trauma (eg, crush injuries)
9. Surgical pain or scarring
10. Obesity
11. Pregnancy
12. Premature birth—hyaline membrane disease

Pulmonary hypertension

Primary pulmonary hypertension
1. Autoimmune dysfunction
2. Vascular dysfunction

Secondary pulmonary hypertension
1. Severe obstructive or restrictive lung disease
2. Severe heart failure

TABLE 9-1 Particular Patient Characteristics Suggestive of a Pulmonary Disorder

Patient Presentation	Underlying Rationale	Pulmonary Disorder
Dyspnea	VPD or VPF	Most pulmonary disorders
Excessive accessory muscle use	Necessary to breathe	Most pulmonary disorders
Cyanosis of skin, lips, or extremities	Poor oxygenation	Many pulmonary disorders, but bronchitis in particular (eg, blue bloater)
Digital clubbing	Chronic poor oxygenation	Many pulmonary disorders
Look of apprehension	Dyspnea and increased work of breathing	Many pulmonary disorders
Nasal flaring	Dyspnea and increased work of breathing	Many pulmonary disorders
Nasal prongs and oxygen tubing with oxygen tank	Necessary to improve oxygenation and comfort	Many pulmonary disorders
Abnormal breathing pattern	VPD or VPF[a]	Many pulmonary disorders, but an abdominal paradoxical breathing pattern is associated with diaphragmatic paralysis (ie, C2 spinal cord injury) or severe diaphragmatic flattening (ie, COPD); both are suggestive of VPF in need of intervention

[a]VPD, ventilatory pump dysfunction; VPF, ventilatory pump failure; C2, second cervical vertebra; COPD, chronic obstructive pulmonary disease.

TABLE 9-2   **Different Methods to Evaluate Dyspnea**

Method	Strengths	Weaknesses	Examination Technique
Borg 1–10	Ratio scale	Patient unfriendly	Number scale with descriptors
Borg 6–20	Ordinal scale	Somewhat patient friendly	Number scale with descriptors
Visual Analog Scale	Patient friendly	?	10-cm line with "no" and "severe dsypnea" written at the ends of the line which can be positioned vertically or horizontally
Dyspnea index	Accurate and physiologically sound	Requires PFTs,[a] Exercise, and peak exercise $\dot{V}E$ to be performed	Peak exercise $\dot{V}E$ is compared to the measured or estimated MVV ($\dot{V}E$/MVV) and if the peak exercise $\dot{V}E$ is ≥ to MVV then dyspnea is likely due to a pulmonary limitation
Questionnaires	More specific	Time consuming, often requires a health care professional to administer, and often patient unfriendly	Questionnaire administered to a patient by a health care professional using specific methods

[a]PFTs, pulmonary function tests; $\dot{V}E$, ventilation; MVV, maximal voluntary ventilation.
?The question mark imply questionable or unknown characteristics.

Auditory Examination
Listening to the Breathing Cycle

Listening to the breathing cycle of a patient, one can provide very important information about other needed patient examinations and treatments. Listening to the baseline inspiratory

TABLE 9-3   **Original and Modified Borg Dyspnea Scales**

Original Borg Dyspnea Scale		Modified Borg Dyspnea Scale	
6		Nothing at all	0
7	Very, very light	Very, very slight	0.5
8			
9	Very light	Very slight	1
10			
11	Fairly light	Slight	2
12			
13	Somewhat hard	Moderate	3
14			
15	Hard	Somewhat severe	4
16			
17	Very hard	Severe	5
18			6
19	Very, very hard	Very severe	7
20			8
		Very, very severe	9
		(almost maximal) maximal	10

Adapted with permission from McGraw-Hill from Cahalin LP. Exercise tolerance and training for healthy persons and patients with cardiovascular disease. Ch. 7 In: Hasson S, ed. *Clinical Exercise Physiology*. St Louis, MO: Mosby-Year Book; 1994:121.

and expiratory cycles of breathing can provide information about the respiratory rate, type of primary lung disease, and the effects of specific maneuvers on the baseline breathing pattern, which may be helpful to direct specific therapeutic interventions.[17]

For example, a rapid respiratory rate with short and shallow inspiratory and expiratory periods heard at rest may indicate a primary lung abnormality. Likewise, a prolonged expiratory portion of the inspiratory–expiratory duty cycle may be suggestive of a primary obstructive lung disease. A rapid respiratory rate with a prolonged expiratory phase may be indicative of a patient with isolated obstructive lung disease or combined obstructive and restrictive lung disease.[17,18] These auditory patterns are described in Table 9-4.

Simple perturbations of the baseline breathing cycle via body position changes, pursed-lip breathing, or therapist-simulated breathing (breathing out loud with the patient in a desired pattern of breathing) can direct further examination techniques or suggest potential treatment techniques.[19,20] Several possible perturbations to the baseline breathing cycle are listed in Table 9-4. Auscultation of the lungs follows the auditory examination and will be presented in the next section.

Auscultation of the Lungs
Proper Use of the Stethoscope

Proper use of the stethoscope is crucial in the examination of patients with cardiopulmonary diseases.[21,22] The stethoscope is a medical tool that is often taken for granted. It was developed in 1816 by Rene Laennec after he observed children with their ears pressed against the end of a long, hollow log, while other children were tapping with stones at the other end of the log. Laennec shortly thereafter used tightly wound newspapers and large wooden tubes to examine the sounds heard in the thorax. He later refined the wooden tubes and while doing so developed a new clinical tool and terminology that is still in

TABLE 9-4   Listening to the Breathing Cycle at Rest and During Perturbations

Listening at Rest			
Respiratory Rate (RR)	**Inspiratory Cycle**	**Expiratory Phase**	**Possible Pulmonary Problem**
Rapid	Short	Short	Restrictive lung disease
Slow	Short	Prolonged	COPD
Rapid	Short	Prolonged	COPD or combined COPD restrictive lung disease

Listening During Perturbations				
RR	**Inspiratory Cycle**	**Expiratory Cycle**	**Perturbation**	**Anticipated Effect**
Rapid	Short	Short	Body position change/MT[a] Auditory stimulus[b]	Lengthened inspiratory and expiratory cycles and decreased RR
Slow	Short	Prolonged	Pursed-lip breathing (PLB), Auditory stimulus	Shortened expiratory cycle and possible lengthened inspiratory cycle
Rapid	Short	Prolonged	PLB, body position change Auditory stimulus	Shortened expiratory cycle and possible lengthened inspiratory cycle and decreased RR

[a]Manual techniques such as tactile stimulation, quick stretches to facilitate inspiratory or expiratory muscles, inhibitory stimulation to excessive accessory muscle use via hand pressure, or other manual techniques with possible addition of biofeedback mechanisms (incentive spirometry, electromyography, or oxygen saturation; these methods will be discussed in greater detail in Chapter 19.

[b]Therapist-simulated breathing (breathing out loud with the patient in a desired pattern of breathing).

use today. The stethoscope has since undergone significant modifications and has enabled health care professionals throughout the past two centuries to enhance physical examinations and determine the effects of medical treatment. Although the clinical utility of auscultation has been questioned and the reliability of auscultation has been observed to be modest to poor, it remains a useful adjunct in the examination of patients with cardiovascular and pulmonary disorders.[21-24] Furthermore, the recent introduction of electronic stethoscopes now provides superior acoustic recognition, digital signal processing, and recording of breath and heart sounds that can be downloaded to personal computers. Auscultation of the heart and lungs with an electronic stethoscope appears to address many of the limitations previously identified with traditional auscultation.

The stethoscope usually consists of a diaphragm and bell as shown in Fig. 9-1. Stethoscopes without the bell exist but are frequently lower-quality stethoscopes with limited auscultatory ability. The stethoscope should be of acceptable quality to enable accurate auscultation of the heart and lungs and should have most of the characteristics that are listed in Box 9-3. The presence of a diaphragm and bell, tubing size of at least 50 cm, and a comfortable earpiece fit are possibly the most important qualities of a good stethoscope. The presence of a diaphragm and bell on the stethoscope ensure that the stethoscope is of a moderate to high quality, and a comfortable and correct earpiece fit will enable longer periods of auscultation.

The earpieces are inserted into the ears with the earpieces facing (pointing toward) the patient. This aligns the earpieces

with the auditory canal. Placing the earpieces into the ears backward (with the earpieces pointing to the therapist) reduces heart and lung sounds and is a common error of students and new clinicians. Optimal auscultation of the lungs can be accomplished by using the helpful hints listed in Box 9-3.[21,22]

Method of Auscultating the Lungs

The method of auscultating the lungs requires proper use of the stethoscope as well as the correct placement of the diaphragm of the stethoscope on the chest. A systematic approach to lung auscultation is important and is always performed in such a manner that allows one side of the chest to be compared to the other side at the same level.[21,22] The traditional sites used for auscultation of the lungs are shown in Fig. 9-1. This figure shows that there are six to eight auscultatory sites on the posterior chest and four to six sites on the anterior chest. Two sites are also present in the left and right axillary areas. Placement of the diaphragm of the stethoscope in these areas in a systematic manner and comparing both sides of the chest will improve lung auscultation efforts.

It is not uncommon for patients to become dizzy and fatigued during continuous auscultation of the chest because of repeated deep breathing. Patients should be instructed to stop and rest during a complete lung auscultatory examination. It is recommended that the patient take two complete deep breaths while the diaphragm of the stethoscope is applied at each site followed by a short rest.[21,22] Figure 9-1 may be helpful in understanding what lobes of the lungs are being auscultated when the diaphragm is placed at each of the sites on

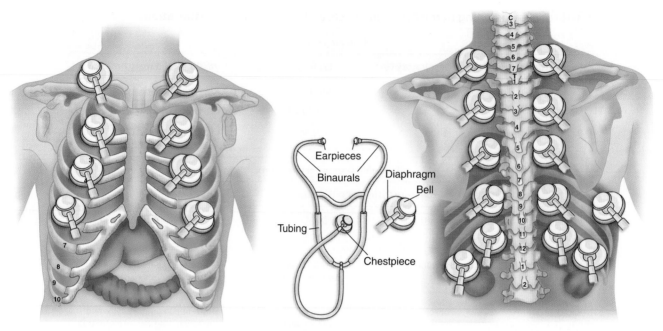

FIGURE 9-1   The stethoscope and sites for optimal auscultation with underlying lung segments.

the chest. The second and third laboratory exercises mentioned at the end of this chapter may also be helpful.

Sounds Heard During Auscultation of the Lungs—Breath Sounds

The sounds heard during auscultation of the lungs can be summarized as tracheal, bronchial, bronchovesicular, or vesicular.[23] Other extra (adventitious) sounds also may be heard during auscultation of the lungs. The different types of breath sounds and the different qualities of the traditional breath sounds are listed in Table 9-5. It is important to note that the four traditional breath sounds are normally heard in the locations listed in Table 9-5. **Breath sounds heard in areas where they are not supposed to be suggest that a pathological**

BOX 9-3

Important Characteristics and Use of the Stethoscope

1. Optimal auscultation can be performed with a stethoscope that has both a bell and a diaphragm (see Fig. 9-1).
2. Use the diaphragm of the stethoscope to auscultate for high-frequency sounds.
3. Use the bell of the stethoscope to auscultate for low-frequency sounds.
4. Optimal tubing length (long enough to allow for adequate distance between patient and therapist, but not too long to cause excessive movement of the tubing, which may interfere with auscultation; approximately 20–26 cm).
5. Comfortable and well-fitting earpieces.
6. Position the earpieces in the ears with both of the earpieces pointing toward the patient or client to be examined (see Fig. 9-1).
7. Ensure correct position of the head of the stethoscope when auscultating with the bell and diaphragm (see Fig. 9-1).*

8. Auscultate directly over the skin with firm pressure on the diaphragm—never auscultate over clothing. Auscultation with the bell should be performed with light pressure on the bell, which will enhance the detection of low-frequency sounds (see Chapter 10 for more information on auscultation with the bell of the stethoscope).
9. Minimize hand movement on the stethoscope and movement of the stethoscope on the skin when auscultating in the areas shown in Fig. 9-1.
10. Encourage patients or clients to take one to two deep breaths at each of the above sites and compare auscultatory findings to the opposite side as shown in Fig. 9-1.
11. Provide patients a rest period after several deep breaths to prevent fatigue, dizziness, or other complaints.
12. Auscultate in a quite environment.

*The head of the stethoscope with both a bell and a diaphragm can rotate so that sound is heard from either the bell or the diaphragm, but never from both at the same time. When the head of the stethoscope is rotated to the bell or diaphragm, a small hole at the base of the metal stethoscope will line up with either the bell or the diaphragm (see Fig. 9-1) and allow sounds to be transmitted through from the head of the stethoscope to the tubing and upward to the ears. Figure 9-1 shows the open hole for use of the bell and the closed hole for use of the diaphragm when auscultating.

TABLE 9-5   **Distinguishing Characteristics of Breath Sounds**[a]

Sound	Location of Sound	Sound Quality	Distinguishing Characteristic
Vesicular	Periphery of lungs	Soft, low-pitched ("gentle rustling sound")	Inspiration is longer and louder than expiration without a pause
Bronchial	Sternum/manubrium	Loud, high-pitched ("hollow-pipe sound")	Expiration is longer and louder than inspiration with a pause
Bronchovesicular	First and second ICS and between scapulae (near mainstem bronchus)	Medium-pitched	Inspiration and expiration are equal in length and loudness
Tracheal	Over the trachea	Loud, harsh	Expiration is slightly longer than inspiration with similar loudness
Adventitious crackles (rales)	Over lungs with disease or disorders	Soft, high-pitched, discontinuous (like hair rubbed between the fingers)	Occur early during inspiration with Bronchitis Emphysema Asthma Occur late during inspiration with Interstitial lung disease Pulmonary edema
Wheeze	Over lungs and airways that are constricted	High-pitched, continuous ("musical")	Heard most often during expiration, but may be heard during inspiration; the result of airway constriction
Transmitted voice sounds Egophony	Over consolidated lung tissue	"E" is heard as "A"	Mass/exudate in the lungs enables greater transmission of the sound of a patient repeating the letter "E"
Bronchophony	Over consolidated lung tissue	"99" is heard clearly	Mass/exudate in the lungs enables greater transmission of the sound of a patient repeating the number "99"
Whispered Pectoriloquy	Over consolidated lung tissue	Whispered sound is heard clearly	Mass/exudate in the lungs enables greater transmission of the sound of a patient whispering

ICS, intercostals space.

[a]The objective of auscultation of the lungs and distinguishing different breath sounds is identifying breath sounds in areas where they should not be located. For example, hearing bronchial breath sounds in the periphery of the lungs is abnormal because vesicular breath sounds should be heard in the periphery of the lungs (bronchial breath sounds should be limited to the sternal area). Specific identification of lung diseases or disorders is difficult via auscultation of the lungs; further tests and measures are needed to identify specific lung disease or disorders.

problem likely exists.[23] Subtle, yet specific, characteristics may accompany the presence of a breath sound in an area where it should not exist. Identifying the presence of a breath sound in an area where it should not be, combined with other specific characteristics, enables the clinician to better understand the pathological process and direct further examination and subsequent treatment. A summary of different breath sounds heard when auscultating the lungs and their pathological implications is listed in Table 9-6.[24]

Chest Wall Excursion and Breathing Patterns

Examination of the baseline breathing pattern is possibly one of the most important and useful examination techniques of patients with pulmonary disease. The absence or presence of an abnormal breathing pattern may better direct other examinations and may be useful to direct specific management efforts (see Chapter 20). Several major types of breathing patterns include normal breathing, abdominal paradoxical breathing, upper-chest paradoxical breathing, and excessive

accessory muscle breathing without abdominal paradoxical breathing.[25] The characteristics and examination techniques of these breathing patterns are listed in Table 9-7.

Identifying an abnormal breathing pattern in a patient with known pulmonary disease may help to direct therapeutic interventions. For example, a patient demonstrating a paradoxical breathing pattern may obtain relief by a change in body position (see Chapter 20).[26,27] Normal and abnormal breathing patterns can be appreciated only after review of the (1) muscles of ventilation, (2) biomechanics of breathing, and (3) tests used to measure breathing patterns. A more detailed review of the ventilatory muscles and the biomechanics of breathing are provided in Chapters 4 and 5, respectively.

Examining the Muscles of Breathing

Inspiratory muscles—The muscles of inspiration consist of primary and secondary (or accessory) muscles. The diaphragm is the primary muscle of inspiration accounting for approximately 75% of the work of inspiration. The secondary or accessory muscles of inspiration include the external intercostals, internal intercostals (the parasternal portion), scalenes, and

TABLE 9-6   Breath Sounds and Other Examination Findings Commonly Associated with Specific Pathologies

Pathology or Condition	Breath Sounds	Adventitious Breath Sounds	Transmitted Voice Sounds	Percussion Sounds	Fremitus	Position of Trachea
Normal Lung	Vesicular	Possibly late-inspiratory crackles at bases which resolve with deep breaths	Absent	Resonant	Normal	Midline
Emphysema	Diminished Vesicular	Usually absent	Absent	Hyperresonant	Decreased	Midline
Bronchitis	Vesicular	Early-inspiratory crackles and possible ronchi and wheezing	Absent	Resonant to hyperresonant	Normal	Midline
Bronchiectasis	Vesicular	Mid-inspiratory crackles	Absent	Resonant	Normal	Midline
Pulmonary fibrosis	Bronchovesicular	Late-inspiratory crackles	Absent	Resonant	Normal or Increased	Midline
Status asthmaticus	Vesicular	Inspiratory and expiratory wheezing	Absent	Hyperresonant	Decreased	Midline
Large pleural effusion	Bronchial sounds immediately above the effusion and absent sounds over the effusion	? Friction rub above the effusion	Possibly present above the effusion, but absent over the effusion	Flat	Absent	Shifted to the side opposite the pleural effusion
Pneumothorax	Absent	Absent	Absent	Tympanic	Absent	Shifted to the side opposite the pneumothorax
Atelectasis with patent bronchi	Bronchial	Absent	All are present	Dull	Increased	Shifted to the same side of the atelectasis
Atelectasis with plugged bronchi	Absent	Absent	Absent	Dull	Absent	Shifted to the same side of the atelectasis
Consolidation (eg, pneumonia)	Bronchial	Late-inspiratory crackles	All are present	Dull	Increased	Midline

TABLE 9-7   Characteristics and Examination Techniques of Different Breathing Patterns

Breathing Pattern	Distinguishing Characteristic	Examination Technique
Normal	Synchronous upward and outward motion of the abdomen and upper chest	Visual, palpation, CWE[a]
Abdominal paradox	Upward and outward motion of the upper chest and inward motion of the abdomen	Visual, palpation, CWE
Upper chest paradox	Upward and outward motion of the abdomen and inward motion of the upper chest	Visual, palpation, CWE
Excessive accessory muscle use	Excessive upper chest motion with increased use of the sternocleidomastoid (STCM) Scalanes, and other accessory muscles of inspiration	Visual, palpation, CWE

[a]CWE, chest wall excursion via tape measure or ruler if patient can assume a supine position.

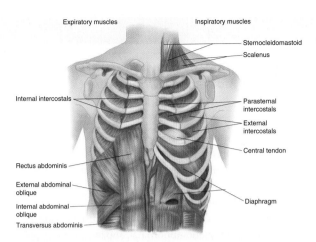

FIGURE 9-2 The muscles of inspiration and expiration. Anterior view of the chest wall depicting the bony cavity formed by the ribs, vertebrae, and sternum. Muscles of expiration (**left**) and inspiration (**right**) are shown.

sternocleidomastoid muscles, which account for approximately 25% of the work of inspiration.[28] Figure 9-2 shows the muscles of inspiration, which should facilitate the examination of these muscles. Observation, palpation, and perturbation of these inspiratory muscles can provide important information about other examination techniques and primary areas of treatment. **For example, a patient with obstructive lung disease observed and palpated to have excessive use of the scalene and sternocleidomastoid muscles with adequate perturbed diaphragmatic descent would likely benefit from inhibitory breathing techniques to the scalene and sternocleidomastoid muscles while facilitating diaphragmatic breathing.**[29] Information such as that obtained during the initial examination of a patient can facilitate specific therapeutic interventions. Methods to measure and determine the degree of accessory muscle use and diaphragmatic activity and movement (or potential for movement) will be discussed in the latter part of this chapter.

Expiratory muscles—Expiration is normally a passive activity, and the muscles of expiration are rarely active except during increased levels of exercise and in several pulmonary diseases. The muscles of expiration consist of the abdominal muscles (rectus abdominis, oblique externus abdominis, oblique internus abdominis, and transversus abdominis) and internal intercostals (except for the parasternal portion). Figure 9-2 also shows the muscles of expiration, which should facilitate the examination of these muscles. Observation, palpation, and perturbation of these expiratory muscles can provide important information about other examination techniques and primary areas of treatment. **For example, a patient with obstructive lung disease observed and palpated to have excessive use of his abdominal muscles, internal intercostals, and paravertebral muscles would likely benefit from inhibitory breathing techniques to the abdominal, internal intercostals, and paravertebral muscles while facilitating different body positions (eg, forward leaning) and breathing techniques (eg, pursed-lip breathing) to assist exhalation.** As in the previous example,

with excessive use of the inspiratory muscles, information such as that obtained during the initial examination of a patient can direct and facilitate specific therapeutic interventions.

Biomechanics of Breathing

The biomechanics of breathing are critical in understanding the results of all examination techniques of patients with pulmonary disorders. A schematic of the biomechanics of breathing is provided in Box 9-4.[30–32] A quick glance at this schematic reveals the simplicity, yet complexity, of breathing.

In normal breathing, it is necessary for the diaphragm to contract against the abdominal contents. As the diaphragm contracts and descends against the abdominal contents, it causes an increase in intra-abdominal pressure. The increase in intra-abdominal pressure produces three distinct motions. One motion is to separate the lower ribs, which essentially expand the lower rib cage. The increased intra-abdominal pressure transmits pressure laterally to the lower ribs, which separate them minimally (yet importantly) at end inspiration.[29]

A second motion is the upward and outward motion of the lower ribs, which is often referred to as the *bucket handle motion*. The bucket handle motion occurs as the diaphragm contracts and descends against the increased intra-abdominal pressure, which produces a fulcrum effect and causes the lower ribs to move upward and outward. This upward and outward motion is the result of the (1) diaphragm's descent on the abdominal contents (increasing the intra-abdominal pressure), producing a fulcrum from which the diaphragm's muscle fibers can *pull* the lower ribs upward and outward and (2) the orientation that the diaphragm's muscle fibers are attached to the ribs in such a way that when they *pull* downward they actually cause the ribs to rotate medially and lift laterally in an upward/outward direction.[29]

BOX 9-4

Biomechanics of Breathing

Diaphragmatic contraction
↓
Compression of abdominal contents, thus increasing intra-abdominal pressure causing
(a) lateral transmission of pressure to the lower ribs laterally = expansion of lower rib cage
(b) upward and outward motion of lower ribs = bucket handle motion
(c) anterior/posterior motion of upper ribs = pump handle motion
↓
Increase in thoracic volume vertically and transversely
↓
Decrease in intrathoracic pressure
↓
Facilitates inspiration and venous return

The best way to picture the diaphragm's descent on the abdominal contents and pull on the lower ribs is to place your hands in front of your body at chest level about 6 in. apart with elbows at your side; then bring you hands together and move them downward, allowing the elbows to move upward and outward away from your body. The outward motion of both arms (with elbows rising upward) represents the upward and outward motion of the lower ribs (bucket handle motion). Combining the inward motion of the clenched hands with upward rising elbows demonstrates how the diaphragm's descent on the abdominal contents produces the bucket handle motion of the lower ribs.

Another way to visualize the bucket handle motion is to use a bucket with two handles: one handle representing the diaphragm and the other handle representing the lower ribs. Position one handle at the top of the bucket (top dead center) and the second handle at the bottom against the side of the bucket. Movement of the top handle downward represents diaphragmatic descent, whereas movement of the bottom handle (the one against the side of the bucket) upward represents bucket handle motion during inspiration. During expiration, these movements are reversed and yield the so-called bucket handle motion of the lower ribs. Observing the amount of diaphragmatic descent as well as the amount of bucket handle motion is critically important in managing patients with cardiopulmonary disorders.

A third motion is the anteroposterior motion of the upper ribs, which is often referred to as *pump handle* motion. Pump handle motion is less related than bucket handle motion to the increase in intra-abdominal pressure. It is more related to the contraction of the accessory muscles of breathing that, upon contraction (shortening), pull the upper ribs in an anterior and outward manner, which move posterior or inward upon relaxation of the accessory muscles. Pump handle motion can be best appreciated by visualizing an old-fashioned water pump (similar to the type used at a campsite). Pushing down on a pump handle is synonymous to the relaxation of the accessory muscles, which produce the posterior or inward motion of the upper ribs. The upward motion of the pump handle is synonymous with the contraction of the accessory muscles of breathing, which moves the upper ribs anterior and outward.[29]

Methods to Measure Breathing Patterns

A variety of methods to measure breathing patterns exist, many of which are listed in Boxes 9-5 and 9-6 and also shown in Fig. 9-3. These methods will be described in the following section.

Observation—Observation of the breathing pattern can be made by focusing on the upper chest wall movement (from the xiphoid process upward) and the lower chest wall movement (abdominal area around the umbilicus). The normal breathing pattern consists of an outward upper and lower chest wall motion during inspiration and inward upper and lower chest wall motion during expiration. The outward lower chest wall motion during inspiration is due to the downward descent of the diaphragm on the abdominal contents, which increases the intra-abdominal pressure and causes the abdominal contents to move forward, or actually, outward. The outward

---

BOX 9-5

Methods to Directly and Indirectly Evaluate Chest Wall Motion and Diaphragmatic Excursion

1. Fluoroscopy
2. Distribution of ventilation via nitrogen washout and xenon distribution (^{133}Xe)
3. Chest wall motion via respiratory inductive plethysmography tape measure or ultrasound
4. Pulmonary function test results
5. Maximal inspiratory and expiratory mouth pressures
6. Transdiaphragmatic, abdominal, and intrathoracic pressures
7. Palpation—placing the fingertips above and under the anterior lower ribs bilaterally, approximately 6–8 cm lateral from the xiphoid process during a sniff; palpation of abdominal and upper chest wall motion (hand placement on the abdomen and upper chest, respectively); palpation of the anterior chest wall with the thumbs over the costal margins and thumb tips meeting at the xiphoid process (with movement of the hands laterally and slightly upward at least 5–8 cm); see Fig. 9-3A
8. Percussion in the anterior and posterior aspects of the thorax between the lowermost ribs and the 12th thoracic vertebrae; see Fig. 9-3B
9. Auscultation of breath sounds
10. Visual observation

---

upper chest wall motion during inspiration is due to increased intra-abdominal pressure (from diaphragmatic contraction) and contraction of the accessory muscles of inspiration.[30–32]

While seated, place one hand on your lower chest (abdominal area) and one hand on your upper chest (midsternal area) and observe and palpate the chest motion during inspiration and expiration.

Palpation—Placement of the hands on the upper and lower chest of a patient while breathing will yield valuable examination information about the principal breathing pattern. Palpation in the abdominal area (for lower chest wall motion) and in the midsternal area (for upper chest wall motion) should direct the examiner to areas of hypermobility or hypomobility of the thorax.

Palpation of the chest wall can also be performed with the hands placed in a manner different from the method mentioned previously. The hands can be placed posteriorly or anteriorly in several different areas of the chest to evaluate the primary breathing pattern. The posterior hand placement locations include the base of the lungs bilaterally, between the scapulae bilaterally, and on the shoulders (on the superior and posterior aspects of the trapezius) bilaterally. The anterior hand placement locations include the base of the lungs bilaterally

BOX 9-6

Chest Wall Excursion Measurements: A Data Sheet

Name _____ Age _____ Gender _____

Activity Level _____

History of Lung Disease _____

Thorax Size: Small   Medium   Large

Tape measurement of chest wall excursion—Wrap a tape measure around the thorax and with a slight tautness bring the end of the tape measure (the 1-cm spot) alongside the other end of the tape measure as shown below. Observe the movement of a reference point on the tape measure (any centimeter line mark that can be easily visualized) during inspiration and expiration. Line up the reference point at the end of expiration and determine the distance the reference point moves during inspiration. The increased distance measured during inspiration subtracted from the starting reference point (at the end of expiration) on the tape measure is the amount of chest wall excursion.

	Supine (land)	**Sitting**	**Standing** (water)
Respiratory Rate	_____	_____	_____
UCWE	_____	_____	_____
MCWE	_____	_____	_____
LCWE	_____	_____	_____

UCWE, upper chest wall excursion; MCWE, middle chest wall excursion; LCWE, lower chest wall excursion.

(immediately below the breasts), just above the breasts bilaterally, and on the shoulders bilaterally (on the superior and anterior aspect of the trapezius). An example of such hand placement is shown in Fig. 9-3.

Such gross examinations are helpful to determine the severity of chest wall motion abnormalities, but more objective measurement techniques exist, which increase the likelihood for correct and accurate examination and management techniques. The remaining sections will present other objective techniques to measure chest wall excursion in patients with pulmonary and even cardiac disorders.

Chest wall excursion via tape measure—Simple measurements of chest wall excursion using a tape measure can quantify motion in different areas of the thorax. We have found the measurement of chest wall excursion at three anatomical sites to be beneficial in better understanding the chest wall excursion of a variety of subjects with and without disease.[33–35] The three anatomical sites include the sternal angle of Louis on the sternum (at the second rib), the xiphoid process, and a midpoint between the xiphoid process and the umbilicus (see Fig. 9-3A). Chest wall excursion measurements made at the sternal angle may best represent upper chest wall motion, whereas measurements made at the xiphoid process site represent middle chest wall motion. Chest wall excursion measurements made at the midpoint between the xiphoid process site and the umbilicus represent lower chest wall motion. In fact, the midpoint between the xiphoid process and the umbilicus appears to be the site at which much of the bucket handle motion can be measured. The sternal angle site as well as the xiphoid

process site likely measures much of the pump handle motion. Therefore, using these three anatomical locations to measure chest wall excursion can provide an objective measure of upper and lower chest wall motion (or the amount of pump handle and bucket handle motion, respectively).

The technique to measure chest wall excursion at the aforementioned anatomical sites involves using a standard tape measure that is pulled taut, but not so tight that it prevents inspiration at the site being measured. Adding a spring-loaded metal phalange to the end of the tape can improve the measurement technique and decrease measurement error. Spring-loaded metal phalanges are quite inexpensive and can be purchased from a variety of medical suppliers.

The tape should be wrapped around the thorax at the level of the anatomical landmark, which can be identified with a marker to ensure similar measurement sites (especially the site for lower chest wall excursion measurements—midpoint between the xiphoid and the umbilicus). After the tape is checked for levelness, the subject is asked to inspire normally (not maximally). The tape measure should move horizontally as the subject inspires and the distance from preinspiration to end of normal inspiration is measured. The method of measuring from the end of expiration to the end of normal inspiration is shown in Fig. 9-3 and further described in Box 9-6.[33–35] A data input sheet for measurements of chest wall excursion is also included in Box 9-6.

The amount (distance) of chest wall motion during normal breathing (which can be referred to as tidal volume [V_T] breathing) should be recorded in centimeters or inches on the data input sheet of Box 9-6 under V_T breathing. This table can be

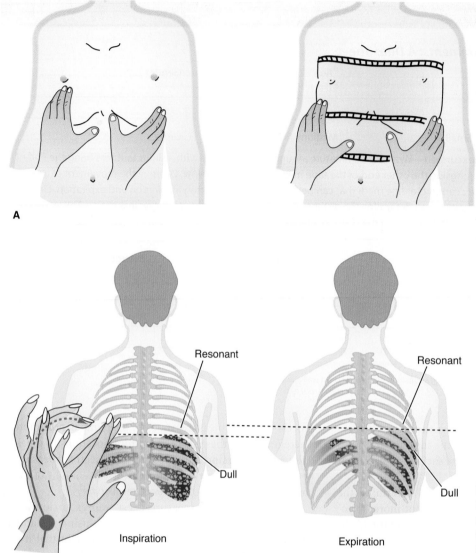

FIGURE 9-3   Methods to measure breathing patterns and diaphragmatic descent. (Modified with permission from Cherniack RM, Cherniack L. *Respiration in Health and Disease*. 2nd ed. Philadelphia, PA: WB Saunders; 1972.)

used during the laboratory session during normal conditions or when students are submerged in water as referred to in Box 9-6.

Chest wall motion during a maximal inspiration should be measured in the manner described previously, and the amount of motion should be recorded in centimeters or inches under vital capacity (VC) breathing in Box 9-6. It may be difficult to measure chest wall excursion at all three anatomical sites, but measurements at the sternal angle and midpoint between the xiphoid process and umbilicus will yield important information related to pump handle and bucket handle motion. This information can be used to direct therapeutic interventions and to evaluate the effectiveness of interventions.

Chest Wall Excursion via Respiratory Inductive Plethysmography

Respiratory inductive plethysmography is considered by some to be the "gold standard" technique to evaluate chest wall excursion and the relationship between upper and lower chest wall excursion.[36] Inductive plethysmography is a technique that requires two elastic bands to be placed around the thorax at two anatomical sites (see Figs. 9-4A and 9-4B). One strap is wound around the thorax at the level of the nipples and the other strap is wound around the thorax at the level of the umbilicus. The straps have electrical wires sewn into the elastic, which enables chest wall motion to be identified as a change in the electrical potential. The change in electrical potentials is relayed to an analog-to-digital converter, which provides accurate analysis and recording of the chest wall motion at the two sites as well as the relationship between the chest wall excursion at the upper and lower chest straps. The chest straps and the resultant data from them (Fig. 9-4C) are also shown in Fig. 9-4B.

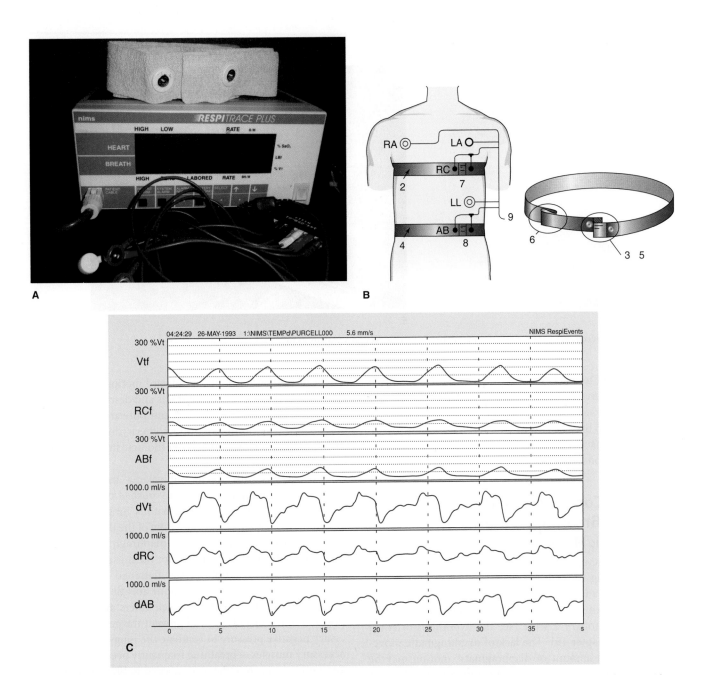

FIGURE 9-4 Respiratory inductive plethysmography unit and ultrasound measurement of chest wall motion. (**A**) Plethysmography unit with elastic bands. (**B**) Placement of the bands around the thorax. (**C**) Resultant graph of measures obtained from the plethysmography unit. *(continued)*

Other Novel Techniques to Measure Chest Wall Excursion

Several other novel techniques to measure chest wall excursion are presently being developed. The use of ultrasound rays emitted from a transducer, which has the capacity to measure motion of the chest and digitize the motion at each site of a transducer (or a series of transducers), can provide information about chest wall motion in a manner that has not been possible before now. The placement of six transducers over the thorax can analyze the motion occurring in all areas of the thorax or individually in the upper, lower, or right/left sides of the thorax. For example, the upper and lower chest wall

excursions can be evaluated by combining the data from the two transducers in the upper right and left quadrant (upper chest wall) and comparing it to the data from the two transducers in the lower right and left quadrant (lower chest wall). However, the chest wall motion of the left upper quadrant can also be compared to the motion in the upper right quadrant as well as to one or both of the transducers over the lower quadrants. The device to measure chest wall motion in this manner is shown in Figs. 9-4D and 9-4E.

Electromyography (EMG) does not measure actual chest wall motion, but it provides important information that is directly related to chest wall motion. The EMG activity of the respiratory muscles can be observed visually and

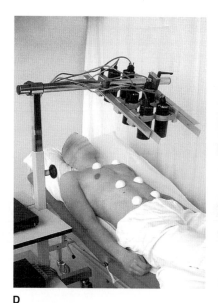
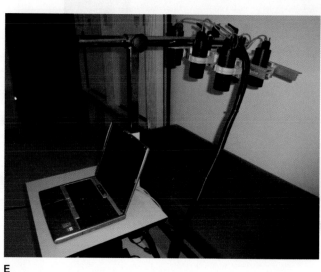

D   E

FIGURE 9-4   *(Continued)* **(D, E)** Ultrasound unit used to measure chest wall motion.

can be analyzed to determine whether the muscle activity is normal, hyperactive, or hypoactive. The EMG can also be used as a biofeedback tool to help patients understand different ways in which to breathe and use the respiratory muscles.[37,38] Such methods have proven to be beneficial for a variety of patient populations.

Important Considerations When Examining Breathing Patterns

Diaphragmatic Movement

The ability of the diaphragm to move is critically important when attempting to understand particular breathing patterns. It is also an important examination technique when utilized to determine the correct intervention for subjects with cardiopulmonary disease (see the hypothesis-oriented algorithm in Chapter 19). The lack of diaphragmatic movement or limited amount of diaphragmatic motion may be responsible for specific abnormal breathing patterns.[29] **For example, if the diaphragm is unable to contract as in spinal cord injury or if it contracts poorly because of moderate-to-severe flattening from obstructive lung disease, particular abnormal breathing patterns are likely to be observed. Likewise, specific interventions can be more confidently provided when diaphragmatic motion, or lack of it, can be determined.**

In patients with complete spinal cord injuries above the third cervical level, the diaphragm is unlikely to receive nervous system signals to contract, and as a result, they will require immediate mechanical ventilation to enable them to breathe. A person with a spinal cord injury below the fifth cervical level will very likely receive nervous system signals for the diaphragm to contract, but will not have abdominal or other accessory muscle function, which will likely result in an *upper chest paradoxical breathing pattern*. This breathing pattern is characterized by a prominent outward motion of the abdominal area (as the diaphragm contracts and descends and pushes the abdominal contents forward and outward) and a prominent inward motion of the upper chest (due to the lack of structural support from paralyzed thoracic musculature) during inspiration (see Fig. 9-5A).[39,40]

In patients with severe emphysema and hyperinflated chests, the diaphragm is frequently pushed downward (from severe air trapping in emphysematous lungs) and is often referred to as flattened. The flattening of the diaphragm places the skeletal muscle fibers of the diaphragm in a shortened position, which makes it difficult for the muscle fibers to optimally contract. In addition, the flattened position of the diaphragm leaves very little room for the diaphragm to descend. Both the shortened muscle fibers and the flattened position of the diaphragm will prevent the generation of necessary negative pressure to ventilate the lungs. As a result, the accessory muscles of breathing frequently become more active and perform much of the work needed to breathe. In fact, the generation of negative pressure needed to ventilate the lungs becomes prominent in the pump handle area of the chest (upper chest), whereas the diaphragm produces very little negative pressure to ventilate and breathe. Under such a condition, the lack of adequate diaphragmatic contraction and descent produces very little generation of negative pressure in the bucket handle area (lower chest), and the negative pressure generated in the upper chest area sucks the abdominal area inward while the upper chest moves outward during inspiration (see Fig. 9-5B). This breathing pattern is termed as the *abdominal paradoxical breathing pattern* and is associated with ventilatory failure.[41-43] Both the previously cited breathing patterns are shown in Fig. 9-5.

Of utmost importance is the examination of diaphragmatic movement or the potential for movement. The following section will review a variety of examination techniques (listed

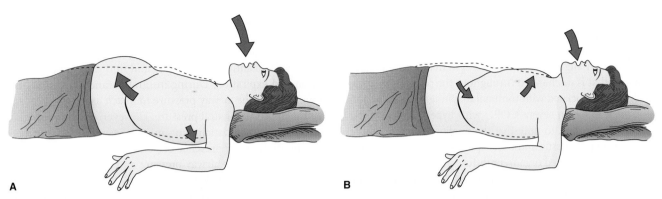

FIGURE 9-5 Paradoxical breathing: (**A**) Upper chest paradoxical breathing, (**B**) abdominal paradoxical breathing. (Modified, with permission, from Massery M. The patient with neuromuscular or musculoskeletal dysfunction. In: Principles and Practice of Cardiopulmonary Physical Therapy. 3rd ed. Mosby Yearbook; 1996.)

in Box 9-5) to determine the amount of diaphragmatic motion and the potential for improvement in motion.

Methods to Directly and Indirectly Measure Diaphragmatic Motion

A number of methods are available to directly and indirectly measure diaphragmatic motion and include fluoroscopy, magnetic resonance imaging (MRI), differences between abdominal and transdiaphragmatic pressures, chest wall excursion measurements, palpation, mediate percussion, and several other methods. A list of all methods to directly and indirectly measure diaphragmatic motion is provided in Box 9-5.[29]

Palpation—In view of the previous discussion, it should be apparent how important it is to evaluate the ability of the diaphragm to move. Palpation of the movement of the diaphragm during breathing can be performed indirectly by placing the hands upon the thorax (one hand on the abdomen and one hand on the upper chest to evaluate abdominal and upper chest wall motion, respectively). However, a more specific indirect method of palpating diaphragmatic motion is to place the fingertips of both hands under the lower ribs anteriorly, placing the fingertips above and under the anterior lower ribs bilaterally, approximately 6 to 8 cm lateral from the xiphoid process (see Fig. 9-3). As the person inspires, the downward descent of the diaphragm can be appreciated as the fingertips of both hands are pushed away from the lower ribs. Patients with no or very little diaphragmatic descent will not push the fingertips away from the lower ribs. If it is difficult to feel the push of the fingertips away from the lower ribs, it is helpful to complete the palpation examination for diaphragmatic movement by asking the patient to sniff forcefully. Sniffing is likely to enhance diaphragmatic contraction, which is necessary to completely understand the amount and potential of diaphragmatic movement.[29]

Examining the descent of the diaphragm in the aforementioned manner can also be helpful in understanding whether both hemidiaphragms are contracting and descending downward. Patients with cerebrovascular accidents may have only one hemidiaphragm functioning and may demonstrate a "pushing away" of the fingertips only on the side that is actively contracting downward.

Another potentially useful method to clinically evaluate diaphragmatic excursion is palpation of the anterior chest wall with the thumbs over the costal margins and thumb tips meeting at the xiphoid process, with normal movement of the hands laterally and slightly upward at least 5 to 8 cm during a deep inspiration (see Fig. 9-3).[29] Patients with severe COPD and hyperinflated lungs may demonstrate very little palpable motion due to very little diaphragmatic excursion.

Mediate percussion and auscultation—Mediate percussion and auscultation are two additional methods to indirectly measure diaphragmatic excursion. *Mediate percussion* is a technique which physicians often use to understand the status of structures inside the body by listening for the quality of sound produced by a fingertip tapped on the middle finger of the opposite hand placed flat against the body. The dullness or lack of dullness identifies the presence or absence of an underlying organ or foreign body. The descent of the diaphragm during inspiration and the ascent of the diaphragm during expiration can be appreciated by performing mediate percussion during the breathing cycle on the posterior aspect of the thorax at the lower ribs.[29]

Mediate percussion in the posterior thorax at the level of the lowermost ribs may yield important differences in sound quality associated with diaphragmatic movement. Movement of resonance (loud or high amplitude, low-pitched, and long-duration sounds heard over air-filled organs such as the lungs) during inspiration and expiration provides an indirect measure of diaphragmatic excursion. Mediate percussion at maximal end inspiration can identify the lowest level of diaphragmatic descent by identifying a resonant tone. Mediate percussion at end exhalation should normally reveal a higher level on the thorax at which the resonant tone is heard. The difference between the levels of higher and lower resonance on the thorax is an indirect measure of diaphragmatic excursion and is normally 3 to 5 cm (see Fig. 9-3B). The change in levels of resonance during the respiratory cycle provides an indirect measure of the caudal and cranial movement of the diaphragm.[29]

Less than 3 cm of audible movement is suggestive of limited diaphragmatic movement. No change in the quality of sound during mediate percussion throughout the respiratory cycle is strongly suggestive of a diaphragm that is not moving. Resonance that is unchanged throughout the respiratory cycle is likely to be associated with minimal diaphragmatic excursion and is often found in severe COPD with hyperinflation of the lungs. It is important to note that the quality of sound will be affected by adipose tissue and other space-occupying structures such as tumors, enlarged organs, or diffuse pulmonary disease.[29]

Finally, auscultation of breath sounds may provide some indirect information regarding diaphragmatic excursion during diaphragmatic breathing (DB) with greater breath sounds in the basilar segments of the lungs occurring with greater diaphragmatic excursion. However, the clinical utility of both of these techniques (auscultation and mediate percussion) requires further investigation.[29]

Another very important adjunct when examining breathing patterns and understanding the reasons for particular patterns of breathing is the strength and endurance of the respiratory muscles. The following sections will address the available methods to measure the strength and endurance of the breathing muscles but will be preceded by an overview of the significance of the strength and endurance of the breathing muscles upon the pressure changes during the breathing cycle.

Pressure Changes During the Breathing Cycle

The importance of pressure changes during the breathing cycle is evident in Box 9-4. During normal breathing, it is necessary for intrathoracic pressure to become more negative during inspiration and more positive (yet still negative) during expiration. These changes in the intrathoracic pressure allow for atmospheric air to move into the lungs during inspiration and for the air to leave the lungs during expiration. Pressure changes within the thorax and lungs also reflect the changes occurring within the intrathoracic area. These pressure changes are shown in Fig. 9-6A.[44]

During inspiration, the intrathoracic pressure decreases, which is also accompanied by a decrease in the intrapleural pressure and alveolar pressure as shown in Fig. 9-6A. As a result of the changes in pressure in each of the aforementioned areas, the volume of air increases and inward flow increases during mid-to-late inspiration. During expiration, the intrathoracic pressure, which is also accompanied by an increase in intrapleural pressure and alveolar pressure, increases. These increases in pressure during expiration cause the volume of air to decrease and outward flow to increase.[44]

The effects of these changes in pressure during the respiratory cycle (preinspiration, inspiration, end inspiration, and forced expiration) are shown in Fig. 9-6B. Intrapleural pressure decreases to a maximal level of -8 cm H_2O at end inspiration, but can quickly rise to $+30$ cm H_2O during a forced expiration. Alveolar pressure decreases to a maximal level of -2 cm H_2O at midexpiration, but increases to 0 cm H_2O at end inspiration.

Alveolar pressure increases much more during a forced expiration. Other very important pressure changes seen in Fig. 9-6 include the airway pressures and the opposing pressures, which significantly affect volume and flow during both inspiration and expiration. During inspiration and expiration, it is important for the airway pressure to match as closely as possible the opposing pleural pressure. However, during expiration it may be difficult to maintain similar pressures due to the force of expiration or the presence of pulmonary disease. If the difference between the airway pressure and the opposing pleural pressure is great, it is possible that the airway will collapse as shown in Fig. 9-6.[44] Such a collapse during expiration will significantly decrease the volume and flow of air leaving the lungs.

Figure 9-6C also shows the typical volume and flow of a single normal alveoli. Note that the flow is characterized by a certain unit of time, which is typically measured in minutes. Normal alveolar ventilation is approximately 5,250 mL/min, whereas normal total ventilation is approximately 7,500 mL/min. The normal volume of alveolar gas is approximately 3,000 mL and the normal VT is approximately 500 mL.[44] Pulmonary disease will markedly change these volumes and flows and will significantly alter the biomechanics of breathing. The altered biomechanics of breathing associated with pulmonary disease are frequently due to abnormal pressures throughout the breathing cycle and throughout the lung.

Pressure Differences Within the Lung

The abnormal pressure differences throughout the breathing cycle of a person with pulmonary disease are often due to abnormal pressure differences throughout the lung. This can be better understood by viewing Fig. 9-7, in which a more normal presentation of the pressure differences within the lung are shown. Because of the weight of the lungs on the abdominal contents, the intrapleural pressure at the base of the lungs is greater than that at the apex. The intrapleural pressure at the base is still negative (-2.5 cm H_2O), but it is less negative than that at the apex of the lung (-10 cm H_2O).[44]

Under conditions like emphysema, or even in aging, the intrapleural pressures at both the base and the apex are less negative than those in the normal person. In fact, at very low lung volumes such as in advanced emphysema, the intrapleural pressure at the base of the lung can actually be positive (see Fig. 9-7B). Therefore, the pressure at the base of the lung exceeds the pressure within the airways, which is likely to collapse the airways at the base of the lungs.[44]

Noninvasive Measurement of Inspiratory and Expiratory Pressures

In view of the preceding discussion, breathing muscle strength is an important examination technique that is critical in understanding abnormal breathing patterns and in directing optimal interventions for persons with cardiopulmonary disease. A number of different techniques exist to measure breathing muscle strength that include manual muscle testing, measurements of maximal inspiratory pressure and maximal expiratory pressure (MIP and MEP, respectively), and tests of breathing

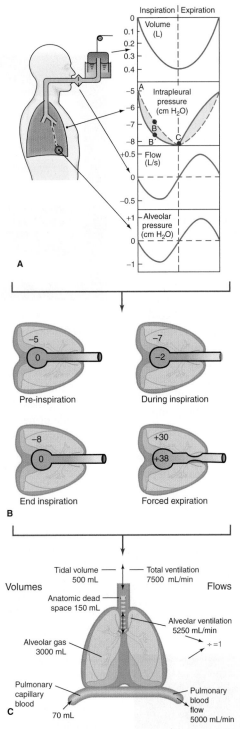

Inspiration | Expiration

Volume (L)
0
0.1
0.2
0.3
0.4

Intrapleural pressure (cm H$_2$O)
−5 A
−6
−7 B
−8 B′ C

Flow (L/s)
+0.5
0
−0.5

Alveolar pressure (cm H$_2$O)
+1
0
−1

A

Pre-inspiration
−5
0

During inspiration
−7
−2

End inspiration
−8
0

Forced expiration
+30
+38

B

Volumes

Tidal volume 500 mL — Total ventilation 7500 mL/min

Anatomic dead space 150 mL

Alveolar ventilation 5250 mL/min

÷ =1

Alveolar gas 3000 mL

Pulmonary capillary blood

70 mL

Pulmonary blood flow 5000 mL/min

Flows

C

FIGURE 9-6   Changes in volume, pressure, flow, and ventilation.

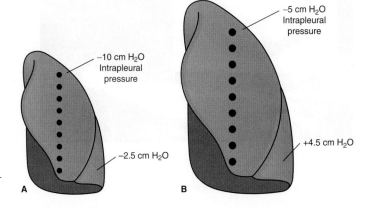

FIGURE 9-7   Pressure differences in the top of the lungs compared to those at the bottom in (**A**) health and (**B**) disease.

−10 cm H$_2$O Intrapleural pressure

−2.5 cm H$_2$O

A

−5 cm H$_2$O Intrapleural pressure

+4.5 cm H$_2$O

B

muscle strength via weighted breathing (ie, weights are added to the abdominal area of a supine patient).[45] Only MIP and MEP measurements provide the specificity and quantification of breathing muscle strength necessary to establish the primary problem and mode of intervention for patients with cardiopulmonary disorders. However, a brief discussion of the other noninvasive techniques will be provided in an attempt to strengthen the clinical utility of MIP and MEP measurements.

Manual muscle testing—Manual muscle testing of the respiratory muscles is difficult, because it is virtually impossible to perform a manual muscle test of the diaphragm, and it is very difficult to quantify the combined strengths of the accessory muscles of breathing and their contribution to the breathing process. However, several of the methods to examine diaphragmatic motion, previously described and listed in Box 9-5, can be adapted in such a way that manual resistance applied during inspiration may provide an indirect measure of inspiratory muscle strength. Attempting to resist the (1) pushing away of the fingertips from under the lower ribs bilaterally, (2) bucket handle motion of the lower ribs bilaterally, or (3) outward movement of the abdomen during inspiration may all provide an indirect manual measurement of diaphragmatic muscle strength.

Maximal inspiratory and expiratory pressure measurements—Measurement of MIP and MEP has increased in popularity in recent years.[46,47] Several different devices are available, which allow for MIP and MEP to be measured. An example of one such device, the *Magnehelic,* is shown in Fig. 9-8. Each device works essentially the same way and measures the amount of negative pressure developed during a maximal inspiration and the amount of positive pressure developed during a maximal expiration. The unit of measure to record the strength of the breathing muscles for MIP and MEP is frequently in centimeters of water (cm H_2O). These electronic devices measure with

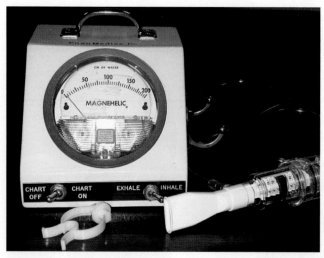

FIGURE 9-8 **Left,** the *Magnehelic,* a device used to measure maximal inspiratory and expiratory pressure. **Right,** a *Threshold* inspiratory muscle loading device to measure ventilatory muscle endurance.

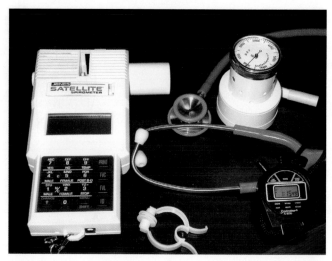

FIGURE 9-9 Examples of two portable spirometers used for pulmonary function testing.

greater accuracy and reliability than do the other devices. However, accurate and reliable measurements can also be achieved when using these less costly devices by carefully observing the magnitude of needle deflection during inspiratory and expiratory measurements of ventilatory muscle strength.

The methods of measuring MIP and MEP are presented in Box 9-7, which also contains a data input sheet. It is very important that measurement of MIP be performed after a maximal expiration (near residual volume [RV]) and that measurement of MEP be performed after a maximal inspiration (total lung capacity [TLC]). It is also important to standardize the testing procedures and to test the patients while seated in a chair with their hips perpendicular to the back.[46,47] The patient should be encouraged during the measurement of both MIP and MEP but should not be allowed to flex forward or to extend backward during testing. An adequate seal at the mouthpiece is also important to obtain accurate and reliable MIP and MEP measurements.

In addition to the measurement of MIP and MEP, spirometric measurement of VC at the patient's bedside can yield additional and important information about the patient's ability to move air into and out of the lungs. Figure 9-9 shows two commonly used spirometer devices for the bedside measurement of PFTs.

Weighted breathing as a test of breathing strength—Placing weights upon the abdominal area of a patient with cardiopulmonary disease has previously been described as a method to test and train the ventilatory muscles.[48] It has been advocated as a method to increase the strength and endurance of the respiratory muscles and has been used extensively for persons with spinal cord injury.[48] Although placing progressively greater weight on the abdominal area during breathing can identify a particular level of strength and point at which a patient may no longer be able to breathe, it actually measures the breathing endurance of a patient. Therefore, weighted breathing is less specific for breathing strength and more

BOX 9-7

Methods to Measure MIP and MEP

Measurement

Measurement device: Several different types of devices are used to measure ventilatory muscle strength. The methods to measure the positive and negative pressure (in centimeters of water) generated by the patient during such testing is by using a manometer or pressure transducer. When using a manometer, a needle is deflected to the point of maximal generated pressure after which the needle may fall back to the resting level of 0. Such devices typically have poorer resolution and reliability. Newer devices have an internal pressure transducer that provides a digital display, which remains illuminated and as a result has desirable resolution and reliability.

Body position: During the measurement of ventilatory muscle strength the patient should wear a nose clip and be seated with the trunk at a 90-degree angle to the hips.

Procedure:

1. MIP

   (a) Have patient expire fully (near residual volume).

   (b) Motivate patient to inspire as forcefully as possible.

   (c) Document the MIP and repeat the above until a stable baseline is observed.

MIP (cm H_2O) _____ _____ _____ _____ _____ _____ _____ _____

2. MEP

   (a) Have patient inspire fully (total lung capacity).

   (b) Motivate patient to exhale as forcefully as possible.

   (c) Document the MEP and repeat the above until a stable baseline is observed.

MEP (cm H_2O) _____ _____ _____ _____ _____ _____ _____ _____

3. Comparing the measured MIP and MEP to previously published "normal" values

   Prediction Equations from Black and Hyatt.[46]

     Men 20–54 years of age:

       MIP = 129 − (age × 0.13)

       MEP = 229 + (age × 0.08)

     Men 55–80 years of age:

       MIP = 120 − (age × 0.25)

       MEP = 353 − (age × 2.33)

     Women 20–54 years of age:

       MIP = 100 − (age × 0.39)

       MEP = 158 − (age × 0.18)

     Women 55–86 years of age:

       MIP = 122 − (age × 0.79)

       MEP = 210 − (age × 1.14)

   Prediction equations from Enright et al.[47]

     Men ≥ 65 years of age:

       MIP = (weight* × 0.131) − (age × 1.27) + 153

       MEP = (Weight* × 0.250) − (age × 2.95) + 347

     Women ≥ 65 years of age:

       MIP = (weight* × 0.133) − (age × 0.805) + 96

       MEP = (weight* × 0.344) − (age × 2.12) + 219

*Weight in pounds.

specific for breathing endurance. The following section will present other methods to test breathing muscle endurance.

Noninvasive Measurement of Ventilatory Muscle Endurance

A number of different methods to measure breathing muscle endurance exist.[49] The most widely used methods and their strengths and weaknesses are listed in Table 9-8. The primary methods to measure ventilatory muscle endurance include (1) the ability to sustain breathing loads (frequently 70%–85% of maximum voluntary ventilation [MVV]) for a particular duration, (2) breathing with an externally applied mechanical load (eg, threshold loading), (3) measurement of sustainable pressure loads in which a subject begins breathing at a load of

TABLE 9-8   Strengths and Weaknesses of Various Methods to Measure Ventilatory Muscle Endurance

Technique	Methods	Strengths	Weaknesses
Weighted breathing	Weights placed on the abdominal area of a supine lying subject	Ease	Patient must be supine to perform the test, which may not accurately measure VME in a patient with lung disease with a mechanical disadvantage to breathing when supine
MVV	Rapid, deep breathing for 10–15 s	Ease	Nonspecific to true VME
Loaded breathing	VT breathing at particular % of MIP	Ease	Can be time consuming and erroneous if MIP is inaccurate
Incremental loaded breathing	VT breathing at particular % of MIP with incremental workloads (ie, 20% of MIP initially for 2 min with 20% increments every 2 min)	Ease	Erroneous if MIP is inaccurate

MVV, maximal voluntary ventilation; VME, ventilatory muscle endurance; VT, tidal volume; MIP, maximal inspiratory pressure.

90% MIP that is gradually decreased in 5% decrements until the load can be sustained for greater than 10 minutes, or (4) progressive incremental breathing against resistance (beginning at approximately 20%–30% of MIP and increasing the load every 2 minutes by 10%–20% increments for as long as possible).[50]

Perhaps the most clinically useful and applicable test of ventilatory muscle endurance is the progressive incremental breathing against resistance. Such inspiratory muscle endurance testing has been described by Martyn et al.[51] The measurement of inspiratory muscle endurance can be performed with a threshold loading device, which will provide a patient resistance during inspiration. An example of the threshold loading device is shown in Fig. 9-8. The test usually begins at 20% of MIP, and the patient is asked to breathe with the device for 2 minutes. If the patient tolerates breathing with resistance set at 20% of MIP, the resistance will be progressed by 20% increments (based on the initial MIP) until exhaustion. End-tidal carbon dioxide and oxygen saturation levels, inspiratory muscle use, and level of dyspnea are often monitored; and testing is terminated if abnormal carbon dioxide levels are observed, if a paradoxical breathing pattern occurs, or if a patient reports of severe dyspnea (Borg-modified dyspnea score of ≥7/10). The measurement of ventilatory muscle endurance using this method has been found to be safe, reproducible, and representative of other measurements, often accepted as a measure of ventilatory muscle endurance.[52–54] The specific methodology of (progressive) incremental ventilatory muscle endurance testing and a data input sheet are provided in Box 9-8.

The pressure changes inside and outside of the lung during breathing are what allow for adequate oxygenation of the blood and the removal of carbon dioxide from the blood. Therefore, it is now necessary to discuss the effects of the previously cited pressure changes during breathing on ventilation and oxygenation of the lungs. The methods to examine ventilation, perfusion, and oxygenation of the lungs are medical examinations that are rarely performed by physical therapists but are used extensively by physical therapists to diagnose, allocate specific interventions, and determine a likely prognosis for patients with cardiovascular and pulmonary disorders.

MEDICAL EXAMINATIONS USED BY PHYSICAL THERAPISTS

Ventilation and Perfusion of the Lungs

Ventilation of the lungs can be simply defined as the *movement of air* into and out of the lungs. *Perfusion* of the lungs can also be simply defined as the *movement of blood* into and out of the lungs. Ventilation of the lungs can be examined in several different ways including auscultation of the lungs, ventilation–perfusion scans, and arterial blood gases.[55–57] Perfusion of the lung can be examined via the aforementioned ventilation–perfusion scan during which a radioisotope is administered by intravenous injection and another isotope is administered via inhalation. The uptake of the inhaled isotope by the lungs and the uptake of the injected isotope by the pulmonary circulation is examined with radiographic techniques (X-rays) that provide detailed information about the areas of the lung and the amount of lung tissue receiving air (ventilation) and circulation (perfusion).[55–57] Deficit areas, or areas of mismatch, are indicative of particular diseases. This method is considered the "gold standard" to measure ventilation and perfusion of the lungs, but other less sophisticated and invasive methods can also provide some information related to the ventilation and perfusion of the lungs; however, they are often less sensitive and specific to certain diseases.[55–57] The other less informative methods include auscultation of the lungs, use of a respirometer, respiratory inductive plethysmography, and arterial blood gases. The methods, strengths, and weaknesses of each of the measurement techniques of ventilation and perfusion of the lungs are presented in Table 9-9.

It is important to note that if the pressure changes during the breathing cycle that were discussed previously are minimal, patients will often suffer from less ventilation, which will result in elevated carbon dioxide levels and poor oxygenation.[55–57] Such abnormalities can be better understood by examining arterial blood gases.

BOX 9-8

Specific Methods to Perform Progressive Incremental Ventilatory Muscle Endurance Test

Pretest Preparation

Monitor oxygen saturation and attempt to visualize the patient's thorax as best as possible to evaluate chest wall motion of the abdominal area and upper chest to examine the level of oxygenation and breathing pattern (to determine if the breathing pattern is synchronous or dyssynchronous) during ventilatory muscle endurance testing. Measurement of end-tidal carbon dioxide is valuable if measurement devices are available to determine if carbon dioxide is retained during ventilatory muscle endurance testing.

Test Procedures

Measurement of inspiratory muscle endurance can be performed with a threshold loading device that will provide resistance to a patient during inspiration (see Fig. 9-8). The test should begin at 20% of MIP, and the patient will be asked to breathe with the device for 2 minutes, after which a Borg rating will be obtained and the patient will be progressed by 20% increments of resistance (based on the initial MIP) until exhaustion. Inspiratory muscle use will be monitored and testing will be terminated if an abnormal breathing pattern (paradoxical) occurs. If the patient desaturates (oxygen saturation < 90%), or shows signs of significant carbon dioxide retention, or if the patient reports dizziness or fatigue that prevents further testing,

1. Measure MIP
2. Repeat measurement of MIP until a stable baseline is established
3. Set threshold inspiratory muscle trainer at 20% of MIP
4. Patient should begin breathing with the inspiratory muscle trainer while wearing a nose clip and with a good seal around the mouthpiece such that inspiration occurs only through the trainer and produces an audible "sucking" sound and visible movement of the valve at the end of the trainer (see Fig. 9.8) during inspiration. This will prevent the patient from breathing around the mouthpiece trainer, which would decrease the work required to breathe and invalidate the test.
5. Breathing with the trainer set at 20% of MIP should continue for 2 minutes after which a Borg rating and visual analog scaling of dyspnea should be obtained, and the patient should be progressed by 20% increments of resistance until exhaustion. Documentation of the minutes completed, breathing pattern, and oxygen saturation for each stage can be done in a format similar to that below.

Stage 1
(20% MIP = _____ cm H$_2$O)
Minutes completed _____
Breathing pattern: Synchronous (normal)   Dyssynchronous (paradoxical)
Oxygen saturation _____
Borg dyspnea score _____
Dyspnea: Visual Analog Scale (VAS)

_____
NONE   VERY SEVERE

Stage 2
(40% MIP = _____ cm H$_2$O)
Minutes completed _____
Breathing pattern: Synchronous (normal)   Dyssynchronous (paradoxical)
Oxygen saturation _____
Borg dyspnea score _____
Dyspnea: Visual Analog Scale (VAS)

_____
NONE   VERY SEVERE

Stage 3
(60% MIP = _____ cm H$_2$O)
Minutes completed _____
Breathing pattern: Synchronous (normal)   Dyssynchronous (paradoxical)
Oxygen saturation _____
Borg dyspnea score _____
Dyspnea: Visual Analog Scale (VAS)

_____
NONE   VERY SEVERE

(continued)

BOX 9-8 *(Continued)*

Stage 4
(80% MIP = _____ cm H_2O)
Minutes completed _____
Breathing pattern: Synchronous (normal)   Dyssynchronous (paradoxical)
Oxygen saturation _____
Borg dyspnea score _____
Dyspnea: Visual Analog Scale (VAS)

_____
NONE   VERY SEVERE

Stage 5
(100% MIP = _____ cm H_2O)
Minutes completed _____
Breathing pattern: Synchronous (normal)   Dyssynchronous (paradoxical)
Oxygen saturation _____
Borg dyspnea score _____
Dyspnea: Visual Analog Scale (VAS) _____

_____
NONE   VERY SEVERE

Arterial Blood Gases

The pressure changes that occur during breathing, which were discussed in several of the preceding sections, allow for alveolar ventilation and oxygenation to occur.[55–57] Arterial blood gases provide the opportunity to examine alveolar ventilation, oxygenation, and the acid–base relationship of the body. Box 9-9 provides an overview of the examination process of arterial blood gases. From Box 9-9 it is apparent that only two blood gas variables are needed to understand basic arterial blood gas status. The two blood gas variables are (1) the level of carbon dioxide in the arterial blood ($Paco_2$) and (2) the blood pH. The level of $Paco_2$ in arterial blood will provide an insight into the level of alveolar ventilation, and the pH level will yield information about the effect of $Paco_2$ on the body's homeostatic environment (acid–base relationship).[58] It is critical to understand that increased levels of $Paco_2$ decrease pH and decreased levels of $Paco_2$ increase the pH.[58] This inverse relationship between $Paco_2$ and pH is the basis for much of arterial blood gas analyses because the carbon molecule is countered by the negative charges of two O_2 molecules. This relationship can be better understood by referring to the Henderson–Hasselbalch equation.[59]

The Henderson–Hasselbalch equation examines the relationship between carbonic acid and bicarbonate ions, which in turn yield the pH:

$$pH = pK + Log\ [HCO_3^-]/H_2CO_3].$$

TABLE 9-9   Measurement Techniques of Ventilation and Perfusion of the Lungs: Methods, Strengths, and Weaknesses

Technique	Methods	Strengths	Weaknesses
Measurement techniques of lung ventilation			
Respirometer	$V_E = TV \times RR$	Ease, rapid, inexpensive	Nonspecific to lung anatomy
Pulmonary function tests	$MVV = FEV_1 \times 35$	Ease, rapid, inexpensive	Nonspecific to lung anatomy
Respiratory inductance plethysmography (RIP)	Special chest straps relay chest wall motion to a computer programmed with regression equations to predict lung ventilation	Ease, rapid, inexpensive	Nonspecific to lung anatomy
Arterial blood gases	$Paco_2$	Ease, rapid, inexpensive	Nonspecific to lung anatomy
Nitrogen washout	Nitrogen is inhaled	Rapid and Specific to lung anatomy	Expensive and specialized equipment
Xenon gas (^{133}Xe)	^{133}Xe is inhaled and serial images of ^{133}Xe distribution via scintigraphy	Rapid and specific to lung anatomy	Expensive and specialized equipment
Measurement techniques of lung perfusion			
Radioactive iodine (^{131}I)	Injection of ^{131}I with serial images of ^{131}I via scintigraphy	Rapid and specific to lung anatomy	Expensive and specialized equipment

BOX 9-9

Methods to Analyze Arterial Blood Gases

Two main pathways can be followed when interpreting arterial blood gas data. The direction of the pathway is determined by the pH. One pathway identifies an acidosis and the other pathway identifies an alkalosis. Identification of a primary respiratory problem versus a primary metabolic problem is accomplished by examining the pH and Paco$_2$ relationship on the second and fourth levels of this figure. The compensatory ability of the body to manage an acidic or alkalotic environment is reflected by the concentration of bicarbonate (HCO$_3^-$ and Paco$_2$)

on the sixth and seventh levels of this figure. A primary respiratory problem is associated with an inverse relationship (opposite directions) between Paco$_2$ and pH. A primary metabolic problem is associated with a direct relationship (in the same direction) between Paco$_2$ and pH. Abnormal bicarbonate levels can provide important information to better distinguish acute versus chronic respiratory and metabolic problems. If the relationship between pH and Paco$_2$ is direct, the problem is likely to be primarily metabolic while an indirect relationship between the two likely identifies a primary respiratory problem.

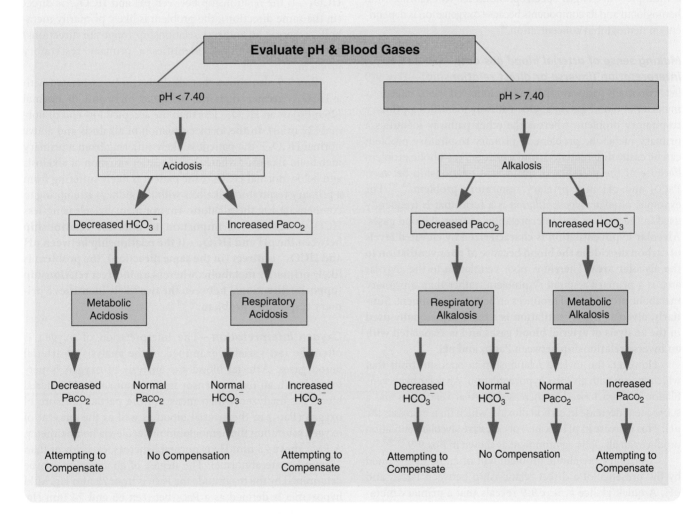

The specific relationship between carbonic acid and bicarbonate ions and calculation of pH using the previous equation is somewhat complex. It is clinically acceptable to replace carbonic acid (H$_2$CO$_3$) with Paco$_2$ to calculate pH.[59] However, the specific calculation of pH is rarely calculated by hand. Automated blood gas analysis systems that have been programmed with the Henderson–Hasselbalch and other equations rapidly calculate the pH and other blood gas measures. **Perhaps one of the most important principles of the aforementioned relationships and equations is that the pH is the negative log of the hydro-**

gen ion concentration.[59] It is this fact that enables the inverse relationship between Paco$_2$ and pH, presented previously, to be applied clinically. An excellent source to learn more about the Henderson–Hasselbalch equation and its role in pH and blood gas analysis can be found at http://www.tmc.tulane.edu/departments/anesthesiology/acid/default.html.

Methods of Measuring Arterial Blood Gases

Obtaining a blood sample—A sample of arterial blood is taken from an indwelling arterial line or an arterial puncture is made that will provide access to arterial blood. Venous blood samples or mixed venous samples can be obtained from a peripheral vein puncture or from a pulmonary artery catheter. Usually one to two test tubes of blood are taken from a patient, and the sample is often immediately sent to the laboratory for analysis.[60]

Arterial blood gas analysis—When arterial blood gases are analyzed, blood samples are subjected to an automated pH–blood gas analyzer, which consists of an oxygen and carbon dioxide sensor. Standardized calibration of the analyzer is performed with reference gases before the sample obtained for study is subjected for analysis. Hemoximetry is usually performed in conjunction with blood gas–pH analysis; it utilizes a multiple wavelength spectrophotometer to examine total hemoglobin and its components because oxygenation is dependent on hemoglobin concentration.[60]

Making sense of arterial blood gas data—pH and Pa_{CO_2} interpretation (inverse or direct relationship)—Box 9-9 lists two main pathways that can be followed when interpreting arterial blood gas data. One pathway identifies a primary respiratory problem, whereas the other pathway identifies a primary metabolic problem. A primary respiratory problem can be easily differentiated from a primary metabolic problem because of the presence of an inverse relationship between Pa_{CO_2} and pH in a primary respiratory problem.[58-60] For example, *alveolar hypoventilation* is a term that is frequently used in the analysis and interpretation of arterial blood gases. **Alveolar hypoventilation is characterized by elevated levels of carbon dioxide in the blood because of poor ventilation to the alveolar area.** Therefore, poor ventilation to the alveolar area is a primary respiratory problem, rather than a primary metabolic problem, and produces an acidic environment. **Similarly, alveolar hyperventilation is a term occasionally used in the analysis of arterial blood gases and is associated with an inverse relationship between Pa_{CO_2} and pH.**

However, the inverse relationship is opposite from that which is seen with alveolar hypoventilation. Alveolar hyperventilation is characterized by increased alveolar ventilation and a subsequent decrease in carbon dioxide, which then increases the pH. This increase in pH because of excessive alveolar ventilation produces an alkalotic environment as shown in Box 9-9.[58-60]

A primary metabolic problem will often be determined by the presence of a direct relationship between Pa_{CO_2} and pH. A quick glance at Box 9-9 reveals that a primary metabolic acidosis or alkalosis is associated with direct relationships between pH and Pa_{CO_2}. The Pa_{CO_2} of a metabolic acidosis is less than the accepted low end of normal (35 mm Hg), and the pH is less than the accepted normal of 7.40; thus, both values are less than the accepted normal value in a similar direction, which produces the direct relationship between Pa_{CO_2} and pH. The Pa_{CO_2} of a metabolic alkalosis is greater than the accepted high end of normal (45 mm Hg), and the pH is also greater than the accepted normal of 7.40; thus, both values are greater than the accepted normal value in a similar direction, which produces the direct relationship between Pa_{CO_2} and pH.[58-60]

Bicarbonate HCO_3^- interpretation—Abnormal bicarbonate levels can provide important information to better distinguish acute versus chronic respiratory and metabolic problems. Box 9-9 shows that acidosis can be associated with a HCO_3^- less than the accepted low end of normal (22 mEq) or an HCO_3^- greater than the accepted high end of normal (26 mEq). In the former situation of acidosis and below normal HCO_3^-, the patient is likely suffering from a primary metabolic acidosis, whereas in the latter situation of acidosis and above normal HCO_3^-, the patient is likely suffering from a primary respiratory acidosis with the kidneys attempting to compensate for the acidic environment by releasing more HCO_3^-. Of note is the relationship between the pH and HCO_3^-. If the relationship between pH and HCO_3^- is direct (in the same direction), the problem is likely primarily metabolic, whereas an indirect relationship (opposite directions) between the two likely identifies a primary respiratory problem.[58-60]

Box 9-9 also shows that alkalosis can be associated with a HCO_3^- greater than the accepted high end of normal (26 mEq) or an HCO_3^- less than the accepted low end of normal (22 mEq). In the former situation of alkalosis and above normal HCO_3^-, the patient is likely suffering from a primary metabolic alkalosis; whereas in the latter situation of alkalosis and below normal HCO_3^-, the patient is likely suffering from a primary respiratory alkalosis with the kidneys attempting to compensate for the alkalotic environment by releasing less HCO_3^-. **Again, it is important to note the relationship between the pH and HCO_3^-. If the relationship between pH and HCO_3^- is direct (in the same direction), the problem is likely primarily metabolic, whereas an indirect relationship (opposite directions) between the two likely identifies a primary respiratory problem.**[58-60]

Oxygen interpretation—The interpretation of oxygen is often the last variable examined in the analysis of arterial blood gases. Arterial blood gas analysis of oxygen is performed with an oxygen sensor in the automated pH–arterial blood gas analyzer, which measures the partial pressure of oxygen (Pa_{O_2}) in the arterial blood as well as the amount of oxygen saturating the hemoglobin molecule via hemoximetry. A Pa_{O_2} above 75 mm Hg is normal, whereas levels lower than 75 mm Hg are abnormal. The degree of abnormality can be determined by the magnitude the Pa_{O_2} is from 75 mm Hg. Mild hypoxemia is defined as a Pa_{O_2} between 65 and 74 mm Hg, whereas moderate hypoxemia is defined as a Pa_{O_2} between 50 and 65 mm Hg. Severe hypoxemia is defined as a Pa_{O_2} less than 45 to 50 mm Hg.

Oxygen status is also evaluated via the amount of oxygen saturating the hemoglobin molecule. Normal oxygen saturation is accepted as 95% or greater, whereas mild hypoxemia is defined as oxygen saturation between 90% and 95%. Moderate and severe hypoxemia are defined as oxygen saturation levels between 80% and 90% and less than 75% to 80%, respectively.[58-60] **Oxygen saturation is related to Pa_{O_2} via the oxyhemoglobin saturation curve as discussed in Chapter 5.**

TABLE 9-10 Relationship Between Pao$_2$ and Oxygen Saturation

Pao$_2$	40	50	60
Oxygen saturation	70	80	90

A simple way to remember the relationship between oxygen saturation and Pao$_2$ is to construct a table with the numbers 40, 50, and 60 on the top row and the numbers 70, 80, and 90 on the bottom row as shown in Table 9-10. The top row represents the Pao$_2$, and the bottom row represents oxygen saturation (Table 9-10). A quick glance at Table 9-10 provides an estimate of the oxygen saturation when the Pao$_2$ is a certain value or vice versa. For example, if the Pao$_2$ is 60 mm Hg, then the oxygen saturation is approximately 90%; and if the oxygen saturation is 80%, the Pao$_2$ is approximately 50 mm Hg.

Pulse oximetry provides a very similar measure to the direct measurement of oxygen saturation, discussed previously. The infrared sensor of a pulse oximeter worn on the finger, earlobe, or any other body part senses the amount of oxygen saturating hemoglobin by interpreting the density of the blood flow through the particular body part with the probe (see Fig. 9-10). The oxygen saturation is then calculated automatically via regression equations within the pulse oximeter. Although the values for normal and specific degrees of hypoxemia are identical to those previously cited, the accuracy of pulse oximetry is less than the direct measurement of oxygen saturation via arterial blood gases. **The degree of error associated with pulse oximetry has been established to be approximately ±3%. Potential causes of less accurate pulse oximetry measurements include darker skin color, poor circulation, Raynaud phenomenon, presence of nail polish, and poor placement of the finger probe, among others.**

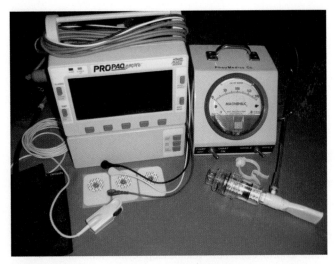

FIGURE 9-10 On the left, a combination pulse oximeter-ECG unit. Note the finger sensor in the lower left portion of the photo.

"Other" related issues—From the previous discussion, it is apparent that arterial blood gas values are frequently influenced by the ability or inability of the breathing muscles to properly ventilate the lungs. **Although the arterial blood gas information is extremely helpful and important in the management of patients with cardiopulmonary disease, identification of a blood gas abnormality is occasionally too late to adequately intervene with physical therapy interventions.** Many of the specific interventions to improve abnormal arterial blood gas findings involve improving the (1) biomechanics of breathing, (2) airway diameter, or (3) alveolar ventilation and oxygenation by removing retained pulmonary secretions or providing mechanical ventilation. **Besides arterial blood gas analysis, observation of the patient's appearance (color, degree of distress, and breathing pattern) and auscultation of the lungs can provide important information about the biomechanics of breathing, airway diameter, and alveolar ventilation and oxygenation, which may direct therapeutic interventions to rapidly improve a patient's status before arterial blood gases deteriorate.** In addition, the methods of perturbating the breathing of a patient with a pulmonary disorder can provide information that may be useful in the implementation of therapeutic interventions (Table 9-4). **However, there does appear to be limited data suggesting that particular patients with markedly abnormal pulmonary function may be unable to improve their biomechanics of breathing.**[29]

Pulmonary function testing can provide important information about both the patient and the lung function.

Pulmonary Function Tests

Pulmonary function tests measure the volume and flow of air during inspiration and expiration. A flow–volume loop provides a graphic display of both inspiratory and expiratory flows and volumes (see Fig. 9-11).[61-63] The flow–volume loop is a standard measure of pulmonary function, and it is useful in interpreting not only inspiratory flow and volumes but also patient effort and somewhat of an accurate graphic depiction of many types of pulmonary disorders including obstructive, restrictive, and interstitial lung diseases. Many pulmonary disorders have a characteristic flow–volume loop (see Fig. 9-11B–E) due to abnormal airway function, lung tissue, biomechanics of breathing, or some combination of these abnormalities.

Many measurements of pulmonary function exist (Table 9-11), but perhaps the two most frequently used and clinically important measurements of pulmonary function are the forced vital capacity (FVC) and the forced expiratory volume in 1 second (FEV$_1$). The FVC is the amount of air expelled during a forceful exhalation from the end of inspiration to the end of expiration. The FEV$_1$ is the amount of air expelled during the first second of a forceful exhalation. Examining just these two values can provide a wealth of information about the presence or absence of pulmonary disease as well as the severity of

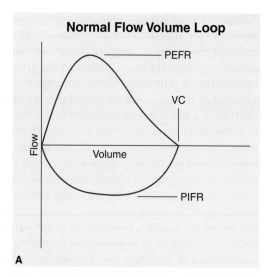

Normal Flow Volume Loop

PEFR

VC

Flow

Volume

PIFR

A

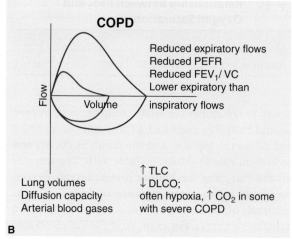

COPD

Flow

Volume

Reduced expiratory flows
Reduced PEFR
Reduced FEV_1/ VC
Lower expiratory than
inspiratory flows

Lung volumes
Diffusion capacity
Arterial blood gases

↑ TLC
↓ DLCO;
often hypoxia, ↑ CO_2 in some
with severe COPD

B

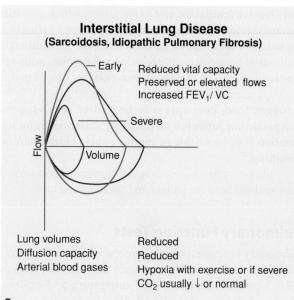

Interstitial Lung Disease
(Sarcoidosis, Idiopathic Pulmonary Fibrosis)

Early

Severe

Flow

Volume

Reduced vital capacity
Preserved or elevated flows
Increased FEV_1/ VC

Lung volumes
Diffusion capacity
Arterial blood gases

Reduced
Reduced
Hypoxia with exercise or if severe
CO_2 usually ↓ or normal

C

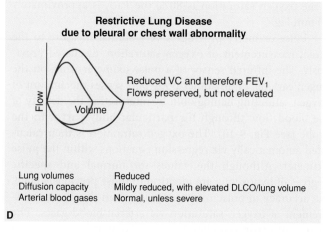

Restrictive Lung Disease
due to pleural or chest wall abnormality

Flow

Volume

Reduced VC and therefore FEV_1
Flows preserved, but not elevated

Lung volumes
Diffusion capacity
Arterial blood gases

Reduced
Mildly reduced, with elevated DLCO/lung volume
Normal, unless severe

D

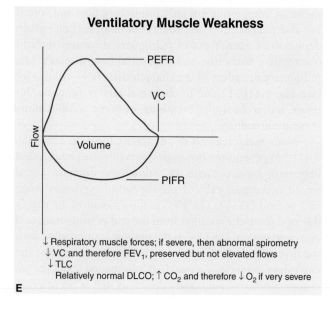

Ventilatory Muscle Weakness

PEFR

VC

Flow

Volume

PIFR

↓ Respiratory muscle forces; if severe, then abnormal spirometry
↓ VC and therefore FEV_1, preserved but not elevated flows
↓ TLC
Relatively normal DLCO; ↑ CO_2 and therefore ↓ O_2 if very severe

E

FIGURE 9-11   Graph of flow–volume loops. (**A**) Normal flow–volume loop. (**B**) COPD flow–volume loop. (**C**) Interstitial lung disease flow–volume loop. (**D**) Restrictive lung disease flow–volume loop. (**E**) Ventilatory muscle weakness flow–volume loop.

TABLE 9-11 Typical Pulmonary Function Test Results in a Patient with Severe Emphysema

Patient Name: Age: 51 y	Date: 6/9/02		
	Gender: F	Height: 163.5 cm	Weight: 48 kg
Spirometry results	**Observed**	**Predicted**	**% Predicted**
FEV$_1$ (L)	0.42	2.7	16
FVC (L)	1.11	3.32	33
FEV$_1$/FVC	35	81	43
Peak expiratory flow (L/s)	1.66	6.07	27
Flow—50% FVC (L/s)	0.13	3.95	3
Flow—75% FVC (L/s)	0.09	1.96	5
FEF$_{25\%-75\%}$ (L/s)	0.11	2.85	4
Peak inspiratory flow (L/s)	1.32	4.25	31
MVV (L/min)	15	95	16
Lung volumes (plethysmography results)			
Total lung capacity (L)	7.17	4.99	144
Residual volume (L)	6.06	1.78	340
RV/TLC	0.85	0.36	237
Functional residual capacity (L)	6.23	2.82	221
Airway resistance (cm H$_2$O/L/s)	0	0.8–2.4	—
Specific conductivity of the airway (L/s/cm H$_2$O/L)	0	>0.12	—

Interpretation

A severe obstructive defect is present in view of the reduced FEV$_1$, FVC, and expiratory flow rates above. The lung volumes are markedly increased, which is also consistent with an obstructive defect. The patient was unable to perform the diffusing capacity for carbon monoxide (DLCO) test due to marked dyspnea. The current test results are essentially unchanged since the previous pulmonary function test on 12/18/01.

pulmonary dysfunction (Tables 9-11 and 9-12).[61–63] The values presented in Table 9-12 are values that have been predicted from the actual volume of air that a person can exhale, which can be used to diagnose the severity of lung disease. This information and measurement of pulmonary function will be discussed in the following sections.

Standard Measurements of Pulmonary Function

Perhaps the best methods to describe the measurement of pulmonary function are to explain how two antiquated measurement devices (a water-sealed spirometer and the Vitalograph) measure pulmonary function (see Fig. 9-12). Although these antiquated systems are seldom used today because of newer automated systems, their mechanism of operation clearly reveals the origin of the measurements obtained during a pulmonary function test. The water-sealed spirometer records a patient's breathing efforts with a pen attached to the spirometer that moves upward or downward as air is blown into or out of the spirometer (see Fig. 9-12A). Actually, as a person inspires and draws air from the spirometer into their lungs, a large metal cylinder that moves within the water-sealed chamber is pulled downward, which causes the attached pen to deflect upward. (A counterweight pulley system seen at the top of the large metal cylinder in Fig. 9-12A produces this inverse relationship.) As a person exhales into the water-filled spirometer, the air has no place to go so the cylinder moves upward causing a downward deflection of a pen that marks the revolving chart paper (allowing each upward and downward excursion of the pen to be recorded). The marks drawn on the chart paper during the upward

TABLE 9-12 American Thoracic Society Classification of Lung Disease

Test	Normal (% of Predicted)	Mild Disease (% of Predicted)	Moderate Disease (% of Predicted)	Severe Disease (% of Predicted)
FVC	≥80	60–80	50–60	≤50
FEV$_1$	≥80	60–80	40–60	≤40
FEV$_1$/FVC	75	—	—	—
DLCO	80	60–80	40–60	≤40

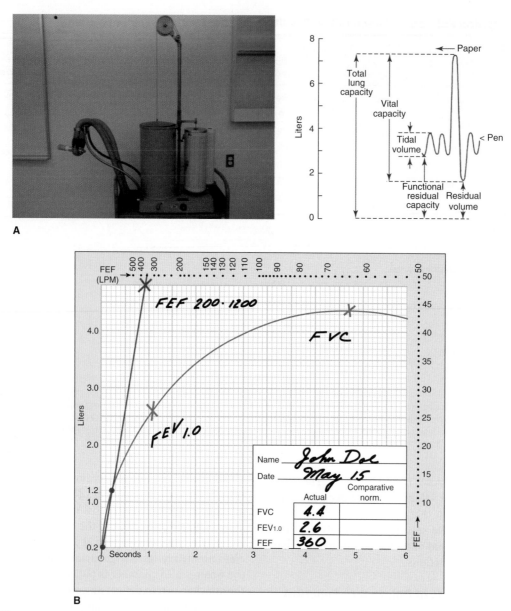

FIGURE 9-12   (**A**) A water-sealed spirometer and the resultant static lung volume curve. (**B**) Recording of an expiratory flow–volume curve on specialized Vitalograph chart paper.

and downward excursions of the pen can be measured and a specific volume and flow of air during the inspiratory and expiratory maneuvers can be calculated. These volumes and flows are shown in Fig. 9-12A.

Several measurements of pulmonary function can be viewed moving from right to left (the actual direction that the pen records on the revolving chart paper) of Fig. 9-12A. The first measurement is the V_T, which is the amount of air moving in and out of the lungs during normal, relaxed breathing (the small cyclical sine wave in the center of the figure displays the V_T; the amount of air moved normally is regular and similar during inspiration and expiration). However, the first large upward deflection above the V_T is the inspiratory reserve volume (IRV). It is the result of a maximal inspiration and reflects the volume of air that can be

moved, which is on reserve above the V_T (to be used during maximal exercise or functional tasks). Adding the V_T to the IRV provides a measure of inspiratory capacity (IC), which is also shown in Fig. 9-12A.[61–63]

The next major deflection below the V_T moving from right to left is the expiratory reserve volume (ERV). It is the result of a maximal exhalation and reflects the volume of air that can be moved, which is on reserve below the V_T (to also be used during maximal tasks). Adding the sum of the V_T and the IRV (the IC, as presented above) to the ERV yields the VC. Two additional measurements displayed in Fig. 9-12A, but not measured with the water-sealed spirometer, are the RV and the functional residual capacity (FRC). The FRC and RV can be measured via body plethysmography, helium dilution, or nitrogen washout methods. Each of these tests and the methods by

TABLE 9-13 **Methods to Measure Functional Residual Capacity and Residual Volume**

Method	Procedure	Strengths	Weaknesses
Body plethysmography	Subject sits in an airtight box that contains pressure transducers that measure alveolar pressure in the known volume and pressure of the box, which enable measurement of FRC and RV.	Quick and relatively patient friendly	Measures total gas in the thorax and may overestimate
Helium dilution method	Subject breathes a known volume and concentration of helium (He) until equilibrium of the He within the subject and a closed-circuit spirometer He source are achieved. At this time the FRC can be calculated from the change in He concentration in the closed-circuit spirometer (less He will be in the spirometer when the patient's lung volume is large and vice versa).	Quick and relatively patient friendly, but may be time consuming in patients with severe COPD	Some patients may find it difficult to be connected to a closed-circuit spirometer for a prolonged period of time.
Nitrogen washout method	Subject breathes pure oxygen from an open-circuit spirometer during which nitrogen (N_2) is "washed out" of the lungs and the amount of N_2 exhaled allows FRC to be calculated (based on N_2 in the lungs and atmosphere is approximately 79%).	Quick and relatively patient friendly	?

?The question mark imply questionable or unknown characteristics.

which they measure FRC and RV are described in Table 9-13. The RV measures the volume of air left in the lungs at the end of a maximal expiration. The RV provides information about air trapped within the lungs. **The RV and other measurements shown in Table 9-11 under the heading "Lung Volumes" also provide information that can help to diagnose the severity of lung disease and to predict treatment outcomes.**[61-63] This is particularly true for patients with lung disease who may need breathing retraining such as diaphragmatic breathing.

The FRC is the sum of the ERV and the RV, and represents the amount of air remaining in the lungs at the end of V_T breathing (see Fig. 9-12A). The FRC also represents the point in the respiratory cycle where the forces expanding the chest wall equal the forces that have the potential to collapse the lungs. Finally, the TLC is the sum of the RV and the VC.[61-63] Patients with severe COPD typically have a very large TLC that greatly exceeds the expected values for age, height, and gender (the percentage of predicted TLC is often greater than 100% of predicted values; see Table 9-11). Measurement

of the FEV_1 and several of the other pulmonary function test results shown in Table 9-11 are unable to be measured with the water-sealed spirometer but can be measured with the Vitalograph.

The Vitalograph works in a manner that is similar to the water-sealed spirometer, but without the water medium. The Vitalograph is constructed with a calibrated flow–volume pen that moves when a person exhales into a mouthpiece. The deflection of the pen records the expiratory flow and volume, which can be calculated from the axes of the special Vitalograph recording paper. A recording of expiratory flow and volume on the Vitalograph paper is shown in Fig. 9-12B. The FVC and FEV_1 can be easily calculated from the specialized chart paper and the recorded data.

Once the measurements of pulmonary function have been made, they can be compared to the pulmonary function results of other people of similar age, height, and gender (Tables 9-11 and 9-14). The actual measured values of a patient can then be evaluated as a percentage of what others have been observed to have in one or more of the pulmonary function test measurements.[61-63]

For example, a 51-year-old female patient who was 163.5 cm in height was measured to have a FVC of 1.11 L (Table 9-11). Many research studies have been performed, which have determined that the average FVC of a 51-year-old female who is 163.5 cm in height is 3.32 L. Therefore, either by using a regression equation or by looking at a chart of normal values from these research studies, we can determine the percentage that the FVC of our subject is to that of the FVC of other 51-year-olds who are 163.5 cm tall. Table 9-13 provides the regression equations and tables to determine the percentage of predicted FVC of this subject and of others with a known age, height, and gender. **Knowing the actual measurement of FVC as well as the percentage of the predicted value can**

TABLE 9-14   Prediction Equations and Charts to Estimate Pulmonary Function Test Results

Prediction equations (height measurements given in centimeters):

FVC (L): Crapo RO, Morris AH, Gardner RM. *Am Rev Respir Dis.* 1981;123:185-190.
  Males: (height $\times$ 0.06) $-$ (age $\times$ 0.0214) $-$ 4.65
  Females: (height $\times$ 0.049) $-$ (age $\times$ 0.0216) $-$ 3.59

FEV_1 (L): Crapo RO, Morris AH, Gardner RM. *Am Rev Respir Dis.* 1981;123:185-190.
  Males: (height $\times$ $-$0.0414) $-$ (age $\times$ 0.0244) $-$ 2.19
  Females: (height $\times$ $-$0.0342) $-$ (age $\times$ 0.0255) $-$ 1.58

FEV_1/FVC: Crapo RO, Morris AH, Gardner RM. *Am Rev Respir Dis.* 1981;123:185-190.
  Males: (height $\times$ 0.13) $-$ (age $\times$ 0.152) + 110.5
  Females: (height $\times$ 0.202) $-$ (age $\times$ 0.252) + 126.58

$FEF_{25\%-75\%}$: Crapo RO, Morris AH, Gardner RM. *Am Rev Respir Dis.* 1981;123:185-190.
  Males: (height $\times$ 0.0204) $-$ (age $\times$ 0.038) + 2.133
  Females: (height $\times$ 0.0154) $-$ (age $\times$ 0.046) + 2.683

DLCO (steady state—mL/min/mm Hg): Bates DV et al. *Med Serv J Canad.* 1962;18:211.
  Males: (height $\times$ 0.0723) $-$ (age $\times$ 0.2793) + 18.17
  Females: (height $\times$ 0.06857) $-$ (age $\times$ 0.252) + 15.86

DLCO (single breath—mL/min/mm Hg): Miller A et al. *Am Rev Respir Dis.* 1983;127:270-277.
  Males: (height $\times$ 0.1646) $-$ (age $\times$ 0.229) + 12.91
  Females: (height $\times$ 0.1602) $-$ (age $\times$ 0.111) + 2.24

DLCO (corrected for hemoglobin—mL/min/mm Hg): Clark EH. *Clin Sci Mol Med.* 1978;54:727.
  Males: value from one of the above methods $\times$ (1.7 $\times$ Hb)/(Hb + 10.91)
  Females: value from one of the above methods $\times$ (1.7 $\times$ Hb)/(Hb + 9.62)

MVV (L/min) for males and females:
  Freedman S. *Respir Physiol.* 1970;8:230-244.
    MVV = 129 + 25 (FEV_1 $-$ 4.01)

  Jones NL, Campbell EJM. *Clinical Exercise Testing.* 2nd ed. Philadelphia, PA: WB Saunders; 1982.
    MVV = FEV_1 $\times$ 0.35

TLC (L): Goldman HI, Becklake MR. *Am Rev Tuberc Pulm Dis.* 1959;79:457-467.
  Males: (height $\times$ 0.094) $-$ (age $\times$ 0.015) $-$ 9.167
  Females: (height $\times$ 0.079) $-$ (age $\times$ 0.008) $-$ 7.49

RV (L): Goldman HI, Becklake MR. *Am Rev Tuberc Pulm Dis.* 1959;79:457-467.
  Males: (height $\times$ 0.027) + (age $\times$ 0.017) $-$ 3.447
  Females: (height $\times$ 0.032) + (age $\times$ 0.009) $-$ 3.9

FRC (L): Crapo RO, Morris AH, Gardner RM. *Am Rev Respir Dis.* 1981;123:185-190.
  Males: (height $\times$ 0.051) $-$ 5.16
  Females: (height $\times$ 0.047) $-$ 4.85

		Charts developed from the preceding equations[a]			
Height (cm)	Age (y)	FVC[b] (L)	FEV_1 (L)	FEV_1/FVC (%)	$FEF_{25\%-75\%}$ (L/s)
Predicted values for adult men					
155	20	4.22	3.74	87.4	4.53
	30	4.01	3.49	85.8	4.16
	40	3.79	3.25	84.3	3.78
	50	3.58	3.01	82.8	3.40
	60	3.37	2.76	81.3	3.02
	70	3.15	2.52	79.7	2.64
165	20	4.82	4.15	86.1	4.74
	30	4.61	3.91	84.5	4.36
	40	4.39	3.66	83.0	3.98
	50	4.18	3.42	81.5	3.60
	60	3.97	3.18	80.0	3.22
	70	3.75	2.93	78.4	2.84
175	20	5.42	4.57	84.8	4.94
	30	5.21	4.32	83.2	4.56
	40	4.99	4.08	81.7	4.18
	50	4.78	3.84	80.2	3.80
	60	4.57	3.59	78.7	3.42
	70	4.35	3.35	77.2	3.04

(continued)

TABLE 9-14 **Prediction Equations and Charts to Estimate Pulmonary Function Test Results** *(Continued)*

Height (cm)	Age (y)	FVC[b] (L)	FEV$_1$ (L)	FEV$_1$/FVC (%)	FEF$_{25\%-75\%}$ (L/s)
185	20	6.02	4.98	83.5	5.15
	30	5.81	4.74	81.9	4.77
	40	5.59	4.49	80.4	4.39
	50	5.38	4.25	78.9	4.01
	60	5.17	4.01	77.4	3.63
	70	4.95	3.76	75.9	3.25
Predicted values for adult women					
155	20	3.59	3.21	90.3	4.15
	30	3.37	2.96	87.8	3.69
	40	3.16	2.70	85.2	3.23
	50	2.94	2.45	82.7	2.77
	60	2.72	2.19	80.2	2.31
	70	2.51	1.94	77.7	1.85
165	20	4.08	3.55	88.3	4.30
	30	3.86	3.30	85.7	3.84
	40	3.65	3.05	83.2	3.38
	50	3.43	2.79	80.7	2.92
	60	3.22	2.53	78.2	2.46
	70	3.00	2.28	75.7	2.00
175	20	4.57	3.90	86.2	4.46
	30	4.35	3.64	83.7	4.00
	40	4.14	3.39	81.2	3.54
	50	3.92	3.13	78.7	3.08
	60	3.71	2.88	76.2	2.62
	70	3.49	2.62	73.6	2.16

[a]The prediction equations used to obtain the values in the above charts provide more specific pulmonary function test results than the above charts, which must be interpreted with a degree of interpolation for height and age since heights and ages are likely to vary from those provided in the charts.

[b]FVC, forced vital capacity; FEV$_1$, forced expiratory volume in 1 second; FEF$_{25\%-75\%}$, forced expiratory flow, midexpiratory phase.

help to categorize the severity of a patient's pulmonary disease as well as the prognosis. This is evident by examining Table 9-12. In fact, using the FVC regression equation in Table 9-13 to determine the predicted FVC for a 51-year-old woman who is 163.5 cm tall, it is clear that the patient's predicted FVC should be 3.32 L. The patient's measured FVC was 1.11 L, which is 33% of the predicted value (1.11/3.32 = 33%). When viewing Table 9-12, it is evident that this patient suffers from severe pulmonary disease based on the percentage of predicted FVC of 33% (an FVC <50% is associated with severe lung disease).[61–64]

Evaluating Chest Radiographs

Evaluation of chest radiographs is frequently performed by physical therapists involved in the direct care of patients in the intensive care unit. A quick overview of the methods to evaluate chest radiographs is presented in the following section and is summarized in Box 9-10. The methods of examining chest radiographs are dependent on identifying the presence of the white and dark areas on radiographs. The white areas are referred to as opacities and the dark areas are referred to as lucencies. **Identifying the correct amount of both opacities and lucencies in the correct location of the chest is the basis for chest radiograph interpretation.**[65,66]

Methods to Evaluate Chest Radiographs

The methods used to examine chest radiographs include orienting oneself to the radiograph, identifying the right from the left side of the chest radiograph, looking for areas of increased or decreased opacity and lucency, identifying the inferior angles of the lungs and the height of the diaphragm, and identifying enlarged or irregular structures on the radiograph. Each of these examination techniques will be briefly reviewed in the following sections and is presented in Box 9-10.

Orienting oneself to the chest radiograph requires the reader of the radiograph to view it as if facing the patient. Examining a frontal chest film on a view box is viewed as if the patient's right side were on your left side. Examining a left lateral chest film on a view box is viewed as if the patient's left side were facing the examiner. The standard chest radiograph consists of a posteroanterior view and a left lateral view, and for patients hospitalized in the intensive care unit, an anteroposterior view is standard. The radiograph is typically performed while the patient is holding his or her breath after a deep inspiration.[65,66]

The left side of the chest radiograph can be appreciated by simply identifying the heart and the great vessels. Once found, the size, shape, and location of the heart and great vessels are

---

BOX 9-10

Methods to Examine Chest Radiographs

1. Begin examining the chest radiograph from the center of the film and examine it outward.
2. Identify the bones, soft tissues, and organs of the body.
   a. Mediastinum from the larynx to the abdomen
   b. Heart, lungs, and vascular tree
   c. Hila
   d. Diaphragm/hemidiaphragm
3. Specific lung field examination: Compare observed chest radiograph images to expected images.
   a. Mediastinum should be a vertical translucent shadow overlying the cervical vertebrae.
   b. Heart and great vessels should occupy the lower two-thirds of the mediastinum with two distinct visible curves on the right side and four distinct curves on the left side of the cardiovascular tree. On the right side, the first curve is formed by the right atrium that begins at the right cardiophrenic angle and proceeds superiorly as well as the inferior vena cava entering the right atrium inferiorly. The second curve on the right side is the ascending aorta and the superior vena cava. The four distinct curves on the left side include the transverse arch and descending aorta, main pulmonary artery, left atrial appendage (which may or may not be visible), and the border of the left ventricle.
   c. Hila should be poorly defined areas of variable density in the medial part of the central portion of the lung fields.
   d. Diaphragm/hemidiaphragm should be visible and the dome of the right hemidiaphragm is normally 1 to 2 cm higher than the left (diaphragm is elevated if during inspiration <9 ribs are visible above the level of the domes and depressed if >10 ribs are visible).
   e. Lung fields should be examined in view of the different lobes of the lungs and the various bronchopulmonary segments of the different lobes. Lesions in the lungs can be localized by a silhouette sign (normal lines of demarcation between different structures are partially or completely obscured) or changed vascular markings (increased vascular markings are associated with venous dilation and decreased markings are often associated with hyperinflation of the lungs).
   1. Search for abnormal density within all lung fields that would be identified by radiopacity (white image) in areas where there should be radiolucency (dark image).
   2. Examine the position of the diaphragms.
   3. Examine the angle of the ribs (normally oriented obliquely; may be oriented horizontally with severe hyperinflation of the lungs as in chronic COPD) and the intercostal spaces.

---

examined. The inferior angles of the lungs and the height of the diaphragm can be found by counting the number of ribs that are visible during breath holding after a deep inspiration. If fewer than 9 ribs are visible above the level of the domes, the diaphragm is elevated; if more than 10 ribs are visible, the diaphragm is depressed.[65,66]

Increased or decreased opacity and enlarged or irregular structures can be found by careful evaluation of the chest radiograph, which usually requires mentoring and experience as well as a good understanding of the anatomy underlying specific bony landmarks.[65,66] Participating in patient rounds at any hospital or clinic where chest radiographs are discussed, will likely provide the mentoring and experience that will enable a physical therapist to interpret and utilize chest radiographs.

"Other" Imaging and Investigational Studies

Other sophisticated methods of examining and evaluating pulmonary pathologies exist and are frequently employed when one or more of the previous tests demonstrate suspected pathologies in need of further investigation. The most common methods of further examination include computed tomography (CT), MRI, ultrafast scanning, lung biopsy, and sputum tests.

Computed Tomography

A CT test is simply digitized radiography, which allows numerous digital images (taken at many different angles) of a specific tissue to be mathematically manipulated based on the characteristics of the tissue being examined. The degrees of radiolucency and radiopacity are quantified, which then allows for the digitized radiograph to be computed and acquired.[67,68]

Magnetic Resonance Imaging

An MRI test is the result of hydrogen nuclei perturbations by a magnet combined with the computation of digitized images as described previously with CT. The magnet of an MRI scanner produces a magnetic field in the area of the body being imaged. The magnetic field makes the hydrogen nuclei resonate and align themselves with the magnetic field. A radio signal is then introduced to the magnetic field, which further stimulates the hydrogen nuclei and allows for a radio antenna in the MRI scanner to digitally record the resonating and realigned hydrogen nuclei. This quantifies and qualifies the tissue being scanned, which then allows for computation and acquisition of the MRI.

Ultrafast Scanning

Ultrafast three-dimensional contrast-enhanced MRI scanning tests are fast becoming an additional method of fully examining patients with suspected pathologies. It is the result of a very rapid MRI with more sophisticated application and computation abilities than the traditional MRI, yielding high-resolution three-dimensional examinations of the entire mediastinum in a single 10- to 30-second breath-hold. Ultrafast scanning can also be done with an angiogram to provide more specific information about arterial and venous disorders.[69,70] A radioactive contrast administered during magnetic resonance angiography improves the delineation of vessel borders and enables three-dimensional reconstruction of the heart and great vessels as well as of the pulmonary vasculature.[69,70]

Bronchoscopy

Bronchoscopy is simply the visualization of the proximal airways of the lungs through a bronchoscope.[71,72] The bronchoscope is a relatively large flexible scope that requires lubrication and some degree of anesthetic before insertion through the mouth into the trachea. The primary reasons for bronchoscopy include the visualization of the proximal airways and the removal of secretions in the proximal airways.[71,72] Occasionally, a physical therapist may assist a physi-

cian who is performing a bronchoscopy by applying a variety of secretion clearance techniques in hope of removing more pulmonary secretions than those obtained via bronchoscopy alone.

Secretion/Sputum Tests

Secretions or sputum removed via bronchoscopy or by a physical therapist is often in need of analysis. Sputum obtained during chest physical therapy is typically collected in a small sputum specimen collection cup using sterile techniques. Sterile techniques include wearing gloves and collecting only the patient's sputum in the collection cup. The time and date as well as the patient's name are recorded on a label that is applied to the collection cup. The collection cup is frequently placed in a plastic bag and brought to the hospital laboratory. The physical therapist often notes the color, consistency, and smell of the sputum as presented in Box 9-11.[73]

Laboratory analysis of the sputum sample includes many different tests for specific pathogens. Box 9-11 lists many of the possible results from the laboratory analysis of sputum. The results of sputum analyses provide physicians with important

---

BOX 9-11

Clinical and Laboratory Analysis of Sputum

Color*: Clear
White
Yellow
Brown
Greenish brown
Green

Consistency: Thin—Patient is often less sick.
Moderately thick—Patient is often slightly more sick than the patient with thin consistency of sputum.
Thick—Patient is often more sick than the patient with thin or moderately thick consistency of sputum.

Smell: No striking smell—Patient is often less sick.
Foul smell—Patient is often more sick.

Laboratory analysis†—Specific pathogen recognition (via culturing of specimens in various cultural media with or without oxygen and carbon dioxide at different temperatures and durations) to diagnose respiratory infections includes the following:

Bacterial pathogens	*Chlamydia*
	Enterobacteriaceae
	Haemophilus influenzae
	Klebsiella pneumoniae
	Legionella
	Mycoplasma pneumoniae
	Pseudomonas aeruginosa
	Streptococcus pneumoniae
	Staphylococcus aureus
Fungal pathogens	*Aspergillus*
	Blastomyces dermatitidis
	Candida
	Coccidioides immitis
	Cryptococcus neoformans
	Histoplasma capsulatum
Protozoa pathogens	*Pneumocystis carinii*
Viral pathogens	Adenoviruses
	Influenza A
	Influenza B
	Parainfluenza viruses
	Respiratory syncytial virus

*A patient with clear sputum is often less sick than a patient with green sputum. Patients with foul-smelling, purulent sputum that separates into three layers (an upper layer of white to slightly greenish brown, a middle mucus layer, and a bottom layer of thick greenish sputum—often plugs) after standing for approximately 20 minutes is characteristic of bronchiectasis. Copious sputum that is clear with occasional mucus is characteristic of chronic bronchitis, especially when there is a chronic productive cough with significant morning expectoration.

†Patients with copious sputum and *P. aeruginosa* and/or *S. aureus* are characteristic of cystic fibrosis.

information about particular pathogens that may be treated with specific medications.[73]

Lung Biopsy

Lung biopsies are performed to examine lung tissue under a microscope. The procedure used for a lung biopsy includes a bronchoscopy followed by the insertion of a special catheter through the bronchoscope. Once the catheter reaches the desired area of lung, a small scissors-like device cuts or crimps away a very small specimen of lung tissue that is removed via the bronchoscope and prepared for microscopic examination.[74]

EXERCISE TESTING

Traditional Exercise Testing

Traditional exercise testing of patients with pulmonary disease appears to be less commonplace in many research and clinical settings. This is likely due to a variety of issues of which the major reasons are the limited exercise performance of persons with pulmonary disease; cumbersome and often uninformative exercise test results; limited measurements and analyses of respiratory gases in patients with pulmonary diseases requiring supplemental oxygen, which are often less clinically useful; and time/reimbursement constraints. Nonetheless, traditional exercise testing on a cycle ergometer or occasionally on a treadmill is performed in patients with pulmonary disease.[75–77]

The most common reasons traditional exercise testing is employed in patients with pulmonary disease are to (1) better understand the causes and severity of dyspnea, (2) better understand the oxygen and carbon dioxide relationships as well as oxygen saturation level at rest and during exercise, (3) determine the level of exercise tolerance, and (4) investigate the presence of heart disease.[78–80] The methods of traditional exercise testing in patients with pulmonary disease will be discussed in the following section and will be followed by a discussion of other types of less traditional exercise tests (eg, walk tests, stair climbing tests), which may be more acceptable and clinically useful for patients with pulmonary disease.

Methods to Administer Traditional Exercise Testing in Pulmonary Disease

The methods employed during traditional exercise testing often include pretest pulmonary function testing; pre-, during, and posttest analysis of arterial blood gases and lactate levels; the evaluation of heart rate, heart rhythm, and signs of myocardial ischemia via electrocardiography before, during, and after exercise; and the measurement of blood pressure, oxygen saturation, respiratory gases, and rating of perceived exertion during exercise.[78–80] Occasionally, evaluation of heart function is also performed via echocardiography or other methods, which will be discussed in Chapter 10.

Preexercise Test Procedures

Before the exercise test, the patient is questioned about risk factors for heart and lung disease, recent and past complaints, recent and past medical history, and the primary problem that they perceive has brought them to seek medical attention. After questioning, a physical examination is performed, which includes the examination of blood pressure, heart sounds, breath sounds, the electrocardiogram, and pulmonary function test results. Comparisons will be made with any past questioning and tests are given with emphasis placed on recent and past complaints, blood pressure measurements, electrocardiogram, and pulmonary function tests. The variables that are very important to measure before exercise testing of patients with pulmonary disease include FEV_1, MVV, oxygen saturation, resting dyspnea level, Borg rating of perceived exertion, and for some patients, measurements of arterial blood gases. Finally, an estimate of the patient's exercise tolerance will be made, which will help to determine the exercise testing protocol and magnitude of workload increments. An estimate of the patient's exercise tolerance is made based on the aforementioned baseline measurements, current levels of activity and exercise, and possibly previous exercise test results.[78–80]

During Exercise Test Procedures

During the exercise test, the patient is provided a short period to "warm up" or the initial workloads of the exercise testing protocol are minimal and are progressed slowly with modest workload increments. Many patients with pulmonary disease will undergo cycle ergometry exercise testing and will be provided a short period of time to warm up by cycling without resistance for 1 to 2 minutes.[78–80]

After warming up, the workload will be gradually increased to a level that will enable the patient to (1) reach several *steady-state* levels until exhaustion or more commonly, until a predetermined submaximal endpoint has been achieved or (2) progressively *ramp* up to workloads that allows for 8 to 12 minutes of exercise before exhaustion. These methods of exercise testing will enable modestly accurate predictions of exercise performance and peak oxygen consumption using steady-state levels of exercise or more accurate measurements of maximal exercise performance using *ramping* protocols.[78–80]

The same measurements performed before exercise testing are frequently repeated during the exercise test (often at one-minute intervals and at peak exercise). Many of these variables and a data input sheet are presented in Chapter 10. The measurements most important to critically examine patients with pulmonary disorders include symptoms (via a Visual Analog Scale or Borg rating of perceived exertion), accurate provision of workloads, oxygenation (via pulse oximetry or PaO_2 from arterial blood gas analyses), ventilation (via CO_2 levels or respiratory gas analyses), electrocardiography (to examine the heart rate, heart rhythm, and signs of myocardial ischemia), and respiratory gas analyses (ventilation [V_E], dyspnea index [peak V_E/MVV], ventilatory threshold, and oxygen consumption).[78-80] Numerous other variables can also be considered during traditional exercise testing with respiratory gas analyses, but which have greater clinical utility for patients with heart disease and will, therefore, be discussed in Chapter 10.

Postexercise Test Procedures

Immediately after exercise testing, the patient will be asked to remain seated on the seat of the cycle ergometer or brought to a more comfortable seat. Laying the patient supine, as is done after exercise testing in patients with known or suspected heart disease, is often impossible in a patient with pulmonary disease. If respiratory gas analysis was performed, the mouthpiece or face mask used for the collection of respiratory gases can be removed immediately after the exercise test. This will likely make the patient more comfortable and allow them to breathe easier. The same previously cited measurements should also be frequently repeated (every 1–2 minutes) until the values return to baseline (or near baseline).[78-80]

Analysis of Exercise Test Results

The analysis of exercise test results in a patient with pulmonary disease involves determining the (1) primary reason(s) for terminating exercise (was the test submaximal and terminated because of attainment of a predetermined endpoint, or was the test maximal and terminated due to symptoms or adverse signs) and whether the peak workload was achieved (and at what percentage of the expected workload did the patient achieve); (2) oxygenation response via oxygen saturation or Pa_{O_2}; (3) ventilation response via respiratory gas analysis, Pa_{CO_2}, or dyspnea index (V_E/MVV); (4) maximal achieved heart rate and what percentage it is of the age-predicted maximal heart rate ($208 - 0.7 \times$ age); (5) maximal blood pressure achieved; (6) "other" respiratory gas analysis measurements such as the ventilatory threshold and peak oxygen consumption; and (7) electrocardiogram for signs of rhythm abnormalities and myocardial ischemia.[78-80] The methods of analyzing respiratory gases and the electrocardiogram as well as examining heart rate and blood pressure will be further discussed in Chapters 10 and 11. However, one respiratory gas analysis measurement that is necessary to discuss for patients with pulmonary disorders is the dyspnea index.

The dyspnea index is of value when analyzing the exercise test results of patients with known or suspected pulmonary disorders. Comparing the calculated MVV ($FEV_1 \times 0.35$) to the peak ventilation achieved during an exercise test can provide insight into the influence of a pulmonary limitation to exercise.

Walk Tests

The short exercise duration, limited amount of information, and difficulty of traditional exercise testing with respiratory gas analysis have resulted in greater research and clinical use of walk tests. The 12-, 6-, and 3-minute walk tests have been used in many clinical research trials and appear to be important tests capable of measuring improvement or deterioration in patients undergoing medical treatment and rehabilitation for pulmonary disorders.[75-77,81-84]

The first walk test was reported by McGavin et al., who evaluated the clinical utility of the 12-minute walk test.[82] These investigators discovered moderate-to-good correlation between the 12-minute walk test distance ambulated and several measures of pulmonary function. Other investigators have demonstrated similar relationships between walk test distances ambulated during different timed tests and measures of pulmonary function, respiratory gases, and arterial blood gases. Therefore, the distance ambulated during 12, 6, or 3 minutes appears to be a good measure of functional performance and is much easier to administer than traditional exercise testing. The only equipment needed include a premeasured hallway in which to walk and a stopwatch to determine when to stop the walking test depending on the duration of the test.[75-77,81-84]

Methods to Administer Walking Tests

Information about the walking test to be administered to a patient can be very helpful for the patient and therapist and can be provided to the patient in writing or verbally a day prior or immediately before the walk test. The information and instructions for therapists and those given to patients before a walking test are provided in Box 9-12. The specific methods to perform a 6-minute walk test, record the walk test results, and analyze the walk test results are provided in Box 9-13. The data input sheet of Box 9-13 can be extremely helpful when administering a walk test.[82-84]

The shuttle walk test is another walking test that is administered in a manner slightly different from that of other walking tests. The shuttle walk test is different from other walking tests in that a metronome is used during the test to which the walking cadence is synchronized. The synchronization of walking to the increased cadence of a metronome is done to increase the walking velocity such

BOX 9-12

Instructions for the 6-Minute Walk Test

Inform patients of the purpose of the test

The purpose of the 6-minute walk test is to understand how far you can walk in 6 minutes. It also gives us both an opportunity to see how you walk and something with which we can compare how you are doing in the future.

Instructions given to the patient

The purpose of the 6-minute walk test is to understand how far you can walk in 6 minutes, giving your best effort possible. The goal of the walking test is for you to walk at a pace that will allow you to walk as far as possible within 6 minutes. You can stop if you need to, but the clock will continue to run and you must stop walking when 6 minutes have elapsed. Remember, the time clock will continue to run if you stop walking for a rest, and the goal of this walking test is for you to walk as far as possible in 6 minutes. Do you understand? Do you have any questions?

We will ask you to walk down this hallway to the end, at which time we want you to turn around and walk back to this line. We want you to continue walking back and forth until 6 minutes have elapsed or until you believe you must stop. Do you have any questions?

We will walk slightly behind you with this monitor, and we will ask you how short of breath you are several times during the walking test. We do not want you to run during this test—the goal is for you to walk as far as possible in 6 minutes. A number of measurements will be made and documented before, during, and after the walk test and include the heart rate, blood pressure, respiratory rate, oxygen saturation, your rating of perceived exertion, possibly electrocardiogram, the number of stops you take if needed, and the total distance walked.

Responsibilities of the test administrator

Provide patients a 5-minute rest period before walking to establish baseline values.

Possibly monitor the electrocardiogram of patients with a history of heart disease, cardiac arrhythmias, palpated irregular pulse, or pulmonary hypertension.

Monitor and document the heart rate, blood pressure, respiratory rate, oxygen saturation, and rating of perceived exertion before and after the walk test as well as minutes 2, 4, and 6 of ambulation.

Repeat several times before and during the walk test that "the goal of the walk is to walk as far as possible in 6 minutes."

Allow the patient to set the walking pace, which can often be accomplished by walking slightly behind the patient.

Document distance ambulated by recording the number of completed laps on a premeasured (premeasuring can be accomplished with a surveyor's wheel, which can also be used to measure final ambulated distances that may be near a premeasured marker) hallway.

Document the number of rest stops needed.

Document the use and amount of supplemental oxygen or walking assists if needed.

Standardize the use or lack of encouragement during the walk test.

Terminate the walk test if

a. the oxygen saturation decreases <80% or if other signs/symptoms of significant desaturation are present (ie, confusion, stupor)
b. dizziness
c. level II/IV angina
d. marked dyspnea
e. marked fatigue
f. severe musculoskeletal pain or vascular insufficiency such as leg claudication
g. greater than moderate discomfort from any cause
h. ataxic gait
i. patients monitored with electrocardiography demonstrate
   i. increasing multifocal premature ventricular contractions (PVCs), coupled PVCs, or ventricular tachycardia (three consecutive PVCs)
   ii. rapid atrial arrhythmias
   iii. signs of myocardial ischemia

---

that patient motivation can be more controlled. As the metronome increases, the walking velocity is expected to increase. However, no method of ensuring increased walking velocity similar to that used with the metronome is mentioned in the methods of performing the shuttle walk test.[85] Therefore, if the shuttle walk test is to be performed properly, it appears that frequent monitoring of the walking velocity is necessary to ensure that it is in keeping with the metronome. However, this is easier said than done. Likewise, patients with hearing difficulty and neurologic or orthopedic problems may find the shuttle walk test difficult due to the figure-of-eight pattern of walking that is needed to perform the shuttle walk test.

"Other" Types of Exercise Tests and Methods of Administration

Other types of exercise tests include step tests and stair climbing tests. The different types of step tests and stair climbing tests as well as the methods to administer them are provided in Table 9-15. Although traditional step tests have been used very little in patients with pulmonary disease, stair climbing tests have been used in several studies and have been helpful in identifying patients with pulmonary pathologies who are most appropriate for thoracic surgery and other medical interventions (Table 9-15).[86-88] Figure 9-13 provides an illustration of these types of tests.

BOX 9-13

Data Sheet to Document Walk Tests

Prewalk test:

How short of breath are you now?

Borg dyspnea score _____

Dyspnea: Visual Analog Scale (VAS)

_____

NONE   VERY SEVERE

Record the resting:

Heart rate _____

Blood pressure _____

Respiratory rate (count the number of breaths in 1 complete minute) _____

Oxygen saturation _____

During the walk test:

Please ask the patient to begin walking and record the number of laps walked and rests taken by crossing out the 1 each time a lap is completed and rest is taken:

Laps: 1   1   1   1   1   1   1   1   1   1   1
                 1   1   1   1   1   1   1   1   1   1   1

Rests: 1   1   1   1   1   1   1   1   1   1

Record the following parameters during and immediately after the walking test:

Minute 2:   HR _____   Sao$_2$ _____   RPE _____

Minute 4:   HR _____   Sao$_2$ _____   RPE _____

Minute 6 (immediately after walking is terminated):   HR _____   BP _____   RR _____

        Sao$_2$ _____   Borg dyspnea score _____

                Dyspnea: Visual Analog Scale (VAS)

_____

NONE   VERY SEVERE

Postwalk test:

Record the following parameters after the walking test:

Minute 2 after walk: HR _____   Sao$_2$ _____   RPE _____

Minute 4 after walk: HR _____   Sao$_2$ _____   RPE _____

Total no. of laps = _____

Total distance walked (each lap = 300 ft): _____

Total no. of rests = _____

Comparing measured 6-minute walk test distance to previously published "normal" values from

Enright PL, Sherrill DL. *Am J Respir Crit Care Med.* 1998;158(1):1384-1387.

Healthy men between 40 and 80 years of age:

Predicted 6' WT = (7.57 × height in cm) − (5.02 × age) − (1.76 × weight in kg) − 309.

Healthy women between 40 to 80 years of age:

Predicted 6' WT = (2.11 × height in cm) − (2.29 × weight in kg) − (5.78 × age) + 667.

TABLE 9-15 Other Types of Exercise Tests[a]

	Methods of Administration
Different types of step tests	
One-step test	One step up and one step down with the same leg followed by one step up and one step down with the other leg; can be performed on any steps
Two-step test	Step up two steps and step down two steps often on a specially built series of four steps (two steps up and two steps down)
Climbing step test	Climb up as many steps as possible during a specific time period; can be performed on any steps and is usually performed in a stairwell with continuous steps
Different types of stair climbing tests	
Stair climbing protocol	Ask the subject to climb as many stairs as possible in the specified time period (eg, 1, 2, 3, or more minutes)
Stair-stepper protocol	Ask the subject to begin stair-stepping for as long as possible or to step as often as possible in a specified time period (eg, 1, 2, 3, or more minutes)

A cursory comparison of submaximal exercise tests on postoperative complications

Investigators	N	Patient population	Measurements	Outcomes
Bagg[86]	22	BC and lung resection	12-min WT	Did not differentiate between patients with and without POC
Holden et al.[87]	16	Lung resection	6-min WT	>1000 ft, less POC
			Stair climbing peak[b]	>44 steps, less POC
			$\dot{V}O_2$[b]	>Did not differentiate between patients with and without POC
Olsen et al.[88]	54	Thoracotomy	Stair climbing	>110 steps, fewer days hospitalized and intubated

N, sample size; WT, walk test; POC, postoperative complications.

[a]See Fig. 9-3 for specific illustrations on step and stair climbing tests.

[b]$\dot{V}O_2$, oxygen consumption.

EXAMINATION OF OUTCOMES AND QUALITY OF LIFE IN PULMONARY DISEASE

Table 9-16 provides an overview of many instruments that can be used to measure outcomes and quality of life in pulmonary disease. A summary of the general health status questionnaires and the disease-specific questionnaires commonly used with persons suffering from pulmonary disease is outlined. Likewise, the strengths and weaknesses of the different instruments are also presented in Table 9-16.[89,90] The most frequently used instruments used to evaluate the quality of life of persons with pulmonary disease appear to be the Saint George's Health Questionnaire, Chronic Respiratory Disease Questionnaire, Living with Asthma Questionnaire, and Pulmonary Functional Status Scale (PFSS). The Medical Outcomes Study Short Form, Health Survey, or MOSSF-36, and the pulmonary functional status scale both appear to be very useful tools for the physical therapist because they examine the general perceived health status (MOSSF-36) and true functional tasks as well as the manner in which they affect dyspnea and other outcome measures (PFSS). The MOSSF-36 is shown in Fig. 9-14.

SUMMARY

The majority of the methods of examination presented in this chapter have focused on those that can be allocated by a physical therapist. The traditional medical tests and measures for a patient with pulmonary disorders have also been presented, but the focus of these tests and measures has been on the clinical application for the patient being examined and treated by a physical therapist. A number of data sheets have been incorporated into the tables of this chapter and an initial patient note has been provided in the Appendix. The key tests and measures presented in this chapter include examining (1) the appearance of the patient, (2) the breathing pattern of the patient, (3) the potential for changing the breathing pattern and diaphragmatic motion, (4) the breath sounds via auscultation, (5) the ventilatory muscle strength and endurance, (6) the pulmonary function test results, (7) the exercise and functional abilities via exercise testing, and (8) the outcome measures and quality of life of patients with known or suspected pulmonary disorders. Of all these examinations, observing the breathing pattern and evaluating the potential for changing abnormal breathing patterns may be the most clinically useful for the physical therapist. The information gained from these examinations can then be used to allocate treatment interventions and determine appropriate outcome measures and effects on quality of life. In fact, a hypothesis-oriented algorithm has been developed for the treatment of patients with pulmonary disorders in which the observation of the breathing pattern is the primary point from which further examinations and treatments follow. This hypothesis-oriented algorithm is presented in Chapter 19 and incorporates many of the examinations presented in this chapter. The results of these examinations have been used to allocate further examinations and treatments based on previously published literature. Such an evidence-based examination is needed in physical therapy.

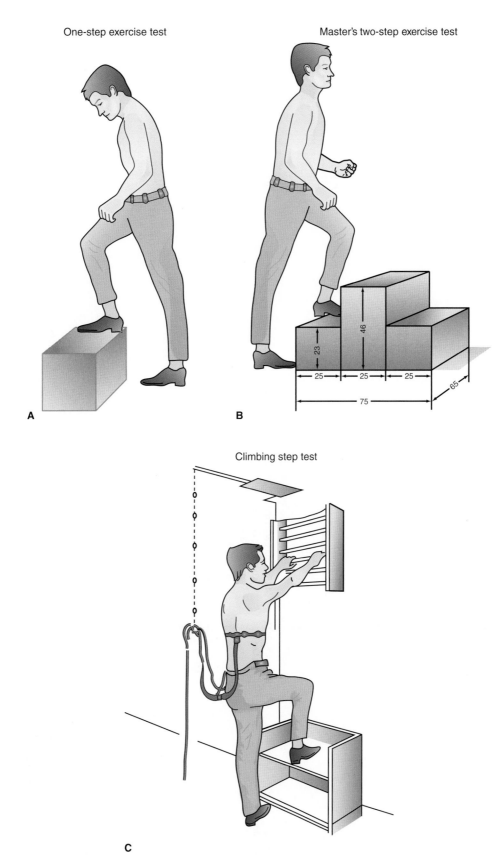

One-step exercise test

Master's two-step exercise test

A

B

Climbing step test

C

FIGURE 9-13 One- and two-step stair climbing tests and a vertical climbing test.

TABLE 9-16 Quality of Life and Health-Related Instruments

Instrument	Reference	What Is Measured?	Patient Population	Test Methods	Time to Complete	Cost to Use Instrument	Source
General health status/quality of life instruments							
Dartmouth Primary Care Cooperative (COOP) Information Project	Wasson J et al. Med Care. 1992;30 (5):42-49.	F, Phys, E, S, P, QOL, OH[a]	Adolescents, adults, and geriatrics	Interviewer or self-administered charts	5–7 min	$15.00	Dartmouth COOP Project, Dartmouth Medical School, Hanover, NH 03756
DUKE Health Profile	Parkerson GR et al. Med Care. 1981; 10:806-828.	Phys, M, S, OH, SE, A, D, P, Di	Adults with acute or chronic illness	Self-administered	2–4 min	?	Dr. Parkerson, Dept. of Community Medicine, Box 3886, Duke University Medical Center, Durham, NC 27710
Illness Effects Questionnaire	?	D, Psy, S	Physical medicine, chronic pain, dialysis, cancer, and cardiac	Self-administered	20 min	None	Dr. Greenberg, Children's Rehabilitation Hospital, Thomas Jefferson University, Ford Road and Fairmount Park, Philadelphia, PA 19131
Medical Outcomes Study Short Form (MOSSF-36)	Stewart AL et al. Med Care. 1988; 724-735.	F, Phys, S, R, M, E/F, OH	U.S. adults with mild to severe chronic medical and psychiatric disorders	Self-administered	10–15 min	$15.00	Health Outcomes Institute, 2001 Killebrew Drive, Suite 122, Bloomington, MN 55425
Nottingham Health Profile (NHP)	Hunt SM et al. J Epid Com Health. 1980; 34:281-295.	QOL, E/F, P, E, Phys, SI, S, ADL	Multiple patient populations	Interview or self-administered	10 min	None	?
Quality of Life Systemic Inventory (QLSI)	Dupuis G et al. Qual Life Cardiovasc Care. 1989; Spring:36-45.	Life domains of QOL	Any patient population and apparently normal subjects	Interview	45–60 min	$250.00 for scoring materials and $100.00 for training	Dr. Dupuis, Montreal Heart Institute, 5000 Belanger East, Montreal, Canada H1T 1C8
Quality of Well-Being Scale (QWB)	Kaplan RA et al. J Chronic Dis. 1984;37(2):85-95.	Mob, Phys, S, SC, Symp	Adults with disease or injury	Interview	10–15 min	$69.00	Dr. Kaplan, Dept. of Community and Family Medicine, University of CA – San Diego, La Jolla, CA 92093
Sickness Impact Profile (SIP)	Gibson BS Gibson JS. Ann Intern Med. 1975;65(12): 1304-1310.	Phys, Psy, and five independent factors	Any patient population and severity of illnesses	Interview or self-administered	30 min	$10.00	Dr. Bergner, Dept. of Health Sciences, School of Hygiene and Public Health, Johns Hopkins University, 624 North Broadway, Baltimore, MD 21205
Symptom Questionnaire	?	D, A, Symp, A/H	Psychiatric patients	Interview or self-administered	2–5 min	$10.00–$25.00	Dr. Kellner, Univ. of New Mexico School of Medicine, Dept. of Psychiatry, 2400 Tucker, Albuquerque, NM 87131

Pulmonary disease-specific quality of life instruments

Instrument	Reference	Domains[a]	Population	Administration	Time		Contact
Chronic Respiratory Disease Questionnaire (CRQ)	Guyatt GH et al. *Thorax.* 1987;42:773-778.	Dys, E/F, E, MD	COPD	Interview	15–30 min	?	Dr. Guyatt, Dept. of Clinical Epidemiology, McMaster Univ. Medical Center, 1200 Main Street, Hamilton, Ontario, Canada L8N 3Z5
Living with Asthma Questionnaire	Hyland ME. *Respir Med.* 1991;85 (suppl B):13-16.	QOL	Patients with asthma	Interview or self-administered	20 min	?	Dr. Hyland, Dept. of Psychology, Polytechnic Southwest, Plymouth, Deron, PL4 8AA, UK
Pulmonary Functional Status and Dyspnea Questionnaire (PFSDQ)	Lareau S et al. *Heart Lung.* 1994;23 (3):242-250.	Dys, F	Moderate-to-severe COPD	Self-administered	15 min	?	Dr. Lareau, Jerry L. Pettis Memorial VA Hospital, 11201 Benton Street, Loma Linda, CA 93457
Pulmonary Functional Status Scale (PFSS)	Weaver TE et al. *Nurs Res.* 1992;41:286-291.	ADL, Dys, D, SC, T, HT, GS, MP, S, A	COPD	Self-administered at patient's home	15–35 min	None	Dr. Weaver, Univ. of Pennsylvania School of Nursing, Nursing Education Building, Philadelphia, PA 19104
Saint George's Respiratory Questionnaire (SGRQ)	Jones PW et al. ARRD 1992;145:1321-1327.	Impact of symptoms on ADL	Asthmatics and COPD	Self-administered	?	None	Dr. Jones, Dept. of Medicine, St. George's Hospital Medical School, London, UK

[a]F, functional status; Phys, physical function; E, emotional function; S, social function; P, pain; QOL, quality of life; OH, overall health; M, mental function; SE, self-esteem; A, anxiety; D, depression; Di, disability; Psy, psychological; R, role limitations attributed to physical and emotional problems; E/F, energy/fatigue; SI, sleep; ADL, activities of daily living; Mob, mobility; SC, self-care; Symp, symptoms; A/H, anger and hostility; Dys, dyspnea; MD, mastery of disease; T, transportation; HT, household tasks; GS, grocery shopping; MP, meal preparation.
?The question marks imply questionable or unknown characteristics.

Health Status Profile — SF-36™

INSTRUCTIONS: This survey asks for your views about your health. This information will help keep track of how you feel and how well you are able to do your usual activities.

Answer every question by marking the appropriate oval. If you are unsure about how to answer a question, please give the best answer you can.

Now begin with the questions below.

1.   **In general**, would you say your health is: (Mark only one.)

- ① Excellent
- ② Very good
- ③ Good
- ④ Fair
- ⑤ Poor

2.   **Compared to one year ago**, how would you rate your health in general now? (Mark only one.)

- ① Much better now than 1 year ago
- ② Somewhat better now than 1 year ago
- ③ About the same as 1 year ago
- ④ Somewhat worse now than 1 year ago
- ⑤ Much worse now than 1 year ago

The following items are about activities you might do during a typical day. **Does your health now limit you** in these activities? If so, how much? (Mark one oval on each line.)

	Yes, Limited A Lot	Yes, Limited A Little	No, Not Limited At All
3. **Vigorous activities**, such as running, lifting heavy objects, participating in strenuous sports	①	②	③
4. **Moderate activities**, such as moving a table, pushing a vacuum cleaner, bowling, or playing golf	①	②	③
5. Lifting or carrying groceries	①	②	③
6. Climbing **several** flights of stairs	①	②	③
7. Climbing **one** flight of stairs	①	②	③
8. Bending, kneeling, or stooping	①	②	③
9. Walking **more than a mile**	①	②	③
10. Walking **several blocks**	①	②	③
11. Walking **one block**	①	②	③
12. Bathing or dressing yourself	①	②	③

During the **past 4 weeks**, have you had any of the following problems with your work or other regular daily activities **as a result of your physical health?** (Mark one oval on each line.)

13. Cut down the **amount of time** you spent on work or other activities	① Yes	② No	
14. **Accomplished less** than you would like	① Yes	② No	
15. Were limited in the **kind** of work or other activities	① Yes	② No	
16. Had **difficulty** performing the work or other activities (for example, it took extra effort)	① Yes	② No	

A

FIGURE 9-14   The MOSSF-36. (Reprinted with permission of QualityMetric, Inc.) *(continued)*

This is Side 2 of this Questionnaire.
Make sure you complete the OTHER side first.

During the **past 4 weeks**, have you had any of the following problems with your work or other regular daily activities **as a result of any emotional problems** (such as feeling depressed or anxious)? (Mark one oval on each line.)

17. Cut down the **amount of time** you spent on work or other activities	① Yes	② No
18. **Accomplished less** than you would like	① Yes	② No
19. Didn't do work or other activities as **carefully** as usual	① Yes	② No

20. During the **past 4 weeks**, to what extent has your physical health or emotional problems interfered with your normal social activities with family, friends, neighbors, or groups? (Mark one oval.)

① Not at all ④ Quite a bit
② Slightly ⑤ Extremely
③ Moderately

21. How much **bodily** pain have you had during the **past 4 weeks?** (Mark one oval.)

① None ④ Moderate
② Very mild ⑤ Severe
③ Mild ⑥ Very severe

22. During the **past 4 weeks**, how much did **pain** interfere with your normal work (including both work outside the home and housework)? (Mark one oval.)

① Not at all ④ Quite a bit
② A little bit ⑤ Extremely
③ Moderately

These questions are about how you feel and how things have been with you **during the past 4 weeks**. For each question, please give the one answer that comes closest to the way you have been feeling. How much of the time during the **past 4 weeks** ... (Mark one oval on each line.)

	All of the Time	Most of the Time	A Good Bit of the Time	Some of the Time	A Little of the Time	None of the Time
23. Did you feel full of pep?	①	②	③	④	⑤	⑥
24. Have you been a very nervous person?	①	②	③	④	⑤	⑥
25. Have you felt so down in the dumps that nothing could cheer you up?	①	②	③	④	⑤	⑥
26. Have you felt calm and peaceful?	①	②	③	④	⑤	⑥
27. Did you have a lot of energy?	①	②	③	④	⑤	⑥
28. Have you felt downhearted and blue?	①	②	③	④	⑤	⑥
29. Did you feel worn out?	①	②	③	④	⑤	⑥
30. Have you been a happy person?	①	②	③	④	⑤	⑥
31. Did you feel tired?	①	②	③	④	⑤	⑥

32. During the **past 4 weeks**, how much of the time has your **physical health or emotional problems** interfered with your social activities (like visiting with friends, relatives, etc.)? (Mark one oval.)

① All of the time ④ A little of the time
② Most of the time ⑤ None of the time
③ Some of the time

How **true** or **false** is **each** of the following statements for you?

	Definitely True	Mostly True	Don't Know	Mostly False	Definitely False
33. I seem to get sick a little easier than other people	①	②	③	④	⑤
34. I am as healthy as anybody I know	①	②	③	④	⑤
35. I expect my health to get worse	①	②	③	④	⑤
36. My health is excellent	①	②	③	④	⑤

37. Are you male or female?	① Male	② Female

38. How old were you on your last birthday?

① Less than 18 ⑤ 45-54
② 18-24 ⑥ 55-64
③ 25-34 ⑦ 65-74
④ 35-44 ⑧ 75+

39. In the past year, have you had 2 weeks or more during which you felt sad, blue, or depressed; or when you lost all interest in things that you usually cared about or enjoyed?

① Yes ② No

40. Have you had 2 years or more in your life when you felt depressed or sad most days, even if you felt okay sometimes?

① Yes ② No

41. Have you felt depressed or sad much of the time in the past year?

① Yes ② No

B

FIGURE 9-14 *(Continued)*

The 36 questions found in the SF-36 are reduced to a profile of scores representing 8 domains of health

Physical functioning	Performance of a range of physical activities such as self-care, walking, climbing stairs, and vigorous activities
Role physical	Impact of physical health on performance of work or other regular daily activities
Bodily pain	Severity of bodily pain and its interference with work inside or outside the home
General health	Evaluations of general health including current health, health outlook, and resistance to illness
Vitality	Frequency of feeling full of energy versus feeling tired and worn-out
Social functioning	Extent and frequency of limitations in social activities with friends/relatives due to health problems
Role emotional	The impact of emotional problems on performance of work or other daily regular daily activities
Mental health	Composite measure of anxiety, depression, and loss of behavioral/ emotional control versus psychological well-being

C

FIGURE 9-14   *(Continued)*

REFERENCES

1. Baum G, Wolinski E. *Textbook of Pulmonary Diseases.* 5th ed. Boston, MA: Little, Brown and Company; 1994.
2. Casaburi R, Petty TL. *Principles and Practice of Pulmonary Rehabilitation.* Philadelphia, PA: WB Saunders; 1993.
3. Murray JF, Jade JA. *Textbook of Respiratory Medicine.* Philadelphia, PA: WB Saunders; 1994.
4. Burton GG, Hodgkin JE, Ward JJ. *Respiratory Care: A Guide to Clinical Practice.* 4th ed. Philadelphia, PA: JB Lippincott; 1997.
5. Fishman A. *Pulmonary Diseases and Disorders.* 2nd ed. New York: McGraw-Hill; 1988.
6. Constant J. *Bedside Cardiology.* Boston, MA: Little, Brown and Company; 1993.
7. Sackner M. *Diagnostic Techniques in Pulmonary Disease.* New York: Marcel Dekker; 1980.
8. Cherniack NS. *Chronic Obstructive Pulmonary Disease.* Philadelphia, PA: WB Saunders; 1991.
9. Badgett RG, Tanaka DJ, Hunt DK, et al. Can moderate chronic obstructive pulmonary disease be diagnosed by historical and physical findings alone? *Am J Med.* 1993;94:188.
10. Haselton PS. *Spencer's Pathology of the Lung.* 5th ed. New York: McGraw-Hill; 1996.
11. Chen R, Tunstall-Pedoe H, Tavendale R. Environmental tobacco smoke and lung function in employees who never smoked: the Scottish MONICA study. *Occup Environ Med.* 2001;58(9):563.
12. Nelson E. The miseries of passive smoking. *Hum Exp Toxicol.* 2001;20(2):61.
13. Borg G. Psychophysical bases of perceived exertion. *Med Sci Sports Exerc.* 1982;14:377.
14. Borg G, Ottoson D. *The Perception of Exertion in Physical Work.* London, UK: Macmillan; 1986.
15. Mahler D. Dyspnea: diagnosis and management. *Clin Chest Med.* 1987;8(2):215.
16. Mahler D. *Dyspnea.* Mount Kisco, NY: Futura Publishing; 1990.
17. O'Donnell DE, Chau LK, Webb KA. Qualitative aspects of exertional dyspnea in patients with interstitial lung disease. *J Appl Physiol.* 1998;84(6):2000.
18. Kostianev S, Hristova A, Iluchev D. Characteristics of tidal expiratory flow pattern in healthy people and patients with chronic obstructive pulmonary disease. *Folia Med (Plovdiv).* 1999;41(3):18.
19. Barach A. Chronic obstructive lung disease: postural relief of dyspnea. *Arch Phys Med Rehabil.* 1974;55:494.
20. Ito M, Kakizaki F, Tsuzura Y, Yamada M. Immediate effect of respiratory muscle stretch gymnastics and diaphragmatic breathing on respiratory pattern. Respiratory Muscle Conditioning Group. *Intern Med.* 1999;38(2):126.
21. Buckingham EB. *A Primer of Clinical Diagnosis.* 2nd ed. New York: Harper Row; 1979.
22. Forgacs P. *Lung Sounds.* London, UK: Cassel and Collier Macmillan Publishers Ltd; 1978.
23. Bettencourt PE, Del Bono EA, Spiegellman D, et al. Clinical utility of chest auscultation in common pulmonary diseases. *Am J Respir Crit Care Med.* 1994;150:1291.
24. Wilkins RL, Hodgkin JE, Lopez B. *Lung Sounds.* St Louis, MO: Mosby; 1988.
25. Tobin MJ, Chadha TS, Jenouri G, et al. Breathing patterns—diseased subjects. *Chest.* 1983;84(3):286.
26. Sharp JT, Druz WS, Moisan T, et al. Postural relief of dyspnea in severe chronic obstructive pulmonary disease. *Am Rev Respir Dis.* 1980;122:201.
27. Delgado HR, Braun SR, Skatrud JB, et al. Chest wall and abdominal motion during exercise in patients with chronic obstructive pulmonary disease. *Am Rev Respir Dis.* 1982;126:200.
28. Reid WD, Dechman G. Considerations when testing and training the respiratory muscles. *Phys Ther.* 1995;75:971.
29. Cahalin LP, Braga M, Matsuo Y, et al. Efficacy of diaphragmatic breathing in persons with chronic obstructive pulmonary disease—a review of the literature. *J Cardiopulm Rehabil.* 2002;22(1):7-21.
30. Tobin MJ, Chadha TS, Jenouri G, et al. Breathing patterns—normal subjects. *Chest.* 1983;84(2):202.
31. De Troyer A, Estenne M. Functional anatomy of the respiratory muscles. *Clin Chest Med.* 1988;9:175.
32. Similowski T, Yan S, Gauthier AP, et al. Contractile properties of the human diaphragm during chronic hyperinflation. *N Engl J Med.* 1991;325:917.

33. Dueker JA, Gabriel RJ, Tretter SM, et al. Intra- and interrater reliability of a method of measuring chest expansion. *Phys Ther.* 1995;65(5):720.

34. Harris J, Johansen J, Pedersen S, et al. Site of measurement and subject position affect chest excursion measurements. *Cardiopulm Phys Ther.* 1997;8(4):12-17.

35. Feldman D, Ouellette M, Villamez A, et al. The relationship of ventilatory muscle strength to chest wall excursion in normal subjects and persons with cervical spinal cord injury. *Cardiopulm Phys Ther J.* 1998;9(4):20.

36. Konno K, Mead J. Measurement of the separate volume changes of rib cage and abdomen during breathing. *J Appl Physiol.* 1967; 22:407.

37. Kossler W, Lharmann H, Brath H, et al. Feedback-controlled negative pressure ventilation in patients with stable severe hypercapnic chronic obstructive pulmonary disease. *Respiration.* 2000;67(4):362.

38. Maarsingh EJ, van Eykern LA, Sprikkelman AB, et al. Respiratory muscle activity measured with a noninvasive EMG technique: technical aspects and reproducibility. *J Appl Physiol.* 2000;88(6):1955.

39. Rochester D. Respiratory effects of respiratory muscle weakness and atrophy. *Am Rev Respir Dis.* 1986;134:1083.

40. Saumarez RC. An analysis of possible movement of the human upper rib cage. *J Appl Physiol.* 1986;60(2):678.

41. Gilmartin JJ, Gibson GJ. Mechanisms of paradoxical rib cage motion in patients with COPD. *Am Rev Respir Dis.* 1986;134:683.

42. Sharp JT, Goldberg NB, Druz WS, et al. Thoraco-abdominal motion in chronic obstructive pulmonary disease. *Am Rev Respir Dis.* 1977;115:47.

43. Ashutosh K, Gilbert R, Auchincloss JH, et al. Asynchronous breathing movements in patients with chronic obstructive pulmonary disease. *Chest.* 1975;67(5):553.

44. West JB: *Pulmonary Pathophysiology—The Essentials.* 4th ed. Baltimore, MD: Williams & Wilkins; 1992.

45. Polkey MI, Moxham J. Clinical aspects of respiratory muscle dysfunction in the critically ill. *Chest.* 2001;119:926.

46. Black LF, Hyatt RE. Maximal respiratory pressures: normal values and relationship to age and sex. *Am Rev Respir Dis.* 1969; 99:696-702.

47. Enright PL, Dronmal RA, Manolio TA, et al. Respiratory muscle strength in the elderly: correlates and reference values. Cardiovascular Health Study Research Group. *Am J Respir Crit Care Med.* 1994;149:430.

48. Wetzel JL, Lunsford BR, Peterson MJ, et al. Respiratory rehabilitation of the patient with spinal cord injury. In: Irwin S, Tecklin JS, eds. *Cardiopulmonary Physical Therapy.* 2nd ed. St Louis, MO: CV Mosby; 1990:519.

49. Epstein SK. An overview of respiratory muscle function. *Clin Chest Med.* 1994;15(4):619.

50. Clanton TL, Diaz PT. Clinical assessment of the respiratory muscles. *Phys Ther.* 1995;75:983.

51. Martyn JB, Moreno RH, Pare PD, et al. Measurement of inspiratory muscle performance with incremental threshold loading. *Am Rev Respir Dis.* 1987;135(4):919.

52. Van't Hul A, Gosselink R, Kwakkel G. Constant-load cycle endurance performance: test–retest reliability and validity in patients with COPD. *J Cardiopulm Rehabil.* 2003;23(2):144-150.

53. Cahalin LP, Callahan B. Measurement of ventilatory muscle endurance: methods and relationships. *Chest.* 1997;112(3):51S.

54. Gosselink R, Decramer M. Peripheral skeletal muscles and exercise performance in patients with chronic obstructive pulmonary disease. *Monaldi Arch Chest Dis.* 1998;53(4):419-423.

55. Corbridge T, Irvin CG. Pathophysiology of chronic obstructive pulmonary disease with emphasis on physiologic and pathologic correlations. In: Casaburi R, Petty TL, eds. *Principles and Practice of Pulmonary Rehabilitation.* Philadelphia, PA: WB Saunders; 1993:18.

56. Schmidt GA, Hall JB. Acute or chronic respiratory failure: assessment and management of patients with COPD in the emergent setting. *JAMA.* 1989;261:3444.

57. Juan G, Calverley P, Talamo C, et al. Effect of carbon dioxide on diaphragmatic function in human beings. *N Engl J Med.* 1984; 310:874.

58. Shapiro BA, Peruzzi WT, Kozelowski-Templin R. *Clinical Application of Blood Gases.* 5th ed. St Louis MO: CV Mosby–Year Book; 1994.

59. Williams AJ. ABC of oxygen: assessing and interpreting arterial blood gases and acid–base balance. *BMJ.* 1998;317:1213.

60. Andrews JL, Copeland BE, Salah RM, et al. Arterial blood gas standards for healthy young nonsmoking subjects. *Am J Clin Pathol.* 1981;75(6):773.

61. Crapo RO, Morris AH, Gardner RM. Reference spirometric values using techniques and equipment that meet ATS recommendations. *Am Rev Respir Dis.* 1981;123:659.

62. Cherniack RM. *Pulmonary Function Testing.* Philadelphia, PA: WB Saunders; 1977.

63. Miller WF, Scacci R, Gast LR. *Laboratory Evaluation of Pulmonary Function.* Philadelphia, PA: JB Lippincott; 1987.

64. American Thoracic Society. Evaluation of impairment/disability secondary to respiratory disorders. *Am Rev Respir Dis.* 1986; 133:1205.

65. Freundlich IM, Bragg DG. *A Radiologic Approach to Diseases of the Chest.* 2nd ed. Baltimore, MD: Williams & Wilkins; 1997.

66. Meholic A, Ketai L, Lofgren R. *Fundamentals of Chest Radiology.* Philadelphia, PA: WB Saunders; 1996.

67. Briggs GM. Chest imaging: indications and interpretation. *Med J Aust.* 1997;166:555.

68. Lillington G. *A Diagnostic Approach to Chest Disease.* Baltimore, MD: Williams & Wilkins; 1987.

69. Bosmans H, Wilms G, Dymarkowski S, et al. Basic principles of MRA. *Eur J Radiol.* 2001;38(1):2.

70. Ferrari VA, Scott CH, Holland GA, et al. Ultrafast three-dimensional contrast-enhanced magnetic resonance angiography and imaging in the diagnosis of partial anomalous pulmonary venous drainage. *J Am Coll Cardiol.* 2001;37:1120.

71. Borchers SD, Beamis JF. Flexible bronchoscopy. *Chest Surg Clin N Am.* 1996;6:169.

72. Wood-Baker R, Burdon J, McGregor A, et al. Fibre-optic bronchoscopy in adults: a position paper of the thoracic society of Australia and New Zealand. *Intern Med J.* 2001;31(8):479.

73. Maestrelli P, Richeldi L, Moretti M, et al. Analysis of sputum in COPD. *Thorax.* 2001;56(6):420.

74. Ryan A, Banks J, Roberts S. Methods for lung cancer biopsy. *Lancet.* 2001;358:1909.

75. Guyatt GH, Thompson PJ, Berman LB, et al. How should we measure function in patients with chronic heart and lung disease? *J Chronic Dis.* 1985;38:517.

76. Jette DU, Manago D, Medved E, et al. The disablement process in patients with pulmonary disease. *Phys Ther.* 1997;77(4):385.

77. Singh SJ, Morgan MD, Hardman AE, et al. Comparison of oxygen uptake during a conventional treadmill test and the shuttle walking test in chronic airflow limitation. *Eur Respir J.* 1994; 7(11):2016.

78. Wasserman K, Hansen JE, Sue DY, et al. *Principles of Exercise Testing and Interpretation.* Philadelphia, PA: Lea Febiger; 1987.

79. Ellestad MH. *Stress Testing—Principles and Practice.* 2nd ed. Philadelphia, PA: FA Davis Co; 1980.

80. Jones NL, Campbell EJM. *Clinical Exercise Testing.* 2nd ed. Philadelphia, PA: WB Saunders; 1982.

81. Solway S, Brooks D, Lacasse Y, et al. A qualitative systematic overview of the measurement properties of functional walk tests used in the cardiorespiratory domain. *Chest.* 2001;19(1):256.

82. McGavin CR, Gupta SP, McHardy GJR. Twelve-minute walking test for assessing disability in chronic bronchitis. *Br Med J.* 1976; 1:822.

83. Cahalin L, Pappas P, Prevost S, et al. The relationship of the six-minute walk test to maximal oxygen consumption in transplant candidates with end-stage lung disease. *Chest.* 1995;108:452.

84. Singh SJ, Morgan MD, Scott S, et al. Development of a shuttle walking test of disability in patients with chronic airways obstruction. *Thorax.* 1992;47(12):1019.

85. Revill SM, Morgan MD, Singh SJ, et al. The endurance shuttle walk: a new field test for the assessment of endurance capacity in chronic obstructive pulmonary disease. *Thorax.* 1999;54(3):213.

86. Bagg LR. The 12-min walking distance: its use in the preoperative assessment of patients with bronchial carcinoma before lung resection. *Respiration.* 1984;46:342.

87. Holden DA, Rice TW, Stelmach K, et al. Exercise testing, 6-min walk, and stair climb in the evaluation of patients at high risk for pulmonary resection. *Chest.* 1992;102:1774.

88. Olsen GN, Bolton JWR, Weiman DS, et al. Stair climbing as an exercise test to predict perioperative complications of lung resection: two years experience. *Chest.* 1991;99:587.

89. Guyatt GH, King DR, Feeny DH, et al. Generic and specific measurement of health-related quality of life in a clinical trial of respiratory rehabilitation. *J Clin Epidemiol.* 1999;52(3):187.

90. American Association of Cardiovascular and Pulmonary Rehabilitation Outcomes Committee. *Guidelines for Pulmonary Rehabilitation Programs.* 3rd ed. Champaign, IL: Human Kinetics; 2004.

APPENDIX 1

I. Initial Patient Note

INITIAL EVALUATION AND PLAN OF TREATMENT

Date _____ Date of Onset _____ Date of Admission _____

Date of Referral _____ Initial Evaluation & Treatment Time _____

Diagnosis _____

Name _____ Patient # _____ Phone # _____

Address _____ City _____ State _____ Zip _____

Age _____ DOB _____ Sex _____ Height _____ Weight _____

Blood Type _____ Virology: CMV _____ Toxo _____

Supplemental O$_2$ _____ ID: HIV _____ Mumps _____ PPD _____

HEP-ABC _____ Other _____

Body Composition: Date: _____ Date: _____

Male: Thigh _____ Abdomen _____ Chest _____ Male: Thigh _____ Abdomen _____ Chest _____

Female: Thigh _____ Suprailiac _____ Triceps _____ Female: Thigh _____ Suprailiac _____ Triceps _____

% Body Fat: _____ % Body Fat: _____

Skeletal Muscle Abnormalities _____

I. <u>MEDICAL HISTORY</u>: _____
_____
_____

II. <u>RISK FACTORS</u>: Family History _____ Hypercholesterolemia _____

Hypertriglycenidemia _____ Smoking (pk./yrs.) _____ HTN _____

DM _____ Sedentary lifestyle _____ Obesity _____

Type A Behavior _____ Elevated FeSO$_4$ _____ Stress _____

III. <u>MEDICATIONS</u>: _____
_____
_____

IV. <u>ECG</u>: Date _____ Interpretation _____

V. <u>CARDIAC CATHERIZATION</u>: Date _____ LVEDP _____ PA _____

EF _____ C.O. _____ C.I. _____

Ventricular Function _____

Coronary Vessels _____

ECG _____

Post:

2 Minutes HR _____ BP _____ RR _____ SaO$_2$ _____

4 Minutes HR _____ BP _____ RR _____ SaO$_2$ _____

Complications _____

XI. <u>PHYSICAL THERAPY PROBLEMS</u>: _____
_____

<u>PHYSICAL THERAPY GOALS</u>: _____
_____

<u>REHABILITATION POTENTIAL</u>:

Poor _____ Fair _____ Good _____ Excellent _____

XII. <u>PLAN</u>:

Exercise: Mode _____ Intensity _____

Duration _____ Frequency _____

Repeat exercise test/6-minute walk test _____

Repeat body composition assessment _____

Suggested frequency of treatment _____

Next appointment _____

Refer to Transplant Daily Exercise Record: Yes _____ No _____

Recommendations: _____
_____
_____
_____

II. Suggested Laboratory Exercises

Laboratory Exercise 1: Evaluation of risk factors for pulmonary disease—Students role-play patients and physical therapists and simulate an initial interview session during which pertinent information is discussed and obtained between the physical therapists and the patients (half of the students role-play patients and the other half role-play therapists; if time permits, students should be paired and switch roles after interview is complete), using Tables 9-1 through 9-6 as reference sources.

Laboratory Exercise 2: Anatomy of the thorax (identifying the bony landmarks of the chest to appreciate the lobes of the lungs)—Students draw bony landmarks and lung lobes with washable markers using specific landmarks described in the following. Drawing the figures by hand in the space provided at the end of this laboratory exercise may facilitate the completion of this lab: **sternum—palpate and draw the manubrium, sternal angle of Louis, body of the sternum, and xiphoid process.**

a. Manubrium: Superiorly begins at the suprasternal notch (horizontal to the level of T2)—outline the suprasternal notch with a washable marker and palpate the junction of the clavicle with the manubrium to locate and draw the lateral aspect of the manubrium. The inferior aspect of the manubrium can be located and drawn by identifying the sternal angle of Louis (horizontal to T4 and T5 and easily located by the raised ridge on the anterior of the sternum).

b. The sternal angle of Louis is found by locating the second rib. The second rib can be found by palpating the sternoclavicular joint (SCJ), moving slightly inferior to the first rib (which may be difficult to palpate because it lies underneath the clavicle), and the next rib inferior to the first is the second rib. Palpating medially toward the center of the sternum will reveal a raised ridge, which is the sternal angle of Louis. The sternal angle is the point where the trachea bifurcates into the right (wider and more vertical) and left mainstem bronchi (narrow and more horizontal). After the trachea bifurcates at the sternal angle of Louis:

   i. The right mainstem bronchus divides into three lobar bronchi:

      1. right upper lobar bronchus that divides into

         a. three segmental bronchi to the right upper lobe

      2. right middle lobar bronchus divides into

         a. two segmental bronchi to the right-middle lobe

      3. right lower lobar bronchus divides into

         a. five segmental bronchi to the right lower lobe

   ii. The left mainstem bronchus divides into two lobar bronchi:

      1. left upper lobar bronchus that divides into

         a. three segmental bronchi to the left upper lobe

      2. left lower lobar bronchus that divides into

         a. four segmental bronchi to the left lower lobe

The divisions of the lobar bronchi and segmental bronchi to the different lobes of the lung are relatively rapid and short and can be hypothetically visualized on the thorax (with the drawings described above and below) as occupying only a small area traveling laterally, superiorly, and inferiorly from the sternum. The rest of the sternum inferior to the sternal angle is the body of the sternum from which the underlying lobar and segmental bronchi travel outward to the different lobes of the lungs.

   c. The body of the sternum should now be easily palpated and drawn as well as the attachments of the ribs 3 through 7.

   d. The xiphoid process should also be easily palpated and drawn at the base of the sternum.

Ribs: Palpate and draw the ribs (12 ribs exist—7 true ribs, which are attached to the sternum anteriorly and vertebrae posteriorly, and 5 false ribs, which are attached to the vertebrae posteriorly but not attached directly to the sternum).

   a. The seven true ribs can be palpated by moving inferiorly along the lateral aspects of the sternum until reaching the xiphoid process. Moving inferior from the xiphoid process will allow for palpation of the remaining false ribs.

   b. The false ribs can be palpated by moving inferiorly from the xiphoid process. Ribs 8, 9, and 10 are attached to a cartilage sheet arising from the sternum anteriorly, while ribs 11 and 12 are free-floating ribs and are not attached anteriorly to the cartilage sheet.

Lungs: Locate the right and left lungs by

a. Drawing a line superior and laterally from the SCJ to a point that is approximately 2.5 cm above the medial one-third of the clavicle and continuing the line to a point that is on the clavicle at one-third the distance from the end of the clavicle at the acromioclavicular joint. This should be done bilaterally. **These lines identify the superior borders of the lungs.**

b. Drawing a line from the right SCJ to the center of the sternal angle down the sternum to the xiphoid process. **This line identifies the anterior border of the right lung.**

c. Drawing a line from the left SCJ to the center of the sternal angle down the sternum to the fourth rib, where the line should be continued laterally along the fourth rib to a point approximately 3 cm from the sternal border from which the line should be continued inferiorly and slightly medially to the sixth rib and then back medially to the sternum. **This line identifies the anterior border of the left lung.**

d. Drawing a line laterally from the inferior end of the above anterior borders of the right and left lungs crossing the midclavicular line (at the 6th rib), midaxillary line (at the 8th rib), midscapular line (at the 10th rib), and finally ending at the spinous process of T10. This should be done bilaterally. **These lines identify the inferior borders of the lungs.**

e. Drawing a line cranially (and approximately 2.0 cm lateral from the thoracic spinous processes) from the level of the T10 spinous process to the level of the C7 spinous process. This should be done bilaterally. **These lines identify the posterior borders of the lungs.**

f. Drawing a line caudally and laterally from the spinous process of T3 to the costochondral junction of the sixth rib. This should be done bilaterally. **These lines identify the oblique fissure, which on the right separates the lower lobe from the upper and middle lobes and on the left separates the lower lobe from the upper lobe.**

g. Drawing a horizontal line from the point where the oblique fissure line crosses the right midaxillary line along the fourth rib to the right anterior border of the lung. **This line identifies the horizontal fissure that separates the right middle lobe from the right upper lobe.**

Students should attempt to draw figures of each previous exercise to complete "Laboratory exercise 2" and to gain a better appreciation for the anatomy of the thorax:

Anterior view of the thorax	Posterior view of the thorax
Lateral view of the thorax—right	Lateral view of the thorax—left

Laboratory Exercise 3: Auscultation of the lungs—breath sounds using Tables 9-4 through 9-6 and Box 9-3.

Laboratory Exercise 4: Arterial blood gases; practice Boxes 9-5 and 9-6.

Laboratory Exercise 5: Examining the effects of body position change on breathing (using Table 9-8 to record respiratory rates and provide structure to the laboratory, but not measuring chest wall excursion with a tape measure until laboratory exercise 6) by

a. observing upper chest motion and the respiratory rate while supine, sitting, and standing

b. observing lower chest motion and the respiratory rate while supine, sitting, and standing

c. observing both upper and lower chest motion and the respiratory rate while supine, sitting, and standing

Laboratory Exercise 6: Chest wall excursion measurements—with a tape measure comparing supine to sitting to standing or chest wall excursion on land and in water using Table 9-8.

Laboratory Exercise 7: Performing measurements of ventilatory muscle strength and endurance using Tables 9-9 and 9-10.

Laboratory Exercise 8: Performing pulmonary function tests with the Vitalograph (use principles introduced in Table 9-9 and information shown in Table 9-11 through Table 9-13 as well as that shown in Fig. 9-10).

Laboratory Exercise 9: Examining chest radiographs—using Table 9-14 and Fig. 9-11.

Laboratory Exercise 10: Exercise testing in pulmonary disease—cycle ergometry exercise testing and walk tests (Boxes 9-11 through 9-13).

Laboratory Exercise 11: Quality of life examination—Practice administering several quality-of-life tools followed by a discussion of the pros and cons of each using Figure 9-14 and Table 9-16.

Cardiovascular Evaluation

Lawrence P. Cahalin & William E. DeTurk

INTRODUCTION

Like the pulmonary system, examination of the cardiac system requires optimal use of auditory, observational, positional, tactile, auscultatory, and medical information. Perturbation of initial examination findings with different body positions or maneuvers may provide important observational, tactile, and auscultatory findings that may yield important information that could (1) direct further examination techniques, (2) direct

treatment techniques, and (3) provide important prognostic information. This chapter will review a variety of practical examination techniques and specific maneuvers that may help to direct and predict the effects of examination and treatment techniques. Much of this information is alluded to in the patient note of Box 10-1.

PHYSICAL THERAPY EXAMINATION

Medical Information and Risk Factor Analysis

The past medical history is very important for the patient with cardiac disease and must be included in the systems review process. This is particularly true of patients with known or suspected cardiac disease. A number of previous medical problems may predispose a person to cardiac disorders. Examples of such previous medical problems are shown in Box 10-2 and include pulmonary disorders, neuromuscular abnormalities, peripheral vascular disease, and treatment of oncologic disorders.

The key medical alerts for cardiac diseases are also listed in Box 10-2 and include environmental and self-imposed risks. The Framingham studies continue to identify key risk factors responsible for the development of heart disease, including a variety of blood test results (homocysteine, glucose, insulin sensitivity, lipids, fibrinogen, and many others) as well as many environmental, societal, and personal risk factors. The early studies from Framingham identified cigarette smoking, hypertension, and hyperlipidemia as the three major risk factors of heart disease. Recent Framingham studies have confirmed the importance of these three risk factors as well as of other risk factors significant for heart disease. The key risk factors for heart disease are listed in Box 10-2. A complete discussion of the risk factors for heart disease is provided in Chapter 15.

Two relatively simple and objective methods to examine cardiovascular risk are shown in Box 10-3. These risk-factor profiles examine cardiovascular risk by questioning and measuring

particular risk factors and assigning the questions and measurements specific scores. Each of the areas of examination can be scored and the scores for each of the areas can be summed. The total summed scores can then be compared to the risk-factor profile of the study population, and the specific degree of risk can be obtained and used as a reference measurement. The second column of Box 10-3 can be used to examine cardiovascular risk at a subsequent examination session. Examination of the body weight question in Box 10-3 requires the calculation of the ideal body weight, which is described in a later section and can be appreciated in Table 10-4. The CD-ROM accompanying this textbook provides prognostic indices of cardiovascular risk. Please use the CD-ROM at this time to see the tremendous amount of prognostic information provided by inputting several simple measurements and answering several pertinent questions. This tool should be useful in primary, secondary, or tertiary settings and can be used to track patient response to physical therapy.

As with pulmonary disease, listening to the patients, past history and primary complaints is critical in the examination process. In fact, a good history can provide very important information that can be very useful in diagnosing a variety of cardiac disorders. Most cardiac and cardiovascular disorders can be grouped or categorized by specific signs and symptoms. Table 10-1 provides a cursory overview of several such signs and symptoms that are helpful to categorize patients with cardiac and cardiovascular diseases. The importance of good listening as the initial part of the auditory examination cannot be underestimated. The remainder of this chapter should provide a better appreciation for the characteristics of specific cardiac and cardiovascular diseases listed in Table 10-1. Of these particular

BOX 10-1

Examination Techniques and Specific Methods to Determine the Disablement of Cardiac Disorders and Direct and Predict Physical Therapy: A Patient Case Example*

1. **Why are you here today?**
2. **Have you been diagnosed with a cardiac disorder in the past?**
3. **Have you had any special tests to examine your heart like an electrocardiogram, stress test, echocardiogram, or cardiac catheterization?**
4. **Do you experience angina or shortness of breath at rest, only with activity/exercise, or both at rest and with activity/exercise?**
5. If you experience angina or become short of breath during activity or exercise, could you please **describe the type of activity or exercise, which produces your angina or shortness of breath?**
6. Can you **describe your angina or shortness of breath?** Can you help me understand your angina or shortness of breath by pointing to the numbers 1 through 4 to describe the level of angina you experience at rest and exercise or by pointing to your level of shortness of breath using this 10-point scale or by marking this Visual Analog Scale?
7. Could I **feel your pulse to determine your heart rate and the strength of your pulse?**
8. Could I **place this finger probe on your index finger to obtain an oxygen saturation measurement?**
9. Could I **place these electrodes on your chest to obtain a simple single-lead electrocardiogram (ECG)?**
10. Could I **take your blood pressure while you are seated and then compare it to the blood pressure while you are lying down and then standing?** I would also like to observe your pulse, oxygen saturation, ECG, and symptoms when you are lying down and standing.
11. Could I **listen to your heart and lungs with my stethoscope?** While I do this **I will concentrate on watching your ECG so that I can identify your heart sounds and**

any changes in the ECG while you are breathing deeply when listening to your lungs.
12. Could I **place one of my hands on your stomach and one hand on your upper chest to determine how you breathe?**
13. Could I **place my hands on the lowermost ribs on each side of your chest to determine how you breathe?**
14. Could I **place my hands on your back to determine how you breathe?**
15. Could I **wrap my tape measure around your chest at several different sites to determine how you breathe?**
16. Now that I understand some very basic information about the manner in which you breathe could you please **breathe in the manner I instruct you via sounds I make, pressure from my hands, methods I show to you, or different body positions?** I will occasionally place my hands on your chest and wrap my tape measure around your chest to determine how you breathe during these simple tests, and I will ask you to identify your level of shortness of breath using the 10-Point Scale or Visual Analog Scale—Is this OK with you?
17. Could I **measure the strength of your breathing muscles** by having you place this mouthpiece in your mouth and breathe in and out as deeply and as forcefully as you are able?
18. I would like you to **now perform the activity or exercise which produces your angina or shortness of breath—** Could you please do this now?
19. Thank you for giving me the chance to examine you today. I will call your physician to get some more information about you like the **electrocardiogram, echocardiogram, and pulmonary function tests that you said were performed last week as well as the arterial blood gas results, chest X-ray, and exercise test results.** In the meantime, I would like you to practice breathing in the manner that we discovered helped you feel less short of breath and produced the best chest wall motion that I felt with my hands and measured with the tape measure. I will see you next week for further examinations and treatments!

*Bolded information identifies important examination procedures for patients with pulmonary disorders.

characteristics, the presence of anginal pain is most important and meaningful.

Angina—Methods to Evaluate Angina from Nonanginal Pain

Angina is often described as "heart pain," "if an elephant is sitting upon my chest," "if someone is squeezing my chest," "substernal burning," "chest pressure," or "chest tightness." It is apparent that many descriptions of angina exist. However, it is almost always due to the same thing—myocardial ischemia. The lack of oxygen to a specific portion of the myocardium is

identified by the central nervous system, and sensory fibers in the thoracic vertebrae refer the identified sensation of a lack of oxygen as a noxious stimulant to nerve fibers in the chest and elsewhere. This noxious stimulation is often referred to the anterior upper chest (substernal area, left pectoral area, or even upward into the neck) or possibly to the left arm or shoulder (Fig. 10-1).

Methods to differentiate angina from nonanginal pain (ie, musculoskeletal pain) exist and are based on several particular characteristics. If a suspected anginal pain changes (increases or decreases) with breathing, palpation in the painful area, or movement of a joint (ie, shoulder flexion and abduction), it is

BOX 10-2

Risk Factors for Cardiovascular Disorders

Previous Medical Problems Predisposing a Person to Cardiovascular Disorders

1. Pulmonary disorders
2. Neuromuscular disorders (eg, muscular dystrophy)
3. Past oncologic disorder treated with chemotherapy or radiation therapy
4. Obesity
5. Premature birth with low birth weight
6. Autoimmune dysfunction
7. Vascular dysfunction
8. Bacterial or viral infections (chlamydia pneumonia, porphyromonas gingivalis, cytomegalovirus)
9. Hypothyroidism
10. Endocrine or metabolic disorder

Risk Factors for Cardiovascular Diseases

1. Smoking
2. Occupational exposure to irritants or allergens (eg, carbon monoxide, chemicals)
3. Residing in locations with high levels of air pollution
4. Hypertension
5. Diabetes (types 1 and 2)
6. Hypercholesterolemia
7. Sedentary lifestyle
8. Family history of heart disease
9. High stress (type "A" personality and type "D")*
10. Age (older age > younger age)
11. Gender (males > females)
12. Altered serum sex hormones
    a. Men: low testosterone and DHEA
    b. Women: low progesterone and possibly estrogen
13. Elevated serum homocysteine
14. Hyperinsulinemia (insulin resistance)
15. Oxidized LDL cholesterol with hypertriglyceridemia
16. Low serum vitamin D
17. Increased serum iron
18. Inadequate dietary mineral intake
19. Inadequate dietary antioxidant intake
20. Inadequate dietary essential fatty acids intake

*Type "A" personality, time urgency with high stress; type "D" personality, suppression of emotions; DHEA, dehydroepiandrosterone.

very likely that the pain is NOT angina. Angina cannot be changed with the aforementioned maneuvers. However, it can be worsened by physical exercise or activity. Therefore, if the suspected anginal pain is unchanged with the previously cited maneuvers and the pain occurred with exertion, this finding MAY BE angina. If the suspected anginal pain is unchanged by these maneuvers, if the pain occurred with exertion, and if the pain decreases or subsides with rest, it is very likely that the pain IS angina. Finally, if the suspected pain decreases or subsides with nitroglycerin, it is even more likely that the pain IS angina. This sequence of tests to differentiate angina from nonanginal pain is listed in Table 10-2. Occasionally, angina is

TABLE 10-1 Particular Patient Characteristics Suggestive of a Cardiovascular Disorder[a]

Patient Characteristic	Rationale	Possible Disorder
Angina	Myocardial ischemia	Coronary artery disease
Dyspnea	VPD, VPF, or anginal equivalent	Pulmonary disease, coronary artery disease, CPF
Resting or easily provoked fatigue	VPD, VPF, CPD, or CPF	Pulmonary disease, coronary artery disease, CPD, or CPF
Cyanosis of skin, lips, or extremities	Hypotension or poor oxygenation	Pulmonary disease or CPF
Dizziness/light-headedness	Hypotension or poor oxygenation	Pulmonary disease, CPD, or CPF
Look of apprehension	Dyspnea and increased work of breathing	Pulmonary disease or CPF
Palpitations	Cardiac dysrhythmias	Pulmonary disease, coronary artery disease, CPD, or CPF
Nasal prongs and oxygen tubing with oxygen tank	Necessary to improve oxygenation and comfort	Pulmonary disease, CPD, or CPF
Abnormal breathing pattern	VPD or VPF	Many pulmonary disorders, but an abdominal paradoxical breathing pattern is associated with diaphragmatic paralysis (ie, C2 spinal cord injury) or severe diaphragmatic flattening (ie, COPD); both are suggestive of VPF in need of intervention
Sense of impending doom	CPF with cardiac dysrhythmias	Pulmonary disease, CPD, CPF

[a]VPD, ventilatory pump dysfunction; VPF, ventilatory pump failure; CPD, cardiac pump dysfunction; CPF, cardiac pump failure; C2, second cervical vertebrae; COPD, chronic obstructive pulmonary disease.

BOX 10-3*

Name _____   Social Security _____

| | | | | | | SCORE |
| | | | | | | 1 2 |

Weight _____   % fat _____   LBW* _____   Ideal wt. _____   Date _____

Age	10–20 y `1`	21–30 y `2`	31–40 y `3`	41–50 y `4`	51–60 y `6`	61+ y `8`	
Heredity: parents and siblings	No family history of CVD `1`	One with CVD older than 60 y `2`	Two with CVD older than 60 y `3`	One death from CVD less than 60 y `4`	Two deaths from CVD less than 60 y `6`	Three deaths from CVD less than 60 y `7`	
Weight	More than 5 lb below standard weight `0`	−5 to +5 lb of standard weight `1`	5 to 20 lb overweight `2`	21 to 35 lb overweight `3`	36 to 50 lb overweight `5`	51 to 65 lb overweight `7`	
Tobacco smoking	Nonuser `0`	Occasional cigar/or pipe `1`	10 cigarettes or less/d `2`	11–20 cigarettes/d `4`	21–30 cigarettes/d `6`	More than 31 cigarettes/d `10`	
Exercise	Intensive occupational and recreational exertion `0`	Moderate occupational and recreational exertion `1`	Sedentary occupation and intensive recreation `2`	Sedentary occupation and moderate recreation `4`	Sedentary occupation and light recreation `6`	Sedentary occupation no special exercise or recreation `8`	
Cholesterol	Below 180 mg% `1`	181–205 mg% `2`	206–230 mg% `3`	231–255 mg% `4`	256–280 mg% `5`	281–300 mg% `7`	
Systolic blood pressure	Below 110 mm Hg `0`	111–130 mm Hg `1`	131–140 mm Hg `2`	141–160 mm Hg `3`	161–180 mm Hg `5`	Above 180 mm Hg `7`	
Diastolic blood pressure	Below 80 mm Hg `0`	80–85 mm Hg `1`	86–90 mm Hg `2`	91–95 mm Hg `4`	96–100 mm Hg `7`	101 and above `9`	
Gender	Female `1`	Female older than 45 y `2`	Male `4`	Bald male `5`	Bald, short male `6`	Bald, short, stocky male `7`	

*LBW, lean body weight; CVD, cardiovascular disease.

J Occupational Health Risk Factor Profile.

Anginal Patterns

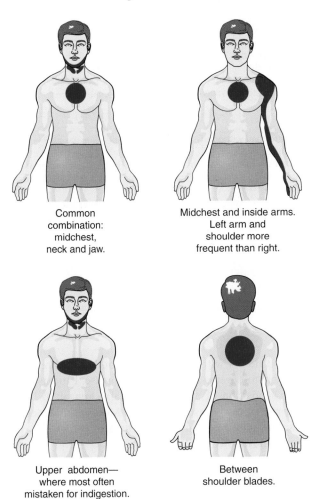

Common combination: midchest, neck and jaw.

Midchest and inside arms. Left arm and shoulder more frequent than right.

Upper abdomen—where most often mistaken for indigestion.

Between shoulder blades.

FIGURE 10-1 Anginal patterns. (Modified with permission from McArdle W, Katch F, Katch V. *Exercise Physiology: Energy, Nutrition, and Human Performance.* 5th ed. Philadelphia, PA: Lippincott Williams & Wilkins; 2001.)

not perceived, despite the fact that a patient may be experiencing myocardial ischemia. The inability to perceive angina when myocardial ischemia is present has been described as *silent myocardial ischemia*. In such cases, the most common

complaint is dyspnea. Dyspnea is occasionally described as an *anginal equivalent*—meaning that, in certain patients, dyspnea is equivalent to the sensation of angina, which again is most often due to myocardial ischemia. Myocardial ischemia may directly or indirectly produce other symptoms, which will be discussed in the following section.

"Other" Symptoms of Heart Disease

Other symptoms of heart disease exist and include dyspnea, fatigue, dizziness, light-headedness, palpitations, and a sense of impending doom (Table 10-1). It is apparent from Table 10-1 that dyspnea is possibly the most common complaint of patients with pulmonary and cardiac disorders. However, the other symptoms listed in Table 10-1 may or may not accompany dyspnea. Often, dyspnea accompanied by one of the other symptoms is suggestive for cardiovascular disease alone or combined cardiovascular and pulmonary disease. However, other measurements besides symptoms are necessary to clearly differentiate dyspnea due to a cardiac origin from a pulmonary origin. These other measurements will be presented later but can be seen in Table 10-14.

Symptom Recognition and Grading
New York Heart Association Classification

The recognition and grading of symptoms were initially described by the New York Heart Association (NYHA) in 1964. This classification schema has been accepted universally and consists of categorizing patients into one of four classes, based on symptoms and the amount of effort required to provoke them (Table 10-3). Patients without symptoms and no limitations in ordinary physical activity are categorized into class I, whereas patients who are unable to perform any physical activity without discomfort are categorized into class IV. Classes II and III are characterized by slight limitation and marked limitation in physical activities due to symptoms, respectively (Table 10-3). The symptoms recognized as limiting physical activity can be due to any of those listed in Table 10-1, but the most common symptoms for cardiovascular disease appear to be angina, dyspnea, and fatigue. The Canadian Heart Association classification

TABLE 10-2   Methods to Differentiate Angina from Nonanginal Pain

Symptoms	Maneuver	Symptoms	Outcome
Suspected angina (eg, chest, arm, shoulder, or neck pain)	Deep breathing, palpation in the painful area, or joint movement	Suspected angina changes (increases or decreases)	Not angina
Suspected angina (eg, chest, arm, shoulder, or neck pain)	Deep breathing, palpation in the painful area, or joint movement	Suspected angina does not change	Possibly angina
Suspected angina (eg, chest, arm, shoulder, or neck pain)	Physical exercise or activity	Suspected angina increases	Likely angina
Suspected angina (eg, chest, arm, shoulder, or neck pain)	Physical exercise or activity followed by a rest period	Suspected angina increases during exercise or activity and decreases with rest	Very likely angina
Suspected angina (eg, chest, arm, shoulder, or neck pain)	Nitroglycerin	Suspected angina decreases	Very likely angina

TABLE 10-3   Symptom Recognition and Grading

Class	Symptoms
	New York Heart Association
I	Ordinary physical activity does not cause undue dyspnea, fatigue, palpitations, pain, or angina.
II	Patients are comfortable at rest, but ordinary physical activity results in dyspnea, fatigue, palpitations, pain, or angina.
III	Patients are comfortable at rest, but less than ordinary physical activity causes dyspnea, fatigue, palpitations, pain, or angina.
IV	Patients may be uncomfortable at rest experiencing dyspnea, fatigue, palpitations, pain, or angina and are unable to perform any physical activity without increased symptoms and discomfort.
	Canadian Heart Association
I	Ordinary physical activity (eg, walking or climbing stairs) can be performed without dyspnea, fatigue, palpitations, pain, or angina. However, strenuous prolonged exertion may produce these symptoms.
II	Slight limitation due to one or more of the previously cited symptoms in ordinary physical activities (eg, walking or climbing stairs rapidly; walking uphill; walking or stair climbing after meals, in cold, or when under emotional stress; walking more than two blocks or climbing more than one flight of ordinary stairs at a normal pace).
III	Marked limitation due to one or more of the previously cited symptoms in ordinary physical activities (eg, walking 1–2 blocks or climbing more than one flight of ordinary stairs).
IV	Unable to perform any physical activity without discomfort from any of the above symptoms.
	Specific Activity Scale
I	Patients can perform activities requiring ≥7 METS[a]
II	Patients can perform activities requiring ≥5 METS, but unable to exceed 7 METS of activity
III	Patients can perform activities requiring ≥2 METS, but unable to exceed 5 METS of activity
IV	Patients cannot perform activities requiring ≥2 METS

[a]METS, metabolic equivalents.

and Specific Activity Scale are two additional measures used to recognize and grade symptoms in regard to performance of functional tasks. These measures are also presented in Table 10-3.

Examinations of Patient Appearance
Specific Patient Characteristics (eg, Skin Color and Body Traits)

As presented in Table 10-1, specific patient characteristics can provide important information about the likelihood or presence of cardiovascular disease. In terms of the likelihood of cardiovascular disease, a simple examination of particular body characteristics can provide helpful information about cardiovascular risk. One such characteristic is the skin color of the peripheral extremities. Pale or cyanotic skin in the legs, feet, arms, and fingers is associated with poor cardiovascular function. Another characteristic is the presence of a diagonal earlobe crease. This phenomenon has been investigated for many years and recently was once again found to be highly predictive of heart disease.[1] Many other patient characteristics can provide helpful diagnostic or prognostic information and include cyanosis, an abnormal breathing pattern, a look of apprehension, or a variety of symptoms such as dizziness, light-headedness, palpitations, or even a sense of impending doom as mentioned earlier. This subjective information combined with particular aspects of a patient's appearance can help to categorize the predominant disorder in need of physical therapy (Table 10-1).

Examination of body type (body habitus or somatotype) can also provide important information about cardiovascular risk. Patients who fall outside the somatotype classification of endomorphs (heavyset), mesomorphs (average body build), or ectomorphs (thinset) appear to have a greater risk for cardiovascular disease followed by endomorphs and meso-morphs. Patients with a pear-shaped body are three times more likely to develop cardiovascular disease. Patients with a greater deposition of abdominal fat also appear to have a greater risk of cardiovascular disease. More specific methods to examine body type and physical characteristics will be presented in the following sections.

Anthropometric Measurements

A variety of anthropometric measurements can be made in subjects suspected to have cardiovascular or pulmonary disease or in subjects with known cardiovascular disease. Likewise, anthropometric measurements can be helpful in predicting the risk of cardiovascular disease. The most common methods to perform anthropometric measurements include body weight, finger pressure on an edematous area, girth measurements, skinfold caliper measurements, calculation of the body mass index (BMI), hydrostatic weighing (underwater weighing), and a variety of quick methods to indirectly measure the percentage of body fat and lean muscle mass (bioimpedance analysis, infrared). Appropriate sites from which to obtain girth measurements are shown in Figs. 10-2A and 10-2B. Each of these methods, the methods to perform them, and the strengths and weakness of each method are presented in Table 10-4. Furthermore, the measurement of waist-to-hip ratio can provide very important information regarding risk of cardiovascular disease. The methods to properly perform the waist-to-hip ratio measurements are shown in Fig. 10-3. Measurement of the waist circumference is made just above the umbilicus while the hip circumference is made near the greater trochanter. The following Web site provides excellent resources for anthropometric measurements: http://www.topendsports.com/testing/anthropometry.htm.

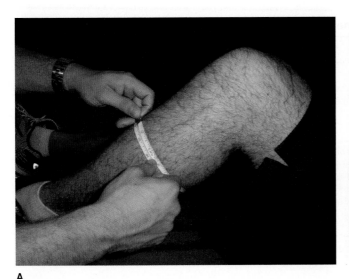

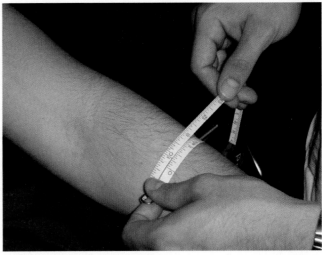

FIGURE 10-2   Methods to measure limb girth. (**A**) midcalf and (**B**) midforearm.

The calculations of ideal body weight and BMI are also described in Table 10-4. In brief, ideal body weight can be calculated by determining body height and frame size (small, medium, large) and assigning a certain amount of weight for body height and frame size (Table 10-4). The BMI is simply the quotient of body weight in kilograms and the square of height in meters (BMI $=$ kg/[m]^2). The BMI is quite easy to calculate, but a very useful Web site (http://www.nhlbisupport.com/bmi/) provides rapid conversions from English to metric and provides helpful information about individual results. An overview of normal (normal BMI is considered to be between 20 and 25) and abnormal values is provided and methods to improve abnormal results are suggested. Figure 10-4 shows several sites for skinfold caliper measurements.

Jugular Venous Distension

Jugular venous distension (JVD) is simply the filling of the jugular vein(s) with excessive fluid such that they become visibly distended. The etiology of JVD is varied, but it is often due to right-sided heart failure. Figure 10-5 shows a patient with right-sided heart failure and visible JVD. It is easily seen in this patient and can be documented by simply indicating that the jugular veins were markedly distended bilaterally. However, not all patients demonstrate such extreme JVD as that shown in Fig. 10-5. Patients with suspected JVD can actually be placed semisupine (lying on a table at a 45-degree angle). This position is the standard initial reference position to measure for JVD. After assuming this body position, the patient is slowly brought to a more upright position, and the angle of the table and the patient's neck are observed for signs of JVD. If JVD is observed, the position of the table and the magnitude of JVD should be measured. The position of the table can be easily read off of the goniometer-like device providing the exact angle of the table. The magnitude of JVD is measured with the base of a small metric ruler placed at the sternal angle of Louis and aligned cranially alongside the jugular vein. The movement of

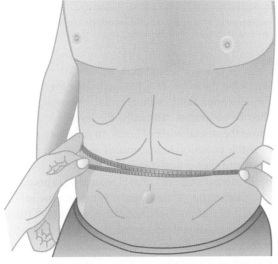

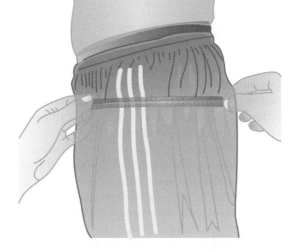

FIGURE 10-3   Methods to measure the waist-to-hip ratio.

TABLE 10-4   Common Methods to Perform Anthropometric Measurements

Method	Procedure	Strengths	Weaknesses
Body weight	Subject stands in the middle of a calibrated scale. A simple calculation of ideal body weight can be made for men and women and compared to the measured body weight.[a] **Men:** Base height and weight of 5 ft and 106 lb, respectively. Add 6 lb for each inch more than 5 ft (ie, a 5 ft 10 in. male has an ideal body weight of 166 lb (based on 106 + [10 × 6]) **Women:** Base height and weight of 5 ft and 100 lb, respectively. Add 5 lb for each inch more than 5 ft (ie, a 5 ft 5 in. female has an ideal body weight of 125 lb (based on 100 + [5 × 5])	Ease of measurement	Scale may not be calibrated producing an inaccurate measurement
Finger pressure	Index finger is pressed into an edematous area, and the time for the indentation to resolve is measured and graded (grade 1+ = barely perceptible indentation; grade 2+ = skin rebounds to original contour within 15 s, grade 3+ = skin rebounds to original contour within 15–30 s, grade 4+ = skin rebounds to original contour in >30 s)	Ease of application—only equipment needed is a watch	Useful only for the measurement of peripheral edema
Girth measurements	Tape measure is wrapped around an edematous area or particular body part (waist and hip, yielding a waist-to-hip ratio)	Ease of application—only equipment needed is a tape measure; can measure edema or particular body parts, which can provide important diagnostic and prognostic information	None that are significant
Skinfold calipers	Specific body parts are positioned. Skinfolds are gathered and subsequently measured with a caliper	Ease of application—only equipment needed is a skinfold caliper; can determine the amount of body fat and lean muscle mass which may provide important diagnostic and prognostic information	Slight discomfort during the gathering of skin folds
Body mass index	Body weight in kg. Body height in m^2 (http://www.nhlbisupport.com/bmi/)	Very easy calculation	Inaccurate if body weight or height or incorrectly measured
Hydrostatic weighing	Subject is completely immersed in water and instructed to exhale completely while the weight of the subject is obtained with a scale attached to a seat upon which the subject is sitting	Considered the gold standard to determine body fat and lean muscle mass	Many opportunities for measurement error and lack of patient cooperation. There is also a need to calculate the subjects' Residual Volume

[a]Ideal body weight calculations should be made in reference to body frame type, such that subjects with a small body frame should undergo a correction of the ideal body weight calculation by multiplying the calculated ideal body weight by 0.90, and subjects with a large body frame should undergo a correction of the ideal body weight calculation by multiplying the calculated ideal body weight by 1.10.

the pulse of JVD can then be measured in centimeters and documented. Observation of an increase or decrease in the pulse of JVD can then be tracked and provides important information about the status of the cardiovascular system. Figure 10-6 provides an overview of the methods to measure JVD.

From Fig. 10-6, it is apparent that more detailed measurements can be obtained by rotating the head slightly away from the vein being examined, and at the point of elevation of the bed at which distention is first observed, pressure should be applied to the external jugular vein just above and parallel to the clavicle for approximately 10 to 20 seconds. This amount of time should allow the lower part of the vein to fill, and after

removing the finger that was occluding the vein, the height of the distended fluid column within the vein will rise and can then be measured. Normally, the level is less than 3 to 5 cm above the sternal angle of Louis. In summary, the highest point of visible pulsation is determined as the trunk and head are elevated and the vertical distance between this level and the level of the sternal angle of Louis is recorded as shown in Fig. 10-6.

Evaluation of the jugular waveforms can also be performed in this position, but catheterization of the pulmonary artery for assessment of pulmonary arterial pressures and waveforms (via Swan–Ganz monitoring) provides the greatest amount of information. A tremendous amount of information

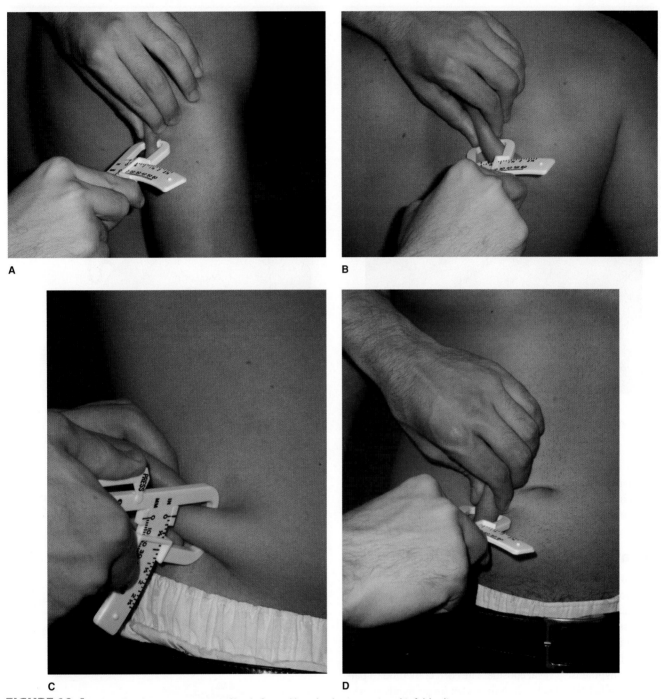

A

B

C

D

FIGURE 10-4   Sites for the measurement of body fat and lean body mass using skinfold calipers.

can be projected to a hemodynamic monitor, where the pulmonary artery pressure and waveforms can be examined. A variety of different waveforms may be identified by this invasive method of monitoring, but a thorough noninvasive examination of the jugular neck veins for particular pulsatile waveforms may allude to specific cardiac disorders. Several examples of this are the wave of venous distention from right atrial systole (that occurs just before the first heart sound [S$_1$]) and the v wave that is frequently associated with a regurgitant tricuspid valve.

Although the assessment of hemodynamic function via Swan–Ganz monitoring is considered an advanced skill, it is relatively simple to interpret the typical intensive care unit (ICU) monitor and thus obtain important hemodynamic information to examine and treat patients in the ICU. Perhaps one of the most important measurements from such monitoring is identifying the pulmonary artery pressure waveform and digital display of the systolic, diastolic, and mean pulmonary artery pressures. A mean pulmonary artery pressure greater than 25 mm Hg is the threshold level that is used to define pulmonary hypertension.

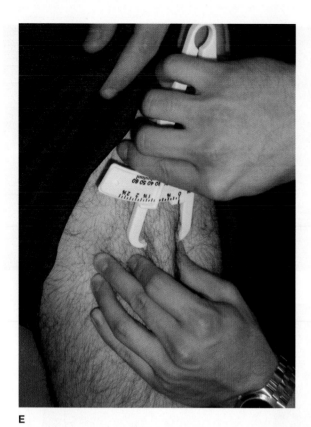

E

FIGURE 10-4   *(Continued)*

This is a very important measurement, because pulmonary hypertension is associated with a variety of life-threatening pathophysiologic phenomena (hypoxia, cardiac arrhythmias, and pulmonary abnormalities).

Palpation of the Radial Pulse

Palpation of the radial pulse can provide important information about the status of the cardiovascular system. The radial pulse is the preferred pulse to palpate because of the possibility of excessive vagal stimulation from excessive palpation (actually searching or massaging) of the carotid artery. Such excessive vagal stimulation may significantly decrease the heart rate and induce a hypotensive vagal eposide. The correct method to palpate the radial artery is to place the index finger lightly on the subject's radial artery just below the thumb on either wrist. The pulse should be examined in both wrists in similar locations.

Much of the information obtained from the palpation of the radial pulse is listed in Table 10-5 and includes the rate of the pulse (the heart rate by counting the number of beats per minute), regularity or lack of regularity of the pulse, strength of the pulse, palpable turbulence, relationship of the pulse to a continuous electrocardiographic tracing and heart sounds, and the relationship of the pulse to the breathing cycle. Palpation of the pulse can provide an enormous amount of information about normal and abnormal physiologic phenomenon. Of particular importance is learning to get the "feel" of the cardiac cycle and determining the heart rate.

Right-Sided Heart Failure in a Patient with Dilated Cardiomyopathy

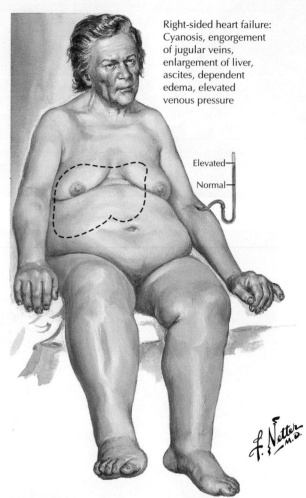

Right-sided heart failure: Cyanosis, engorgement of jugular veins, enlargement of liver, ascites, dependent edema, elevated venous pressure

Elevated

Normal

FIGURE 10-5   Patient demonstrating signs and symptoms of right-sided heart failure. Copyright (2004) Icon Learning Systems, LLC. A subsidiary of MediMedia, Inc. US. All rights reserved. (Reprinted with permission from *The CIBA Collection of Medical Illustrations*, by Frank H. Netter, MD.)

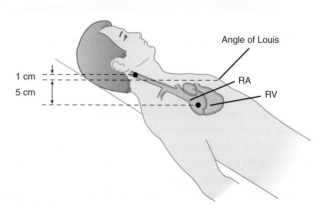

Angle of Louis

1 cm

5 cm

RA

RV

FIGURE 10-6   Measurement of jugular venous distension. (Reproduced, with permission, from McPhee SJ. *Pathophysiology of Disease: An Introduction to Clinical Medicine*, 6th ed. New York: McGraw-Hill, 2010:265.)

TABLE 10-5 Information Obtained from Palpation of the Radial Pulse[a]

Variable	Normal	Abnormal	Clinical Correlate
Presence of a pulse	Pulse is palpated	Pulse is not palpated	Inability to palpate the pulse may be due to PVD or compromised cardiovascular function.
Pulse rate	60–100 bpm	<60 bpm, >100 bpm	Too rapid or slow of a pulse rate may decrease the cardiac output.
Pulse regularity	Regular (even pulse)	Irregular (uneven pulse)	An irregular pulse may decrease the cardiac output.
Pulse strength	Consistent and strong	Inconsistent and weak	An inconsistent and weak pulse may signify poor cardiac performance.
Palpable turbulence ("thrill")	No palpable thrill	Palpable thrill	Turbulent blood flow from a variety of disorders that are associated with a hyperdynamic circulation or abnormal valvular function.
Relationship of the pulse to the ECG	Pulse palpated at the same time the R wave of the ECG is displayed.	Pulse not palpated at the same time the R wave of the ECG is displayed.	A pulse that is not consistently palpated when the R wave of the ECG is displayed is suggestive of compromised cardiovascular function.
Relationship of the pulse to auscultation of the heart	Pulse is palpated shortly after S_1.	Pulse is not palpated shortly after S_1.	A pulse that is not consistently palpated shortly after S_1 is suggestive of compromised cardiovascular function.
Relationship of the pulse to breathing	Pulse may alter during the breathing cycle.	Pulse is unchanged during the breathing cycle.	A pulse that is unchanged during the breathing cycle may be normal, but is likely associated with a less healthy cardiovascular system. A pulse that decreases with inspiration may be normal, but may also be associated with a compromised cardiovascular system.
Relationship of the pulse to BP	Pulse is absent.	Pulse is not absent.	The pulse should become obliterated during inflation of the BP cuff and will remain obliterated until the pressure in the artery being compressed exceeds the pressure in the BP cuff. A pulse that is palpated during BP cuff inflation indicates that the cuff is insufficiently inflated which will result in an inaccurate BP measurement.

[a]PVD, peripheral vascular disease; ECG, electrocardiogram; S_1, first heart sound; BP, blood pressure.

Feeling the Cardiac Cycle and Determining the Heart Rate

Palpation of the radial pulse allows for a quick examination of the contraction and relaxation characteristics of the heart. The contraction of the heart is associated with the blood being ejected from the heart into the peripheral vasculature yielding an arterial pulse. The relaxation of the heart is that period of time between palpated arterial pulses and is called diastole. Palpation of the arterial pulse identifies systole, whereas the absence of a pulse identifies diastole. Palpation of the radial pulse, therefore, yields very specific information about the cardiac cycle and can provide information about the actual heart rate and other important findings (Table 10-5).

The method to determine the heart rate from the radial pulse basically involves counting the number of palpated pulses in 1 minute. In addition to determining the heart rate, it is critically important to palpate for differences in the strength and regularity of the pulses at rest during the breathing cycle (examining the strength and regularity of the pulses during inspiration and during expiration), during different body positions, and during physical activity or exercise. Differences in these parameters during the aforementioned perturbations can identify normal or abnormal physiologic function (Table 10-5).

One particular palpable parameter is the presence of excessive turbulence in an artery. Turbulent blood flow can be easily palpated by applying light pressure on a suspected artery and feeling for the turbulent blood flow. Turbulent blood flow in an artery is referred to as a thrill. The presence of a thrill is often associated with different types of heart disease, which produce an abnormal degree of turbulent blood flow because of hyperdynamic circulations or abnormal valvular function. Finally, it is also important to examine the pulse and the relationship of the pulse to other cardiovascular examinations such as auscultation of the heart, a continuous electrocardiogram, or even while taking the blood pressure. The examination of the pulse as it pertains to the electrocardiogram will be discussed in Chapter 11. The examination of the pulse as it pertains to the blood pressure and auscultation of the heart will be discussed in the following sections.

Blood Pressure Examination
Measurement of Systolic Blood Pressure

Arterial blood pressure can be measured in a variety of methods, but the standard examination of arterial blood pressure utilizes a sphygmomanometer (either aneroid or a mercury

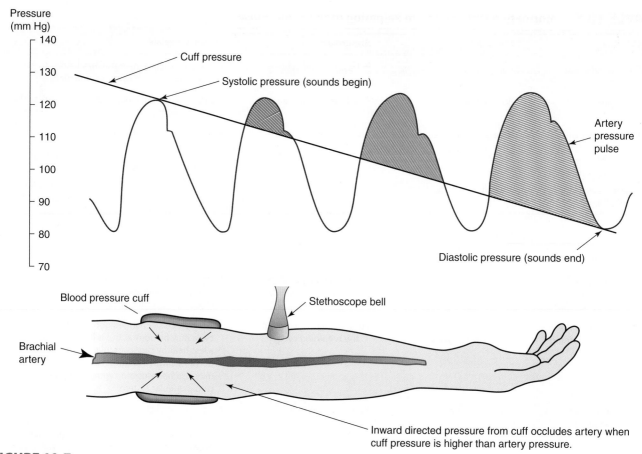

FIGURE 10-7 Measurement of blood pressure with the resultant arterial pressure waveform.

column) and blood pressure cuff, which occludes blood flow (by filling the cuff with air) at the site the blood pressure cuff is inflated (Fig. 10-7). The occlusion of blood flow at a particular site of the body is identical to a tourniquet. Arterial blood flow is stopped at the site of the blood pressure cuff. When the air filling the cuff is slowly released from the cuff, the stopped blood will forcefully flow past the blood pressure cuff when the arterial blood pressure is greater than the pressure in the blood pressure cuff. The forceful and rapid flow of blood past the site of cuff occlusion produces turbulence and yields the sounds heard with a stethoscope (often referred to as Korotkoff sounds). The Korotkoff sounds and the manner that they are used to measure blood pressure are described in Table 10-6. Using the methods described in Table 10-6 should provide accurate and reliable measurements of the systolic and diastolic blood pressure using a sphygmomanometer. Figure 10-7 graphically portrays the previously cited methods and changes when measuring arterial blood pressure.

The relationship of the pulse to blood pressure is that the pulse will be absent when the blood pressure cuff is inflated. In fact, this relationship is very important because it is the method used to determine the maximal cuff inflation pressure needed to measure the blood pressure (Table 10-6) and because it can provide an indirect measurement of the systolic blood pressure when a stethoscope is unavailable. Inflating a blood pressure cuff at the brachial artery will stop blood flow distal to the

brachial artery. Thus, the radial pulse will be absent—no pulse will be palpated due to the occluded blood flow at the brachial artery. As air is slowly released from the blood pressure cuff, there will be a time when the pressure within the artery exceeds that in the cuff. When this occurs, blood will flow past the brachial artery and can be palpated in the radial artery. The initial pulse that is palpated after such an occlusion is essentially the systolic blood pressure. Observing a mercury column or aneroid sphygmomanometer as air is being released from the blood pressure cuff and identifying the point on the sphygmomanometer that the radial pulse is palpated provide an indirect estimate of the systolic blood pressure. Auscultation of the turbulent blood flowing past the deflating blood pressure cuff is the preferred method to measure arterial blood pressure.

Measurement of Diastolic Blood Pressure

The measurement of arterial blood pressure involves the pressure not only during systole but also during diastole. As inferred from Table 10-6, the measurement of the diastolic blood pressure is made using one of two different criteria. The main two criteria are the absence of sound during the release of air from the blood pressure cuff and the muffling of sound during the release of pressure from the cuff. As previously mentioned, diastole is that period of time when there is no palpated pulse and essentially represents the resting phase of the

TABLE 10-6 Measurement of Blood Pressure

Proper equipment
1. Calibrated sphygmomanometer without air leaks in sphygmomanometer or tubing
2. Correct cuff size (see Fig. 10-11)[a]
   a. Standard cuff sizes are 12 cm (adult cuff), 15 cm (large adult cuff), and 18 cm (thigh cuff)
   b. The **ideal arm circumference for the 12-, 15-, and 18-cm cuffs are 30-, 37.5-, and 45-cm,** respectively. Measure a patient's arm circumference and use a cuff size that is closest to the ideal arm circumference. (For example, a 12-cm cuff should be used for a patient with an arm circumference at or near 30 cm, whereas an 18-cm cuff should be used for a patient with an arm circumference at or near 45 cm.)
   c. A patient with an arm circumference measured to be below or above the ideal circumference for a 12-, 15-, or 18-cm cuff should have the systolic and diastolic blood pressure measurements taken with these incorrect cuff sizes undergo a simple arithmetic correction to yield a true systolic and diastolic blood pressure (see following).
3. **Arithmetic correction for an incorrect cuff size**—The actual measured arm circumference is used to determine the amount of mm Hg to add or subtract from the blood pressure measured with an incorrect cuff size. For example, using the following Table, a patient with a measured arm circumference of 26 cm and who had their blood pressure taken with a 12-cm cuff should have 5 mm Hg added to the systolic blood pressure and 3 mm Hg added to the diastolic blood pressure. Conversely, a patient with a measured arm circumference of 40 cm and who also had their blood pressure taken with a 12-cm cuff should have 10 mm Hg subtracted from the systolic blood pressure and 7 mm Hg subtracted from the diastolic blood pressure (American Heart Association. *Recommendations of Human Blood Pressure Determinations by Sphygmomanometers.* New York; AHA: October 1951).

Ideal Arm Circumference	12-cm Cuff (30 cm)		15-cm Cuff (37.5 cm)		18-cm Cuff (45 cm)	
Measured Arm Circumference (cm)	**SBP**	**DBP**	**SBP**	**DBP**	**SBP**	**DBP**
26	5	3	7	5	9	5
28	3	2	5	4	8	5
30	0	0	4	3	7	4
32	−2	−1	3	2	6	4
34	−4	−3	2	1	5	3
36	−6	−4	0	1	5	3
38	−8	−6	−1	0	4	2
40	−10	−7	−2	−1	3	1
42	−12	−9	−4	−2	2	1
44	−14	−10	−5	−3	1	0
46	−16	−11	−6	−3	0	0
48	−18	−13	−7	−4	−1	−1
50	−21	−14	−9	−5	−1	−1

4. Proper use of an optimal stethoscope (see Chapter 9)

Proper methods
1. Place patient in a quiet environment with the arm resting at heart level.
2. Place the manometer (mercury, aneroid, or electronic) at eye level to accurately see numbers and markings on the manometer.
3. Place the most appropriate-sized cuff (see above) on the patient's left arm approximately 2.5 cm above the antecubital space alongside the brachial artery and wrap it smoothly and snugly around the arm.
4. Identify (visually) and palpate the brachial pulse.
5. **Identify the maximal cuff inflation pressure needed to measure blood pressure.** Rapidly inflate the cuff and identify (visually) and palpate for the absence of the brachial pulse. Observe the pressure on the manometer when the brachial pulse is absent (this is the cuff pressure needed to occlude blood flow in the brachial artery) and then release the air in the cuff. The cuff pressure needed to measure the blood pressure must exceed the pressure, occluding blood flow in the brachial artery by approximately 30 mm Hg. Therefore, adding 30 mm Hg to the cuff pressure noted when the brachial pulse became absent is the level of maximal cuff inflation needed to measure blood pressure.
6. Wait 15–30 seconds after identifying the maximal cuff inflation pressure needed to measure blood pressure.
7. Place the bell of the stethoscope with light pressure on the brachial artery which was identified and palpated earlier in no. 4.
8. Rapidly inflate the cuff to the maximal cuff inflation pressure needed to measure blood pressure determined in no. 5.
9. Release the air in the cuff so that the pressure falls at a rate of 2 to 3 mm Hg/s.
10. Listen for the Korotkoff sounds which are described as phases:
    a. Phase I—The pressure level at which the first faint, clear tapping sounds are heard = systolic blood pressure.
    b. Phase II—The phase associated with swishing sounds (or murmurs) that are heard while the cuff continues to be deflated.
    c. Phase III—The phase associated with crisper and more intense tapping and/or swishing sounds that are heard as the cuff continues to be deflated.
    d. Phase IV—The phase associated with a distinct, abrupt, muffling of sound (with a blowing quality) that is heard as the cuff continues to be deflated.
    e. Phase V—The pressure level when the last sound is heard = **diastolic blood pressure.**
11. In certain situations, **the Korotkoff sounds** do not disappear and **may be heard until the pressure in the cuff falls to or near 0 mm Hg. Phase IV should be used to identify the diastolic blood pressure when this occurs.**

[a]Cuff width should be approximately 50% of the upper arm circumference and cuff length should be approximately 80% of the upper arm circumference. Measurement of the arm circumference with a tape measure can be easily and reliably performed. Measurement of blood pressure should be made bilaterally, beginning with the left arm. The same procedures described in the Table for blood pressure measurement at the brachial artery using the upper arm can also be applied to the posterior tibial and dorsalis pedis arteries at the ankle, bilaterally. Measurement of the ankle circumference should be applied to the same criteria described in Table for the 12-, 15-, and 18-cm cuffs. The measurement of blood pressure at the ankle is identical to the methods described for the measurement of blood pressure at the brachial artery. Figure 10-5 shows the sites and methods to measure and compare ankle and brachial blood pressures yielding the ankle–brachial index (ABI). Box 10-4 provides a practice sheet to document the arm and ankle blood pressures as well as the ankle–brachial index.

heart. During this resting phase of the heart, the ventricles are filling with blood, which will subsequently be ejected during the next systolic period. The pressure within the cardiovascular system can be identified by the point at which blood flow traveling through the arteries produces less turbulence such that sound is no longer heard with the stethoscope.

As mentioned previously, the relationship of the pulse to the blood pressure is that the pulse will be absent when the blood pressure cuff is inflated and felt when the blood pressure cuff is deflated to a level that is less than the pressure within the artery. The pulse first palpated after the cuff is deflated is an indirect estimate of the systolic blood pressure. Unfortunately, no indirect relationship can be obtained for the diastolic blood pressure. Its measurement is dependent on the absence (essentially, the last sound heard) or muffling of sound as air is released from the blood pressure cuff. In view of this, the practice of listening to the Korotkoff sounds and using the methods described in Table 10-6 and shown in Fig. 10-7 is essential to obtain valid and reliable measurements of both systolic and diastolic blood pressure.

Measurement of Systolic and Diastolic Blood Pressure

Systolic and diastolic blood pressures provide important information to detect, categorize, and treat hypertension. The American Heart Association and American College of Cardiology (AHA/ACC) have developed strict guidelines to classify blood pressure. These stages are shown in Table 10-7 and consist of optimal, normal, and hypertensive classifications.[2] Both systolic and diastolic blood pressures are important and can contribute to a diagnosis of hypertension separately or in combination (Table 10-7). This table also lists particular treatment strategies according to the hypertension classification consisting of lifestyle modification and drug treatment.

Another important aspect of measuring the systolic and diastolic blood pressure is calculating the pulse pressure. The pulse pressure is the difference between the systolic and the diastolic blood pressure and is considered the force or pressure responsible for the perfusion of organs and tissues. Therefore, it is preferable to have a wide pulse pressure like 50 mm Hg compared to a narrow pulse pressure like 10 mm Hg. It can be assumed that the wider the pulse pressure, the better organs and tissues are perfused, whereas the more narrow the pulse pressure, the poorer organs and tissues are perfused.

The examination of blood pressure described previously pertains to adults. Examination of blood pressure in children and adolescents is performed using methods similar to those described in Table 10-6, but the categorization and classification of hypertension are different. Appendix 1 of this chapter shows the expected systolic and diastolic blood pressures of children, adolescents, and young adults at specific ages (above which a child, adolescent, or young adult would be recognized to have hypertension). See the CD-Rom activity for Chapter 5 to review and practice taking blood pressures.

MEASUREMENT OF THE SYSTOLIC BLOOD PRESSURE AND PULSE DURING BREATHING AND SIMPLE PERTURBATIONS OF THE BREATHING CYCLE

As previously suggested, it is important to examine the pulse and blood pressure during the breathing cycle. This is because the examination of the systolic blood pressure and pulse during breathing can provide important diagnostic and prognostic information about cardiovascular performance. For example, an alternating strong and weak pulse can identify severely depressed cardiac function. Such an alternating strong then weak pulse has been referred to as *pulsus alternans* and has been specifically described as a mechanical alteration of the femoral or radial pulse characterized by a regular rhythm and alternating strong and weak pulses. If such an alternating

TABLE 10-7   Classification of Systolic and Diastolic Blood Pressure and Recommended Treatments

Category	Systolic BP (mm Hg)		Diastolic BP (mm Hg)	Treatment by Risk Stratification[a]		
				A	**B**	**C**
Optimal	<120 and <80			No treatment recommended		
Normal	<130 and <85			No treatment recommended		
High-normal	130–139	Or	85–89	LM[b]	LM	LM, DT
Stage 1 HTN	140–159	Or	90–99	LM[c]	LM[c]	LM, DT
Stage 2 HTN	160–179	Or	100–109	LM, DT	LM, DT	LM, DT
Stage 3 HTN	>180	Or	>110	LM, DT	LM, DT	LM, DT

[a]Treatment of risk stratification is based on the presence of risk factors, organ damage, and cardiovascular disease, such that group A has no risk factors, organ damage, or cardiovascular disease; group B has at least 1 risk factor (other than diabetes) and no organ damage or cardiovascular disease; and group C has organ damage or cardiovascular disease, with or without risk factors.

[b]LM, lifestyle modification; DT, drug treatment; HTN, hypertension.

[c]Lifestyle modification should be attempted for up to 12 months for patients in group A and for up to 6 months for patients in group B. If the systolic or diastolic blood pressures do not improve after these time periods, drug treatment is recommended.

Reproduced, with permission, from Levy D, Bairey-Merz CN, Cody RJ, et al. Hypertension detection, treatment, and control—a call to action for cardiovascular specialists. *J Am Coll Cardiol.* 1999;34(4):1360.

pulse is suspected, the suggested method to further examine the pulse is to use light pressure on the radial artery (as one would obtain the radial pulse) with the patient's breath held in midexpiration (to avoid the superimposition of respiratory variation on the amplitude of the pulse previously mentioned). If during midexpiration breathholding the pulse is observed to alternate from strong to weak, the patient is identified to have *pulsus alternans,* which is associated with cardiac pump failure.

Sphygmomanometry can more readily recognize this phenomenon, which commonly demonstrates ≥20 mm Hg alternating systolic blood pressure. Characteristically, if pulsus alternans exists, a 20 mm Hg or greater decrease in systolic blood pressure occurs during breath holding because of increased resistance to left ventricular ejection. It should be noted that a difference exists between *pulsus alternans* and *pulsus paradoxus,* the latter of which is characterized by a marked reduction of both systolic blood pressure (−20 mm Hg) and strength of the arterial pulse during inspiration. Pulsus paradoxus can also be detected by sphygmomanometry and is occasionally seen in cardiac pump failure. However, it is associated more frequently with cardiac tamponade and constrictive pericarditis primarily due to increased venous return and right heart volume, which bulges the interventricular septum into the left ventricle, thus decreasing the amount of blood present in the left ventricle and the amount of blood ejected from it (because of a decreased left ventricular volume and opposition to stroke volume from the bulging septum).

Finally, the integrity of the autonomic nervous system can be examined by measuring the pulse or an electrocardiogram before and after 1 minute of deep breathing at a rate of approximately 6 breaths per minute. While seated, the resting pulse should be obtained after which a subject is asked to breathe deeply and slowly. The patient should be encouraged to breathe at a respiratory rate of approximately 6 breaths per minute. After breathing in this manner for approximately 1 minute, the pulse should again be measured. Normally, the pulse should decrease by approximately 15 to 20 beats per minute with deep, slow breathing. If the pulse rate decreases less than 15 to 20 beats from the resting pulse before deep, slow breathing, it is suggestive that an autonomic nervous system disturbance exists.[3] A more rigorous perturbation of breathing with measurement of pulse and blood pressure has been found to be highly predictive of cardiovascular function and will be discussed later in this chapter.

MEASUREMENT OF THE SYSTOLIC AND DIASTOLIC BLOOD PRESSURE AND PULSE IN DIFFERENT BODY POSITIONS—SUPINE VERSUS STANDING

The examination of heart rate and arterial blood pressure before, during, and after a change in body position is clinically useful because it can (1) alert a clinician to the status of the cardiovascular system, (2) enable the cardiovascular system to be perturbated to determine the health of the cardiovascular system, and (3) help the clinician to predict the likelihood of cardiovascular

pathology developing in the future. Each of these areas will be discussed in the following section. It is clinically important to evaluate the changes in both *systolic* and *diastolic* blood pressure as well as the subsequent change in pulse during body position changes. Of particular importance is the understanding that arterial blood pressure is the product of cardiac output and total peripheral resistance (BP = cardiac output × TPR). It is also important to make several rather broad assumptions about the previous equation to enhance one's understanding of blood pressure and the changes accompanying positional change. First, although BP in this equation defines overall arterial blood pressure, it is possibly easier to understand the physiology of blood pressure by assuming that BP (in the previous equation) is equivalent to the systolic blood pressure. Second, although TPR in this equation defines overall total peripheral resistance, it is likely easier to more thoroughly understand the influence of positional changes on blood pressure by assuming that TPR (again, in the previous equation) is equivalent to the diastolic blood pressure. The reason for this latter assumption is that the changes in diastolic blood pressure appear to be quite reflective of the changes occurring in the peripheral vasculature (either peripheral vascular constriction or relaxation). These two assumptions and the rationale for them will become more apparent in the following sections. Also, utilization of Table 10-8 should enable a better appreciation for the previous assumptions and examinations described in the following section.

EXAMINATION OF THE PULSE AND ARTERIAL BLOOD PRESSURE WITH BODY POSITION CHANGE TO DETERMINE THE STATUS OF THE CARDIOVASCULAR SYSTEM

The status of the cardiovascular system can be easily determined by examining the change in heart rate and blood pressure while changing the position of the body from supine to standing and vice versa.

CLINICAL CORRELATE

The observation of a reduction in both the systolic and diastolic blood pressure upon standing suggests that the cardiovascular system may be impaired and is unable to produce the necessary peripheral vascular constriction needed to increase venous return and subsequently maintain or increase the systolic blood pressure.

Although venous pooling may be responsible for a decrease in venous return when standing from a supine or seated position, the forward movement of blood back to the heart can only occur with an increase in peripheral vascular constriction or, essentially, with an increase in diastolic blood

TABLE 10-8   Heart Rate and Blood Pressure Measurements: A Data Sheet

Name _____ Age _____ Gender _____

Activity level _____

History of lung disease _____

Arm circumference _____

Choose the correct cuff size based on the measured arm circumference and use the following table for correction of measured blood pressure if necessary.

Ideal Arm Circumference	12-cm Cuff (30 cm)		15-cm Cuff (37.5 cm)		18-cm Cuff (45 cm)	
Measured Arm Circumference (cm)	SBP	DBP	SBP	DBP	SBP	DBP
26	5	3	7	5	9	5
28	3	2	5	4	8	5
30	0	0	4	3	7	4
32	−2	−1	3	2	6	4
34	−4	−3	2	1	5	3
36	−6	−4	0	1	5	3
38	−8	−6	−1	0	4	2
40	−10	−7	−2	−1	3	1
42	−12	−9	−4	−2	2	1
44	−14	−10	−5	−3	1	0
46	−16	−11	−6	−3	0	0
48	−18	−13	−7	−4	−1	−1
50	−21	−14	−9	−5	−1	−1

Arm (brachial artery) blood pressure

	Supine *(land)*	Sitting	Standing *(water)*
Heart rate	_____	_____	_____
Systolic BP	_____	_____	_____
Diastolic BP	_____	_____	_____
Respiratory rate	_____	_____	_____

Ankle (pedal artery) blood pressure

	Supine *(land)*	Sitting	Standing *(water)*
Heart rate	_____	_____	_____
Systolic BP	_____	_____	_____
Diastolic BP	_____	_____	_____
Respiratory rate	_____	_____	_____

Ankle–brachial artery index = _____

pressure. When such an increase in peripheral vascular constriction is delayed or does not occur, the compensatory response of the cardiovascular system is to increase the heart rate in hope of increasing the cardiac output (because cardiac output is the product of heart rate and stroke volume; cardiac output = HR × stroke volume; see Chapter 5).

In fact, observation of a decrease in systolic and diastolic blood pressure without a subsequent increase in heart rate when changing body position from supine to standing is considered a positive sign for autonomic nervous system dysfunction.[4,5] Several studies have examined the heart rate and systolic and diastolic blood pressure responses to body position change and observed that subjects with a significant decrease in both systolic and diastolic blood pressure (greater than 20–30 mm Hg)

and an unchanged heart rate suffered from autonomic nervous system dysfunction that was often the result of diabetes.

EXAMINATION OF THE PULSE AND ARTERIAL BLOOD PRESSURE WITH BODY POSITION CHANGE TO DETERMINE THE HEALTH OF THE CARDIOVASCULAR SYSTEM

The health of the cardiovascular system can also be determined by examining the change in heart rate and arterial blood pressure while changing the body position from supine to standing and vice versa. **A cardiovascular system that responds rapidly to body position change is likely in a better state of health than a cardiovascular system that responds sluggishly.** This is apparent from the previous section. However, one patient population who seems to be a contradiction to this phenomenon is the extremely well-conditioned athlete. Subjects who are well conditioned have been observed to have greater parasympathetic versus sympathetic nervous system activity. The parasympathetic predominance of a well-trained athlete may limit or delay the heart rate response and peripheral vascular constriction needed when moving from a supine to standing position. Therefore, the time that it takes for the heart rate and blood pressure to increase in an athlete is delayed and is similar to the response of a person who has an unhealthy cardiovascular system. **Methods to differentiate the delayed cardiovascular response of persons with a healthy versus unhealthy cardiovascular system can be done with several simple questions. Questions about activity and exercise habits as well as past medical history should enable a quick differentiation of a healthy versus unhealthy cardiovascular system based on a delayed cardiovascular response to body position change.** Insufficient data exist to identify a normal time period for the cardiovascular system to respond to body position change. However, it has been suggested that a pulse rate taken approximately 30 seconds after standing which is less or greater than a pulse rate taken immediately after standing is indicative of autonomic nervous system dysfunction. This measurement of pulse rate at approximately 30 seconds after standing (or the 30th pulse beat or ECG complex after standing) compared to the pulse rate immediately after standing (or the 15th pulse beat or ECG complex after standing) has been referred to as the "30:15" ratio.[6] The 30:15 ratio reflects the change in heart rate at approximately 30 seconds compared to that at approximately 15 seconds after moving from supine to standing. A heart rate that is unchanged would yield a 30:15 ratio of 1, whereas a heart rate that decreases after 30 seconds of standing would be less than 1.0. Both an unchanged or decreased heart rate after standing for 30 seconds (compared to the heart rate at 15 seconds) is suggestive of autonomic dysfunction. This phenomenon has been observed primarily in persons with diabetes but likely has direct application in the examination of persons with known or suspected cardiovascular disease.

Additionally, a sluggish or *hypoadaptive (less than normal)* heart rate and blood pressure response during a change in body position from supine to standing should be considered abnormal and suggestive of an unhealthy cardiovascular system. Conversely, a more *adaptive* rapid increase in heart rate and blood pressure after moving from a supine to standing position (approximately 30 seconds) is likely associated with a healthier cardiovascular system which should probably respond favorably to increased functional tasks and therapeutic exercise which will be discussed in a subsequent section.

EXAMINATION OF THE PULSE AND ARTERIAL BLOOD PRESSURE WITH BODY POSITION CHANGE TO DETERMINE THE PRESENCE OR LIKELIHOOD OF CARDIOVASCULAR PATHOLOGY DEVELOPING IN THE FUTURE

The presence or likelihood of future development of cardiovascular pathology has been found to be related to the heart rate and blood pressure response during a change in body position from supine to standing. Nardo et al.[7] observed in 13,340 men and women aged 45 to 65 years that the mean change in systolic blood pressure from supine to standing was a very slight decrease of approximately 0.5 mm Hg. Unfortunately, no data were provided on the diastolic blood pressure response from supine to standing. However, it is likely that the diastolic blood pressure increased to prevent a more substantial decrease in the systolic blood pressure.

Several important findings were observed in this study of one of the largest cohorts to date including mean positional changes in systolic blood pressure of white and black men and women as well as analyses of the systolic response to cardiovascular morbidity, sociodemographic factors, and cigarette smoking. Table 10-9 presents the mean positional changes in systolic blood pressure of black and white men and women. It is apparent that black men were the only subset to have an increase in the mean systolic blood pressure when moving from supine to stand.

The change in systolic blood pressure during the aforementioned positional change was also categorized into deciles and the top and bottom 30% of the distribution were compared

TABLE 10-9 Mean Change in Systolic Blood Pressure of Black and White Men and Women

Variable N[a]	All Participants (13,340)	Black Women (2242)	Black Men (1385)	White Women (5091)	White Men (4622)
Mean change in SBP	−0.45	−0.07	1.10	−0.37	−1.19
SD of change in SBP	10.8	12.5	11.9	10.5	9.87
Median change in SBP	0.08	0.67	1.67	0.15	−0.55
Range of change in SBP	(−63 − 54)	(−63 − 48)	(−52 − 37)	(−56 − 54)	(−55 − 36)

[a]N, number of subjects; SBP, systolic blood pressure.

Reproduced, with permission, from Nardo CJ, Chambless LE, Light KC, et al. Descriptive epidemiology of blood pressure response to change in body position—The ARIC Study. *Hypertension.* 1999;33:1123.

with the individuals in the middle 40% of the distribution. **It is important to note that a larger proportion of the participants in the top 30% of the distribution (having an increase in systolic blood pressure when standing) were black, had a mean seated blood pressure that was greater, and had a predicted risk of developing coronary heart disease after 8 years that was greater than the middle 40% or bottom 30% of the distribution.**

EXAMINATION OF THE PULSE AND ARTERIAL BLOOD PRESSURE DURING FUNCTIONAL TASKS AND EXERCISE

The examination of the pulse and arterial blood pressure during functional tasks is occasionally performed by physical therapists, but not to the extent that these measurements are used to determine the exercise prescription or functional exercise training session. Application of the examination processes described previously during functional or exercise training can provide an indirect measurement of cardiovascular function, which is frequently the primary system affected in many patients seen by a physical therapist (eg, neurological disorders from stroke, heart diseases, pulmonary diseases, or endocrine/metabolic disorders). Frequent monitoring of the heart rate and blood pressure may be the best way to examine the safety of exercise and help to establish guidelines and procedures for functional or exercise training. The heart rate and blood pressure responses during exercise and functional training can determine the mode, intensity, duration, and frequency of functional and exercise training as well as determine the need to terminate or continue training. For example, a patient with a recent coronary artery bypass graft surgery seen for progressive exercise and functional training may be limited to several minutes of hallway ambulation due to an abnormally high heart rate and low systolic blood pressure. The abnormally high heart rate and low systolic blood pressure may or may not be accompanied with symptoms of dizziness or light-headedness which would also alert a clinician to modify or terminate training, but often the subjective complaints of dizziness or light-headedness are too late and results in a syncopal or near syncopal episode.

Observation of specific changes in the diastolic blood pressure can also be valuable. The diastolic blood pressure should decrease or remain unchanged during functional or exercise training. If the diastolic blood pressure is observed to increase during increased activity, it is a strong indication that the cardiovascular system is dysfunctional. An increase in the diastolic blood pressure of 10 mm Hg or more is an indication to modify or terminate functional or exercise training. Likewise, an increase in the diastolic blood pressure when the diastolic blood pressure should be decreased (or low) is a strong indicator of cardiovascular dysfunction. An example of this is when the diastolic blood pressure is higher in the supine position compared to the standing position. Such a finding is highly suggestive of a failing cardiovascular (rather than dys-

functional) system. In fact, it is well documented that increased diastolic blood pressure in the supine position (which should promote peripheral vascular dilation) after a maximal exercise test (when the peripheral vasculature is maximally dilated) is highly predictive of ischemic heart disease. In this scenario, ischemic heart disease decreases the pumping ability of the heart (because of myocardial ischemia from maximal exercise) making it difficult for the heart to eject blood from the left ventricle (resulting in elevated left ventricular filling pressures and volume) that is worsened in the supine position (because of increased venous return). Thus, a decreased volume of blood is ejected into the periphery. To compensate for this, the body attempts to return more blood back to the heart (interpreting that the decreased ejection of blood is due to inadequate blood volume and that there is a need for greater venous return). The body subsequently increases venous return by increasing the peripheral vascular resistance (resulting in an increased diastolic blood pressure). The body's assumption that an increase in venous return will improve cardiovascular function is incorrect and only worsens cardiac pumping leading to further increases in the diastolic blood pressure and subsequent decreases in systolic blood pressure as cardiac pumping continues to fail. Therefore, examination of the pulse and systolic and diastolic blood pressure at rest and during exercise can provide very important diagnostic, prognostic, and therapeutic information.

Auscultation of the Heart

Auscultation of the heart is considered an advanced skill, but listening for several select heart sounds can provide important diagnostic, prognostic, and therapeutic information. The sounds that are likely most important to recognize when auscultating the heart are the first heart sound (S_1) and second heart sound (S_2), the third heart sound (S_3) and fourth heart sound (S_4), and a loud S_2. These sounds will be presented in the following section.

Proper Use of the Stethoscope

As discussed in Chapter 9, the stethoscope frequently consists of a diaphragm and bell as shown in Fig. 9-1 and should have many of the characteristics that are listed in Box 9-3. The presence of a diaphragm and bell is critically important when auscultating the heart. Similarly, correct insertion of the earpieces into the ears (with the earpieces pointing to the patient we want to examine) is possibly more important when auscultating the heart because a proper fit will improve the identification and differentiation of the high- and low-frequency sounds of the heart. Optimal auscultation of the heart can be accomplished by using the helpful hints listed in Box 9-3.

From Box 9-3 it is apparent that the bell is used extensively when auscultating the heart. The bell is used with light pressure and identifies low-frequency sounds such as the Korotkoff sounds when measuring blood pressure or when listening for abnormal heart sounds (eg, the S_3 and S_4).

BOX 10-4

Methods of Auscultation of the Heart

1. Identify a reference point in the cardiac cycle:
   a. Listen for the difference in the time interval between S_1 and S_2 (shorter duration) and S_2 and S_1 (longer duration).
   b. Palpate the pulse—the sound heard at or near the time the radial pulse is palpated is the S_2.
   c. Observe the ECG—the sound heard at the time the R wave is displayed is the S_1.
2. Use the stethoscope properly:
   a. Diaphragm—designed to identify high-frequency sounds and should be used with firm pressure.
   b. Bell—designed to identify low-frequency sounds and should be used with light pressure. However, firm pressure applied to the bell of the stethoscope transforms the bell into a diaphragm. Alternating light and firm pressure

to the bell of the diaphragm can help to differentiate normal from abnormal heart sounds.
3. Auscultate with a "systematic standard" utilizing different chest wall locations and body positions (ie, left side-lying, sitting, squatting, and standing):
   a. Aortic area = second ICS, right sternal border—S_2 is best heard in this area.
   b. Pulmonic area = second ICS, left sternal border—pulmonic valve closure (P_2) of the second heart sound is best heard in this area.
   c. Tricuspid area = fifth ICS, right sternal border—tricuspid valve closure (T_2) of the first heart sound is best heard in this area.
   d. Mitral area = fifth ICS, midclavicular line near the left nipple—mitral valve closure (M_1) of the first heart sound is best heard in this area.

Method of Auscultating the Heart

The method of auscultating the heart is similar to that when auscultating the lungs and requires proper use of the stethoscope as well as the correct placement of the diaphragm and bell of the stethoscope on the chest (Box 10-4). A logical and systematic sequence of placing the diaphragm and bell on the chest is necessary. The standard sites used for auscultation of the heart are shown in Fig. 10-8. It is apparent from Fig. 10-8 that there are six to eight sites on the anterior chest that are used for diaphragm and bell placement. The axillary area can

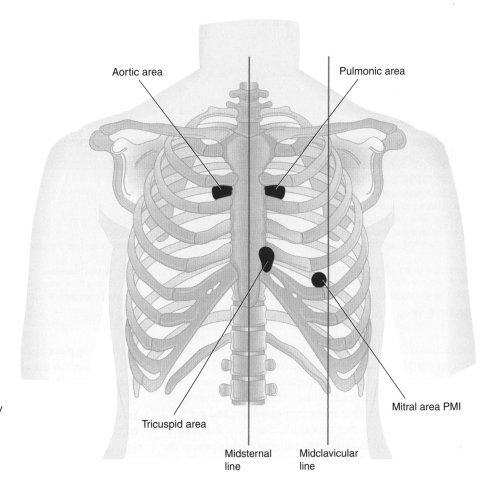

FIGURE 10-8 Cardiac auscultatory areas. (Used with permission from Hillegass E, Sadowsky S. *Essentials of Cardiopulmonary Physical Therapy.* 2nd ed. Philadelphia, PA: WB Saunders; 2001:124.)

Aortic area

Pulmonic area

Tricuspid area

Mitral area PMI

Midsternal line

Midclavicular line

Performing the ABI Test

The ABI measurement is performed with the patient resting in a supine position. The examiner should make all arm and leg blood pressure measurements with an appropriately sized blood pressure cuff and the Doppler device. The systolic blood pressure is determined in both arms, and the ankle systolic blood pressure is determined for the right and left posterior tibial (PT) and dorsalis pedis (DP) arteries. The ABI for each leg is determined by using the higher of the two readings from either the PT or the DP arteries, and the higher of the two brachial readings. The lower ABI of the two is used for diagnostic purposes. An ABI measurement can usually be performed in less than 10 minutes. (See sample ABI worksheet.)

ABI Procedure

Step 1. Have the patient lie in a supine position with shoes and stockings removed for at least 10 minutes prior to obtaining blood pressure measurements.

Step 2. Apply the blood pressure cuff snugly on the upper arm with the lower edge of the cuff 1 in above the antecubital fossa. Usually the cuff that is the appropriate size for the patient's arm will also be suitable for the ankle pressure measurement. In the rare instance that upper arm and ankle pressures are markedly different, choose cuff sizes that are appropriate for each site.

Step 3. Apply a 1- to 2-cm ribbon of Doppler gel to the antecubital area. Be sure to use enough gel.

Step 4. Turn the Doppler probe on and place it at the antecubital area at approximately a 60-degree angle to the surface of the skin. Move the probe around until the clearest arterial pulse sounds are heard and keep the probe at that position.

Step 5. Inflate the blood pressure cuff to approximately 20 mm Hg above the numerical reading where the pulse sounds cease.

Step 6. Deflate the cuff at a rate of 2 mm Hg/s until the first arterial pulse sound is heard. When this number is determined, deflate the cuff completely and record this systolic reading. Remove the gel from the patient's skin with a tissue.

Step 7. Apply the same blood pressure cuff snugly to the ankle on the same side of the body.

Step 8. Palpate the area around the medial malleolus to find the posterior tibial (PT) arterial pulse.

Step 9. If this pulse is palpable, apply a 1- to 2-cm ribbon of Doppler gel to the area. If there is no palpable pulse, apply gel to the general area, turn on the Doppler probe, and move the probe around until the clearest arterial sound is heard. Keep the probe in that position. Continue inflating the blood pressure cuff as before, followed by deflation and reading (steps 5-6).

Step 10. Palpate the dorsal arch of the same foot for the dorsalis pedis (DP) arterial pulse. Apply the Doppler gel and use the Doppler probe as before (step 9).

Step 11. Apply the blood pressure cuff to the opposite ankle and record the PT and DP pressures as before (steps 8–10).

Step 12. Then repeat steps 2–6 on the other arm.

Use the ABI worksheet page to figure the patient's ABI. Measurements should be noted in the patient's medical record.

Both the DP and the PT arterial pressures are measured to provide a complete assessment of the extent of PAD in each limb. Additionally, some patients may have a congenitally absent dorsalis pedis pulse.

Other patients, particularly some older and diabetic individuals, have calcification in their arteries that prevents occlusion of flow by the pressure cuff. This will cause an abnormally high reading. Typically any reading greater than 1.50 is considered abnormal. Such patients should be referred for additional testing in a vascular laboratory.

Helpful Hints

- Follow the instructions specific to the Doppler probe you are using.
- Be sure to use enough gel.
- Use a cuff size that is right for both the arm and the ankle of the patient.
- Be sure you are centered on the pulse when you take the reading; if you are off to the side, the reading will be low.
- Be aware of known diabetics with calcified vessels and abnormally high ABI.
- In a small percentage of patients, 1 of the ankle pressures will be nondetectable; use the detectable pressure for calculating the ABI.

Patients with an ABI value of 0.90 or less are diagnosed as having Peripheral Arterial Disease and considered at increased risk for cardiovascular ischemic events. Prompt investigation and risk-reducing treatments are then warranted.
Don't be discouraged if measuring the ABI seems slow or clumsy at first. Like any procedure, the ABI becomes easier to do with practice.

FIGURE 10-9   Procedure for performing and recording the ankle–brachial index.

also be used (often just the left, but the right may also be examined for particular heart sounds). Placement of the diaphragm and bell of the stethoscope in these areas in a systematic manner and comparing the sounds heard in the different areas can provide much information about the physiologic and mechanical events occurring within the cardiac chambers. Referring to Fig. 10-9 will be helpful in understanding what chambers of the heart are being auscultated and what mechanical events are

likely taking place underneath the sites where the diaphragm or bell is placed on the chest. A review of laboratory exercises 2 and 3 may also be helpful. See Appendix 1.

Sounds Heard During Auscultation of the Heart—Heart Sounds

The sounds heard during auscultation of the heart can be cursorily summarized as being one of five possible sounds.

BOX 10-5

Normal and Abnormal Heart Sounds

Normal Heart Sounds

First heart sound (S_1)—due to closure of the mitral (M_1) and tricuspid (T_1) valves—that is heard as a high-frequency sound.

Second heart sound (S_2)—due to closure of the aortic (A_1) and pulmonic (P_2) valves—that is heard as a high-frequency sound.

Abnormal Heart Sounds

Third heart sound (S_3)—due to poor ventricular compliance and subsequent turbulence—that is heard as a low-frequency sound in early diastole.

Fourth heart sound (S_4)—due to an exaggerated atrial contraction and subsequent turbulence—that is heard as a low-frequency sound in late diastole.

Ejection sound—due to the forceful and rapid ejection of blood, often past an obstruction—that is heard as a harsh higher-frequency sound most often during systole.

Systolic click—due to a prolapsed mitral or tricuspid valve that falls backward into the atria with regurgitant blood flowing forcefully past the prolapsing valve causing turbulence—that is heard as single or multiple "clicking" sounds during systole.

Opening snap—due to the forceful opening of a stenotic mitral valve—that is heard as a harsh "snapping" sound in early diastole.

Pericardial friction rub—due to increased pericardial fluid in the pericardial sac—that impairs filling of the ventricles during diastole and during which the filling ventricles "rub" against the engorged pericardial sac producing a "leathery to squeaky-door" sound during diastole. A pericardial friction rub can also be heard in systole with marked pericardial inflammation or fluid.

Heart murmurs—due to rapid and forceful blood flow or blood flowing past a site of stenosis or regurgitation, all of which produce turbulence—that is heard as a "swishing" sound in systole, diastole, or both systole and diastole.

These sounds include the normal S_1 and S_2, the abnormal S_3 and S_4, and adventitious heart sounds such as murmurs, clicks, and snaps. The different types of heart sounds and the different characteristic qualities of each of the sounds are listed in Box 10-5 and Tables 10-10 through 10-13. Subtle, yet specific characteristics may accompany the presence of a heart sound in a specific area that allows for specific diagnostic, prognostic, and therapeutic information to be obtained. These specific characteristics enable the clinician to better understand the pathological processes and the need for further examination and subsequent treatment. A summary of different heart sounds heard when auscultating the heart of individuals with known or suspected cardiac pathologies are listed in Table 10-11, and specific methods to differentiate the various types of heart sounds are provided in Table 10-12.

The bell of the stethoscope is used when attempting to distinguish abnormal from normal heart sounds. S_3 and S_4 are abnormal heart sounds that occur because of elevated filling pressures. The elevated filling pressure of the left ventricle (with elevated left ventricular volume) causes blood entering the left ventricle in early diastole to produce a low-frequency sound of turbulence (S_3, which results from blood entering a high-pressure and high-volume system). The same elevated ventricular filling pressure causes the atria to contract forcefully near the end of diastole to complete ventricular filling. The forceful contraction of the atria sends a final surge of blood into the ventricles to complete ventricular filling, but if the pressure and volume in the ventricle are elevated, turbulence is produced yielding a low-frequency sound in late diastole (the S_4). Auscultatory areas for the appreciation of abnormal heart sounds are shown in Fig. 10-8.

Potential Indirect Measures of Cardiac Function

A number of potential indirect measures of cardiac function exist, which can help to categorize and treat patients with cardiac and cardiovascular disease (Table 10-13). Some of these measurements are more sensitive and specific to cardiac function than others, but combining measurements may be helpful to better understand the degree of cardiac and cardiovascular dysfunction or failure. The majority of these measurements will assist in the differentiation of a failing versus normal or dysfunctional cardiac pump. The following section will provide the rationale for these measurements as potential measures of cardiac function.

Symptoms and Functional Classification

Symptoms and functional classification using one or more classification methods (eg, NYHA classes I–IV as shown in Table 10-4) can provide an indirect measure of cardiac function. Patients with greater symptoms and lower levels of function have been repeatedly observed to suffer from poorer cardiac function (refs of GSHFA). Similarly, paroxysmal nocturnal dyspnea (PND) and orthopnea are two symptoms that are commonly associated with poorer cardiac function.

Cold, Pale, and Possibly Cyanotic Extremities

Individuals with cold, pale, and possibly cyanotic extremities may suffer from cardiovascular dysfunction or failure, which is frequently due to the profound sympathetic nervous system activation associated with cardiac dysfunction and failure. Peripheral vascular constriction in the extremities is likely

TABLE 10-10   Systolic and Diastolic Murmurs

Type of Murmur	Characteristics of Murmur	Possible Accompanying Heart Sounds	Possible Additional Physical Examination Findings
Systolic murmurs			
Mitral insufficiency (MI)	Loud murmur that may radiate to the axillary areas in a bandlike fashion which decreases with inspiration or sudden squatting and increases with standing or the Valsalva maneuver. The intensity of the murmur is unchanged with PVCs	Loud S_3 and S_2	Brisk upstroke of the carotid pulse Jerky, hyperdynamic PMI Occasionally a prominent substernal impulse
Tricuspid insufficiency (TI)	Variable quality murmur at the left lower sternal border that increases with inspiration and often has a varying intensity from day to day (which may be associated with Afib)	None of significance	Swan–Ganz measurements: Absent × descent Prominent V wave with inspiration Giant C wave with each ventricular systole
Aortic stenosis (AS)	Harsh crescendo-decrescendo murmur at the left sternal border and aortic area, which often radiates into the neck and possibly the right shoulder. The intensity of the murmur is increased with PVCs	Ejection sound Soft S_2 if AV is calcified Possible S_3 or S_4 Possible high-pitched "seagull" sound to murmur	Small delayed carotid pulse Nondisplaced sustained PMI Possible left ventricular heave Possible rales from pulmonary edema Possible JVD
Pulmonic stenosis (PS)	Nonspecific murmur that radiates to the left shoulder area	Soft, widely split S_2 If severe PS, no S_2	Giant A wave in jugular venous pulse
Ventriculoseptal defect (VSD)	Loud murmur and palpable "thrill" in the 3rd and 4th ICS, LSB	None of significance	Possibly a loud S_2 Brisk carotid pulse Jerky hyperdynamic PMI Occasionally a prominent substernal impulse
Diastolic murmurs			
Mitral stenosis (MS)	Harsh "rumble" murmur heard best at the LSB that begins shortly after S_2. The intensity of the murmur increases with exercise and coughing	Loud S_1 and S_2 Opening snap	Diastolic thrill at apex Giant A wave Possible rales Increased respiratory rate Dyspnea on exertion If severe = mitral facies (dilated cheek veins)
Tricuspid stenosis (TS)	Harsh "rumble" murmur heard well at LSB, xiphoid area, and possibly RSB. The intensity of the murmur increases	None of significance	Prominent A waves in the jugular venous pulse Flushed cheeks Usually no dyspnea on exertion
Aortic insufficiency (AI)	"Blowing" murmur heard best at the aortic area.	Possible ejection sound S_3 If severe AI: AS murmur Soft S_1 Separate apical-presystolic murmur = Austin Flint murmur	Possible head movement with heartbeat Prominent carotid pulsations Throbbing peripheral arteries Prominent left ventricular impulse If severe AI: Wide pulse pressure
Pulmonic insufficiency (PI)	High-pitched murmur heard best at base	None of significance	Giant A wave in jugular venous pulse Thrill radiating to the left shoulder Substernal heave due to right ventricular contraction Lack of symptoms If severe PI signs of PH: JVD Prominent right ventricular heave Cyanosis Systemic edema Rales

TABLE 10-11 Heart Sounds and Physical Examination Findings Associated with Specific Diseases

Disease	Heart Sounds	Physical Examination Findings
HTN	S_4, possibly a loud S_1 and S_2	BP > 140/90 mm Hg
CAD (eg, myocardial ischemia or MI)	Myocardial ischemia: possibly S_4 Myocardial infarction: S_4, possibly S_3 if large MI	Angina with ECG ST-segment depression for ischemia or elevation for MI; elevated serum enzymes (ie, CK-MB, LDH, SGOT, troponin)
Valvular heart disease	Systolic, diastolic, or combined systolic and diastolic murmurs (see Table 10-12)	Palpable thrills, chest motion (substernal heaves) and valvular closure, abnormal jugular venous pulse waves, dyspnea, fatigue, and possibly rales
Heart valve replacement	Metallic "click" or prosthetic valve sound of artificial valve	None of significance
Pericarditis or myocarditis	Pericardial friction rub	Pulsus alternans and pulsus paradoxus, chest pain, dizziness and light-headedness
CHF	S_3	Dyspnea, fatigue, rales from pulmonary edema, JVD
IHSS	Systolic murmur similar to murmur of AS and MI which increases with the Valsalva maneuver or standing (because of decreased left ventricular volume and cavity size that increases the subaortic obstruction) and decreases with maneuvers that increase venous return (eg, squatting, lying supine with legs elevated): **Innocent murmurs typically decrease with the Valsalva maneuver because of decreased venous return.**	Dyspnea, fatigue, dizziness, light-headedness, blood pressure may be lower in the lower extremities
MVP	Late systolic murmur often with systolic clicks which move closer to S_1 with decreased venous return (ie, standing, Valsalva maneuver)	Chest pain that is similar to angina, but not due to to myocardial ischemia, palpitations
Congenital heart disease	Murmur of ASD (see Table 10-12): loud systolic murmur	Signs of pulmonary HTN, brisk carotid pulse, jerky hyperdynamic PMI, occasionally a prominent substernal impulse, and thrill in the third and fourth ICS
Pulmonary hypertension	Loud S_2 (particularly P_2) that may be markedly split, systolic click(s), soft systolic ejection murmur, possibly a right ventricular S_4 at LSB, systolic murmur of TI at LLS. If severe pulmonary hypertension, early diastolic murmur of PI (Graham-Steele murmur)	Left parasternal lift from RVH, palpable systolic impulse of the pulmonary artery, and palpable closure of the pulmonic valve in the second left ICS
Cardiac dysrhythmias	Irregular sequence of S_1 and S_2—difficult to determine S_1 and S_2, which requires utilization of ECG or palpation of the pulse to identify the location of heart sounds in the cardiac cycle (this makes it extremely difficult to interpret abnormal heart sounds).	Dyspnea, fatigue, palpitations, and possibly chest pain
Right bundle branch block	Abnormal wide splitting of S_2 during inspiration due to delayed pulmonic valve closure	Classic ECG findings (see Chapter 11)
Left bundle branch block	Reversed splitting of S_2 (paradoxical splitting; the split decreases with inspiration and increases with expiration) due to delayed aortic valve closure.	Classic ECG findings (see Chapter 11)
Pacemaker	Paradoxical splitting of S_2 due to right ventricular pacing with subsequent initial right-sided electrical and mechanical activity (P_2 followed by A_2 rather than the normal sequence of A_2 followed by P_2).	Classic ECG pacemaker spike (see Chapter 11)
Obstructive lung disease	Decreased intensity of heart sounds due to hyperinflated lungs. If severe, pulmonary HTN signs such as a loud S_2 and other sounds (see above).	Increased accessory muscle use, cyanosis, decreased oxygen saturation, and decreased breath sounds

TABLE 10-12 **Distinguishing Characteristics of Heart Sounds**[a]

Sound	Location of Sound	Sound Quality	Distinguishing Characteristic
First heart sound (S_1)	Best heard in mitral area	High frequency	First high-frequency sound after the longer pause of diastole
Second heart sound (S_2)	Best heard in aortic area	High frequency	Second high-frequency sound after the shorter pause of systole
Third heart sound (S_3)	Best heard at LSB, in 5th ICS or mitral area	Low frequency	Low-frequency sound heard early in diastole
Fourth heart sound (S_4)	Best heard at LSB, in 4th ICS or mitral area	Low frequency	Low-frequency sound heard late in diastole
Split S_1	Best heard in mitral area	High frequency	Two high-frequency sounds heard after the longer pause of diastole (the same high-frequency sound is the key characteristic differentiating the split S_1 from the S_4)
Split S_2	Best heard in the aortic area	High frequency	Two high-frequency sounds heard after the shorter pause of systole (the same high-frequency sound is the key characteristic differentiating the split S_2 from the S_3)
Systolic click(s)	Best heard at LSB	High-frequency "click"	The high-frequency click(s) in mid- to late systole are a higher frequency than S_1 and S_2 and have a characteristic "clicking" sound that is different from S_1 and S_2 distinguishing a systolic click(s) from (1) a split S_1 or split S_2 (both of which would have the same high-frequency sound without the slightly higher-frequency "clicking" sound and (2) a S_3 (which is a low-frequency sound without the high-frequency "clicking" sound)
Opening snap of MS	Best heard in mitral area	High-frequency "snap"	The high-frequency "snap" in early diastole is a higher frequency than S_2 and has a characteristic "snapping" sound that is different from S_2, distinguishing an opening snap of MS from (1) a split S_2 (which would have a slightly lower frequency identical to the preceding sound) and (2) a S_3 (which is a low-frequency sound without the high-frequency "snapping" sound)
Pericardial friction rub	Possibly best heard alongside the LSB	"Leathery to squeaky-door" like sound	The distinguishing characteristic of the pericardial friction rub is the "leathery to squeaky-door" sound heard most often in diastole, but may be heard in systole
Heart murmur	May be heard throughout the entire thorax often dependent on the location of the incompetent or stenotic valve	"Swishing" sound	The distinguishing characteristic of a heart murmur is the "swishing" sound that is frequently more prolonged than many of the aforementioned heart sounds (often occupying all of systole or diastole)

[a]The objective of auscultation of the heart and distinguishing different heart sounds is identifying the location of the heart sounds, the quality of the sound, where it occurs in the cardiac cycle, and other characteristic physical findings (see Table 10-18).

more common in patients with cardiac pump failure and can be a potential sign of poor cardiac function. However, other disorders such as peripheral vascular disease can produce similar findings, which decrease the specificity of this measure as a true measure of cardiac function.

Jugular Venous Distension and Peripheral Edema

Jugular venous distension and peripheral edema are indirect measures of cardiac function because they represent the end result of poor cardiac function. Good cardiac function is asso-ciated with a jugular venous measurement of 3 to 5 cm above the sternal angle of Louis and an absence of peripheral edema (at least due to a cardiac origin). The greater that the JVD is above 5 cm from the sternal angle, the poorer the cardiac pumping ability and the greater the venous congestion (which may or may not be associated with peripheral edema). Therefore, JVD is more specific for poor cardiac function, whereas peripheral edema is associated with poor cardiac performance but is less specific due to the many etiologies of peripheral edema.

TABLE 10-13 **Potential Indirect Measures of Cardiac Function**

Potential Measurement	Strength	Weakness
Symptoms and functional class	Ease, standardized, and universally accepted	Unknown sensitivity and specificity
Cold, pale, and possibly cyanotic extreme	Ease and physiologically sound	Unknown sensitivity and specificity
JVD and peripheral edema	Ease and physiologically sound	Unknown sensitivity and specificity
Heart sounds	Ease, but clinical experience needed	Unknown sensitivity and specificity
Pulse	Ease and physiologically sound	Intermediate sensitivity and specificity
Electrocardiography	Ease, but ECG equipment needed	Intermediate to high sensitivity and specificity
Blood pressure	Ease and physiologically sound	Intermediate to high sensitivity and specificity when properly performed
Blood pressure during the breathing cycle	Ease and physiologically sound	Intermediate sensitivity and specificity when properly performed
Pulse and BP during positional change	Ease and physiologically sound	Intermediate to high sensitivity and specificity when properly performed
Pulse and BP during the Valsalva maneuver	Ease and physiologically sound	Intermediate to high sensitivity and specificity when properly performed
BP during supine to standing	Ease and physiologically sound	Unknown sensitivity and specificity

Heart Sounds

Heart sounds are another indirect measure of cardiac function.

CLINICAL CORRELATE

The presence of a third heart sound (S_3) has been considered a hallmark for heart failure and as such identifies a poor cardiac pump.

Furthermore, an S_4 appears to be commonly associated with myocardial infarction (MI) and hypertension, which provide it a certain degree of predictive ability for MI and hypertension. The presence of a combined S_3 and S_4 is suggestive of a poor cardiac pump, and a loud S_2 is suggestive of pulmonary hypertension (which would be associated with either the potential or the presence of a poor cardiac pump).

Pulse

As previously discussed, much of the information obtained from the palpation of the radial pulse is listed in Table 10-5 and includes the rate of the pulse (the heart rate by counting the number of beats per minute), regularity or lack of regularity of the pulse, strength of the pulse, palpable turbulence, relationship of the pulse to a continuous electrocardiographic tracing and heart sounds, and the relationship of the pulse to the breathing cycle. Palpation of the pulse can provide an enormous amount of information about normal and abnormal physiologic phenomena. A pulse that is relatively regular

with a normal rate, strength, relationship to heart sounds, electrocardiogram, and breathing cycle and absence of turbulence is a pulse that is likely associated with a good cardiovascular system and normal cardiac pump. However, a pulse that is accompanied by palpable turbulence or lacking one or more of the previously cited normal characteristics is a pulse that is likely associated with a dysfunctional or failing cardiac pump. For example, if during midexpiration breath holding the pulse is observed to alternate from strong to weak, the patient is identified to have pulsus alternans, which is associated with cardiac pump failure. Furthermore, a decrease in the strength of the pulse during inspiration may be associated with pulsus paradoxus, which is also associated with cardiac pump failure.

Electrocardiography

Electrocardiography will be discussed in detail in the following chapter, but several electrocardiographic (ECG) measurements have been found to be associated with cardiovascular function and cardiac performance and include the presence of an irregular ECG rhythm, unchanged R-R wave interval, Q waves, lack of R waves, where R waves should be present, ST-T wave abnormalities such as ST-T wave depression or elevation, prolonged PR, QRS, and QT intervals, excessive voltage, and single-chamber pacer spikes. All of these ECG findings are associated with poorer cardiac and cardiovascular function. More specific ECG findings and the methods to examine them are described in Chapter 11.

Blood Pressure

As previously presented, the systolic and diastolic blood pressures can provide important information to detect, categorize, and treat hypertension (Table 10-7). The American Heart Association and American College of Cardiology guidelines to classify blood pressure were developed to detect, categorize, and treat blood pressure that is observed to be too high. Minimal data exist for blood pressure that is too low, but poor cardiac pumping may eventually progress to low systolic blood pressure and higher diastolic blood pressure (thus decreasing the pulse pressure). It is generally assumed that a patient's systolic blood pressure can be as low as they can tolerate—once a patient becomes symptomatic (eg, dizziness, light-headedness, dyspnea, fatigue) due to a low blood pressure, attempts should be made to increase the systolic blood pressure. Often this is done by decreasing the dosage or timing of antihypertensive drugs. However, if after decreasing the dosage or frequency of antihypertensive drugs, the systolic blood pressure and pulse pressure are abnormally low and producing symptoms, it may be that the cardiac pump is failing and unable to maintain adequate cardiac output (remember BP = cardiac output × TPR).

Blood Pressure During the Breathing Cycle

As previously discussed, blood pressure changes during the breathing cycle may be suggestive of cardiac dysfunction or failure. In fact, the palpated pulsus alternans associated with cardiac failure that was presented earlier can also be measured via sphygmomanometry. If pulsus alternans exists, a 20 mm Hg or greater decrease in systolic blood pressure will occur during breath holding because of increased resistance to left ventricular ejection. Likewise, a marked reduction in the systolic blood pressure of 20 mm Hg or more during inspiration is associated with pulsus paradoxus, which is also associated with cardiac pump failure.

Pulse and Blood Pressure During Positional Change

Methods to examine the status of the cardiovascular system via pulse rate and blood pressure response while changing the position of the body from supine to standing and vice versa were presented earlier. It is important to remember that an observation of a reduction in both the systolic and the diastolic blood pressure upon standing without subsequent increase in pulse rate suggests that the cardiovascular system may be impaired and is unable to produce the necessary (1) peripheral vascular constriction needed to increase venous return or (2) chronotropic response. Without peripheral vascular constriction to increase venous return and without an increase in pulse rate to compensate for the reduction in venous return, symptoms of dizziness, light-headedness, and even syncope or near-syncope may occur. Such findings are often the result of overmedication with antihypertensive drugs (in particular large doses of β-blockers), but if antihypertensive drugs are not a possible cause, autonomic nervous system dysfunction and a poor cardiac pump are the most likely culprits.

Pulse and Blood Pressure During the Valsalva Maneuver

Examination of the pulse and blood pressure response to the Valsalva maneuver has been studied extensively and has been found to reliably distinguish between a failing and a dysfunctional cardiac pump with a high degree of sensitivity and specificity. It is important to understand the physiologic changes accompanying the Valsalva maneuver, which can be appreciated by viewing Box 9-4, which displays the biomechanics of breathing. It is helpful to view this table, because the changes taking place within the intrathoracic area during the Valsalva are opposite those occurring during normal breathing (which as shown in Table 9-11 are associated with a decrease in intrathoracic pressure). **During a Valsalva maneuver, the intrathoracic pressure is increased.** This increase in intrathoracic pressure produces an opposite reaction to venous return. It is seen in Box 9-4 that the decrease in intrathoracic pressure facilitates inspiration and venous return (increasing venous return because blood at the superior and inferior vena cava sense a low-pressure area within the thorax to which it will readily move). The opposite is true of the Valsalva maneuver. **The increased intrathoracic pressure from the Valsalva decreases venous return because the movement of blood from the vena cava now encounters a high-pressure system, which makes the movement of blood into the thorax less facilitated (decreasing the venous return).**

The decrease in venous return and subsequent physiologic changes accompanying the Valsalva maneuver can be appreciated in Fig. 10-10. Figure 10-10A shows the normal pulse and arterial blood pressure response to the Valsalva via

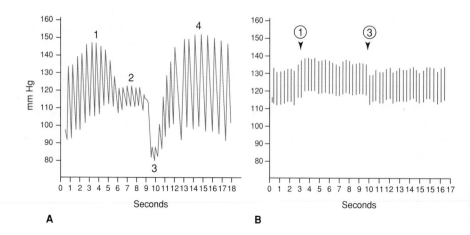

FIGURE 10-10 Arterial blood pressure response to the Valsalva maneuver. (**A**) Normal response. (**B**) Abnormal response.

an arterial line tracing. The blood pressure is observed to increase initially (stage I), but after it peaks, it drops precipitously to a rather stable level (stage II). After the Valsalva has been held for approximately 10 seconds, it is released (and subjects inspire) and a characteristic negative spike is observed which represents a slight decrease in arterial pressure (stage III). This slight decrease in arterial pressure is the result of inspiration and the development of negative pressure within the thorax. During inspiration the venous return is facilitated (or increased; see Box 9-4), which increases diastolic filling and results in an improved stroke volume and an increase in blood pressure (stage IV) with subsequent reduction in pulse. (This also should be apparent in the tracing of Fig. 10-10A as each spike represents a pulse and the distance between these spikes is greater indicating a lower pulse.)

Figure 10-10B shows an abnormal pulse and arterial blood pressure response to the Valsalva maneuver. The initial increase in blood pressure seen in the normal response of Fig. 10-10A remains elevated and does not decrease during stages II or III as seen normally. In fact, when the Valsalva is terminated, the blood pressure returns to the pre-Valsalva level. Additionally, the pulse rate (or pressure spikes from the arterial line) does not change in Fig. 10-10B. The graphic depiction in Fig. 10-10B is a classic arterial blood pressure response associated with cardiac pump failure. Identification of such a response is highly suggestive of cardiac pump failure.

The methods to measure the blood pressure and pulse during the Valsalva maneuver are shown in Box 10-6. Adhering to these methods should enable accurate and safe measurements of the pulse and blood pressure during the Valsalva maneuver. It is important to note that no complications have been reported in more than 50 studies of the Valsalva maneuver with more than 5,000 patients being examined. Nonetheless, the term *Valsalva* has a bad connotation and as such we have referred to this examination technique as a controlled expiratory maneuver, because the methods described in the literature and in Box 10-6 are best represented (and possibly better accepted) by a controlled expiratory maneuver during which one exhales through a blood pressure manometer. The methods to perform and interpret the controlled expiratory maneuver are also described on the CD-ROM included with this textbook.

Blood Pressure During Supine to Standing

The aforementioned changes in systolic blood pressure during the Valsalva maneuver may also be apparent during a simple change in body position from supine to standing. As previously discussed in this chapter, body position change can produce dramatic changes in the cardiovascular system. Likewise, the observed response of the cardiovascular system to positional change can identify present or future cardiovascular and cardiac disorders. Because of this, it may also be possible to identify current cardiovascular function by examining the changes in systolic and diastolic blood pressure during a position change from supine to standing.

Like the Valsalva maneuver, a position change from supine to standing produces a reduction in venous return. The

---

BOX 10-6

Methods to Measure Blood Pressure and Pulse During the Valsalva Maneuver

1. **Obtain the resting systolic blood pressure.**
2. **Inflate the blood pressure cuff approximately 30 to 40 mm Hg above the resting systolic blood pressure.** Immediately before the Valsalva maneuver, inflate the sphygmomanometer cuff pressure approximately 30 to 40 mm Hg above the resting systolic blood pressure.
3. **Valsalva maneuver:** Forceful exhalation into a mouthpiece connected to an aneroid sphygmomanometer with sufficient strength to maintain the pressure steadily at approximately 40 mm Hg for approximately 10 seconds (see CD-ROM).
4. **Listen for the Korotkoff sounds at the higher blood pressure cuff pressure.** The systolic blood pressure should be greater during phase 1 of the Valsalva maneuver and should ***normally*** decrease approximately 10 to 20 mm Hg during phase 2 of the Valsalva maneuver (because of a decrease in venous return from the increase in intrathoracic pressure during the Valsalva maneuver). This can be heard by closing the sphygmomanometer valve to release air when the first Korotkoff sound is heard. In the normal person or person with dyspnea due to pulmonary disease, the following Korotkoff sounds will fade and eventually disappear because of the decrease in systolic blood pressure due to the decreased venous return from the increased intrathoracic pressure. In the person with dyspnea due to cardiac muscle dysfunction the Korotkoff sounds following the first Korotkoff sound will not fade and will not disappear because the systolic blood pressure does not decrease during phase 2 of the Valsalva maneuver, because the elevated end-diastolic volume and pressure of CHF find the 10-second decrease in venous return favorable.

---

specific changes in the systolic and diastolic blood pressure can provide important indirect information about cardiac and cardiovascular function. The decrease in venous return accompanying a change in position from supine to standing can possibly provide information that is similar to that obtained during the Valsalva maneuver; understanding whether the cardiac pump is normal, dysfunctional, or failing. Normally, the diastolic blood pressure will be lower in the supine position (compared to that in the standing position) because of the positional related increase in venous return and subsequent decrease in peripheral vascular constriction (remember, BP = cardiac output × TPR). However, if the diastolic blood pressure is observed to be higher in the supine position compared to that in the standing position, it is likely that the heart is failing and prefers to have a decreased venous

BOX 10-7

Methods to Distinguish a Normal from Abnormal Cardiovascular System Using the Supine to Standing Test

Method to perform test

1. Measure supine systolic and diastolic blood pressure (patient should lie supine for 5 minutes) and record (see Box 10-4).
2. Measure standing systolic and diastolic blood pressure (immediately upon standing)* and record (see Box 10-4).

Method to distinguish a normal from an abnormal response

Normal response

1. A lower diastolic blood pressure in supine compared to standing

2. A higher diastolic blood pressure standing compared to supine
3. Maintenance of the systolic blood pressure as a result of the higher diastolic blood pressure in standing compared to supine.

Abnormal response

1. A higher diastolic blood pressure in supine compared to standing
2. A lower diastolic blood pressure standing compared to supine
3. Maintenance of the systolic blood pressure (despite a lower diastolic blood pressure in standing compared to supine).

*The blood pressure cuff and stethoscope should be in place and immediately ready to use when the patient initially stands (the cuff of the sphygmomanometer should be inflated when the patient initially stands).

return. A change in body position from supine to standing should normally cause the diastolic blood pressure to increase to maintain the systolic and mean arterial blood pressures. A diastolic blood pressure that decreases with standing and is associated with a systolic blood pressure that is similar to that observed in supine is indicative of a heart that has a poor pumping capacity and pumps better with less of a venous return (such as that when standing). Therefore, signs of a failing cardiac pump are (1) a higher diastolic blood pressure in a supine position compared to that in a standing position, (2) a lower diastolic blood pressure standing compared to that when supine, and (3) maintenance of the systolic blood pressure (despite a lower diastolic blood pressure in standing compared to that when supine). Signs of a more normal cardiac pump are (1) a lower diastolic blood pressure in supine compared to that when standing, (2) a higher diastolic blood pressure standing

compared to that when supine, and (3) maintenance of the systolic blood pressure as a result of the higher diastolic blood pressure in standing compared to that when supine. These characteristics are shown in Box 10-7.

Differentiation of Dyspnea due to a Cardiac Origin from Pulmonary Origin

Dyspnea is possibly the most common complaint of patients. It may be due to a variety of disorders, but the two major categories producing dyspnea are of cardiac and pulmonary origins. A variety of examination techniques may provide important information to differentiate dyspnea of a cardiac origin from that of a pulmonary origin (Table 10-14). The etiology of dyspnea is important to know so that optimal treatment interventions can be allocated. Often, the etiology of dyspnea is apparent from

TABLE 10-14   Differential Diagnosis of Dyspnea: Cardiac or Pulmonary Origin?

	Cardiac	**Pulmonary**
Past history:	CHF, CAD, and DM, cardiac RF[a]	Pulmonary disease, pulmonary RF
Symptoms:	Dyspnea on exertion	Resting dyspnea and dyspnea on exertion
Signs:		
Appearance	Less accessory muscle use	More accessory muscle use
Heart rate	Significantly increased	Less significantly increased
Blood pressure	SBP often lower than expected	SBP often greater than expected
	DBP often greater than expected	DBP often greater than expected
	<so>	<so>
Pulse pressure	Lower pulse pressure	Greater pulse pressure
Respiratory rate	Increased respiratory rate	Significantly increased respiratory rate
O$_2$ saturation	Likely normal	Decreased
Valsalva[b]	Delayed/absent fall of phase II-SBP	Normal fall of phase 2-SBP

[a]CHF, congestive heart failure; CAD, coronary artery disease; DM, diabetes mellitus; RF, risk factors; SBP, systolic blood pressure; DBP, diastolic blood pressure.

[b]Valsava maneuver should be performed in the manner described in Box 10-6.

the patient history. The patient history can help to differentiate the shortness of breath of pulmonary disease from heart disease and the shortness of breath of congestive heart failure versus anginal equivalents such as that in patients with diabetes mellitus. Table 10-14 presents the distinguishing characteristics of shortness of breath in pulmonary and cardiac disease. The three main categories represent the past history, symptoms, and signs. The information important in the category of patient history includes a past history of (1) congestive heart failure (CHF), (2) cardiac disease (or risk factors for cardiac disease/dyspnea), (3) combined coronary artery disease and diabetes mellitus (diabetes may impair the sensation of angina to be perceived), or (4) pulmonary disease (or risk factors for pulmonary disease/dyspnea).

The methods used to evaluate dyspnea in patients with known or suspected pulmonary disorders (Chapter 9) can also be used for patients with known or suspected cardiac disease. Tables 9-2 and 9-3 show several different methods that can help to measure and quantify dyspnea. However, often other important tests and measurements are necessary to fully understand the true etiology and treatment of dyspnea. Several such measurements are described in Table 10-14. The differentiating signs include the appearance, heart rate, blood pressure, pulse pressure, respiratory rate, oxygen saturation level, and the blood pressure response during the Valsalva maneuver. The distinguishing characteristics of each of these measurements are described in Table 10-14. These characteristics are broad generalizations that can be cautiously applied to both resting and exercising conditions.

Of these characteristics, the heart rate and blood pressure observations may be the most confusing and in greatest need of clarification. Persons with known cardiac disease who experience dyspnea will likely have a poorer stroke volume than patients with pulmonary disease (because of damaged myocardium from myocardial infarction [MI]). Because of this, the patient with cardiac disease must increase the resting and exercise heart rate to maintain an optimal cardiac output. Therefore, the heart rate of a patient with cardiac disease may be greater than that of a patient with pulmonary disease. However, a patient with pulmonary disease may suffer from poor oxygenation and may need to increase the resting and exercise heart rate to maintain optimal oxygenation. Therefore, the heart rate category of Table 10-14 is less specific in distinguishing cardiac from pulmonary dyspnea. The systolic blood pressure may be only slightly better at distinguishing cardiac from pulmonary dyspnea. As shown in Table 10-14, the systolic blood pressure of a patient with dyspnea due to a cardiac disorder is likely to be lower than the systolic pressure of a patient with dyspnea due to a pulmonary disorder. The lower systolic blood pressure of the patient with a cardiac disorder appears to be the result again of damaged myocardium, which in the long term reduces the overall cardiac output and responsiveness of the autonomic nervous system (resulting in a reduced cardiac output and total peripheral resistance). Reducing both cardiac output and total peripheral resistance will subsequently decrease the arterial blood pressure because BP = cardiac output × TPR (yielding a lower systolic blood pressure at rest and during exercise in a patient with dyspnea due to a cardiac origin). A quick glance at Table 10-14 also reveals that the diastolic blood pressure does not distinguish cardiac from pulmonary dyspnea, but the pulse pressure appears to be a distinguishable characteristic (being lower in a patient with dyspnea due to a cardiac origin) that is modestly supported in the literature.

Patients suffering from shortness of breath due to heart disease will likely have congestive heart failure or anginal equivalents represented as shortness of breath. The differentiation of dyspnea between heart and lung disease as well as the primary cause of shortness of breath in heart disease (anginal equivalent vs CHF) are relatively simple. However, it may be difficult to distinguish the shortness of breath of pulmonary disease from cardiac disease because of combined heart and lung disease, a poor medical history or similar signs, symptoms, and risk factors for cardiac and pulmonary disease. Another method to examine shortness of breath is by performing the Valsalva maneuver. The Valsalva maneuver has been observed to differentiate the shortness of breath of heart disease from that of pulmonary disease. In this case, it may be helpful to perform a controlled Valsalva maneuver and evaluate the arterial blood pressure response and pulse during the Valsalva.

CLINICAL CORRELATE

A blood pressure and pulse response similar to that in Fig. 10-10A is indicative of dyspnea due to a pulmonary origin. A blood pressure response like that in Fig. 10-10B is indicative of dyspnea due to a cardiac origin of congestive heart failure.

MEDICAL EXAMINATIONS USED BY PHYSICAL THERAPISTS

This section will briefly review the medical examinations that are used by physical therapists. They will include the traditional tests of cardiovascular and cardiac function as well as other less traditional measurements of cardiac function. Table 10-15 provides an overview of the different methods of examination (and treatment) that may be employed in heart diseases. A categorization of the nine most common forms of heart disease and methods to examine them are provided in Table 10-15.

Examination of Cardiac Function
Standard Measurements of Cardiac Function

The standard measurements of cardiac function, perfusion, and viability, as well as the strengths and weaknesses of each method, are listed in Table 10-16. Each method will also be presented in the following sections.

TABLE 10-15 **Methods to Examine and Manage Heart Disease**

Major Types of Heart Disease	Examination Techniques	Medical Interventions	Physical Therapy
1. "High risk"	History; question (naire); blood test (eg, lipids, **homocysteine**); body weight; exercise; blood pressure body fat/LBM/BMI[a]	Risk-factor reduction Lipid-lowering drugs Weight loss programs Antihypertensive drugs	Risk-factor reduction Diet eval./ex. Exercise Diet eval./ex.
2. **Hypertension**	Blood pressure; echocardiogram; ECG; symptoms	Antihypertensive drugs	Diet eval./ex. stress Reduction
3. **Coronary artery disease** **Angina**	Symptoms; ECG; ex. test with ECG; thallium rest or exercise test; cardiac catheterization; transesophageal echocardiogram	Antianginal drugs; PTCA; stenting; CABG surgery; Mid-CABG; laser	Properly prescribed ex. diet eval. Stress reduction **Rest if unstable angina**
MI	Symptoms; ECG; serum enzymes; echocardiogram cardiac catheterization with ventriculography; transesophageal echocardiogram	Antianginal drugs; PTCA; stenting; CABG surgery; mid-CABG; TPA/streptokinase; aspirin	Properly prescribed ex. Diet eval. Stress reduction **Rest Days 1–2 after MI and decrease of cardiac enzymes**
4. **Cardiac dysrhythmias**	Symptoms; ECG; ex. test with ECG; Holter monitoring; **EP studies**	Antidysrhythmic drugs; pacemakers; AICD; **ablation**	Properly prescribed ex. Diet/drug eval. Stress reduction **Rest if a rapid or slow rhythm**
5. **Valvular disease**	Symptoms; auscultation; Echocardiogram; cardiac catheterization with ventriculography; transesophageal echocardiogram	Vasodilators and anticoagulants; valvuloplasty; valve replacement	Properly prescribed ex. Diet/drug evaluation
6. **Myocarditis/ pericarditis**	Symptoms; auscultation; echocardiogram; cardiac catheterization with ventriculography; transesophageal echocardiogram	Vasodilators/anticoagulants and anti-inflammatory drugs; pericardial tap	Properly prescribed ex. Diet/drug evaluation
7. **Cor pulmonale**	Symptoms; ECG; echocardiogram; cardiac catheterization with ventriculography; transesophageal echo	Vasodilators/antihyperten sives/O_2	Properly prescribed ex. Diet/drug evaluation
8. **Cardiomyopathy**	Symptoms; echocardiography; cardiac catheterization with ventriculography transesophageal echocardiogram	Vasodilators/diuretics Digoxin and β-blockers; IABP; LVAD; **cardiac transplantation**	Properly prescribed ex. Diet/drug evaluation
9. **Heart failure**	Symptoms; echocardiography; cardiac catheterization with ventriculography transesophageal Echocardiogram	Vasodilators/diuretics digoxin and β-blockers; IABP; LVAD; **cardiac transplantation**	Properly prescribed ex. Diet/drug evaluation

[a]LBM, lean body mass; BMI, body mass index (kg/m^2); ECG, electrocardiogram; PTCA, percutaneous transluminal coronary angioplasty; CABG, coronary artery bypass grafting; MID-CABG, minimally invasive direct-coronary artery bypass grafting; ex., exercise; eval., evaluation; AICD, antidysrhythmic implantable cardiodefibrillator; TPA, tissue plasminogen activator; LAVD, left ventricular assist device; IABP, intra-aortic balloon pump.

Cardiac catheterization—*Cardiac catheterization* is considered the gold standard to examine cardiac function, blockage in coronary arteries, and the status of cardiac valves and structures. It is an invasive technique that requires a small incision in the femoral artery through which a catheter is introduced and carefully moved through the femoral artery to the common iliac and then to the descending aorta. From here the catheter is progressed to the ascending aorta and then positioned at the base of the coronary sinus where radioactive dye is injected into the coronary arteries after which radiographic films are made of the dye in the coronary arteries. These films are often referred to as angiograms. Areas of blockage can be readily observed, and decisions can then be made on the type of intervention (angioplasty, bypass surgery, or medicine). Repeat catheterizations are often done to examine the efficacy of an intervention. Cardiac catheterization may be immediately performed after an angioplasty or weeks to months after bypass surgery or medical therapy. Ventricular performance can also be examined as measurements of the dye injected into the ventricles are made during systole and diastole that are then used to calculate the ejection fraction and wall motion abnormalities.

Figures 10-11A to 10-11D show the catheter and other equipment needed for the cardiac catheterization. It also shows the progression of a cardiac catheterization from the initial incision to the final injection of dye into the coronary arteries. Dye can also be injected into the left ventricle and examination of the radiographic films can provide fairly accurate measurements of stroke volume, cardiac output, and ejection fraction. In addition to the visual information from a catheterization, information about the pressures within the cardiac chambers can be obtained from a pressure transducer positioned at the tip of the catheter. Figures 10-11E show the pressure data from

TABLE 10-16   Direct Measures of Cardiac Function: Methods, Strengths, and Weaknesses

Technique	Methods	Strengths	Weaknesses
Measurement techniques of cardiac contraction			
Ventriculography (via catheterization)	Radioactive dye	Accurate	Expensive, invasive, possible allergy to radioactive dye
Echocardiography	Ultrasound to heart	Ease, rapid, relatively inexpensive, noninvasive	None of significance except possible less precise than ventriculography
Technitium-99M (sestamibi and teboroxime)	Injection of technitium with serial imaging	Rapid and specific to cardiac anatomy	Relatively expensive and specialized equipment with occasional allergy to technetium
Bioimpedance analysis	Special ECG electrodes relay impedance data to a computer programmed with regression equations to predict cardiac output and other cardiac measurements	Ease, rapid, inexpensive	Less precise than other measurements
Swan–Ganz catheterization	Balloon floatation catheter that rests in the pulmonary artery or capillary	Rapid, accurate right heart measurements that reflect left heart function	Invasive with potential for infection and limited mobility due to catheter and associated lines
Arterial line	Indwelling catheter in the radial artery	Rapid, accurate measurements of arterial blood pressure	Invasive with potential for infection and limited mobility due to catheter associated lines
Central venous pressure	Indwelling catheter in the vena cava or right atrium	Rapid, accurate measurements of right heart function and fluid volume	Invasive with potential for infection and limited mobility due to catheter associated lines
Measurement techniques of cardiac perfusion			
Thallium-201	Injection of thallium with serial imaging	Rapid and specific to cardiac anatomy	Relatively expensive and specialized equipment with occasional allergy to thallium
Technitium-99M (sestamibi and teboroxime)	Injection of technitium with serial imaging	Rapid and specific to cardiac anatomy	Relatively expensive and specialized equipment with occasional allergy to technetium
Measurement techniques of cardiac viability			
FDG	FDG is absorbed by living tissue	Rapid estimate of living myocardium	Questionable sensitivity specificity
[^{11}C]-Acetate	Coupled with oxidative metabolism	Accurately reflects oxidative metabolism	None of significance
Technitium-99M Pyrophosphate	Combines with calcium which is released with cell death	High sensitivity	Low specificity because other disorders can produce a positive scan (eg, trauma, aneurysm)

a catheterization that can then be compared to the normal (ie, expected) values within the cardiac chambers (the normal values for the cardiac chambers are also shown in Fig. 10-11E).

Several drawbacks to cardiac catheterization exist and include in some an allergic reaction to the radioactive dye, a high cost (approximately $3,000.00), and the fact that it is an invasive technique which carries a potential risk of complications (eg, stroke, MI, death) in 1 out of every 10,000 individuals. However, specialized centers where catheterizations are frequently performed have lower complication rates.

Finally, another indirect measure of cardiac function can be obtained at the same time a catheterization is performed. This indirect measure is a biopsy of the endocardium of the left or right ventricle. Biopsy of the ventricular endocardium can provide important information related to myocardial cell structure (to diagnose particular types of cardiomyopathy), presence of myocarditis, or myocardial rejection in patients with cardiac transplantation.

Echocardiography—*Echocardiography* is fast becoming one of the most common examinations of persons with known or suspected cardiopulmonary disorders. It involves placing a handheld transducer that emits sound waves through the chest wall to the heart. Sound waves introduced to the heart bounce back to the transducer and produce images that often look similar to the structures underlying the transducer. The extensive amount of information that can be obtained noninvasively via echocardiography is exceptional. In fact, today's technology has improved the acquisition, processing, and analysis of data obtained from echocardiography and novel modes of echocardiographic imaging (ie, transesophageal [TEE]) appears to provide information about the patency (openness) of the coronary arteries that is similar to that obtained from cardiac catheterization. Nonetheless, perhaps the major variables obtained from echocardiography are the stroke volume, cardiac output, and ejection fraction both at rest and during exercise. Exercise echocardiography is

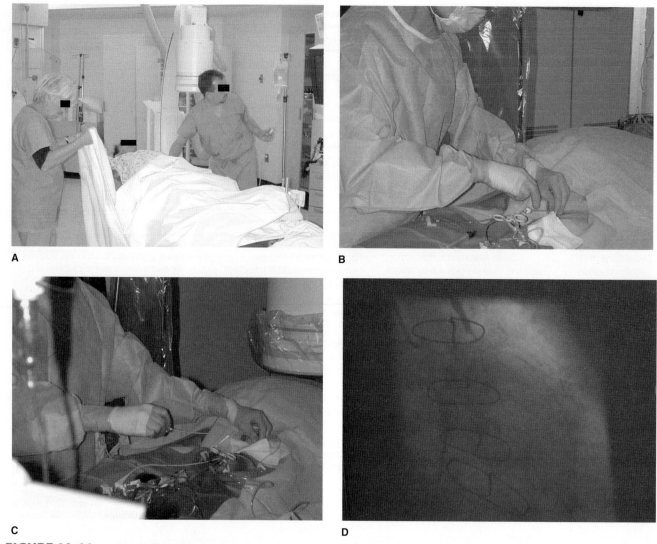

A   B

C   D

FIGURE 10-11   (**A–E**) Cardiac catheterization. (**A–D**) The procedure. *(continued)*

becoming a common technique to diagnose and prognosticate persons with suspected and known heart disease. Different methods used in echocardiography include Doppler, color flow Doppler, two-dimensional (2-D), M-mode, and TEE echocardiography.

Swan–Ganz catheterization—*Swan–Ganz catheterization* was first introduced by the doctors Swan and Ganz in the 1960s. They developed a special balloon flotation catheter that currently provides much of the data that are projected to an ICU monitor such as the pulmonary artery pressure and pulmonary capillary wedge pressure. The procedure used for Swan–Ganz catheterization includes a small incision in the jugular artery through which a catheter is introduced and progressed to the common carotid and then to the superior vena cava. The catheter is then progressed into the right atrium past the tricuspid valve and into the right ventricle. From here the catheter is moved into the pulmonary artery and the balloon tip is allowed to float and essentially wedge itself into the pulmonary capillaries (thus providing a pulmonary capillary wedge pressure).

The information obtained from Swan–Ganz catheterization is pressure and temperature related. The key pressure variables are those mentioned previously (eg, pulmonary artery and pulmonary capillary wedge pressures), and oximetry and the key temperature variable is the cardiac output. The temperature probe of the Swan–Ganz catheter is used to measure the time it takes for a known amount of cold injectate (between $0°C$ and $5°C$) to move within the cardiovascular system, yielding the thermodilution measurement of cardiac output. Dye is also used to measure the cardiac output and requires a spectrophotometer to examine the dye dilution to measure cardiac output. All of the data obtained via Swan–Ganz catheterization provide direct information relevant to cardiac function.

Arterial line—An *arterial line* is simply an indwelling catheter with a pressure transducer attached to the end of a catheter. It is commonly placed at the radial artery and is used primarily to (1) measure the arterial pressure and (2) as a site to obtain frequent arterial blood gases. Therefore, the arterial line indirectly measures cardiac performance via the blood

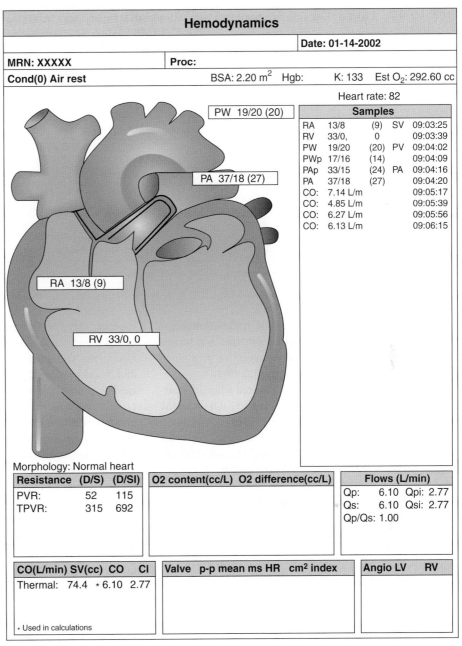

Hemodynamics

Date: 01-14-2002

MRN: XXXXX   Proc:

Cond(0) Air rest   BSA: 2.20 m² Hgb: K: 133   Est O₂: 292.60 cc

Heart rate: 82

PW 19/20 (20)

PA 37/18 (27)

RA 13/8 (9)

RV 33/0, 0

Samples				
RA	13/8	(9)	SV	09:03:25
RV	33/0,	0		09:03:39
PW	19/20	(20)	PV	09:04:02
PWp	17/16	(14)		09:04:09
PAp	33/15	(24)	PA	09:04:16
PA	37/18	(27)		09:04:20
CO:	7.14 L/m			09:05:17
CO:	4.85 L/m			09:05:39
CO:	6.27 L/m			09:05:56
CO:	6.13 L/m			09:06:15

Morphology: Normal heart

Resistance	(D/S)	(D/SI)
PVR:	52	115
TPVR:	315	692

O2 content(cc/L) O2 difference(cc/L)

Flows (L/min)	
Qp:	6.10 Qpi: 2.77
Qs:	6.10 Qsi: 2.77
Qp/Qs: 1.00	

CO(L/min) SV(cc) CO	CI
Thermal: 74.4 * 6.10 2.77	

* Used in calculations

Valve p-p mean ms HR cm² index

Angio LV   RV

FIGURE 10-11 *(Continued)*
(**E**) The formal report.   **E**

pressure and blood gas information. The arterial line travels from the arm of the patient to a monitor where the arterial blood pressure waveform and digital readout are displayed. Often, the noninvasive automatic blood pressure is digitally displayed just above or below the arterial blood pressure on the standard ICU monitor. The proximity of one to the other is a check mechanism for the clinician. Both the arterial line and noninvasive automatic blood pressures should be similar. If a discrepancy exists, it is an indication that a potential problem may exist (eg, arterial line displacement or automatic blood pressure cuff unattached).

Central venous pressure—The *central venous pressure* (CVP) is obtained via a catheter introduced at a vein and

advanced to the inferior or superior vena cava or right atrium. It reflects right-sided heart function and is frequently used to examine blood volume, vascular tone, and venous return. The differences between the CVP and the arterial line include the initial access via a vein versus artery and more detailed information regarding cardiac function than that obtained from the arterial line alone.

Cardiac enzymes—*Cardiac enzymes* can provide a measurement of cardiac function by identifying the presence of myocardial damage. Myocardial damage and cardiac function examined by cardiac enzymes alone, however, are somewhat incomplete. However, it is generally accepted that a large release of cardiac enzymes from necrotic myocardial fibrils

TABLE 10-17   Cardiac Enzymes Associated with Myocardial Injury and Infarction

Enzyme	Normal Level	Minor Cardiac Dysfunction Is Likely When the Measured Level Is Near the Level Given Below	Major Cardiac Dysfunction Is Likely When the Measured Level Is Near the Level Given Below
CPK[a]	5–75 mU/mL or 55–71 IU	100–500 mU/mL	≥1000 mU/mL
CK-MB	0%–3%	5%	10%
LDH	100–225 mU/mL or 127 IU	300–750 mU/mL	≥1000 mU/mL
SGOT	24 IU	50 IU	≥100 IU
AST	10–40 mU/dL	100–200 mU/dL	≥500 mU/dL
Troponin	0–0.2 µg/mL	5 µg/mL	≥10 µg/mL
Myoglobin	<100 ng/mL	200 ng/mL	≥500 ng/mL
Myoglobin/ carbonic anhydrase	<3.2	Myoglobin/carbonic anhydrase > 5.0	Myoglobin/carbonic anhydrase > 10.0

[a]CPK, creatine phosphokinase; CK-MB, creatine kinase-myocardial band isoenzyme; LDH, lactic dehydrogenase; SGOT, serum glutamate oxalocetate transaminase; AST, aspartate aminotransferase; FDG, fluorodeoxyglucose.

can indirectly identify the degree of cardiac dysfunction that is likely to be associated with myocardial damage. A minimal release of cardiac enzymes is usually suggestive of a small myocardial infarction and less cardiac dysfunction.

The cardiac enzymes commonly measured when myocardial damage is suspected are listed in Table 10-17. Of these, the most specific enzymes for myocardial tissue are the myocardial band of creatine kinase (CK-MB) and troponin T. Levels that are observed to be greater than the accepted normal range are indicative of myocardial damage. Furthermore, a cardiac enzyme level that is markedly elevated is associated with a greater degree of myocardial damage and dysfunction, whereas a minimal elevation is associated with a slight degree of myocardial damage and dysfunction. This is an important characteristic and is best seen in the enzyme troponin-t, which has been observed to be elevated in not only myocardial infarction but also the failing cardiac pump. Despite this apparent degree of nonspecificity, troponin-t is perhaps one of the most sensitive and specific markers of myocardial infarction and cardiac pump failure. Patients with myocardial infarction will have markedly elevated levels that will decrease within 7 to 14 days, whereas the less elevated level of troponin-t of cardiac failure will not subside and will enzymatically profile a failing cardiac pump. It is apparent that each enzyme is released from the dying cardiac tissue at different times and with different durations to reach peak concentration and reabsorption (uptake) of the released enzymes. Therefore, identification of the time post injury and the relationship of time post injury to the observed cardiac enzymes should further improve the examination of cardiac function via cardiac enzymes.

Atrial Natriuretic Peptide and Brain Natriuretic Peptide

Atrial natriuretic peptide (ANP) is a regulatory hormone that is released from the atrial myocytes when atrial volume and pressure are elevated. It is the body's initial attempt to decrease excess fluid volume via natriuresis (excretion of sodium) and

diuresis (excretion of water). ANP also suppresses the secretion of renal renin and aldosterone that increases the excretion of electrolytes and water and subsequently decreases fluid volume and blood pressure. Elevated levels of ANP are associated with cardiac pump failure and increased morbidity and mortality rates.[8,9] *Brain natriuretic peptide* (BNP) also reflects increased pressure within the cardiovascular system (commonly due to a poor cardiac pump) and is released from the brain when cardiovascular pressures and volumes are elevated. The specific values of pressure or volume that cause ANP and BNP to be released are unknown, but the release often suggests poor cardiac function.

Radiologic Evidence (eg, Heart Size, Pulmonary Edema)

Indirect measures of cardiac function can be obtained from radiographic methods such as a chest radiograph. Evidence of poor cardiac function can be ascertained when the chest radiograph shows (1) a dilated heart, (2) pulmonary edema, (3) increased size of the pulmonary artery, and (4) other findings suggestive of abnormal structural or compensatory abnormalities. For example, the poor cardiac function responsible for coronary heart failure (CHF) can be appreciated via radiography by the size and shape of the cardiac silhouette as well as via the presence of interstitial, perivascular, and alveolar edema (evaluating fluid in the lungs). Interstitial, perivascular, and alveolar edema are the radiologic hallmarks of CHF, but the size and shape of the cardiac silhouette provide evidence about the etiology of the pulmonary edema. A review of the radiologic examination process described in Chapter 9 will enable a better understanding of the previous information.

Examination of Cardiac Perfusion

Examination of *cardiac perfusion* is often used to assist in the diagnosis, prognosis, and understanding of the effectiveness of treatment of heart disease. The examination of cardiac perfusion is essentially the measurement of blood flow to myocardial tissue. Perhaps the best example of this is thallium scanning immediately after exercise and then several hours after exercise. Thallium-201 is often used in conjunction with an exercise test, and at peak exercise it is injected intravenously. Areas of the heart receiving less blood flow are identified by either decreased areas of thallium uptake that become reperfused or areas of thallium uptake that remain underperfused long after exercise has ended. The former scenario is associated with myocardial ischemia, whereas the latter is associated with a past myocardial infarction.

Areas of the heart with coronary blockage may be observed to receive less blood flow at peak exercise because of the greater work of the heart (due to higher heart rates and blood pressures which increase the myocardial oxygen demand). As the work of the heart decreases after exercise, the areas of the heart observed to have diminished blood flow at peak exercise now have a return of blood flow to the areas observed to be deficit of blood flow at peak exercise. These changes are reflected in the absence of thallium uptake at peak exercise and in the presence of thallium uptake after resting. This scenario is associated with myocardial ischemia and blockage in the coronary arteries. These thallium findings are often referred to as signs of reversible ischemia. A sign of irreversible ischemia (where thallium uptake is diminished at peak exercise and long after exercise testing; thallium is not absorbed after exercise or at peak exercise) is indicative of a past myocardial infarction. Irreversible ischemia is actually somewhat of a misnomer because the area showing this finding is not really ischemic; it is dead. It is an area where blood flow no longer travels (often because of a complete obstruction of a coronary artery). Such areas are often referred to as fixed defects where the lack of thallium uptake is consistent immediately after exercise and hours after exercise.

Cardiac perfusion measurements such as those mentioned here can be performed with other radioisotopes such as technetium, and they can be performed with pharmacologic methods to increase the work of the heart. Patients unable to exercise (ie, patients with severe orthopedic or peripheral vascular disorders) are often provided drugs such as persantine, adenosine, or dobutamine to increase the work of the heart. The same procedures described previously can be employed at peak pharmacologic effect and several hours after the peak pharmacologic effect. In this manner, areas of reversible or irreversible ischemia can be examined.

Examination of Cardiac Viability

Cardiac viability is essentially the examination of the heart's metabolism. It is an examination of life or death in particular regions of the heart. In fact, examination of cardiac viability has gained new importance since the discovery of stunned or hibernating areas of myocardium associated with myocardial injury and the development of newer therapeutic interventions for heart disease (eg, feasibility of angioplasty and thrombolytic therapy based on salvageable tissue). Several different techniques are used to examine the viability of cardiac tissue, but all

appear to incorporate positron-emitting tomography (PET). PET acquires information related to tissue metabolism. The main methods of PET include perfusion-FDG metabolism imaging, $[^{11}C-]$ acetate oxidative metabolism scanning, and technetium-99M-pyrophosphate scanning. The strengths and weakness of each method are presented in Table 10-16.

Examination of Cardiovascular Function and Risk

Examination of the peripheral cardiovascular system is not dissimilar to that for central cardiac function. In fact, many of the same methods and principles apply to both central and peripheral examination of the cardiovascular system. The following sections will describe some of the similarities and differences and will present several other examination techniques that may be quite useful to the physical therapist attempting to diagnose, categorize, and treat patients with peripheral vascular disease.

Arterial and Venous Angiography

Arterial and *venous angiography* are simply angiograms of the arterial and venous systems in the periphery compared to the central angiograms of the heart discussed previously. The same radioactive dye injected into the coronary arteries is injected into the peripheral arteries and veins, and a radiograph of the dye within the vessels provides a radiograph similar to that of the coronary arteries. The same concerns with angiography of the heart exist with peripheral angiography and include the invasive nature of the procedure and the potential for infection as well as the possibility of an allergic reaction to the radioactive dye.

Doppler Ultrasound

Doppler ultrasound is also used to examine cardiovascular function. It utilizes the same methodology and principles used to examine cardiac function via echocardiography. Sound waves are directed to areas suspected of being blocked, and the underlying structures can be visualized by the reflected sound wave. Evidence of blockage can be quantified and results of therapeutic interventions can be reexamined. Another benefit of ultrasound is the clinical utility of the auditory aspect of the circulation as it flows past a Doppler transducer. Blood flow can be heard and visualized by the interruption of sound waves from the transducer. In fact, Doppler velocimetry uses the methods and principles described previously to identify pulses that are difficult to palpate and is helpful in the bedside diagnosis of peripheral vascular disease.

Peripheral Limb Pressure Measurements

Peripheral limb pressure measurements can be made with a standard sphygmomanometer cuff (by inflating the cuff 20 to 40 mm Hg above the systolic blood pressure at a number of sites such as the thigh, knee, calf, and ankle) or via special plethysmographic pressure cuffs at the thigh and ankle. The actual blood pressure measurements are obtained with the sphygmomanometer cuff (possibly using a Doppler device), and a pulse volume recording is made with the special plethysmographic pressure cuffs at the thigh and ankle. The pulse volume recording can be examined for signs of peripheral artery disease that may include an absent waveform in severe complete or near-complete occlusion of the peripheral arteries of the legs or simply minor alterations in the rapid systolic upstroke and downstroke of the pulse volume recording.

Ankle–Brachial Index

Although the *ankle–brachial index* (ABI) is relatively easy to perform and analyze, it is only seldom performed by physical therapists. The methods to perform and analyze the ABI are provided in Fig. 10-9 and simply consist of measuring the systolic blood pressure in the arms and ankles and developing a ratio of the highest ankle pressure and the highest arm pressure (highest ankle systolic BP/highest arm systolic BP), bilaterally. It is important to note that an ABI above 0.90 is normal, whereas an index less than 0.40 is associated with severe arterial obstruction.

Systolic Blood Pressure Response After Exercise

The systolic blood pressure response to exercise can also be used to diagnose peripheral artery disease. Observation of a decrease in ankle systolic blood pressure after exercise is strongly related to peripheral artery disease.

Venous Filling Time and Rubor Dependency Tests

Body position and cardiovascular response to change in body position can help to diagnose and categorize patients with known or suspected peripheral vascular disease. For both the *venous filling time* and *rubor dependency tests,* patients are positioned supine on a table with the legs elevated to approximately 45 degrees. After several minutes with the legs in this position they are brought down to rest on the table in a dependent position, which should promote increased blood flow back to the legs. Patients with peripheral artery disease will be observed to have a deep red color in the feet (the "rubor" of the rubor dependency test) and delayed filling (>15 seconds) of the veins.

Homan's Sign and Trendelenburg Test of Venous Insufficiency

Homan's sign is simply a test for deep vein thrombophlebitis and consists of squeezing the gastrocnemius muscle while the foot is dorsiflexed. Elicitation of pain in the gastrocnemius strongly suggests thrombophlebitis. A positive Homan's sign with signs of thrombophlebitis (rubor, warmth, and swelling) confirms thrombophlebitis but requires further examination via Doppler ultrasound, plethysmographic pressure recordings, venograms (dye injected into the venous system), and possibly immediate treatment.

The Trendelenburg test is a test to examine the valvular competence of the venous system. It requires the patient to lie supine with the legs elevated to 45 to 90 degrees. After lying in this position for several minutes, a tourniquet is placed around the thigh to occlude venous flow. The patient then stands and the time for venous filling is measured. Venous filling should normally occur within 30 seconds, and filling taking longer than this is associated with venous insufficiency. Furthermore, filling of the superficial veins within or after 30 seconds suggests that the veins are incompetent, whereas further filling of the superficial veins after the tourniquet is removed suggests that the valves of the saphenous veins are incompetent.

Catecholamines (Norepinephrine and Epinephrine)

The measurement of *catecholamines* can provide an indirect measurement of cardiovascular function. The release of *norepinephrine* and *epinephrine* is stimulated by cardiovascular stress (ie, often due to the so-called fight or flight response). In cardiovascular and cardiac disease, these catecholamines are released to compensate for impaired cardiac and cardiovascular function. The measurement of catecholamines can be easily performed with a sample of blood that can provide accurate measures of sympathetic nervous system activity.

Lipids

The examination of *lipids* is routinely done in subjects with suspected and known heart disease. It has also become a common screening tool to predict the likelihood of cardiovascular disease. Lipid tests have become almost as commonplace as having blood pressure measured. The lipids that appear to be most important to examine include the total cholesterol, low-density lipoprotein, high-density lipoprotein, apolipoproteins, and triglycerides. The specific lipids, normal values, and rationale for these lipids contributing to cardiovascular disease are provided in Table 10-18.

EXERCISE TESTING

Exercise testing is an important method to examine the cardiovascular, pulmonary, and muscular systems. Perhaps the best example of this is Fig. 10-12, which was first introduced by Wasserman and Whipp in 1975. Figure 10-12 shows the relationship of these systems and the potential methods to distinguish a disorder in 1 system from the others. In brief, the three major wheels shown in this Figure represent the interrelatedness among the muscular, cardiovascular, and pulmonary systems. Defects in one or more of these major "wheeled" systems may produce observable signs and symptoms that may be best observed during a controlled bout of exercise—during an exercise test. Furthermore, defects in one or more of the cogs in one or more of the wheels may also produce observable signs and symptoms that may best be observed during exercise testing (Fig. 10-12). Defects in one system may produce defects in another. The observation of particular signs and symptoms during exercise testing combined with other tests

TABLE 10-18   Examination of Lipids

Lipid	Optimal Value	Rationale for the Association with Cardiovascular Disease
Total cholesterol	160–199 mg/dL	Higher levels are associated with greater deposition of cholesterol in artery walls
Very low-density lipoprotein[a]	Not established	Higher levels may associated with greater deposition of cholesterol and fats in artery walls and other diseases or abnormalities that increase atherosclerosis
Low-density lipoprotein	<100 mg/dL	Higher levels are associated with greater deposition of cholesterol in artery walls
High-density lipoprotein	≥40 mg/dL for men; ≥50 mg/dL for women	Higher levels are associated with less heart disease and lower levels of other lipids
Apolipoprotein A	<30 mg/dL	Higher levels are associated with greater deposition of cholesterol in artery walls and the inhibition of thrombolysis
Apolipoprotein B[b]	Not established	Higher levels are associated with greater deposition of cholesterol in artery walls
Triglycerides	<150 mg/dL	Higher levels may associated with greater deposition of cholesterol and fats in artery walls and other diseases or abnormalities that increase atherosclerosis
Total cholesterol/HDL	<5.0	Lower levels of total cholesterol and higher levels of HDL yield a lower total cholesterol/HDL ratio which is associated with less heart disease

[a]Optimal very low-density lipoprotein levels do not appear to be established.

[b]Optimal apolipoprotein B levels have been difficult to identify because of different apolipoprotein B component isoforms (apo B_{48} and apo B_{100}), but higher levels are directly associated with increased risk of coronary artery disease. Also, exercise and diet interventions appear to favorably alter apolipoprotein B levels in a manner that is similar to the changes in LDL cholesterol.

and measures can provide a wealth of information about the cardiac, pulmonary, and muscular systems.

The following sections will attempt to briefly distinguish cardiac dysfunction and failure from pulmonary, vascular, and muscular dysfunctions and failures. Furthermore, they will also attempt to outline the pertinent information that can be obtained from an exercise test. The primary reason patients with known or suspected heart disease undergo an exercise test

is to examine the electrocardiogram for signs of myocardial ischemia. Although this is the primary reason for the administration of an exercise test, much more important information can be obtained from a properly performed exercise test. Diagnostic and prognostic information can be obtained from exercise testing with and without electrocardiographic interpretation and analyses. The goals of this section are to review the methods and results of exercise testing in patients with

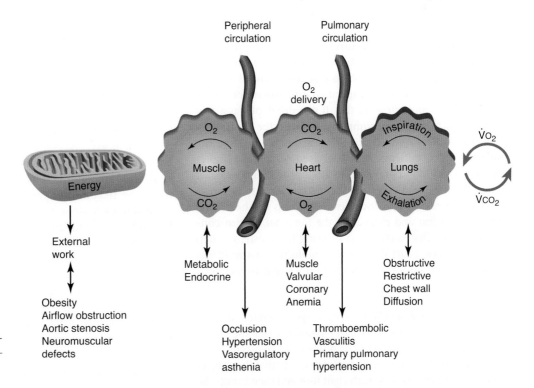

FIGURE 10-12 The interrelationship among cardiac, pulmonary, and muscular systems.

known or suspected heart disease and to highlight the diagnostic and prognostic information obtained from an exercise test. The methods of electrocardiographic interpretation and analysis will be presented in the following chapter.

Traditional Exercise Testing

Exercise testing in the United States has undergone a significant history. A variety of modes to exercise patients and protocols to follow when performing an exercise test have been used over the years. The first mode of exercise used in exercise testing was the step test from which other similar and more sophisticated methods were employed. Today in the United States, the most common mode of exercise to administer an exercise test is the treadmill ergometer (or simply, the motorized treadmill). The most common protocol is likely the Bruce, which was first introduced in 1973 by Robert Bruce. Table 10-19 provides a historical perspective of exercise testing in the United States. It is striking how the development of particular modes, methods, and protocols were dependent on the initial work of Master, in 1920, who introduced the first exercise test, the step test.

Step Tests

Step tests were the first mode to administer exercise to subjects with known or suspected heart disease. The first step test appears to have been developed by Leo Master and resulted in the Master's 2-Step Test. However, Master developed the step test from reports by his contemporaries who had subjects ascend a certain number of steps in a specific time period. A brief description of the step tests will be presented below with the equipment, methods, and use of results.

Master's 2-Step Test—Master's 2-Step Test is a step test that was developed to quickly examine large groups of subjects for health screening. The 2-Step Test is simply a test in which subjects ascend and descend two steps in synchrony with a metronome. Figure 9-13 in Chapter 9 shows the procedure used to perform the Master 2-Step Test and the need for specially constructed steps (with specified dimensions for height and width) to standardize the test. It was developed as a tool to first predict oxygen consumption, but with the clinical use of electrocardiography in the 1950s it quickly became the mode by which patients were exercised to achieve higher heart rates and blood pressures to attempt to diagnose heart disease. Figure 10-13 describes the method used to interpret the step test results and includes measuring the heart rate after the step test and estimating the maximal oxygen consumption. The first such report of using the Master's 2-Step Test to diagnose heart disease was published in the 1950s. From this point on, exercise testing underwent tremendous growth.

1-Step Test—The *1-Step Test* was developed from the Master's 2-Step Test and appears to have developed because the 2-Step Test was too time consuming. The procedure consists of 1 step that is ascended and descended in such a way that the subject initially steps onto the step with right foot and then brings the left foot onto the step. The right foot is then removed from the step and placed on the floor that is followed by the left foot. The stepping sequence begins again, but the left foot is initially placed on the step followed by the right foot. This reciprocal sequence of right foot up followed by left foot, right foot down followed by left foot, left foot up followed by right foot, and left foot down followed by right foot down is done in synchrony with a metronome. The heart rate at the end of the step test was then used to estimate oxygen consumption (Fig. 10–13).

Climbing-Step Test—The *Climbing-Step Test* was an extension of the aforementioned step tests and appears to have been developed to again decrease the time required of 1- and 2-step tests. The Climbing-Step Test was developed by the German physician Kaltenbach, who found the standard step tests too time consuming. Therefore, he added a component of arm exercise to increase the heart rate and blood pressure response. This method of testing was done primarily to diagnose heart disease and examine the electrocardiogram for evidence of myocardial ischemia. The Climbing-Step Test also utilized standardized steps and arm heights, which were used in the manner shown in Fig. 9-13 in Chapter 9. The results of the Climbing-Step Test were then used to estimate fitness level, oxygen consumption, and presence or absence of heart disease.

Cycle Ergometry Tests

Shortly after step tests became an accepted method to diagnose heart disease, European physiologists began studying the physiologic response to cycle ergometry. The most prolific and noteworthy investigator of the exercise response to cycling was Per Olif Astrand. Astrand standardized cycle ergometry testing and developed normal values that could be estimated based on a given level of work. These standardized estimated values for healthy individuals are still in use today. A number of cycling protocols exist, but the most common appear to be the Astrand–Rhyming protocol, the YMCA protocol, and ramping protocols.

Treadmill Tests

As European and American physicians and physiologists continued to use cycling ergometry exercise tests and step tests to diagnose heart disease, the treadmill ergometer was fast becoming a mode of exercise that no longer was limited to specialized laboratories. Physicians in the United States began using the treadmill ergometer almost exclusively after the seminal work of Robert Bruce was published in April of 1973. Robert Bruce was the co-director of cardiology at the University of Washington in Seattle, Washington. He had experimented with treadmill testing for approximately 10 years during which time he gathered extensive data and examined the cardiorespiratory response to treadmill exercise in healthy persons and patients with heart disease. In 1973, he published the article Maximal Oxygen Intake and Nomographic Assessment of Functional Aerobic Impairment in Cardiovascular Disease in the *American Heart Journal.* This paper described the Bruce exercise testing protocol, which is still likely the most popular

TABLE 10-19 History of Exercise Testing

Date	Historical Figure	Contribution
1908	Einthoven	Published the first ECG tracing of ST segment depression, but did not comment on the cause of the depression
1918	Bousfield	First to record ST-segment depression in the 3 standard ECG leads during a spontaneous episode of angina
1928	Feil and Siegal	First to exercise patients with known angina and simultaneously record an ECG. The exercise consisted of sit-ups without and with pressure applied to the patient's chests. Pressure applied to the chests was done to increase the resistance and work of sitting up. They also hypothesized that the ST segment depression was due to decreased coronary blood flow and published ECG tracings showing the ST segments return to normal after the pain had subsided and also after the administration of nitroglycerin.
1929	Master	First to develop an exercise test protocol using a stepping test and recognized the importance of monitoring heart rate and blood pressure, but not the ECG.
1931	Wood and Wolferth	Described ST-segment changes during exercise and indicated its usefulness in the diagnosis of coronary artery disease (especially precordial lead 4). However, they believed it was too dangerous to exercise test patients with known coronary disease.
1932	Goldhammer and Scherf	First to publish that a significant percentage of patients with angina had ST-segment depression (75% of 40 patients) during exercise testing, but also discussed the notion of false-negative and -positive exercise test results.
1935	Katz and Landt	Found precordial lead 5 to better discriminate coronary artery disease than lead 4 using a standardized exercise test of lifting dumbbells while lying supine. They also hypothesized that pain and ischemia were related to catabolism in the myocardium and studied the effects of anoxia and intravenous epinephrine on the ST segment.
1938	Missal	Possibly the first person to perform a maximal exercise test by having patients run up 3 to 6 flights of stairs, but later elected to use Master's 9-in. steps. He exercised patients to the point of pain and emphasized the importance of recording the ECG at the point of pain. He also was the first person to document the increase in exercise tolerance after administration of nitroglycerin.
1940	Riseman, Waller, and Brown	First to publish a review article comparing a test of anoxia to exercise testing in which they emphasized the importance of continuous ECG monitoring, that ST-segment depression usually appeared before the onset of angina and usually persisted after the pain had subsided, that mild ST-segment depression (1.0 mm or less) may occur in normal subjects while patients were likely to have more ST-segment depression (2.0–7.0 mm), and that a test of anoxia was of greater practical value than exercise testing.
1941	Master and Jaffe	Proposed for the first time that an ECG could be obtained before and immediately after his step test described 12 years earlier to improve the diagnosis of coronary artery disease.
1941	Liebow and Feil	First to report that digitalis produced ST-segment depression, which could confuse the diagnosis of ischemia in the exercise ECG.
1942	Johnson, Brouha, and Darling	They developed the Harvard Step Test while working at the Harvard Fatigue Laboratory that was used widely among athletic programs to document fitness level based upon the heart rate response during recovery.
1943	Brouha and Heath	First to use the Harvard Step Test to evaluate the cardiovascular response to various occupations and environmental conditions.
1949	Hellerstein and Katz	First to study the direction of the ECG vector and confirmed that ST segment depression is primarily a diastolic injury current manifested during the TQ interval.
1949	Hecht	Reported 90% sensitivity in diagnosing coronary artery disease with the anoxia test and that previous myocardial necrosis is likely to mask ECG signs of ischemia.
1950	Wood et al.	First to establish several important exercise testing points including the likelihood that the amount of work performed should not be fixed, but adjusted to a patient's capacity; the more strenuous the exercise, the greater the number of true positive tests in patients with known coronary disease; and different exercise test protocols demonstrated different levels of reliability, sensitivity, and specificity. Their test consisted of having patients run up 84 steps adjacent to their laboratory at London's National Heart Hospital.
1951	Yu et al.	First to report an exercise test protocol performed on a motor-driven treadmill elevated to a 10% or 20% grade.
1952	Yu and Soffer	Using the Master's Step Test they identified several important ECG findings indicative of myocardial ischemia including 1.0 mm or more of ST-segment depression, T-wave alterations (upright to inverted or vice versa and increased amplitude), and prolonged QT/TQ ratios.
1954	Astrand and Rhyming	First to document that peak oxygen consumption was correlated to heart rate during submaximal exercise.
1956	Bruce	Presented a treadmill exercise test with standardized guidelines that was used to group patients into the New York Heart Association classifications 1–4.
1959	Balke and Ware	First to establish the importance of exercise testing military personnel and developed a formula to estimate oxygen uptake associated with treadmill walking.

(continued)

TABLE 10-19   **History of Exercise Testing (***Continued***)**

Date	Historical Figure	Contribution
1959	Hellerstein	First to demonstrate to employers that employees with cardiac disease could safely return to work based on his investigation of the oxygen cost of various activities and onset of ischemia related to various workloads and types of work. This work led to the beginning of cardiac rehabilitation.
1966	Blackburn	Important contribution to exercise testing by reporting on the clinical utility of ECG monitoring using V5 or CM5 which enabled exercise testing to be performed outside of the research laboratory.
1967	Robb and Marks	First to present the predictive value of ST-segment depression in 2224 males applying for life insurance. They identified that horizontal and down-sloping ST-segment depression was most predictive of coronary disease.
1968	Najmi et al.	First to correlate ST-segment changes with coronary arteriography.
1971	Rochmis and Blackburn	First to examine the safety of exercise testing reporting a morbidity rate of 2.4/10,000 exercise tests and a mortality rate of 1/10,000 exercise tests.
1975	Wasserman and Whipp	Possibly the first to describe how exercise test results could be used to differentiate different diseases and disorders.
1980	ACSM[a]	Established guidelines for graded exercise testing.
1987	CIGNA Study	First to examine the safety of independent exercise testing by physical therapists reporting a morbidity rate of 3.8/10,000 exercise tests and a mortality rate of 0.9/10,000 exercise tests.
1997	Franklin et al.	Reported on the clinical efficacy of independent nonphysician exercise testing.

[a]ACSM = American College of Sports Medicine.

protocol for testing patients with known or suspected heart disease. The reasons it likely remains the most popular treadmill protocol even today are because it (1) is dynamic exercise of large muscle groups using a functional task (walking and running if necessary), (2) begins with relative submaximal exertion and provides progressive increments of work until exhaustion, (3) is safe and relatively acceptable to patients, (4) requires minimal time to perform (perhaps this is one of the most important reasons), and (5) has established normal standard values of oxygen consumption and functional impairment based on the duration of exercise. These same reasons were given as rationale for the development of this protocol by Dr. Bruce at the time of the 1973 publication in the American Heart Journal.

Bruce protocol—The Bruce protocol is a relatively straightforward exercise testing protocol consisting of 3-minute intervals of incremental workloads beginning with a speed of 1.7 mph and a 10% grade and progressing to increased tread-mill speeds and grades every 3 minutes until exhaustion or a predetermined endpoint is attained. The Bruce treadmill exercise testing protocol is shown in Table 10-20. Corresponding to this protocol are the data shown in Fig. 10-14, which show the cardiorespiratory response of normal men and women and cardiac men. It is clear from this figure that there is a relatively linear response to oxygen consumption using the Bruce protocol. This figure also shows the slight differences in submaximal and maximal oxygen consumption among normal men and women and cardiac men. In fact, close examination of Fig. 10-14 reveals that women without heart disease who exercised more than 10 minutes were observed to have a higher level of oxygen consumption than men without heart disease. This is typically not the case (men usually have a higher level of peak oxygen consumption), but Bruce suggested that the reason for this finding in his study was the fact that the women were well-trained athletes.

Other important results of this study are shown in Table 10-20 and Fig. 10-15. Table 10-20 provides a simple equation to estimate maximal oxygen consumption based on the amount of time completed during the Bruce protocol. Maximal oxygen consumption $\dot{V}O_{2max}$ *for healthy men and women* was estimated with the following equation: $\dot{V}O_{2max} = 6.70 - 2.82$ (gender factor of 1 for men and 2 for women) $+ 0.056$ (time completed during the Bruce protocol in seconds). Maximal oxygen consumption *for cardiac men* was estimated with the following equation $\dot{V}O_{2max} = 10.5 + 0.035$ (time completed during the Bruce protocol in seconds). Figure 10-15 shows three nomograms developed with the data from this study by Bruce. The three nomograms allow for the prediction of the functional aerobic impairment (FAI), which is defined as the difference between the predicted and the measured maximal oxygen consumption divided by the predicted oxygen consumption (FAI = predicated $\dot{V}O_{2max}$ − measured $\dot{V}O_{2max}$/predicated $\dot{V}O_{2max}$). Using a ruler, the FAI can be determined by

TABLE 10-20   **A Comparison of the Bruce and Naughton Exercise Test Protocols**

Stages	Bruce Protocol	Naughton Protocol
1	1.7 mph, 10% grade × 3 min	1.2 mph, 0% grade × 2 min
2	2.5 mph, 12% grade × 3 min	1.5 mph, 0% grade × 2 min
3	3.4 mph, 14% grade × 3 min	1.5 mph, 3% grade × 2 min
4	4.2 mph, 16% grade × 3 min	1.5 mph, 6% grade × 2 min
5	5.2 mph, 18% grade × 3 min	1.5 mph, 9% grade × 2 min
6	6.0 mph, 20% grade × 3 min	2.0 mph, 12% grade × 2 min

Data from Fox S, Naughton J, Haskell W. Physical activity and the prevention of coronary heart disease. *Ann Clin Res*. 1971;3(6):404-432.

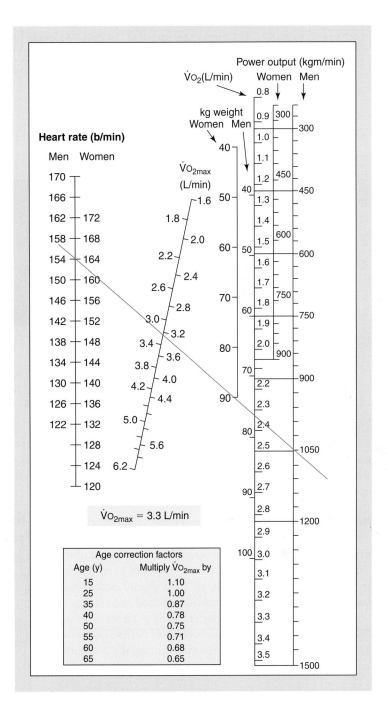

FIGURE 10-13 Nomogram utilizing measurement of heart rate and the results of the step test to predict oxygen consumption. (Used with permission from Robergs R, Roberts S. *Exercise, Physiology: Exercise, Performance and Clinical Applications*. The McGraw-Hill Companies; 1997.)

placing 1 end of the ruler at the point representing age (on the A axis) and the other end of the ruler on the point representing the duration of exercise (in minutes) on the Bruce protocol (on the B axis). The FAI is then evaluated based on the activity level of the individual that can be interpreted as either sedentary or active. No specific definition of either sedentary or active was described by Bruce, so this parameter is left to the interpretation of the examiner. The range for FAI using these nomograms is between −20% and +70%. An FAI of −20% is associated with no FAI (actually, no FAI is measured at 0%, and −20% represents a person with an aerobic capacity above the normal standard), whereas an FAI of +70% represents a person with significantly impaired aerobic capacity.

The results of the 1973 Bruce article provided a standardized format for exercise testing of healthy men and women and for men with cardiac disease. He did not study women with cardiac disease and subsequently was unable to provide data to estimate oxygen consumption of FAI of women with heart disease. Overall, the Bruce exercise testing protocol was observed to be acceptable for many patients. However, the rather large and rapid workload increments of the Bruce protocol were found to be less acceptable by patients who were debilitated. Additionally, the amount of useful information was limited because the muscular systems of the debilitated patients fatigued before the cardiac, pulmonary, or cardiovascular systems were taxed, thus yielding

I 1.7 mph, 10% grade	II 2.5 mph, 12% grade	III 3.4 mph, 14% grade	IV 4.2 mph, 16% grade

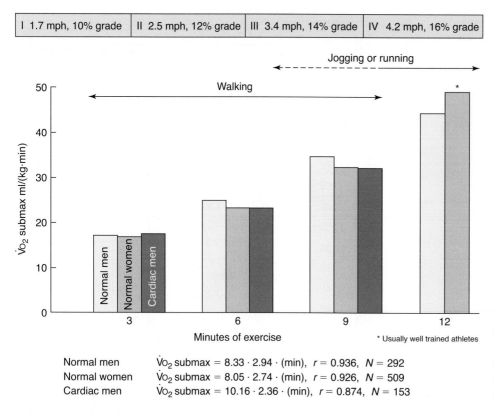

FIGURE 10-14   Aerobic requirements for multistage treadmill exercise stress test (submaximal only). (Modified with permission from Bruce RA, Kusumi F, Hosmer D. Maximal oxygen intake and nomographic assessment of functional aerobic impairment in cardiovascular disease. *Am Heart J.* 1973;85(4):546-560.)

Normal men	$\dot{V}O_2$ submax = 8.33 · 2.94 · (min), $r = 0.936$, $N = 292$
Normal women	$\dot{V}O_2$ submax = 8.05 · 2.74 · (min), $r = 0.926$, $N = 509$
Cardiac men	$\dot{V}O_2$ submax = 10.16 · 2.36 · (min), $r = 0.874$, $N = 153$

little useful information about these other systems (which likely was the reason for the test). Therefore, exercise testing protocols with more gradual and lower increments of work were developed. One such protocol was the Naughton.

Naughton protocol—*The Naughton protocol* is a lower-level exercise testing protocol developed by John Naughton. It is somewhat difficult to find the actual first description of the complete Naughton protocol, but the protocol as performed today is also outlined in Table 10-20. It should be apparent from Table 10-20 that the gradual workload increments of the Naughton protocol are preferred by patients who are debilitated. For this reason and because of perhaps a greater linearity in cardiorespiratory response during the Naughton

protocol, it is the exercise testing protocol most often used in patients who are debilitated such as those with heart failure.

Distinguishing Characteristics From Exercise Test Results

Earlier in this section it was suggested that a distinction between or among the cardiac, pulmonary, and muscular systems could be made using exercise test results. This section will describe several important distinguishing characteristics based on information provided in Chapter 3 and presented earlier in this chapter. Of major importance is once again appreciating

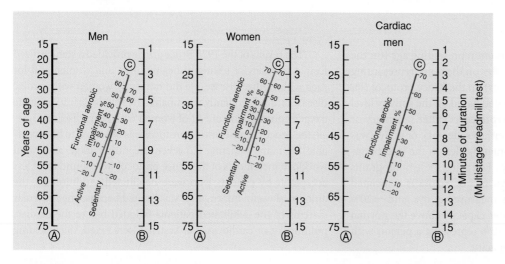

FIGURE 10-15   Bruce nomograms of functional aerobic impairment (FAI) for (A) men, (B) women, and (C) cardiac men. (Reprinted with permission from Bruce RA, Kusumi F, Hosmer D. Maximal oxygen uptake and nomographic assessment of functional aerobic impairment in cardiovascular disease. *Am Heart J.* 1973;85:545.)

the Fick equation ($\dot{V}O_2$ = heart rate × stroke volume × arteriovenous oxygen difference). This equation and several other variables will be used to distinguish between and among cardiac and pulmonary disease, cardiac and cardiovascular disease, cardiac and muscular disease, pulmonary and muscular disease, cardiovascular and muscular disease, and cardiovascular and pulmonary disease.

Distinction Between Cardiac and Pulmonary Disease

The distinction between cardiac and pulmonary disease may be the simplest of all the distinctions listed previously. This is because a distinction can be made by examining the heart rate alone during standardized exercise testing. Figure 10-16A shows the relationship of the heart rate and oxygen consumption during exercise testing in octogenarians, normal subjects, and patients with cardiac and respiratory diseases. It should be clear that the heart rate response of the cardiac patients is much greater at lower workloads than that of the patients with respiratory disease and the other two groups (octogenarians and normal subjects). The reason that this was observed is due to the Fick equation ($\dot{V}O_2$ = heart rate × stroke volume × arteriovenous oxygen difference). Because patients with cardiac disease have a reduced stroke volume during exercise (because of myocardial ischemia or infarction), the heart rate must be greater to maintain cardiac output and the work performance. This particular finding is also shown in Fig. 10-16B, where the oxygen pulse (milliliters of oxygen consumed per heart rate) is lower in the patients with cardiac disease compared to that in the other groups. The oxygen pulse is generally accepted as an indirect measure of stroke volume and in keeping with the common finding of a reduced stroke volume with heart disease, the oxygen pulse is also observed to be lower in heart disease than in pulmonary disease in the other groups shown in Fig. 10-16. Other distinguishing characteristics are presented in Table 10-21.

Distinction Between Cardiac and Cardiovascular Disease

The distinction between cardiac and cardiovascular disease is difficult because both often accompany each other. However, depending on the type of cardiovascular disease, particular signs or symptoms may be present that can help to distinguish cardiac from cardiovascular disease. Several signs and symptoms suggestive of cardiovascular disease include attainment of only low levels of exercise and work due to intermittent claudication in the calf musculature, a hypertensive blood pressure response, attainment of a low peak heart rate, an attenuated or blunted heart rate response, and a decreased systolic blood pressure in the lower extremities after exercise. This last finding of a decreased systolic blood pressure at the ankle after exercise and several other findings consistent with cardiovascular disease (eg, a low ankle–brachial index, delayed venous filling time, and a positive rubor dependency test) can be found in several earlier sections of this chapter. Other distinguishing characteristics are shown in Table 10-21.

Distinction Between Cardiac and Muscular Disease

The distinction between cardiac and muscular disease is not that dissimilar from the distinction discussed for cardiac and cardiovascular disease. The characteristics of muscular disease would be associated with many of the same signs during exercise testing (low levels of exercise and work due to muscular fatigue, attainment of a low peak heart rate, or an attenuated or blunted heart rate response). Other characteristics are presented in Table 10-21.

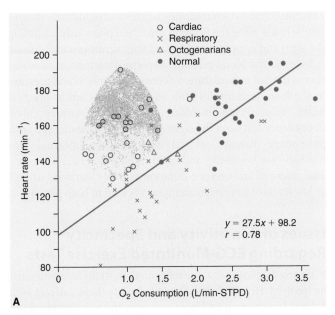

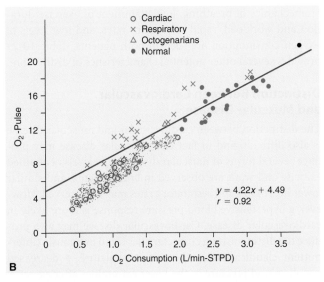

FIGURE 10-16 Wasserman and Whip plots of the (**A**) relationships of heart rate and (**B**) oxygen pulse to oxygen consumption. (Used with permission from Wasserman K, Whipp B. Exercise physiology in health and disease. *Am Rev Respir Dis.* 1975;112(2):219-249.)

TABLE 10-21   **Distinguishing Characteristics Among Cardiac, Pulmonary, Cardiovascular, and Muscular Diseases Using Exercise Test Results**[a,b]

	Cardiac Disease	Pulmonary Disease	Cardiovascular Disease	Muscular Disease
Cardiac disease	—	Lower HR, Sao$_2$, and peak $\dot{V}o_2$; Higher O$_2$ Pulse **and RR; ABP**	Lower WKL, peak HR and peak $\dot{V}o_2$; Lower ABI	**Lower WKL, peak HR, peak $\dot{V}o_2$, and skeletal mm strength and endurance;** possibly ABP and rapid RR
Pulmonary disease	Higher HR and peak $\dot{V}o_2$; lower O$_2$ Pulse and RR; **often no ABP, VLE, and normal Sao$_2$**	—	Often similar WKL, HR, and peak $\dot{V}o_2$; **no ABP and lower ABI**	Often similar WKL, HR, and peak $\dot{V}o_2$; **often lower RR and higher Sao$_2$; often less ABP and skeletal mm strength and endurance**[a]
Cardiovascular disease	Higher WKL, peak HR, peak $\dot{V}o_2$, and **ABI**	Often similar WKL, HR, and peak $\dot{V}o_2$; ABP; **Higher RR and ABI; Lower Sao$_2$**	—	Often similar WKL, HR, and peak $\dot{V}o_2$; **higher ABI; often less skeletal mm strength and endurance**[c]
Muscular disease	**Higher WKL, peak HR, peak $\dot{V}o_2$;** often greater skeletal mm strength and endurance[c]	Often similar WKL, HR, and peak $\dot{V}o_2$; **ABP;** often higher RR and lower Sao$_2$; **often greater skeletal mm strength and endurance**[c]	Often similar WKL, HR, and peak $\dot{V}o_2$; **lower ABI;** often greater skeletal mm strength and endurance	—

[a]To use this table in an attempt to distinguish one disease from others, it is necessary to use the top portion of this table as the disease being distinguished. For example, cardiac disease is distinguished from pulmonary disease by the findings in the cell under the bolded **Cardiac Disease** (on the top portion). The other diseases bolded in the top portion are similarly distinguished from the other disease in the unbolded section in the far-left hand column.

[b]The most likely significant distinguishing characteristic between diseases is bolded. HR, heart rate; Sao$_2$, oxygen saturation; $\dot{V}o_2$, oxygen consumption; O$_2$, oxygen; RR, respiratory rate; ABP, abnormal breathing pattern; VLE, ventilatory limit to exercise; WKL, workload; ABI, ankle–brachial index; mm, muscle.

[c]The skeletal muscle strength of patients with chronic heart and lung diseases may develop myopathic abnormalities due to several reasons including a chronic debilitating condition that decreases exercise abilities, decreased oxygenated blood flow to the skeletal muscles, and mitochondrial abnormalities due to a variety of causes.

Distinction Between Pulmonary and Muscular Disease

The distinction between pulmonary and muscular disease is difficult because many of the signs and symptoms of pulmonary disease are the same as those of muscular disease. Several possible distinguishing characteristics are signs of arterial desaturation with pulmonary disease. However, abnormal biomechanics of breathing, low attainment of exercise duration and workload, rapid respiratory rates, and low levels of oxygen consumption are seen in both patients. Table 10-21 provides several other potential characteristics of distinction.

Distinction Between Cardiovascular and Muscular Disease

The distinction between cardiovascular and muscular disease is also difficult, and in fact cardiovascular disease may produce several forms of muscular disease. Low levels of attained exercise and work are observed in both patients, and similar lower heart rates and respiratory rates may be observed. However, a hypertensive blood pressure response is more likely in cardiovascular disease. Cardiovascular disease may also produce the distinguishing characteristics listed previously (intermittent claudication in the calf musculature, a decreased systolic blood pressure in the lower extremities after exercise, a low ankle–brachial index, delayed venous filling time, and a positive rubor dependency test). Again, the specific methods to perform these examinations can be found in the previous sections, and other possible distinguishing characteristics are shown in Table 10-21.

Distinction Between Cardiovascular and Pulmonary Disease

The distinction between cardiovascular and pulmonary disease can be made using the findings discussed previously, including the signs and symptoms associated with cardiovascular disease (a hypertensive blood pressure response, intermittent claudication in the calf musculature, a decreased systolic blood pressure in the lower extremities after exercise, a low ankle–brachial index, delayed venous filling time, and a positive rubor dependency test) and the signs and symptoms associated with pulmonary disease (arterial desaturation, abnormal biomechanics of breathing, and rapid respiratory rates). However, attainment of low exercise duration and low workload as well as low levels of oxygen consumption is seen in both patients.

Issues of Sensitivity and Specificity Regarding ECG-Monitored Exercise Tests

With any diagnostic test, the following questions arise and must be resolved: How well does the test identify those patients with disease (*sensitivity*); and how well does the test identify those patients without disease (*specificity*)? In order to answer these questions, test results must be compared to some sort of a benchmark or gold standard. In the case of diagnostic stress tests, that benchmark is coronary angiography, which allows direct visualization of the coronary anatomy and exposes lesions of atherosclerosis which is the etiology of coronary artery disease. Coronary angiography is both risky and costly: Clearly, it is to both the patient's and the clinician's advantage to substitute (whenever possible) coronary angiography for a test that possesses both good sensitivity and good specificity. An ECG-monitored stress test is noninvasive, relatively inexpensive, and easy to administer. The hallmark of myocardial ischemia is depression of the ST segment that comes on with exercise and resolves with rest. Use of ECG monitoring during exercise testing maximizes both sensitivity and specificity when the ECG criterion for a positive test is established at 1.0 mm of ST-segment depression.

In order to understand the clinical implications of sensitivity and specificity, we will consider two scenarios:

1. Let us arbitrarily set the ECG diagnostic criterion at 0.5 mm of ST-segment depression. It should be obvious that setting the criterion at such a low level will cause a lot of subjects to rule in for coronary disease. However, if they subsequently undergo coronary angiography, very few of these subjects will show evidence of coronary artery disease. This is an example of a test with *very high sensitivity*.
2. Now let us arbitrarily set the ECG diagnostic criterion at 2.0 mm of ST-segment depression. It should be obvious that setting the criterion at such a high level will cause very few subjects to rule in for coronary disease. However, if they subsequently undergo coronary angiography, almost all of these subjects will show evidence of coronary artery disease. This is an example of a test with *very high specificity*.

Clearly, sensitivity and specificity are reciprocal to each other and, within any given test, need to be balanced so that the test accurately identifies not only those individuals who have the disease, but also those people who do not.

It turns out that sensitivity and specificity are maximized when the ECG criterion is set at 1.0 mm of ST-segment depression. Indeed, when data from multiple studies are pooled, meta-analysis of noninvasive ECG exercise testing demonstrates a sensitivity of 68% and a specificity of 77%.[10]

Walk Tests

Walk tests have also been used in patients with heart disease. They have been used extensively in the examination of patients with heart failure. The same methods described in Chapter 9 can be used when performing a walk test in a patient with heart disease. The 6-minute walk test appears to provide information about the functional status, exercise tolerance, oxygen consumption, and survival of persons with cardiac pump failure. Although the exercise performed during the 6-minute walk test is considered submaximal, it nonetheless closely approximates the maximal exercise of persons with cardiac pump failure and is correlated to peak oxygen consumption (Fig. 10-17A). Additionally, information obtained from the 6-minute walk test has been used to predict peak oxygen consumption and survival in persons with advanced heart failure

BOX 10-8

Prediction Equations for Peak Oxygen Consumption and expected 6-Minute Walk Test Distance Ambulated in Persons with Cardiac Pump Failure

Prediction equations for peak oxygen consumption in patients with heart failure using 6-minute walk test results

1. Distance

$$\text{Peak } \dot{V}_{O_2} = 0.03 \times \text{distance (m)} + 3.98$$
$$r = 0.64; r^2 = 0.42; P < 0.0001; \text{SEE} = 3.32^*$$

2. Distance + age + weight + height + RPP

$$\text{Peak } \dot{V}_{O_2} = 0.02 \times \text{distance (m)} - 0.191 \times \text{age (y)}$$
$$- 0.07 \times \text{weight (kg)} + 0.09 \times \text{height (cm)}$$
$$+ 0.26 \times \text{RPP} (\times 10^{-3}) + 2.45$$
$$r = 0.81; r^2 = 0.65; P < 0.0001; \text{SEE} = 2.68$$

3. Distance + age + weight + height + RPP + FEV$_1$ + FVC

$$\text{Peak } \dot{V}_{O_2} = 0.02 \times \text{distance (m)} - 0.14 \times \text{age (y)} - 0.07$$
$$\times \text{weight (kg)} + 0.03 \times \text{height (cm)} + 0.23 \times \text{RPP}$$
$$(\times 10^{-3}) + 0.10 \times \text{FEV}_1 (1) + 1.19 \times \text{FVC} (1) + 7.77$$
$$r = 0.83; r^2 = 0.69; P < 0.0001; \text{SEE} = 2.59$$

4. Distance + age + weight + height + RPP + LVEF + PAP + CI

$$\text{Peak } \dot{V}_{O_2} = 0.02 \times \text{distance (m)} - 0.15 \times \text{age (y)} - 0.05$$
$$\times \text{weight (kg)} + 0.04 \times \text{height (cm)} + 0.17 \times \text{RPP}$$
$$(\times 10^{-3}) + 0.03 \times \text{EF (\%)} - 0.04 \times \text{PAP (mm Hg)}$$
$$+ 0.31 \times \text{CI (mL/min/m}^2) + 8.43$$
$$r = 0.85; r^2 = 0.72; P = 0.0001; \text{SEE} = 2.06$$

Prediction equation to determine the expected 6-minute walk test distance ambulated by heart failure patients

$$\text{SMWT (m)} = (\text{gender [1 = male, 0 = female]} \times 89) - (\text{age}$$
$$[\text{y}] \times 3) - (\text{HFdur [y]} \times 7.3) + 401$$
$$r^2 = 0.34; P < 0.0001$$

*r, correlation coefficient; r^2, coefficient of determination; SEE, standard error of the estimate; $\dot{V}_{O_{2max}}$, maximal oxygen consumption; RPP, rate–pressure product; LVEF, left ventricular ejection fraction; PAP, pulmonary artery pressure; CI, cardiac index; HFdur, heart failure duration.

awaiting cardiac transplantation (Box 10-8). Patients unable to ambulate greater than 300 m during the 6-minute walk test appear to have poorer survival (Fig. 10-17B).

Finally, the equations provided in Box 10-8 can be used to estimate peak oxygen consumption of patients with heart failure who are being examined for possible heart transplantation and who have undergone a 6-minute walk test. However, the predicted values of peak oxygen consumption have a relatively high standard error of the estimate (approximately

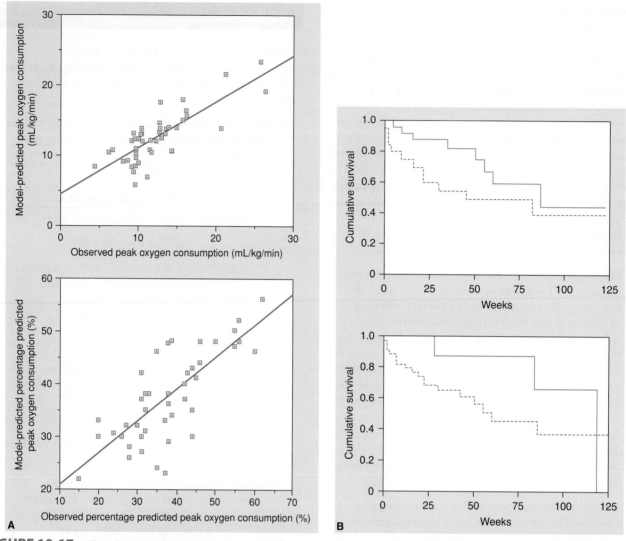

FIGURE 10-17   The relationship between the 6-minute walk test distance ambulated to (**A**) peak oxygen consumption and (**B**) survival. (Reprinted with permission from Cahalin LP, Mathier MA, Semigran MJ, Dec GW, DiSalvo TG. The six-minute walk test predicts peak oxygen uptake and survival in patients with advanced heart failure. *Chest.* 1996;110:325-332.)

2.0–3.0 mL/kg/min). Nonetheless, the ability to predict peak oxygen consumption from the 6-minute walk test can be helpful in categorizing and possibly treating patients with heart failure. Finally, we have developed a prediction equation to determine the normal or expected 6-minute walk test distance ambulated by heart failure patients. This equation is also shown in Box 10-8.

EXAMINATION OF OUTCOMES AND QUALITY OF LIFE IN HEART DISEASE

Table 10-22 provides an overview of many instruments that can be used to measure outcomes and quality of life in cardiac disease. The general health status questionnaires that can be used in patients with cardiac disease are the same general health questionnaires previously presented in Chapter 9 Table 9-16. The disease-specific questionnaires commonly used in persons suffering from heart disease are outlined in Table 10-22. Likewise, the strengths and weaknesses of the different

instruments are also presented in Box 10-8 and Table 10-22.[11,12] The most frequently used instruments used to evaluate the quality of life of persons with heart disease appear to be the general heart disease and the Minnesota Living with Heart Failure Questionnaire. The MOSSF-36 appears to be one of the most useful tools to examine general perceived health status (MOSSF-36) of patients with heart disease. The MOSSF-36 is shown in Fig. 9-14A to 9-14C, Chapter 9. The MLWHFQ is a 21-item questionnaire that evaluates socioeconomic, psychologic, and physical characteristics of patients with heart failure by using a Likert scale of 0 to 5. A score of 0 indicates that a patient has not been affected by heart failure within the past month, whereas a score of 5 indicates that the patient has been "very much" affected by heart failure within the past month. The higher the total score from the 21 questions, the poorer the quality of life. The worst quality of life would be associated with a total score of 105 (the maximum score of 5 on each of the 21 questions).

Finally, Box 10-9 shows the relationships among the MLWHFQ and several other instruments used to examine the

TABLE 10-22 Quality of Life and Health-Related Instruments Specific for Cardiac Disease

		Cardiac Disease Specific Quality of Life Instruments				
Instrument	Reference	What Is Measured?	Patient Population	Test Methods	Time to Complete	Source
Seattle Angina Questionnaire	Spertus J et al. *J Am Coll Cardiol.* 1995;25:333.	Phys, Symp, P (anginal)	CAD	Self-administered	4 min	Spertus J et al. *J Am Coll Cardiol.* 1995;25:333
Quality of Life after Acute MI Questionnaire	Oldridge N et al. *Am J Cardiol.* 1991;67:1084.	Phys, E, SE	CAD after MI	Interview	10 min	Oldridge N et al. *Am J Cardiol.* 1991;67:1084
MacNew Quality of Life after Acute MI Questionnaire[a]	Lim LY et al. *J Clin Epidemiol.* 1993; 46:1249.	QOL, Phys, E, S	CAD after MI	Self-administered	10 min	Lim LY et al. *J Clin Epidemiol.* 1993; 46:1249
Quality of Life Index-Cardiac Version III Questionnaire	Ferrans CE et al. *ANS Adv Nurs Sci.* 1985;8:15.	OH, F, S, Phys, SEC, QOL	CAD	Self-administered	10 min	Ferrans CE et al. *ANS Adv Nurs Sci.* 1985;8:15
Outcomes Institute Angina Type Specification Questionnaire	Rogers W et al. *J Am Coll Cardiol.* 1994;23:393.	QOL, P&PO	CAD	Self-administered	2–3 min	Rogers W et al. *J Am Coll Cardiol.* 1994;23:393
Minnesota Living with Heart Failure Questionnaire	Rector T et al. *Heart Failure.* 1987 Oct/Nov: 198–209.	QOL, Phys, S, Psy, SEC	CHF	Self-administered	15 min	Rector T et al. *Heart Failure.* 1987 Oct/Nov: 198–209.

[a]MacNew Quality of Life after Acute MI Questionnaire was adapted from the Quality of Life after Acute MI Questionnaire. CAD, coronary artery disease; MI, myocardial infarction; F, functional status; Phys, physical function; E, emotional function; S, social function; P, pain; QOL, quality of life; OH, overall health; SE, self-esteem; SEC, socioeconomic; P&PO, patient & physician outcomes; Psy, psychological.

BOX 10-9

Relationships Among Several Functional Classification Schemes Used in Congestive Heart Failure*

	NYHA†	SAS	CCSFCS	BDI	DFI	O_2CD	6WT	Ex. Dur.	$\dot{V}O_{2max}$	MLWHFQ
NYHA	×									
SAS		×								
CCSFCS			×							
BDI			0.55	×						
DFI*					×					
O_2CD				0.42	0.58	×				
6'WT	−0.45	0.47‡			0.59	0.49	×			
Ex. Dur.	−0.54	0.11p	−0.64	0.29P‖	0.30*	0.02p	0.57x¶	×		
$\dot{V}O_{2max}$								0.57§	×	
MLWHFQ		0.60 v#								×

*Although no correlations were developed among these classification schemes, the change in exercise duration after pharmacologic treatment (ACE inhibition via Captopril and Lisinopril) was correlated to the change in each of the three categories of the DFI (functional impairment, magnitude of task, and pace of task) and the total aggregate score with correlation coefficients of 0.21 to 0.37.

†NYHA, New York Heart Association Functional Classification Scheme; SAS, Specific Activity Scale; CCSFCS, Canadian Cardiovascular Society Functional Classification Scheme; BDI, baseline dyspnea index; DFI, dyspnea-fatigue index; O_2CD, oxygen cost diagram; 6'WT, 6-minute walk test; Ex. dur., exercise test exercise duration; $\dot{V}O_{2max}$, maximal oxygen consumption.

‡The relationship of the 6'WT to the SAS was also observed to be an indirect relationship with a correlation coefficient of −0.37 (See Guyatt G, Thompson P, Berman L, et al. How should we measure function in patients with chronic heart and lung disease? J Chronic Dis. 1985; 38(6): S17–S24.)

§The 6'WT was also found to be able to differentiate between the NYHA classification levels (I–IV) and the level of oxygen consumption.

¶Guyatt also found a significant correlation between these 2 variables that was slightly less than that in the Table ($r = 0.42$).

‖The correlation coefficients between these variables were not statistically significant (ex. dur. and SAS $p = 0.47$, ex. dur. and BDI $p = 0.06$, and ex. dur. and O_2CD $P = 0.89$).

#An important finding of the Rector study was the significant correlation ($r = 0.80$) between a question asked after the MLWHFQ was administered ("Overall, how much did your heart failure prevent you from living as you wanted during the last month?") and the total MLWHFQ score.

health status of persons with cardiac pump failure. It is important to note that of these instruments the 6-minute walk test was consistently found to be modestly correlated to other measures of health status and quality of life. This is an important characteristic in an examination tool and makes the 6-minute walk test an important test for persons with heart failure and possibly other cardiac diseases.

SUMMARY

The majority of the methods of examination presented in this chapter, like those presented in the pulmonary examination chapter, have focused on those that can be allocated by a physical therapist. The traditional medical tests and measures for a patient with cardiac disorders have also been presented, but the focus of these tests and measures has been on the clinical application for the patient being examined and treated by a physical therapist. A number of data sheets have also been incorporated into the tables of this chapter and an initial patient note has been provided in Appendix 1 of this textbook. The key tests and measures presented in this chapter include examining the (1) appearance of the patient, (2) feel of the pulse, (3) resting systolic and diastolic blood pressures, (4) systolic and diastolic blood pressures' response to a variety of perturbations, (5) heart sounds via auscultation, (6) specific signs and symptoms of cardiac and cardiovascular diseases, (7) direct and indirect measurements of cardiac and cardiovascular function, (8) exercise and functional abilities via exercise testing, and (9) outcome measures and quality of life of patients with known or suspected cardiac disorders. Of all these examinations, observing the signs and symptoms of cardiac and cardiovascular disease may be the most clinically useful for the physical therapist. Of the signs presented in this chapter, the manner in which the systolic and diastolic blood pressures respond to a variety of perturbations may be the most simple and informative in terms of examining the status of the cardiac and cardiovascular system. Furthermore, the arterial blood pressure response to the Valsalva maneuver appears to have the strongest supportive literature supporting its role in distinguishing a normal from failing cardiac pump. This simple test will be the basis for the hypothesis-oriented algorithm presented in Chapter 17. The information gained from this and other examinations presented in this chapter can then be used to allocate treatment interventions and determine appropriate outcome measures and effects on quality of life. The results of these examinations have been used to allocate further examinations and treatments based on previously published literature. Again, such evidence-based examination is needed in physical therapy.

APPENDIX 1

I. Expected systolic and diastolic blood pressures of children, adolescents, and young adults at specific ages (above which a child, adolescent, or young adult would be recognized to have hypertension).

II. Suggested laboratory exercises for cardiac examination

Laboratory Exercise 1—Evaluating Risk Factors for Heart Disease Risk-Factor Profiles

Laboratory Exercise 2—Effects of Body Position Change on Heart Rate and Blood Pressure

Laboratory Exercise 3—Effects of the Valsalva Maneuver on Heart Rate and Blood Pressure

Laboratory Exercise 4—Electrocardiography Practice

Laboratory Exercise 5—Auscultation of the Heart Practice

Laboratory Exercise 6—Echocardiography and Other Medical Tests Review via CD-ROM, World Wide Web, and Video

Laboratory Exercise 7—Exercise Testing Practice

Laboratory Exercise 8—Quality of Life Examination

Heads Up!

This chapter contains a CD-ROM activity.

REFERENCES

1. Kuri M, Hayashi Y, Kagawa K, et al. Evaluation of diagonal earlobe crease as a marker of coronary artery disease: the use of this sign in preoperative assessment. *Anaesthesia.* 2001;56(12):1160-1162.
2. Levy D, Bairey-Merz CN, Cody RJ, et al. Hypertension detection, treatment, and control—a call to action for cardiovascular specialists. *J Am Coll Cardiol.* 1999;34(4):1360.
3. Ewing DJ. Cardiac autonomic neuropathy. In: Jarrett RL, ed. *Diabetes and Heart Disease.* New York: Elsevier Science; 1984:1107.
4. Clements RSJ, Bell DS. Diabetic neuropathy: peripheral and autonomic syndromes. *Postgrad Med.* 1982;71:50.
5. Clements RSJ, Bell DS. Complications of diabetes. Prevalence, detection, current treatment, and prognosis. *Am J Med.* 1985;79:2.
6. Ewing DJ. Cardiac autonomic neuropathy. In: Jarrett RL, ed. *Diabetes and Heart Disease.* New York: Elsevier Science; 1984:1107.
7. Nardo CJ, Chambless LE, Light KC, et al. Descriptive epidemiology of blood pressure response to change in body position—The ARIC Study. *Hypertension.* 1999;33:1123.
8. Wallen T, Landahl S, Hedner T, et al. Atrial natriuretic peptides predict mortality in the elderly. *J Intern Med.* 1997;241:269.
9. Iivanainen AM, Tikkanen I, Tilvis R, et al. Associations between atrial natriuretic peptides, echocardiographic findings and mortality in an elderly population sample. *J Intern Med.* 1997;241:261.
10. Gibbons RJ, Balady GJ, Bricker J, et al. ACC/AHA 2002 guideline update for exercise testing: a report of the American College of Cardiology/American Heart Association Task Force on Practice Guidelines (Committee on Exercise Testing). 2002. American College of Cardiology Web site. http://www.ncbi.nlm.nih.gov/sites/entrez. Accessed December 22, 2009.
11. American Association of Cardiovascular and Pulmonary Rehabilitation Outcomes Committee. *Guidelines for Cardiac Rehabilitation and Secondary Prevention Programs.* 4th ed. Champaign, IL: Human Kinetics; 2004.
12. Guyatt GH, King DR, Feeny DH, Stubbing D, Goldstein RS. Generic and specific measurement of health-related quality of life in a clinical trial of respiratory rehabilitation. *J Clin Epidemiol.* 1999;52(3):187.

11

Electrocardiography

William E. DeTurk & Lawrence P. Cahalin

INTRODUCTION

The electrocardiogram (ECG) is a graphic representation of the depolarization of the heart. The physiology of depolarization of the heart is described in Chapter 5, and the particular pathways for conduction of the wave of depolarization are

Myocardial contraction (*systole*) and relaxation (*diastole*) are caused by myocardial cell depolarization and repolarization, respectively. The vector, or sum total, of all the electrical forces during any given cardiac cycle is called a *wave of depolarization*. This wave of depolarization moves down the normal conduction pathway from the atria to the ventricles, causes myocardial contraction, and produces deflections of the ECG waveform. **Three of the most important concepts regarding interpretation of the ECG are that (1) as the wave of depolarization moves *toward* a positive electrode, a *positive* deflection is observed on the ECG; (2) as the wave of depolarization moves *away from* a positive electrode, a *negative* deflection is observed on the ECG; and (3) as the wave of depolarization moves *perpendicular* to a positive electrode, an *isoelectric* deflection is observed on the ECG (ie, a deflection with both positive and negative components).** The ECG electrode and wires that attach to the electrodes transmit the heart's electrical activity to an ECG recorder or display and are shown in Fig. 11-1. The ECG electrode is very simple in construction, yet yields much important information about the cardiovascular system. For the correct interpretation of single- and multiple-lead ECGs, it is essential to remember the three rules listed previously.

Single-lead ECGs, or *rhythm strips*, are the graphic depiction of cardiac electrical activity from one particular view of the heart using two to three electrodes. Multiple-lead ECGs are the graphic depiction of cardiac electrical activity from multiple views of the heart using many electrodes. Multiple views are typically 12 in number and are grouped as *limb leads* and *precordial leads*. The standardized electrode placement for a typical 12-lead ECG recording is shown in Fig. 11-2.

The pathway for the conduction of the wave of depolarization initiated by the sinoatrial (SA) node is shown in

shown in Fig. 11-3. The ECG has undergone tremendous development and use since it was first applied to humans in 1887 by Augustus D. Waller.[1] A brief history of the ECG is presented in Table 11-1.[1-6]

Fig. 11-3. This pathway includes the intranodal pathways, atrioventricular (AV) node, AV bundle of His, right and left bundle branches, and Purkinje fibers, from which the final wave of depolarization spreads across the ventricles in an inferolateral direction. Normally, the SA node initiates the wave of depolarization. **However, it is important to note that, under certain conditions, other areas along the conduction pathway are capable of initiating an action potential and causing a wave of depolarization.** The following sections will describe (1) the basic construct of the ECG, (2) skills required for ECG interpretation, (3) common ECG rhythm disturbances and methods to interpret them, (4) 12-lead ECG interpretation, and (5) cardiac pacemakers.

BASIC CONSTRUCT OF THE ELECTROCARDIOGRAM

An electrocardiograph machine is an ECG recording unit consisting of a signal amplifier, filter, writing unit, and paper printout unit. A motor pulls special heat-sensitive paper across a set of heated styluses, which "burn" a series of ECG complexes onto the paper. The paper has a grid printed on the surface, consisting of small and large boxes. The small boxes are 1.0 mm square; five small boxes form one large box (see Fig. 11-5A).

The *X* axis, or horizontal axis, is *time*. The paper moves under the styli at a precise standardized speed, typically 25 mm/s. This dictates the value of one little box as 0.04 seconds, or 40 milliseconds. Similarly, the value of one big box is 0.20 seconds, or 200 milliseconds. There are five big boxes in 1 second. Many brands of ECG paper have marks placed on the top of the grid at 3-second intervals. As you will see, these marks can be used to measure heart rate (HR).

TABLE 11-1   **History of the Electrocardiogram**

Date	Historical Figure	Contribution
1842	Carlo Matteucci	First to find that an electric current accompanies each heart beat
1843	Emil Dubois-Reymond	First to find that an "action potential" accompanies muscular contraction
1872	Gabriel Lippmann	Invented a capillary electrometer (a thin glass tube with a mercury column beneath sulfuric acid—mercury was observed to move with an action potential)
1876	E. J. Marey	First to record a frog's electrical activity using a capillary electrometer
1878	John Burden Sanderson Frederick Page	First to describe that the heart's electrical activity consists of two phases, which later were labeled as the QRS and T waves
1887	Augustus D. Waller	Published the first human ECG
1890	G. J. Burch	Devised a mathematical correction for the sluggish fluctuations of the electrometer
1891	William Bayliss	Improved the electrometer and identified three Edward Starling phases of the heart's electrical activity, which were later called the P, QRS, and T waves
1893	Willem Einthoven	Introduced the term *electrocardiogram*
1895	Willem Einthoven	Improved the electrometer and identified five distinct deflections, which he names P, Q, R, S, and T waves
1897	Clement Ader	Developed an amplification system called a string galvanometer
1901	Willem Einthoven	Modified the string galvanometer to produce ECGs
1905	Willem Einthoven	Began transmitting ECGs via telephone cable from the hospital to his laboratory approximately 1.5 km away[a]
1906	Willem Einthoven	Published the first report on normal and abnormal ECGs[2]
1910	Walter James Horatio Williams	Published the first American review of electrocardiography and also transmitted ECGs from one location to another[3a]
1912	Willem Einthoven	Published the first report on an equilateral triangle formed by his standard limb leads (I, II, and III), which was later called Einthoven's triangle[4]
1920	Harold Pardee	Published the first ECG of an acute myocardial infarction[5]
1924	Willem Einthoven	Wins the Nobel Prize for inventing the electrocardiograph
1928	A. C. Ernstine and S. A. Levine	First to use vacuum tubes to apply the ECG, rather than the string galvanometer
1928	Frank Sanborn	Developed the frst portable ECG machine weighing 50 lb
1932	Charles Wolferth and Francis Wood	First to introduce and describe chest leads (V_1 through V_6)
1938	American Heart Association and Canadian General Standards Board	Published ECG standards[6]
1942	Emmanuel Goldberger	First to introduce and describe augmented limb leads (aVR, aVL, aVF), which together with Einthoven's three limb leads and Wolferth and Wood's chest leads completed the current 12-lead ECG[7]

[a]The first transtelephonic ECG systems that today is becoming somewhat of a common method to examine the ECG of a patient at a distant site.

The *Y* axis, or vertical axis, is *voltage*. The amount of electricity generated by myocardial cells is quite small and is measured in millivolts. The height of any given waveform is a function of the amount of muscle mass it represents. Thus, voltage from atrial depolarization is quite small relative to the voltage generated by the larger ventricles and produces a small deflection of the waveform.

Correct ECG interpretation assumes that the machine is calibrated and is running in a standardized mode. *Calibration marks* should be included in any given ECG tracing. These marks provide a known voltage for a known period of time. When present, they will appear on the ECG paper as either a boxlike upward, horizontal, and downward deflection or a vertical spike that separates one group of leads from the other (see Fig. 11-26). **An ECG machine that is calibrated to a standard moves ECG paper at 25 mm/s; a 1.0 mV signal deflects the stylus by 10 mm (10 mm/mV).**

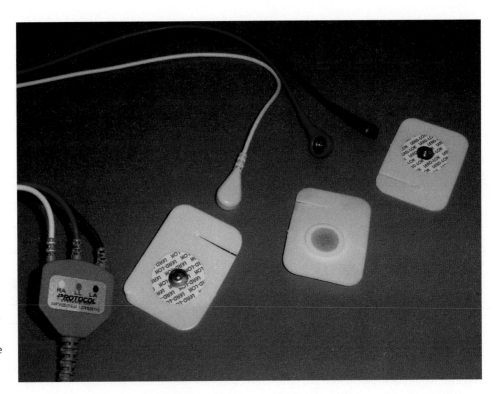

FIGURE 11-1 ECG electrodes consisting of a foam pad with an aggressive adhesive, a highly conductive electrolyte medium of silver–silver chloride, nipple clip onto which the wires attach, and the wires relaying the electrical activity of the heart to an ECG recorder or display.

DEPOLARIZATION OF THE HEART

Atrial Depolarization

Depolarization of the atria normally begins at the SA node. The SA node consists of a bundle of specialized neural conduction fibers, which spontaneously depolarizes and generates an action potential as ions move from one area to another. Once a critical concentration of sodium ions moves into the sarcoplasmic reticulum of the SA node, threshold is reached and an action potential is released. A wave of depolarization spreads downward to the AV node, bundle of His, bundle branches, and Purkinje fibers. This propagation of electrical activity can be captured with ECG electrodes and recorded on ECG recording paper with the equipment shown in Figs. 11-1 and 11-2. The typical ECG waveform representing one wave of depolarization (or one cardiac cycle) is shown in Fig. 11-4. The P wave represents atrial depolarization. Several specific aspects of the SA node give the P wave and PR interval their characteristic appearance. These aspects include the location, ion concentrations, and inherent atrial pathways down which the SA node action potential propagates.[8,9] The P wave is the result of sodium and calcium ion influx that produces atrial depolarization and contraction.

Atrioventricular Depolarization

Like the SA node, the AV node is also composed of a bundle of specialized neural conduction fibers, but they differ in construction from those of the SA node and therefore yield a different shaped action potential (Fig. 11-3). The PR segment represents conduction from the AV node through the bundle of His. Conduction velocity through AV node fibers is slower than that of the SA node. This contributes to the flat piece of baseline that separates the P wave from the QRS complex. The slow conduction velocity, which is due to differing ion concentrations and myocardial tissues, decreases the rapidness of the upslope for action potential development and slightly increases the time for repolarization, as fewer potassium ions move into the sarcoplasmic reticulum of the AV node.[8,9] This slowing of conduction through the AV node allows time for the atria to contract, and "top off" blood in the ventricles, which will in turn provide a "quick stretch" to the ventricles and enhance ventricular contraction.

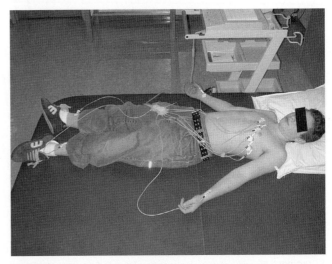

FIGURE 11-2 Placement of ECG electrodes on the limbs (for limb leads) and across the chest (for precordial leads).

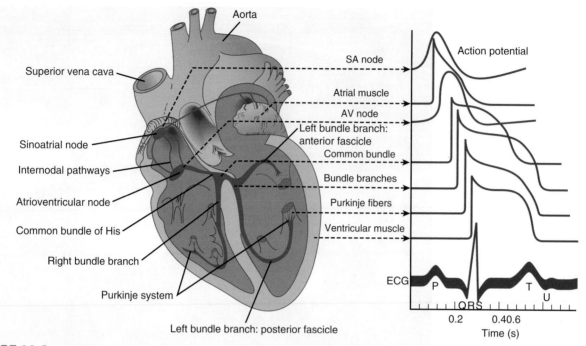

FIGURE 11-3   Conduction pathway that the wave of depolarization takes to elicit first atrial depolarization and subsequent contraction, and then ventricular depolarization and subsequent contraction. (Reproduced with permission from McPhee SJ. *Pathophysiology of Disease: An Introduction to Clinical Medicine.* 6th ed. New York: McGraw-Hill; 2010:250. Redrawn with permission from Ganong WF. *Review of Medical Physiology.* 22nd ed. McGraw-Hill; 2005.)

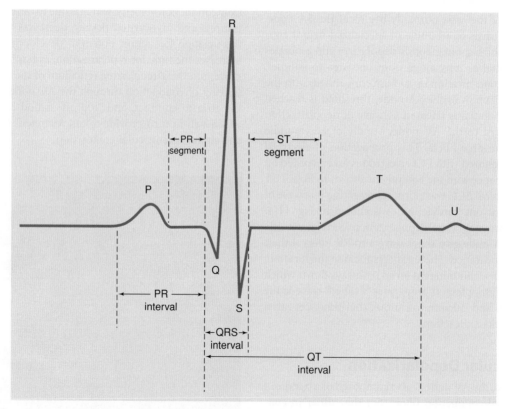

FIGURE 11-4   The typical ECG basic construct of the ECG with P, Q, R, S, T, and U waves; time intervals for the PR, QRS, and QT intervals; and ST segment. (Reproduced with permission from Tintinalli JE. *Emergency Medicine: A Comprehensive Study Guide.* 6th ed. New York: McGraw-Hill; 2004:181.)

Ventricular Depolarization

The ventricles of the heart propagate an action potential that is, again, different in appearance from SA and AV node action potentials. The QRS complex represents ventricular muscle depolarization. This waveform is typically *wide*, reflecting depolarization of nonspecialized, slow-conducting myocardium, and *tall*, reflecting the large amount of muscle mass present in the ventricles and the large voltage that such muscle mass generates. The morphology of the QRS complex is primarily due to ion concentrations within ventricular myocardium, which decrease the rapidness of the upslope for action potential development and increase the time for repolarization. Both of these aspects produce a wider and taller waveform.[8,9] The Q wave is the result of an influx of sodium and calcium ions into ventricular muscle (producing the negative deflection) that initiates ventricular contraction. The R and S waves are the result of greater levels of ion exchange in ventricular muscle during ventricular contraction.

The ST segment represents early ventricular repolarization. The T wave represents later ventricular repolarization. These waveforms are the result of an increase in potassium ion concentration within the sarcoplasmic reticulum of the myocardial fibrils and produce diastolic depolarization (needed for myocardial relaxation). The U wave is only occasionally seen on ECG and is the result of abnormal electrolyte and ion concentrations (either depleted or excessive concentrations).[8,9] Each of these waveforms represents areas that are very important for myocardial performance and will be discussed in greater detail in the following sections.[9-12]

ELECTROCARDIOGRAPHIC INTERPRETATION—BASIC SKILLS NEEDED

The basic skills needed for ECG interpretation include determination of (1) heart rate and rhythm for the recognition of rhythm disturbances, (2) relationships among the different waves of an ECG complex and the rhythm for the recognition of some rhythm disturbances, and (3) presence of myocardial ischemia, because most disturbances in cardiac rhythm are due to myocardial irritability from myocardial ischemia.[9-12] The following sections will review each of these essential skills.

Determining the Heart Rate

The heart rate can be measured using the methods already presented in Chapter 10. These include arterial palpation, cardiac auscultation, and use of a heart rate digital display watch. The ECG is considered the gold standard for determination of heart rate and as such is a good reference to measure the accuracy of these other heart rate measurements and to identify location of the cardiac cycle for these other examination techniques.[9-12] Measuring the heart rate from an ECG tracing can be performed using a heart rate ruler, estimating the heart rate using the 6-second marks on the ECG recording paper, or using a counting mnemonic representative of the mathematical calculations used to measure heart rate. The heart rate ruler method is simplest, whereas the counting mnemonic becomes less accurate at high and low heart rates.

Heart Rate Ruler Method

Measurement of the heart rate with a heart rate ruler simply requires one to place the reference point of a heart rate ruler on one of the waves of an ECG complex (often the R wave because it is large and observable) and identify the point where the same wave of a subsequent ECG complex falls (either two or three ECG complexes to the right of the original ECG complex, see Fig. 11-5A). This method quickly and accurately measures the number of beats per minute by measuring the number of cardiac cycles (ECG complexes) that fall between the reference point and heart rate reference points that have been plotted on the heart rate ruler based on mathematical calculations. **It is important to note that the use of the heart rate ruler presupposes a regular rhythm.** Inaccuracies result if the interval between complexes changes from beat to beat.[9-12] If such is the case, use of the 6-second mark will yield more accurate results.

Six-Second Mark Method

Measurement of the heart rate using the 6-second marks on ECG recording paper can also be done quickly but may be less accurate in determining the true heart rate. The method simply involves counting the number of ECG complexes between two 3-second marks on the ECG paper and multiplying this number by 10, which yields the number of ECG complexes in 60 seconds (or the number of cardiac cycles/min) (see Fig. 11-5A). Inaccurate heart rates may be measured if the number of ECG complexes between the 6-second markers is incorrectly counted or if over the course of a minute the rhythm changes. However, the measurement of heart rate in an ECG with frequent rhythm disturbances is best accomplished using the 6-second mark method. Rhythm disturbances that would be appropriate for this method of heart rate measurement include atrial fibrillation (afib) and occasional to frequent premature atrial or ventricular contractions.[9-12] **It should be noted that slight inaccuracies in one 6-second strip become magnified by 10 when the heart rate is expressed in beats per minute. Therefore, multiple 6-second strips yield more accurate results.**

Counting Mnemonic Method

The measurement of heart rate via counting mnemonic can also be used by applying the mnemonic scale shown in Fig. 11-5B. This counting mnemonic is based on the same mathematical calculations that allow the heart rate to be measured using the heart rate ruler. The mnemonic is very simple and requires that the student memorize the numeric sequence "300-150-100-75-60-50." These numbers represent the heart rates obtained when the next consecutive waveform falls on a heavy

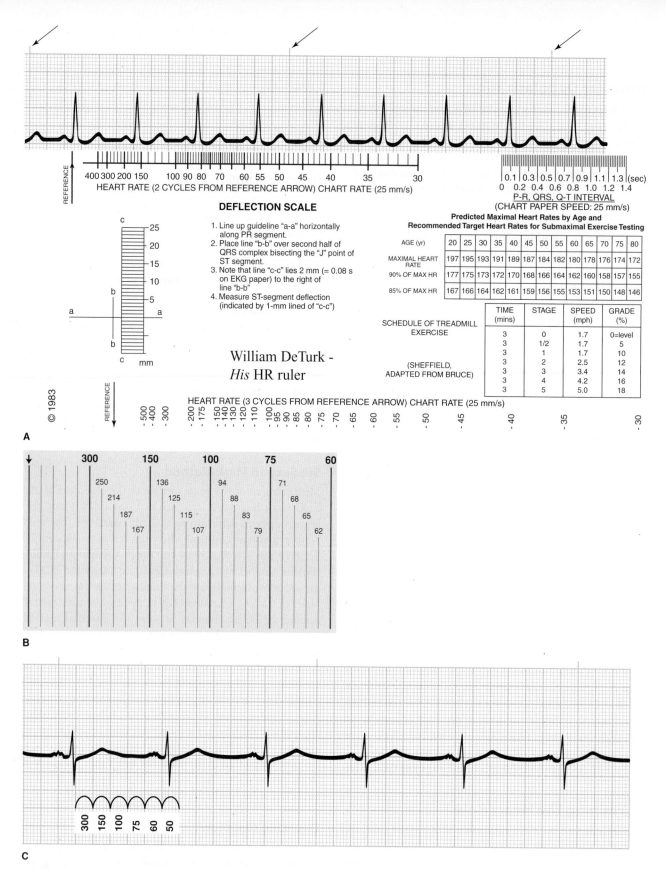

FIGURE 11-5 Three methods of measuring the heart rate from an ECG. Note the small boxes (1 mm square) and large boxes (5 mm square) that form a grid. (**A**) Use of a heart rate ruler and 3-second marks to form a 6-second strip. Note that the reference arrow is aligned with the beginning of the R wave. The heart rate is measured at 84 complexes per minute. Use of the two 3-second marks (arrows), counting the number of complexes between these marks and extrapolating the results yields approximately the same value. (**B**) The counting mnemonic. (**C**) Use of the mnemonic to measure the heart rate. Note that the value of each little box between 50 and 60 is 2. Thus, counting backward from "50" to the R wave yields an approximate heart rate of 56 complexes per minute. ((**C**) Reprinted with permission from Dubin D. *Rapid Interpretation of ECGs.* 5th ed. Tampa, FL: Cover Publishing Company; 1996.)

black line, that is, the edge of a large box. Note that the difference between 300 and 150 is 150; the "value" of each of the five little boxes between 300 and 150 is 30. Similarly, the difference between 75 and 60 is 15; the "value" of each little box is 3. **The "value" of each little box changes as a function of your location in the mnemonic.**

This information is useful when the next consecutive complex fails to fall on a heavy black line and will "fine-tune" your heart rate. The application of the counting mnemonic is as follows:

1. Identify a waveform of the ECG complex that falls on or near the heavy black line of a large box. Often the R wave is used because it is large and identifiable, but it need not be so—Q waves and S waves are also acceptable.
2. Identify the same wave in the next consecutive ECG complex (the next complex to the right of the first complex).
3. Apply the counting mnemonic by counting *cycles* across the big boxes until the next consecutive waveform is crossed; then stop counting.
4. The point where the same wave of the second consecutive complex falls (often near a large box) in the counting mnemonic yields the approximate heart rate in beats per minute.
5. Count backward (to the left) from the heavy black line of the large box just to the right of the second consecutive waveform using the value of each *little* box until you land on the second waveform. This final number represents the most accurate estimation of heart rate.[9–12] See Fig. 11-5C for an example of the application of the counting mnemonic method.

Determining the Heart Rhythm

Determining the rhythm of the heart is critically important when attempting to interpret different types of rhythm disturbances. Determination of the rhythm of the heart simply involves evaluating the regularity of the heart's discharge of electrical activity (or ECG complexes), which can be accomplished via palpation of the arterial pulse (see Chapter 10), observation of the regularity of the ECG complex on an ECG screen (which can also be heard with a "beep" when the ECG complex appears on the screen), or actual measurement on a recorded ECG. The rhythm of the heart can be measured on a recorded ECG using one of the three different methods, including a quick glance at the regularity between ECG complexes, use of a caliper, and use of marks on paper.[9–12] Heart rhythm is expressed as either "regular" or "irregular." Sometimes an irregular rhythm has a recurring pattern within it; for example, every third impulse is missing. These rhythms are then expressed as "regularly irregular." This will be discussed in greater detail later in this chapter.

Quick Glance of the Regularity Between ECG Complexes

As mentioned earlier, a quick glance at an ECG screen or a recorded ECG can provide important information about the

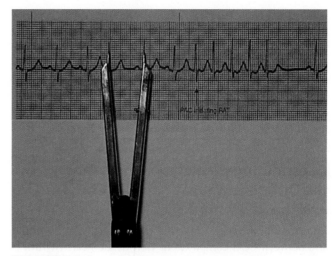

FIGURE 11-6 Use of calipers to assess heart rhythm. Note that once the R-R interval is obtained the calipers are simply "marched out" across the tops of the remaining R waves. This ECG reflects a grossly irregular rhythm. (Used with permission from J. Huff, *ECG Workout: Exercises in Arrhythmia Interpretation*, 3rd ed., Lippincott Williams & Wilkins, 1997.)

regularity between ECG complexes and whether or not a rhythm disturbance exists. Almost all rhythm disturbances display (or audibly "beep") irregularity between ECG complexes. The time period between ECG complexes is unpredictable and not consistently equal. An example of a cardiac rhythm irregularity can be seen in Fig. 11-6.

Use of a Caliper

A cardiac caliper is similar to the long legs of a compass and can be positioned on the same waves of two consecutive ECG complexes (see Fig. 11-6). Some cardiac calipers allow for the measured distance between waves to be locked into the measured distance (by turning a small set screw at the end of the caliper that keeps the legs of the caliper from moving). This locked position represents the distance between two consecutive ECG complexes. This interval can then be used to plot the distance between remaining ECG complexes, termed *marching out* the rhythm.[9–12] Perfect alignment of ECG complexes with the points of the caliper across the rhythm strip signifies a regular rhythm. The inability to march out successive ECG complexes signifies an irregular rhythm.[9–12]

Use of Marks on Paper

A "crude" method that can be used to examine regularity between ECG complexes involves identifying a specific wave in one ECG complex (again, often the R wave is chosen because it is largest and easily identified), marking its location on a piece of paper, and then identifying the same wave in the next consecutive ECG complex and marking its location on the same piece of paper. These two marks are then marched out between the next two consecutive ECG complexes, and the marks are examined for alignment within the two consecutive ECG complexes. Examining the alignment of the marks on paper with pairs of ECG complexes is continued until all pairs of ECG complexes have been measured. If the heart rhythm is regular, the marks on the paper will line up in perfect alignment with each subsequent pair of ECG complexes. If, however, the rhythm is irregular, the marks on paper would not line up; for example, they would be lined up with the first ECG complex and not the second (because of irregularity between the complexes).

Determining the Relationships Among the Different Waves of an ECG Complex and the Rhythm

Determining the relationships of different waveforms within and between ECG complexes in view of the heart rhythm is helpful in identifying some disturbances in cardiac rhythm. The position of the waves on an ECG tracing should always follow the sequence presented in Fig. 11-4. The P wave should be first, followed by the QRS complex, T, and U waves (if present). When this order is not observed, it is very likely that a cardiac rhythm disturbance exists.[9–12] Of equal importance are the *intervals* between these waves. Each of these waves has a specified interval of time between it and the next wave (Fig. 11-4). If the intervals between one or more of these waves is not within normal limits or if it is irregular (changing from one ECG complex to another), it is also very likely that a cardiac rhythm disturbance exists.[9–12] For example, the normal specified time interval between the P wave and the R wave (PR interval) should be no greater than 0.20 seconds (or one big box). If the time interval between these two waves is greater than 0.20, a cardiac rhythm disturbance exists. Likewise, if the time interval between these two waves changes from one ECG complex to another, then another type of cardiac rhythm disturbance exists. Examples of specific rhythm disturbances will be presented immediately after the next section. The next section will provide a brief overview of methods to recognize the primary cause of cardiac rhythm disturbances and that of myocardial ischemia.

Determining the Presence of Myocardial Ischemia

Myocardial ischemia is the most common cause of cardiac rhythm disturbances.[9–12] It can be observed on ECG by examining the position of the ST segment of the ECG (Fig. 11-4). Myocardial ischemia typically produces ST-segment depression, which can be measured with a ruler or any straight-edged device. The process is as follows:

1. The PR intervals of two successive complexes are identified. A ruler is placed horizontally from one PR interval to the next PR interval. This horizontal line from two successive PR intervals can be marked with a pencil and identifies the *isoelectric line* (the line of equal charge or the midpoint of depolarization and repolarization).

2. The *J point* of the complex to be evaluated is identified. The J point is defined as the *break point* between the end of the QRS complex and the beginning of the ST segment.

3. The examiner moves to the right, away from the J point 2 little boxes, or 0.08 seconds.

4. It is at this point that the magnitude of ST segment depression is measured by counting the number of boxes vertically from the point of the ST segment, that is, two little boxes to the right of the J point to the isoelectric line.

5. A measured value of depression of the ST segment that is greater than 1.0 mm is highly suggestive of myocardial ischemia.

See Chapter 12 for an additional description, figures, and examples of ST-segment measurement.

CLINICAL CORRELATE

It is important that physical therapists develop assessment skills for the presence of myocardial ischemia through accurate measurement of ST-segment changes. These changes typically come on with exercise and go away with rest, as the demand for oxygen by the myocardium outstrips the supply. These ECG changes are usually, but not always, accompanied by complaints of chest pressure. Once evidence of myocardial ischemia is obtained, exercise should be terminated.

It should be noted that the morphology, or shape, of the ST segment also contributes to the diagnosis of ischemia. Downsloping or horizontal ST segments are more diagnostic than ST segments that are upsloping. Fig. 11-16 demonstrates downsloping ST-segment depression. Additionally, a number of other things may cause ST-segment depression and are listed in Box 11-1. The presence of one or more of the items listed in Box 11-1 may decrease the likelihood that ST-segment depression is due to myocardial ischemia. See Chapter 12 for further discussion of ST-segment interpretation and the clinical application of these data.

Myocardial ischemia due to coronary artery spasm may present with ST-segment elevation. The method to measure ST-segment elevation is similar to the measurement of ST-segment depression, only measuring from the isoelectric line to the top of the elevated ST segment, 0.08 seconds to the right of the J point. Finally, ST-segment elevation is also associated with acute myocardial infarction, which will be discussed later in this chapter.

BOX 11-1

Causes of ST-Segment Depression or Elevation

1. Myocardial ischemia or infarction
2. Coronary artery spasm
3. Electrolyte abnormalities
4. Left ventricular hypertrophy
5. Interventricular conduction delays (eg, bundle branch blocks)
6. Atrial fibrillation or flutter
7. Digoxin
8. Pacemaker

DISTURBANCES IN CARDIAC RHYTHM

Whereas heart rate is *quantified* as beats per minute, heart rhythm is *qualified* as either *regular* or *irregular*. Regular rhythms, like music, are predictable in nature—we know when the next beat will fall. Irregular rhythms are either irregularly irregular (completely random) or regularly irregular—there is a pattern to the irregularity.[9-14]

Heart rhythm may be assessed through cardiac auscultation or through peripheral pulse palpation. Indeed, palpation of peripheral pulses is frequently where rhythm disturbances are first discovered. Detection of arrhythmias through peripheral pulse palpation presumes a normal vascular system.

CLINICAL CORRELATE

Advanced atherosclerosis, which occludes the brachial artery, can preclude accurate assessment of rhythm. This should prompt the physical therapist to an assessment of rhythm through cardiac auscultation.[9-14]

Alterations in rhythm may originate from within the normal conduction pathway, specifically, from normal pacemakers of cardiac depolarization: the SA node or the AV node. These normal pacemakers possess their own intrinsic firing rates. The normal rate of spontaneous depolarization of the SA node is between 60 and 100 bpm. The normal rate of the AV node is between 40 and 60 bpm. If, for whatever reason, the AV node becomes dysfunctional and fails to fire, even the ventricles can assume pacemaker control, at their own inherent rate of 20 to 40 bpm. As we shall see, **the pacemaker with the highest rate of discharge assumes pacemaker control of the heart.**

This principle of the highest-order pacemaker acts as a safety net, which turns on as a progressive fallback system when human viability is threatened.[9-14]

Rhythm disturbances may also arise from outside the normal conduction pathway. These *ectopic foci* consist of areas of irritable myocardium, which can spontaneously depolarize. This wave of depolarization spreads outward and in the process, depolarizes the normal conduction pathway.

Rhythm disturbances can arise from the atria, from the junctional (AV nodal) area or from the ventricles. This section will describe commonly encountered arrhythmias in order from the top, at the level of the atria, and down to the bottom, at the level of the ventricles.[9-14]

Sinus Node Rhythm Disturbances

In a healthy normal subject at rest, the sinoatrial node (SA node) spontaneously depolarizes at a rate between 60 and 100 bpm. This positive wave of depolarization proceeds down the normal conduction pathway, depolarizing first the atria, then the ventricles. The rhythm is regular; that is, the distance between R and R intervals is fixed. Assuming normal excitation–contraction coupling, ventricular depolarization causes ventricular contraction. Ventricular contraction expels a bolus of blood from the chamber of the left ventricle, such bolus traveling down the arterial tree and giving rise to a *peripheral pulse* that can be palpated at any of the several sites where the artery travels close to the skin surface. The term *normal sinus rhythm* (NSR) implies both a heart rate between 60 and 100 bpm and a spontaneous depolarization initiated by the SA node[9-14] (see Fig. 11-7).

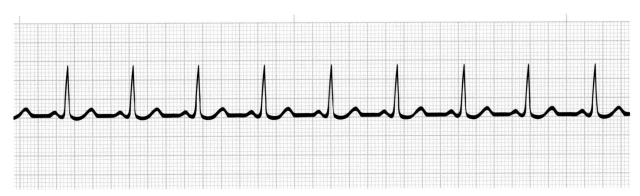

FIGURE 11-7 Normal sinus rhythm, rate 86 bpm.

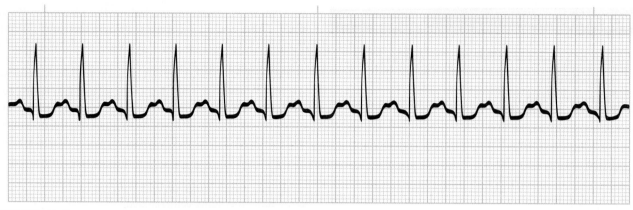

FIGURE 11-8   Sinus tachycardia, rate 120 bpm.

A sinus rate may exceed 100 bpm and is termed *sinus tachycardia* (ST) (see Fig. 11-8). Sinus tachycardia may pose a threat to the patient, depending on the rate. Rapid ST narrows diastolic filling time and reduces stroke volume; this in turn may reduce cardiac output and cause the patient to become dizzy or even lose consciousness. Although rare, sinus tachycardia may come on suddenly and have a sudden termination. This is termed *paroxysmal atrial tachycardia* (PAT), and is sometimes associated with digitalis toxicity (see Fig. 11-9). Patients may experience palpitations, accompanied by feelings of light-headedness or even syncope. Many patients respond favorably to *carotid sinus massage*. This maneuver involves direct massage of the area over the bifurcation of the carotid artery in an effort to enhance parasympathetic nervous system activity and "break" this rapid, runaway rate.[9–14]

Sinus tachycardia is normal during exercise, as the demand for blood and oxygen by working skeletal muscle is normally met by increases in both heart rate (HR) and stroke volume.

A sinus rate may fall below 60 bpm and is thus termed *sinus bradycardia* (SB) (see Fig. 11-10). Sinus bradycardia may also pose a danger to the patient, particularly if the HR is very low. This time the reduction in cardiac output is due to diminished HR, which also cause dizziness and syncope. Sinus bradycardia is normal in athletes where SB is compensated by enhanced stroke volume, which is due to an exercise-induced increase in left ventricular muscle mass and better contractility.[9–14]

Yet another sinus node disturbance in rhythm is caused by changes in intrathoracic pressure and is termed *sinus arrhythmia* or *respiratory arrhythmia*. Alterations between inspiration and expiration produce phasic increases and decreases in intrathoracic pressure that impacts on venous return and thus heart rate. Sinus arrhythmia is better thought of as a normal heart rhythm variant. Many healthy individuals demonstrate sinus arrhythmia on routine ECG, and it rarely has any clinical relevance because there is no hemodynamic compromise[9–14] (see Fig. 11-11).

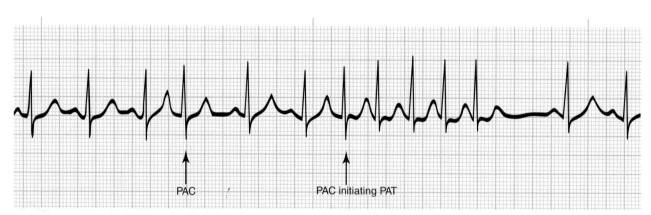

PAC   /   PAC initiating PAT

FIGURE 11-9   Paroxysmal atrial tachycardia (PAT), rate 167 bpm of the PAT. Note the sudden onset and termination.

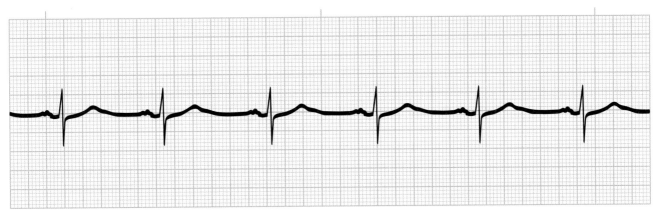

FIGURE 11-10 Sinus bradycardia, rate 54 bpm.

CLINICAL CORRELATE

The significance of normal sinus rhythm, sinus tachycardia, and sinus bradycardia resides within the context of additional data. Normal sinus rhythm at rest is a normal finding; NSR at a high level of exercise is abnormal. Similarly, sinus bradycardia in a patient with an acute MI is quite different from SB in a 24-year-old athlete. Physical therapists should avoid evaluating a single piece of data in isolation; rather, ECGs should be evaluated within the context of the total patient, and a clinical decision should be made on that basis.

Occasionally the SA node becomes lazy; the ECG demonstrates an abnormally long cycle between complexes. This phenomenon is called *sinoatrial block*, or, more commonly, *sinus pause*. Although it is difficult to determine the etiology, short sinus pauses are rarely problematic. Prolonged sinus pauses, however, can predispose to dizziness and syncope and require intervention, usually pacemaker implantation (see Fig. 11-12). A prolonged sinus pause should give rise to an *escape beat* or an *escape rhythm*. An escape beat may originate from the atrium, the AV node, or the ventricles. An escape beat responds to flat pieces of baseline that are void of electrical activity by spontaneously depolarizing the myocardium and is yet another safety net that is activated to help restore a normal rhythm and maintain cardiac output[9-14] (see Fig. 11-12).

Premature Atrial Contractions

Sinus tachycardia, SB, and sinus arrhythmia all originate from spontaneous depolarization of the SA node. However, in certain individuals and in some circumstances, a spontaneous wave of depolarization can originate from outside the normal conduction pathway. An *ectopic focus* (pleural, *foci*) is an area within the myocardium that, in certain circumstances, can spontaneously depolarize. When it does so, it "jumps ahead" of SA node depolarization and is thus premature. Indeed, prematurity is one of the

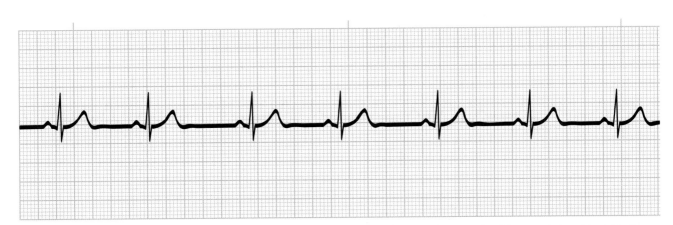

FIGURE 11-11 Sinus arrhythmia, rate 60 bpm. Note the gradual shortening and prolongation of the R-R interval, consistent with the respiratory cycle.

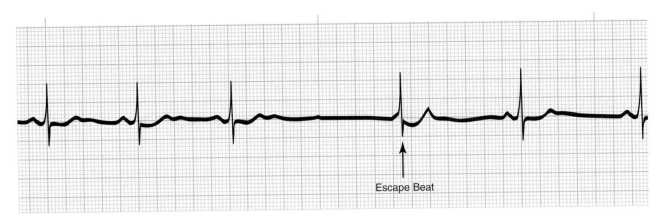

FIGURE 11-12   Sinus pause, following NSR at a rate of 60 bpm. Note the junctional escape beat, which reestablishes the rhythm.

hallmarks of a *premature atrial contraction* (PAC). PACs originate from areas of irritable, sometimes ischemic, myocardium that form the wall of the atrium. The P wave of a PAC may look different from the P wave of sinus node origin; this is because the P wave comes from a different place within the atrium. However, the atria are relatively small compared to the ventricles; thus, failure to detect a different looking P wave should not in and of itself eliminate the presence of a PAC. Because the SA node is briefly "silenced" as a pacemaker by the PAC, the SA node must *reset* itself in order to restore a new normal sinus rhythm. The reset of the SA node is another hallmark of a PAC. Once the AV node has been depolarized, the ventricular response to a PAC is usually normal. Therefore, most of the time, the QRS complex looks the same as a normal ECG complex[9–14] (see Fig. 11-13).

PACs are characterized as *isolated* if they occur as a single ECG event. They are classified as *bigeminal* if every other ECG event is a PAC. *Trigeminy* indicates that two ECG events are normal for every premature complex. Two PACs in a row are termed *paired PACs* or *couplets*. Occasional isolated PACs pose no threat to patients. There is no

significant alteration in heart rate and thus no reduction in cardiac output.[9–14]

Atrial Flutter

A single irritable ectopic focus can fire occasionally and capture the ventricle, giving rise to a PAC. However, a single ectopic focus also can fire repetitively and so rapidly that the slow-conducting AV node fails to conduct every impulse. This arrhythmia gives rise to an ECG complex characterized by multiple P waves to every QRS response. In *atrial flutter (aflutter)*, the P waves have a typical "saw-tooth" pattern (see Fig. 11-14). This shows four P waves for every QRS complex. In general, the rate of the flutter waves is between 200 and 300 bpm, and the P waves–QRS complex ratio is commonly 2:1. This ratio can change, however, sometimes to 3:1, which slows the ventricular response and decreases cardiac output. Atrial flutter is commonly found in patients with ischemic heart disease or with patients recovering from any acute illness; it may appear transiently after heart surgery.[11] The variability in ventricular response makes atrial flutter somewhat unstable and requires treatment.[9–14]

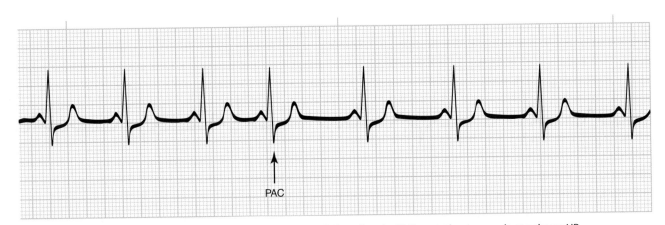

FIGURE 11-13   Normal sinus rhythm, rate 74 bpm, with one PAC. Note that the PAC resets the sinus node at a slower HR.

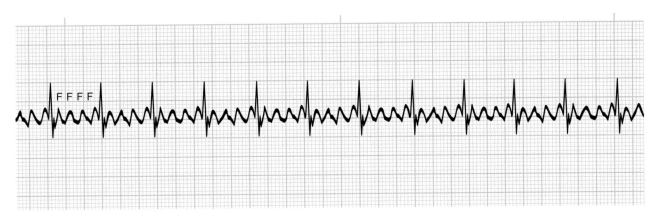

FIGURE 11-14   Atrial flutter, with an atrial rate of 428 bpm and a rapid ventricular response of 110 bpm. Note the 4:1 AV conduction.

Atrial Fibrillation

Atrial flutter is characterized by repetitive firing of a single ectopic atrial focus, with periodic transmission of the depolarization wave through the AV node down to the ventricles. The P waves are well-formed and similar in morphology, implying that there is a high degree of organization in both atrial depolarization and atrial contraction. In *atrial fibrillation (afib),* this high degree of organization is lost. An afib is characterized by multiple ectopic foci, all firing at random throughout the cardiac cycle. There is no single, unified wave of depolarization in the atria and thus no organized myocardial contraction. Indeed, the atria have been characterized as "quivering like a bag of worms (anon)." The ventricular response is extremely variable; occasionally, enough voltage will summate to depolarize the AV node, which will then propagate the impulse down the His bundle to the ventricles and cause ventricular depolarization in the usual manner[9-14] (see Fig. 11-15). **Afib is characterized by an irregular, jagged baseline and an irregular ventricular response, and it can be identified by (1) a constantly changing R-to-R wave interval, (2) absence of a P wave, and (3) jagged (fibrillatory) baseline.**

Because the ventricular response is so variable, it is desirable to calculate the ventricular rate. This requires that the practitioner count the number of QRS complexes in a 6-second strip and multiply by 10. Heart rates in afib may be categorized and documented as

> 60 to 100 bpm = afib with moderate ventricular response (MVR),

> \> 100 bpm = afib with rapid ventricular response (RVR),

and

> < 60 bpm = afib with slow ventricular response (SVR).

Afib is produced by a variety of disease processes, including rheumatic heart disease, ischemic heart disease, hypertensive heart disease, and heart failure.[11] *New-onset afib* requires treatment, either by medications that slow conduction through the AV node by prolonging refractoriness (eg, digitalis, verapamil) or by electrical stimulation (eg, DC defibrillation). *Chronic afib* is well-tolerated by many patients. The "atrial kick" provided by an atrium contracting in syncytium tops off an already full ventricle and thus contributes

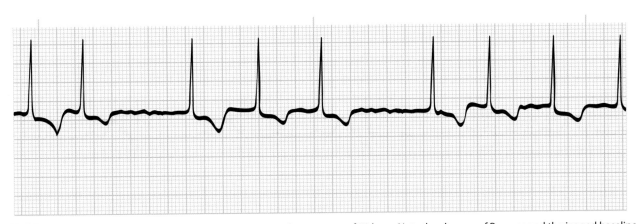

FIGURE 11-15   Atrial fibrillation, with an irregular ventricular response of 70 bpm. Note the absence of P waves and the jagged baseline.

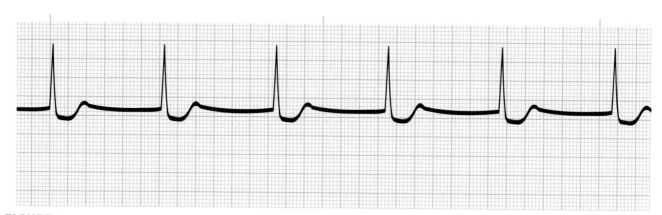

FIGURE 11-16   Junctional rhythm, rate 50 bpm. Note the absence of P waves and the narrow, normal looking QRS complex. Note the presence of ST-segment depression.

only a small additional amount of blood to stroke volume. Additionally, the risk of conversion to NSR outweighs the benefits of such a procedure.[9–14]

Atrioventricular Node Rhythm Disturbances (Junctional Rhythms)

As mentioned previously, in circumstances where the SA node becomes electrically silent, the AV node can take over pacemaker function. The AV node can also spontaneously depolarize, giving rise to a *junctional premature contraction* (JPC). Because the AV node is part of the supraventricular conduction system, the QRS complex in a JPC appears normal, that is, is of normal width. The P wave is absent, which is consistent with the loss of SA node input from above[9–14] (see Fig. 11-16).

The normal resting rate of depolarization of the AV node is 40 to 60 bpm. The AV node, however, does respond to exercise by increasing its rate, and physical therapists may be called on to develop an exercise prescription in patients with junctional rhythms to attain a training effect.

Junctional premature contractions are best thought of as an escape rhythm due to loss of the SA node, rather than to true arrhythmias. Causes of JPCs include those of suppression

of SA node function, for example, myocardial ischemia and particularly right coronary artery lesions that supply the SA node. Treatment is directed toward treating the cause of default to a lower order pacemaker.[9–14]

Heart Blocks

Heart blocks occur when conduction from the SA node to the AV node gets altered. This alteration typically occurs at the level of the AV node and can present either as a delay in conduction or as a complete block. Heart blocks are graded by levels of severity from first degree, through second degree, to third degree.[9–14]

First-Degree Heart Block

Recall that the normal PR interval is short, that is, less than 0.20 seconds long. In first-*degree AV block*, conduction from the atria to the ventricles is delayed, causing prolongation of the PR interval (see Fig. 11-17). Note that while the PR interval is prolonged, conduction proceeds through the AV node and down the common bundle of His, and the ventricles are still captured. First-degree AV block is frequently benign and commonly occurs in endurance-trained athletes. These

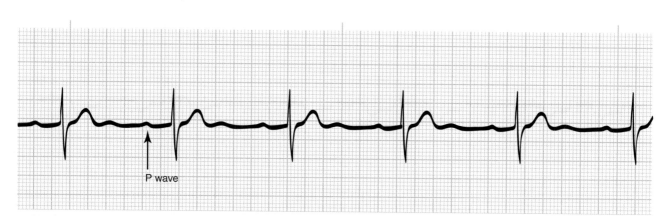

P wave

FIGURE 11-17   First-degree AV block, rate 48 bpm. Note the prolonged PR interval measuring 0.30 seconds.

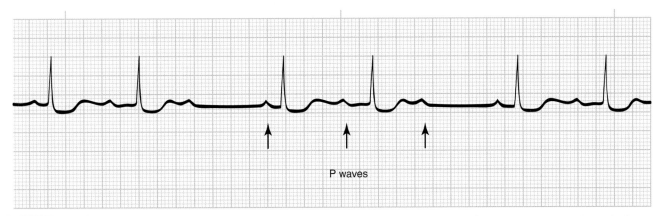

FIGURE 11-18 Second-degree AV block, Mobitz type I; atrial rate 72 bpm, ventricular rate approximately 55 bpm. Note the gradual prolongation of the PR interval, until a QRS complex is dropped.

individuals also demonstrate a shift toward vagal tone, producing sinus bradycardia coupled with a slowing of conduction through the AV node.[9-14]

Second-Degree Heart Block

There are two types of second-*degree AV block*. In *Mobitz type I* heart block there is gradual prolongation of the PR interval until a QRS complex is dropped. After the dropped QRS complex, the next beat recaptures the ventricles with a shortened PR interval, and then gradual prolongation of the PR interval repeats (see Fig. 11-18). Also known as *Wenckebach phenomenon*, the lesion is usually located within the AV node and is usually caused by an excess in parasympathetic output to the AV node or medications that cause parasympathetic effects. Wenckebach is usually innocuous and frequently occurs transiently in the setting of acute MI.[9-14]

Second-degree AV block, Mobitz type II, is also characterized by dropped QRS complexes. However, the PR interval is fixed and remains unchanged throughout consecutive cardiac cycles[9-14] (see Fig. 11-19).

Both second-degree AV blocks are associated with rheumatic fever, acute inferior wall MI, and digitalis toxicity. They rarely progress to *complete heart block* (CHB).

Third-Degree Heart Block

A third-degree heart block is a complete heart block and is characterized by complete AV dissociation, with atrial and ventricular rhythms functioning independently[9-14] (see Fig. 11-20). This figure shows a fixed P-to-P interval and a fixed R-to-R interval, with resultant variation in PR interval, confirming complete AV dissociation and complete heart block. CHB is frequently compensated for by an escape rhythm that originates at a site distal to the lesion. However, if these escape beats are not forthcoming, the patient could lose consciousness, or worse. Therefore, CHB usually requires the insertion of an artificial pacemaker.[9-14]

Premature Ventricular Contractions and Ventricular Tachycardia

Many of the same issues that guided discussion of premature atrial contractions hold true for *premature ventricular*

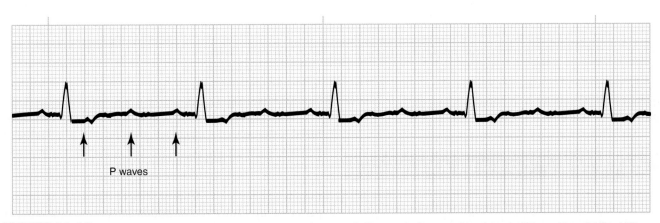

FIGURE 11-19 Second-degree AV block, Mobitz type II; atrial rate 130 bpm, ventricular rate approximately 41 bpm. Note the fixed PR interval, with every third P wave capturing a QRS complex.

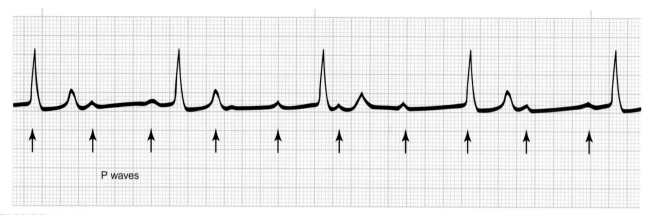

FIGURE 11-20   Third-degree AV block, atrial rate 88 bpm, ventricular rate approximately 38 bpm. Note the relatively fixed P–P interval, the fixed R–R interval, and the variable PR interval, indicating complete dissociation between the atria and ventricles.

contractions (PVCs). The irritable ectopic focus described earlier now resides in the myocardium of the ventricle. This focus consists of irritable, usually ischemic, myocardium that spontaneously depolarizes and "jumps the gun" ahead of the wave of depolarization traveling down the normal conduction pathway from the atria. As in PACs, prematurity is also the hallmark of the PVC. However, the QRS complex of most PVCs is wide and bizarre looking. PVCs are wide because they travel through slower conducting myocardium; they are frequently tall because the muscle mass that they travel through generates more voltage than neural elements found in conduction tissue. PVCs do not reset the SA node; the atria are relatively "protected" from spontaneous depolarization originating from the ventricles by the common bundle of His. The maintenance of normal, undisturbed P wave activity across the PVC establishes complete AV dissociation at that point in time and is a hallmark of the PVC.[9–14]

PVCs take on added significance because their presence, in the setting of ischemic heart disease, places the patient at higher risk for reinfarction and sudden death. PVCs are also problematic because they can be hemodynamically compromising and can degenerate into a lethal arrhythmia. It is helpful, therefore, to describe PVC activity in terms of frequency, morphology, and relationship to the cardiac cycle.[9–14]

Like PACs, PVCs can be described as isolated, bigeminal, trigeminal, and paired. However, PVCs arise from the much larger muscle mass of the ventricles and thus may compromise stroke volume and cardiac output. For this reason, the frequency of PVC activity is important as well as their relative proximity to each other.

PVCs can arise from multiple foci within the ventricle. These are termed *multifocal* PVCs (see Fig. 11-22). This figure shows two bizarre, premature complexes that look different from each other. This is because they originate from different areas of the ventricles. Multifocal PVCs are more significant than unifocal PVCs because their activity can summate and produce more PVCs per minute.[9–14]

PVCs can also be evaluated on the basis of their relationship to the previous ECG cycle. Occasionally, a PVC is so premature that it appears on the T wave of the preceding ECG complex. This is called an *R-on-T* PVC (see Fig. 11-23). The presence of R-on-T PVCs is of particular concern because they depolarize the myocardium during its relative refractory period. This is a particularly vulnerable period in the repolarization phase and can set up a series of rapid sequential depolarizations termed *ventricular tachycardia* (vtach or VT).[9–14] VT is defined as three or more PVCs in a row at a rate of >100 bpm (see Fig. 11-24). Chapter 12 will describe the significance of PVC behavior as it relates to exercise.

Ventricular Fibrillation

Ventricular tachycardia can degenerate into a lethal arrhythmia known as *ventricular fibrillation* (vfib). Like afib, vfib is caused by multiple ectopic foci, all firing at random. There is no organization to the ECG waveform, and there is no organized wave of depolarization. The ventricles thus fail to contract in syncytium and instead "quiver like a bag of worms" (anon)[9–14] (see Fig. 11-25).

Vtach can be restored to NSR through the use of synchronized cardioverters, machines that deliver a preselected amount of energy by way of paddles applied over the chest. These devices "read" the patient's ECG waveform and time the delivery of countershock to the patient's R wave. In this way, the practitioner avoids delivery of shock during the refractory period of myocardial repolarization and prevents the onset of vfib. Ventricular fibrillation, on the other hand, is corrected using a defibrillator device.[9–14]

CLINICAL CORRELATE

Movement from ventricular trigeminy through ventricular bigeminy to PVC pairs increases PVC significance, especially in the setting of an acute MI or during exercise[9–14] (see Fig. 11-21).

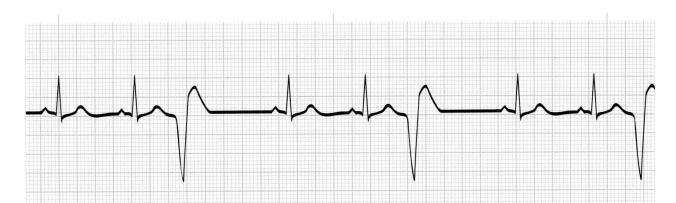

FIGURE 11-21 Unifocal PVCs, presenting as ventricular trigeminy. Note that the sinus node is not reset and continues to depolarize "on time" through the PVCs.

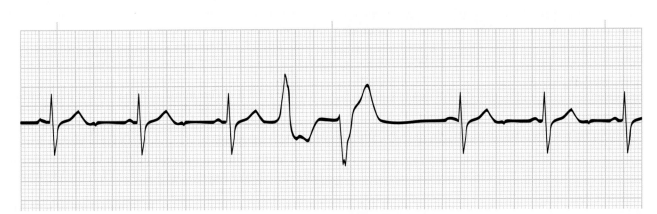

FIGURE 11-22 Multifocal PVCs, presenting as a PVC pair or couplet. The underlying sinus rate is 63 bpm. Note the P wave in the negative limb of the first PVC.

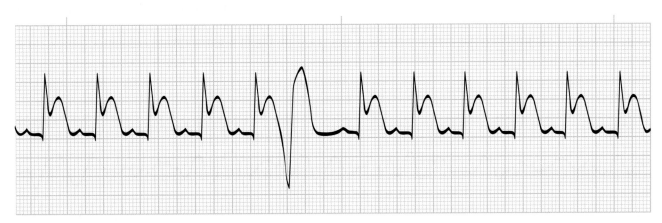

FIGURE 11-23 R-on-T PVC. The underlying sinus rate is 105 bpm.

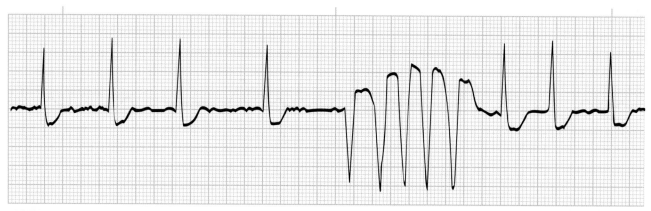

FIGURE 11-24   A self-limited burst of ventricular tachycardia. This should be documented by the clinician as five PVCs in a row at a rate of 210 bpm. Note the profound ST-segment depression, indicating myocardial ischemia that sets the stage for this dangerous arrhythmia.

CLINICAL CORRELATE

It should be noted that it is easier to bring patients back from vtach than it is from vfib. Physical therapists encountering a patient in sustained vtach should initiate emergency procedures by calling a code. This will hopefully reduce the likelihood that the patient will degenerate in a lethal vfib.[9–14]

TWELVE-LEAD ELECTROCARDIOGRAPHY

The actual 12-lead ECG that we know today was developed by Emmanuel Goldberger in 1942 (refer to the history of the ECG in Table 11-1 to appreciate the efforts of many others)[1–7] and allows for a more detailed and systematic examination of the ECG and specific disorders that may affect the ECG. As previously mentioned, each ECG electrode provides a view of the electrical activity of the heart under which the ECG electrode lies.

The ECG leads that produce the 12-lead format include the *limb leads* (leads I through III, aVR, aVL, aVF) and the *precordial leads* (V_1 through V_6), which are shown in an ECG from a normal heart in Fig. 11-26. Note that they are arranged upon the page in a systematic, standardized manner. The limb leads occupy the left half of the page, and the precordial leads occupy the right half of the page. Note also that three heat styluses are vertically arranged one on top of the other, which allows the simultaneous recording of three leads. Leads I, II, and III (reading from top to bottom) are recorded at the same time; then, aVR, aVL, and aVF (reading from top to bottom). V_1, V_2, and V_3 and V_4, V_5, and V_6 are clustered in the same manner. **It is important to note that this simultaneous recording allows the three different views of the same electrical event. This allows the practitioner to make judgment calls and clinical decisions about a particular ECG complex based on information obtained from three sources, and not just one.** A simple count of these leads reveals that 12 different views of the heart's electrical activity are provided in a typical 12-lead ECG. An ECG profile of a normal heart without a cardiac rhythm

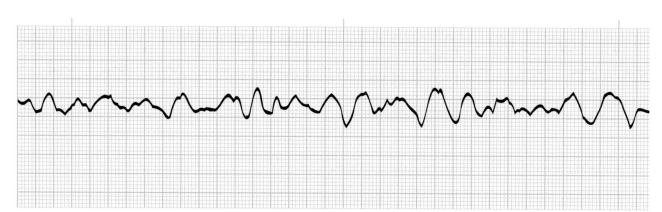

FIGURE 11-25   Coarse ventricular fibrillation. Note the loss of electrical organization in the irregularly shaped waveforms that reflect multiple ventricular foci firing randomly in vfib. This lack of organization prevents measurement of heart rate.

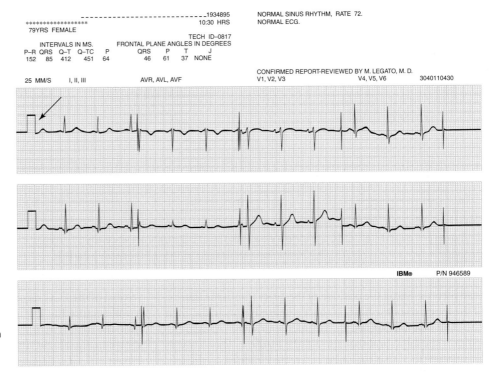

------------------------------------1934895
10:30 HRS

****
79YRS FEMALE

TECH ID-0817

NORMAL SINUS RHYTHM, RATE 72.
NORMAL ECG.

INTERVALS IN MS.   FRONTAL PLANE ANGLES IN DEGREES

P–R	QRS	Q–T	Q–TC	P	QRS	P	T	J
152	85	412	451	64	46	61	37	NONE

CONFIRMED REPORT-REVIEWED BY M. LEGATO, M. D.

25 MM/S   I, II, III   AVR, AVL, AVF   V1, V2, V3   V4, V5, V6   3040110430

IBM®   P/N 946589

FIGURE 11-26 The ECG leads that produce the 12-lead ECG include the limb leads (leads I through III, aVR, aVL, aVF), and the precordial leads (V_1 through V_6). Note the presence of calibration marks (arrow) and the notation "25 mm/s" reflecting a machine that is set to standard calibration.

disturbance or disease is shown in Fig. 11-26. Each of these views was obtained from an ECG–electrode interface (a lead) that picked up the electrical activity of the heart and transported it through a series of wires to a circuit box (the proverbial "black box"), which processed the electrical activity so that it could be graphically displayed.[9–13]

VIEWS OF THE HEART: EINTHOVEN'S TRIANGLE

In order to understand the area of the heart that each limb lead looks at, it is important to understand something about Einthoven's triangle. Willem Einthoven placed electrodes on both arms and both legs and used leads to connect them to a simple ECG recorder. He manipulated the polarity of each lead relative to the other leads and developed a triangle of polarity as shown in Fig. 11-27A. Each face of the triangle was given a numeric lead assignment, either I, II, or III. If the leads are all collapsed around an imaginary center, one develops a different figure, as shown in Fig. 11-27B. Note that each of these leads has a positive pole and a negative pole. Each of these leads is configured to "look toward" the positive pole. Thus, lead I "looks toward" the patient's left, lead II "looks toward" the patient's left leg, and lead III "looks toward" the patient's right leg.

Now conceptualize a 360-degree circle that is superimposed on your own chest. Let us arbitrarily designate 0 degrees as looking toward the left arm, +90 degrees as looking straight down toward the floor, and +/−180 degrees as looking toward the right arm. Similarly, −90 degrees looks straight up

toward your head, and 0 degrees looks once again toward your left arm and completes the circle.

The previous exercise allows the practitioner to assign a value in degrees to each of Einthoven's three leads. Lead I looks toward 0 degrees, lead II looks toward 60 degrees, and lead III looks toward 120 degrees. This system allows the practitioner a view of the heart every 60 degrees.

The problem with Einthoven's original scheme was that it was not specific enough to accurately pinpoint cardiac pathology. The development of the augmented lead system in 1942 changed that. The augmented lead system uses more than one lead as the negative pole and thus splits the difference between leads I, II, and III. This allows a view of the heart every 30 degrees.

As can be appreciated from Fig. 11-27C, lead aVR looks over the right shoulder, lead aVL looks over the left shoulder, and lead aVF looks straight down. An augmented lead thus alternates with an Einthoven lead.

In order to identify the location of cardiac pathology, it is important that the clinician learn where each of the six limb leads "looks." This can be accomplished by recalling the 360-degree circle that was constructed over the anterior chest and the assignment of degrees beginning at 0 degrees on the left and moving to +/−180 degrees on the right. By recalling that an Einthoven lead alternates with a limb lead, it should be easy to divide the circle into 30-degree units and rotate around the lower hemisphere of the 360-degree circle, reciting "I-aVR-II-aVF-III-aVL" (see Fig. 11-27C).

Knowledge of the position of the heart within the chest is essential in understanding the area of the heart that each ECG

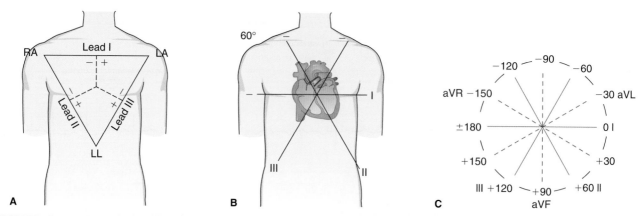

FIGURE 11-27   (**A**) Einthoven's triangle. (**B**) The three limb leads derived from this triangle. (**C**) The current 6-lead system consisting of Einthoven and augmented leads, providing a view of the heart's electrical activity every 30 degrees. (Only A reproduced with permission from Barrett KE, Barman SM, Boltano S, et al. *Ganong's Review of Medical Physiology*. 23rd ed. New York: McGraw-Hill; 2010, Fig. 30-8.)

lead records. Recall the position of the heart within the thorax. If the long axis of the heart is conceptualized as an arrow, then the shaft is a line formed by the interventricular septum, the point is the apex, and the atria are the feathers. This arrow is positioned such that the point is directed inferior, to the left, and anterior, while the feathers are directed superior, to the right, and posterior, toward the back. The heart is rotated on its long axis such that the left ventricle is to the left and the right ventricle is an anterior structure. The position of the heart is such that a large portion of the left ventricle is in direct contact with the diaphragm (called the *inferior*, or *diaphragmatic*, portion of the left ventricle).

Recall that the limb leads look at the heart's electrical activity in the frontal plane and reflect cardiac electrical activity that lies beneath these leads. Thus, leads I and aVL look at the high lateral wall of the left ventricle; leads II, III, and aVF look at the inferior wall of the left ventricle; and lead aVR looks toward the right atrium. The previous information is vital in appreciating pattern recognition in patients with myocardial ischemia or infarct.

Data Acquisition from the 12-Lead ECG

The student should have some understanding of the manner in which a 12-lead ECG is obtained. This is best accomplished by reviewing the operation of a typical ECG recorder. Two such recorders are shown in Fig. 11-28.

Limb Leads

The limb leads consist of leads I, II, III, aVR, aVL, and aVF and are obtained from the electrode–wire interfaces shown in Fig. 11-29A. **The limb leads look at the heart's electrical activity in the frontal plane.** The electrodes of the ECG recorder are actually spring-loaded plastic grips, which have a small metal piece inside the plastic grip. Placing conductive gel on these metal pieces and then placing the grips on the limbs allow the electrical activity of the heart to be acquired. If

the dial of the ECG recorder is set on limb lead I (Fig. 11-29B), it will acquire the electrical activity of the heart as it travels from the right arm to the left arm and will produce the tracing shown in Fig. 11-29C that is characteristic of limb lead I. Lead I *looks toward* 0 degrees and *looks at* the high lateral wall of the left ventricle. Similarly, if the dial of the ECG recorder is set on limb lead II, it will acquire the electrical activity of the heart as it travels from the right arm to the left leg and will produce a different tracing characteristic of limb lead II. Lead II *looks toward 60* degrees and *looks at* the inferior wall of the left ventricle. Finally, if the dial of the ECG recorder is set on limb lead III, it will acquire the electrical activity of the heart as it travels from the left arm to the left leg and will produce the tracing that is characteristic of limb lead III. Lead III *looks toward* 120 degrees and also *looks at* the inferior wall of the left ventricle.[9-13]

Leads aVR, aVL, and aVF form the augmented leads that subdivide Einthoven's leads and provide a view of the heart's

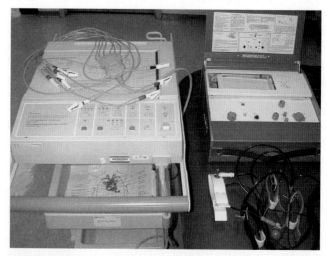

FIGURE 11-28   Left, a modern 12-lead ECG machine. Right, the Hewlett-Packard 1500B 12-lead ECG system.

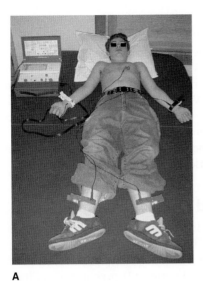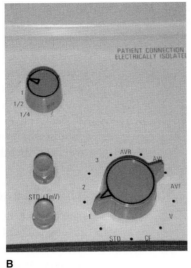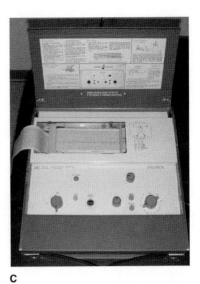

FIGURE 11-29 (**A**) Placement of the limb leads on a subject. (**B**) Setup of ECG acquisition in order to obtain lead I. (**C**) The resultant paper printout of lead I.

electrical activity every 30 degrees. When the dial of the ECG recorder is set on aVR, it will acquire the electrical activity of the heart as it travels to the right arm and will produce a tracing that is characteristic of lead aVR. It should be noted that in a normal tracing (Fig. 11-26), all the ECG waveforms in aVR are inverted. This is because the positive electrode of aVR looks over the right shoulder; because the vector is moving down and to the left (ie, down the normal conduction pathway), the vector is moving away from a positive electrode and therefore inverts the P, QRS, and T waves. When the dial of the ECG recorder is set on aVL, it will acquire the electrical activity of the heart as it travels to the left arm and will produce a tracing that is characteristic of lead aVL. Finally, when the dial of the ECG recorder is set on aVF, it will acquire the electrical activity of the heart as it travels to the left foot and will produce a tracing that is characteristic of lead aVF. It should be noted that normally the waveforms in aVF are strongly positive; this is because the positive electrode of aVF looks straight down; because the vector is moving down and to the left (ie, down the normal conduction pathway), the vector is moving toward a positive electrode and therefore produces upright P, QRS, and T waves.[11]

Precordial Leads

The precordial leads are unipolar leads like the augmented voltage leads and consist of V_1, V_2, V_3, V_4, V_5, and V_6. **The precordial leads look at the heart's electrical activity in the horizontal (transverse) plane.** The value of the precordial leads is the proximity each has to the heart (rather than the large distance in the augmented voltage leads presented immediately above) as well as the different views of the heart's electrical activity that can be acquired as each lead traverses the left upper quadrant of the thorax. The position of each of the precordial leads is presented in Table 11-2 as well as Fig. 11-30.

Acquisition of V1 is accomplished by setting the dial of the ECG recorder on "V" and placing the suction cup in the fourth intercostal space, right parasternal border, as shown in Table 11-2. The ECG machine will acquire the electrical activity of the heart from the location of the suction cup. The suction cup is placed at each of the six standard precordial placement sites provided in Table 11-2 and will acquire the electrical activity from each of these sites. The acquired electrical activity of the heart from these six sites will produce the characteristic ECG complexes shown in Fig. 11-26, right side of the panel.

For the interpretation of the 12-lead ECG, it may be best to group the six precordial leads by their anatomical location (eg, the part of the heart that they overlie and from which the heart's electrical activity is acquired).[9-13] Precordial leads V_1 through V_2 are typically considered to represent the electrical activity of the heart from an anterior perspective (or view) of the left ventricle, leads V_3 through V_4 are considered to

TABLE 11-2 Location of the Precordial Electrodes on the Chest Wall

Precordial Electrode	Location on the Chest Wall
V_1	Just to the right of the sternum in the fourth intercostal space
V_2	Just to the left of the sternum in the fourth intercostal space
V_3	Halfway between V_2 and V_4
V_4	Midclavicular line in the fifth intercostal space
V_5	Halfway between V_4 and V_6
V_6	Midaxillary line in the fifth intercostal space

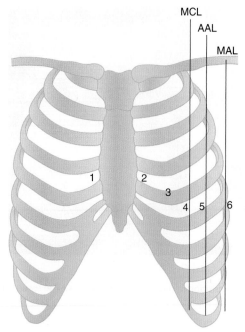

FIGURE 11-30 Standardized placement of the precordial leads across the chest in order to obtain V_1 through V_6.

provide an anteroseptal view of the electrical activity from the left ventricle, and leads V_4 through V_6 are considered to provide lateral views of the electrical activity from the left ventricle. A posterior view of the heart's electrical activity is acquired from leads V_1 through V_2 by examining these leads for inverse or reciprocal changes (often referred to as a mirror image) associated with the posterior wall of the left ventricle.[9-13] The inferior wall of the left ventricle is the only area of the left ventricle not represented by the precordial leads. The inferior wall of the left ventricle can be examined in leads II, III, and aVF.[9-13] The right ventricle can be appreciated by viewing right (rather than left) precordial leads.[15,16] Several right precordial leads that have been used in the past include precordial leads V_3 through V_6, but on the right of the sternum, as well as a right precordial lead, CR_{4R}. The standard left precordial leads V_1 and V_2 as well as lead aVF have also been used to examine the right ventricle via electrocardiography. The ability to examine different aspects of the heart and different diseases by viewing specific ECG leads and characteristics will be further discussed in the following section.

The 12-Lead Electrocardiogram

The 12-lead ECG shown in Fig. 11-26 and in Figs. 11-31 through 11-34 is performed for many reasons. These include assessing the (1) likelihood of cardiovascular, pulmonary, or other diseases; (2) presence of cardiac rhythm disturbances; (3) likelihood of an acute or old myocardial infarction; (4) likelihood of atrial or ventricular hypertrophy; and (5) possibility of ECG changes over a certain period of time due to one or more of the aforementioned or other conditions (see Table 11-3). The methods to examine and interpret these particular findings are presented in the following section.

Use of the 12-Lead Electrocardiogram in Physical Examination

The preceding section highlights the important role the 12-lead ECG can play in the physical examination of patients seen by a physical therapist. Although these skills have been considered to be advanced,[17] they are easily acquired and can aid in the examination and management of all types of patients seen in physical therapy. These clinical skills are particularly important for the Doctor of Physical Therapy (DPT) student and practitioner. The areas worthy of further attention include

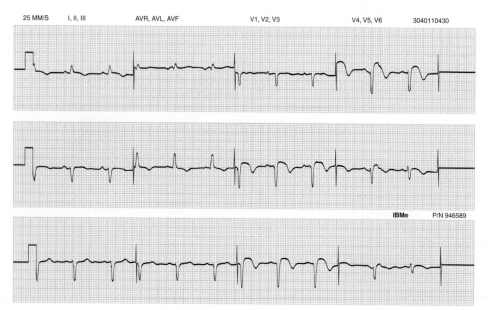

FIGURE 11-31 Twelve-lead ECG representing an acute anteroseptal and lateral wall MI. Note the ST-segment elevation and the loss of R waves in V_2 through V_6 coupled with deep T wave inversions. Note also the loss of R waves in leads II, III, and aVF (a probable old inferior wall MI) with the resultant left axis deviation (LAD) of −60 degrees.

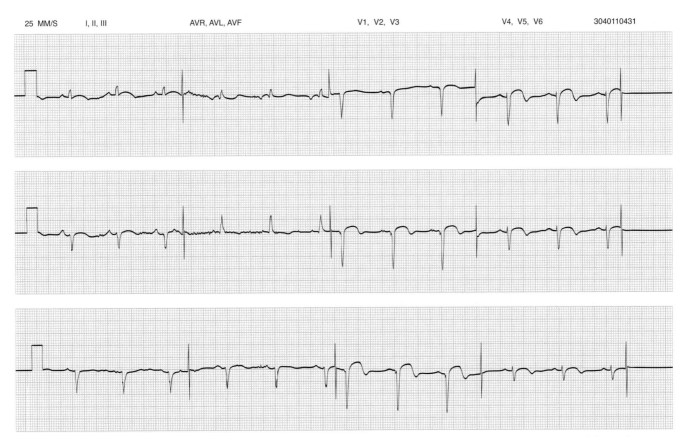

FIGURE 11-32   Inferior wall MI, age indeterminate. Note the loss of R waves in II, III, and aVF. Note also the new anteroseptal wall MI, as evidenced by the deep Q waves in leads V_1 through V_3. This individual clearly has multivessel disease of both the right and the left coronary arteries.

methods to (1) calculate the axis of the heart, (2) evaluate the likelihood of atrial and ventricular hypertrophy, and (3) identify signs of myocardial injury or infarction. These areas will be presented in the following sections.

Axis of the heart—The *axis* represents the sum total of all the electrical forces during any given cardiac cycle and the direc-

tion that the positive wave of depolarization takes as it travels from the SA node to the terminal fibers of the Purkinje system. The reader will recall the 360-degree circle superimposed on the patient's chest that forms the landmarks against which the limb leads are derived. The positive electrode of lead I "looks at" the patient's left, representing 0 degrees; aVF "looks" straight down at 90 degrees. These two landmarks will provide

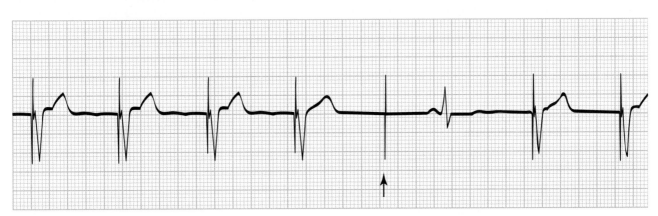

FIGURE 11-33   ECG rhythm strip showing a pacemaker spike initiating a ventricular response. Note the failure to capture the ventricle (arrow) and the native rhythm that follows.

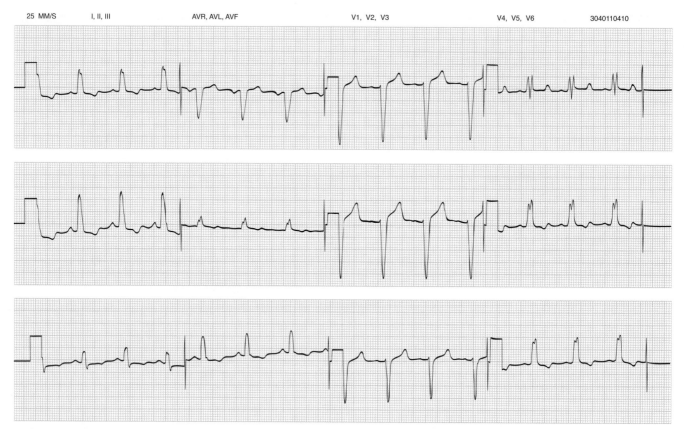

25 MM/S   I, II, III   AVR, AVL, AVF   V1, V2, V3   V4, V5, V6   3040110410

FIGURE 11-34   Twelve-lead ECG showing left bundle branch block. Note the wide QRS complexes that look like PVCs. Note also that each QRS complex is preceded by a P wave, which rules this possibility out.

the basis for determination of axis. The procedure for this determination is represented in Box 11-2.

The mechanisms responsible for the axis of the heart include the position of the heart in the chest, the size of the heart, and the viability of the myocardium. As mentioned previously, the vector, or sum total of all the electrical forces developed during depolarization, travels through the normal conduction pathway in a downward and leftward direction. If a 360-degree circle is superimposed over the anterior chest, the normal axis of the heart is approximately 60 degrees or anywhere between 0 degrees and 90 degrees. The direction of the heart's electrical axis can deviate from the normal value. Individuals who are unusually tall can have a "vertical heart" that places their axis at 90 degrees or more; obese individuals

BOX 11-2

Estimation of Axis

1. Examine lead I (0 degrees). If the R wave is mostly positive, then it means that the positive wave of depolarization is heading *toward* lead I and that the axis must lie in the hemisphere whose center is 0 degrees.
2. Examine lead aVF (90 degrees). If the R wave is mostly positive, then it means that the positive wave of depolarization is heading *toward* lead aVF, and that the axis must lie in the hemisphere whose center is 90 degrees.
3. The area that both hemispheres have in common is a half-hemisphere wedge between 0 and 90 degrees. Therefore, the axis must lie somewhere between 0 and 90 degrees.
4. Examine all six limb leads. Find the lead that is the most isoelectric (ie, that demonstrates a balance between upward and downward deflection of the QRS complex.)
5. Recall that if the positive wave of depolarization travels perpendicular to a positive electrode, an isoelectric waveform is the result.
6. Construct the perpendicular to this lead. Use only that portion of the construct that falls between 0 and 90 degrees. The position toward which this new constructed lead points is an approximation of the true axis. See Fig. 11-31 for an example of an axis shift.

TABLE 11-3   Reasons to Perform a 12-Lead Electrocardiogram

Reason	Possible ECG Finding
Cardiovascular disease	Signs of hypertension, myocardial ischemia, or infarction or disturbance in rhythm
Pulmonary disease	Signs suggestive of pulmonary hypertension and air trapping
Metabolic/endocrine disease	Signs of electrolyte imbalance

may have a "horizontal heart" that places their axis at 0 degrees or less because of the upward displacement of the heart and diaphragm brought about by expansion of the abdomen. Ventricular hypertrophy due to hypertension can increase left ventricular muscle mass and its electrical activity and can cause an axis deviation to the left, *toward* the hypertrophy. Finally, myocardial infarction can cause significant myocardial cell muscle death, which is replaced by nonconducting scar tissue. This causes an axis shift *away* from the lesion. Each of these mechanisms has a major influence of the determination of axis, but the position of the heart in the chest and the size of the heart and its respective chambers will have the greatest influence on the development and direction of the heart's electrical activity. See Fig. 11-31 for an example of an axis shift away from an old inferior wall MI.

Atrial and ventricular hypertrophy—The likelihood of atrial and ventricular hypertrophy can be evaluated using a variety of methods that were presented in Chapter 10. Table 11-4 provides an overview of the different methods to evaluate atrial and ventricular hypertrophy using the ECG. Close examination of this table reveals that the key methods to evaluate the likelihood of atrial or ventricular hypertro-phy are to measure the (1) duration of particular ECG intervals or segments and (2) magnitude of voltage in the R and S waves. The greater the hypertrophy, the greater the amount of time required for electrical activity to traverse hypertrophied myocardium, thus producing a prolonged or abnormal ECG interval or segment. Similarly, a greater amount of myocardial muscle mass will generate a greater amount of voltage and produce taller R waves or deeper S waves in particular ECG leads. It is also apparent from Table 11-4 that specific methods to differentiate left from right ventricular hypertrophy exist, but no such specific method exists to differentiate left from right atrial hypertrophy. However, it has been suggested that it may be possible to identify left atrial hypertrophy by the observation of a biphasic P wave in V_1 that is characterized by the terminal portion of the P wave being 1.0 mm or more in depth and 0.04 seconds in duration.[11]

Table 11-5 provides two methods to quantify these measurements using the criteria established by Estes and Scott.[17,18] Estes's method assigns a certain number of points based on particular ECG findings, whereas Scott's criteria simply use the voltage measurements of the R and S waves in the limb leads and several of the precordial leads.[17,18] **The practicing**

TABLE 11-4 Methods to Evaluate Atrial and Ventricular Hypertrophy via Electrocardiography

Evaluation Technique	Methods
Atrial hypertrophy[a]	
P waves of limb lead II or III	Examine the P wave for a biphasic pattern (upward and downward phases of at least 1.0 mm and width of 1.0 mm)
P waves of V_1	Examine the P wave for a biphasic pattern (upward and downward phases of at least 1.0 mm and width of 1.0 mm)
Left ventricular hypertrophy (LVH)	
R or S waves in limb leads	Measure the magnitude of voltage in mm (>20 mm)
R waves in V_4, V_5, or V_6	Measure the magnitude of voltage in mm (>25 mm)
S waves in V_1, V_2, or V_3	Measure the magnitude of voltage in mm (>25 mm)
ST-T wave abnormalities	Examine the ST segments and T waves for abnormalities such as ST-segment depression or elevation or T-wave inversion or flattening
Prolonged QRS interval duration	Measure the QRS interval duration for signs of prolongation (>0.10–0.12 s)
Prolonged Q wave to peak of R wave in V_1 and V_6	Measure the distance from the Q wave to the peak of the R wave in V_1 and V_6 for signs of prolongation (> 0.02 s and > 0.04 s, respectively)
Atrial hypertrophy	Examine the P wave in leads II, III, and V_1 for a biphasic pattern (upward and downward phases of at least 1.0 mm and width of 1.0 mm)
Left axis deviation (LAD)	Measure the axis of the heart's wave of depolarization (if −15 degrees or more negative, then LAD)
Right ventricular hypertrophy (RVH)	
Tall R waves in V_1 and V_2	Measure the magnitude of voltage in mm[b]
Deep S waves in V_5 and V_6	Measure the magnitude of voltage in mm[b]
ST-T wave abnormalities, especially in leads V_1, V_2, II, III, and Avf	Examine the ST segments and T waves for abnormalities such as ST-segment depression or elevation or T-wave inversion or flattening
Prolonged QRS interval duration, especially an incomplete right bundle branch block	Measure the QRS interval duration for signs of prolongation (>0.10–0.12 s)
Prolonged Q wave to peak of R wave in V_1 and V_2	Measure the distance from the Q wave to the peak of the R wave in V_1 and V_2 for signs of prolongation (>0.02 s)
Atrial hypertrophy	Examine the P wave in leads II, III, and V_1 for a biphasic pattern (upward and downward phases of at least 1.0 mm and width of 1.0 mm)
Right axis deviation (RAD)	Measure the axis of the heart's wave of depolarization (if +90 degrees or more positive, then RAD)

[a]Differentiation of right versus left atrial hypertrophy is difficult to distinguish based on ECG criteria alone.

[b]If the R-to-S wave ratio (R wave/S wave) is > 1.0, then RVH likely exists. The R wave/S wave ratio is determined by measuring the height of the R wave in V_1 or V_2 and the depth of the S wave in V_1 or V_2.

TABLE 11-5   **Scoring Methods to Predict Left Ventricular Hypertrophy**

Evaluation Technique	Estes' Scoring Method		
	Methods		Points
R or S waves in limb leads	If the magnitude of voltage is > 20 mm		
R waves in V_4, V_5, or V_6	If the magnitude of voltage is > 25 mm	THEN	3
S waves in V_1, V_2, or V_3	If the magnitude of voltage is > 25 mm		
ST-T-wave abnormalities	If any sign of ST-segment or T-wave abnormalities	THEN	3
Prolonged QRS interval duration	If the QRS interval duration is > 0.10–0.12 s	THEN	1
Prolonged Q wave to peak of R wave in V_1 and V_6	If the distance from the Q wave to the peak of the R wave in V_1 or V_6 is > 0.02 s or > 0.04 s, respectively	THEN	1
Atrial hypertrophy	If the P wave in leads II, III, and V_1 is biphasic with upward and downward phases of at least 1.0 mm and a width of 1.0 mm	THEN	3
Left axis deviation (LAD)	If the axis is −15 degrees or more negative	THEN	2
LVH is likely to exist if 5 points	Total number of points		13
	Scott's Scoring Method		
Limb-lead criteria			
R-wave voltage in lead I and S-wave voltage in lead III	If combined voltage > 25 mm	THEN	LVH
R-wave voltage in aVL	If voltage > 7.5 mm	THEN	LVH
R-wave voltage in aVF	If voltage > 20 mm	THEN	LVH
S-wave voltage in aVR	If voltage > 14 mm	THEN	LVH
Precordial lead criteria			
R-wave voltage in V_5 or V_6 and S-wave voltage in V_1 or V_2	If combined voltage > 35 mm	THEN	LVH
R-wave and S-wave voltage in any precordial lead	If combined voltage > 45 mm	THEN	LVH
R-wave voltage in V_5 or V_6	If voltage > 26 mm	THEN	LVH

physical therapist may find that Scott's precordial lead criteria offer the easiest way to assess for the presence of left ventricular hypertrophy.

Myocardial injury or infarction—Identification of myocardial injury or infarction is also an ECG skill considered to be advanced, but simple observation of the ST segment and a few other ECG abnormalities can provide a wealth of information about injury or infarction to the myocardium.

CLINICAL CORRELATE

Physical therapists working with patients who have suffered a recent acute MI should follow the evolution or resolution of this event using serial ECG reports, which can provide valuable information that can be used to direct subsequent exercise strategies.

Table 11-6 provides an overview of the process used to examine the ECG for signs of myocardial injury or infarction. Identification of ST-segment depression and elevation as well as the significance and implications of both have been presented in the earlier portion of this chapter. Table 11-6

expands the role of measuring ST-segment depression or elevation in one single ECG lead presented earlier and presents the methods to characterize and group these and other measurements to localize specific areas of the heart that have been damaged, both acutely and long ago.

TABLE 11-6   **Patterns of Recognition of Myocardial Injury/Infarction[a]**

Pattern ECG Leads	Coronary Arteries Likely Responsible
Anterior V_1 and V_2	Left main and LAD
Anteroseptal V_2 and V_3	Left main and LAD
Lateral V_4, V_5, and V_6	Circumflex and diagonal divisions of LAD
Posterior V_1 and V_2	RCA
Inferior II, III, aVF	Posterior descending of the RCA
Superior I, II, aVR, aVL	Circumflex and diagonal divisions of LAD

[a]An acute myocardial injury or infarction is identified by elevation of the ST segments in the ECG leads overlying or associated with particular myocardial anatomy. An old transmural myocardial infarction can be identified by deep, wide Q waves in the ECG leads overlying or associated with particular myocardial anatomy or circulation. Because of this, the location of myocardial injury or infarction as well as the coronary artery that is likely responsible for the insult can be identified. However, because of inherent differences in coronary anatomy and coronary artery dominance, the actual identification of the artery(ies) responsible for myocardial injury or infarction is made via cardiac catheterization. Nonetheless, the actual location of myocardial insult can be made with the ECG.

It should be clear from Table 11-6 that particular *patterns* of injury or infarction can be observed with a 12-lead ECG. These patterns are dependent on the anatomy of the coronary arteries and the location of the ECG electrodes. In brief, these patterns of injury or MI include locations in the anterior, posterior, anteroseptal, lateral, and inferior areas of the heart. Some evidence exists that a superior pattern can also be identified, but this pattern is not universally accepted. These patterns of recognition, the ECG leads, and the underlying coronary anatomy that appear to be responsible for the aforementioned patterns are provided in Table 11-6.

The aforementioned process of pattern recognition can be appreciated in Fig. 11-31 in which the 12-lead ECG displays an acute MI and the evolutionary changes after several days of recovery. The acute MI is apparent in the anteroseptal precordial leads (V_2, V_3) and lateral precordial leads (V_4, V_5, V_6) of Fig. 11-31 by the ST-segment elevation, representing a zone of injury. Also of note is the presence of T-wave inversions in I, II, and aVL, representing a zone of ischemia. This zone of ischemia represents jeopardized myocardium that could become necrotic over the next few days as the MI continues to evolve. Fortunately, the ischemic changes in this example normalized approximately 4 days later. Figure 11-32 demonstrates the presence of an older inferior wall MI, with characteristic changes in leads II, III, and aVF. Note the presence of deep Q waves in these leads, coupled with loss of the R waves. The Q waves represent areas of full-thickness myocardial necrosis, a change that usually evolves subsequent to the earlier ST-segment displacements seen in Fig. 11-31. In Fig. 11-32, note also the newly evolving MI in the anteroseptal area, as evidenced by the dramatic ST-segment elevations in the early and midprecordial leads, and the *poor R-wave progression* as one moves from V_1 to V_6.

CARDIAC PACEMAKERS

Cardiac pacemakers play an important role in the treatment of heart disease due to cardiac rhythm disturbances. They have the ability to *pace* the heart (ie, discharge an electrical stimulus to initiate a wave of depolarization throughout the heart). Pacemakers have a characteristic pattern that is easy to recognize on an ECG. The pacemaker produces its own wave of depolarization that marks the ECG with a *pacer spike* as shown in Fig. 11-33. Improved technologies have increased the application of pacemakers and pacemaker principles to the treatment of other types of heart disease including coronary artery disease and heart failure. Because the use of pacemakers has increased (and will likely further increase as technological advancements continue), as well as the potential role of physical therapy for persons with cardiac pacemakers, this section will be devoted to the cardiac pacemaker. This potential role includes assisting with the (1) establishment of pacing parameters (with electrophysiologic physicians) to obtain optimal functional and exercise outcomes and (2) establishment of safe functional and exercise activities for patients with pacemakers and automatic implanted cardioverter-defibrillators (AICDs).

BOX 11-3

Indications for a Cardiac Pacemaker

1. Sick sinus syndrome
2. Complete heart block
3. Cardiac denervation as in cardiac transplantation
4. Severe cardiac rhythm disturbances
5. Easily provoked angina
6. Congestive heart failure

The indications for a pacemaker, types of pacemakers, as well as pacemaker codes and pacing modes will be presented so that the physical therapist can provide optimal physical therapy to patients with cardiac pacemakers.

Indications for a Cardiac Pacemaker

The indications for a cardiac pacemaker are listed in Box 11-3 and include a sick sinus syndrome, complete heart block, or cardiac denervation as in cardiac transplantation. Several other indications exist and for each of these reasons the primary goal is to improve the synchrony of myocardial mechanics (chamber filling and emptying) to enhance cardiac function such as the stroke volume, cardiac output, and ejection fraction.

Types of Pacemakers

The types of pacemakers that are currently available are listed in Table 11-7. Four basic types of pacemakers exist and include fixed-rate pacemakers, demand pacemakers, atrial-triggered pacemakers, and ventricular-triggered pacemakers. The most common pacemakers are demand pacemakers, which pace the heart on demand and most frequently will pace the ventricle. To fully understand the pacemakers listed in Table 11-7, it is necessary to review the three-letter pacemaker codes, which have been expanded over the years to five-letter codes.

Pacemaker Codes

The coding of pacemakers began in 1974 and outlined a three-letter coding sequence, which made it easy for one to understand the cardiac chamber being *paced* (the first letter of the code and can be an A for atrium, V for ventricle, or D for dual atrium and ventricle), the cardiac chamber being *sensed* (the second letter of the code and can be an A for atrium, V for ventricle, D for dual atrium and ventricle, or O for none), and the *mode* of response (the third letter of the code and can be I for inhibited, T for triggered, D for atrial triggered and ventricular inhibited, R for reverse, or O for none). Because the initial 3-letter code was introduced, two additional codes have been added to keep pace with the technological advancements applied to pacemakers. The two additional codes represent *programmability* (the fourth letter of the code and can be a P

TABLE 11-7   Different Types of Pacemakers

Type of Pacemaker	Pacemaker ICHD Code[a]	Response to Sensed Activity
Fixed-rate ventricular[b]	VOO	None
P-triggered ventricular	VAT	Triggered
QRS-triggered ventricular	VVT	Triggered
QRS-inhibited ventricular	VVI	Inhibited
Fixed-rate atrial[b]	AOO	None
Demand AV sequential	DVI	Inhibited
Fixed-rate AV sequential[b]	DOO	None
Fixed-rate AV simultaneous[b]	DOO	None
Atrial synchronous	VDD	Atria triggered
Ventricular-inhibited		Ventricle inhibited
Universal, fully automatic	DDD	Inhibited on channel Sensed (either the atria or the ventricle) and triggered on alternate channel (either the atria or the ventricle)

[a]The Pacemaker ICHD Code provides specific information about the pacemaker such that the position of each letter (first, second, or third) and the letter itself (V, A, D, O, T, or I) informs a clinician about the cardiac chamber being paced (first letter), the cardiac chamber being sensed (second letter), and the mode of pacemaker response (the third letter). The letters are abbreviations for the following words: V, ventricle; A, atrium; D, atrium and ventricle; O, none; T, triggered; I, inhibited.

[b]The fixed-rate atrial, ventricular, and AV sequential pacemakers are currently obsolete. However, a few older patients may still have such a pacemaker implanted. These pacemakers are obsolete because the fixed rate does not allow for optimal physiologic function (cardiac or functional activities).

for programmable rate and/or output, M for multiprogrammable, or O for none) and *tachyarrhythmia* functions (the fifth letter of the code and can be a B for burst, N for normal rate competition, S for scanning, E for externally activated, or O for none). It is now apparent that adding these two additional codes to the original 3-letter code system produces a 5-position pacemaker code.

Each of the specific letters within each of the code positions after the second letter is related to specific actions of the pacemaker, which gives it greater or lesser clinical utility. Table 11-7 alludes to this, but further discussion of the actual pacing modes is needed to fully appreciate pacemaker capabilities and the role of the physical therapist when working with patients who have received a permanent pacemaker.

Pacing Modes

The available pacing modes can be interpreted from Table 11-7. A quick review of the actual available modes of pacing should facilitate a better appreciation for the pacemaker. Table 11-7 identifies three of the listed pacemakers as obsolete. The reason for this is due to the rather primitive mode of pacing, a fixed rate of pacing of either the atria or the ventricle.

The second type of pacemaker listed in Table 11-7 is the P-triggered ventricular pacemaker that has a VAT coding. The V indicates that the cardiac chamber being paced is the ventricle, A indicates that the cardiac chamber sensing the electrical activity in the heart is the atria, and T indicates that the mode of response is to trigger a paced beat in the ventricle when the atrium senses the SA node's wave of depolarization that cannot proceed past the AV node. This type of pacemaker is used in patients with normal SA node function and without bradycardia or atrial tachyarrhythmias (because with this type of pacemaker it is the role of the atria to signal the pacemaker to discharge an action potential to the ventricle). When the pacemaker sensor in the atria senses electrical activity, it triggers the pacemaker to pace the ventricle at a rate commensurate with the normal and needed atrial rate of discharge from the SA node. This is truly a physiologically favorable pacing mode. It is also easy to understand why a patient with bradycardia or atrial tachyarrhythmias would not be a good candidate for such a pacemaker, because the pacemaker would be pacing the ventricle either too slow or too fast. The atrial-synchronized, ventricular-inhibited pacemaker (with an ICHD code of VDD) and the QRS-triggered and -inhibited ventricular pacemakers (with ICHD codes of VVT and VVI, respectively) function in much the same way as the P-triggered ventricular pacemaker (with VAT code), only they sense from the atrium and ventricle (for the VDD pacemaker) or the QRS wave from the ventricle (for the VVT and VVI pacemakers), but all similarly pace the ventricle.

The demand AV sequential pacemaker with an ICHD coding of DVI is another type of pacemaker that attempts to provide more physiologically sound pacing (like the P-triggered ventricular pacemaker). It attempts to synchronize the atrial and ventricular electrical activity of the heart, which may result in better mechanical activity of these cardiac chambers and improved cardiac function. This pacemaker is used in patients with atrial bradyarrhythmias with or without impaired AV node function. It is not used in patients with prolonged bouts of atrial fibrillation or flutter. When a patient with this DVI coded pacemaker experiences sinus bradycardia, the ventricle senses a need to pace the atrium and ventricle (the "D" code) and inhibits pacing when the ventricle no longer senses sinus bradycardia. Despite the fact that this pacemaker attempts to pace the heart in a truly physiologic manner, it is unable to (1) alter the paced rate (the heart rate) to increased physiologic demands and (2) maintain AV synchronous pacing during periods of normal sinus rhythm and AV block.

The last pacemaker listed in Table 11-7 is the universal, fully automatic pacemaker with DDD coding. The DDD pacemaker is used in patients with (1) atrial bradyarrhythmias with or without impaired AV node conduction and (2) normal sinus node function, but with impaired AV node conduction. When a patient with this DDD-coded pacemaker experiences sinus bradycardia or impaired AV node conduction, either the atrium or ventricle senses (the second "D" code) the abnormality and inhibits pacing where pacing was sensed and then

triggers either the atria or ventricle to pace in the chamber where no electrical activity was sensed (the first "D" code). Although there are really no significant disadvantages to the universal, fully automatic pacemaker, the other pacemakers presented previously have several important advantages and disadvantages that are worthy of further discussion. This discussion will hopefully further clarify the modes and mechanism of action of pacemakers.

Advantages and Disadvantages of Available Pacing Modes

The advantages and disadvantages of the currently available pacing modes are listed in Table 11-8. It is apparent from this table that the patient with a pacemaker other than the universal, fully automatic pacemaker will likely have limited cardiac function due to suboptimal AV contraction (and other characteristics inherent in the different types of pacemakers), which is likely to affect functional activities. Because of this and other pacemaker issues, the next section will present a more complete listing of pacemaker modes and functions (rate modulation, cardiac resynchronization therapy [CRT], and implantable cardioverter defibrillator [ICD] therapy).

Additional Pacemaker Modes and Functions

Table 11-9 provides an overview of the pacemaker codes previously reviewed as well as two additional symbols that have become increasingly important in the management of patients requiring a pacemaker. The two additional symbols sit in the fourth and fifth positions of the pacemaker code. The fourth symbol identifies the programmable rate modulation function of the pacemaker while the fifth symbol identifies the antitachyarrhythmia function of the pacemaker. Pacemakers with

letters in these positions have one of more of the functions listed in Table 11-9.

Rate modulation—Rate modulation refers to the pacemaker's ability to modulate heart rate based on activity or physiologic demands.[19-23] Pacemakers usually are fit with one or two (dual) sensors including various derivatives of two methods consisting of (1) activity or motion based and (2) physiological based with the most common sensor being one that measures minute ventilation. The sensors and pacemaker attempt to promote a normal sinus node response to increasing HR with exertional demands.[24]

The type of sensor(s) utilized may impact the ability of the pacer to respond to various exercise modalities.[25] Motion/activity sensors result in sluggish HR response to activities that are smooth such as on the bicycle ergometer or with supine, seated, or standing exercise, and rapid response to ambulation. However, these pacers have poor proportionality (ie, faster rates when descending stairs than when ascending) and poor specificity (ie, inappropriate high rates when riding over a bumpy road).[26] In patients with motion sensors, activities that promote movement of the thorax (hallway ambulation) or treadmill protocols that include increases in both speed and grade, should be utilized to trigger an increase in HR. QT sensors and ventilatory driven sensors may require longer warm-up periods because of delayed responses to activity; however, these sensors have good proportionality and specificity. QT sensors are the only sensors that respond to emotional stress; however, medication and electrolyte level changes may impact responsiveness of HR with QT interval sensors.[26]

Combinations of sensors, or dual sensor rate modulation pacers, seem to offer the best HR response to immediate activity

TABLE 11-8 Advantages and Disadvantages of Different Pacemakers

Type of Pacemaker	Advantages	Disadvantages
Fixed-rate ventricular[a]	?	Fixed rate of pacing
P-triggered ventricular	Maintains normal sinus rhythm	Does not maintain control of the ventricular synchronous AV rate contraction, because the atria are not paced
QRS-triggered ventricular QRS-inhibited ventricular	Long history of use	Does not maintain synchronous AV contraction because the atria are not paced
Fixed-rate atrial	?	Fixed rate of pacing
Demand AV sequential	Maintains synchronous AV contraction during sinus bradycardia	Does not maintain synchronous AV contraction when normal sinus rhythm with AV block
Fixed-rate AV sequential[a]	?	Fixed rate of pacing
Fixed-rate AV simultaneous[a]	?	Fixed rate of pacing
Atrial-synchronous, ventricular-inhibited	Maintains normal sinus control of the ventricular rate	Does not maintain synchronous AV contraction, because the atria are not paced
Universal, fully automatic	Maintains synchronous AV contraction and normal sinus control of the ventricular rate during NSR and during sinus bradycardia	?

[a]Likely currently obsolete.

AV, atrioventricular; NSR, normal sinus rhythm.

TABLE 11-9 Pacemaker Code Classification[a]

First Symbol Pacing Location	Second Symbol Sensing Location	Third Symbol Response to Pacing	Fourth Symbol Programmability/ Modulation	Fifth Symbol Antitachyarrhythmia Function
O = none	N = none	N = none	O = none	O = none
A = atrium	A = atrium	I = inhibited	S = simple programmable	P = pacing
V = ventricle	V = ventricle	T = triggered	M = multiprogrammable	S = shock
D = dual	D = dual	d = dual	C = communicating	D = dual
			R = rate modulation	

Definitions:

Dual: atrium and ventricle can be sensed and/or paced independently.

Inhibited Response: pending stimulus is inhibited when a spontaneous stimulation is detected.

Triggered Response: detection of stimulus produces an immediate stimulus in the same chamber.

Simple Programming: either or both rate and output adjustment.

Multiprogrammable: can be programmed more extensively.

Communicating: has telemetry capabilities.

Rate Modulation: can adjust rate automatically based on one or more other physiological variables.

[a]Bernstein AD, Camm AJ, Fletcher RD, et al. The NASPE/BPEG generic pacemaker code for antibradyarrhythmia and adaptive pacing and antitachyarrhythmia devices. *Pacing Clin Electrophysiol*. 1987;10:795.

demands by exploiting strengths and counteracting weaknesses of individual sensors. Ventilation sensors provide the predominant contribution during intense effort with activity sensors failing to reach required HRs for optimal hemodynamic response.[27–30]

The upper limit of the pacemaker rate modulation should be known since blood pressure may not be adequately maintained if the upper limit is exceeded. Thus, blood pressure should be properly monitored in patients with pacemakers that have been programmed to provide rate modulation. Increases in heart rate above the upper limit of the pacemaker modulation rate will stimulate the pacemaker to introduce a Wenckebach (Mobitz I) atrioventricular heart block rhythm that can result in reductions in blood pressure and shortness of breath. The best mechanism to identify such a phenomenon may be to simply monitor the ECG during exercise.[31]

While the majority of pacemakers implanted in the United States generate a rate response, not all pacers are equipped with rate modulation, and therefore some patients have heart rates that may not change with activity. In patients with pacemakers not equipped with rate modulation, low-level activity with small incremental increases in metabolic demand are preferred. Assessment of RPE, blood pressure, and symptoms should be utilized to monitor tolerance to exercise.

Implantable cardioverter-defibrillators—The use of pacemakers and implantable cardioverter defibrillator (ICD) therapy has increased considerably over the past decade because of the lifesaving defibrillation provided to patients with fatal arrhythmias as well as one or more of the indications listed in Table 11-10.[19,32–44] Despite the mostly favorable effects of ICD therapy (defibrillating a patient who experiences a life-threatening cardiac arrhythmia), patients with ICD have significant psychological ramifications from the possibility of sudden defibrillation and frequently limit their functional and exercise activities in fear of defibrillation.[32–34] Support groups for patients with ICD appear to help decrease the anxiety and fear associated with ICD therapy.

TABLE 11-10 Indications for an Implantable Cardioverter-Defibrillator

1. Cardiac arrest due to VT or VF

2. Spontaneous sustained VT with structural heart disease

3. Spontaneous sustained VT without structural heart disease that is not amenable to other treatments

4. Nonsustained VT in patients with coronary disease, prior MI, left ventricular dysfunction, and inducible VF or sustained VT at EPS that is not suppressible by a class I antiarrhythmic drug

5. Left ventricular dysfunction with an ejection fraction ≤ 30% at least 1 month post-MI and 3 months post–coronary artery revascularization surgery

6. Severe symptoms (eg, syncope) attributable to ventricular tachyarrhythmias in patients awaiting cardiac transplantation

7. Ventricular tachyarrhythmias due to a transient or reversible disorder that is likely to substantially reduce the risk of recurrent arrhythmia

8. Syncope with
   a. unexplained etiology with typical or atypical right bundle branch block and ST-segment elevations
   b. advanced structural heart disease without clear etiology
   c. unexplained etiology without inducible VT and without structural heart disease

VT, ventricular tachycardia; VF, ventricular fibrillation; EPS, electrophysiological services.

Adapted from Gregoratos G, Abrams J, Epstein JE, et al. ACC/AHA/ NASPE 2002 guideline update for implantation of cardiac pacemakers and antiarrhythmia devices: summary article: a report of the American College of Cardiology/American Heart Association Task Force on Practice Guidelines (ACC/AHA/NASPE Committee to Update the 1998 Pacemaker Guidelines). *Circulation*. 2002;106:2145-2161.

TABLE 11-11 Potential Role of Physical Therapists for Patients with Implantable Cardioverter-Defibrillators

1. Identify the reasons for ICD implantation.

2. Identify the ICD discharge heart rate for defibrillation.

3. Identify the level of anxiety and fear associated with the ICD.

4. Identify the patient's functional and exercise abilities while monitoring symptoms, heart rate, blood pressure, and the electrocardiogram and not allowing the heart rate to exceed the ICD discharge heart rate for defibrillation.

5. Communicate functional and exercise results with the patient's primary physician and the EPS team.

EPS, electrophysiologic services.

Only through the actual performance of functional and exercise tasks can a patient realize their functional and exercise abilities, which highlights the important role for physical therapists in the care of persons receiving ICD therapy.[24-34,45-47] The physical therapist's role in the examination and management of patients with ICD can be substantial and could include one or more of the tasks outlined in Table 11-11. Of these tasks the most important are likely to understand the reasons for ICD implantation and each patient's ICD discharge heart rate for defibrillation. Maintaining the patient's heart rate below the ICD discharge heart rate will prevent defibrillation that may occur accidentally due to the increase in heart rate from exercise. However, newer and more sophisticated pacemakers with ICD capacity are able to interrogate the morphology of the heart rhythm and differentiate an expected sinus tachycardia during exercise from a fatal ventricular tachycardia.

Finally, it has been reported that inappropriate discharge of an ICD may occur from transcutaneous electrical nerve stimulation (TENS) and other electromagnetic therapy that may be provided by a physical therapist.[36-39] Thus, it is important to obtain a comprehensive history of a patient known to have a pacemaker to determine if it has ICD capacity. Physical therapists should consult with referring physicians before providing patients with an ICD pacemaker with any form of electromagnetic therapy.

For example, several case reports exist whereby neuromuscular electrical stimulation (NMES) has resulted in electromagnetic interference causing false sensing and leading to inappropriate defibrillation in patients with AICDs, which results in cardiac arrhythmias or painful shocks.[36-39] Interference has been observed during both NMES of the trapezius and the quadriceps of patients, indicating that individual testing for interference is warranted before NMES should be utilized in patients with ICDs. Electromagnetic energy (EME) from household devices, airport security, and cell phones can also cause inappropriate shocks and interfere with pacemaker function by either creating a sensed beat or delaying the sequence of a paced beat. Patients should be advised to discuss the possibility of EME with their cardiologist since the major

determinant of response is based on the manufacturer of their device. Some general guidelines include the following: the potential for EME is proportional to the strength of the environmental source; the closer the source to the implantable device, the greater the risk (with <10 cm distance even cell phones can create EME—therefore, patients are advised to use cell phones on the side opposite of the implantable device); security systems are usually safe as long as the patient does not linger at the source; and security staff should be advised of the location of an implantable device to avoid bringing a electromagnetic wand within close proximity.[36-39]

Cardiac resynchronization therapy—Cardiac resynchronization therapy (CRT) is a medical treatment that is used to synchronize the electrical, physiologic, and mechanical events of the heart via a pacemaker.[48-52] It has become useful in the management of patients with heart failure.

A simplified explanation of CRT is the process that is used to synchronize AV as well as right and left ventricular depolarization and contraction in hopes of eliciting a more efficient and effective cardiac contraction. Although CRT has been a potential therapeutic modality for the past 6 to 8 years, it is only now receiving greater clinical use. This is surprising in view of the benefits that have been observed in much of the CRT literature, which has been summarized in Table 11-12.[48-52] Furthermore, several important predictors of mortality have also been improved with CRT including left ventricular size, norepinephrine levels, heart rate and heart rate variability, peak oxygen consumption, New York Heart Association classification, and 6-minute walk test distance ambulated.[48-52] Although the improvements in these important indices of survival in CHF are noteworthy, investigation of the specific effects of CRT on mortality are needed. Nonetheless, the improvements in many of the manifestations of CHF shown in Table 11-12 are likely to improve the functional abilities and quality of life of individuals with CHF.[48-52]

The beneficial effects of CRT in persons with CHF are likely due to the combined effects of numbers 1 to 5 in Table 11-12. The improvements in atrioventricular conduction; ventricular filling, activation and contraction; and improved ventricular wall motion likely produce the remaining beneficial effects (numbers 6–12) in Table 11-12.[17-22] Despite the potential beneficial effects of CRT on the manifestations of CHF, there are several potential adverse effects of CRT in persons with CHF including infection, bleeding disorders, pacemaker dysfunction, and possibly increased arrhythmias.

Pacemakers and Physical Therapy

As mentioned previously, the potential role of physical therapy in the care of persons with pacemakers includes assisting with the (1) establishment of pacing parameters (with electrophysiological physicians [EP]) to obtain the best functional and exercise outcomes and (2) establishment of safe functional and exercise activities for patients with pacemakers and AICDs. An additional role for the physical therapist may be consultation

TABLE 11-12 **Potential Beneficial Effects of Cardiac Resynchronization Therapy on the Manifestations of Chronic Heart Failure**

Adverse Manifestation of CHF	Potential Beneficial Effect
1. Prolonged AV conduction delay	Improved AV conduction delay
2. Delayed ventricular activation	Improved ventricular activation
3. Disorganized ventricular contraction	Improved ventricular contraction
4. Impaired ventricular filling (eg, MR, limited filling period, suboptimal atrial systole)	Improved ventricular filling
5. Abnormal ventricular wall motion	Improved ventricular wall motion
6. Abnormal ventricular size	Improved ventricular size
7. Abnormal myocardial O_2 consumption	Improved myocardial O_2 consumption
8. Abnormal catecholamine levels	Improved catecholamine levels
9. Abnormal heart rate and HRV	Improved heart rate and HRV
10. Poor functional status (eg, 6MWT)	Improved functional status
11. Low levels of peak O_2 consumption	Improved peak O_2 consumption
12. Poor NYHA classification (eg, classes 3–4)	Improved NYHA classification
13. Frequent hospitalization	Less frequent hospitalization

AV, atrioventricular; MR, mitral regurgitation; O_2, oxygen consumption; HRV, heart rate variability; 6MWT, 6-minute walk test; NYHA, New York Heart Association.

with an EP to determine the type of pacemaker to be implanted in a patient based on functional and exercise tasks examined by the physical therapist. The methods by which a physical therapist may provide optimal physical therapy to patients with cardiac pacemakers and AICDs are presented in Table 11-13. The typical pacemaker ECG tracing is shown in Fig. 11-33. It is important to note that the pacemaker is easy to identify by the presence of one or more pacer spikes such as those shown in Fig. 11-33. **The absence of a pacer spike in a patient who previously demonstrated such a spike may indicate pacemaker malfunctioning or pacing alterations. Likewise, pacer spikes in locations of the cardiac cycle where they should not be may be suggestive of pacemaker malfunctioning.** If such ECG findings are observed and are accompanied by increased symptoms and decreased functional abilities, pacemaker malfunctioning is highly likely. In either case, consultation with EP physicians may be needed to better understand the goals of the EP physicians and to contribute to a patient's overall care.

Much of the methodology presented in the cardiac examination chapter (Chapter 10) applies to the patient with a cardiac pacemaker, but evaluation of symptoms and the cardiovascular response to exercise or functional tasks is critically important in the pacemaker patient. In fact, examination of symptoms and the cardiovascular response of a patient with a pacemaker can provide important information to EP to help to establish optimal pacemaker-sensing and pacing modes. Observing a patient's symptoms, cardiovascular response, and achieved workloads or duration of exercise, we can identify the best pacemaker settings for a particular patient. This type of direct physical therapist–physician consultation and teamwork are likely to maximize a patient's full potential in the realms of cardiovascular and functional outcomes.

"OTHER" IMPORTANT APPLICATIONS OF THE ELECTROCARDIOGRAM

Segmental/Interval Analysis

Specific segments or intervals of the ECG complex have significant clinical utility that provides important diagnostic, prognostic, and possibly even therapeutic information (ie, identification of a particular ECG pattern within the interval may guide physical or medical therapies). Because of this, a cursory overview of several of these segments and intervals will be provided below.

PR Interval

As previously mentioned, the PR interval provides information about the wave of depolarization traveling from the SA

CLINICAL CORRELATE

Perhaps the best methods of contributing to the care of patients with pacemakers are to monitor (1) the ECG for signs of pacemaker failure, (2) the ECG at rest and during exercise or functional tasks, (3) symptoms (eg, shortness of breath, Borg rating of perceived exertion) at rest and during exercise or functional tasks, and (4) the systolic and diastolic blood pressure at rest and during exercise or functional tasks.

TABLE 11-13 **Methods to Provide Optimal Physical Therapy to Patients with Pacemakers**

Method	Procedure	Potential Outcome
Observation	Observe patient and ECG[a]	Recognition of optimal pacemaker function evidenced by a comfortable, healthy looking patient with appropriate pacing spikes at appropriate intervals and locations of the cardiac cycle or pacemaker malfunction evidenced by an uncomfortable, apprehensive patient without appropriate pacing spikes at appropriate intervals and locations of the cardiac cycle
Question and measure	Use a dyspnea or angina scale or Borg RPE[a]	Recognition of optimal pacemaker function evidenced by less dyspnea or angina and lower Borg RPE or pacemaker malfunction evidenced by increased dyspnea or angina and higher Borg RPE
Measure	Measure ECG, SBP, DBP, PP, exercise tolerance, and achieved workload[a]	Recognition of optimal pacemaker function evidenced by increased exercise tolerance and greater workloads, greater SBP, lower DBP, and a wider PP or pacemaker malfunction evidenced by decreased exercise tolerance and attainment of lower workloads, lower SBP, greater DBP, and a narrow PP

[a]See Chapters 9 and 10 for further information regarding the measurements in the Table.

ECG, electrocardiogram; RPE, rating of perceived exertion; SBP, systolic blood pressure; DBP, diastolic blood pressure; PP, pulse pressure (SBP–DBP).

node to the AV node. It can provide information about conduction that is too fast or too slow and is measured in the manner shown in Fig. 11-5. The PR interval is measured by simply placing a heart rate ruler with a special PR interval ruler section, using a calipers, or counting the number of boxes between the beginning of the P wave to the beginning of the QRS complex as shown in Fig. 11-5. The measured PR interval can then be compared to the normal range for a PR interval (0.12–0.20 seconds). Conduction that is too slow is represented by a prolonged PR interval and was discussed earlier. Conduction that is too fast is represented by a shortened PR interval (<0.12 seconds). This shortened PR interval may produce rapid rhythm disturbances that may be life-threatening. In fact, this characteristic ECG abnormality has been given the name Wolff–Parkinson–White syndrome (WPW).

Wolff–Parkinson–White syndrome—WPW is caused by the presence of fast conducting accessory tracks that bypass the AV node. It is a syndrome characterized by rapid depolarization and is evident by a shortened PR interval that may or may not have an upward slope (*delta wave*). The presence of WPW is associated with rapid atrial rhythm disturbances and the identification of the shortened PR interval and delta wave should alert the clinician that rapid atrial rhythm disturbances may occur during physical therapy examinations or treatments.

QRS Interval

The QRS interval provides information specific to the manner by which the wave of depolarization travels through the ventricles, culminating in ventricular depolarization and contraction. Several specific abnormalities of the QRS interval can be identified in the ECG and can help to provide important diagnostic and prognostic information. Some of this information was alluded to in the earlier discussion of hypertrophy and the axis of the heart. The QRS interval can provide information about interventricular conduction delays (IVCD) and bundle branch blocks (BBB).

Interventricular conduction delays—Interventricular conduction delays (IVCD) simply indicate that the wave of depolarization through the ventricles is slowed, which may be due to a number of factors but commonly is due to scarring and blocked electrical pathways or abnormal routing of the wave of depolarization via other pathways.

Bundle branch blocks—Bundle branch blocks (BBB) are an extension of an IVCD with a very characteristic pattern seen best on 12-lead ECG. The right BBB is best identified by examining leads V_1 and V_2 for a "rabbit-ear" appearance in the R wave. In fact, the "rabbit-ear" appearance is the result of two distinct R waves that are displayed on the ECG in leads V_1 and V_2 because the blocked right bundle branch causes the wave of depolarization to travel to only the left bundle, which causes the anterior precordial leads on the chest (V_1 and V_2) to receive two interrupted waves of depolarization (the first one from the left bundle branch and the second from the blocked right bundle branch), which is delayed and traverses the right bundle area through an alternate route and arrives after the initial wave of depolarization via the left bundle branch.

Figure 11-34 displays a left BBB. The left BBB is best identified by examining leads V_5 and V_6 for a wide, bizarre-looking QRS complex (resembling a PVC). When a wide, bizarre QRS complex is seen in leads V_5 and V_6 and is accompanied by an IVCD, the subject is diagnosed with a left bundle branch block (Fig. 11-34). The IVCD and a wide, bizarre QRS complex are the result of a blocked left bundle branch that requires the wave of depolarization to travel through the right bundle branch, which takes a longer period of time that is best seen in the lateral precordial ECG leads (V_5 and V_6).

QT Interval

The QT interval is another parameter that provides important information about the effects of particular medications on the electrical activity of the heart as well as a patient's prognosis. The QT interval is measured by placing a heart rate ruler with a special QT interval ruler section, using a

TABLE 11-14   **Estimated QT Intervals Based on a Given Heart Rate**

Heart Rate (bpm)	Estimated QT Interval (s)
60	0.33–0.43
70	0.31–0.41
80	0.29–0.38
90	0.28–0.36
100	0.27–0.35
>100	<0.27–0.35

calipers, or counting the number of boxes between the Q wave and the end of the T wave as shown in Fig. 11-4. The measured QT interval should then be compared to the estimated QT interval, which is closely related to the heart rate. The QT interval decreases as heart rate increases. Therefore, the measured QT interval should be compared to the estimated QT interval for a particular heart rate. Table 11-14 provides the estimated QT intervals for a given heart rate. The estimated QT interval for heart rates greater than 100 bpm should be less than 0.27 to 0.35 seconds.

R wave height—As previously mentioned in the myocardial injury and infarction section of this chapter, the height of the R wave can provide information about damaged myocardial tissue. The sudden disappearance of an R wave in an ECG lead that had consistently been observed to have an R wave is a sign suggestive of an MI. This sign is due to the inability of the area of the MI to generate and transmit a wave of depolarization.

In addition to this sign of MI, the actual height of the R wave has been suggested to yield important information regarding myocardial contractility and filling pressures of the chambers of the heart. It has been hypothesized that the R wave of a heart that is contracting poorly (and producing elevated filling pressures within the cardiac chambers) will increase, whereas the R wave of a heart that is contracting normally will not change appreciably or will decrease. It is quite easy to measure the height of the R wave before and after an exercise test, a bout of exercise, or a functional task. Simply measuring the height of the R wave from the isoelectric line to the top of the R wave will yield a measurement that can be recorded and compared before and after an exercise session. It is important to note that the R-wave measurements of one session should not be compared to those of another session during which the ECG electrodes have been replaced. Replacement of the ECG electrodes may be responsible for changes in the height of the R wave when comparing the results of one exercise session to another session. The clinical significance of the change in height of the R wave appears to have some clinical utility in the examination of patients with suspected heart disease. It is another ECG finding that may be helpful in evaluating the likelihood of heart disease in an

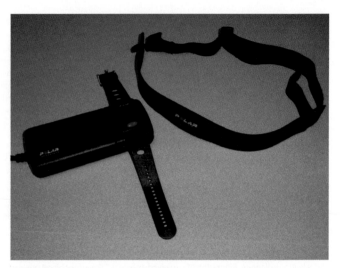

FIGURE 11-35   The *Polar Heart Rate Monitor* can provide the physical therapist with the mechanisms needed to measure and assess a patient's cardiovascular risk before, during, and after exercise as well as using the mode to measure heart rate variability. *(Manufactured by Polar Electro, Inc., Woodbury, NY.)*

exercising patient and should be examined with many of the other variables previously presented in this chapter and in Chapter 10 (such as ST-segment depression, heart rate, blood pressure, and symptoms).

Heart Rate Variability

Heart rate variability involves the examination of fluctuation between ECG complexes. The fluctuation between ECG complexes is the result of several interrelated dynamic processes including breathing, nervous system activation, and cardiovascular performance. **Perhaps the most important finding from heart rate variability research is that a healthier heart has greater fluctuation between ECG complexes, whereas an unhealthier heart has less fluctuation between ECG complexes.** The simplest and first method used to examine heart rate variability is obtained by measuring the regularity between the ECG complexes using the caliper method previously described and shown in Fig. 11-6. Today, many ECG devices such as Holter monitors, ECG acquisition systems, and even the Polar Heart Rate Monitor can examine the fluctuations between ECG complexes and provide useful output data to evaluate a patient's cardiovascular risk. Examining heart rate variability via either the caliper method (previously described) or the *Polar Heart Rate Monitor* may be the most clinically efficacious methods for a physical therapist. The methods previously described and shown in Fig. 11-5 and the equipment shown in Fig. 11-35 (the Polar HR Monitor) should provide the physical therapist with the mechanisms needed to measure and assess a patient's cardiovascular risk using heart rate variability.

SUMMARY

This chapter has provided an overview of electrocardiography. It has been presented from a clinical perspective with valuable techniques for acquiring the electrical activity of the heart. Newer methods of acquiring the electrical activity of the heart (via the Polar Heart Rate Monitor) have also been presented in hope that these techniques may be employed by physical therapists interested in better understanding patient prognosis and response to therapeutic interventions. The most important principles of ECG interpretation are likely the measurement of heart rate, rhythm, and axis as well as the evaluation of myocardial injury, infarction, and hypertrophy. The methods to perform these relatively easy and basic skills have been described in the text and outlined for clarity within the tables of this chapter. Numerous examples of single-lead and 12-lead ECGs and methods to interpret them have also been provided.

REFERENCES

1. Waller AD. A demonstration on man of electromotive changes accompanying the heart's beat. *J Physiol (Lond)*. 1887;8:229.
2. Einthoven W. *Am Heart J*. 53;602,1957 (English translation and publication of the original paper first published in *Arch Int de Physiol*. 1906;4:132-164).
3. James WB, Williams HB. The electrocardiogram in clinical medicine. *Am J Med Sci*. 1910;140:408.
4. Einthoven W. The different forms of the human electrocardiogram and their significance. *Lancet*. 1912;1:853.
5. Pardee HEB. An electrocardiographic sign of coronary artery obstruction. *Arch Intern Med*. 1920;26:244.
6. Barnes AR, Pardee HEB, White PD, et al. Standardization of precordial leads. *Am Heart J*. 1938;15:235.
7. Fye WB. A history of the origin, evolution, and impact of electrocardiography. *Am J Cardiol*. 1994;73:937.
8. Tsien RW, Hess P. Excitable tissues. The heart. In: Andreoli TE et al., eds. *Physiology of Membrane Disorders*. New York: Plenum Publishing; 1986.
9. Zipes DP. Genesis of cardiac arrhythmias: electrophysiological considerations. In: Braunwald E, ed. *Heart Disease—A Textbook of Cardiovascular Medicine*. Philadelphia, PA: WB Saunders; 1988.
10. Dubin D. *Rapid Interpretation of EKG's*. 6th ed. Tampa, FL: Cover Publishing Company; 2001.
11. Marriott HJL. *Practical Electrocardiography*. 10th ed. Baltimore, MD: Williams & Wilkins; 2001.
12. Fisch C. Electrocardiography and vectorcardiography. In: Braunwald E, ed. *Heart Disease—A Textbook of Cardiovascular Medicine*. Philadelphia, PA: WB Saunders; 1988.
13. Froelicher VF. *Exercise and the Heart—Clinical Concepts*. 2nd ed. Chicago, IL: Year Book Medical Publishers Inc; 1987.
14. Wagner G. *Marriott's Practical Electrocardiography*. 10th ed. Philadelphia, PA: Lippincott Williams & Wilkins; 2001.
15. Kinch JW, Ryan TJ. Right ventricular infarction. *N Engl J Med*. 1994;330(17):1211-1217.
16. Setaro JF, Cabin HS. Right ventricular infarction. *Cardiol Clin*. 1992;10(1):69-90 Review.
17. Estes EH. Electrocardiography and vectorcardiography. In: Hurst JW, Logue RB, eds. *The Heart*. 3rd ed. New York: McGraw-Hill; 1974:chap 21.
18. Scott RC. The electrocardiographic diagnosis of left ventricular hypertrophy. *Am Heart J*. 1960;59:155.
19. Gregoratos G, Abrams J, Epstein JE, et al. ACC/AHA/NASPE 2002 guideline update for implantation of cardiac pacemakers and antiarrhythmia devices: summary article. *Circulation*. 2002;106:2145.
20. Mallela VS, Ilankumaran V, Srinivasa Rao N. Trends in cardiac pacemaker batteries. *Indian Pacing Electrophysiol J*. 2004;4(4):201-212.
21. Martinez C, Tzur A, Hrachian H, Zebede J, Lamas GA. Pacemakers and defibrillators: recent and ongoing studies that impact the elderly. *Am J Geriatr Cardiol*. 2006;15(2):82-87.
22. Bernstein AD, Camm AJ, Fletcher RD, et al. The revised NASPE/BPEG generic pacemaker code for antibradyarrhythmia and adaptive rate and multiscale pacing. *Pacing Clin Electrophysiol*. 2002;25:260-264.
23. Leung S, Lau C. Developments in sensor driven pacing. *Cardiology Clin*. 2000;18:113-155.
24. Wilkoff BL, Corey J, Blackburn B. A mathematical model of the cardiac chronotropic response to exercise. *J Electrophysiology*. 1989;3:176-180.
25. Sharp CT, Busse EF, Burgess JJ, Haennel RG. Exercise prescription for patients with pacemakers. *J Cardiopulm Rehabil*. 1998;18:421-431.
26. Trohman R, Kim M, Pinski S. Cardiac pacing: the state of the art. *Lancet*. 2004;364(9446):1701.
27. Page E, Defaye P, Bonnet JL, Durand C, Amblard A. Comparison of the cardiopulmonary response to exercise in recipients of dual sensor DDDR pacemakers versus a healthy control group. *Pacing Clin Electrophysiol*. 2003;26(pt II):239-243.
28. Alt E, Combs W, Fotuhi P. Initial clinical experience with a new dual sensor SSIR pacemaker controlled by body activity and minute ventilation. *Pacing Clin Electrophysiol*. 1995;18:1487-1495.
29. Ovsyshcher I, Guldal M, Karaoguz R. Evaluation of a new rate adaptive ventricular pacemaker controlled by double sensors. *Pacing Clin Electrophysiol*. 1995;18:386-390.
30. Lascault G, Pansard Y, Scholl JM. Dual chamber rate responsive pacing and chronotropic insufficiency: comparison of double and respiratory sensors. *Arch Mal Coeur Vaiss*. 2001;94:190-195.
31. Collins SM, Dias KJ, Cahalin LP. Pacer settings and exercise tolerance in heart failure: a case presentation [Abstract]. *Cardiopulm Phys Ther J*. 2004;15(4):36.
32. Mehta D, Langan MN, Banker J. Pacemakers and defibrillators for congestive heart failure. *Curr Cardiol Rep*. 2001;3(2):119-123.
33. Higgins S. Automatic implantable cardiac defibrillators. *Curr Treat Options Cardiovasc Med*. 2002;4:287-293.
34. Duru F, Buchi S, Klaghofer R, et al. How different pacemaker patients are recipients of implantable cardioverter-defibrillators with respect to psychosocial adaptation, affective disorders and quality of life? *Heart*. 2001;85:375-379.
35. Aydemir O, Ozmen E, Kuey L. Psychiatric morbidity and depressive symptomatology in patients with permanent pacemakers. *Pacing Clin Electrophysiol*. 1997;20:1628-1632.
36. Philbin DM, Marieb MA, Aitwal KH. Inappropriate shocks delivered by an implantable cardioverter-defibrillators as a result of sensed potentials from a TENS unit. *Pacing Clin Electrophysiol*. 1998;21:2010-2011.
37. Vlay SC. Electromagnetic interference and implantable cardioverter-defibrillators discharged related chiropractic prescription. *Pacing Clin Electrophysiol*. 1998;21:2009.

38. Curwin H, Coyne RF, Winfes SL. Inappropriate defib(ICD) implantable cardioverter-defibrillators shocks caused by transcutaneous electron nerve stimulation (TENS) unit. *Pacing Clin Electrophysiol*. 1999;22:692-693.

39. Crevenna R, Stix G, Pleiner J, et al. Electromagnetic interference by transcutaneous neuromuscular electrical stimulation in patients with bipolar sensing implantable cardioverter defibrillators: a pilot safety study. *Pacing Clin Electrophysiol*. 2003;26(pt I):626-629.

40. Vanhees L, Schepers D, Heidbuchel H, Defoor J, Fagard R. Exercise performance and training in patients with implantable cardioverter-defibrillators and coronary heart disease. *Am J Cardiol*. 2001;87:712-715.

41. Vanhees L, Kornaat M, Defoor J, et al. Effect of exercise training in patients with an implantable cardioverter defibrillator. *Eur Heart J*. 2004;25:1120-1126.

42. Fitchet A, Doherty P, Bundy C, Bell W, Fitzpatrick A, Garratt C. Comprehensive cardiac rehabilitation programme for implantable cardioverter-defibrillator patients: a randomized controlled trial. *Heart*. 2003;89:155-160.

43. Bardy GH, Lee K, Mark D, et al. Amiodarone or an implantable cardioverter–defibrillator for congestive heart failure. *New Engl J Med*. 2005;352:225-237.

44. Ambrus L, Norris J. Patients with cardiac pacemakers: considerations for physical therapy. *Phys Ther*. 1967;47(3):193-199.

45. Freedman R, Hopper D, Mah J, Hummel J, Wilkoff BL. Assessment of pacemaker chronotropic response: implementation of the Wilkoff mathematical model. *Pacing Clin Electrophysiol*. 2001;24:1748-1754.

46. Kindermann M, Schwaab B, Finkler N, Schaller S, Bohm M, Frohlig G. Defining the optimum upper heart rate limit during exercise: a study in pacemaker patients with heart failure. *Eur Heart J*. 2002;23:1301-1308.

47. Boland J, Scherer M, Hartung W. Clinical evaluation of an automatic sensor response algorithm in patients with DR pacemakers: a multi-center study [abstract]. *Pacing Clin Electrophysiol*. 1999;(pt II): A102.

48. Philippon F. Cardiac resynchronization therapy: device-based medicine for heart failure. *J Card Surg*. 2004;19:270-274.

49. Saxon LA, DeMarco T, Schafer J, et al. Effects of long-term biventricular stimulation for resynchronization on echocardiographic measures of remodeling. *Circulation*. 2002;105:1304-1310.

50. Young JB, Abraham WT, Smith AL, et al. Combined cardiac resynchronization and implantable cardioversion defibrillation in advanced heart failure—the MIRACLE ICD Trial. *JAMA* 2003;289(20):2685-2694.

51. Grassi G, Vincenti A, Brambilla R, et al. Sustained sympathoinhibitory effects of cardiac resynchronization therapy in severe heart failure. *Hypertension*. 2004;44:727-731.

52. Adamson PB, Smith AL, Abraham WT, et al. Continuous autonomic assessment in patients with symptomatic heart failure. *Circulation*. 2004;110:2389-2394.

Evaluation of Patient Intolerance to Exercise

12

William E. DeTurk & Lawrence P. Cahalin

INTRODUCTION

The reader may recall that Chapters 9 and 10 presented information on pulmonary and cardiac evaluations. This information included tests and measures appropriate for diagnosis and measurement of cardiac and pulmonary status. Heart rate and blood pressure (BP) determination as well as pulse oximetry and evaluation of ventilatory muscle function were also included. Chapter 11 introduced electrocardiography, which provided another important measurement tool. However, knowledge of examination, instrumentation, and procedures is only part of the picture: During an exercise session, the clinician must also interpret these data and decide what to do with the information once it is acquired. Use of this information may be confined to deciding whether or not to stop exercise. Certainly this would be an appropriate first consideration. Just as important is the synthesis of this information with therapeutic interventions that optimizes outcomes. Examination and

intervention are thus dynamic processes that are not only restricted to the therapist–patient relationship. Appropriate documentation and consultation may also bring in other members of the multidisciplinary team—the nurse, cardiologist, and social worker, for example. **A physical therapy program that utilizes ongoing continuous evaluation, blended with treatment, and integrated with documentation that incorporates other members of the health care team would appear to optimize results.** Indeed, such an approach is of benefit in at least three ways: (1) It enhances the physical therapist's ability to develop an effective exercise prescription, (2) it provides the referral source with information elicited during an exercise state; information that might not be otherwise available, and (3) it ultimately benefits the patient, the recipient of the combined care of both the physical therapist and the other members of the health care team.

This chapter* has two sections. The first portion will present pathophysiological processes that limit exercise capacity. These processes will be summarized in two cardiopulmonary hypothesis–oriented algorithms—one for patients with cardiovascular disease and the other for patients with pulmonary disease. These can be used to direct the physical therapist's actions by assignment of exercise response into categories subsumed under them. The second part of the chapter will apply the algorithms to two case studies of patients with cardiopulmonary disease. **In this way, the chapter will provide a systematic approach to patient management during an exercise session and will highlight hypothesis testing as a means of identifying impairments and functional limitations in patients who are limited by cardiovascular or pulmonary disease.** This chapter will also prepare the reader for subse-

quent discussion of patient management strategies for an overall plan of care, found in the six preferred practice pattern chapters.

This chapter will serve to reinforce an important point: Ongoing, systematic examination and evaluation during treatment may be important determinants for an overall plan of care. Practical tips on how to make accurate measurements and how to document the findings are also included.

HYPOTHESIS TESTING AND THE ALGORITHMS

As discussed in Chapter 2, a diagnosis of "ischemic heart disease" or "chronic obstructive pulmonary disease" does not provide specific information about the nature of the disablement as it relates to the status and location of the impairment. Neither do such diagnoses guide the practitioner toward specific treatment interventions. The exercise response categories found in the hypothesis-oriented algorithms in this chapter

---

*Portions of this chapter were modified and reprinted from DeTurk WE. Exercise and the intolerant heart. *Clin Manag.* 1992;12(1):67-73 and DeTurk WE. Exercise and the intolerant heart, part 2. *Clin Manag.* 1992;12(2):32-39, with the permission of APTA.

are designed to be used during individual treatment sessions. They include sets of questions that are appropriate to each of the categories. A positive response to any given question assists the therapist in "ruling in" the patient to that category and is part of a general hypothesis-testing approach that is integral to the proper use of the algorithms. In this chapter, *hypothesis testing* is defined as an approach to patient care whereby the therapist applies the algorithm to the patient through the formulation of questions about findings that, when answered, either supports or refutes the inclusion of the finding in the appropriate exercise response category. Hypothesis testing may begin at the level of subjective complaints of chest pain or shortness of breath (SOB) during exercise, for example. It may continue as additional information is gathered through the use of an electrocardiogram (ECG) telemeter or pulse oximeter. Hypothesis testing culminates in the synthesis of all the obtained data, at which point the therapist places the patient in the most appropriate exercise response category and reaches conclusions about the feasibility of exercise continuance. Along the way, additional information is obtained as regards the location of impairments and the nature of the functional limitations. This information is then used to direct subsequent treatment. **Hypothesis testing may be used to direct a total plan of care. However, the hypothesis testing that drives the algorithms in this chapter is part of a dynamic, ongoing process that occurs during an exercise session.**

EXERCISE DOSAGE

It is not uncommon for the physical therapist to receive referrals for patients who are in need of "exercise conditioning" or "endurance training." These patients may or may not be patients whose primary diagnosis is cardiac or pulmonary disease; however, all should undergo some sort of an initial exercise test. This need not be a formal treadmill protocol with cardiologists in attendance. It can be, and often is, performed by the physical therapist and may consist of climbing up flights of stairs, walking down the hall, or exercising with an arm-crank ergometer. Although not traditionally interpreted as an exercise test, examination of the cardiovascular and pulmonary responses during bouts of physical exertion yields information that may be just as important as traditional exercise testing.

CLINICAL CORRELATE

The concept of both exercise testing and training, however, is that exercise should be treated like a drug: A measured "dose" should be administered to the patient, and future "doses" should be based on the patient's response to exercise.

It is important to *quantify* the amount of exercise that a patient is given. This can be expressed in a number of ways. It may be simply the total distance walked, usually coupled with the time it takes. It may be the workload, for example, watts on a cycle ergometer, and the time spent exercising. The data obtained during such testing should include heart rate (HR) and systolic blood pressure (SBP), which, when multiplied, is expressed as the rate–pressure product (RPP). The RPP is highly correlated with both myocardial oxygen consumption, systemic oxygen consumption, and cardiac output. Measurement of HR and BP at rest, peak exercise, and at periodic points along the way (depending on the patient) will help ensure patient safety and be used later to write the exercise prescription. Use of pulse oximetry, the dyspnea index (DI), and measurement of respiratory rate may be important additions to HR and BP when monitoring patients with pulmonary disease.

Information obtained from the exercise evaluation can be used to place the patient into any or multiple categories of exercise intolerance that may be subsequently used to direct treatment interventions. For patients with cardiac disease, these categories include arrhythmia, ischemia, cardiovascular pump failure, and cardiovascular pump dysfunction. For pulmonary disease, these categories include poor oxygenation, ventilatory pump dysfunction, ventilatory pump failure, and pulmonary hypertension.

EXERCISE LIMITATIONS IN CARDIAC DISEASE

Arrhythmia

It is not uncommon to find that a patient's pulse is irregular prior to exercise. Some therapists may dismiss this finding as unimportant, and place the patient in an unmonitored exercise program, thereby exposing the patient to unnecessary risk. Other therapists may be tempted to make a guess as to the origin of the "skipped beats." This temptation should be resisted. The most common arrhythmias include premature atrial complexes (PACs), premature ventricular complexes (PVCs), and atrial fibrillation. There is no way of knowing the true cause of the irregularity—unless the patient is hooked up to an ECG machine. Many therapists do not have access to an ECG telemeter (a device consisting of a radiotransmitter and an oscilloscope that enables one to look at the ECG complexes). However, most therapists can borrow a standard 12-lead unit with a paper printout. What is seen may very well determine how the patient is treated. In general, PACs are not as significant as PVCs: Loss of adequate filling and contraction of the atria are not as hemodynamically disruptive as premature contractions within the ventricles. Occasional isolated PACs present no particular problem to the patient—*unless* those PACs are hemodynamically compromising. Patients *can* present with very rapid (200–300 beats per minute [bpm]) atrial arrhythmias that produce reduction of forward blood flow and decreased BP. Symptoms of dizziness, light-headedness, or even syncope can result. Physical therapists should check with the patient for the presence of symptoms when irregular pulse rhythms are palpated. **In order to maximize accuracy, physical therapists should measure the HR for 1 full minute by palpating the peripheral pulse. Electrocardiography/radiotelemetry should be utilized, when available, to determine the exact type of arrhythmia.**

Evaluating the Significance of PVCs

PVCs are quite common in the setting of coronary artery disease and require further discussion. They are characterized by complexes that are usually wide, bizarre looking, and premature. PVCs originate from an ectopic focus (or multiple foci) within the ventricles (see Chapter 11). Like PACs, these complexes do not necessarily present a problem: PVCs are present in roughly half of healthy normal adults. In this population, PVCs may present themselves during times of emotional stress, upon lying down at night, or after caffeine ingestion. Occasional PVCs in a normal population are usually well tolerated because the myocardium is healthy and nonischemic. The significance of PVCs in patients with heart disease is more ominous. The myocardium from which these PVCs arise is oxygen deprived. These PVCs occur as a result of spontaneous depolarization of irritable foci, through either reentry or blocked conduction[1] (see Chapter 11). **The following are key concepts in understanding the significance of PVCs:**

1. PVCs can present a problem to the patient for two reasons. When they occur as a run of PVCs at a rapid rate (ventricular tachycardia, or VT), they can be *hemodynamically compromising*. This rhythm can also degenerate into a lethal arrhythmia (ventricular fibrillation) that is difficult to terminate.

2. *The significance of PVCs is based on the company they keep.* Healthy, normal hearts can tolerate an occasional PVC very well without sacrifice of forward blood flow or degeneration into ventricular fibrillation. PVCs in the presence of ischemic heart disease, however, take on added significance, and some physicians might treat frequent PVCs in this latter group with anti-ischemic or antiarrhythmic drugs.[1]

The first appearance of PVCs may be at rest, when the patient is first connected to the ECG machine or radiotelemeter. The question that may be asked by the physical therapist when confronted by PVCs at rest is as follows: What happens to them during exercise? It is an important question and one that the physical therapist is in perhaps a unique position to answer. There are three possibilities:

1. *The PVCs decrease with exercise.* This is a good response to exercise. It indicates that the PVCs get suppressed by a higher-order pacemaker (overdrive suppression) as physical activity (and HR) increases.

2. *The PVCs increase with exercise.* This is a less desirable response, as it indicates that the PVCs may be ischemic in origin. Normally quiescent foci become irritable and fire

as myocardial O_2 demand outstrips the supply of oxygen available to it.

3. *There are PVCs at rest and with exercise that do not change during exercise.* The most that can be said about these PVCs is that they are unrelated to exercise.

To document this response, resting PVC activity should be *quantified and qualified*. The clinician should take a moment to examine the resting rhythm. The number of PVCs per minute should be counted. The characteristics of the waveforms should then be evaluated. PVCs may be *unifocal* or *multifocal,* or *interpolated,* or appear as an *R-on-T phenomenon*. They may occur in a regularly recurring pattern, for example, *trigeminy, bigeminy,* or PVC *pairs*. Categorization of PVC activity will help to determine their overall significance. Multifocal complexes are more significant than unifocal complexes; R-on-T phenomenon can predispose to ventricular tachycardia; closely coupled (eg, paired) PVCs are more significant than distant (eg, trigeminal) PVCs[2] (see Fig. 12-1).

Following the evaluation of resting PVC activity, the physical therapist may elect to evaluate PVC behavior during exercise. As the patient begins to exercise, there may be an increase in ectopic activity, another ectopic focus may manifest itself and the form of the PVC may change, or the PVCs may become coupled closer together. Once it is clearly established that PVC activity does increase, exercise should be terminated. Document these findings, and refer the patient back to the physician or other referral source on the same day. It should be noted that there may be diurnal variability to PVC frequency; therefore, the time of the day of the treatment session and the relationship of the session to the last meal should also be noted. It is important not to draw hasty conclusions about the importance of PVC activity. However, it should be

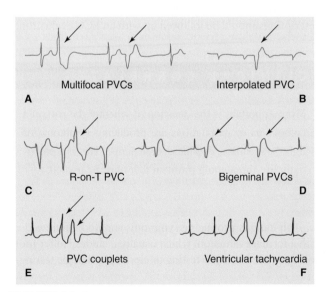

FIGURE 12-1   Examples of PVC morphologies. (**A**) Multifocal PVCs; (**B**) interpolated PVC; (**C**) R-on-T PVC; (**D**) bigeminal PVCs; (**E**) PVC couplets; (**F**) ventricular tachycardia. (Reprinted from DeTurk WE. Exercise and the intolerant heart. *Clin Manag*. 1992;12(1):67-73, with permission of the American Physical Therapy Association. Guide to Physical Therapist Practice. 2nd ed. *Phys Ther*. 2001 Jan;81(1):9-746.)

noted that PVCs in the setting of an acute myocardial infarction (MI) are always significant. The physician may follow up the findings obtained during the treatment session with 24-hour ECG Holter monitoring.

Ventricular tachycardia deserves special mention. This is defined as three or more consecutive PVCs that occur at a rate of at least 100 bpm. Its appearance at rest or during exercise is a contraindication to further effort. It is important to document the number of complexes in the run, calculate the rate at which the complexes occur, and notify the referral source. The patient should be observed for further arrhythmias and seen by a physician as soon as possible.

In general, the therapist's response to ventricular ectopy is a function of two factors. The therapist's experience in cardiopulmonary physical therapy and their own "comfort level" should be taken into account. Recent graduates, more so than therapists with more experience, tend to be more hesitant in working with patients having ventricular ectopy, and this is appropriate. The work setting is an important factor also. Hospital-based therapists working with a crash cart down the hall and an arrest team close by can evaluate and treat patients more aggressively than those who are employed by an outpatient clinic in a shopping plaza. In both settings, however, the question remains the same: What happens to PVCs during exercise?

Palpitations

Many patients with arrhythmia may complain of skipped beats or "fluttering" of the heart. Therapists should pursue description of this symptom. By inquiring whether the palpitations are rapid, forceful, or irregular in nature, the therapist may gain some insight into their origin. Rapid palpitations are often associated with supraventricular arrhythmias, forceful with exercise, and irregular with ventricular ectopy. These descriptions should be followed up with an ECG evaluation.

CLINICAL CORRELATE

More important is the question of whether the patient's complaints of palpitations are producing symptoms of light-headedness, dizziness, or syncope. This is a potentially life-threatening problem that must be treated.

Palpitations producing symptoms should be followed up with a formal evaluation, which usually includes Holter monitoring, graded exercise testing or electrophysiologic testing.

Ischemia

Myocardial ischemia occurs when the demand for oxygen by cardiac muscle outstrips the supply of oxygen available to it. This situation frequently arises during exercise with the onset of chest pain or angina. It is usually relieved by rest. There are electrocardiographic changes as well, typically presenting as a downward shift in the position of the ST segment (see Chapters 6 and 11).

Myocardial ischemia produces classic symptoms that can be obtained through a comprehensive patient history. It is typically described as crushing or squeezing in quality and is either precordial or substernal in location. It comes on with exercise and is relieved by rest. There are wide variations in this presentation; the discomfort may go up into the jaw, neck, back, or down to one or both arms; the "chest pain" may present as SOB, particularly among the elderly (see Chapter 6 and the CD-ROM representation for that chapter).

It should be noted that other pathologies may present with similar symptoms. Gastrointestinal disturbances can radiate pain into the chest; musculoskeletal problems (eg, arthritis) can involve pain in the costochondral or sternoclavicular joints. These symptoms, although coming on with exercise, are related to the mechanics of heavy breathing and can be elicited through palpation of the chest wall, thus ruling out chest pain of cardiac origin. Because so many things produce chest pain, it is helpful to know the typical presentation of angina and differential maneuvers that the therapist can perform to rule out other causes. An examination of the patient via electrocardiography can provide additional information and "cinch" the clinical impression.

Various bipolar lead systems have been described.[3] Placement of the positive electrode over the apex of the heart and the negative electrode over the sternum, right shoulder, or on the back under the inferior angle of the right scapula usually provide adequate waveform differentiation and maximum sensitivity to changes in the ST segment.

Most facilities recognize a 1.0 mm (0.1 mV) of horizontal or downsloping depression of the ST segment as a criterion for a positive exercise test indicative of myocardial ischemia.[4] Upsloping ST-segment depression is usually considered positive when it exceeds 1.5 mm. The measurement is made as shown in Fig. 12-2.

In addition to *quantifying* the amount of ST-segment depression that occurs during exercise, the response should be *qualified.* The shape of the ST segment is as important as the amount of depression. Three morphologies of ST segments have been described: horizontal, upsloping, and downsloping (Fig. 12-3). In general, downsloping ST-segment depression is more significant than horizontal ST-segment depression; similarly, upsloping ST-segment depression is less significant than horizontal ST-segment depression. ST-segment elevation that occurs during exercise (a rare finding) could signify coronary artery spasm and/or transmural ischemia and should prompt immediate termination of exercise (see Chapter 6).

There is a moderate relationship between the time spent in exercise and the severity of ischemic heart disease.[5,6] Patients who experience ST-segment depression early in an exercise test tend to have more severe ischemic heart disease than patients who become ischemic later in the exercise test, as measured by the number of coronary vessel involvement via

FIGURE 12-2 Measurement of ST segment changes as a criterion for a positive ECG stress test indicative of myocardial ischemia. (Reprinted from DeTurk WE. Exercise and the intolerant heart. *Clin Manag.* 1992;12(1):67-73, with permission of the American Physical Therapy Association. Guide to Physical Therapist Practice. 2nd ed. *Phys Ther.* 2001 Jan;81(1):9-746.)

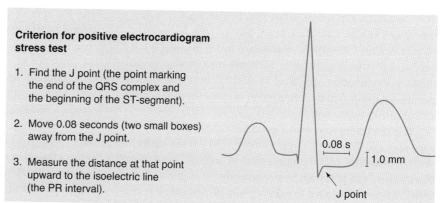

Criterion for positive electrocardiogram stress test

1. Find the J point (the point marking the end of the QRS complex and the beginning of the ST-segment).

2. Move 0.08 seconds (two small boxes) away from the J point.

3. Measure the distance at that point upward to the isoelectric line (the PR interval).

0.08 s

1.0 mm

J point

angiography. Physical therapists encountering this situation should treat these patients conservatively. Additionally, patients who become ischemic during exercise may remain ischemic for a protracted period of time in the postexercise recovery period. It may take many minutes before myocardial blood flow is fully restored. Therefore, the time of recovery from ST-segment depression should also be noted. These patients need more conservative management, as they tend to demonstrate more advanced disease.[6,7]

CLINICAL CORRELATE

If the patient develops chest discomfort during exercise, it is important that exercise be terminated at once if other possible causes of the chest discomfort have already been ruled out.

The patient should be positioned in a semifowlers or seated position if such positions are tolerated without light-headedness. A supine body position should be avoided, as this position will enhance venous return, which is likely to increase the work of the heart, thereby increasing myocardial ischemia. The level of exertion that provokes symptoms is called the *anginal threshold*. **The workload and/or HR at which the patient becomes symptomatic should be noted.** This is important to the physical therapist because this information

can be used to formulate a safe exercise program. The physical therapist may also decide to teach the patient how to take his or her own pulse and then instruct the patient not to exceed the HR at which myocardial ischemia becomes manifest. Documentation of the anginal threshold is also useful to the referral source who may want to prescribe, or adjust, cardiac medications to enhance the patient's tolerance to exercise.

Documentation

If the patient is monitored via electrocardiography, it is important to obtain a paper printout at both rest and peak exercise. Therapists should measure the amount of ST-segment depression, characterize the morphology, note the HR and BP, and state what the patient was doing. For example:

Ms. R terminated treadmill walking because of the onset of chest pain and 1.5 mm of downsloping ST-segment depression in the lateral precordial leads. Peak exercise HR was 134 bpm and BP was 158/84 mm Hg.

Cardiovascular Pump Failure

The third category, which may be responsible for intolerance to exercise, is cardiovascular pump failure, which is combined with cardiovascular pump dysfunction to form the *Guide's* preferred Practice Pattern 6D.[8] In the setting of the acute response to exercise, cardiovascular pump dysfunction is often a sequela to cardiovascular pump failure. Therefore, heart failure will be discussed separately from dysfunction.

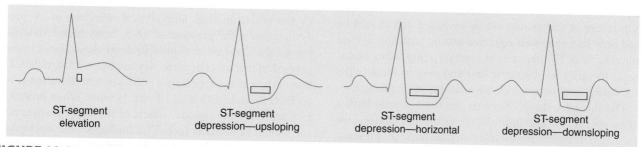

ST-segment elevation

ST-segment depression—upsloping

ST-segment depression—horizontal

ST-segment depression—downsloping

FIGURE 12-3 Diagnostic shapes of ST segments. (Reprinted from DeTurk WE. Exercise and the intolerant heart. *Clin Manag.* 1992;12(1):67-73, with permission of the American Physical Therapy Association. Guide to Physical Therapist Practice. 2nd ed. *Phys Ther.* 2001 Jan;81(1):9-746.)

Cardiovascular pump failure may be abbreviated to pump failure and is also known as heart failure (HF). Many therapists associate SOB with this pathology, but SOB alone is not a very specific finding, because SOB can also be due to pulmonary dysfunction, physical inactivity, or even anxiety. Additional information is required to rule out the other causes and to rule in pump failure.

It is important to obtain a good patient history. The therapist may ask, "Do you ever get unusual SOB?" If the answer is yes, the response may be quantified by asking "How many blocks/stairs can you walk before you have to stop because of SOB?" Responses limited to a description of SOB may be of little help, because patient responses vary widely, from "air hunger" to panting. It is helpful to ascertain the presence of SOB at rest, using the methods described in Chapter 9. Ask about the number of pillows the patient slept on at night, and whether, if those pillows were removed, the patient would then get SOB. The presence of *paroxysmal nocturnal dyspnea* (PND) should also be ascertained. The patient goes to sleep without symptoms but wakes up several hours later acutely short of breath and has to sit up for relief. The feeling subsides and the patient returns to bed. This scenario is typical of patients with paroxysmal nocturnal dyspnea and is most likely associated with pump failure.

Common causes of cardiovascular pump failure include MI, cardiomyopathy, and valvular heart disease. It is useful to differentiate between left-sided and right-sided pump failure. In left-sided failure, the left side of the heart cannot pump out all the blood that is delivered to it by the right side. The pressure builds up in the left ventricle and is reflected backward, up through the left atrium and into the lungs. The lungs become wet, stiff, soggy, and difficult to move, hence, the feeling of SOB. In patients with heart disease, right-sided failure is usually the result of left-sided failure. The pressure, due to a restriction in forward flow, now passes through the lungs and gets reflected through the right ventricle and right atrium and into the venous circulatory system. However, patients with pulmonary disease can have pump failure confined to the right side.

Signs and Symptoms of Cardiovascular Pump Failure

Patients can present in chronic pump failure at rest or can develop transient pump failure during exercise. Before proceeding with exercise, it is important to check for signs and symptoms of left-sided pump failure at rest. Patients with pump failure at rest should not be exercised and should be tested only in a safe, well-equipped setting with appropriate medical backup. The objective of a resting pump failure evaluation is to verify its absence at rest and then to identify the point during exercise at which the patient goes into failure.

The therapist should listen to the heart sounds with a stethoscope, at rest, and immediately following exercise. One of the hallmarks of cardiovascular pump failure is the presence of an S_3 *heart sound*. It is a very low-pitched sound, heard best with the bell of the stethoscope placed lightly on the chest wall over the apex of the heart. S_3 follows close on the heels of the second heart sound. It is, at best, difficult to hear, but its presence is highly significant. The lungs should be auscultated for the presence of *crackles*. These adventitious sounds are discrete, popping sounds that are heard primarily during inspiration. Unlike pulmonary crackles, they do not clear with a cough. Crackles, like the S_3 heart sound, can be absent at rest but come on during exercise, indicating that the workload is too strenuous and producing transient pump failure. The therapist's clinical response is similar to that of arrhythmia and ischemia: Mark the onset of these signs by noting the workload, HR, and BP, and then stop exercise and adjust the exercise regimen accordingly.

CLINICAL CORRELATE

It is important to avoid placement of a patient with cardiovascular pump failure in supine during recovery; this will increase the volume of blood that the heart has to pump out and exacerbate the patient's symptoms. Rather, the patient's upper chest and head can be propped up with pillows, or the head of the bed can be cranked up, or the patient can be seated in a chair.

Cardiovascular pump failure will be discussed in greater detail in Chapter 18.

Cardiovascular Pump Dysfunction

The fourth classification of exercise intolerance is specific to patients with overt, manifest heart disease, usually those patients recovering from MI. The term *dysfunction* refers to residual mechanical pathology as the result of myocardial necrosis or ischemia. Radionuclide imaging recognizes three kinds of pump dysfunction: left ventricular (LV) wall *hypokinesis, akinesis,* and *dyskinesis.* Normal myocardial fibers contract together in a spiral, corkscrew fashion around a given volume of blood to effect systolic ejection. Damaged myocardium contracts only slightly (hypokinesis), fails to contract (akinesis), or balloons out the other way (dyskinesis). This latter category represents ventricular wall aneurysm.

Patients in the early recovery period of MI are subject to LV pump dysfunction. One clinical reflection of LV pump dysfunction is the presence of an S_3 heart sound, described previously. Three other clinical findings should be of interest to physical therapists because they can be exercise related. The first of these is the appearance of ST-segment elevation at rest on ECG in leads with a significant Q wave. When present, it may represent the residual effects of the MI (eg, aneurysm) and should be noted as such. This finding should not be confused with ST-segment elevation during exercise in non–Q-wave leads, which represents a markedly positive test for ischemic heart disease, because of coronary artery vasospasm (see Chapter 6).

The second finding is the *murmur of mitral regurgitation,* appreciated during auscultation of the heart. It is an adventitious, blowing type of sound that occurs between S_1 and S_2. It is relatively high pitched and therefore heard best with the diaphragm of the stethoscope applied to the apical area of the heart. In the setting of MI, it frequently represents papillary muscle dysfunction. In this latter case, the murmur is invariably associated with an S_4 heart sound and often with a loud S_1.

ST-segment elevations and murmurs may be absent at rest. The physical therapist who can detect these findings during exercise and report their presence to the physician or other referral source is making a substantial contribution to the care and well-being of the patient.

The third finding is more problematic because it requires not only accurate assessment but also immediate response. This is a fall in SBP during exercise. Although both diastolic and SBPs are important when making a resting determination of the presence of hypertension, during exercise the SBP assumes preeminence. This is because the SBP more accurately reflects the functional state of the left ventricle.

When a patient first begins to exercise, there may be an early, transient drop in SBP. This is most likely due to regional changes in blood distribution (shunt); as exercise continues, pressure will usually rise. One should be particularly concerned when an increase in exercise workload fails to elicit a normal SBP response (usually 10–20 mm Hg per stage), or if there is a fall in SBP during moderate exercise. Absence of a rise in SBP during exercise, or a "flat response," may also signify evolving cardiovascular pump dysfunction.

When the patient complains of dizziness during exercise, the therapist should protect the patient from injury and document the findings. Instruct the patient to tell you if these symptoms become more severe; then immediately take the BP again. If SBP is dropping, continue to monitor and check with the patient and take serial BPs until a definite, inexorable trend has been established. Then stop exercise and place the patient supine.

The previous protocol requires that the therapist become proficient in taking rapid, accurate SBPs. This can be done with practice. The benefits in doing so can be significant: The patient is not "undertreated," useful information about exercise-induced cardiac function is obtained, and patient safety is assured.

Accurate measurement of diastolic blood pressure (DBP) can be problematic during exercise. During strenuous exercise, the "thump" representing DBP frequently becomes audible "all the way down" the column of mercury and thus loses significance. In this situation, the therapist should use the fourth Karotkoff sound as the measure of DBP. Documentation of this event in the following manner communicates to the reader that the fifth sound was heard all the way down the column of mercury:

Blood pressure on treadmill at 3 mph, 5% grade = 168/85/0.

Elevation of DBP during exercise is a pathologic finding and probably reflects evolving stiffness of the myocardium as a result of ischemia. An elevation in DBP coupled with a fall in SBP with increasing exercise causes a narrowing of *pulse pressure* and is particularly ominous. If allowed to continue, the patient could lose consciousness. Once again, the physical therapist must protect the patient from injury by terminating exercise and document the findings (see Chapter 10).

Four categories of cardiac effort intolerance have been identified, consisting of arrhythmia, ischemia, cardiovascular pump failure, and cardiovascular pump dysfunction. Figure 12-4 summarizes these response categories as a hypothesis-oriented algorithm that can be used to classify patients with cardiac disease into categories which then may be used to direct treatment.

EXERCISE LIMITATIONS IN PULMONARY DISEASE

Four categories of exercise intolerance will now be presented that are appropriate to patients with pulmonary disease. These categories consist of poor oxygenation, ventilatory pump dysfunction, ventilatory pump failure, and pulmonary hypertension. These response categories are summarized in Fig. 12-5 as a hypothesis-oriented algorithm. Like the cardiac algorithm, this figure subsumes signs and symptoms of pulmonary decompensation under their appropriate headings.

The reader may note that SOB is a symptom that is shared by all four categories and, therefore, is of little value in differentiating one response category from the other, or even pulmonary disease from cardiac disease. Nevertheless, the hallmark of pulmonary disease is SOB. This abnormality may be present at rest; however, it may become more pronounced during exercise. Similarly, the decrease in oxygen saturation (SaO_2) and resultant cyanosis are shared by all four response categories. Clearly, the best discriminators between categories are those unique to them: retained secretions for poor oxygenation, accessory muscle use and costal retractions for ventilatory pump dysfunction, paradoxical breathing for ventilatory pump failure, and the abrupt onset of symptoms and reduction in oxygen saturation found in patients with pulmonary hypertension.

As noted previously, the decrease in SaO_2 and cyanosis are global symptoms of pulmonary disease. Use of a pulse oximeter can be particularly helpful in evaluating the pulmonary system's ability to transfer oxygen to the blood and then to peripheral tissues. This device consists of a small, portable control unit that is battery powered and a finger sensor connected to the control unit by a cable. The oximeter determines SaO_2 by passing two wavelengths of light, one red and one infrared, through the finger to a photodetector. The intensity of the light sources and the differential absorption of light of arterial and venous blood allows calculation of saturation of oxygen on the hemoglobin molecule.[9] The accuracy of this device depends on adequate perfusion of the selected finger,

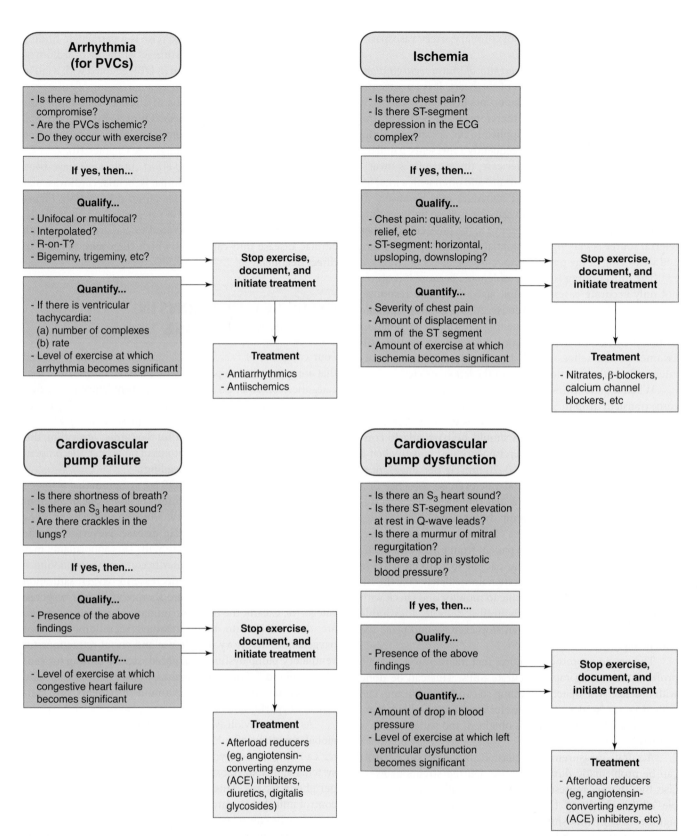

FIGURE 12-4   Hypothesis-oriented algorithm describing an evaluation approach for classifying patients with cardiovascular disease through the collection of data obtained during exercise. (Modified from DeTurk WE. Exercise and the intolerant heart, part 2. *Clin Manag.* 1992;12(2):32-39, with permission of the American Physical Therapy Association. Guide to Physical Therapist Practice. 2nd ed. *Phys Ther.* 2001 Jan;81(1):9-746.)

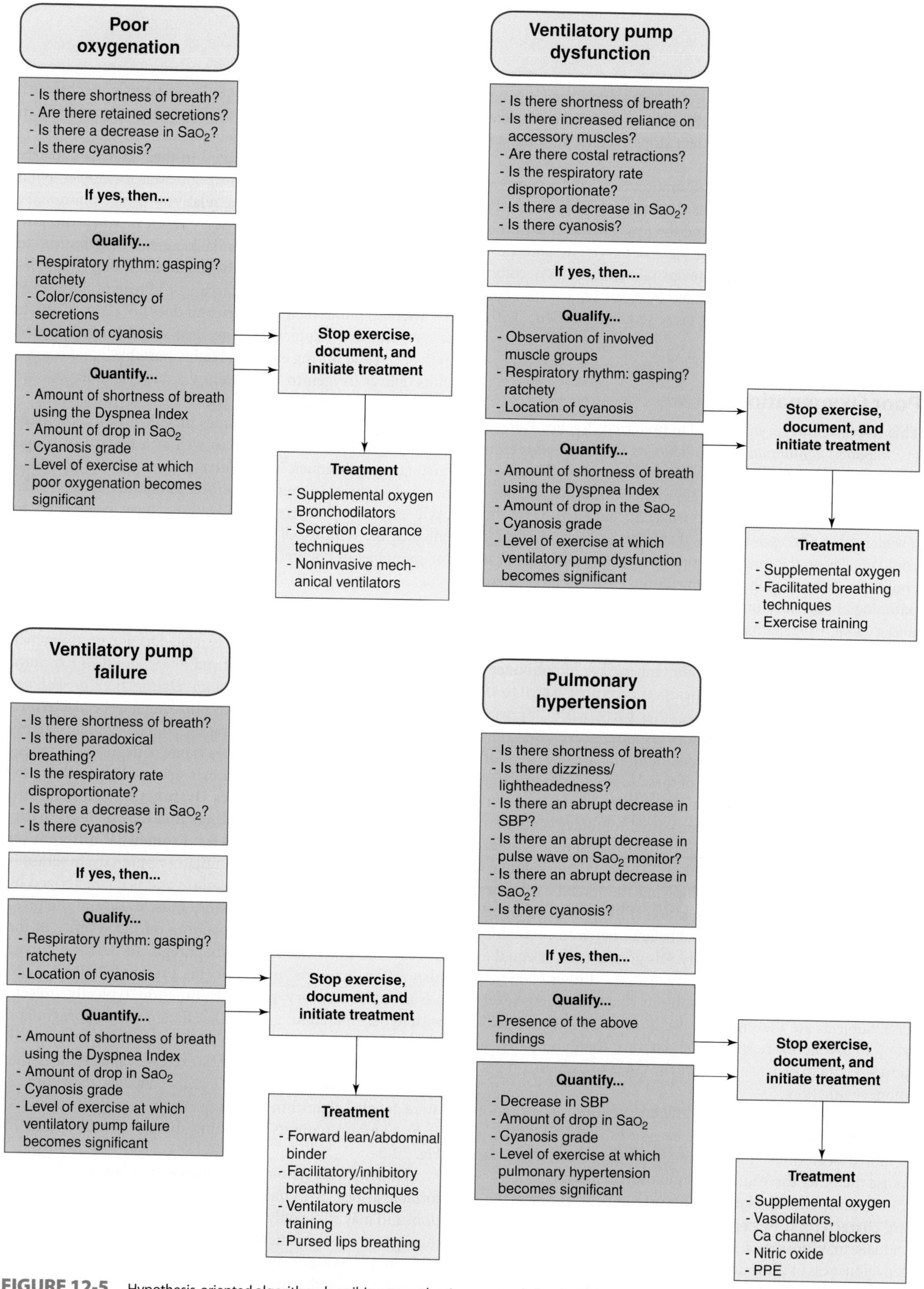

Poor oxygenation

- Is there shortness of breath?
- Are there retained secretions?
- Is there a decrease in SaO_2?
- Is there cyanosis?

If yes, then...

Qualify...

- Respiratory rhythm: gasping? ratchety
- Color/consistency of secretions
- Location of cyanosis

Quantify...

- Amount of shortness of breath using the Dyspnea Index
- Amount of drop in SaO_2
- Cyanosis grade
- Level of exercise at which poor oxygenation becomes significant

Stop exercise, document, and initiate treatment

Treatment

- Supplemental oxygen
- Bronchodilators
- Secretion clearance techniques
- Noninvasive mechanical ventilators

Ventilatory pump dysfunction

- Is there shortness of breath?
- Is there increased reliance on accessory muscles?
- Are there costal retractions?
- Is the respiratory rate disproportionate?
- Is there a decrease in SaO_2?
- Is there cyanosis?

If yes, then...

Qualify...

- Observation of involved muscle groups
- Respiratory rhythm: gasping? ratchety
- Location of cyanosis

Quantify...

- Amount of shortness of breath using the Dyspnea Index
- Amount of drop in the SaO_2
- Cyanosis grade
- Level of exercise at which ventilatory pump dysfunction becomes significant

Stop exercise, document, and initiate treatment

Treatment

- Supplemental oxygen
- Facilitated breathing techniques
- Exercise training

Ventilatory pump failure

- Is there shortness of breath?
- Is there paradoxical breathing?
- Is the respiratory rate disproportionate?
- Is there a decrease in SaO_2?
- Is there cyanosis?

If yes, then...

Qualify...

- Respiratory rhythm: gasping? ratchety
- Location of cyanosis

Quantify...

- Amount of shortness of breath using the Dyspnea Index
- Amount of drop in SaO_2
- Cyanosis grade
- Level of exercise at which ventilatory pump failure becomes significant

Stop exercise, document, and initiate treatment

Treatment

- Forward lean/abdominal binder
- Facilitatory/inhibitory breathing techniques
- Ventilatory muscle training
- Pursed lips breathing

Pulmonary hypertension

- Is there shortness of breath?
- Is there dizziness/ lightheadedness?
- Is there an abrupt decrease in SBP?
- Is there an abrupt decrease in pulse wave on SaO_2 monitor?
- Is there an abrupt decrease in SaO_2?
- Is there cyanosis?

If yes, then...

Qualify...

- Presence of the above findings

Quantify...

- Decrease in SBP
- Amount of drop in SaO_2
- Cyanosis grade
- Level of exercise at which pulmonary hypertension becomes significant

Stop exercise, document, and initiate treatment

Treatment

- Supplemental oxygen
- Vasodilators, Ca channel blockers
- Nitric oxide
- PPE

FIGURE 12-5 Hypothesis-oriented algorithm describing an evaluation approach for classifying patients with pulmonary disease through the collection of data obtained during exercise. (Modified from DeTurk WE. Exercise and the intolerant heart, part 2. *Clin Manag.* 1992;12(2):32-39, with permission of the American Physical Therapy Association. Guide to Physical Therapist Practice. 2nd ed. *Phys Ther.* 2001 Jan;81(1):9-746.)

the absence of nail polish, and absence of motion artifact. Although determination of SaO_2 can be accomplished during exercise, it is recommended that the actual measurement take place immediately after the patient stops exercise in order to minimize faulty readings.

Loss of peripheral oxygen saturation is usually accompanied by increasing cyanosis. This cyanosis may be particularly evident in the fingernail beds and the lips. Indeed, one of the first clinical signs that herald the onset of oxygen desaturation occurs during exercise when the lips take on a "dusky" color. Oxygen desaturation, cyanosis, and SOB are typical findings that cause early termination of exercise among patients with pulmonary disease.

Poor Oxygenation

This response category is related to preferred Practice Pattern 6C: *Impaired Ventilation, Respiration/Gas Exchange, and Aerobic Capacity Associated with Airway Clearance Dysfunction.* The site of the lesion could be anywhere within the alveolar–pulmonary capillary unit. For example, it could appear on the alveolar side as excessive mucus that impedes gas exchange. It could appear on the interstitial side as a pneumoconiosis, or it could appear more globally as pneumonia. Any or all of these pathologies can account for the findings that are subsumed under poor oxygenation that limit exercise capacity—SOB, retained secretions, decreased SaO_2, and cyanosis.

Because SOB is such an important marker of pulmonary dysfunction, its quantification deserves comment. The 0 to 10 category ratio scale used by Borg[10] has particular utility, as it relates to the immediate ventilatory response to exercise.[11] The DI has also been used to document the degree of SOB obtained during exercise. Both of these scales are described in Chapter 9. The DI is the ratio of the ventilation obtained during exercise (numerator) to the maximal voluntary ventilation (MVV, denominator). The ventilation during exercise is measured via closed-circuit gas analysis. The maximal voluntary ventilation is obtained by multiplying the forced expiratory value in the first second of expiration (FEV_1), in liters, by 35. DIs around 0.70 reflect a normal balance between ventilatory demand and ventilatory capacity. DIs greater than or equal to 1.0 are associated with pulmonary disease.[12] Either scale may be administered as a pretest to subjects about to undergo exercise. Subjects are then retested using the same scale immediately following exercise. Pretest data are then compared to posttest data in order to measure the effect of exercise on pulmonary function.

The singular finding that differentiates poor oxygenation from the other three response categories is the presence of retained secretions. Indeed, retained secretions alone can cause the other three and thus limit exercise performance.

Disease entities like cystic fibrosis and chronic bronchitis are characterized by copious mucus production. These individuals may possess a strong cough, but the thickness and tenaciousness of the mucus make the cough ineffective in raising secretions. Patients with an ineffective cough are thus dou-

bly jeopardized, in that the excessive mucous production is not matched by an optimal secretion clearance mechanism. Thus, the presence of an ineffective cough may contribute to poor oxygenation.

Many patients who are limited in their exercise capacity because of poor oxygenation respond well to supplemental oxygen. These patients have a relatively intact pulmonary anatomy that allows the increased oxygen to reach the pulmonary artery circulation for subsequent distribution to working skeletal muscle. Those who fail to respond to supplemental oxygen do so because scarring or fibrosis at the level of the alveolar–pulmonary capillary unit does not allow adequate oxygen transfer. Supplemental oxygen may be administered both at rest and during exercise. Highly portable liquid oxygen units deliver oxygen to the patient via nasal cannula and are well tolerated for even 24-hour use.

Secretion clearance techniques include postural drainage with percussion and vibration as well as a myriad of cough facilitation techniques. These interventions may be provided routinely or prior to exercise. Aerobic endurance activities like cycle ergometry or treadmill walking have been used to enhance the removal of secretions by lowering the threshold for spontaneous cough (see Chapter 17).

Ventilatory Pump Dysfunction

This exercise response category is related to preferred Practice Pattern 6E: *Impaired Ventilation and Respiration/Gas Exchange Associated with Ventilatory Pump Dysfunction or Failure.* Patients with ventilatory pump dysfunction may be placed on a continuum with those demonstrating ventilatory pump failure. The difference between categories is one of degree or advancement of the disease. **The hypothesis-oriented algorithm presented in Fig. 12-5 separates dysfunction from failure because there are clinical findings that may be used to differentiate them and each calls for a somewhat different set of treatment interventions.** Ventilatory pump dysfunction is typically a precursor of pump failure and is characterized by the increased reliance on accessory muscle use and the presence of costal retractions. Depending on the severity of the disease, the potential for the diaphragm to descend during inspiration may or may not be present. Patients with advanced ventilatory pump dysfunction typically present with hyperinflated lung fields that flatten the diaphragm and restrict further descent during inspiration. This finding will negatively influence the patient's exercise capacity. It is this phenomenon that is reflected in this chapter's algorithm. A more detailed algorithm reflecting breathing patterns obtained at rest among patients with lung disease can be found in Fig. 20-3.

Patients with ventilatory pump dysfunction may be comfortable at rest, with only a slight decrease in oxygen saturation, and may show only mild accessory muscle use. However, during exercise the patient may complain of increasing SOB. If not already present at rest, this symptom will usually be accompanied by the appearance of costal retractions, a further decrease in oxygen saturation, and concomitant cyanosis. Physical therapists should be attentive to the onset of these findings and terminate exercise when they become prohibitive to further exercise.

Immediately upon exercise termination the patient should be placed supine with the head of the bed gatched up, or the patient may be placed in the seated position with his or her arms supported. The flat-lying position places the ventilatory muscles at a mechanical disadvantage and contributes to SOB and should be avoided. Supplemental oxygen administered immediately following exercise usually restores oxygen saturation levels quickly and relieves SOB. Oxygen use during exercise may also be beneficial. As before, **the workload and/or HR at which ventilatory pump dysfunction becomes apparent should be noted. Subsequent exercise "doses" should be administered at an intensity below the threshold that evokes symptoms. Most facilities recognize an oxygen desaturation level less than 85% to 90% as a criterion for exercise discontinuance.**

Ventilatory Pump Failure

Like ventilatory pump dysfunction, this exercise response category is related to preferred Practice Pattern 6E: *Impaired Ventilation and Respiration/Gas Exchange Associated with Ventilatory Pump Dysfunction or Failure.* Ventilatory pump failure may be thought of as the advancement of ventilatory pump dysfunction, as the accessory muscles of ventilation and the diaphragm continue to weaken, which in turn cause further declines in oxygen saturation. It is not surprising that exercise tolerance in these individuals tends to be less than that for those in ventilatory pump dysfunction.

The algorithm in Fig. 12-5 contains signs and symptoms that are found in patients with ventilatory pump failure. The finding that helps to differentiate dysfunction from failure is *paradoxical breathing.* The reader may recall that, in patients with chronic lung disease, the shortened muscle fibers of the diaphragm and its flattened position prevent the generation of enough negative pressure required to adequately ventilate the lungs. Because the diaphragm has become ineffective, contraction of the muscles of the upper chest must provide the negative pressure to draw air into the lungs. In doing so, the upper chest sucks the abdominal area *inward,* while the upper chest moves *outward* during inspiration. This is termed *paradoxical breathing.* This breathing pattern is characteristic of ventilatory pump failure. Ventilatory failure is usually accompanied by deterioration in arterial blood gases, most notably an increase in carbon dioxide and a fall in oxygen tensions.

Paradoxical breathing may be improved by leaning the seated patient forward in a chair or by applying an abdominal binder. If the paradox resolves, the patient may be a candidate for exercise training, and hence appears in this chapter's hypothesis-oriented algorithm (Fig. 12-5). If paradoxical breathing continues in spite of the forward lean posture, the patient's level of function is quite low and may require mechanical ventilation. See Chapter 20, Fig. 20-3, which pres-

ents an algorithm that provides analysis of this breathing pattern in a resting patient.

Paradoxical breathing may be absent at rest but becomes manifested during exercise. It may also be present at rest and increase in severity with exercise. As before, **the workload and/or HR at which ventilatory pump dysfunction becomes apparent should be noted. Future exercise training sessions should occur at an intensity somewhat below the onset of symptoms.**

Pulmonary Hypertension

The fourth category of pulmonary intolerance to exercise is pulmonary hypertension. This pathology is not found as a preferred practice pattern per se. However, it is actually a common element in both ventilatory pump dysfunction and failure. Indeed, most patients with chronic obstructive lung disease develop pulmonary hypertension as their disease progresses. It is represented in the hypothesis-oriented algorithm in Fig. 12-5 because, although it may be occult at rest, it will become manifested during exercise.

Patients with chronic bronchitis and emphysema typically demonstrate chronic hypercapnia and hypoxia. Hypoxic pulmonary vasoconstriction causes chronically elevated pulmonary artery pressures—the hallmark of pulmonary hypertension. Right ventricular hypertrophy and some degree of right heart failure are commonly observed with pulmonary hypertension. Right ventricular hypertrophy develops over time as a compensatory mechanism in response to scarring and disruption of the pulmonary capillary bed, which creates a chronically high afterload against which the right ventricle must pump. These limitations may reach critical mass during exercise, as the demand for oxygen by metabolically active (skeletal muscle) tissues outstrips the pulmonary system's ability to load oxygen. Therefore, a patient with pulmonary hypertension may experience a sudden decrease in exercise capacity, which is caused by a cascade of events. (1) Increasing hypoxia during exercise causes increasing pulmonary vasoconstriction. (2) As pulmonary vascular resistance increases, right ventricular stroke volume decreases. (3) A reduction in blood volume from the right side of the heart causes a reduction in oxygenated blood volume to the left side of the heart. (4) This causes a reduction in left side of the heart's cardiac output. (5) BP falls and the patient becomes dizzy and lightheaded.

If exercise is allowed to continue, the patient will likely lose consciousness. The physical therapist must accurately and rapidly evaluate the situation, collect useful data, and protect the patient from injury. Exercise should be terminated immediately. The patient may be seated if BP can be maintained, or he or she may be placed supine with the head and upper trunk propped up with pillows. **The workload and/or HR at which pulmonary hypertension becomes apparent should be noted.** An exercise prescription should be developed that emphasizes steady-state, aerobic activities at an intensity below the symptom threshold.[13] The use of low-flow supplemental oxygen may significantly improve exercise tolerance.

SUMMARY

Four categories of effort intolerance for patients with cardiovascular disease have been identified: arrhythmia, ischemia, cardiovascular pump failure, and cardiovascular pump dysfunction. Similarly, patients with pulmonary disease may be limited by poor oxygenation, ventilatory pump dysfunction, ventilatory pump failure, or pulmonary hypertension. Categorization of exercise intolerance is appropriate for patients with documented cardiac or pulmonary disease, but it is also useful for patients at risk for their presence: the elderly, or those with multiple risk factors for cardiopulmonary disease, for example. Figures 12-4 and 12-5 summarize the evaluation approach for classifying patients into categories that then may be used to direct procedural interventions.

The following are three closing thoughts on cardiopulmonary evaluation obtained from the patient's acute response to exercise:

1. Physical therapists should be alert to the presence of other, more general signs of effort intolerance that may appear during therapeutic intervention. Some patients may demonstrate unusual pallor or diaphoresis, for example. The therapist should take note of the onset of these signs and make an assessment of the appropriateness of that response given the workload. Other patients may adopt a dull, fixed stare as exercise progresses, or fail to initiate conversation or respond to questions. **Although admittedly these responses are "soft" data, they may be the earliest, and most important, indication of effort intolerance.** They should be followed up with an evaluation to determine their etiology. With or without the other objective parameters discussed previously, these observations must not be ignored. Appropriate clinical responses include cautious continuance of exercise or its termination. It should be noted that these general signs of effort intolerance may be due to metabolic problems, pain (eg, visceral, orthopedic, neurologic), or comorbid disease (eg, cancer, multiple sclerosis).

2. Proper exercise evaluation and subsequent training challenge the cardiovascular and pulmonary systems with a progression of workloads applied over time, which should be both quantified and qualified by the physical therapist. Patient safety should be ensured through the use of the monitoring techniques outlined previously. **The patient should not be encouraged to continue exercise in order to provoke symptoms; provocative testing should be performed only in an exercise laboratory with emergency equipment and personnel close by.**

3. As the hypothesis-oriented algorithms demonstrate, the clinical evaluation of a patient's cardiovascular and pulmonary status should not rest on one or two isolated findings; all the available data should be examined and a clinical impression should be developed out of that total.

CASE STUDIES

The following case studies will use the system for evaluation and classification of patient intolerance to exercise, as just described, and place this system in the context of a comprehensive cardiopulmonary rehabilitation service. Two patients referred to physical therapy will be described—one for "early mobilization cardiac rehabilitation" and the other for "pulmonary rehabilitation and evaluation for supplemental oxygen."

Case Study

John Speed is a 57-year-old advertising executive who was admitted to the emergency department of a local community hospital on January 28, 2001, at 3:00 in the morning following 1½ hours of severe, unremitting precordial chest pressure. He was admitted to the cardiac intensive care unit (CICU) to rule out an MI. Data collected during the initial examination of Mr. Speed while in the CICU are summarized in Box 12-1.

Mr. Speed ruled in for an inferior wall MI. His 36-hour course in the CICU was unremarkable, and he was subsequently transferred to a private room, at which time he was referred to physical therapy for "cardiac rehabilitation."

Magda Nuchal, PT, was assigned to the patient on day 2 post-MI. She reviewed the chart. She noted that the patient's course in the CICU was characterized by the absence of ongoing chest pain, arrhythmia, or CHF. She examined the latest ECG and noted the presence of significant Q waves in leads II, III, and aVF indicative of a full-thickness inferior wall MI. She also noted that the patient had been placed on β-blockade and was anxious to begin physical therapy. After introducing herself to the patient, she began her physical assessment of Mr. Speed by obtaining resting baseline data (Table 12-1). These data show no evidence of ischemia, CHF, or LV dysfunction at rest, but do not preclude the onset of these findings with exercise. Magda palpated a slow, irregular pulse that she thought could be indicative of either atrial or ventricular arrhythmia. She decided to connect the patient to a portable ECG radiotelemeter to assess the origin of the skipped beats. She

---

BOX 12-1

Mr. Speed: Results of the Coronary Intensive Care Unit Evaluation

Blood pressure	110/72 mm Hg
Pulse	88 bpm, regular
Lungs	Clear to auscultation
Heart	No S_3, no arrhythmia; ECG shows Q waves and ST-segment elevations in II, III, aVF; ST-segment depression in V_1 through V_3
Enzymes	CPK = 2500; MB+

TABLE 12-1   Mr. Speed: Results of the Preexercise Resting Examination

Blood pressure	120/60 mm Hg
Pulse	55 bpm irregular
Lungs	No crackles
Heart	No S_3, S_4; no murmurs

Reprinted from DeTurk WE. Exercise and the intolerant heart, part 2. *Clin Manag.* 1992;12(2):32-39, with permission of the American Physical Therapy Association. Guide to Physical Therapist Practice. 2nd ed. *Phys Ther.* 2001 Jan;81(1):9-746.)

placed the negative electrode over the patient's sternum and the positive one just under the patient's left nipple. Figure 12-6 illustrates what Magda saw. The rhythm strip shows multifocal PVCs at an intrinsic HR of 60 bpm. These resting PVCs are worrisome for three reasons. (1) They probably originate from two areas within the ventricles and thus increase the likelihood of becoming more frequent. (2) They were absent during the patient's CICU stay. (3) They occur in the presence of known ischemic heart disease.

Her initial resting evaluation now complete, Magda formulated two questions to be answered by the patient's response to exercise: "What happens to the PVCs during exercise?" and "Is occult myocardial ischemia present?"

Comment

It should be noted that the patient is in the early recovery period of an MI and as such is vulnerable to reinfarction, or extension, or in some cases myocardial rupture. This situation does not preclude mild exercise, but cardiovascular training at high levels is a contraindication. Exercise prescription during this period is characterized by the administration of a known "dose" of exercise that is usually identified by the HR and SBP response to that exercise and expressed as the RPP. Future doses are based on the patient's response to the prior session. Early mobilization exercises tend to be dynamic as opposed to static and progress from a low level to a moderate level, compatible with most activities of daily living by the time of hospital discharge to the home. There is no

"exercise test" per se at the beginning of an early mobilization rehabilitation program; each exercise session becomes, in effect, a "mini-stress test."

Progressive Exercise Sessions

Magda began her initial exercise session with some low-level calisthenics designed to provoke a modest increase in HR, generally no more than 10 bpm above the resting level. The patient remained connected to a radiotelemeter throughout the exercise session. She noted that the PVC frequency stayed about the same during exercise and thus appeared to be unrelated to mild levels of exertion. She also noted that the ST segment did not change its position with the exercise, and the patient did not complain of any chest discomfort, indicating an absence of myocardial ischemia.

Over the next few days, Mr. Speed increased his activities, from bed level through self-care activities to ambulation down the hall and back. He was taken off β-blockade. His PVCs went away. As the time of hospital discharge approached, the patient was able to walk 200 ft down the hall and back fairly rapidly, at a HR not exceeding 98 bpm and a SBP of 134 mm Hg (RPP of 13.1×10^3) without any signs or symptoms of effort intolerance.

On day 4 post-MI, Magda decided to simulate the patient's home environment by allowing him to walk up and down a flight of stairs followed by ambulation down the hospital corridor. After climbing the flight of stairs, Mr. Speed complained of mild chest pain and palpitations. Magda terminated exercise immediately but was able to get a peak exercise paper printout from the telemeter before doing so (Fig. 12-7). Magda took an immediate postexercise BP measurement and listened to the heart and lungs. The patient was placed in a wheelchair and taken back to his room. His chest pain subsided after approximately 2 minutes. Magda paged the physician and wrote the following note in the patient's chart:

Progress note: Day 4 post-MI. The patient experienced mild precordial chest pressure and palpitations after walking up and down a flight of stairs, associated with

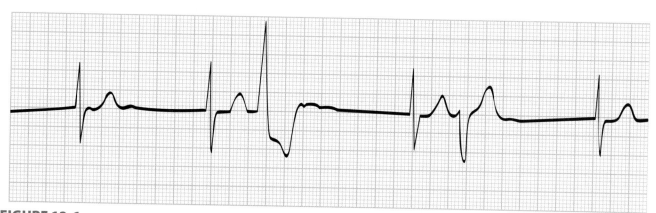

FIGURE 12-6   Mr. Speed: Telemetered ECG rhythm strip obtained at rest.

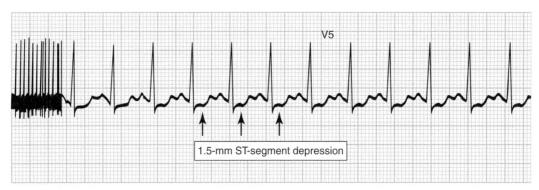

FIGURE 12-7   Mr. Speed: Telemetered ECG rhythm strip obtained during ambulation.

1.5 mm of horizontal ST-segment depression in lead CM5 via telemeter. Maximum HR was 140 bpm and BP was 148/80 mm Hg. No arrhythmia, S_3, S_4, murmur, or crackles before, during, or after exercise. Pain subsided with rest within 2 minutes. See attached ECG telemeter strip.

Ischemia at a Distance

The rhythm strip (Fig. 12-7) documents for the health care team the inappropriately high HR during exercise off beta-blockade and the exercise-induced ischemic event. This is a significant finding. Mr. Speed suffered an inferior wall MI as evidenced by significant Q waves in leads II, III, and aVF. This usually results from occlusion of the right coronary artery. The ST-segment depression in lead CM5 implicates high lateral wall ischemia that is supplied by branches of the left coronary artery. The patient is at risk for an ischemic event from another, distant source, frequently the left circumflex artery. The physical therapist responded appropriately by not only terminating exercise immediately but also correctly documenting and reporting her findings to the physician. She protected the patient from potential injury at home by identifying a problem while the patient was still in the hospital.

Postscript

Mr. Speed was kept in the hospital by his physician and referred to the cardiac catheterization laboratory for coronary angiography. The results of that test showed a totally occluded right coronary artery and a 90% lesion of the circumflex artery. The ejection fraction was 45%. The patient subsequently underwent coronary artery bypass grafting of the circumflex artery, thus saving the lateral wall of the heart. He was placed back on beta-blockade and enjoyed an uneventful postoperative hospital course. (Magda married the attending physician.)

Case Study

Charlene Posey is a 51-year-old retired laboratory technician with a 66 pack year smoking history, which she discontinued 13 years ago. She was diagnosed with chronic bronchitis and emphysema 2 years ago. Her chief complaint has been exer-

tional SOB and early onset of fatigue. Until recently these symptoms were predictable and relatively stable, until the afternoon of August 16, 2000, when she developed an acute attack of SOB while pulling weeds in the garden in her backyard. Her local physician had prescribed Atrovent (ipratropium) to be taken as needed for relief of SOB due to bronchospasm. Usually two metered doses were sufficient, but this time it took four. This event caused Ms. Posey to call her physician. The physician scheduled her for pulmonary function testing. This procedure revealed further deterioration in her pulmonary status. He recommended that the patient enroll in the pulmonary rehabilitation program at the local community hospital and be evaluated for supplemental oxygen use.

One week later Ms. Posey was referred to outpatient physical therapy for endurance training. In order to substantiate the medical diagnosis, Walt Early, the physical therapist, scheduled her for a maximum symptom-limited exercise test to be performed by the Division of Pulmonary Medicine. Recognizing her severe exercise limitations, this laboratory chose a bicycle ergometer exercise test protocol. This protocol is characterized by 2-minute stages and small increments in exercise intensity between stages. It is designed to increase both the HR and systemic O_2 transport mechanism slowly up to a maximum exercise level. Testing is terminated if the patient demonstrates early signs and symptoms of exercise intolerance. Otherwise, the test is terminated when the patient reaches 90% of their age-related maximum heart rate (ARMHR). This HR is calculated by the following revised formula (see Chapter 3):

$$ARMHR = 208 - 0.7 \times age.$$

Ms. Posey was 51 at the time of her test; her ARMHR was thus 172 bpm. The goal of testing was to increase the subject's HR up to the onset of signs and symptoms of exercise intolerance or 90% of 172 bpm, whichever came first.

The test was performed on September 1, 2000. Expired gas analysis was performed using a closed-circuit metabolic cart. Ms. Posey's performance is presented as a formal report (see Box 12-2).

BOX 12-2

MS. Posey: Report of the Results of the Community Hospital Protocol Bicycle Ergometer Exercise Test

The patient exercised for 4.0 minutes, 2.0 minutes into stage II of the Community Hospital protocol bicycle ergometer exercise test. She achieved a maximum HR of 140 bpm with an SBP of 112 mm Hg and SaO_2 of 80%. Exercise was terminated because of the onset of shortness of breath and dizziness, coupled with a fall in blood pressure and oxygen saturation. There was no anginal pain, no change in the position of the ST segments, and no ectopic activity. Immediately following exercise, physical examination revealed an increase in both peripheral cyanosis and crackles in the lung bases. Functional aerobic capacity, as measured by closed-circuit gas analysis, was 4.0 MET, less than that predicted for sedentary women of this age. Results of this test suggest a diagnosis of pulmonary hypertension secondary to chronic obstructive lung disease.

Comment

Ms. Posey's tests did not perform well. The exercise test results in Box 12-2 confirm the reduced functional capacity (4 MET) that accounts for the patient's complaint of early fatigue. The test suggests that, although there are no symptoms of pulmonary decompensation at rest, the patient is limited by pulmonary hypertension during exercise. This is evidenced by increasing SOB, coupled with sudden decreases in both oxygen saturation and SBP, that was accompanied by feelings of light-headedness. The SOB, although a nonspecific finding by itself, takes on added significance when coupled with the other data. Taken together, these data confirmed a diagnosis of exercise-limiting pulmonary hypertension.

Before pulmonary rehabilitation could begin, the patient was referred back to the physician for medical management. The physician suspected that there was an exercise-induced bronchospastic component to her disease. She was placed on Proventil (albuterol) tablets for the prevention of bronchospasm and Flovent inhalation aerosol to use as an anti-inflammatory. She was referred back to pulmonary rehabilitation almost 2 weeks later, with a request to begin exercise trials using supplemental oxygen.

A Dilemma

Walt Early was faced with a dilemma. Initially, Ms. Posey received a maximum symptom-limited exercise test for the purpose of rendering a diagnosis, while on Atrovent. However, before Walt could develop an exercise program, her medications had been expanded to include Proventil and Flovent. This change made the bicycle ergometer exercise test no longer useful in developing an exercise prescription. Additionally, Walt noted that the diagnosis of pulmonary hypertension was based on an exercise test characterized by increasing levels of physical exertion on a bicycle. Walt wondered what her tolerance to exercise would be if the workload was maintained at one level of intensity. Finally, Walt also questioned the validity of applying a bicycle ergometer test to a patient whose goal was to resume walking with her friends. Because of the change in medications, and the inappropriateness of the bicycle test for the purpose of developing an exercise prescription, Walt decided to conduct his own exercise test.

Walt chose the 6-minute walk test. He felt that this test would have more functional relevance to Ms. Posey, as much of her time is spent in walking. This test is different from the bicycle ergometer exercise test. In the 6-minute walk test, the patient walks down a corridor or other flat area, where distance is mapped out, for a period of 6 minutes. The patients are instructed to cover as much ground as possible during this time. The patients are allowed to stop walking if they have to rest, but then must resume walking if they are still within the 6-minute period. Ambulation down a corridor represents a relatively constant workload; the intensity of effort is based on how fast the patient chooses to walk and is thus controlled by the patient (see Chapter 10).

Comment

Walt's dilemma and his resolution to the problem are not atypical in cardiopulmonary rehabilitation settings. Stress tests ordered for the purpose of rendering a medical diagnosis or clearing the patient for cardiovascular training frequently reveal residual pathology that require medical intervention, but may be inappropriate for use in developing an exercise program. **The patient who comes back to physical therapy after alterations in cardiopulmonary medication is not the same patient who left.** Fiscal restraints or full laboratory appointment schedules make it impractical to formally test repeat patients in the same circumstances with the same protocol. The physical therapist must utilize the resources available within his or her department without sacrificing patient safety. The 6-minute walk test is a test that meets these criteria. It is safe, economical, and requires only a measured corridor and a stopwatch. It also matches the type of activity that Ms. Posey engages in on a daily basis—and the workload is relatively constant.

After introducing himself to the patient and conducting an initial interview, Walt proceeded to perform a physical examination. He then connected Ms. Posey to an ECG telemeter and collected pretest resting baseline data (Table 12-2). He also connected her to a pulse oximeter. The abnormal DI and the decreased oxygen saturation values suggest some nonspecific pulmonary decompensation at rest. However, although the physical examination, ECG, and pulse oximeter data show no evidence of ventilatory pump dysfunction, ventilatory pump failure, or pulmonary hypertension at rest, they do not preclude the onset of these findings with exercise.

The results of Ms. Posey's 6-minute walk test are also shown in Table 12-2. Ms. Posey covered 500 ft in 6.0 minutes

TABLE 12-2   Ms. Posey: Results of the First 6-Minute Walk Test

Pretest	
Blood pressure	132/80 mm Hg
Heart rate	102 bpm, regular
Rate–pressure product	13.5×10^3
Dyspnea index	1.31
Heart	No S_3 or S_4; no murmurs
Lungs	Clear to auscultation
O_2 saturation	91%
Immediate posttest	
Distance covered	500 ft
Number of stops	4
Immediate postexercise blood pressure	152/82 mm Hg
Immediate postexercise heart rate	132 bpm, regular
Rate–pressure product	20.1×10^3
Dyspnea index	1.45
Heart	No S_3 or S_4; no murmurs
Lungs	Crackles present bilateral lung bases
O_2 saturation	84%

Reprinted from DeTurk WE. Exercise and the intolerant heart, part 2. *Clin Manag.* 1992;12(2):32-39, with permission of the American Physical Therapy Association. Guide to Physical Therapist Practice. 2nd ed. *Phys Ther.* 2001 Jan;81(1):9-746.)

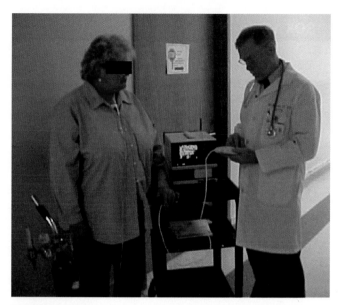

FIGURE 12-8   Ms. Posey: Just before her second 6-minute walk test. Note the presence of the pulse oximeter, oxygen tank, nasal cannula, and ECG telemeter. (Courtesy of Dr. W. E. DeTurk.)

with 4 rest stops. At the end of 6 minutes, she was markedly short of breath but maintained her BP and had no complaints of dizziness. Her oxygen saturation dropped to 84%. Ms. Posey was placed supine on a treatment table, and her head and chest were propped up with four pillows. She was given supplemental O_2 at 2.0 L/min. These signs and symptoms resolved after approximately 5 minutes of rest. Her O_2 saturation normalized within 2 minutes. The patient felt exhausted following the test and further evaluation was deferred until the next treatment session.

Walt evaluated the findings and recognized that the patient was experiencing some of the findings obtained during the bicycle ergometer test, but that, while the bicycle test elicited symptomatic hypotension, the 6-minute walk test did not. The bicycle test brought the patient up to a *maximal* level of exertion as measured by the HR response. The 6-minute walk test was a *submaximal* test that allowed the patient to walk at their own, self-selected pace at a relatively constant workload. Use of the walk test is consistent with literature that suggests that steady-state aerobic exercise may be of benefit in patients with pulmonary hypertension.[13] Walt documented his findings in the chart and sent the patient back to the referring physician. Two weeks later, Ms. Posey returned to the Pulmonary Rehabilitation Program for her second visit. The patient reported feeling unusually fatigued for the rest of the afternoon and evening, following her initial visit but felt "back to normal" at present.

This time Walt decided to repeat the same test using supplemental oxygen. Walt proceeded to administer the second 6-minute walk test in the same way as he had administered the first. However, this time Ms. Posey wore a nasal cannula connected to an E cylinder supplemental O_2 source set at 2 L/min (see Fig. 12-8). A physical therapy aide trundled the

unit behind Ms. Posey as she walked down the hall and progressed through the test. The results of this test are shown in Table 12-3. This second test is notable for the increase in distance ambulated, combined with a higher oxygen saturation both pre- and postexercise, a lower DI, and a lower HR response.

The beneficial effect of oxygen on cardiac function in the second test is apparent both at rest and during exercise

TABLE 12-3   Ms. Posey: Results of the Second 6-Minute Walk Test[a]

Pretest	
Blood pressure	130/84 mm Hg
Heart rate	88 bpm, regular
Rate–pressure product	11.4×10^3
Dyspnea index	1.20
Heart	No S_3 or S_4; no murmurs
Lungs	Clear to auscultation
O_2 saturation	99%[a]
Immediate posttest	
Distance covered	620 ft
Number of stops	3
Immediate postexercise blood pressure	150/80 mm Hg
Immediate postexercise heart rate	128 bpm, regular
Rate–pressure product	20.2×10^3
Dyspnea index	1.38
Heart	No S_3 or S_4; no murmurs
Lungs	Crackles present bilateral lung bases
O_2 saturation	87%

[a]The patient is receiving supplemental O_2 at 2.0 L/min both at rest and during exercise.

Reprinted from DeTurk WE. Exercise and the intolerant heart, part 2. *Clin Manag.* 1992;12(2):32-39, with permission of the American Physical Therapy Association. Guide to Physical Therapist Practice. 2nd ed. *Phys Ther.* 2001 Jan;81(1):9-746.)

when compared to the first test. The patient was able to walk for a longer period of time with fewer rest periods. Most importantly, SBP was maintained and Ms. Posey was less symptomatic. The beneficial effect of oxygen therapy is due to its direct action on pulmonary vasculature causing decreased pulmonary vascular resistance and enhanced arterial oxygen content, providing more oxygen to the heart, brain, and other organs. This also indicates that, with supplemental oxygen, the heart does not have to work hard to supply blood to working skeletal muscles during the 6-minute walk test.

The Exercise Prescription

Ms. Posey began exercise training on the treadmill with 2.0 L of supplemental oxygen soon after her second exercise test. There were five components to her exercise prescription.[14] (1) The *intensity* of exercise was determined as a percentage of the maximum HR attained on the second 6-minute walk exercise test, while Ms. Posey was on low-flow oxygen. Walt found, through trial and error, that Ms. Posey could comfortably sustain an HR that was 75% of 128 bpm, or 96 bpm. (2) The *total duration* of training at this intensity was approximately 20 minutes. However, Ms. Posey could not sustain 20 minutes of *continuous* exercise; therefore, she trained for 4 minutes in the training window and rested for 2 minutes, and then repeated this sequence 5 times for a total of 20 minutes in the training window. The training period was preceded by 5 minutes of stretching and calisthenic warm-up exercises and concluded with 5 minutes of slower walking. (3) The *frequency* of training was three times a week. Ms. Posey was able to undergo training as an outpatient for a period of 10 weeks. (4) The *modality* of choice was the treadmill, set at 1.2 mph at a 0% grade. (5) This last component of the exercise prescription took into consideration the *patient's goals and level of motivation;* both Walter and the patient felt that cardiovascular training should be geared toward return to household activities such as gardening and recreational walking with her friends.

Postscript

Eleven weeks later, Walt assessed the results of the patient's training program with another 6-minute walk test, again with supplemental O_2 set at 2.0 L/min (see Table 12-4). This test showed a reduction in both the patient's resting HR and the HR immediately following completion of the test. Ms. Posey was able to increase her ambulation distance to 1,060 ft. These data demonstrate successful acquisition of a cardiopulmonary training effect. The use of oxygen combined with a program of aerobic endurance exercise training were key elements in her rehabilitation.

Upon discharge from the Pulmonary Rehabilitation Program, Ms. Posey was prescribed very high dose calcium channel blockade[15] and continuous supplemental oxygen to be used during the day. She was outfitted with a nasal cannula and a highly portable liquid O_2 system that was attached to a

TABLE 12-4 Ms. Posey: Results of the Third 6-Minute Walk Test After a 9-Week Aerobic Endurance Training Program[a]

Pretest	
Blood pressure	128/86 mm Hg
Heart rate	82 bpm, regular
Rate–pressure product	10.5×10^3
Dyspnea index	1.1
Heart	No S_3 or S_4; no murmurs
Lungs	Clear to auscultation
O_2 saturation	98%[a]
Immediate posttest	
Distance covered	1060 ft
Number of stops	2
Immediate postexercise blood pressure	150/80 mm Hg
Immediate postexercise heart rate	122 bpm, regular
Rate–pressure product	18.3×10^3
Dyspnea index	1.25
Heart	No S_3 or S_4; no murmurs
Lungs	Crackles present bilateral lung bases
O_2 saturation	93%[a]

[a]The patient is receiving supplemental O_2 at 2.0 L/min both at rest and during exercise.

belt that she wore around her waist. Ms. Posey feels that the combination of pulmonary rehabilitation and supplemental O_2 have given her a new lease on life. She has rejoined the walking club with her friends and continues to pull weeds in her garden.

CLOSING

This chapter has summarized some of the examination tools and techniques found in the pulmonary and cardiac evaluation chapters and in the electrocardiography chapter. It has structured these tools and techniques to form an evaluation approach for classifying patients into categories that are summarized as hypothesis-oriented algorithms in Figs. 12-4 and 12-5. This classification system was applied to two case studies. **An ongoing evaluation approach that is applied during a therapeutic intervention session that utilizes such a classification system will direct the therapist to respond in ways that are appropriate for optimum patient management.** Additionally, **an understanding of this process will provide the reader with a proper background with which to appreciate the complexity inherent in monitoring patient progress, not only during a treatment session but also over the course of a total plan of care.**

Management plans for patients exemplifying the Cardiopulmonary Preferred Practice Patterns will be covered in detail in Chapters 15 through 22.

Heads Up!

This chapter contains a CD-ROM activity.

REFERENCES

1. American Heart Association. Guidelines 2000 for Cardiopulmonary Resuscitation and Emergency Cardiovascular Care. *Circulation.* 2000;102(suppl):158.

2. Pollock ML, Wilmore JH. *Exercise in Health and Disease.* 2nd ed. Philadelphia, PA: WB Saunders; 1990.

3. Froelicher VF. *Exercise and the Heart: Clinical Concepts.* 2nd ed. Chicago, IL: Year Book Medical Publishers; 1987:18.

4. American Heart Association. *Exercise Standards: A Statement for Health Care Professionals from the American Heart Association.* Dallas, TX: American Heart Association; 1996.

5. Goldschlager H, Selzer Z, Cohn K. Treadmill stress tests as indicators of presence and severity of coronary artery disease. *Ann Intern Med.* 1976;85:277.

6. Ellestad MH. *Stress Testing: Principles and Practice.* 4th ed. Philadelphia, PA: FA Davis; 1996.

7. American Heart Association. ACC/AHA guidelines for exercise testing: executive summary. *Circulation.* 1997;96:345-354.

8. American Physical Therapy Association. Guide to Physical Therapist Practice. 2nd ed. *Phys Ther.* 2001 Jan;81(1):9-746.

9. *Oximeter Operation Manual, version 3.* Watford, Hertfordshire, United Kingdom: SIMS BCI Inc; 2000.

10. Borg G. Psychophysical bases of perceived exertion. *Med Sci Sports Exerc.* 1982;14:377-381.

11. Ramirez-Venegas A, Ward J, Olmstead E, et al. Effect of exercise training on dyspnea measures in patients with chronic obstructive pulmonary disease. *J Cardiopulm Rehabil.* 1997;17:103-109.

12. Jones N, Moran Campbell E. *Clinical Exercise Testing.* 2nd ed. Philadelphia, PA: WB Saunders; 1982.

13. Cahalin L. Pulmonary hypertension and exercise. *Cardiopulm Phys Ther.* 1995;6:3-12.

14. Rich S, Kaufmann E, Levy P. The effect of high doses of calcium-channel blockers on survival in primary pulmonary hypertension. *N Engl J Med.* 1992;327:76-81.

15. American College of Sports Medicine. *Guidelines for Exercise Testing and Prescription.* 6th ed. Philadelphia, PA: Lippincott Williams & Wilkins; 2000.

Cardiopulmonary Concerns in the Patient with Musculoskeletal and Integumentary Deficits: An Evidence-Based Approach

John S. Leard* & Chris L. Wells

INTRODUCTION

The purpose of this chapter is to describe common musculoskeletal and integumentary pathologies and the evidence found in the literature regarding their influence on the cardiopulmonary system. Impairments of bony structures, joints, skin, fascia, and musculature of the thorax may lead to a decrease in cardiopulmonary function. These impairments will lead to impaired circulation, aerobic capacity/endurance, ventilation, and respiration/gas exchange by restriction of movement of structures in the body. This results in decreased functional mobility of the patient and disability. This chapter will also describe the evidence in the literature as it relates to the interventions commonly associated with these pathologies.

MUSCULOSKELETAL CONDITIONS

Osteoporosis (Practice Patterns 4A, 4B, 4C, 4F, 4G; *ICD-9-CM* Code: 733.0)

Introduction

Osteoporosis is a general term for a decrease in the mass of normal bone per unit volume and leads to an increase risk of fracture. Many conditions and diseases may be involved in the etiology of developing osteoporosis including metabolic disorders of osteoclastic versus osteoblastic activity, endocrine disease, bone disuse, genetic factors, and postmenopausal state. Bone loss is generally associated with advancing age in both sexes but proceeds at a faster rate in women, especially following menopause.[1,2]

The current intervention strategy is prevention of normal bone loss per unit volume by increasing peak bone mass by the third decade through diet, weight-bearing exercise, and cessation of smoking. Inherited factors account for an estimated 60% to 80% of the variability in peak bone mass. Diet, physical activity, and hormonal status are important modifiers of bone accrual.[3] Reversal of widespread osteoporosis is extremely difficult to achieve.

Classic spinal deformities associated with osteoporosis are increased kyphosis with loss of height, thoracic vertebral body fractures, and back pain.[4,5] The increased kyphosis is related to thoracic wedge fractures but also has nonskeletal contributing factors.[6] One of these factors is the intervertebral disc shape.[7] The loss of height does not seem to be due to the patient having small vertebral bodies but instead is due to the wedging, which causes an increase in the kyphosis.[8] Besides osteoporosis, there are many reasons why thoracic vertebral body fractures occur in patients older than 50 years . Metastases, multiple myeloma, and trauma[9,10] are associated with these fractures as well. In Finland, fractures occur in men and women with equal frequency, and gradually

TABLE 13-1   Summary of Studies Comparing Pulmonary Function and Bony Deformities

Author	Subjects	Measurements	Results
Culham et al. (1994)[17]	15 women	Motion sensors	Greater kyphotic angles produced greater reductions in pulmonary function.
Leech et al. (1990)[14]	74 women	Cobb angle	Kyphosis reduced FVC.[a]
Mellin et al. (1987)[16]	185 men, 87 women	Cobb angle inclinometer	Greater kyphotic angles produced greater reductions in pulmonary function.
Schlaich et al. (1998)[15]	34 osteoporotic Fxs, 51 chronic LBP	Measures of body stature (height reduction, distance from lowest rib to iliac crest, distance of occiput from wall)	PFTs are reduced in patients with osteoporotic Fxs, but not in patients with LBP.

[a]FVC, forced vital capacity; Fxs, fractures; LBP, low back pain; PFTs, pulmonary function tests.

increase with age. At age 65, the frequency sharply increases in women. This is attributed to the pattern of age-related osteoporosis between the sexes due to menopause. In a study of 942 women in Rochester, Minnesota, increasing age was also associated with vertebral fractures.[11] The level of peak frequency for spinal fractures occurs at T7-T8 and T11–T12.[8] Vertebral body fractures have radiological characteristics that are different from fractures associated with osteoarthritis. Osteoporotic fractures have a greater height difference posterior to anterior in the saggital plane than fractures in patients with osteoarthritis.[12]

Back pain in patients suffering from osteoporosis is associated with the number of vertebral body fractures and the severity of the kyphotic curve.[13] The literature is not conclusive regarding the pathomechanics of the increased kyphotic curve. Poor posture, decreased strength of the muscles that extend the thoracic spine, and the spinal fractures themselves are all possible beginnings to this increased curve.

Impairments That Influence Cardiopulmonary Function

There appears to be no literature that supports the notion that back pain leads to pulmonary dysfunction. However, pulmonary function loss is associated with women suffering from osteoporosis due to their increased kyphotic curve and thoracic compression fractures. Kyphosis and thoracic compression fractures caused by osteoporosis produce some predictable declines in vital capacity in women.[14] Schlaich et al. noted that pulmonary function is reduced in patients who have spinal osteoporotic fractures and not in patients suffering from chronic low back pain.[15] It is questionable as to whether this decrease in pulmonary function is only related to the spinal hypomobility, causing a decrease in the ability to expand the chest, or whether it is related to osteoporosis which is progressive with age, such that older patients experience more severe impairments. In 1987, Mellin and Harjula studied 187 men and 87 women and concluded that patients with increased spinal curves had decreased vital capacities and forced expiratory volumes.[16] Culham et al. studied 15 women with kyphosis and found a significant negative correlation

among kyphotic angle and inspiratory capacity, vital capacity, and lateral expansion of the thorax.[17] Table 13-1 summarizes the findings of these articles, which examined cardiopulmonary function and bone deformities.

Interventions to Improve Cardiopulmonary Function

No treatment effectiveness studies have been found that have examined the benefits of physical therapy on pulmonary function with osteoporotic patients. A group of physical therapists did study the effects of physical therapy on chronic pain and performance associated with osteoporotic patients. Treatments included balance training, muscle strength training, and lumbar stabilization exercises. They concluded that the program improved balance and level of daily function, decreased pain, decreased the use of analgesic medication, and improved quality of life after the active training period.[18]

Associated Conditions With Osteoporosis

If the musculoskeletal impairments described previously are associated with other comorbidities, such as congestive heart failure (CHF) or cardiovascular disease, the pulmonary function of the patient and the outcomes of interventions may be negatively influenced. Vogt et al.[19] studied 1,492 older white women with osteoporosis and found no relationship between the incidence and the prevalence of vertebral fractures and cardiovascular disease. However, they discovered that women with cardiovascular disease had more disabling back pain than women without cardiovascular disease. A single case report of an older woman with osteoporosis and congestive heart failure (CHF), who required mitral valve replacement, suggests that osteoporosis may have a role in the morbidity and mortality of patients. This subject had a profound collapse of the thoracic spine that resulted in pulmonary insufficiency and death.[20] Although this was a single case study, such situations may occur to a greater extent in older patients with cardiovascular and pulmonary diseases and may require further investigation.

Summary

The relationship between osteoporosis and cardiopulmonary impairments is difficult to identify, because osteoporosis has many associated impairments that could affect cardiopulmonary function. Osteoporosis affects older men and women and is associated with an increased kyphotic curve, thoracic compression fractures, and decreased lateral chest expansion. It is difficult to separate these factors individually to identify whether the overall decrease in chest wall size or expansion is altering cardiopulmonary function or whether other comorbidities are influencing function. No treatment effectiveness studies have been found that have examined the effects of physical therapy on pulmonary function with patients diagnosed with osteoporosis.

Ankylosing Spondylitis (Practice Patterns 4E, 4F; *ICD-9-CM* Code: 720)

Introduction

Ankylosing spondylitis is a chronic inflammatory disease that primarily affects the sacroiliac joint and the spine. The shoulder and hip, as well as other lower extremity joints, may be affected. It is a form of chronic seronegative spondyloarthritis. The disease results in progressive stiffening of the joints, typically beginning with the spine and sacroiliac joints. It attacks the site of insertion of tendons, ligaments, fascia, and fibrous joint capsules.[2] There is also a high risk of cardiomyopathy, arrhythmias, pericarditis, and aortic valvular disease associated with ankylosing spondylitis. Males are afflicted at a rate of 10:1, male-to-female ratio, and Caucasians are afflicted more frequently than Afro-Americans. The onset of the disease occurs between 20 and 40 years of age.[21,22] The cause of ankylosing spondylitis is unknown, but its etiology may be a hyperreactivity response of the immune system.

Initially, the patient may present with complaints of poorly localized back pain that is provoked by sudden movements. The back pain is differentiated from "mechanical low back pain" because movement relieves the symptoms, the symptoms do not diminish with rest, and the patient experiences night pain. The progression of these signs and symptoms is either continuous or intermittent, spreading cephalically along the spine. In the most severe cases, the spine and hips will become stiff, a spinal flexion deformity develops, and pathological vertebral fractures occur. Only one-third of the patients diagnosed will progress to these severe symptoms.[2]

Impairments That Influence Cardiopulmonary Function

Pulmonary involvement affecting the upper lobes of the lungs has been documented in 1.2% of patients with ankylosing spondylitis. Histological findings can include nonspecific fibrosis, dilated bronchi, and bulla formation and occur at a rate of 50:1, male-to-female ratio.[22]

Over time, the stiffening and straightening of the spine cause a decrease in chest wall compliance and result in a *mechanical restrictive process.* This chest wall restriction is associated with an increase in pneumothorax, atelectasis, and aspiration due to esophageal dysfunction that can lead to pulmonary infection. In the presence of fibrotic changes, the recurrence of infection can lead to progressive pulmonary fibrosis.[21]

Pulmonary involvement is documented by abnormal findings on standard laboratory tests. Pulmonary function tests show a decline in vital capacity and total lung volumes. Maximal expiratory and inspiratory efforts are reduced. Radiological examination demonstrates small apical nodules, infiltrates, and pleural thickening. There is an increase in B lymphocytes and a lower level of neutrophils upon bronchoalveolar lavage.[21,23] As the disease progresses, the spine becomes hypomobile at the costovertebral joints, resulting in decreased chest expansion and sometimes provoking pain with deep breathing.[2]

Interventions to Improve Cardiopulmonary Function

Treatment for pulmonary involvement includes general spinal and rib cage mobility intervention, such as general trunk stretching, soft tissue mobilization, and deep breathing exercises to improve mobility. Modalities and medications can be used to control pain and spinal inflammation. Corticosteroids may be utilized if intrinsic pulmonary disease impairs function.[21,23] Depending on the severity of the disease, aerobic exercises are prescribed to maintain cardiopulmonary conditioning and trunk range of motion. Diaphragmatic breathing or inspiratory hold-breathing can be used as a breathing strategy when the patient has a high respiratory rate, anxiety, or signs of oxygen desaturation with exertion. An incentive spirometer may also be used as visual feedback in order to facilitate larger tidal volumes. In severe cases, the patient may not be able to generate a large enough lung volume to manage his or her own secretions; therefore, chest physical therapy and postural drainage will be indicated to address these impairments. If the patient is retaining carbon dioxide, he or she may need mechanical ventilatory support (see Table 13-2).

TABLE 13-2 Common Interventions for Ankylosing Spondylitis

Impairment	Interventions
Spinal immobility	Stretching of thoracic spine, soft tissue mobilization
Rib immobility	Deep breathing, joint mobilization, aerobic conditioning
Spinal pain and inflammation	Modalities, corticosteroids, aerobic conditioning
Anxiety or high respiratory rate with exertion	Diaphragmatic breathing, relaxation
Reduced lung volumes	Incentive spirometer, postural drainage, chest physical therapy, mechanical ventilator support

Prognosis varies considerably. Approximately 35% of patients with ankylosing spondylitis will succumb to deadly arrhythmias. Infection and fractures of the cervical spine are also leading causes of death. These occur once the disease has progressed and has produced a brittle and rigid cervical spine that is susceptible to injury, even after minimal trauma. Death from pulmonary involvement is rare, but when it occurs, it is usually associated with infection and respiratory failure secondary to cervical spine injury.[21]

Summary

Pulmonary function is altered with patients suffering from ankylosing spondylitis, mainly due to restriction of chest wall movement. This results in decreased chest expansion and sometimes provokes pain with deep breathing. As the disease progresses, the restriction of chest wall movement and stiffening of the spine cause other impairments such as pneumonia, inability to remove secretions, small apical nodules, infiltrates, and pleural thickening. Initial intervention is aimed at maintaining or increasing chest wall movement.

Idiopathic Scoliosis (Practice Pattern 4B; *ICD-9-CM* Code: 737.3)

Introduction

Scoliosis is the development of an abnormal lateral curvature of the spine. Approximately 80% of all abnormal lateral curvatures of the spine have mechanisms that are unknown, so they are classified as idiopathic. The onset generally appears in childhood or adolescence and has a 10:1 female-to-male ratio.[24] The curve may progress from mild to severe, particularly during rapid stages of growth, and can be located in the lumbar, thoracic, or both regions of the spine.[2] The lateral curve usually presents with rotation and increased kyphosis. **The lateral curve plus the rotation of the involved thoracic vertebrae around a vertical axis causes a decrease in lung function.**[25]

Impairments That Influence Cardiopulmonary Function

The scoliosis results in a compression of the lung on the concave side of the abnormal thoracic curve and may decrease lung volumes.[24,26] The greater the lateral curve of the spine, the more likely the patient will have pulmonary symptoms. As the curve progresses, the first indication of pulmonary limitation occurs during exercise with breathlessness.[27] Upon examination, there is a decrease in diaphragmatic excursion and breath sounds on the concave side. These impairments are related to the severity of the curve.[28] **If the curvature becomes greater than 60 degrees, which is classified as** *severe*, **the skeletal deformity begins to affect pulmonary function and the patient will present with more respiratory complaints.** It is difficult to determine how much of the dyspnea is associated with deconditioning.[27] In some cases, the deformity actually causes a pulmonary restrictive breathing pattern when the

PFTs are examined. There is a decrease in vital capacity; forced vital capacity; forced expiratory volume in 1 second (VC, FVC, FEV_1), and an elevation of the FEV_1/FVC ratio. **When the curve is more than 90 degrees, there is mechanical impairment of inspiratory muscles and decreased lung compliance leading to a decrease in inspiratory muscle strength.**[24,29] **With patients having curves between 100 and 136 degrees, the pattern of respiratory muscle activation is similar to that in patients with severe chronic obstructive pulmonary disease (COPD).** This pattern does not use the sternocleidomastoid at rest but has a stronger than normal recruitment of the rib cage inspiratory muscles, the abdominal muscles, and the diaphragm with less mechanical efficiency.[30] In both COPD and severe kyphoscoliosis, abnormal biomechanics are the major causes in abnormal pulmonary function. Patients with COPD have increased lung compliance and decreased chest wall compliance, whereas patients with severe kyphoscoliosis have marked reduction in lung and chest wall compliance. The acute decompensation occasionally seen in patients with severe kyphoscoliosis appears to be primarily due to the marked reduction in lung and chest wall compliance and less to airway resistance and positive end-expiratory pressure.[31] Patients with severe scoliosis are more susceptible to developing atelectasis, pneumonia, and a reduction in exercise tolerance. Pulmonary complications are a contributing factor to the death of 82% of patients with clinically significant scoliosis.[29]

Kyphoscoliosis is most frequently associated with respiratory complications due to increased chest wall stiffness. Patients will present with low lung volumes particularly VC and expiratory reserve volume with little change in the right verticle (RV). This is consistent with a restrictive pattern. If the tidal volume is significantly impaired, hypoventilation may occur. Hypoventilation is associated with hypoxemia and ventilation–perfusion mismatch. Pulmonary vascular resistance is elevated because of the distortion and compression of vascular tissue caused by this skeletal deformity.[32] Severe kyphoscoliosis can lead to bronchial torsion, which will obstruct the airway and cause moderate to severe air trapping.[33] Boyer et al.[34] found moderate-to-severe air trapping in 46% of 44 children with idiopathic scoliosis.

Surgical Interventions to Improve Cardiovascular Function

Surgical correction of the deformity is the intervention of choice in cases of severe scoliosis. Severe lateral curves are usually greater than 40 degrees, as measured by the Cobb method[2] (see Fig. 13-1). The surgery may be done through either an anterior and/or a posterior approach. Both approaches involve bone grafts from the ribs or the iliac crest and utilization of spinal instrumentation. **Surgical intervention has an impact on pulmonary function.** In long-term follow-up, it has been reported that the *posterior approach* restores pulmonary function to normal predicted levels, whereas the anterior approach does not correct the restrictive pulmonary pattern.[35] In a study with long-term follow-up of patients who had undergone the

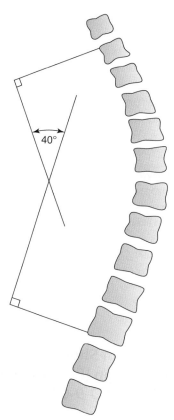

FIGURE 13-1 The Cobb method is used to measure this 40-degree lateral thoracic spinal curvature of the spine seen on an AP radiograph.

anterior approach, there was a small decrease in forced vital capacity. The authors concluded that improvement in pulmonary function could not be achieved with this surgery.[36] The anterior approach is also associated with an increased incidence of pulmonary complication in the postoperative period because one lung must be deflated in order to achieve surgical access. Harvesting bone grafts from the ribs also has a longer-term negative effect in restoration of PFTs than grafts taken from the pelvis. Patients who have undergone the placement of spinal instrumentation (Harrington rod) demonstrate little to no improvement in the restrictive pulmonary process.[35]

Nonsurgical Interventions to Improve Cardiopulmonary Function

Sixty-eight percent of patients with idiopathic scoliosis do not have pulmonary symptoms because the curve is not great enough either to cause symptoms or to have surgery.[27] These less severe curves are often treated with *bracing* to decrease progression of the curve. A meta-analysis of the efficacy of nonoperative treatment found brace wear for 23 hours a day was significantly more effective than brace wear, or paravertebral electrical surface stimulation, for shorter periods of time.[37]

Some bracing may be a concern in the nonsurgical treatment of these patients.[24,29,38] The Boston brace, a common thoracolumbosacral (TLSO) brace, was shown to have reduced

lung volume and pulmonary compliance in patients wearing this brace for treatment of idiopathic scoliosis.[39] Bracing increased respiratory effort, NVD, and dyspnea scores during progressive-cycle ergometry exercise.[40] However, long-term effects of wearing a TLSO brace for 2 years showed no harm to lung function, in contrast to the short-term effects of bracing which showed impaired pulmonary function.[41]

Physical therapy interventions do not appear to reverse the lateral curvature but are aimed at slowing the progression of the curve. Treatments include stretching of soft tissue, strengthening on the convex side of the curve, lower extremity flexibility, and postural instruction.

Patients with severe kyphoscoliosis with ventilatory insufficiency requiring nocturnal nasal ventilation delivered by volume-cycled or pressure-cycled ventilators have been observed to improve symptoms, pulmonary function, and arterial blood gasses.[42] Long-term noninvasive ventilation for patients with thoracic cage abnormalities appears to improve hypoventilation and functional abilities and decreases the need for tracheostomy.[43]

Treatment of mild idopathic scoliosis has included aerobic training and has been shown to be effective in maintaining and improving pulmonary function. Athanasopoulos et al.[44] observed improved forced vital capacity, FEV$_1$/FVC, and exercise tolerance after 2 months of cycling exercise performed 4 times per week for 30 minutes. A control group was observed to have reductions in the FVC, VC, respiratory rate, and exercise tolerance.

Summary

The greater the lateral curve of the spine, the more likely the patient will have pulmonary symptoms. Interventions for idiopathic scoliosis can be classified as *nonsurgical* for the less severe curves (less than 40 degrees) and as *surgical* for the more severe curves. The posterior surgical approach to decrease the lateral curve has many advantages over the anterior approach and demonstrates better return of pulmonary function postoperatively. Sixty-eight percent of the patients with idiopathic scoliosis with less than a 40-degree curve do not have pulmonary symptoms. These less severe curves are often treated with bracing to decrease progression of the curve. Some bracing has been shown to cause pulmonary impairments and may be of concern during the nonsurgical treatment of these patients. Aerobic conditioning has improved the cardiopulmonary function of patients with less severe scoliosis.

Pectus Deformities (Practice Patterns 4B, 4C, 4D, 4F, 4I; *ICD-9-CM* Code: 733)
Introduction

Pectus excavatum, which is commonly referred to as *funnel chest*, is the most common of all the chest wall deformities. It results from an overgrowth of costal cartilage with depression of the sternum, usually the lower portion.

Pectus carinatum or pigeon breast is a less common deformity that is caused by abnormal growth of the costal cartilage or abnormal fusion of the sternal body and manubrium that causes an anterior protrusion of the sternum. This deformity is not associated with respiratory difficulty, but dysplasia and cardiac defects may present as pulmonary symptoms.[24]

Impairments That Influence Cardiopulmonary Function

With pectus excavatum, there is often right sternal rotation as well as depression. This results in more depression on the right side and causes rotation and displacement of the heart to the left side. Heart murmur from altered blood flow is common due to the shift of the mediastinum. Occasionally patients may report dyspnea, chest pain, and palpitations. If pectus excavatum is severe, there is a decrease in stroke volume and respiratory reserve.

Surgical Interventions to Improve Cardiopulmonary Function

Surgical intervention is performed primarily for cosmetic reasons. Surgery is also warranted in the severe case where the deformity is interfering with cardiac output and causing significant pulmonary restrictions.[24]

A surgically produced deformity, a median sternotomy, is a common surgical approach for open heart procedures, such as coronary artery bypass graft and valvular repair or replacement. When compared to nonsternotomy procedures, patients who undergo sternotomy demonstrate a greater decrease in FEV_1, FVC, PaO_2, and $PaCO_2$ in the early postoperative phase. The decline in lung volumes is correlated with pain level. Patients who undergo surgical intervention involving the chest wall generally have a transient decrease in chest wall compliance and increase their risk of pulmonary complications, including atelectasis and pneumonia.[45]

Sternal Precautions

Postoperatively, a patient is provided with sternal precautions in order to protect the incision site, enhance healing, and decrease pain. Many sternal precaution protocols exist and appear to be institution specific. In general, they last from postoperative day 1 until weeks 6 to 8. The goals of these protocols are to prevent shear and distraction forces across the surgical incision site. See Box 13-1 for one example of a sternal precaution protocol.

Summary

Pectus deformities are usually treated surgically for cosmetic reasons or because of impairments in cardiopulmonary function. Postoperatively, cardiopulmonary function is decreased because of pain or decrease in chest wall compliance. Specific postoperative guidelines are given for the first 21 days, and general guidelines, for 8 weeks.

BOX 13-1

Sternal Precaution Protocol

For the first 6 to 8 weeks after surgery, patient may perform
- Bilateral shoulder exercises in forward flexion and extension, but below shoulder level
- Gentle upper-extremity isometric exercises

Patient must avoid
- Bilateral horizontal shoulder abduction, external rotation, and scapular retraction
- Unilateral arm exercises
- Lifting weights greater than 10 lb
- Pushing and pulling heavy objects
- Heavy housework
- Driving a car

The Relationship of Shoulder Motion to Pulmonary Function (Practice Patterns 4D, 4E, 4F, 4G, 4H, 4I; *ICD-9-CM* Codes: 726, 810, 811, 812)

Introduction

Shoulder hypomobility is an impairment that is theorized to influence pulmonary function. The premise of this theory is that a relationship exists between shoulder motion and rib cage motion. This theory posits that shoulder motion influences rib cage and spinal movement and eventually influences pulmonary function. Therefore, treatment techniques have been developed using breathing to facilitate shoulder movement and shoulder movement to facilitate breathing.

Literature Supporting Theoretical Relationship

There appears to be no literature that directly associates shoulder immobilization or dysfunction with a decrease in pulmonary function, although many of the muscles of the shoulder share a respiratory function as well as an arm positional function. Patients suffering from lung disease and athletes recovering from workouts will often use their arms for support in order to facilitate accessory muscle breathing and to assist in ventilation. Studies show that there is an increase in metabolic and ventilatory requirements in patients who breathe at tidal volume with arms elevated and unsupported. It appears that the diaphragm contributes more to ventilatory pressure changes when the arms are unsupported and flexed to shoulder level.[46] Mackey et al. agreed with this study and felt that the intercostals and accessory respiratory muscles act to stabilize the arms and torso, impeding chest wall movement and placing more emphasis on the diaphragm.[47] These studies seem to indicate that there is a direct relationship between the position/support of the arms and pulmonary function. Hodges et al.

found that predictable, anticipatory postural trunk motions occur during unilateral upper arm movement.[48] The trunk movements are synergistic to the direction of the shoulder motion. The authors indicated that the trunk did not simply provide stabilization but worked with the shoulder muscles to facilitate movement. This also provides evidence to suggest that there is a direct relationship between shoulder motion and trunk/rib cage motion that is predictable and synergistic with movement of the glenohumeral joint. With movement of the glenohumeral joint above 160 degrees of flexion, Kapanji noted that thoracic spine extension is necessary in order to allow the scapula to fully depress and full shoulder range of motion to be attained.[49] With thoracic spine extension, there is an increase in chest expansion and a subsequent increase in thoracic volume. This also provides evidence directly connecting the motion of the glenohumeral joint to thoracic cavity expansion.

Intervention to Improve Pulmonary Function

Massery has obtained positive results when utilizing different shoulder positions in order to facilitate breathing. This approach uses breathing, the motions of the trunk, and the motions of the shoulder in a coordinated fashion to facilitate synergistic trunk/shoulder motion and restore shoulder or pulmonary function. Such a treatment technique combines shoulder flexion and trunk extension with inhalation and shoulder extension and trunk flexion with expiration. Improved inspiratory and expiratory capacities have been obtained with this technique.[50] This technique is currently being investigated but enjoys widespread use. More research is needed to determine its effectiveness in treating pulmonary and glenohumeral dysfunction.

INTEGUMENTARY CONDITIONS

Sarcoidosis (Practice Pattern 6H; *ICD-9-CM* Code: 457)

Introduction

Sarcoidosis is a systemic granulomatous disease that primarily affects the lungs and the lymphatic system.[51] Noncaseating tumor-like epitheloids or granulomas are the hallmark of sarcoidosis. There is difficulty in collecting epidemiological information on this disease because of the inconsistency in the definition, variable methods for diagnosis, and variable presentation of disease.[52] There appear to be two peaks for onset of sarcoidosis. One peak is in the third decade of life, followed by another peak in the sixth decade of life. The incidence is estimated at 6 per 100,000. There is a three times higher incidence in Afro-Americans than in Caucasians.[52,53]

Etiology of Pulmonary Involvement

It has been suggested that the granulomas are formed in response to a persistent and poorly degradable immune response that stimulates a T-cell–mediated response to some unidentified stimulus. This chronic immune activity results in fibrosis. There are other theories that have been proposed about the etiology of sarcoidosis. There appears to be a genetic predisposition underlying this disease with an abnormal regulation of antigen recognition. Patients who have been exposed to certain infections, talc, or clay, have a higher incidence of sarcoidosis than does the general population. Approximately 60% of patients who are diagnosed with sarcoidosis will have complete resolution of the granulomas. In the remaining patients, the disease will cause some degree of pulmonary dysfunction. At the site of the granulomas there is an accumulation of T-helper cells that chronically stimulates ongoing inflammation. There is also the detrimental effect of chronic inflammation with the release of enzymes that degrades the delicate tissue of the lungs to create more granulomas and fibrosis.[51–53]

Other Systems Affected

Other systems besides the lungs can be affected from the infiltration of granulomas and fibrosis. Twenty percent of the patients will have kidney involvement, which can extend from interstitial nephritis, and fibrosis that interferes with filtration, kidney stones, and urinary obstruction. Twenty to thirty percent of patients will have cardiac involvement, but most are asymptomatic. There may be fibrosis of the myocardium that both impairs contractility and causes arrhythmias and sudden death. There may be granuloma formation that predominantly affects the meninges, particularly the posterior fossa of the central nervous system (CNS). Sarcoidosis of the CNS can mimic tumors with progressive hydrocephalus and cranial nerve impairment. The gastrointestinal system may be impaired, as well as the liver and the eyes, and the skin, which typically clears.[54]

Diagnosis

The disease is usually diagnosed by both clinical presentation and radiological findings. There is typically bilateral lymphadenopathy in 90% of the cases. This disease can be placed into a staging classification (Table 13-3)[51] that has become helpful in advancing the understanding of sarcoidosis and medical management.

TABLE 13-3 Staging Classification of Sarcoidosis

Staging	Pathology
0	No visible findings
1	Bilateral hilar lymphodenopathy
2	Bilateral hilar lymphodenopathy plus pulmonary infiltration
3	Pulmonary infiltrates with hilar abnormalities
4	Pulmonary fibrosis

Adapted from statement on sarcoidosis. *Am J Resp Crit Med.* 1999;160:736-755.

Open lung biopsy is used to confirm the diagnosis by identifying the presence of granulomas.[55] Pulmonary function tests typically demonstrate a restrictive pattern but may reveal an obstructive pattern if the granulomas are obstructing the airways. As in many fibrotic diseases, the PFTs in the presence of sarcoidosis show a decrease in total lung capacity, vital capacity and a decrease in diffusion capacity.[55]

Patients typically present with nonspecific constitutional symptoms that include fever, fatigue, and malaise; and weight loss, which usually occurs before any other symptom. If there is pulmonary involvement, 95% of the patients' primary complaint will be dyspnea and decreased exercise tolerance. There may be a nonproductive cough and chest pain with exercise that is typically associated with efforts to increase tidal volume. Approximately half of the patients will have clubbing and one-third will have palpable lymph nodes. Upon auscultation there will be basilar crackles associated with fibrosis and arrhythmias. Thirty to sixty percent of patients will be asymptomatic if there is no significant pulmonary involvement.[52,55,56]

Intervention

It is recommended that patients be medically monitored closely for at least two years for signs of remission or progression so that medications can be adjusted as necessary. As with many of the other restrictive diseases that have been discussed in this chapter, corticosteroids are the most common medications administered initially. It has been documented that corticosteroids can actually shrink the size of the granulomas and contribute to remission. Cytotoxic drugs such as methotrexate and azathioprine may suppress the progression of disease but do not cause remission.

Two-thirds of those with the diagnosis will have complete remission without any pulmonary dysfunction. The remaining patients will have some degree of pulmonary dysfunction, and approximately 10% will develop progressive pulmonary fibrosis. Prognosis depends on the stage of the disease at the time of diagnosis. Patients in stage 1 or stage 2 typically have a 70% remission rate. Only 10% to 20% of patients in stage 3 will go into remission, and it is rare to have any recovery when diagnosis is made in stage 4.[52] Almost 90% of patients die from sarcoidosis because of pulmonary failure. A patient who presents with acute symptoms has a higher incidence of recovery than a patient who has an insidious onset with multiple-organ involvement.[51]

Systemic Lupus Erythematosus (Practice Patterns 4D, 7C, 7D, 7E; *ICD-9-CM* Codes: 695.4, 710.0)

Etiology

The etiology of systemic lupus erythematosus (SLE) is unknown, but it has been suggested that there are genetic, environmental, and hormonal influences. Autoantibodies are activated against various nuclear antigens. These autoantibodies and the stimulated immune response are believed to mediate many of the manifestations of SLE. Lupus tends to affect women predominately in their childbearing years. Patients who develop interstitial pulmonary disease tend to be 45 to 50 years of age. Drug-induced SLE typically presents in the older patient, and there appears to be no gender differences. In general the prevalence is 50 per 100,000.[57]

Pulmonary Involvement and Clinical Presentation

Lupus affects the pulmonary system more frequently than any other collagen vascular disease. Pulmonary involvement may present as infectious pneumonia, pleuritis, pleural effusion, alveolar hemorrhage, pulmonary fibrosis, pulmonary hypertension, and obstructive airway disease. It can also be associated with muscular weakness that impairs ventilation. In approximately 5% to 10% of patients, it is suggested that the onset of SLE may be due to exposure to the following drugs: procainamide, penicillamine, quinidine, and hydralazine.[58]

The *pleura* is the most commonly affected tissue within the pulmonary system. The incidence of pleuritis is more common in men and in African Americans. The pleura becomes infiltrated with lymphocytes and plasma cells. A fibrotic process can develop from the inflammatory responses that cause pleural adhesions. This may result in a reduction in diaphragmatic excursion and chest wall expansion. These patients complain of chest pain with dyspnea, cough, and fever. Pleural effusion is usually present but will vary in size; therefore, signs and symptoms will also vary.[56-58] Pleural effusion may present alone or may also be associated with infection, pulmonary embolism, congestive heart failure, or renal dysfunction.[58]

Pneumonitis that is associated with SLE will be associated with acute onset of dyspnea, hypoxia, fever, and hemoptysis. There will be patchy, diffuse infiltrates on chest X-ray, with a predilection for lower-lobe involvement. It often mimics the clinical presentation of adult respiratory distress syndrome. Acute lupus pneumonitis is associated with a 50% mortality rate.[57,58]

Pulmonary interstitial fibrosis primarily affects the lower lobes. It has been suggested that it may be a sequela of pneumonitis with a chronic insidious onset. These patients will present with a restrictive pattern on pulmonary function tests, low diffusion capacity, moderate to severe desaturation with exertion, and pleuritic chest pain with increased tidal volumes.[57,58]

Pulmonary hypertension may be associated with pulmonary fibrosis or may be the primary presentation of the pulmonary disease. It is associated with muscular hypertrophy, intimal proliferation, and capillary fibrosis and thrombus. These patients present with progressive dyspnea, exercise intolerance, and signs of right heart failure.[57,58]

Lupus may be associated with *shrinking lung disorder*. Upon radiographic examination there is a progressive loss of lung volume with basilar atelectasis. Shrinking lung disease is associated with diaphragmatic dysfunction that is not related to peripheral muscle weakness. This results in a decrease in lung compliance and a decrease in expiratory pressure that exceeds inspiratory weakness. Dyspnea is the most pronounced symptom, with many patients also reporting orthopnea.[57,58]

Finally, patients with SLE may present with alveolar hemorrhage that results in dyspnea, cough, and a decline in hemoglobin/hematocrit levels. A low-grade fever may also be present. Alveolar hemorrhage is uncommon but is highly life threatening with a 70% mortality rate. It resembles pneumonitis with infiltrates, but also encompasses alveolar necrosis, edema, and microvascular thrombus. There is a higher prevalence in young women.[57,58]

Diagnosis

Diagnosis of SLE depends on the clinical presentation. Analysis of pleural effusion will show a high concentration of glucose, and the antinuclear antibody test will be positive. The majority of diagnoses will be made on the basis of open lung biopsy.[57,58]

Intervention and Prognosis

Thalidomide and cyclosporine are the leading medications for the management of lupus. Ninety percent of patients will report an improvement in their symptoms, and 60% will go into remission. Ultraviolet A (UV-A) phototherapy is also used where it is suggested to promote DNA repair and enhance cell-mediated immunity. Methylprednisone, plasmaphoresis, azathioprine, and methotrexate can also be utilized to suppress the chronic immune and inflammatory processes that are progressively destroying pulmonary function.[56]

When there is pulmonary involvement with SLE, there is an approximate 50% mortality rate due to pneumonitis, fibrosis, and hemorrhage. Infection is the most common, accounting for the high mortality rate.[58]

Summary

Systemic lupus erythematosus, more frequently than any other collagen vascular disease, affects the pulmonary system. Pulmonary involvement may present as infectious pneumonia, pleuritis, pleural effusion, alveolar hemorrhage, pulmonary fibrosis, pulmonary hypertension, and obstructive airway disease. The majority of diagnoses will be made on the basis of open lung biopsy. Intervention is determined by clinical presentation along with medications for the management of lupus.

Scleroderma and Crest Syndrome (Practice Pattern 7E; *ICD-9-CM* Code: 710.1)
Introduction

Scleroderma or systemic sclerosis is a rare disease that affects multisystems and is characterized by intense fibrosis. It affects 2 to 10 people per 1 million. There is a higher incidence in women with a 7:1 female-to-male ratio, which decreases after the fifth decade of life. There is a slightly higher prevalence in Afro-Americans, 1.6% in males and 4.3% in females. Patients with scleroderma have twice the incidence of breast and bronchoalveolar cancer than the general population.[23,59]

Clinical Presentation and Etiology

Scleroderma is characterized by tightness and thickening of the skin, digital pitting and loss of pulp of the fingertips, and sclerodactyly and pulmonary fibrosis. The etiology of this disease is unknown, but several theories exist. It has been suggested that there is a hormonal influence, because there is an increased onset during pregnancy. It is possible there is a genetic link, but this theory has little evidence. There appears to be an immunological basis for both scleroderma and CREST. It has been documented that there is an increased incidence of scleroderma in males who have been exposed to silica, coal dust toxic oil, and organic solvents.[59,60]

CREST syndrome stands for a cluster of clinical presentations: calcinosis, Raynaud phenomenon, esophageal dysfunction, sclerodactyly, and telangiectasia. The incidence is 4 to 5 per million. Patients with CREST or limited systemic sclerosis typically suffer from Raynaud phenomenon a long time before any other symptoms appear. Raynaud phenomenon involves the vasoconstriction of the digits that leads to local hypoxia and cyanosis, pallor skin, and cold skin temperature. Distal ulcers of fingers and toes are common and frequently result in infections and autoamputation of distal digital segment.[23,59,60] Scleroderma typically has a more acute onset that is associated with fatigue, arthralgias, carpal tunnel syndrome, swelling of hands and feet, and skin thickening.[60]

Pulmonary Involvement

Interstitial pulmonary fibrosis occurs in 74% of the cases of scleroderma, but the pathogenesis is not clearly defined. The incidence of pulmonary fibrosis is lower in CREST, but the pathology is believed to be similar. It may be mediated by growth factors and cytokines that are chemoattractants for fibroblasts, which enhance the synthesis and deposition of collagen within the alveolar walls. Through the inflammatory process, alveolar macrophages also stimulate various chemicals that stimulate fibroblastic activity and collagen formation. There is also a disruption of the capillary permeability that allows protein from the blood to leak into the interstitium that also contributes to collagen production. Typically the bases of the lungs are predominantly affected with alveolar space and capillary obliteration. The alveolar walls are infiltrated with edema and collagen. There is also a risk of further pulmonary fibrosis caused by aspiration of gastric acid from gastroesophageal reflux disease.[23]

With the presence of capillary destruction, there is a risk for the development of pulmonary hypertension. Up to 65% of the diagnosed cases of scleroderma will have pulmonary hypertension. There is a decrease in lumen size in the pulmonary vessels and obliteration due to hypertrophy of the medial layer of the blood vessels with collagen and plaque deposition within the intimal layer and vascular spasm.[23] Patients may also be diagnosed with pleural thickening and effusion, which are usually found incidentally, but the presence of a pneumothorax may cause symptoms.[60]

Other Systems Involved

CREST syndrome and scleroderma can also affect other organs. The skin thickens and tightens, and the patient also suffers from Raynaud phenomenon. Patients may also have difficulty with secretory glands that reduce saliva and tears as well as cause sexual dysfunction. Anorexia, malnutrition, diarrhea, reflux, and osteoporosis are associated with involvement of the gastrointestinal system. Renal dysfunction and failure are associated with vascular insufficiency due to fibrosis. Finally, a small percentage of patients may present with cardiac involvement, pericarditis, pericardial effusion, arrhythmias, and on rare occasions left ventricular heart failure. Right heart failure is more frequently seen in this patient population and is associated with moderate-to-severe pulmonary hypertension.[60]

Diagnosis

The majority of patients will present for medical intervention due to skin changes and Raynaud syndrome. Sixty percent of the patients present with dyspnea. If the chest X-ray is normal in the presence of dyspnea, there must be a concern for pulmonary hypertension. Approximately 20% of patients will complain about a persistent nonproductive cough that usually worsens with exertion. If the cough is productive or occurs with ingestion, aspiration pneumonia must be considered in the differential diagnosis. Pulmonary fibrosis is associated with crackles and desaturation with exertion. Pleural disease may present with pleuritic chest pain.

Chest X-ray will depict interstitial opacities particularly within the lower lobes, which will progress to other lung segments as the disease progresses, decreasing lung volumes. Chest X-ray and a high-resolution computed tomographic (CT) scan will illustrate honeycombing in end-stage disease. The pulmonary function tests will be consistent with a restrictive process. There will be a decrease in total lung volume, FVC, and residual volume if interstitial fibrosis exists. If the primary pulmonary dysfunction is associated with hypertension, PFTs may be normal, but the patient may present with signs and symptoms of right heart failure. Disruption in gas exchange is common and associated with a decrease in diffusion capacity and may be the earliest sign of pulmonary involvement.[23]

Intervention and Prognosis

Many patients will go untreated until the lung disease has caused significant functional impairments. The standard medical intervention includes corticosteroids and cytotoxic drugs such as cyclophosphamide, D-penicillamine, and cyclosporine to decrease the immune response. Lung transplantation is becoming an accepted medical intervention in certain cases.[23]

The prognosis of patients with pulmonary involvement secondary to scleroderma or CREST is very dismal. If the diffusion capacity is less than 40% there is a 95% mortality rate at 5 years as opposed to 75% if diffusion capacity is greater than 40%. With progressive pulmonary hypertension, survival rates are even lower.[23,61,62]

Mixed Tissue Connective Disease (Practice Patterns 4D, 7E; *ICD-9-CM* Codes: 710, 714)
Etiology

The etiology of mixed tissue connective disease (MTCD) is unknown but is classified as a rheumatological disease. The clinical features are a combination of lupus, scleroderma, and polymyositis. There is a female prevalence to this disease, but there appears to be no ethnic or racial preponderance. The onset is typically in the mid-thirties.[63]

Eighty-five percent of patients diagnosed with MTCD have pulmonary involvement; but nearly 70% are asymptomatic, even though many of them will have a low diffusion capacity. Pulmonary involvement can involve pneumonitis, pneumonia, interstitial fibrosis, pleural effusion, pulmonary hypertension, and diaphragmatic dysfunction.[64]

Pulmonary Involvement and Clinical Presentation

The patient usually presents with insidious complications that have been present for an average of 4.5 years prior to seeking medical intervention. The most common signs and symptoms are sclerodactyly, and a nonproductive cough, Raynaud phenomenon, polyarthritis, and dyspnea on exertion. Occasionally, the patient may present acutely with severe hypoxemia, hemoptysis, or acute heart failure.[63]

The clinical presentation will vary based on the pulmonary involvement. If the underlying pulmonary disease is interstitial fibrosis, the peripheral parenchymal layer in the lower lobes is the first affected, and the fibrosis extends superiorly in an asymmetrical pattern as the disease worsens. Clinically the patient will suffer from severe hypoxemia. Pulmonary hypertension may develop secondary to hypoxemia from significant interstitial fibrosis. Pulmonary hypertension may also be caused by thromboembolic disease or pulmonary arteriopathy that leads to the reduction of arteriole lumen size from thrombosis, vasoconstriction, and hypertrophy of the arterial walls.[64]

Dyspnea on exertion, chest discomfort, and light-headedness are common signs of hypertension. As the hypertension increases the patient may present with signs and symptoms of right-heart failure. PFTs will demonstrate a decline in total lung capacity (TLC) and VC and a reduced diffusion capacity associated with hypoxemia. Examination of cardiac function will demonstrate elevations in pulmonary arterial pressure and reduced right ventricular function, which is consistent with pulmonary hypertension. Closer inspection of bronchoalveolar fluid shows an elevation of neutrophils that can lead to further fibrotic changes.[22]

Intervention and Prognosis

As with other diseases that lead to pulmonary fibrosis, the mainstay of treatment involves corticosteroids and the use of immunosuppressive medications. These drugs also increase the risk of infections. Research has begun to analyze the effectiveness of prostacyclin medications such as Flolan and UT15, which are potent vasodilatators that are delivered to the pulmonary arterial system to reduce the pulmonary arterial pressure.

Prognosis depends on the progression of fibrosis or hypertension, the response to treatment, the minimizing adverse effects of medications, and the extent of other tissue involvement such as the kidneys. Death from pulmonary involvement is the result of end-stage pulmonary fibrosis, infection, heart failure, or severe hemoptysis due to pulmonary hypertension.[22]

Sjögren Syndrome (Practice Patterns 4A, 4C, 4D, 4H, 5B, 6B; *ICD-9-CM* Code: 714)
Etiology

Sjögren syndrome is a chronic autoimmune inflammatory disease that causes exocrinopathy and epithelitis. Sjögren syndrome is one of the most common systemic rheumatic diseases and affects 1% of the general population and 3% of the elderly.[65,66] Exocrinopathy involves the infiltration of T- and B-cell lymphocytes that progressively destroy salivary and lacrimal glands. Similar infiltrates may also invade visceral organs including the lungs. Sjögren syndrome is characterized by the infiltration of lymphocytes in the lungs; pancreas; gastrointestinal, hepatobiliary, and renal systems; and bone marrow. There have been several theories to explain the pathology of this syndrome. There appears to be a genetic predisposition, which is supported by the expression of certain antigens in the salivary epithelial cells. It also appears that herpes viruses and retrovirus may contribute to the pathology of this syndrome.[65]

The onset of Sjögren syndrome peaks in the fourth and fifth decades of life. Nine percent of the patient's diagnosed with Sjögren Syndrome will suffer from pulmonary involvement. This syndrome is more pronounced in females with a 9:1 female-to-male ratio. Sjögren syndrome is classified as primary if it occurs without other connective tissue disease and secondary if Sjögren syndrome is associated with another connective tissue disease. It commonly occurs with rheumatoid arthritis.[65]

Pulmonary Involvement and Clinical Presentation

The pulmonary involvement includes various etiologies such as interstitial pneumonitis and fibrosis. Pleural disease—thickening, effusion, or pleuritis—and lymphoproliferative disorders are also associated with Sjögren Syndrome. Sjögren syndrome is also associated with *shrinking lung syndrome* that may be linked to phrenic nerve neuropathy, intrinsic diaphragm muscle weakness, or another unknown cause.[66]

Dryness in the upper airways leads to impairment of smell and taste, epistaxis, and perforation of the nasal septum. Dysfunction of the small peripheral airways leads to obstruction and the potential of hyperactivity of the airways. The end result may be mild obstructive pattern due to small airway disease, to subclinical alveolitis to pneumonitis, or to interstitial fibrotic disease.[65]

Many of the signs and symptoms are nonspecific for many other pulmonary diseases, but classic complaints for Sjögren syndrome include complaints of dry mouth and eyes, and arthritic symptoms. The signs and symptoms related to pulmonary involvement include a nonproductive cough, dyspnea on exertion and at rest, and ill-defined chest pain.[65] In the presence of shrinking lung syndrome, the chest X-ray will illustrate small clear lung fields without evidence of intrinsic or pleural disease and an elevated right diaphragm. This disease is associated with a restrictive breathing pattern on pulmonary function tests.[66]

Diagnosis

The diagnosis of Sjögren syndrome is made based on clinical presentation of dry eyes and mouth and elevation of IgM, presence of a rheumatoid factor, or elevated antinuclear antibodies. The patient should be worked up for other connective tissue disorders, such as rheumatoid arthritis, lupus, or scleroderma.[66]

Intervention and Prognosis

Patients may respond to corticosteroids, but generally speaking, immunosuppressive medications are ineffective. Medications are given for palliative treatment of dryness of mucous lining, and in the presence of hyperreactive airways, bronchodilators are prescribed. Supplemental oxygen will be utilized when hypoxemia is documented.[65–67]

Prognosis is poor if the bronchoalveolar fluid contains excessive neutrophils. Prognosis is also dependent on the presence and progression of other connective diseases.

Summary

Diseases that affect the integumentary system do not just affect the skin. Multiple system involvement is quite common. The cardiopulmonary system is often a target of these diseases, with significant impairments to structures leading to functional limitations and disabilities for the patient.

SUMMARY

We have seen that impairments of bony structures, joints, fascia, skin, and musculature can result in decreases in cardiopulmonary function. The nature of these impairments is usually restrictive, which in turn can lead to decreased pulmonary function and poor exercise tolerance. Diminished movement of air into and out of the lungs may produce secretion retention, thus predisposing the patient to lung infection. Early physical therapy interventions should be directed toward maintaining long expansion, mobilizing secretions (if present) and improving exercise tolerance. These interventions may prevent many of these impairments and keep them from becoming functional limitations or disabilities.

REFERENCES

1. Wolf RL, Zmuda JM, Stone KL, Cauley JA. Update on epidemiology of osteoporosis. *Curr Rheumatol Rep*. 2000;2(1):74-86.
2. Salter RB. *Textbook of Disorders and Injuries of the Musculoskeletal System*. 3rd ed. Baltimore, MD: Williams & Wilkins; 1999.
3. Bachrach L. Acquisition of optimal bone mass in childhood and adolescence. *Trends Endocrinol Metabol*. 2001;12(1):22-28.
4. Enstrud KE, Black DM, Harris F, Ettinger B, Cummings SR. Correlates of kyphosis in older women. The fracture intervention trial research group. *Am Geriatr Soc*. 1997;45(6):682-687.
5. Ismail AA, Cooper C, Felsenberg D, et al. Number and type of vertebral deformities: epidemiological characteristics and relation to back pain and height loss. European vertebral osteoporosis study group. *Osteoporos Int*. 1999;9(3):206-213.
6. De Smet AA, Robinson RG, Johnson BE, Lukert BP. Spinal compression fractures in osteoporotic women: patterns and relationship to hyperkyphosis. *Radiology*. 1988;166(2):497-500.
7. Goh S, Price RI, Leedman PJ, Singer KP. The relative influence of vertebral body and intervertebral disc shape on thoracic kyphosis. *Clin Biomech (Bristol, Avon)*. 1999;14(7):439-438.
8. Hedlund LR, Gallagher JC, Meeger C, Stoner S. Change in vertebral shape in spinal osteoporosis. *Calcif Tissue Int*. 1989;44(3):168-172.
9. Biyani A, Ebraheim NA, Lu J. Thoracic spine fractures in patients older than 50 years. *Clin Orthop*. 1996 July;(328):190-193.
10. Harma M, Heliovaara M, Aromaa A, Knekt P. Thoracic spine compression fractures in Finland. *Clin Orthop*. 1986;205:188-194.
11. Melton LJ, Atkinson EJ, Khosla S, O'Fallon WM, Riggs BL. Secondary osteoporosis and the risk of vertebral deformities in women. *Bone*. 1999;24(1):49-55.
12. Abdel-Hamid Osman A, Bassiouni H, Koutri R, Nijs J, Geusens P, Dequeker J. Aging of the thoracic spine: distinction between wedging in osteoarthritis and fracture in osteoporosis—a cross-sectional and longitudinal study. *Bone*. 1994;15(4):437-442.
13. Ryan PJ, Blake G, Herd R, Fogelman I. A clinical profile of back pain and disability in patients with spinal osteoporosis. *Bone*. 1994;15(1):27-30.
14. Leech JA, Dulberg C, Kellie S, Pattee L, Gay J. Relationship of lung function to severity of osteoporosis in women. *Am Rev Respir Dis*. 1990;141(1):68-71.
15. Schlaich C, Minne HW, Bruckner T, et al. Reduced pulmonary function in patients with spinal osteoporotic fractures. *Osteoporos Int*. 1998;8(3):261-267.
16. Mellin G, Harjula R. Lung function in relation to thoracic spinal mobility and kyphosis. *Scand J Rehabil Med*. 1987;19(2):89-92.
17. Culham EG, Jimenez HA, King CE. Thoracic kyphosis, rib mobility, and lung volumes in normal women and women with osteoporosis. *Spine*. 1994;1(11):1250-1255.
18. Malmros B, Mortensen L, Jensen MB, Charles P. Positive effects of physiotherapy on chronic pain and performance in osteoporosis. *Osteoporos Int*. 1998;8(3):215-221.
19. Vogt MT, Nevitt MC, Cauley JA. Back problems and atherosclerosis—the study of osteoporotic fractures. *Spine*. 1997;22(23):2741-2747.
20. Blansfield HN, Andrew CB. Osteoporosis—a factor in mortality following cardiac surgery. *Comm Med*. 2000;64(2):71-73.
21. Lee-Chiong T. Pulmonary manifestations of ankylosis spondylitis and relapsing polychondritis. *Clin Chest Med*. 1998;19(4):747-757.
22. Wiedemann H, Matthay R. Pulmonary manisfestations of the collagen vascular disease. *Clin Chest Med*. 1989;10(4):677-715.
23. Fishman A, ed. *Pulmonary Diseases and Disorders: Companion Handbook*. 2nd ed. New York: McGraw-Hill; 1994.
24. Grissom L, Harcke H. Thoracic deformities and the growing lung. *Semin Reontgenol*. 1998;33(2):199-208.
25. Leong JC, Lu WW, Luk KD, Karlberg EM. Kinematics of the chest cage and spine during breathing in healthy individuals and in patients with adolescent idiopathic scoliosis. *Spine*. 1999;24(13):1310-1315.
26. Aaro S, Ohlund C. Scoliosis and pulmonary function. *Spine*. 1984;9(2):220-222.
27. Vedantam R, Crawford A. The role of preoperative pulmonary function tests in patients with adolescent idiopathic scoliosis undergoing posterior spinal fusion. *Spine*. 1997;22(23):2731-2734.
28. Giordano A, Fuso L, Galli M, Calcagni M, Aulsia L. Evaluation of pulmonary ventilation and diaphragmatic movement in idiopathic scoliosis using radioaerosol ventilation scintigraphy. *Nucl Med Commun*. 1997;18:105-111.
29. Widmann R, Bitan F, Laplaza J, Burke S, DiMaio M. Spinal deformity, pulmonary compromise, and quality of life in osteogenesis imperfecta. *Spine*. 1999;24(16):1673-1678.
30. Estenne M, Deroom E, DeTroyer A. Neck and abdominal muscle activity in patients with severe thoracic scoliosis. *Am J Resp Crit Care Med*. 1998;158(2):452-457.
31. Conti G, Rocco M, Antonelli M, et al. Respiratory system mechanics in the early phase of acute respiratory failure due to severe kyphoscoliosis. *Intensive Care Med*. 1997;23(5):539-544.
32. Krachman S, Criner G. Hypoventilation syndrome. *Clin Chest Med*. 1998;19(1):139-156.
33. Al-Katten K, Simonds A, Chung KF, Kaplan DK. Kyphoscoliosis and bronchial torsion. *Chest*. 1997;111(4):1134-1137.
34. Boyer J, Amin N, Taddonio R, Dozor AJ. Evidence of airway obstruction in children with idiopathic scoliosis. *Chest*. 1996;109(6):1532-1535.
35. Vedantam R, Lenke L, Bridwell K, Haas J, Linville D. A prospective evaluation of pulmonary function in patients with adolescent idiopathic scoliosis relative to the surgical approach used for spinal arthrodesis. *Spine*. 2000;25(1):82-90.
36. Wong CA, Cole AA, Watson L, Webb JK, Johnston ID, Kinnear WJ. Pulmonary function before and after anterior spinal surgery in adult idiopathic scoliosis. *Thorax*. 1996;51(5):534-536.
37. Rowe DE, Bernstein SM, Riddick MF, Adler F, Emans JB, Gardner-Bonneau D. A meta-analysis of the efficacy of non-operative treatments for idiopathic scoliosis. *J Bone Joint Surg Am*. 1997;79(5):664-674.
38. Cline CC, Coast JR, Arnall DA. A chest wall restrictor to study effects on pulmonary function and exercise. Development and validation. *Respiration*. 1999;66(2):182-187.
39. Katsaris G, Loukos A, Valavanis J, Vassiliou M, Behrakis PK. The immediate effect of a Boston brace on lung volumes and pulmonary compliance in mild adolescent idiopathic scoliosis. *J Eur Spine*. 1999;8(1):2-7.
40. Ferrari K, Goti P, Sanna A, et al. Short term effects of bracing on exercise performance in mild idiopathic thoracic scoliosis. *Lung*. 1997;175(5):299-310.
41. Korovessis P, Filos KS, Georgopoulos D. Long-term alterations of respiratory function in adolescents wearing a brace for idiopathic scoliosis. *Spine*. 1996;21(17):1979-1984.

42. Ferris G, Servera-Pieras E, Vergara P, et al. Kyphoventilatory insufficiency: noninvasive management outcomes. *Am J Phys Med Rehab.* 2000;79(1):24-29.

43. Leger P. Long-term noninvasive ventilation for patients with thoracic cage abnormalities. *Resp Care Clinic North Am.* 1996; 2(2):241-252.

44. Athanasopoulos S, Paxinos T, Tsafantakis E, Zachariou K, Chatziconstantinou S. The effect of aerobic training in girls with idiopathic scoliosis. *Scand J Med Sci Sports.* 1999;9(1):36-40.

45. Aris A, Camara M, Casan P, Litvan H. Pulmonary function following aortic valve replacement: a comparison between ministernotomy and median sternotomy. *J Heart Valve Dis.* 1999;8: 605-608.

46. Couser JI, Martinez FJ, Celli BR. Respiratory response and ventilatory muscle recruitment during arm elevation in normal subjects. *Chest.* 1992;101(2):336-340.

47. Mackey M, Ellis E, Nicholls M. Breathing patterns and heart rate during simulated occupational upper limb tasks in normal subjects. *Physiother Res Int.* 1998;3(2):83-99.

48. Hodges PW, Cresswell AG, Daggfeldt K, Thorstensson A. Three dimensional preparatory trunk motion precedes asymmetrical upper limb movement. *Gait Posture.* 2000;11(2):92-101.

49. Kapandji IA. *The Physiology of the Joints.* Vol 1. 2nd ed. Edinburgh, UK: Churchill Livingstone; 1970.

50. Massery M. A patient with neuromuscular and musculoskeletal dysfunction. In: Frownfelter D, Dean E, eds. *Principles and Practice of Cardiopulmonary Physical Therapy.* 3rd ed. St Louis, MO: Mosby; 1996:679.

51. Anonymous. Statement on sarcoidosis. *Am J Resp Crit Med.* 1999; 160:736-755.

52. Nagai S, Shigematsu M, Hamada K, Izumi T. Clinical courses and prognoses of pulmonary sarcoidosis. *Curr Opin Pulm Med.* 1999;5:293-298.

53. Costabel U, Hunninghake G. ATS/ERS WASOG statement on sarcoidosis. *Eur Resp J.* 1999;14:735-737.

54. Belfer M, Stevens R. Sarcoidosis: a primary care review. *Am Fam Physician.* 1998;58(9):2041-2052.

55. Sheffield E. Pathology of sarcoidosis. *Clin Chest Med.* 1997;18(4): 741-750.

56. Lynch J, Kazerooni E, Gay S. Pulmonary sarcoid. *Clin Chest Med.* 1997;18(4):755-780.

57. Godfrey T, Khamashta M, Hughes G. Therapeutic advances in systemic lupus erythematosus. *Curr Opin Rheumatol.* 1998;10(5): 435-441.

58. Murin S, Weidemann H, Matthay RA. Pulmonary manifestations of systemic lupus erythematosus. *Clin Chest Med.* 1998;19(4): 641-665.

59. Minai O, Dweik R, Arroliga A. Manifestations of scleroderma pulmonary disease. *Clin Chest Med.* 1998;19(4):713-727.

60. Silman A. Epidemiology of scleroderma. *Ann Rheum Dis.* 1991;50:846-853.

61. Steen V. Clinical manifestations of systemic sclerosis. *Semin Cutan Med Surg.* 1998;17(1):48-54.

62. Bulpitt K, Clements P, Lachenbruch P, Paulus H, Peter J. Early undifferentiated connective tissue disease: III. Outcome and prognostic indicators in early scleroderma (systemic sclerosis). *Ann Int Med.* 1993;118:602-609.

63. Prakash U. Respiratory complications in mixed connective tissue disease. *Clin Chest Med.* 1998;19(4):733-745.

64. Corley D, Winterbauer R. Collagen vascular disease. *Semin Resp Infect.* 1995;10(2):78-85.

65. Cain H, Noble P, Matthay R. Pulmonary manifestations of Sjögren's Syndrome. *Clin Chest Med.* 1998;19(4):687-697.

66. Mialon M, Barthelemy L, Sebert P, LeHenaff C, Sarni D. A longitudinal study of lung impairment in patients with primary Sjögren's syndrome. *Clin Exp Rheumatol.* 1997;15(4):49-54.

67. Tavoni A, Cirigliano C, Frigelli S, Stampacchia G, Bombardieri S. Shrinking lung in primary Sjögren's syndrome. *Arthritis Rheum.* 1999;42(10):2249-2250.

Cardiopulmonary Concerns in the Patient with Neurological Deficits: An Evidence-Based Approach

Sue Ann Sisto

INTRODUCTION

Physical therapists are responsible for the exercise prescription and management of patients with neurological disorders. Physical therapists can best treat patients with neurological illnesses by focusing on neurological impairments, functional limitations, and participation outcomes while considering the cardiopulmonary system. The cardiopulmonary system plays an important role in functional activities because of its role in transporting oxygen to skeletal muscle. Abnormalities in the cardiopulmonary system can produce limitations in movement and thus functional outcomes.

Patients with neurological deficits have a particular problem of deconditioning due to hospitalization or inactivity as a result of their disease or illness. This deconditioning could mean the difference between independence and dependence in activities of daily living (ADL). Physical therapists are the first health care professionals to note the functional impact of cardiopulmonary limitations because of the way that their patients are challenged through exercises and position changes in the provision of physical therapy.

Furthermore, physical therapists can contribute to the prevention of cardiopulmonary complications of immobility, weakness, and exercise intolerance. Individuals with neurological injuries, who are within age ranges where cardiac risk factors are high, may be even more at risk during activity or exercise. In the existing health care environment, these neurological patients may be discharged from the acute care hospital in a fragile cardiopulmonary state. Therefore, significant focus must be placed on the cardiopulmonary status of patients with neurological illnesses who demonstrate activity and exercise risk factors.

It is ultimately the intent of this chapter to make the reader familiar with the *Guide to Physical Therapist Practice* (2nd ed.) as it relates to evidence-based treatment of cardiopulmonary disorders for neurological patients. Therapists must select the primary practice pattern that is evident at the time of intervention, taking into account all comorbid conditions. When patients with neurological disorders are "triaged" into the cardiopulmonary practice patterns, it is assumed that the cardiopulmonary status becomes the primary focus of the intervention. With this in mind, this chapter provides guidelines regarding the factors associated with activity and exercise that influence the exercise ability for patients with neurological impairments. This chapter also makes recommendations for common tests and measures used for exercise testing and describes the physiological responses to exercise, including the effect of medications. Finally, the intent is to make recommendations for exercise training interventions and identify other benefits of exercise for patients with neurological disorders.

NEUROLOGICAL DIAGNOSTIC CATEGORIES

Stroke (Practice Patterns 5A, 5D, 5I, 7A; ICD-9-CM Code: 342)

Stroke, or cerebrovascular accident (CVA), is the result of a thrombus or hemorrhage in the brain, producing an area of infarct. This region produces neurological impairments that may result in significant disability. Indeed, stroke is the leading cause of serious, long-term disability in the United States, where 15% to 30% of stroke survivors are permanently disabled[1] with $3.8 billion paid to Medicare beneficiaries.[2] According to the World Health Organization (2002), 15 million people suffer stroke worldwide each year.[1]

There are nearly 4.7 million stroke survivors alive in the United States and 2.3 million are men and 2.4 million are women. There are approximately 700,000 new strokes annually where 500,000 are new strokes and 200,000 are recurrent strokes. Approximately 15% to 30% of individuals who sustain a stroke are permanently disabled (Survey of Income and Program Participation [SIPP]).[2] When considered separately from other cardiovascular diseases (CVDs), stroke ranks as the third leading cause of death after diseases of the heart and cancer. The mean age of onset of stroke is 66 years, and 28% of people who suffer a stroke in a given year are younger than 65 years. At all ages, more women die of stroke than do men. Compared with white men 45 to 54 years old, African American men in the same age group have a threefold greater risk of ischemic stroke. The proportion of strokes that result in death within 1 year is approximately 29% and is less if the stroke occurs before the age of 65 years.[3]

Physical activity, including moderate-intensity exercise such as walking, is associated with a substantial reduction in risk of ischemic stroke in women.[4] Studies have found an association between physical inactivity and the risk of stroke[5,6] and have estimated that 79% of strokes could be averted through regular exercise and avoidance of both smoking and obesity. Walking for the prevention of CVD, in particular ischemic stroke, was related to the higher walking duration, distance, pace, and energy expenditure.[7] A study of 37,000 women aged 45 years and older participating in the Women's Health Study (2006) suggests that a healthy lifestyle consisting of a low body mass index (BMI), regular exercise to name a few, significantly reduced the risk of total and ischemic stroke but not hemorrhagic stroke.[8] A meta-analysis of reports of 31 observational studies conducted mainly in the United States and Europe found that moderate and high levels of leisure time and occupational physical activity protected against all stroke types.[9]

CVD is the most common cause of death in long-term survivors of stroke, which argues for the importance of exercise and activity when guided by an optimal cardiopulmonary examination.[10] Because atherosclerosis is typically the underlying disease process, coronary artery disease (CAD) frequently coexists in patients with stroke. Approximately 75% of individuals who have had a stroke have heart disease[11] (*ICD-9-CM* Code 411). Besides cardiac disease, other risk factors for developing CVA include hypertension (*ICD-9-CM* Code 401), abnormal plasma lipid profiles (*ICD-9-CM* Code 272), obesity (*ICD-9-CM* Code 278), and insulin resistance, potentially resulting in diabetes (*ICD-9-CM* Code 250).[12] Reduction of these risk factors could be addressed through the use of Practice Pattern 6A, *Primary Prevention/Risk Reduction for Cardiovascular/ Pulmonary Disorders.*

The *Guide to Physical Therapist Practice* (2nd ed.) focuses on the practice patterns for stroke in the neuromuscular section (Patterns 5A, 5D, and 5I). This is because, early after a stroke, interventions primarily address the paralysis involving the neuromuscular system. However, a patient who sustained a stroke beyond 3 to 6 months will continue a downward course of deconditioning, requiring greater focus on the cardiopulmonary system practice patterns. Practice Pattern 6B would address those patients with stroke whose aerobic capacity and endurance were limited because of deconditioning. If comorbid conditions such as a previous myocardial infarction or ventilatory pump dysfunction were also present, Practice Patterns 6C, D, and E should be considered.

Factors That Influence Ability to Exercise

There are morphological changes that exist with aging and that affect the stroke population because of the average age of onset (66 years). Cardiac-related changes affect cardiac tissue and chambers, the conduction system, and the coronary arteries. Cardiac function in healthy older people may be adequate to meet the body's need while at rest and is maintained by increases in stroke volume and ejection fraction because of increased cardiac filling (preload).[13] This, however, may be inadequate for patients with neurological disorders when participating in exercise tasks such as ambulation that is commonly prescribed by physical therapists. The energy demands placed on individuals who have suffered a stroke are thought to be at least 50% greater for walking because of the biomechanical challenges of gait.[14] Standard exercise, such as ambulation training, may place a significant demand on an already-compromised cardiovascular system. Therapists must be aware of the potential for patients with stroke who have a compromised cardiovascular system and provide proper monitoring of exercise intensity.

Changes in muscle composition following stroke may also limit exercise participation. Ryan and associates observed a strong relationship of $\dot{V}O_{2peak}$ to thigh lean tissue mass as measured by dual X-ray absorptiometry (DXA). There was gross muscular atrophy and metabolic and muscle phenotype changes that were reported to possibly predispose patients with stroke to fatigue. Computed tomography (CT) scans of the mid-thigh muscle area in 30 patients with stroke were 20% lower in the hemiparetic thigh, with a 25% relatively higher fat content, compared with those of the non–hemiparetic thigh ($P < 0.001$).[15] Heydrick identified, based on a shift to a lower frequency and higher amplitude, spectral profile of electromyography signals. This change corresponded with improved muscle recruitment after treadmill training, a loss of slow-twitch (oxidative) muscle fibers, and anaerobic metabolism in the hemiparetic leg.[16] However, more research is needed to demonstrate the effects of strength training on muscle adaptation in patients with hemiparesis and its effect on exercise capacity. Gerrits and colleagues (2009) studied the strength of the knee extensors bilaterally after stroke by using maximal voluntary torque and half relaxation time compared with controls.[17] The authors reported that aside from bilateral weakness in the stroke group, the knee extensors showed a lower rate of torque development and relaxation bilaterally compared with controls and concluded that these changes may be related to changes in the muscle reported in other studies.

The level of motor impairments is a definitive factor for patients with stroke participating in exercise. For example, patients with stroke frequently demonstrate flaccid and/or spastic limbs with sensory impairments. Walking on a treadmill the sound limb may propel the paretic limb because of the cyclical nature of walking and the use of momentum; however, the contribution of the paretic limbs can be limited. In more severe cases of motor impairment, treadmill walking is limited by reduced trunk balance. In this case, seated ergometry may be used. Furthermore, the hemiparetic/hemiplegic leg may make very little contribution to the walking or cycling motion. Despite the lesser contribution of the hemiparetic limb to exercise, there still may be enough work output to produce aerobic conditioning.

Other comorbid pathologies common to this age group may limit exercise participation. Endocrine abnormalities, in the form of insulin resistance, have been reported to further potentiate the risk of CVD.[18] Almost all patients with neurological dysfunction have a form of restrictive lung disease due to decreased chest wall movement resulting from the paralysis. Patients with neurological disease are, therefore, at risk for atelectasis and pneumonia. Osteoarthritis may limit an individual's ability to ambulate, propel a stationary bicycle, or climb stairs. Peripheral vascular disease may limit walking or cycling ability due to leg pain or swelling. Diabetes or hypertension will put the patient with stroke at greater risk of cardiac pathology or exercise intolerance. The practice patterns and *ICD-9-CM* codes of the potential comorbid conditions of patients with stroke are summarized in Table 14-1.

Impairments such as the loss of proprioception may not only limit motor performance during exercise but also lead to injury. For example, the patient may lack awareness that the ankle is excessively inverted during gait, which may predispose the patient to an ankle sprain. Mental confusion or dementia may be present in addition to the cognitive limitations that are coincident with stroke. This often limits a patient's ability to either follow directions during exercise or adhere to an unsupervised exercise program. Special attention must be paid to these age- or diagnostic-related changes that are noncardiopulmonary precautions during exercise.

Tests and Measures for Exercise Testing

A few studies have measured peak exercise capacity in patients with stroke, resulting in lower functional capacities.[14,19] This is most likely due to the reduced number of motor units available for recruitment during exercise. Additionally, reduced oxidative capacity and overall poor endurance further limit functional capacity. Patients with stroke are unable to achieve the same workload as age-matched control subjects during leg ergometry.[20,21]

Exercise testing is necessary to determine the presence and severity of cardiac disease and resultant functional limitation, if any. A few studies have examined the exercise capacity of hemiparetic populations. MacKay-Lyons et al.[22] evaluated exercise capacity in 29 patients with acute stroke (<1 month), using open-circuit spirometry during maximal treadmill walking effort with 15% body weight support. Mean $\dot{V}O_{2peak}$ was 14.4 mL/kg/min or 60% of age-predicted normative values for sedentary individuals. These values were similar to past values reported for patients with myocardial infarction.[20-26] Comparisons are difficult when the modes of exercise used for testing are different (ie, leg ergometry vs arm or supine ergometry). A summary of published data of the acute peak exercise responses in patients with hemiparesis can be found in Table 14-2.

Because of the presence of CAD, a physician trained in using continuous electrocardiogram (ECG) monitoring should supervise exercise testing. The reasons for implementing an exercise test for patients with stroke would be either to determine the presence and severity of heart disease and/or to determine functional status. If there is a previous history of myocardial infarction with resultant myocardial ischemia, ST-segment depression will appear on the ECG during the test. The level of exercise, at which these ECG changes become significant, can provide guidelines for a safe exercise prescription.

CLINICAL CORRELATE

Exercise testing should be coupled with Borg's[28] ratings of perceived exertion (RPE) at each workload (see Chapter 9).

This will allow the therapist and the patient to use this perceived intensity rating during subsequent exercise training sessions or when ECG monitoring is not possible. As the patient's fitness level increases, the ratings of perceived exertion (RPE) will diminish at the same submaximal exercise level. This should signal the therapist to increase the training workload, while maintaining the target RPE level.

If peak or maximal exercise cannot be accomplished during the test, a submaximal exercise test can be used to determine a safe level for the patient's exercise program. Nomograms[29] can be used to determine estimates of maximal aerobic power ($\dot{V}O_{2max}$) from the submaximal oxygen consumption. Some caution must be taken because this nomogram applies to healthy individuals. Because nomograms are not available for patients with stroke, exercise capacities are likely to be overestimated. However, Birkett and Edwards[30]

TABLE 14-1 Common Comorbid Pathologies, Practice Patterns, and *ICD-9-CM* Codes Associated with Stroke

Comorbid Conditions	Practice Patterns	*ICD-9-CM* Codes
Pulmonary insufficiency	6F	518.82
Osteoarthritis	4C, 4D, 4E, 4F, 4G, 4H, 4I, 6B	715
Peripheral vascular disease	4C, 4J, 6B, 6D, 7A, 7D, 7E	443
Diabetes	4C, 4J, 5G, 6A, 6B, 7A, 7B	250
Hypertension	6B, 6D	402

TABLE 14-2   Cardiovascular Responses at Peak Exercise Testing in Stroke

Author	Exercise Mode	$\dot{V}o_{2peak}$ (mL/kg/min)	Mean Heart Rate	Endpoints
Duncan[27]	Leg ergometry	11.2	NT	90% predicted maximum heart rate
MacKay-Lyons and Makrides[22]	Treadmill w/15% body weight support	14.4	NT	NT
Macko et al.[19]	Treadmill	15.2	NT	Exhaustion
Potempa et al.[26]	Leg ergometer	16.7	142	Exhaustion, RER > 1.15 or 90% maximal predicted heart rate
King et al.[24]	Wheelchair ergometer	NT	121	Exhaustion; unable to maintain power output
Monga et al.[20]	Leg and arm ergometer	NT	104	Exhaustion and 70% predicted values for maximal heart rate and unable to maintain exercise rate
Moldover et al.[21]	Supine ergometer	NT	102	Exhaustion and unable to maintain 50 rpm

RER, Respiratory exchange ratio; NT, not tested or reported; rpm, revolutions per minute.

determined that unilateral arm-cranking exercise could be used to predict an individual's upper-body aerobic exercise capacity by using heart rate (HR). This is particularly helpful in hemiplegia when arm-crank exercise is accomplished by a single arm. Furthermore, a comparison of the HR at the same submaximal workload before and after an exercise training program can document changes in cardiorespiratory fitness. A decrease in the HR after exercise training for the same workload as prior to training is interpreted as improvement in aerobic capacity or fitness. See Chapters 9 and 10 for general guidelines for exercise testing.

The choice of exercise modality will be dependent on the degree of motor impairment. Treadmill walking, for example, may be appropriate only for patients with mild-to-moderate functional impairments. However, the recent introduction of overhead harness devices enables severely involved patients to be treadmill tested. These devices support the patient by means of a metal frame surrounding the treadmill, from which is suspended a canvas vest. The patient is fitted into the vest, which is used to unweigh the body. Harness devices allow the patient with hemiplegia to ambulate safely on a treadmill and also facilitate gait training. Patients should be able to walk independently with a cane or be able to sustain independent ambulation with the support of a treadmill handrail. Walking speeds are typically much slower, and energy expenditure usually is approximately 55% to 65% higher than that in age-matched healthy subjects. It is recommended that the workload increments are organized so that the total exercise time is between 8 and 12 minutes. Therefore, exercise protocols may need to increase the intensity very gradually using protocols such as the Naughton–Balke or modified Balke,[31] where the velocity remains constant and only the grade is increased gradually. Target velocity can be determined by a preliminary treadmill exercise test.[14]

In target cases where patients fatigue easily, an intermittent protocol may be appropriate. This protocol intersperses brief rests between progressively increasing workloads. For example, a patient with stroke may begin a treadmill exercise test at 1 mph for 2 minutes. After a 1-minute rest, the treadmill may be advanced to the next workload, 1.5 mph, again followed by a rest. This progression/rest approach allows for the HR to progress to the highest possible rate, while accommodating for those neuromuscular deficits requiring intermittent rest.

For leg cycle ergometry, a pedaling rate of 50 rpm, starting at 20 W and increasing by 20 W per stage is the general guideline; however, test protocols may have to be determined individually. Maximal HR is similar to the treadmill walking protocol, but the peak oxygen uptake is 10% to 15% higher with treadmill testing.[32]

Combined arm and leg ergometry can be used when spasticity and weakness prohibit sufficient elevation of the HR by using a single upper or lower limb individually. When combining the arm and leg, patients can use both limbs to achieve a maximal effort. Because of muscle fatigue, an intermittent protocol again may be advisable. If the person has poor sitting balance, arm ergometry can be done from the wheelchair and leg ergometry can be done in the supine or semireclined position.[33]

To estimate the workload for leg ergometry, several equations have been proposed.[34-37] These equations involve the use of specific anthropomorphic information to estimate the maximal workloads. For example, Jones and associates[34] determined that maximal power output could be estimated by the following equations:

Work capacity (kpm/min) for males
= 1,506 × [height (m) × 2.7] × [age − 0.46];

Work capacity (kpm/min) for females
= 969 × [height (m) × 2.8] × [age − 0.43].

Caution must be taken when using these equations to estimate maximal workloads for arm ergometry. These equations may overestimate the maximal workload because arm ergometry work capacity is less than that accomplished by the legs. Furthermore, these equations are based on samples of healthy men and women without neurological disability. Therefore, these equations could significantly overestimate the work capacity of individuals with stroke. Workload is often determined empirically, in which case the tester identifies a comfortable workload and increases the workload until the person can no longer continue.

The functional disability of stroke is compounded by the presence of CAD in some individuals. In some cases, patients with stroke and cardiac pathology may wear a Holter monitor, a portable device that is worn around the neck with chest electrode attachments that records continuous 24-hour ECGs. Cardiac monitoring could then be conducted during physical therapy. This would enable the physician to determine the HRs of functional tasks that produce either ischemia or arrhythmia.[11] Continuous ECG monitoring can thus provide the physical therapist with an HR limit to the exercise prescription that is specific to functional tasks.

Assessment of peak oxygen consumption ($\dot{V}O_{2peak}$) by using traditional modes of testing such as treadmill or cycle ergometer can be difficult in individuals with stroke due to balance deficits, gait impairments, or decreased coordination. Billinger et al. (2008) found that a total-body recumbent stepper may be a safe, feasible, and valid exercise test to obtain measurements of $\dot{V}O_{2peak}$ and prescribe aerobic exercise in people with stroke.[38] Eleven participants performed two maximal-effort–graded exercise tests on separate days to assess cardiorespiratory fitness. The authors reported a strong relationship between the total-body recumbent stepper and the cycle ergometer exercise test for $\dot{V}O_{2peak}$ and peak HR ($r = 0.91$ and 0.89, respectively); however, the mean $\dot{V}O_{2peak}$ was significantly higher for the total-body recumbent stepper. Therefore, the mode of testing must be considered when comparing changes in cardiorespiratory fitness within patients and across studies. A summary of exercise testing guidelines can be found in Table 14-3.

Potential Physiological Responses to Exercise

Hemiparesis resulting from stroke produces physiological changes in muscle fibers and muscle metabolism during exercise. One study found that there was a greater percentage of type 2 fibers of the anterior tibialis muscle of 10 ambulatory patients with hemiparesis and spastic gait compared with young and older healthy controls.[39] This study suggested that many motor units are never recruited in the paretic muscle during slow walking. This reduced proportion of type 1 fibers leads to diminished capacity for oxidative metabolism and low endurance. High-intensity aerobic exercise has the potential to minimize these effects by enhancing motor unit recruitment favoring the development of high-oxidative muscle fibers. Ambulatory persons with stroke may be able to perform approximately 70% of the peak power output that can be achieved by age-matched persons without CVA. Paretic muscles are deconditioned and demonstrate increased lactate production, reduced blood flow, and altered fiber-type composition. These physiological changes could be due to changes in the relative proportion of fiber types.[40] However, Sunnerhagen and colleagues[41] did not find major differences in fiber-type composition between the affected and the less-affected legs in high-functioning patients with stroke. These individuals did, however, demonstrate underlying weakness, and the authors concluded that strength training might be indicated. At present, we do not completely understand the effects that exercise has on fiber-type proportion poststroke. It may be possible to impact the muscle fiber–type proportion of patients with stroke as a result of strengthening exercises with more severely involved patients.

Interventions for Exercise Training

Clinical evidence of CVD may delay intensive exercise and limit functional recovery. However, when patients with stroke have progressed beyond the initial rehabilitation phase, a monitored aerobic training program may not only improve endurance and functional capacity but also reduce the risk for subsequent cardiovascular and cerebrovascular events. Therefore, endurance training is recognized as an important component of rehabilitation and long-term maintenance of health.

Potempa and colleagues reported approximately a 13% increase in $\dot{V}O_{2max}$ after a 10-week supervised aerobic training program. The improvements were related to improvements in sensory motor function, therefore suggesting that aerobic training can also improve these neuromuscular impairments.[25] Fletcher and colleagues[42] demonstrated an increase in exercise endurance and reduction in resting HR as a result of a home exercise program consisting of arm ergometry for 5 days a

TABLE 14-3 Summary of Exercise Testing Guidelines for Stroke

	Duration of Test (min)	Rate (mph or rpm)	Workload Progression	Heart Rate (bpm)
Treadmill	8–12	0.5–3 mph	Gradual or intermittent	Age-predicted maximal heart rate[a]
Leg ergometry	4–8[b]	50 rpm	10 W/stage	10% to 15% higher than treadmill exercise
Arm and leg ergometry	4–8[b]	50 rpm	Gradual or intermittent	Age-predicted maximal heart rate[a]

[a]Age-predicted maximal heart rate is determined to be 220 − age. Most stroke patients will stop before this heart rate is reached because of either cardiac pathology or neuromuscular fatigue.

[b]Arm or leg ergometry produce local muscle fatigue earlier than treadmill walking, therefore, the protocols are shorter.

week for 6 months. Using an adapted bicycle ergometer, Fletcher and colleagues found that a 10-week long, gradually progressive training program produced an increase in maximal oxygen consumption, workload, exercise duration, and a reduction in systolic blood pressure (BP) at submaximal workloads.[26] Duncan et al.[27] studied 100 patients with subacute stroke for recovery of function. She stratified them according to whether they received structured, physiologically based exercise or "usual care." The exercise group showed improvement in $\dot{V}O_{2peak}$, duration of exercise, 6-minute walk velocity, and gait velocity.

Survivors of stroke exhibit a peak oxygen uptake of about half their age-matched counterparts, leaving tremendous room for improvement. Peak fitness levels have been reported to be 44% lower than that of age- and gender-matched sedentary controls[10] with $\dot{V}O_{2peak}$ levels of 14.7 ± 4 mL/kg/min. Furthermore, Macko et al.[14] reported that 31 patients with stroke used 66% of peak oxygen capacity to walk on a treadmill with handrail support at a pace that is 75% slower than their self-selected floor-walking velocity. If patients with stroke could participate in exercise training, emerging studies project that there would be as much as a 60% to 70% increase in $\dot{V}O_{2peak}$ and a 100% to 150% increase in self-selected walking speed. Additionally, an overall reduction in the amount of assistive devices and physical assistance needed would result from participating in exercise training.[33]

Macko et al.[19] studied fitness reserve in 21 patients with chronic stroke to evaluate whether treadmill training reduced the energy cost and improved peak fitness during gait. $\dot{V}O_{2peak}$ increased from 15.4 to 17.0 mL O_2/kg/min and lowered oxygen demand at submaximal levels. Patients were able to use 20% less peak exercise capacity to accomplish more work.

Rimmer et al. (2009) compared the effects of three different exercise training regimens on cardiorespiratory fitness and coronary risk factor reduction in subjects with unilateral stroke. Participants exercised three times per week on either a stationery bike or a recumbent stepper.[43] Participants were assigned to a moderate-intensity, shorter duration (MISD) exercise group where they gradually increased exercise intensity while keeping exercise duration constant or to a low-intensity, longer duration (LILD) exercise group where they gradually increased the duration to 60 minutes while keeping exercise intensity constant or to a conventional therapeutic exercise (TE) group consisting of strength, balance, and ROM activities. The MISD group attained improvements in BP and total cholesterol (TC) compared with the other groups and both MISD and LILD groups showed significant reductions in total cholesterol compared with the TE group. However, in this study there was no significant change in $\dot{V}O_{2peak}$ and submaximal $\dot{V}O_2$ in any of the groups despite the significant gains in coronary risk reduction compared with TE group. Thus, aerobic exercise after stroke may reduce cardiac risk factors even if there is no significant change in fitness. This approach could have potential to reduce the occurrence of recurrent strokes and other neurological events.

Training modality—The training modality depends on the severity of the motor impairments. Typical modalities include treadmill, arm- or leg-crank ergometry, or a combination of the two. Body weight–supported (BWS) ambulation may be useful for moderate to severely impaired patients with stroke, where the body weight is supported by an overhead harness while walking on a treadmill or overground if the harness system is mobile. As the patient progresses in their ambulation independence, more body weight can progressively be assumed by the patient by decreasing the overhead support. However, Hesse and associates[44] compared a machine BWS device to a standard treadmill with support provided by two therapists. The machine providing the partial BWS that allowed for the improved ambulation of severely disabled patients with hemiparesis and requiring only one therapist for assistance.

Treadmill training with partial body weight support in subjects with hemiparesis allows practice of gait characterized by greater balance, higher symmetry, and less spasticity as compared with floor walking. Visintin and colleagues[45] reported better mobility outcomes with BWS treadmill training when compared with traditional treadmill training with full weight bearing of 100 patients with stroke. Walking speed and overground walking endurance improved significantly after 6 weeks of training.

Electrical stimulation (ES) on a recumbent bicycle has been explored in chronic stroke. Janssen et al. (2008) demonstrated that a short cycling training program on a semirecumbent cycle ergometer could markedly improve cycling performance, aerobic capacity, and functional performance of people with chronic stroke.[46] The authors evaluated whether leg cycling training in 12 subjects with chronic stroke can improve cycling performance, aerobic capacity, muscle strength, and functional performance and determined whether ES to the contralateral (paretic) leg during cycling has additional effects when performed twice a week for 6 weeks compared with a group who also received ES but with no visible contraction. Aerobic capacity and maximal power output significantly increased but muscle strength was not significantly enhanced after training. The use of ES had no additional effects in this specific group of subjects with chronic stroke and it should be noted that the aerobic and cycling performance effects were not related to functional performance.

Duration—The duration of training will depend on initial fitness level and may initially require intermittent bouts during each session. Cardiopulmonary exercise may last 20 minutes for 10 to 12 weeks. Most exercise programs demonstrate their efficacy by improving fitness, increasing oxygen utilization by muscle, decreasing the need for myocardial work, and reducing the progression of CAD using a frequency of exercise for 3 to 5 times per week.[26,42]

Intensity—HR, as a percentage of the age-predicted maximum, is a useful guide to establish the intensity of exercise. The window to produce aerobic training effects is approximately 60% to 85% of this predicted maximum. This guideline

TABLE 14-4 Exercise Training Studies for Patients with Stroke

Author	Pathology	Impairments	Functional Limitations	Disability
Rimmer et al.[43]	CVA	Peak oxygen consumption Submaximal oxygen consumption Lipid panel Resting BP	NT	NT
Duncan et al.[27]	CVA	Flexibility Strength Balance Peak aerobic capacity Upper limb function	10-m walk test 6-minute test	NT
Macko et al.[19]	CVA	Peak oxygen consumption Economy of gait Peak workload capacity	Gait speed	NT
Teixeira-Salmela et al.[47]	CVA	Muscle strength Leg spasticity	Gait speed and cadence	Human activity and Nottingham Health Profile
Duncan et al.[48]	CVA	Motor function Balance	Gait Speed Barthel ADL Lawton IADL	Medical outcome survey (physical functioning)
Macko et al.[14,23]	CVA	Energy expenditure Oxygen consumption	NT	NT
Potempa[26]	CVA	Maximal oxygen consumption, heart rate, workload, exercise time Blood pressure Sensorimotor function	NT	NT

CVA, cerebrovascular accident; ADL, activities of daily living; IADL; instrumental activities of daily living; NT, not tested or reported.

should be adhered to provided the patient is not on medication that restricts HR, in which case RPE should be used. If a $\dot{V}O_{2max}$ or $\dot{V}O_{2peak}$ was obtained, the HR at 40% to 60% of the measured $\dot{V}O_{2max}$ or $\dot{V}O_{2peak}$ of continuous or discontinuous exercise would be recommended. The training intensity should be increased as tolerated. Wearing a portable chest-worn HR monitor allows for continuous monitoring of HR during training and has the benefit of feedback to the patient as to the gains in fitness. As fitness improves, patients will either be able to walk faster or farther at the same absolute HR. Sufficient warm-up and cool-down periods (10 minutes each) should be included to prevent negative musculoskeletal and cardiovascular effects. A summary of the exercise training for cardiovascular fitness is found in Table 14-4.

Influence of medications on ability to exercise—Patients on vasodilators will require a longer cool-down period after exercise to prevent hypotension. Patients on medications to reduce cardiac output by reducing HR will demonstrate lower peak HRs during exercise. Patients using diuretics may exhibit arrhythmias due to lower fluid volume that alters electrolyte balance. Interactions of all pharmacological agents to each other during exercise must be understood. For a complete review of medications that impact on the cardiovascular and pulmonary systems, see Chapter 8.

Other responses to exercise—Exercise risk factors such as hypertension can be reduced through exercise intensities of 40% to 70% peak O_2 consumption.[49] There is a discrepancy between the self-perception of physical activity that was measured using self-report questionnaires, step activity monitors, self-efficacy expectations related to exercise, and $\dot{V}O_{2peak}$ from treadmill testing. Resnick reported that there were significant discrepancies between subjective (self-efficacy expectations) and objective findings $\dot{V}O_{2peak}$ helping to understand the perspective of stroke survivors with regard to physical activity.[50]

The effects of exercise on patients with stroke may also have an effect on the immune system. Physical exercise has been reported to activate the immune system. Therefore, exercise should be considered for its possible prevention of infectious diseases that are often complications for patients with stroke.[51] Approximately 33% of these patients suffer from depression during their rehabilitation period.[52] The benefits of exercise for patients with depression in general have been established.[53] Therefore, it is likely that exercise will ameliorate depression in patients with stroke. Although no studies have published the effects of exercise on bone mineral density, we know that bone mineral density decreases with age and inactivity for patients with CVA.[54] Therefore, it is reasonable to expect that exercise would reduce this loss in these patients who are at increased risk of osteoporotic fractures.

General Effects of Exercise Training on Impairment, Disability, and Quality of Life

Studies have demonstrated a very positive effect of exercise in patients with stroke, including improvements in gait and endurance. One study examined the effect of 6 months of low-intensity aerobic exercise in patients with chronic stroke and found a substantial and progressive decrease in energy cost and cardiovascular demands.[14] Six weeks of treadmill training with up to 40% body weight support for approximately 15 minutes, four times per week, resulted in better gait and overground walking endurance. Walking speed was measured by taking the middle 3-m velocity while subjects walked on a 10-m walkway. Walking endurance was recorded as the amount of distance an individual could walk until they could no longer continue, up to a maximal distance of 320 m.[45] BWS treadmill training, in addition to neurological physical therapy, was also reported to improve functional gait and walking velocity in seven nonambulatory patients with stroke.[44]

Another 8-week study of supervised home exercise, three times a week, produced an increase in median gait velocity, an increase in the 6-minute walk test time, and an increase in the health-related effects impact physical functioning on quality of life (QOL).[48] Perceived quality impact life relating to health factors was also improved after 10 weeks, three times a week, of aerobic exercise and lower extremity strengthening in patients with chronic stroke (post 9 months). This was in addition to improved gait speed, rate of stair climbing, and increased activity.[47] Silver and colleagues[55] reported an improvement with patients in the get up and go test, whereas Smith and colleagues[56] demonstrated an increase in torque-generating capacity across the knee of patients with chronic stroke who participated in treadmill training.

The activity profiles of walking for patients with stroke are 571 steps/d; 99% of the time is spent at less than 99 steps/min as measured by a step activity monitor. This activity profile may be compared to the findings of Gardner and associates,[57] who found that healthy subjects completed 8,672 steps/d compared with those with peripheral arterial occlusive disease. Therefore, general real-world activity is significantly reduced in stroke.

Exercise appears to have great benefit on patients with stroke, provided it is implemented cautiously. Screening for the appropriateness of exercise must be made on patients with unstable cardiopulmonary symptoms: respiratory distress, hypo- or hypertension, dyspnea, unstable angina, congestive heart failure, or unstable arrhythmias. HR and BP should be monitored before, during, and after exercise. If exercise is progressed prudently, it may also have additional health benefits through the reduction of significant cardiac risk factors.

Traumatic Brain Injury (Practice Patterns 5D; *ICD-9-CM* Codes: 800, 801, 803, 804, 850, 851, 852, 853, 854, 994)

Traumatic brain injury (TBI) occurs at a rate of approximately 500,000 new cases per year in the United States. The most frequent cause of TBI is motor vehicle accidents closely followed by gunshot wounds. TBI can result in motor impairments similar to that which occurs in stroke; however, the major difference is that patients with TBI are primarily young people who usually do not have underlying medical problems. Cognitive disturbances are the primary disability resulting from TBI and may include agitation, memory disturbances, and learning difficulties. One retrospective 10-year follow-up study of recovery of function following patients with severe TBI demonstrated continued improvement in social, cognitive, physical, and emotional functioning for at least 10 years postinjury. This implies that exercise intervention could promote improvement of function throughout this extended recovery period.[58]

Factors That Influence Ability to Exercise

As in all cases of neurological disease or illness, the ability to exercise depends on the severity of neurological impairment and cognitive disturbance. Factors that might affect exercise performance are listed in Box 14-1.

Significant cognitive limitations can cause intellectual deficits, making exercise instructions difficult to comprehend and therefore, limiting compliance. Behavioral/emotional problems can impede the success of an exercise intervention program because of the patient's inability to maintain stable emotions, making communication during exercise training difficult. Dysautonomia or dysregulation of the autonomic nervous system because of severe diffuse axonal injury and brain hypoxia is associated with a poorer outcome,[59] limiting the effectiveness of an exercise program because of the severity of brain damage. TBI can result in significant orthopedic deficits occurring at the time of the injury, which can impair the patient's ability to exercise or require modifications to the exercise modality.[33]

Most individuals who had suffered a TBI had been intubated and had a subsequent tracheostomy during the acute and subacute phases of recovery. The tracheostomy tube may remain in place for some time because of ongoing build-up of pulmonary secretions or because of sleep apnea. Ideally, the tracheostomy tube decreases both dead space and resistance from the oral cavity, making exercise more tolerable. However, a patient with a tracheostomy tube may find it uncomfortable

---

BOX 14-1

Summary of Factors That Influence Exercise Performance in Patients with TBI

- Cognitive deficits
- Emotional lability
- Communication deficits
- Dysautonomia
- Orthopedic deficits
- Respiratory difficulties
- Malnutrition
- Seizure disorder

to exercise because of the expulsion of secretions through the tracheostomy tube brought about by increased ventilation. In some cases, adequate respiration can be accomplished by temporarily closing the tube with the cap to achieve full ventilation by mouth. However, in other cases, it may be necessary to refrain from excessive exertion until the tracheostomy tube is removed.

Another factor associated with TBI that can influence exercise performance is relative malnutrition. A marked catabolic response with a negative nitrogen balance can result in subsequent dietary muscle wasting. Therefore, the appropriate fuel substrate may not be available during exercise training to enhance fitness or the development of muscle mass. This relative malnutrition may persist for a number of months after injury and may require dietary supplementation.

Patients with TBI also may be prone to seizures, especially during exercise testing where hyperventilation is usually induced. Although there is little evidence of the effect of exercise on seizure activity in TBI, one study of 204 patients with epilepsy determined that in a majority of the patients physical exercise had no adverse effects.[60] A considerable proportion (36%) claimed that regular exercise contributed to better seizure control. However, in approximately 10% of the patients, exercise appeared to be a seizure precipitant. The authors concluded that for individuals with epilepsy, the risk of sustaining serious seizure-related injuries during exercise seemed modest. Because similar studies have not been conducted in TBI, caution is advised to ensure appropriate therapeutic anticonvulsant medication levels before exercise testing and training. Appropriate medical supervision should be present during initial testing when rigorous exercise is involved, even when anticonvulsant medications have been taken.

Tests and Measures for Exercise Testing

A consensus statement by rehabilitation professionals from Quebec identified four health-related risk factors that should be included in fitness screening for patients with TBI.[61,62] These include angina pectoris, aortic stenosis, and exertional syncope. Outward aggression, pulmonary embolism, uncontrolled epilepsy, and ventricular arrhythmias can also be exacerbated by exercise. Identifying these risk factors prior to the implementation of an exercise program may help either to exclude inappropriate candidates for exercise or to trigger increased medical supervision during the initial prescription period.

There are few exercise studies that have evaluated the effects of exercise on cardiopulmonary function for patients with TBI. Hunter and colleagues[63] performed progressive exercise tests on 12 subjects with closed TBI by using a treadmill, a bicycle ergometer, and mechanical stairs. The treadmill and stairs produced the higher oxygen consumption and may be a more accurate measure of maximal exercise performance in this population. Jankowski and colleagues[64] tested 14 sedentary adults with TBI for submaximal peak rate of oxygen consumption. These authors determined that the TBI patients demonstrated a subnormal oxidative capacity and an above-average oxygen cost of locomotion.

The 20-m shuttle walk/run test has been demonstrated as a reliable field test for aerobic capacity of patients with TBI.[61] This is a cardiovascular field test that involves walking or running a 20-m shuttle course while maintaining the pace determined by signals from an audiotape (see Chapter 9). The initial slow walking pace of 2.4 km/h was gradually increased each minute until the patient could no longer continue. The shuttle walk/run test, when compared with ergometer and treadmill tests,[65] has been reported to produce an underestimation of peak $\dot{V}O_2$ for healthy fit males. However, when standardized exercise testing equipment may not be available, the shuttle walk/run test may be the most reliable alternative. The key to the reliability of all walk tests is the standardization of testing methods and instructions.

In general, the considerations in exercise testing in TBI that may be different from those in stroke are that motor impairments may involve all limbs rather than affecting one side. In addition, cognitive behavior may limit a patient's ability to understand the purpose of a maximal exercise test. If agitation is present, patients with TBI may not be willing to wear a face mask or mouthpiece necessary for metabolic testing. Finally, there may be significant dysautonomia due to involvement of the subcortical and brainstem structures at the time of the brain trauma. These autonomic problems may present with abnormal HR and BP responses during exercise testing. Careful monitoring with the supervision of a physician is recommended.

Otherwise, an incremental graded exercise test will be sufficient to achieve a maximal effort because CVD is likely not a problem in this population, who generally are young and not at risk. A discontinuous protocol is usually not required because of the young age but may be required if there are significant motor impairments. In this case, other modes of exercise testing such as bicycle or leg ergometry may allow the patient to reach a higher workload.

Interventions for Exercise Training

Few studies exist that evaluate the effect of exercise training in TBI. This is likely due to the wide variability in physical performance across patients and because of the important focus on the cognitive behavior of these patients in the earlier stages of recovery. The physical impairments generally are not as severe as the cognitive. However, Hunter and colleagues[63] evaluated a 3-month conditioning program in 12 patients with TBI and closed head injury. The exercise consisted of aerobic and flexibility exercises for 50 minutes for 12 weeks. Maximal power output increased on the treadmill, bicycle ergometer, and mechanical stairs and resting HR decreased. Maximal oxygen consumption increased to 75% to 85% of their predicted values.

Jankowski and colleagues[64] conducted a 16-week circuit-training program of moderate intensity (2 hours) and prolonged duration (three times a week for 6 weeks). The aerobic stations of the circuit consisted of cycling, rope skipping, jogging, and stair climbing. While there was an increase in oxidative capacity, there was a failure to reduce oxygen cost

TABLE 14-5   Summary of Evidence for Exercise Training for Patients with TBI

Author	Pathology	Impairments	Functional Limitations	Disability
Mossberg et al.[67]		$\dot{V}O_2$, HR, total ambulation time	NT	NT
Wolman et al.[66]	TBI	Exercise duration Maximal workload	NT	NT
Hunter[57]	TBI	Power output Resting heart rate Maximal oxygen consumption	NT	NT
Jankowski and Sullivan[64]	TBI	Oxidative capacity Oxygen cost of walking	NT	NT

HR, heart rate; NT, Not tested or reported; TBI, traumatic brain injury.

while walking. Wolman and associates[66] found improvements in exercise duration and maximal workload for patients with TBI who participated in a 6-week program of biking. However, Mossberg et al.[67] evaluated the cardiorespiratory response to treadmill exercise on admission and discharge in 40 individuals with acquired brain injury. Total ambulation time increased and submaximal HR decreased, suggesting improved aerobic capacity. Peak HR and $\dot{V}O_2$ did not change. Mossberg et al. later (2008) studied the effect of body weight–supported treadmill training (BWSTT) on cardiorespiratory adaptations on two patients with TBI.[68] Each patient received two to three sessions of BWSTT per week. Aerobic capacity was measured while they ambulated on a treadmill without BWS before and after BWSTT and both patients' submaximal and peak responses improved including treadmill work performed, peak oxygen uptake, and estimated cardiac stroke volume (oxygen pulse). This case report suggests that BWSTT has the potential to favorably change cardiorespiratory capacity after TBI.

The results of these studies indicate that patients with TBI can tolerate and benefit from intense exercise training programs.[69] For this reason, exercise training is warranted in TBI to overcome the general deconditioning for the injury and recovery period. Patients with TBI often complain of fatigue that may be central in origin; however, exercise training may cause a reduction of these complaints of fatigue and allow for greater involvement in social and occupational activities. More studies are needed to address the efficacy of exercise training in TBI, particularly those that include measurements of functional limitations and disability. A summary of these exercise training studies is given in Table 14-5.

Influence of Medications on Ability to Exercise

No studies have addressed the pharmacological effects of medications taken by patients with brain injury as they relate to exercise performance. Although most patients with TBI are on many medications to manage brain damage during the early stages after the injury, many patients are on few, if any, medications for the long term.

The primary condition that distinguishes TBI from brain injury associated with stroke is the common use of medications to control seizures and agitation. These medications are

often taken for the long term. Further discussion of medications and their effects on exercise can be found in Chapter 8.

General Effects of Exercise Training on Impairment, Disability, and Quality of Life

Gordon and colleagues[70] conducted a retrospective study of a community-based sample of 240 individuals with TBI (64 exercisers and 176 nonexercisers) and 139 individuals without a disability (66 exercisers and 73 nonexercisers). The researchers found that the exercisers with TBI were less depressed, reported fewer symptoms, and their self-reported health status was better than that of the nonexercising individuals with TBI. There were no differences between the two groups of individuals with TBI on measures of disability and handicap. These findings suggest that exercise improves mood and aspects of health status and also improves aspects of disability and handicap for patients with TBI.

Spinal Cord Injury (Practice Patterns 5H, 5A, 5E, 7A; *ICD-9-CM* Codes: 344, 806, 952, 741, 336)

Spinal cord injury (SCI) produces neuromuscular, skeletal, hormonal, and psychological changes in the injured individual. Injury at the highest level (C1 through C7) causes tetraplegia with impairment of the arms, trunk, legs, and pelvic organs. Injury to the thoracic segments leads to paraplegia with impairments of the legs and pelvic organs.

CLINICAL CORRELATE

SCI leads to partial or complete loss of volitional control of muscles innervated below the level of the lesion resulting in loss of muscle strength and endurance. This loss also alters the cardiopulmonary system's response to exercise because local fatigue of remaining intact musculature often prevents patients from maintaining prescribed workloads.

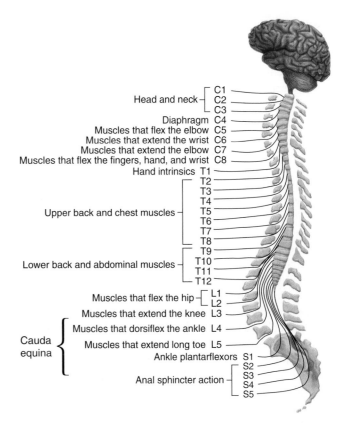

FIGURE 14-1 Spinal cord injury lesion levels and resultant functional limitations. (C = Cervical; T = Thoracic; L = Lumber; S = Sacral)

Stimulation of the cardiopulmonary system is also impaired in SCI due to lack of innervation to the autonomic nervous system, thereby reducing the ability to support higher rates of aerobic metabolism. Regular exercise through either voluntary activity or ES of paralyzed muscles can increase the strength and endurance of these muscles. However, the potential benefits from exercise are drastically altered. Injuries below C7 result in paraplegia. Certain patients with paraplegia may suffer from loss of autonomic control (T6 and above) similar to that in tetraplegia (C1 through C7). Figure 14-1 illustrates lesion levels and resultant functional limitations. A summary of the practice patterns and *ICD-9-CM* codes for SCI are given in Table 14-6.

Factors That Influence Ability to Exercise

SCI impairs thermoregulation due to loss of autonomic nervous system control for vasomotor (vascular dilation/constriction) and sudomotor (sweating) responses in the areas of lost

sensation. Therefore, a person with SCI has a reduced ability to handle thermal extremes and to perform aerobic exercise. Because patients with SCI must rely on their upper body for locomotion, they may be at a thermal risk.[71]

Other factors, including relatively small muscle mass and deficient cardiovascular reflex and inactivity of the venous skeletal muscle pump (resulting in hypokinetic circulation), can cause early onset of fatigue during arm exercise in patients with SCI. Exercise responses to arm-crank ergometry (ACE) are significantly related to the level of lesion of SCI. **The higher the lesion level, the lower the physical work capacity and mean exercise systolic and diastolic blood pressure.**[72]

Tests and Measures for Exercise Testing

In general, wheelchair ergometry (WCE) is less metabolically efficient than arm-crank ergometry at submaximal intensities.[73] However, arm-crank ergometry imposes a

TABLE 14-6 Summary of Spinal Cord Injury Practice Patterns and *ICD-9-CM* Codes

Diagnosis	Practice Pattern(s)	*ICD-9-CM* Codes
Paralytic syndromes	4A, 5H, 6B, 6E, 7A, 7B, 7C	344
Fracture of vertebral column with spinal cord injury	5H	806
Spinal cord injury without evidence of spinal bone injury	5H	952
Spina bifida	5B, 5C	741
Other diseases of the spinal cord	5A, 5E, 5H, 7A	336

greater central circulatory stress. Higher peak HRs are elicited by arm-crank ergometry than by WCE, suggesting that exercise testing needs to be ergometer specific when the results are to be used for exercise prescription.[74] If the subject's neurological level of injury is T10 through L2, the maximal exercise test will progress as conducted for an able-bodied individual. If the injury level is T6 or above, exercise performance may be influenced by lack of sympathetic outflow to the adrenal medulla, resulting in impaired release of catecholamines during exercise. For these individuals, the Borg Perceived Exertion Scale should be applied (see Chapter 9).

McClean and colleagues[75] found that an RPE of 10 to 12 was both linearly related to a 50% to 60% peak power output in tetraplegia and associated with a higher power output than that predicted by HR or oxygen consumption. Therefore, a Borg RPE of 14 to 15 is most often used to represent a sufficient intensity to terminate the test for patients with tetraplegia when other cardiac and metabolic measures are unobtainable due to impaired cardioregulatory responses. However, in 2007 Lewis et al. contradicted the well-accepted relationships between RPE and both HR and $\dot{V}O_2$ during exercise by people without disabilities and challenged its use as a valid index of perceived exertion in persons with SCI.[76] Their study examined the relationship between HR, $\dot{V}O_2$, minute ventilation ($\dot{V}E$), and RPE (Borg categorical 6–20 scale) during a peak-graded arm ergometry in persons with paraplegia and tetraplegia. There were inconsistent associations for subjects with tetraplegia, where the RPE related positively to HR at the initial work rate, but there were no other significant correlations and for subjects with paraplegia where RPE did not correlate significantly with HR, $\dot{V}O_2$, or $\dot{V}E$. In general, HR, $\dot{V}O_2$, and $\dot{V}E$ increased as the exercise intensity increased and were more pronounced in subjects with paraplegia. While RPE values increased with increasing work rates for each group, no differences between groups were found. Therefore, RPE does not appear to be a valid surrogate for physiological stress in SCI during a maximal exercise test.

Generally, subjects whose neurological level is thoracic (T1) and lower can propel a manual wheelchair and complete a maximal wheelchair treadmill exercise test to deter-

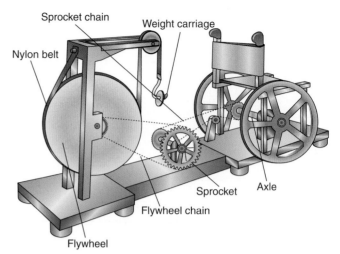

FIGURE 14-2   Wheelchair ergometry modality for exercise testing or training. (From Keyser RE, Rodgers MM, Gardner ER, Russell PJ. Oxygen uptake during peak-graded exercise and single-stage fatigue tests of wheelchair propulsion in manual wheelchair users and the able-bodied. *Arch Phys Med Rehabil.* 1999;80:1289. Used with permission from WB Saunders Company and Randall E. Keyser.)

mine aerobic capacity. However, subjects whose neurological level is cervical (C5 through C8) usually require arm-crank ergometry to determine aerobic capacity, securing the upper extremities as needed. Subjects should refrain from food, caffeine, nicotine, or alcohol for a 4-hour period before testing. The exercise test protocols usually consist of incremental graded workloads of 3-minute stages with the initial power output at 10 or greater for paraplegia. The workload should be progressed by 6 W per stage with the WCE and progressed to 12 W per stage for the arm-crank ergometry because it elicits a higher maximal power output when compared with the wheelchair exercise.[77,78] For tetraplegia, the initial power output is 1 to 3 W with a work rate progression of between 4 and 6 W.[79] The testing protocols for paraplegia and tetraplegia are summarized in Table 14-7. Cycling rates for both exercise modalities can be maintained by a metronome. Figures 14-2 and 14-3 illustrate wheelchair and arm-crank ergometry systems for exercise testing and training.

TABLE 14-7   **Summary of Suggested Guidelines for Exercise Testing in Paraplegia and Tetraplegia**

	Duration of Test (min)	Rate	Workload Progression	Heart Rate (bpm)
			12 W/stage (ACE)	
Paraplegia	12	60 rpm	6 W/stage (WCE)	Age-predicted maximal heart rate[a]
Tetraplegia	6	60 rpm	4–6 W/stage	RPE of 13–15

RPE, Ratings of perceived exertion; ACE, arm-crank ergometry; WCE, wheelchair ergometry.

[a]Age-predicted maximal heart rates are determined to be 220−age.

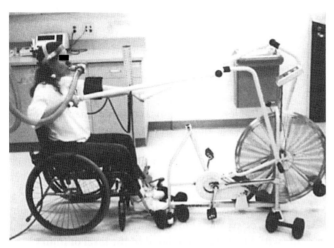

FIGURE 14-3 Arm-crank ergometry modality for exercise testing or training. (Reprinted with permission from Lamont LS, Going A, Kievit J. A comparison of two arm exercises in patients with paraplegia. *Cardiopulm Phys Ther J.* 1996;7:3.)

CLINICAL CORRELATE

Because of the absence of thermoregulatory sweating and vasoconstriction below the level of the lesion, a fan and spray-water system can be used to facilitate heat loss by convection and production of a cooling effect through vaporization of "artificial sweat." Blankets should also be used during the cool-down and postexercise periods to avoid hypothermia. To avoid problems associated with autonomic hyperreflexia such as hyper- or hypotension and venous pooling, subjects with neurological injury of T6 and above should wear an abdominal binder and leg-compressive stockings. In some cases, where hypotension due to venous pooling is persistent, arm-crank ergometry with the legs either elevated or in a semi-reclined position can facilitate venous return and make additional blood available to the exercising arms.[73]

King and colleagues[24] studied exertional hypotension in four lesion levels of patients with SCI who performed a continuous maximal arm ergometry exercise test. Exertional hypotension, defined in this case as a maximal BP lower than the highest submaximal BP, was present in all patients with SCI regardless of lesion level. Patients who experience hypotension can report a sense of dizziness, nausea, visual changes, and/or sweating. Still other patients with SCI who experience hypotension do not report any symptoms. Therefore, it is important to monitor BP throughout the test. This is typically done during arm-crank ergometry by therapist-assisted cranking, while the arm remains still to measure BP.

Aerobic power during maximal exercise was studied in 58 males with traumatic spinal cord lesions from C4 through L4. Twenty-five well-trained "world-class athletes" and 33 untrained subjects were compared with five arm-trained and five arm-untrained able-bodied subjects.[80] During maximal wheelchair exercise, the aerobic power ($\dot{V}O_{2peak}$), pulmonary ventilation, and blood lactate concentration were higher in subjects with lower levels of SCI. At each injury level above C6 through C7, nearly all trained subjects reached a higher $\dot{V}O_{2peak}$ than did untrained subjects with the corresponding level of lesion. The peak HR in the tetraplegia groups was lower than that in the paraplegia group with no or only small differences between trained and untrained subjects at the same level of SCI. Therefore, the expectations of individuals with paraplegia are much the same as that of a healthy group; however, significant limitations in cardiorespiratory responses occur with tetraplegia ergometry; therefore, a Borg perceived exertion scale should be used.

Other studies have demonstrated that exercise capacity is dependent on spinal injury level. Yamasaki and colleagues[81] determined that individuals with high paraplegia (T3 through T8) compared with those with low paraplegia (T10 through L2) who performed arm-crank exercise had low work efficiency. This was attributed to increased ventilation, which yielded an increase in oxygen uptake. In 1998, Yamasaki and colleagues[82] later found that years since injury are not as important in determining cardiorespiratory responses during maximal arm cranking as is level of SCI and training. Gass and colleagues[83] compared arm-crank and treadmill wheelchair propulsion in a homogeneous group of nine men with paraplegia (T4 through T6). This study found that, unlike previous studies, there were no significant differences in oxygen consumption, ventilation, or HR between the two modes of ergometry during the last minute of incremental exercise to exhaustion. This conclusion was most likely due to the study of paraplegics versus tetraplegics and to the fact that the lesion level was homogeneous.

Interventions for Exercise Training

With the growing interest in exercise and sport and the significance of CVD in the spinal cord–injured population, the role of endurance training in improving cardiovascular health is of particular interest. Ordinary daily activities of those with SCI are usually not adequate to maintain cardiovascular fitness, and lack of participation in a regular activity program may result in a debilitative cycle.[84] As this occurs, there is a reduction in functional work capacity that may limit independence, and the reduction in cardiovascular fitness may increase the risk for CVD.

Work capacity in those with SCI is limited by loss of functional muscle mass and sympathetic control. Sympathetic nervous system impairment limits control of regional blood flow and cardiac output, and maximum HR following cervical lesions may be reduced to 110 to 130 beats per minute (bpm). However, endurance training in patients with tetraplegia and paraplegia can elicit improvements in exercise performance similar to those observed in able-bodied individuals.

A HR chest monitor (Polar CIC, Inc; Port Washington, NY) should be worn during all training periods to ensure maintenance of target HR during each training session. Subjects should be progressed from 60% of target HR up to 85% over the course of the training period, usually lasting between 8 and 12 weeks. Training targets will also depend on whether subjects have a neurological level of injury at or above T6 or below T6 because of the potential for autonomic dysreflexia. BP should be measured at intervals throughout exercise. In subjects with tetraplegia, HR may rise to a limited degree during arm-crank ergometry.

A review of 13 cardiorespiratory training studies involving subjects with SCI[84] revealed average improvements of 20% in $\dot{V}O_{2max}$ and 40% in physical work capacity after 4 to 20 weeks of training. On the basis of the positive results of these studies, the general endurance training guidelines for the normal population appear also to be appropriate for the spinal cord–injured population. These guidelines can be followed during participation in a number of different activities and sports including wheelchair pushing, arm-crank ergometry, aerobic swimming, ambulation training, canoeing, and wheelchair basketball.

There is no evidence that intense training and competition are harmful, but special areas of risk as a result of impairments in sensation, cardiovascular function, autonomic function, and temperature regulation must be considered. The long-term benefits of endurance training in those with SCI have not been adequately studied, but there is suggestion that similar physiological and psychological changes may occur in able-bodied individuals.

Taylor and colleagues[85] studied the effects of an arm-crank ergometry training program on several physiological variables of recreational wheelchair subjects. Ten subjects with paraplegia (five experimental and five control) were tested prior to and immediately after a 2-month exercise regimen at 80% of peak HR (30 min/d, 5 d/wk, for 8 consecutive weeks). The results demonstrated significant increases in $\dot{V}O_{2max}$ and workload but only mild improvements in maximal HR and postexercise blood lactate levels. The results indicate that physiological variables of subjects with paraplegia following an arm ergometer endurance training program are similar to changes previously observed in healthy subjects. These values, when compared with those of healthy individuals, are low as a result of the relative inactivity.

Eight men with tetraplegia participating in an 8-week arm-crank ergometry training program demonstrated improved cardiopulmonary function including exercise HR, physical work capacity, and maximal oxygen uptake. Additionally, wheelchair propulsion endurance improved as evidenced by distance covered in 12 minutes on a circular track.[86] Different exercise effects among persons with paraplegia and tetraplegia have been noted. After a training protocol, subjects with paraplegia had cardiorespiratory responses that were similar to those of individuals without SCI, whereas subjects with tetraplegia exhibited increased resting HR and systolic BP.

Twenty individuals with SCI were tested for $\dot{V}O_{2peak}$ by using a WCE.[87] The subjects were divided into four groups: (1) a group with tetraplegia (four subjects); (2) an untrained female group with paraplegia (five subjects); (3) an untrained male group with paraplegia (seven subjects); and (4) a trained male group with paraplegia (four subjects). $\dot{V}O_{2peak}$ for the group with tetraplegia was significantly lower than that for the other groups. $\dot{V}O_{2peak}$ for the untrained female group was significantly lower than that for both the untrained male group with paraplegia and the trained male group with paraplegia. The untrained male group with paraplegia had a $\dot{V}O_{2peak}$ significantly lower than the trained male group with paraplegia. **The present study, combined with the findings from research, gives strong evidence that $\dot{V}O_{2peak}$ in untrained patients with SCI is highly related to the level of injury.**

Hjeltnes and colleagues[88] studied 10 male patients with tetraplegia who completed arm-crank ergometry three times per week. Aerobic capacity was compared to 10 patients with paraplegia who received traditional rehabilitation. Peak workload increased in the group with quadriplegia, but oxidative capacity did not. It was not surprising that peak oxygen capacity was greater in the group with paraplegia and significantly increased as a result of the training.

Price and Campbell[89] examined the thermoregulatory responses of able-bodied athletes, athletes with paraplegia, and athletes with tetraplegia at rest, during prolonged upper-body exercise, and recovery. Exercise was performed on an arm-crank ergometry at 60% $\dot{V}O_{2peak}$ for 60 minutes. Peak oxygen uptake values were greater for the able-bodied individuals when compared with that of the subjects with paraplegia and least for the subjects with tetraplegia.

Dallmeijer and colleagues[90] studied the effect of rehabilitation on physical capacity, mechanical efficiency of manual wheelchair propulsion, and performance of standardized ADL. Nineteen recently injured subjects with SCI were tested on a WCE for peak oxygen uptake and performance time at the beginning and at the end of the active rehabilitation period. Mechanical efficiency of submaximal wheelchair exercise was significantly higher after rehabilitation compared with that before. Performance time showed a significant decrease for most tasks. The results of this study show considerable improvements in physical capacity, mechanical efficiency of manual wheelchair propulsion during rehabilitation, and a concomitant lower performance time during standardized ADL. The higher mechanical efficiency and the decrease in performance time during standardized ADL suggest improvement in wheelchair propulsion techniques.

Bernard and colleagues[91] characterized the influence of neurological lesion level on the cardiorespiratory and ventilatory responses of two groups of athletes with paraplegia during incremental exercise on a treadmill and under the usual conditions for wheelchair exercise. Cardioventilatory responses were evaluated in two groups of wheelchair sports—men with paraplegia designated as athletes with high paraplegia and in athletes with low paraplegia. With the exception of respiration, there were no significant differences in the classic cardiorespiratory parameters ($\dot{V}O_2$, $\dot{V}CO_2$, HR, $\dot{V}E$) between the two groups. For the ventilatory parameters, there were significant differences between the two groups. A ventilatory disturbance was observed that was manifested by values of breathing frequency and tidal volume during exercise that were significantly different between groups.

During maximal exercise, no significant differences between the two groups concerning cardiorespiratory and ventilatory values were observed. The achievement of a greater number of workload levels and the higher maximal values indicated a better capacity for adaptation to exercise in the group with lower thoracic paraplegia. These results raise questions about the influence of neurological level, and further research is needed to define with more precision the capacities of readaptation of cardiovascular and respiratory functions as well as the training methods best adapted to the optimization of physical capacities.

Barstow and colleagues[92] studied the peak and submaximal responses of oxygen uptake and HR in patients with SCI performing arm-crank ergometry and functional electrical stimulation (FES) leg cycling exercise. The purpose was to test whether the blunted HR response and slower rate of adjustment of oxygen uptake seen by using FES leg cycling exercise are also characteristic of arm exercise in these patients. Eight patients with paraplegia performed incremental and constant work rate (CWR) exercise with the legs and arms. Peak HR was higher during incremental arm exercise and was not correlated with that observed during incremental FES leg cycling.

For the same increase in $\dot{V}O_2$, constant work rate arm exercise was associated with faster (and normal) $\dot{V}O_2$ kinetics, greater increase in HR, and lower end-exercise blood lactate compared with FES leg cycling. Therefore, the consistently higher peak HR and $\dot{V}O_2$ and faster $\dot{V}O_2$ kinetics for voluntary arm exercise compared with FES leg cycling exercise suggest no intrinsic dysfunction of HR control in subjects with paraplegia. Rather, these data suggest that during FES leg cycling, the changes seen are due to some characteristic specific to the injury, such as reduced muscle mass and/or deconditioning of the remaining muscle.

Muraki and colleagues[93] studied the main factors that influence physical work capacity (PWC) in wheelchair-dependent subjects with paraplegia by using multivariate analysis. Thirty-two male subjects with paraplegia performed a submaximal arm exercise test on an arm-crank ergometry to determine their physical work capacity at 150 bpm and level of physical activity, occupation, level of SCI, and time since SCI. There was a high correlation between physical work capacity and the level of SCI and physical activity level compared to other factors. These results indicate that the level of SCI and physical activity are the most important factors in determining physical work capacity in wheelchair-dependent males with paraplegia.

Other forms of exercise training, such as ES, have emerged as promising interventions for improving fitness in SCI. Janssen et al. (2008) found that interval training using a modified versus a standard ES leg cycle ergometry can elicit marked improvements, not in peak metabolic and cardiorespiratory responses in men with SCI.[94] Modifications to a standard ES protocol included increasing the current amplitude, adding shank muscle activation, and increasing angular motion. The training consisted of a 6-week interval training program with both experienced and novice riders. The modified protocol elicited significantly higher peak values for oxygen uptake, carbon dioxide production, pulmonary ventilation, cardiac output, HR, and blood lactate concentration. These changes occurred even with the experienced riders who had plateaued with a standard ES protocol. Frotzler et al. (2008) also reported a partial reversal of bone loss in chronic SCI after high-volume ES cycling, especially at the location of the distal femur where the bone is actively loaded during cycling versus the proximal tibia that was passively loaded.[95]

On the subject of dosing, Valent and colleagues (2008) found that regular hand cycling (once a week or more) appeared to be beneficial for improving aerobic physical capacity in persons with paraplegia during clinical rehabilitation.[96] The authors investigated the influence of hand cycling use (questionnaire) on outcome measures of physical capacity during and after rehabilitation and 1 year later in 162 persons with paraplegia and tetraplegia. Peak oxygen uptake and peak power output determined in a hand-rim wheelchair peak exercise test, peak muscle strength of the upper extremities (triceps), and pulmonary function showed a significantly larger increment in paraplegia, not in tetraplegia and not at 1-year follow-up. A summary of parameters of exercise training studies in SCI can be found in Table 14-8.

Influence of Medications on Ability to Exercise

The primary medication that may influence exercise performance in subjects with spasticity is Baclofen. This medication has a tendency to make patients with SCI tired and weak. If possible, physicians often try to reduce or discontinue this medication if spasticity can be maintained under control. In some cases, patients have reported a decrease in spasticity as a result of FES of the lower limbs or even during upper-body exercise. Any medication change should be monitored and recorded to evaluate the influence on exercise capacity and training.

Other Responses to Exercise

Musculoskeletal changes such as decreased rate or possible cessation of bone loss[97] occur as a result of exercise. From a neurological point of view, reports by Daly and colleagues[98] have reported a decrease in spasticity and accelerated peripheral nerve regeneration as a result of exercise. Research also indicates that exercise in SCI produces an enhanced insulin sensitivity, which can lead to the prevention of diabetes.[99] Daly et al. (1996) also reports accelerated wound healing. Kocina[100] demonstrated an increase in weight loss and an increase in fat loss and lean body mass for patients with SCI who participated in an exercise training protocol.

TABLE 14-8   Summary of Parameters of Exercise Training Studies in SCI

Author	Pathology	Impairments	Functional Limitations	Disability
Hoffman[84]	Paraplegia and tetraplegia	Maximal oxygen consumption Physical work capacity	NT	NT
Taylor et al.[85]	Paraplegia	Maximal oxygen consumption Maximal heart rate Blood lactates	NT	NT
DiCarlo[86]	Tetraplegia	Exercise heart rate Physical work capacity Maximal oxygen consumption Systolic blood pressure	Distance covered during propulsion on a circular track	NT
Burkett et al.[87]	Paraplegia and tetraplegia	Peak oxygen consumption	NT	NT
Hjeltnes and Wallberg-Henriksson[88]	Paraplegia and tetraplegia	Peak workload Peak oxygen consumption	NT	NT
Price and Campbell[89]	Paraplegia and tetraplegia	Peak oxygen consumption	NT	NT
Dallmeijer et al.[90]	Paraplegia and tetraplegia	Physical capacity Mechanical efficiency of wheelchair propulsion	ADL performance times	NT
Bernard et al.[91]	Paraplegia	Oxygen consumption Heart rate Ventilation Respiratory quotient Maximal workloads	NT	NT
Barstow et al.[92]	Paraplegia	Peak and submaximal oxygen uptake Heart rate End-exercise lactate	NT	NT
Muraki et al.[93]	Paraplegia	Physical work capacity	Physical activity	Occupation
Valent et al.[96]	Paraplegia and tetraplegia	Peak oxygen uptake, peak power output, pulmonary function	NT	NT

ADL, activities of daily living; NT, not tested or not reported.

During exercise, aural temperature changes in patients with SCI are important to monitor. One study of athletes with tetraplegia demonstrated a gradual rise of 0.9°C in aural temperature throughout exercise. During 30 minutes of passive recovery, the able-bodied athletes demonstrated greater decreases in aural temperatures than those for the athletes with paraplegia. Aural temperatures for the patients with tetraplegia increased, peaking at 5 minutes of recovery and remained elevated until the end of the recovery period. Fluid consumption and weight loss were similar for the able-bodied subjects and patients with paraplegia, whereas changes in plasma volume were greater for the able-bodied athletes. The results of this study suggest that under experimental conditions, athletes with paraplegia are at no greater thermal risk than able-bodied athletes. A relationship between the available muscle mass for heat production and sweating capacity appears evident for the maintenance of thermal balance. During recovery from exercise, decreases in aural temperature were greatest for the able-bodied athletes with the greatest capacity for heat loss and lowest for the athletes with tetraplegia with a lesser capacity for heat loss. A summary of other responses to exercise in patients with SCI can be found in Box 14-2.

General Effects of Exercise Training on Impairment, Disability, and Quality of Life

Noreau et al.[101] found an increased employability and independence in ADL without assistance in patients with SCI who exercised. Spinal cord lesions with paresis reduce the total active skeletal muscle mass. This can cause physical

BOX 14-2

Summary of Other Responses to Exercise in Patients with SCI

- Reduced bone-density loss
- Decrease in spasticity
- Enhanced insulin sensitivity
- Accelerated wound healing
- Weight loss
- Decrease in fat mass
- Increase in lean body mass

inactivity, medical complications, and social isolation. As a consequence, cardiovascular disorders as a cause of death are higher in this group compared with the general population. Therefore, one aim of rehabilitation is to increase the individual's performance in daily life activities. It has been shown that the normal daily life activities of individuals with tetra- and paraplegia with no additional physical training are not intense enough to maintain a satisfactory level of physical fitness.

Manns and Chad[102] studied 38 individuals with paraplegia and tetraplegia to determine the relationships among fitness, physical activity, subjective QOL, and handicap. Physical activity, measured by a leisure time exercise questionnaire, played an important role in the determination of handicap, measured by the Craig Handicap Assessment Reporting Technique (CHART) in SCI. It appears that the greater the time spent in leisure activity, the greater the likelihood that the associated handicap will be lower.

Tawashy et al. (2009) studied 49 individuals with SCI who were community dwellers and were primarily wheelchair users to determine the relationship of self-report physical activity and secondary conditions such as pain, fatigue, and depression.[103] The authors found that those who engaged in heavy-intensity activity within the community had lower pain and fatigue and higher levels of self-efficacy, whereas high amounts of mild-intensity activity led to less depression. Therefore, even mild activity has QOL gains such as less depression and if we can encourage higher-intensity activities, there is potential to thwart pain and fatigue.

Multiple Sclerosis (Practice Patterns 5A, 5E, 6C, 6E, 7A; *ICD-9-CM* Code: 340)

Multiple sclerosis (MS) is an autoimmune demyelinating disease of the central nervous system. The loss of myelin reduces the speed of nerve conduction, thus interfering with smooth, rapid, and coordinated movement. Therefore, MS is associated with minimal-to-severe levels of disability as defined by the expanded disability rating scale (EDSS).[104] MS has an estimated prevalence of 58 per 100,000 in the United States, occurring most frequently in women who are in their third and fourth decades of life. Three patterns of MS have been identified: (1) relapsing/remitting, (2) progressive, and (3) a combination of relapsing/remitting and progressive.[105] Symptoms vary depending on the type and severity of MS and on the location of lesions. Symptoms include spasticity, tremor, weakness, fatigue, visual disturbances, bowel and bladder dysfunction, and pain. The most common and debilitating symptom of MS is a generalized sense of fatigue, frequently resulting from heat sensitivity.

Factors That Influence Ability to Exercise

It has been reported that 75% to 95% of persons with MS have fatigue, whereas 50% to 60% report that fatigue is their worst symptom. Fatigue in MS has been described as different from normal fatigue in that it comes on easily, prevents sustained physical functioning, is worsened by the heat, interferes with physical functioning, and causes frequent problems.[106] Freal and colleagues[107] found that fatigue was most likely to occur in the afternoon and evening as opposed to in the morning. This may be related to the body's core temperature being the lowest in the morning. **To avoid fatigue, the morning may be the best time to perform exercise.**

Surprisingly, the severity of the illness (EDSS score) is not related to the severity of the fatigue. Therefore, even individuals with milder MS might suffer as much from fatigue as those who are more severe. Furthermore, MS fatigue has been found to be separate from depression because if depression is present, it is not related to the presence or severity of fatigue.[106] Iriarte and colleagues[108] found that fatigue was a symptom in 118 out of 155 patients with clinically diagnosed MS (76%). Twenty-two percent had fatigue at rest (asthenia), 72% described fatigue with exercise, and 6% described worsening of symptoms with effort. Finally, some authors have suggested that local skeletal muscle changes may contribute to the global sense of fatigue. These changes may include decreased oxidative capacity, slowed relaxation time, and a decrease in the number of slow-twitch muscle fibers. These changes may be due to inactivity resulting from the CNS dysfunction, leading to deconditioning and disuse. However, reconditioning by increasing the oxidative capacity of skeletal muscles may be warranted.

An estimated 80% of patients with MS are sensitive to changes in core body temperature, either from external environmental factors or from vigorous exercise. Aerobic exercise increases body heat due to an increase in metabolic rate. Without normal thermoregulatory responses from the autonomic nervous system, such as sweating, hyperthermia can result. The change in body temperature that elicits neurological signs varies between 0.1°C and 2.3°C. This rise in temperature causes a decrease in nerve conduction and is directly related to the degree of nerve conduction loss.[109] Therefore, it is important that physical therapists assess temperature sensitivity prior to the beginning of an exercise regimen. Dysautonomia can also cause cardiac acceleration and reduction in the BP response.[110]

Neurological signs such as spasticity, muscle weakness or paralysis, and sensory loss may contribute to an inability to participate in exercise. Additionally, impaired balance and tremor may require modifications to traditional exercise modes. Fear of fatigue or worsening of symptoms can lead patients with MS to avoid exercise, which can lead to deconditioning and disuse atrophy. If the physical therapist can communicate an understanding of the pathophysiology of MS and the expected response to exercise to the patient, the patient's concerns will be put to rest and allow for greater compliance with the exercise program. Box 14-3 summarizes the factors that can influence exercise performance in MS.

Summary of Factors That Can Influence Ability for Patients with MS to Exercise

- Fatigue
- Depression
- Pain
- Temperature insensitivity
- Spasticity
- Muscle weakness
- Sensory loss

Tests and Measures for Exercise Testing

Treadmill testing is often impossible for patients with MS who exhibit motor and sensory impairments of the lower limb such as spasticity or paresis. Therefore, as in severe stroke or head injury, upright or recumbent leg ergometry or a combination of arm and leg ergometry may be more practical. As in all exercise testing, arm ergometry often produces arm muscle fatigue before a cardiopulmonary maximum is reached. Recommendations for exercise testing[110] include the use of a discontinuous protocol of 3- to 5-minute stages, beginning with a warm-up of unloaded pedaling. The work rate should be increased at each stage by approximately 12 to 25 W for legs and 8 to 12 W for arms. Foot stabilization may be necessary to counteract spasms or tremor.

There is very little research on the exercise capacity of patients with MS, most likely due to the wide variability of severity and disease fluctuation. However, most indications are that in the absence of severe paresis and cardiovascular dysautonomia, many individuals have been able to reach 85% to 90% of their age-predicted maximal HR. For physical therapists who may not have access to metabolic testing apparatus, HR is often a more feasible way of measuring maximal exercise capacity.[110]

Tantucci and colleagues[111] found that there was no significant increase in the metabolic cost of exercise for patients with mild MS (EDSS score 0–2). This may have been attributed to minimal spasticity or ataxia. However, there was a significant increase in $\dot{V}E$ at rest and during exercise that could not be explained. In addition, Morrison et al. (2008) found that despite greater reported fatigue levels, participants with MS showed similar RPE and physiologic responses to submaximal and maximal exercise compared with controls.[112] All participants underwent a graded aerobic exercise test on a cycle ergometer with breath-by-breath gas measurements and continuous HR monitoring. After completing the modified fatigue impact scale, participants rated their effort sense every 30 seconds during exercise using the modified Borg 10-point scale. The two study groups showed similar baseline characteristics except for higher fatigue scores in the MS group. There were no significant differences for any fitness measure, including oxygen cost slope. Neither HR nor RPE—measured at 25%,

50%, 75%, and 100% of $\dot{V}O_{2peak}$ peak—differed between groups. Therefore, the Borg 10-point scale may help improve evidence-based exercise prescriptions, which otherwise may be limited by fatigue, motor impairment, heat sensitivity, or autonomic dysfunction.

Temperature sensitivity should be assessed before exercise testing and training. This can be done through patient interviews to determine a past history of temperature sensitivity or through tympanic membrane thermometry during moderate-to-high exercise intensities. Measures should be taken before, during, and after exercise. This will allow for the determination of tolerable exercise intensities. HR and BP should be monitored because of the potential presence of autonomic cardioregulatory dysfunction.

Interventions for Exercise Training

There is a paucity of information in the literature concerning appropriate exercise rehabilitation for individuals with MS. Previous reports have indicated that there are no deleterious effects of exercise on the disease course of MS,[113] implying that individuals with MS can participate in exercise. In fact, limited studies of aerobic exercise in patients with MS have shown increases in cardiorespiratory and muscular functioning.[110] Although incorrect exercise may increase fatigue in subjects with MS, it also may decrease fatigue if performed at an appropriate intensity.

Exercise programs have also not been shown to improve the course of the disease process in most patients. This may be due to the generalized nonspecific low-intensity exercise programs that are typically given to patients with MS.[80] These individuals may begin exercising too late in the progression of the disease, exercise at too low or too high intensity, or perform the exercise incorrectly. It has been shown that persons with MS can lose up to 75% of their muscle strength before typical clinical tools detect it.

If possible, exercises should be initiated early on in the disease process when the greatest gains in strength and endurance can be achieved before the onset of severe disability. Exercises should focus on maintenance and when possible, on increasing flexibility, strength, and endurance. It appears that these kinds of exercises can be performed safely and should help to combat the effects of deconditioning.

The manner in which an exercise program progresses or regresses varies among individuals. During a remission, patients can generally maintain and even increase the intensity of the exercise program, and a new exercise baseline should be established for each remission. Likewise, if a patient is undergoing an exacerbation, the exercise intensity should be reduced. The use of an HR monitor can be an easy guide to help the patient maintain the appropriate exercise intensity. If a patient has significant dysautonomia, other ratings, such as RPE, may be useful for the patient to use in guiding exercise intensity; however, these ratings may not be valid when there are significant cognitive deficits.

Patients should be encouraged to hydrate before, during, and after exercise and should be provided fans when needed to prevent overheating. Precooling, or immersing heat-sensitive patients in cool water before exercise, tends to produce greater increases in physical work and greater comfort, when compared with a noncooled control group.[114] The Schwinn Air-Dyne cycle may be useful because it blows cool air on the user. However, the rise in temperature should not exceed approximately 9°F. Aquatic exercise may also be useful if the water temperature is maintained around 90°F. Considerations should be made for possible cognitive deficits such as memory loss. Writing home instructions will ensure better compliance with prescribed exercises.[110] Expiratory muscle function may also improve if respiratory muscle training is a part of the exercise program. This may subsequently improve exercise capacity and cough efficiency, thus preventing pulmonary complications associated with MS.[115]

Exercise intensity should fall between 60% and 85% of peak HR and between 50% and 70% $\dot{V}O_{2peak}$ for three sessions a week at 30 minutes each for 4 to 6 months.[101] Generally, those patients who have minimal impairments have the best exercise tolerance. Complaints of muscular or general fatigue should not last longer than 30 minutes. If it does, this may indicate that the exercise intensity was too high, indicating a need for subsequent adjustment of intensity at the next session.

The effectiveness of a home aerobic exercise program on exercise capacity was studied by Schapiro and colleagues.[116] The 50 subjects with mild-to-moderate MS participated in 16 weeks of a home program for 15 to 30 minutes per day, 4 to 5 times per week. The exercises were not supervised and their intensity was not controlled. The results showed that there was a 10% increase in maximal workload on the bicycle ergometer test following the intervention. It was noted that those subjects with lower baseline EDSS scores (1.0–3.5) had better results (greater peak workloads and exercise times) than those subjects with EDSS scores greater than 3.5.

Gehlsen and colleagues[117] studied the effects of a 10-week aquatic exercise program on 10 ambulatory subjects with MS. Lower extremity peak torque, work, and fatigue in knee flexors and extensors were determined with a Cybex dynamometer. Upper-limb muscular force, work, fatigue, and power were determined using a biokinetic swim bench. After subjects participated in freestyle swimming and shallow-water calisthenics three times per week for 1 hour per session, an increase in peak knee extensor torque from baseline to the midpoint of the training was measured. No such training effect at the knee was found at 10 weeks. However, reduction in systemic fatigue and total work improved significantly after 10 weeks. The upper limbs showed increased muscle function from pre- to postintervention; however, there was no change in upper-limb fatigue levels.

One uncontrolled study reported on five patients with MS who completed a 4- to 6-week lower-limb endurance training program.[118] Very low resistance was used by all subjects, who performed three sets of 10 repetitions of knee flexion at each exercise session. The results showed that subjects demonstrated

a decreased perception of peripheral fatigue, an increased perception of well-being, and higher peak knee flexor torque levels after the exercise program.

Petajan and colleagues[119] conducted a randomized controlled trial of 15 weeks of aerobic exercise on 54 subjects with mild-to-moderate MS (EDSS ≤ 6.0) to examine its effects on $\dot{V}O_{2max}$ and isometric strength. The exercise group exercised three times per week for 40 minutes per session. The exercise group showed significant increases in $\dot{V}O_{2max}$ (22%), physical work capacity (48%), and upper- and lower-extremity strength. Typically, in the MS population, decreased $\dot{V}O_{2max}$, HR_{max}, and workload are affected by the disease process.[120]

Gappmaier and colleagues[121] studied the effect of a 15-week aerobic exercise program on fitness, strength, body composition, and lipid profiles in patients with MS. There was a 20% increase in maximal exercise capacity and maximal isometric force of the prime movers activated during cycle ergometry. The authors recommended exercise that combines upper- and lower-limb work because it appears to allow patients to compensate for deficits involving primarily the lower limbs. Table 14-9 summarizes exercise training studies relevant to patients with MS.

Influence of Medications on Ability to Exercise

Patients with MS may have amantadine HCL prescribed to temporarily reduce fatigue. Amantadine HCL, fluoxetine HCL, and hyoscyamine sulfate may also cause muscle weakness. Baclofen is often prescribed to reduce spasticity but in high doses may worsen muscle weakness and fatigue. Prednisone, prescribed as an anti-inflammatory, may also cause muscle weakness, reduced sweating, hypertension, diabetes, and/or osteoporosis. Consideration of these medications, as they relate to exercise prescription, is important. Questioning the patient and confirming with the neurologist optimize care when monitoring medications for patients with MS.

Other Responses to Exercise

There may be attenuated HR, BP, or sudomotor responses that require careful monitoring and hydration during exercise. Such exercise should take place in a temperature-controlled room. Also, it has been shown that physical activity may decrease the risk of developing other chronic health conditions[119] such as CAD. There is usually significant weight gain after the onset of MS because of inactivity and sudomotor medications. Exercises that maintain or increase muscle mass may halt weight gain and reduce fat mass. Gappmaier and colleagues[121] found favorable body composition changes with 15 weeks of exercise training, which was sufficient to achieve or maintain proper body weight and a normalization of certain lipid profiles. Weight loss has a psychological benefit but also has an important functional benefit. Patients with MS who are overweight or obese and are moderately to severely disabled have a greater chance of exacerbating fatigue due to the effort required for mobility. Depression may affect exercise

TABLE 14-9   Summary of Exercise Training Studies for Patients with MS

Author	Pathology	Exercise Modality	Exercise Intensity	Exercise Frequency and Duration
Mulcare[110]	MS	NT[a]	60% to 85% peak HR	3 ×/wk for 30 min for 4–6 mo
Schapiro et al. (1988)[116]	MS	Home exercises and bicycle ergometry testing	NT	4–5 ×/wk for 15–30 minutes for 16 wk
Gehlsen et al.[117]	MS	Aquatic exercise	NT	3 ×/wk for 1 h 10 wk
Svensson et al.[118]	MS	Lower-limb strengthening	Low resistance	3 sets of 10 repetitions for 4–6 wk
Petajan et al.[119]	MS	Aerobic exercise and oxygen capacity and isometric strength tests	NT	3 ×/wk for 40 min for 15 wk
Gappmaier et al.[121]	MS	Aerobic exercise Isometric and exercise capacity tests	NT	15 wk

HR, heart rate; MS, multiple sclerosis; NT, not tested or not reported.

adherence, so constant reinforcement to sustain the exercise regimen is necessary for some patients.

General Effects of Exercise Training on Impairment, Disability, and Quality of Life

Fatigue often leads to a reduction in physical activity. This leads to muscle atrophy and weakness, decreases in flexibility, cardiovascular deficits, sleep abnormalities, increases in depression and anxiety levels, and ultimately, more fatigue. By increasing physical activity levels, even in a chronic disabling disease, improvements in physical and psychosocial factors can be obtained.

Petajan and associates[119] demonstrated that there was a decrease in depression, anger, and fatigue after aerobic exercise. This controlled study demonstrated that moderate aerobic exercise could improve physiological function, emotional behavior, fatigue levels, and daily activity functioning.

Aerobic exercise and strengthening have the potential of benefiting patients with MS. Although aerobic exercise can cause an increase in temperature and strengthening muscles can cause muscle fatigue, these effects can be minimized when the exercises are performed correctly. Therefore, it is important to develop exercises that take into consideration the symptoms (especially muscular fatigue and weakness) and pathophysiology of the disease, while maintaining or increasing the functional independence and functional capabilities of the individuals. Because of the early age of onset of MS, the goal should be to maintain functional independence, limit disability, and maintain a high QOL.

Parkinson Disease (Practice Patterns 5A, 5E, 6B, 6E, 7A; *ICD-9-CM* Code: 332)

Parkinson disease (PD) is a progressive neurological disease of the extrapyramidal system. There is an associated reduc-tion in endogenous dopamine, a neurotransmitter primarily located in the substantia nigra of the basal ganglia. Loss of dopamine results in *bradykinesia* (slowness of movement), tremor at rest, rigidity, and gait and postural deformities. Gait is usually described as slow, shuffling, and *festinating* (involuntary hurrying). With more severe PD, freezing or the inability to continue or initiate walking, especially when passing through doors and narrow spaces, is predominant. Standing posture is characterized by increased kyphosis, and the hips, knees, and elbows are maintained in the flexed position. The Hoehn and Yahr[122] scale is used to classify severity of PD. This scale is illustrated in Table 14-10. The Unified Parkinson's Disease Rating Scale (UPDRS) is a PD behavioral rating scale consisting of four categories: (1) mentation, behavior, and mood, (2) ADL both on and off medication, (3) motor examination, and (4) complications of therapy in the previous week. This scale is used to track PD longitudinally and is evaluated by interview. Total disability is 199 and 0 represents no disability. This scale, although more complicated, has supplanted the Hoehn and Yahr scale.

Factors That Influence Ability to Exercise

Exercise response studies are fraught with the problem of both significant variability between patients and medication levels. The autonomic nervous system can be dysfunctional in PD, where there may be problems with thermoregulation. Therefore, sweating patterns as well as HR and BP responses should be monitored during exercise.

Muscular rigidity can reduce exercise efficiency. Walking limitations can even produce falls during treadmill exercise. Overground walking where rapid turns are involved can result in loss of balance in more severe cases. Because of inefficient gait patterns, higher HRs and increased oxygen consumption may be evident during exercise. If a patient is severely kyphotic,

TABLE 14-10   Hoehn and Yahr Grades

Stage I	Unilateral involvement only, usually with minimal or no functional impairment.
Stage II	Bilateral or midline involvement, without impairment of balance.
Stage III	First sign of impaired righting reflexes. This is evident by unsteadiness as the patient turns, or is demonstrated when he or she is pushed from standing equilibrium with feet together and eyes closed. Functionally, the patient is somewhat restricted in his or her activities but may have some work potential, depending on type of employment. Patients are physically capable of leading independent lives, and their disability is mild to moderate.
Stage IV	Fully developed, severely disabling disease; the patient is still able to walk and stand unassisted but is markedly incapacitated.
Stage V	Confinement to bed or wheelchair unless aided.

Hoehn MM, Yahr MD. Parkinsonism: Onset, progression, mortality. *Neurology.* 1967;17:427-442.

lung capacity and thereby exercise capacity may be further reduced.

Tests and Measures for Exercise Testing

Patients who have balance or freezing problems should not be tested on a treadmill; a cycle ergometer is a safe alternative unless there is an overhead harness support to prevent injury from potential near falls. When metabolic exercise testing is indicated, it may be advisable to use a mask rather than a mouthpiece because of the patient's inability to coordinate oral musculature. If patients with PD are in the age group where they are at risk for CVD, appropriate precautions regarding ECG and physician monitoring should be considered. Most importantly, if more than one exercise test is going to be conducted, the time of day and time after medication during "on" or "off" periods should remain consistent. Preferably, testing should begin 45 minutes to 1 hour after medication has been taken. Some patients experience peak-dose tachycardia and dyskinesias. Appropriate cardiac and physical supervision is necessary. Skidmore et al. reported in a pilot study an asymptomatic drop of >20 mm Hg during treadmill exercise in 8 of 9 patients with PD participating in treadmill exercise, indicating a need for autonomic monitoring.[123] Caution should be used when testing individuals who have had a recent change in medication because their physiological performance may be unpredictable. Optimally, if the exercise performance of patients with PD fluctuates significantly on medication, testing should be done both on and off medication to determine exercise response ranges.

Reuter and colleagues[124] studied the cardiovascular performance and metabolic response in 15 patients with PD after exercise training using a cycle ergometer ramp protocol exercise test. The results did not show differences in cardiovascular adaptation to physical work in these patients compared with their healthy counterparts. Therefore, it should be possible to improve cardiovascular endurance in patients with PD.

Stanley and colleagues[125] compared the cardiopulmonary function of individuals with PD to that of healthy normals (HN) on a stationary bicycle by using an incremental exercise protocol. For men and women, there were no significant differences in $\dot{V}O_{2max}$ between those having PD and the HN. Likewise, there was no significant difference in time to achieve a maximal effort. Patients with PD reached their $\dot{V}O_{2max}$ earlier than did HN, indicating that individuals with PD may be less efficient during exercise.

Canning and associates[126] evaluated the exercise capacity of 16 subjects with mild-to-moderate PD to determine whether abnormalities in respiratory function and gait affect exercise capacity. Subjects were categorized according to exercise history, disease severity, and presence/absence of upper airway obstruction. Subjects performed a maximum exercise test on a cycle ergometer, together with respiratory function tests and a walking test. $\dot{V}O_{2peak}$ and peak workloads achieved by subjects with PD were not significantly different from normal values, despite evidence of respiratory and gait abnormalities typical of PD. Sedentary subjects produced scores lower than exercising subjects. Despite their neurological deficit, individuals with mild-to-moderate PD have the potential to maintain normal exercise capacity with regular aerobic exercise.

Protas and colleagues[127] studied the aerobic capacity of eight individuals with PD. This study (1) compared maximal exercise performance in individuals with and without PD, (2) compared exercise performance during upper and lower extremity exercise, and (3) described submaximal exercise responses. Subjects performed a lower extremity ergometer test (LE test) and an arm-crank ergometry test. Peak power was less for the PD group than for the control group for both tests. Submaximal HR and oxygen consumption were higher for the PD group than for the control group. The authors concluded that individuals with mild-to-moderate PD can be tested with both exercise protocols to peak exercise capacity and that there are differences in upper and lower extremity peak power and submaximal responses among persons with and without PD.

Werner et al. (2006) studied differences in vital signs and RPE between 16 individuals with PD compared with a group of healthy individuals during treadmill exercise test (modified Bruce protocol).[128] HR, systolic BP, and the RPE were measured at submaximal exercise (defined as stage 2 of the modified Bruce protocol) and at peak exercise (defined as 85% of age-predicted target HR). During submaximal exercise, no significant differences were found between the PD group and the control group; however, at peak exercise, one half of the subjects with PD exhibited blunted cardiovascular responses (HR, BP, or RPE), despite reaching a comparable intensity of exercise thus displaying abnormal cardiovascular responses at the higher exercise intensities. This exercise protocol could help guide the exercise prescription using BP, HR, and RPE as the rate-limiting parameters.

Interventions for Exercise Training

Exercise training is generally designed to reduce the indirect effects of inactivity and immobility associated with PD but may not affect the disease process directly, for example, tremor and rigidity. Because this disease is progressive, exercise interventions should not be short-term; rather, exercise should become part of the everyday lifestyle. Most clinicians and researchers believe that physical therapy should begin as soon as the diagnosis is made to prevent muscle atrophy, weakness, and reduced exercise capacity.[118]

CLINICAL CORRELATE

In some cases, patients with PD may display bradycardia in response to aerobic exercise activity, making it difficult to reach the target heart rate. Heart rates can be extremely variable and should be monitored closely during exercise. In this case, the rating of perceived exertion should be used to identify exercise intensity. Exercise is best planned at the same time after medication intake to maximize its benefit. In some cases, motor planning and memory may be impaired and repeated demonstrations along with written and visual cues are needed to ensure adherence. Exercise groups can also avoid the feelings of isolation so prevalent in patients with PD.[127]

Koseoglu and colleagues[129] studied the effects of exercise training, as a part of a pulmonary rehabilitation program, on pulmonary function tests and exercise tolerance including subjective RPE among patients with PD and nine age-matched healthy controls. After the training program, there was an improvement in some pulmonary function test parameters, exercise tolerance, and RPE for patients with PD.

Skidmore et al. (2008) conducted a pilot study where they evaluated the safety and feasibility of a 3-month progressive treadmill aerobic exercise (TM-AEX) program for persons with PD with gait impairment.[123] Eight subjects underwent a treadmill stress test to determine eligibility, of which three were referred for further cardiac evaluation and five were

enrolled. In 136 subjects, treadmill aerobic exercise sessions significantly improved the subjects' total UPDRS scores and peak ambulatory workload capacities. The results of this study suggested that an aerobic exercise program is feasible for persons who have PD and gait impairments as long as precautions are taken to prevent falls through the use of an overhead harness. Thus, this pilot study shows promise that treadmill aerobic exercise may reduce symptom severity and improve fitness for persons with PD.

Kurtais et al. (2008) studied whether gait training on a treadmill would improve functional tasks of lower extremities in patients with PD.[130] Twenty-four patients diagnosed with idiopathic PD were enrolled in group I, where they attended a training program on a treadmill for 6 weeks, or group II that served as the control group. Both groups were instructed in home mobility exercises. The primary study outcome measures were timed functional lower extremity tasks and the secondary outcome measures were exercise tests and patient's global assessment. Graded exercise tests (Naughton protocol) were performed on a treadmill. There were significant improvements in exercise test parameters in the exercise group only which carried over to the functional lower extremity activities. Specifically, $\dot{V}O_2$, exercise duration, and METS improved significantly in the exercise group, indicating a benefit of treadmill training on fitness in persons with PD.

Schenkman and colleagues (2008) described three case reports of patients with early PD who completed 4 months of supervised endurance exercise training and 12 months of home exercise, with monthly clinic follow-up sessions for 16 months.[131] The main outcome measure was economy of movement (rate of oxygen consumption during gait) measured at four treadmill speeds. One secondary outcome measure included the UPDRS among others. Economy of movement improved for all three patients and remained above baseline at 16 months. Two patients also had scores that were above baseline for UPDRS total score, even at 16 months. The authors concluded that their study suggested that gains might occur with a treadmill training program that is coupled with specific strategies to enhance adherence to exercise.

Influence of Medications on Ability to Exercise

Medications have been the best way to treat PD to correct dopamine imbalances, decreased epinephrine and norepinephrine, and increased acetylcholine. The most common drugs are dopaminergics like Sinemet, anticholinergics, and monoamine oxidase type B inhibitors. Side effects include upset stomach, confusion, delusional states, and insomnia. Long-term use can actually produce movement disorders such as dyskinesias. Unfortunately, there is a declining effect of these drugs over the years. Drug absorption can be reduced by strenuous exercise, use of anticholinergic drugs, autonomic nervous system dysfunction, food intake, protein and iron supplements, and aerobic fitness.[132]

Enhanced fatigue on performance of motor tasks is a very frequent and disabling complaint of patients with PD and is poorly characterized and understood. Ziv and colleagues[133] found that increased muscle fatigue should be recognized as an integral part of the spectrum of motor impairment of PD and is associated with a central dopamine deficiency.

LeWitt and colleagues[134] studied weakness, easy fatiguing, and lack of endurance perceived by patients with PD. Although the slowed motor repertoire in PD may underlie these experiences, other abnormalities in skeletal muscle utilization may also be involved. The authors investigated whether an index of metabolic efficiency during a continuous exercise task, the latency until anaerobic threshold (AT), is altered by levodopa (LD) while pedaling a bicycle ergometer against a uniform workload. When compared to an unmedicated state, LD treatment delayed anaerobic threshold. Subjects did not differ in their perceived exertion upon reaching anaerobic threshold. In addition to relief of symptoms by LD, the efficiency of energy utilization in exercising skeletal muscle is also increased.

Goetz and colleagues[135] studied 10 regular exercising men with PD on LD under two conditions—at rest and during vigorous exercise started 1 hour after LD ingestion. There was a high degree of agreement between plasma LD level and the patients' disability scores 30 minutes later under both conditions, with no difference between the two. The authors concluded that LD levels accurately reflect disability and motor function in these patients and that vigorous exercise, started 1 hour after LD ingestion, does not influence LD or motor scores.

Carter and colleagues[136] studied the effect of exercise, using cycle ergometry on LD absorption in 10 patients with PD. Oral LD was administered during exercise and at rest on separate days. Exercise-delayed LD absorption in five patients increased it in three and did not influence it in two. The authors concluded that exercise can either increase or decrease LD absorption. Further research is needed on the exercise effects of CD in PD.

Other Responses to Exercise

Comella and colleagues[137] conducted a randomized, single-blind, crossover study, evaluating physical disability in patients with moderately advanced PD after 4 weeks of normal physical activity and after 4 weeks of an intensive physical rehabilitation program. Following physical rehabilitation, there was significant improvement in ADL and motor scores, but there was no change in the mentation score. During the 6 months following physical rehabilitation, patients did not exercise regularly, and the disability scores returned to baseline. The authors concluded that physical disability in patients with moderately advanced PD objectively improves with a regular physical rehabilitation program, but this improvement is not sustained when normal activity is resumed.

Inzelberg et al. (2005) found a reduction in the perception of dyspnea (POD) of individuals with PD when inspiratory muscle training was performed six times per week for 30 min-

utes for 3 months compared with a control group who received a sham treatment.[138] The investigators evaluated the effect of this inspiratory muscle training on pulmonary functions, inspiratory muscle performance, dyspnea, and QOL in patients with PD. Following the training period, there was a significant improvement in the training group but not in the control group, in inspiratory muscle strength, inspiratory muscle endurance, and the perception of dyspnea. Patients with PD who can achieve reductions in dyspnea may improve their QOL or the willingness to engage in activity without experiencing shortness of breath, especially for those activities that require a large effort.[139]

General Effects of Exercise Training on Impairment, Disability, and Quality of Life

Reuter and colleagues[140] studied the influence of intensive exercise training on motor disability, mood, and subjective well-being in patients with PD over a 20-week period. Sixteen slightly to moderately affected idiopathic patients with PD received intensive exercise training twice weekly. They found that motor disability as well as mood and subjective well-being can be significantly improved by intensive sports activities in early- to medium-stage PD patients.

Kuroda and colleagues[141] reported on data obtained from public health nurse visits, including a 1-year follow-up for 438 patients with PD living in Japan. The follow-up period averaged 4.1 years, during which 71 deaths were observed. The patients were classified according to the degree of physical exercise they performed, and the ratios of observed to expected deaths were calculated. The exercising group showed the lowest ratio for patients able to walk independently compared with that for those who could not.

Sasco and colleagues[142] conducted a case control study of patients with PD. Physical exercise was conducted in a cohort of 50,002 men who attended either Harvard College or the University of Pennsylvania between 1916 and 1950, and who were followed up in adulthood for morbidity and mortality. Cases of PD were identified from responses to mailed questionnaires and death certificates through 1978. The association between physical activity at the time of college and subsequent risk of PD was evaluated. Those playing on a varsity sports team or participating in regular physical exercise in college were associated with a lower though nonsignificant risk of PD. In adulthood, participation of moderate or heavy sports activities was linked to a reduced risk. These results, which require further confirmation, are compatible with a slight protective effect of physical exercise on the risk of PD, although the lack of association cannot be refuted.

Schenkman and colleagues[143] reported that task-specific training in addition to aerobic exercise may be more beneficial than standard exercise training. Future research is needed to evaluate the effects of adding external cues, cognitive strategies, task-specific training, and environmental modifications to aerobic exercise for people with PD.

Rodriques de Paula et al. (2006) evaluated changes in different domains of QOL for 20 persons with PD (stages 1–3 on the Hoehn and Yahr scale) after a program of physical activity consisting of 36 group sessions of aerobic conditioning and muscular strengthening.[144] QOL was measured using the Nottingham Health Profile, a generic questionnaire composed of six domains. There were significant gains associated with the program on the total score and those related to emotional reactions (ER), social interactions (SI), and physical ability (PA). Social interaction was the domain that showed the greatest program gains (41.4%). The authors concluded that a light-to-moderate intensity program of physical activity resulted in improvements in their perception of QOL.

Herman et al. (2007) conducted a study of QOL with nine patients with PD who participated in intensive treadmill training four times per week for 30 minutes, each session for 6 weeks. QOL was measured using the Parkinson's Disease Questionnaire (PDQ-39). The PDQ-39 is the most widely used PD-specific measure of health status. It contains 39 questions, covering eight aspects of QOL including mobility, ADL, emotions, stigma, social support, cognitions, communication, and bodily discomfort. The instrument was developed on the basis of interviews with people diagnosed with the disease. Herman and colleagues found that the PDQ significantly improved as a result of the intensive treadmill training from a score of 32 to 22.[145]

Guillain–Barré Syndrome (Practice Patterns 4A, 5E, 5H, 6B, 6E, 7A, 7B, 7C; *ICD-9-CM* Codes: 341, 344)

Guillain–Barré syndrome (GBS) is an autoimmune disorder of the peripheral nervous system causing progressive weakness of limbs with diminished/absent tendon reflexes and has no known etiology. This inflammatory process affects the Schwann cells. The process of remyelination occurs rapidly. The patient may also experience secondary axonal damage. The regrowth rate is slow: approximately 1 mm/d. Despite profound deficits and paralysis, there is a 65% chance of full recovery.[146]

Factors That Influence Ability to Exercise

Physical therapists must consider issues of overwork, avoidance of eccentric contractions, and performance of antigravity muscle training before progressing to the addition of weights. Overwork weakness is a prolonged deficit in the absolute strength and endurance of a muscle as a result of excessive activity.[147] Because GBS affects the peripheral nerve, motor unit recruitment is impaired, leaving fewer muscle fibers available to provide sufficient force during exercise. This puts these muscle fibers at risk for overwork.

Tests and Measures for Exercise Testing

To avoid muscle damage or overuse weakness, maximal exercise testing is not recommended. Submaximal tests like those recommended by Noonan and Dean[148] may be possible once a patient has passed the acute phase of recovery. Testing

should include rest intervals and evaluation of reports of muscle soreness. For example, a therapist should compare reports of muscle soreness immediately after exercise and after a weekend of rest. Repeated muscle testing across days should corroborate whether muscle weakness is increasing, thus requiring additional rest. Initially, rest periods should be frequent. As the patient continues to recover, demonstrated by a reduction in complaints of soreness and weakness, rest periods may be withdrawn and continuous exercise instituted.

There should be a general avoidance of eccentric muscle strengthening and an emphasis on fast-twitch muscle fiber recruitment, such as that obtained from fast contraction concentric exercise on an isokinetic dynamometer. Other functional tasks often involve eccentric contractions and should be avoided if soreness and weakness increase.

Potential Physiological Responses to Exercise

Ropper and Wijdicks studied a 76-year-old man with severe GBS, who demonstrated extremes of hypotension alternating with hypertension.[149] The BP paralleled both systemic vascular resistance and cardiac output. HR, rather than stroke volume, was the major determinant of cardiac output over a wide range of BPs. These findings suggest that hypotension resulted from a vasodepressor response with a vagotomized heart and that hypertension was the result of increased sympathetic activity. Both extremes were caused by parallel changes in vascular resistance and HR. Dysfunction of baroreflex buffering may have accounted for the rapid swings in pressure. The authors caution that BP should be monitored before, during, and after exercise to avoid hypo- or hypertensive reactions.

Interventions for Exercise Training

Pitetti et al.[150] reported a case study of an individual who had residual deficits following an acute incidence of GBS to determine if there would be improved physiological adaptations following aerobic endurance training. A 57-year-old man, who for 3 years needed the aid of a crutch for walking, following an acute bout of GBS, participated in this study. Peak work level (W), oxygen consumption, and ventilation were determined on a bicycle ergometer, a Schwinn Air-Dyne ergometer (SAE), and an arm-crank ergometry before and after exercise training. The subject trained for 16 weeks at an approximate frequency of 3 d/wk at an average duration of 30 minutes and at an average intensity of 75% to 80% of pretraining peak HR.

Approximately a 10% improvement was seen in $\dot{V}O_{2peak}$ for the SAE and bicycle ergometer, respectively. For peak ventilation, a 23% and 11% improvement was seen for the SAE and bicycle ergometer, respectively. For the arm-crank ergometry, a 16% increase in peak ventilation was seen, with no improvement in aerobic capacity. Total work capacity on the bicycle ergometer was improved by 29% following training. This study demonstrated that patients with GBS may be able to improve cardiopulmonary function and work capacity following a supervised training program using the SAE. The subject also reported improvements in ADL.

It is the peripheral denervation process that links GBS to polio and peripheral neuropathy. Irreversible weakness is believed to be due to muscle damage in patients who are postpolio following strenuous activity. In fact, animal studies have demonstrated short-term detrimental responses to intense exercise on the reinnervation of myelinated fibers. Therefore, physical therapists are cautioned against overworking skeletal muscles of patients with GBS.

Postpolio Syndrome (Practice Patterns 4A, 5H, 5G, 6B, 6E, 7A, 7B, 7C; *ICD-9-CM* Codes: 344, 357.4)

Poliomyelitis is an acute viral disease that attacks the brain and the ventral horn of the spinal cord. Damage to the lower motor neurons usually results in atrophy and weakness of muscle groups, perhaps paralysis and possibly deformity. A second type, bulbar poliomyelitis, infects the medulla oblongata and may result in dysfunction of the swallowing mechanism along with respiratory and circulatory distress. Minor forms of poliomyelitis result in fever, sore throat, headache, and upper-body stiffness, but leave no significant atrophy or paralysis.

The most common features of *postparalytic syndrome* (PPS) for more than 350,000 afflicted survivors include general fatigue, weakness, and joint/muscle pain. The primary reasons for these symptoms include (1) destruction of the anterior horn cells by the polio virus, leaving fewer motor neurons to induce muscle contraction; (2) unaffected motor unit enlargement by reinnervation through terminal sprouting; and (3) defective transmission at the neuromuscular junction secondary to failure of terminal axonal sprout.

Postpolio syndrome is a group of related signs and symptoms occurring in people who had paralytic poliomyelitis years earlier. New weakness, fatigue, poor endurance, pain, reduced mobility, increased breathing difficulty, intolerance to cold, and sleep disturbance in various degrees and expressions make up the syndrome. The reported incidence is between 25% and 80%. The origins are multifactorial and can be associated with underexertion, overexertion, inactivity due to intercurrent illness or injury, hypo-oxygenation, sleep apnea, deconditioning, and the failure of sprouted, compensatory large motor units. The exercise question in postpolio syndrome is related to the experience of new weakness or loss of muscle function due to overuse, which is often associated with injudicious repeated challenges to weakened musculature. Carefully prescribed exercise can be used for increasing strength and endurance and improving cardiopulmonary conditioning.

Birk (1993) reviewed the literature involving postpolio syndrome and exercise. The authors concluded that acute responses to resistive exercise suggest significant muscle strength decrements in the knee extensors of individuals with polio compared with similar-aged people without polio. Although there is extremely limited research on training studies, there is a suggestion that low-level training induces significant strength increases for the following at least 6 weeks of training. This should not imply that only the knee extensors are weakened in the lower extremities; however, training research is limited to this muscle group. Birk also reported that acute aerobic responses of individuals with polio also differ significantly from those observed in age-matched control studies. Studies of aerobic training suggest the potential of significant elevations in maximal oxygen uptake.[151]

The manifestations of postpolio syndrome typically occur between 20 and 40 years after an acute episode of poliomyelitis and are confined to previously affected muscles. Because of motor unit remodeling and direct mechanical damage, weakness increases in individual muscles until it exceeds their narrow margin of reserve and becomes clinically apparent. Although the exact cause is not clear, generalized weakness often occurs when several muscles are affected and various postural limb strategies used by the patient are no longer able to compensate for the loss of muscle strength. **The mainstays of treatment are lifestyle changes to avoid overexertion and use of lightweight orthoses and assistive aids to unload the extremities.**[152]

Factors That Influence Ability to Exercise

Weinberg and colleagues[153] evaluated the factors limiting exercise performance and analyzed the respiratory strategies adopted during exercise in five patients postpolio with severe inspiratory muscle dysfunction at rest and during leg or arm cycle exercise. Gas exchange was measured by arterial blood gas analysis and mass spectrometry of expired air. Ventilatory mechanics were studied by measurement of esophageal and gastric pressures. Blood gases at rest were found to be normal, except for subnormal partial pressure of oxygen (Po_2) levels in three patients. In all but one patient, ventilatory insufficiency was the limiting factor for exercise. A compensatory breathing pattern with abdominal muscle recruitment during expiration was present at rest in three of the patients. The pressures generated by the diaphragm were below the fatigue threshold, that is, the level that can be sustained for at least 45 minutes in healthy subjects. The extent of ventilatory dysfunction was evident in blood gas values during the exercise test. In summary, diaphragmatic fatigue seems to be avoided, but at the cost of impaired blood gases.

Willen and Grimby[154] described pain and its relationship to the effects of polio, physical activity, and disability of 32 individuals with late effects of polio. More than 50% of the individuals had pain every day, mostly during physical activity. In the lower limbs, cramping pain was the most common pain characteristic in both polio-affected and non–polio-affected limbs. In the upper limbs and in the trunk, aching pain was the most common pain characteristic, especially in the polio-affected areas. The degree of muscle weakness had no correlation to pain experience. The walking test demonstrated a relatively small difference between self-selected and maximal walking speed. Pain and physical mobility were both strongly correlated with energy expenditure. There is a relationship between physical activity in daily life and experience of pain. In many postpolio individuals who experience a high level of pain, self-selected and maximal walking speeds are approximately the same. **It is strongly recommended that individuals with late effects of polio, experiencing aching and especially cramping pain, modify their level of physical activity.**

Stanghelle et al.[155] studied subjective symptoms, medical and social situations, pulmonary function, and physical work capacity during a period of 3 to 5 years in patients with post-polio syndrome. The patients answered a questionnaire about their subjective symptoms and medical and social situations and underwent spirometry as well as symptom-limited exercise stress testing. Most patients experienced increasing symptoms and physical disability related to their polio, and the majority reported that their mental health was unchanged or improved. Lung function was, on average, moderately reduced and of the restrictive type, and only minor changes were found during 3 to 5 years. A pronounced reduction in peak oxygen uptake was seen at the first evaluation, especially among the women.

At the second examination, peak oxygen uptake was further decreased, especially in men, more than that predicted from increasing age. The patients increased their BMI significantly during the same period. These results indicate that subjective symptoms and physical disability related to polio increased with increasing age in these patients with the post-polio syndrome, and cardiorespiratory deconditioning and weight gain also became increasing problems in most patients. However, the mental status of the patients remained stable or improved, possibly due to a comprehensive re-rehabilitation and educational program.

Tests and Measures for Exercise Testing

Willen and associates[156] studied the physical performance in individuals with late effects of polio; specifically, they evaluated the effects of reduced muscle strength in the lower limbs. Thirty-two individuals performed a bicycle exercise test. Muscle strength in the quadriceps and the hamstrings was measured on an isokinetic dynamometer. Reductions in peak workload, peak oxygen uptake, and predicted HR were seen. The AT was within or slightly lower than normal limits in relation to predicted maximal oxygen uptake, indicating that the cardiorespiratory system was not limiting performance. Muscle testing of the test group demonstrated a significantly lower ability to perform muscle actions compared with individuals from a reference group, and strong correlations were found among muscle strength, peak $\dot{V}O_2$, and peak workload. It appears that adjusted peripheral muscle endurance training might improve the work capacity in those individuals with weak leg muscles and low oxygen uptake, whereas individuals with relatively good muscle strength would improve their aerobic fitness in a general fitness program.

Stanghelle and colleagues[155] studied 68 subjects who were admitted to a rehabilitation hospital with a presumptive post-polio syndrome who were examined with pulmonary function and symptom-limited exercise stress testing to study how many of these subjects could be classified as suffering from

cardiorespiratory deconditioning. The subjects had moderately reduced lung function of the restrictive type, and none of the subjects had forced expiratory volume for 1 second below 30% of predicted value, indicating that hypoventilation would probably not occur. A pronounced reduction in maximal oxygen uptake was seen, especially in women. The maximal HR values were above 70% of predicted values in all but one subject, indicating that subjects might benefit from endurance training. Fifteen subjects had a suspected pulmonary limitation due to the exercise, with the ratio of ventilation to maximal voluntary ventilation greater than 70%. These results indicate that cardiorespiratory deconditioning was considerable in most of the subjects with postpolio syndrome.

Interventions for Exercise Training

Recent studies have shown that judicious exercise can improve muscle strength, cardiorespiratory fitness, and the efficiency of ambulation in postpolio patients. It may also add to the patient's sense of well-being. These benefits appear to occur when patients stay within reasonable bounds while exercising to avoid overuse problems. In particular, patients should be instructed to avoid activities that cause increasing muscle or joint pain or excessive fatigue, either during or after their exercise program.

Patients seen in postpolio clinics frequently complain of new fatigue, weakness, muscle pain, and/or joint pain. The most frequent complaints involving ADL include new difficulties with walking and stair climbing. The therapeutic benefit of exercise to these patients is to minimize or reverse decline in function.

Patients with postpolio syndrome have unique problems, which need to be considered when prescribing an exercise program for an individual patient. A number of functional etiologies for declining function have been hypothesized including disuse weakness, overuse weakness, weight gain, and chronic weakness. Because of the variability in which the motor neurons to different muscle groups may have been affected in a particular patient, both asymmetric and scattered weaknesses may be present. The challenge in prescribing exercise for the patient with postpolio syndrome comes in recognizing these unique factors in each patient and modifying the prescription accordingly.

One must protect muscles and joints experiencing the adverse effects of overuse, and body areas with very significant chronic weakness, while exercising areas experience the deleterious effects of disuse. Weight gain is to be avoided if at all possible in this population because increased weight only leads to further difficulty in the performance of daily activities.

Kriz and colleagues[157] studied the cardiorespiratory responses of 10 subjects postpolio participating in a 16-week upper-extremity aerobic exercise program and compared them with 10 nonexercised controls. The subjects trained three times a week for 20 minutes per session. Exercise intensity was prescribed at 70% to 75% of HR reserve plus resting HR. After training, the exercise group had higher oxygen consumption, carbon dioxide production, $\dot{V}E$, power, and exercise time. There was no reported loss of muscle strength. It was concluded that subjects postpolio can safely achieve an increase in aerobic capacity with a properly modified upper-extremity exercise program. This improvement is comparable to that demonstrated by able-bodied adults.

Many individuals with disabilities may be unable to achieve maximal oxygen uptake in an exercise test, and maximal exercise testing may cause increased fatigue, pain, and muscle weakness. Sasco et al.[142] examined the role of submaximal exercise testing and training based on objective as well as subjective parameters in survivors of polio. Subjects participated in a 6-week exercise training program for 30 to 40 minutes, three times a week. The program consisted of treadmill walking at 55% to 70% of age-predicted maximum HRs; however, exercise intensity was modified to minimize discomfort/pain and fatigue. Neither objective nor subjective exercise responses were significantly different in the control group over the 6 weeks. No change was observed in cardiorespiratory conditioning in the experimental group. However, movement economy, which is related to the energy cost of walking, was significantly improved and walking duration was significantly increased at the end of training. Modified aerobic training may have a role in enhancing endurance and reducing fatigue during ADL in polio survivors.

A final study of clinically stable patients with dermatomyositis/polymyositis who underwent a long-term physical training program (6 months) improved muscle strength and increased aerobic capacity by 28% compared with untrained patients. The authors point out that physical training should be a part of their comprehensive rehabilitation management, particularly in view of the cardiopulmonary risk in these patients.[158]

General Effects of Exercise Training on Impairment, Disability, and Quality of Life

Oncu and colleagues (2009) were one of the first to investigate the impact of a hospital and a home exercise program on functional capacity ($\dot{V}O_2$), fatigue (fatigue severity score), and QOL (Nottingham Health Profile) on 32 patients with postpolio syndrome in Izmar, Turkey.[159] Half the patients each received either hospital or home aerobic exercise programs. Parameters of fatigue and QOL improved in both the home- and hospital-based exercise program, but the energy subscore on the Nottingham Health Profile improved only in the hospital exercise. Furthermore, the functional exercise capacity improved only in the hospital-based environment. This may have been attributable to the PT supervision of the program. Thus the authors concluded that the physical exercise with the goal of increasing functional capacity that leads to positive changes in fatigue and QOL should be conducted under supervision in a hospital environment. Since this health care delivery model may not be feasible in the United States, certainly the implementation of such an exercise program on an outpatient basis might have similar effects.

SUMMARY

Evidence of the potential effectiveness of exercise for neurological populations has been presented. Therapists should consider cardiopulmonary testing and training as part of their therapeutic armamentarium. Training neurological patients with respect to their cardiopulmonary system should lead to a reduction in coronary heart disease risk factors and improvement in other secondary conditions. This improvement in energetics will likely lead to improved functional status, community mobility, and QOL.

REFERENCES

1. World Health Organization. *The World Health Report: Reducing Risk and Promoting Healthy Life*. Geneva, Switzerland: World Health Organization; 2002:61-169.
2. Centers for Disease Control and Prevention. *Prevalence of Disabilities and Associated Health Conditions Among Adults—United States, 1999*. Atlanta, GA: Centers for Disease Control and Prevention; February 23, 2001.
3. D'Agostino RB, Russell MW, Huse DM, et al. Primary and subsequent coronary risk appraisal: new results from the Framingham study. *Am Heart J.* 2000;139:272-281. Erratum in: *Am Heart J* 2002 Jan;143(1):21.
4. Hu FB, Stampfer MJ, Colditz GA, et al. Physical activity and risk of stroke in women. *JAMA.* 2000;283(22):2961-2967.
5. Gillum RF, Mussolino ME, Ingram DD. Physical activity and stroke incidence in women and men. The NHANES I Epidemiologic Follow-up Study. *Am J Epidemiol.* 1996;143(9):860-869.
6. Shinton R. Lifelong exposures and the potential for stroke prevention: the contribution of cigarette smoking, exercise, and body fat. *J Epidemiol Community Health.* 1997;51(2):138-143.
7. Boone-Heinonen J, Evenson KR, Taber DR, Gordon-Larsen P. Walking for prevention of cardiovascular disease in men and women: a systematic review of observational studies. *Obes Rev.* 2009;10(2):204-217.
8. Kurth T, Moore S, Gaziano J, et al. Healthy lifestyle and the risk of stroke in women. *Arch Intern Med.* 2006;166(13):1403-1409.
9. Wendel-Vos G, Schuit A, Feskens E, et al. Physical activity and stroke: a meta-analysis of observational data. *Int J Epidemiol.* 2004;33(4):787-798.
10. Stein J. Stroke. In: Frontera WR, ed. *Exercise in Rehabilitation Medicine*. 1st ed. Illinois: Human Kinetics; 1999:306.
11. Roth EJ. Heart disease in patients with stroke: incidence, impact, and implications for rehabilitation. Part 1: classification and prevalence. *Arch Phys Med Rehabil.* 1993;74(7):752-760.
12. Bronner LL, Kanter DS, Manson JE. Primary prevention of stroke. *N Engl J Med.* 1995;333(21):1392-1400.
13. Ribera-Casado J. Aging and the cardiovascular system. *Z Gerontol Geriatr.* 1999;32(6):412-419.
14. Macko RF, Katzel LI, Yataco A, et al. Low-velocity graded treadmill stress testing in hemiparetic stroke patients. *Stroke.* 1997;28(5):988-992.
15. Ryan A, Nicklas B. Age-related changes in fat deposition in mid-thigh muscle in women: relationships with metabolic cardiovascular disease risk factors. *Int J Obes Relat Metab Disord.* 1999;23(2):126-132.
16. Heydrick D. In: Proceedings of the National Institutes of Health Conference on Engineering and Rehabilitation; 2001; Bethesda, MD.

17. Gerrits KH, Beltman MJ, Koppe PA, et al. Isometric muscle function of knee extensors and the relation with functional performance in patients with stroke. *Arch Phys Med Rehabil*. 2009;90(3):480-487.

18. Albers GW, Alberts MJ, Broderick JP, Lyden PD, Sacco RL. Recent advances in stroke management. *J Stroke Cerebrovasc Dis*. 2000;9(3):95-105.

19. Macko RF, Smith GV, Dobrovolny CL, Sorkin JD, Goldberg AP, Silver KH. Treadmill training improves fitness reserve in chronic stroke patients. *Arch Phys Med Rehabil*. 2001;82(7):879-884.

20. Monga TN, Deforge DA, Williams J, Wolfe LA. Cardiovascular responses to acute exercise in patients with cerebrovascular accidents. *Arch Phys Med Rehabil*. 1988;69(11):937-940.

21. Moldover JR, Daum MC, Downey JA. Cardiac stress testing of hemiparetic patients with a supine bicycle ergometer: preliminary study. *Arch Phys Med Rehabil*. 1984;65(8):470-473.

22. Mackay-Lyons MJ, Makrides L. Exercise capacity early after stroke. *Arch Phys Med Rehabil*. 2002;83(12):1697-1702.

23. Macko RF, DeSouza CA, Tretter LD, et al. Treadmill aerobic exercise training reduces the energy expenditure and cardiovascular demands of hemiparetic gait in chronic stroke patients. A preliminary report. *Stroke*. 1997;28(2):326-330.

24. King ML, Lichtman SW, Pellicone JT, Close RJ, Lisanti P. Exertional hypotension in spinal cord injury. *Chest*. 1994;106(4):1166-1171.

25. Potempa K, Braun LT, Tinknell T, Popovich J. Benefits of aerobic exercise after stroke. *Sports Med*. 1996;21(5):337-346.

26. Potempa K, Lopez M, Braun LT, Szidon JP, Fogg L, Tincknell T. Physiological outcomes of aerobic exercise training in hemiparetic stroke patients. *Stroke*. 1995;26(1):101-105.

27. Duncan P, Studenski S, Richards L, et al. Randomized clinical trial of therapeutic exercise in subacute stroke. *Stroke*. 2003;34(9):2173-2180.

28. Borg G. Psychological basis of physical exertion. *Med Sci Sports Exerc*. 1982;14:377.

29. Astrand I. Aerobic work capacity in men and women with special reference to age. *Acta Physiol Scand Suppl*. 1960;49(169):1-92.

30. Birkett WA, Edwards DF. The use of one-arm crank ergometry in the prediction of upper body aerobic capacity. *Clin Rehabil*. 1998;12(4):319-327.

31. Medicine ACoS. *ACSM Guidelines for Exercise Testing and Prescription*. 6th ed. Baltimore, MD: Williams & Wilkins; 1999.

32. Myers J, Buchanan N, Smith D, et al. Individualized ramp treadmill. Observations on a new protocol. *Chest*. 1992;101 (5 suppl):236S-241S.

33. Palmer-McClean K, Wilberger JE. *Exercise Management for persons with Chronic Diseases and Disabilities*. Champaign, IL: Human Kinetics; 1997.

34. Jones NL, Summers E, Killian KJ. Influence of age and stature on exercise capacity during incremental cycle ergometry in men and women. *Am Rev Respir Dis*. 1989;140(5):1373-1380.

35. Hansen JE, Sue D, Wasserman K. Predicted values for clinical exercise testing. *Am Rev Respir Dis*. 1984;129(2, pt 2):S49-S55.

36. Jones N, Makrides L, Hitchcock C. Normal standards for an incremental progressive cycle ergometer test. *Am Rev Respir Dis*. 1988;131:700-708.

37. Sue DY, Hansen JE. Normal values in adults during exercise testing. *Clin Chest Med*. 1984;5(1):89-98.

38. Billinger SA, Tseng BY, Kluding PM. Modified total-body recumbent stepper exercise test for assessing peak oxygen consumption in people with chronic stroke. *Phys Ther*. 2008;88(10):1188-1195.

39. Jakobsson F, Edstrom L, Grimby L, Thornell LE. Disuse of anterior tibial muscle during locomotion and increased proportion of type II fibres in hemiplegia. *J Neurol Sci*. 1991;105(1):49-56.

40. Tipton CM. Exercise, training and hypertension: an update. *Exerc Sport Sci Rev*. 1991;19:447-505.

41. Sunnerhagen KS, Svantesson U, Lonn L, Krotkiewski M, Grimby G. Upper motor neuron lesions: their effect on muscle performance and appearance in stroke patients with minor motor impairment. *Arch Phys Med Rehabil*. 1999;80(2):155-161.

42. Fletcher BJ, Dunbar SB, Felner JM, et al. Exercise testing and training in physically disabled men with clinical evidence of coronary artery disease. *Am J Cardiol*. 1994;73(2):170-174.

43. Rimmer JH, Rauworth AE, Wang EC, Nicola TL, Hill B. A preliminary study to examine the effects of aerobic and therapeutic (nonaerobic) exercise on cardiorespiratory fitness and coronary risk reduction in stroke survivors. *Arch Phys Med Rehabil*. 2009;90(3):407-412.

44. Hesse S, Uhlenbrock D, Sarkodie-Gyan T. Gait pattern of severely disabled hemiparetic subjects on a new controlled gait trainer as compared to assisted treadmill walking with partial body weight support. *Clin Rehabil*. 1999;13(5):401-410.

45. Visintin M, Barbeau H, Korner-Bitensky N, Mayo NE. A new approach to retrain gait in stroke patients through body weight support and treadmill stimulation. *Stroke*. 1998;29(6):1122-1128.

46. Janssen TW, Beltman JM, Elich P, et al. Effects of electric stimulation-assisted cycling training in people with chronic stroke. *Arch Phys Med Rehabil*. 2008;89(3):463-469.

47. Teixeira-Salmela LF, Olney SJ, Nadeau S, Brouwer B. Muscle strengthening and physical conditioning to reduce impairment and disability in chronic stroke survivors. *Arch Phys Med Rehabil*. 1999;80(10):1211-1218.

48. Duncan P, Richards L, Wallace D, et al. A randomized, controlled pilot study of a home-based exercise program for individuals with mild and moderate stroke. *Stroke*. 1998;29(10):2055-2060.

49. Tipton CM. Exercise training for the treatment of hypertension: a review. *Clin J Sport Med*. 1999;9(2):104.

50. Resnick B, Michael K, Shaughnessy M, et al. Inflated perceptions of physical activity after stroke: pairing self-report with physiologic measures. *J Phys Act Health*. 2008;5(2):308-318.

51. Kurabayashi H, Kubota K, Machida I, Tamura K, Take H, Shirakura T. Effects of physical therapy on immunological parameters in patients with cerebrovascular diseases. *J Med*. 1996;27(3-4):171-175.

52. Mast BT, MacNeill SE, Lichtenberg PA. Geropsychological problems in medical rehabilitation: dementia and depression among stroke and lower extremity fracture patients. *J Gerontol A Biol Sci Med Sci*. 1999;54(12):M607-M612.

53. Yoshida T, Kohzuki M, Yoshida K, et al. Physical and psychological improvements after phase II cardiac rehabilitation in patients with myocardial infarction. *Nurs Health Sci*. 1999;1(3):163-170.

54. Hamdy RC, Moore SW, Cancellaro VA, Harvill LM. Long-term effects of strokes on bone mass. *Am J Phys Med Rehabil*. 1995;74(5):351-356.

55. Silver KH, Macko RF, Forrester LW, Goldberg AP, Smith GV. Effects of aerobic treadmill training on gait velocity, cadence,

and gait symmetry in chronic hemiparetic stroke: a preliminary report. *Neurorehabil Neural Repair*. 2000;14(1):65-71.

56. Smith GV, Silver KH, Goldberg AP, Macko RF. "Task-oriented" exercise improves hamstring strength and spastic reflexes in chronic stroke patients. *Stroke*. 1999;30(10):2112-2118.

57. Gardner AW, Sieminski D, Montgomery PS. Physical activity is related to ankle/brachial index in subjects without peripheral arterial occlusive disease. *Angiology*. 1987;48(10):883-891.

58. Sbordone RJ, Liter JC, Pettler-Jennings P. Recovery of function following severe traumatic brain injury: a retrospective 10-year follow-up. *Brain Inj*. 1995;9(3):285-299.

59. Baguley IJ, Nicholls JL, Felmingham KL, Crooks J, Gurka JA, Wade LD. Dysautonomia after traumatic brain injury: a forgotten syndrome? *J Neurol Neurosurg Psychiatry*. 1999;67(1):39-43.

60. Nakken KO. Physical exercise in outpatients with epilepsy. *Epilepsia*. 1999;40(5):643-651.

61. Vitale AE, Jankowski LW, Sullivan SJ. Reliability for a walk/run test to estimate aerobic capacity in a brain-injured population. *Brain Inj*. 1997;11(1):67-76.

62. Rehabilitation of Persons with Traumatic Brain Injury. NIH Consensus Statement Online 1998 October 26-28, 2010;16(1):1-41.

63. Hunter M, Tomberlin J, Kirkikis C, Kuna ST. Progressive exercise testing in closed head-injured subjects: comparison of exercise apparatus in assessment of a physical conditioning program. *Phys Ther*. 1990;70(6):363-371.

64. Jankowski LW, Sullivan SJ. Aerobic and neuromuscular training: effect on the capacity, efficiency, and fatigability of patients with traumatic brain injuries. *Arch Phys Med Rehabil*. 1990;71(7):500-504.

65. Grant S, Corbett K, Amjad AM, Wilson J, Aitchison T. A comparison of methods of predicting maximum oxygen uptake. *Br J Sports Med*. 1995;29(3):147-152.

66. Wolman Rl, Cornall C, Fulcher K. Aerobic training in brain-injured patients. *Clin Rehabil*. 1994;8:253-257.

67. Mossberg KA, Kuna S, Masel B. Ambulatory efficiency in persons with acquired brain injury after a rehabilitation intervention. *Brain Inj*. 2002;16(9):789-797.

68. Mossberg KA, Orlander EE, Norcross JL. Cardiorespiratory capacity after weight-supported treadmill training in patients with traumatic brain injury. *Phys Ther*. 2008;88(1):77-87.

69. Guiliani C. Strength training for patients with neurological disorders. *Neuro Rep*. 1995;19(3):29-34.

70. Gordon WA, Sliwinski M, Echo J, et al. The benefits of exercise in individuals with traumatic brain injury: a retrospective study. *J Head Trauma Rehabil*. 1998;13(4):58-67.

71. Sawka MN, Latzka WA, Pandolf KB. Temperature regulation during upper body exercise: able-bodied and spinal cord injured. *Med Sci Sports Exerc*. 1989;21(5 suppl):S132-S140.

72. Drory Y, Ohry A, Brooks ME, Dolphin D, Kellermann JJ. Arm crank ergometry in chronic spinal cord injured patients. *Arch Phys Med Rehabil*. 1990;71(6):389-392.

73. Smith PA, Glaser RM, Petrofsky JS, Underwood PD, Smith GB, Richard JJ. Arm crank vs handrim wheelchair propulsion: metabolic and cardiopulmonary responses. *Arch Phys Med Rehabil*. 1983;64(6):249-254.

74. Sedlock DA, Knowlton RG, Fitzgerald PI. Circulatory and metabolic responses of women to arm crank and wheelchair ergometry. *Arch Phys Med Rehabil*. 1990;71(2):97-100.

75. McLean KP, Jones PP, Skinner JS. Exercise prescription for sitting and supine exercise in subjects with quadriplegia. *Med Sci Sports Exerc*. 1995;27(1):15-21.

76. Lewis JE, Nash MS, Hamm LF, Martins SC, Groah SL. The relationship between perceived exertion and physiologic indicators of stress during graded arm exercise in persons with spinal cord injuries. *Arch Phys Med Rehabil*. 2007;88(9):1205-1211.

77. Wicks JR, Oldridge NB, Cameron BJ, Jones NL. Arm cranking and wheelchair ergometry in elite spinal cord-injured athletes. *Med Sci Sports Exerc*. 1983;15(3):224-231.

78. Glaser RM, Sawka MN, Brune MF, Wilde SW. Physiological responses to maximal effort wheelchair and arm crank ergometry. *J Appl Physiol*. 1980;48(6):1060-1064.

79. Lasko-McCarthey P, Davis JA. Protocol dependency of VO_{2max} during arm cycle ergometry in males with quadriplegia. *Med Sci Sports Exerc*. 1991;23(9):1097-1101.

80. Eriksson P, Lofstrom L, Ekblom B. Aerobic power during maximal exercise in untrained and well-trained persons with quadriplegia and paraplegia. *Scand J Rehabil Med*. 1988;20(4):141-147.

81. Yamasaki M, Irizawa M, Ishii K, Komura T. Work efficiency of paraplegics during arm cranking exercise. *Ann Physiol Anthropol*. 1993;12(2):79-82.

82. Yamasaki M, Komura T, Tahara Y, et al. Relationship between physical characteristics and physiological responses during maximal arm cranking in paraplegics. *Spinal Cord*. 1998;36(8):579-583.

83. Gass EM, Harvey LA, Gass GC. Maximal physiological responses during arm cranking and treadmill wheelchair propulsion in T4–T6 paraplegic men. *Paraplegia*. 1995;33(5):267-270.

84. Hoffman MD. Cardiorespiratory fitness and training in quadriplegics and paraplegics. *Sports Med*. 1986;3(5):312-330.

85. Taylor AW, McDonell E, Brassard L. The effects of an arm ergometer training programme on wheelchair subjects. *Paraplegia*. 1986;24(2):105-114.

86. DiCarlo SE. Effect of arm ergometry training on wheelchair propulsion endurance of individuals with quadriplegia. *Phys Ther*. 1988;68(1):40-44.

87. Burkett LN, Chisum J, Stone W, Fernhall B. Exercise capacity of untrained spinal cord injured individuals and the relationship of peak oxygen uptake to level of injury. *Paraplegia*. 1990;28(8):512-521.

88. Hjeltnes N, Wallberg-Henriksson H. Improved work capacity but unchanged peak oxygen uptake during primary rehabilitation in tetraplegic patients. *Spinal Cord*. 1998;36(10):691-698.

89. Price MJ, Campbell IG. Thermoregulatory responses of spinal cord injured and able-bodied athletes to prolonged upper body exercise and recovery. *Spinal Cord*. 1999;37(11):772-779.

90. Dallmeijer AJ, van der Woude LH, Hollander AP, van As HH. Physical performance during rehabilitation in persons with spinal cord injuries. *Med Sci Sports Exerc*. 1999;31(9):1330-1335.

91. Bernard PL, Mercier J, Varray A, Prefaut C. Influence of lesion level on the cardioventilatory adaptations in paraplegic wheelchair athletes during muscular exercise. *Spinal Cord*. 2000;38(1):16-25.

92. Barstow TJ, Scremin AM, Mutton DL, Kunkel CF, Cagle TG, Whipp BJ. Peak and kinetic cardiorespiratory responses during arm and leg exercise in patients with spinal cord injury. *Spinal Cord*. 2000;38(6):340-345.

93. Muraki S, Tsunawake N, Tahara Y, Hiramatsu S, Yamasaki M. Multivariate analysis of factors influencing physical work capacity in wheelchair-dependent paraplegics with spinal cord injury. *Eur J Appl Physiol*. 2000;81(1-2):28-32.

94. Janssen TW, Pringle DD. Effects of modified electrical stimulation-induced leg cycle ergometer training for individuals with spinal cord injury. *J Rehabil Res Dev.* 2008;45(6):819-830.

95. Frotzler A, Coupaud S, Perret C, et al. High-volume FES-cycling partially reverses bone loss in people with chronic spinal cord injury. *Bone.* 2008;43(1):169-176.

96. Valent LJ, Dallmeijer AJ, Houdijk H, Slootman HJ, Post MW, van der Woude LH. Influence of hand cycling on physical capacity in the rehabilitation of persons with a spinal cord injury: a longitudinal cohort study. *Arch Phys Med Rehabil.* 2008;89(6):1016-1022.

97. Hangartner TN, Rodgers MM, Glaser RM, Barre PS. Tibial bone density loss in spinal cord injured patients: effects of FES exercise. *J Rehabil Res Dev.* 1994;31(1):50-61.

98. Daly JJ, Marsolais EB, Mendell LM, et al. Therapeutic neural effects of electrical stimulation. *IEEE Trans Rehabil Eng.* 1996;4(4):218-230.

99. Burstein R, Zeilig G, Royburt M, Epstein Y, Ohry A. Insulin resistance in paraplegics—effect of one bout of acute exercise. *Int J Sports Med.* 1996;17(4):272-276.

100. Kocina P. Body composition of spinal cord injured adults. *Sports Med.* 1997;23(1):48-60.

101. Noreau L, Shephard RJ, Simard C, Pare G, Pomerleau P. Relationship of impairment and functional ability to habitual activity and fitness following spinal cord injury. *Int J Rehabil Res.* 1993;16(4):265-275.

102. Manns PJ, Chad KE. Determining the relation between quality of life, handicap, fitness, and physical activity for persons with spinal cord injury. *Arch Phys Med Rehabil.* 1999;80(12):1566-1571.

103. Tawashy AE, Eng JJ, Lin KH, Tang PF, Hung C. Physical activity is related to lower levels of pain, fatigue and depression in individuals with spinal-cord injury: a correlational study. *Spinal Cord.* 2009;47(4):301-306.

104. Kurtzke JF. Rating neurologic impairment in multiple sclerosis: an expanded disability status scale (EDSS). *Neurology.* 1983;33(11):1444-1452.

105. Matthews WB, Compston A, Allen IV, Martyn CN. *McAlpine's Multiple Sclerosis.* Edinburg, Scotland: Churchill Livingstone; 1991.

106. Krupp LB, Alvarez LA, LaRocca NG, Scheinberg LC. Fatigue in multiple sclerosis. *Arch Neurol.* 1988;45(4):435-437.

107. Freal JE, Kraft GH, Coryell JK. Symptomatic fatigue in multiple sclerosis. *Arch Phys Med Rehabil.* 1984;65(3):135-138.

108. Iriarte J, Subira ML, Castro P. Modalities of fatigue in multiple sclerosis: correlation with clinical and biological factors. *Mult Scler.* 2000;6(2):124-130.

109. Guthrie TC, Nelson DA. Influence of temperature changes on multiple sclerosis: critical review of mechanisms and research potential. *J Neurol Sci.* 1995;129(1):1-8.

110. Mulcare J. *Exercise Management for Persons with Chronic Diseases and Disabilities.* Champaign, IL: Human Kinetics; 1997.

111. Tantucci C, Massucci M, Piperno R, Grassi V, Sorbini CA. Energy cost of exercise in multiple sclerosis patients with low degree of disability. *Mult Scler.* 1996;2(3):161-167.

112. Morrison EH, Cooper DM, White LJ, et al. Ratings of perceived exertion during aerobic exercise in multiple sclerosis. *Arch Phys Med Rehabil.* 2008;89(8):1570-1574.

113. Poser C, ed. *The Diagnosis of Multiple Sclerosis.* New York: Thieme-Stratton Inc; 1984.

114. White AT, Wilson TE, Davis SL, Petajan JH. Effect of precooling on physical performance in multiple sclerosis. *Mult Scler.* 2000;6(3):176-180.

115. Gosselink R, Kovacs L, Decramer M. Respiratory muscle involvement in multiple sclerosis. *Eur Respir J.* 1999;13(2):449-454.

116. Schapiro R, Petajan J, Kosich D. Role of cardiovascular fitness in multiple sclerosis: a pilot study. *J Neurol Rehabil.* 1988;2:43-49.

117. Gehlsen GM, Grigsby SA, Winant DM. Effects of an aquatic fitness program on the muscular strength and endurance of patients with multiple sclerosis. *Phys Ther.* 1984;64(5):653-657.

118. Svensson B, Gerdle B, Elert J. Endurance training in patients with multiple sclerosis: five case studies. *Phys Ther.* 1994;74(11):1017-1026.

119. Petajan JH, Gappmaier E, White AT, Spencer MK, Mino L, Hicks RW. Impact of aerobic training on fitness and quality of life in multiple sclerosis. *Ann Neurol.* 1996;39(4):432-441.

120. Ponichtera-Mulcare JA. Exercise and multiple sclerosis. *Med Sci Sports Exerc.* 1993;25(4):451-465.

121. Gappmaier E, White A, Mino L, et al. Aerobic exercise in multiple sclerosis. *Phys Ther Neurol Rep.* 1995;19(2):41-42.

122. Hoehn MM, Yahr MD. Parkinsonism: onset, progression and mortality. *Neurology.* 1967;17(5):427-442.

123. Skidmore FM, Patterson SL, Shulman LM, Sorkin JD, Macko RF. Pilot safety and feasibility study of treadmill aerobic exercise in Parkinson disease with gait impairment. *J Rehabil Res Dev.* 2008;45(1):117-124.

124. Reuter I, Engelhardt M, Stecker K, Baas H. Therapeutic value of exercise training in Parkinson's disease. *Med Sci Sports Exerc.* 1999;31(11):1544-1549.

125. Stanley RK, Protas EJ, Jankovic J. Exercise performance in those having Parkinson's disease and healthy normals. *Med Sci Sports Exerc.* 1999;31(6):761-766.

126. Canning CG, Alison JA, Allen NE, Groeller H. Parkinson's disease: an investigation of exercise capacity, respiratory function, and gait. *Arch Phys Med Rehabil.* 1997;78(2):199-207.

127. Protas EJ, Stanley RK, Jankovic J, MacNeill B. Cardiovascular and metabolic responses to upper- and lower-extremity exercise in men with idiopathic Parkinson's disease. *Phys Ther.* 1996;76(1):34-40.

128. Werner WG, DiFrancisco-Donoghue J, Lamberg EM. Cardiovascular response to treadmill testing in Parkinson disease. *J Neurol Phys Ther.* 2006;30(2):68-73.

129. Koseoglu F, Inan L, Ozel S, et al. The effects of a pulmonary rehabilitation program on pulmonary function tests and exercise tolerance in patients with Parkinson's disease. *Funct Neurol.* 1997;12(6):319-325.

130. Kurtais Y, Kutlay S, Tur BS, Gok H, Akbostanci C. Does treadmill training improve lower-extremity tasks in Parkinson disease? A randomized controlled trial. *Clin J Sport Med.* 2008;18(3):289-291.

131. Schenkman M, Hall D, Kumar R, Kohrt WM. Endurance exercise training to improve economy of movement of people with Parkinson disease: three case reports. *Phys Ther.* 2008;88(1):63-76.

132. Morris ME. Movement disorders in people with Parkinson disease: a model for physical therapy. *Phys Ther.* 2000;80(6):578-597.

133. Ziv I, Avraham M, Michaelov Y. Enhanced fatigue during motor performance in patients with Parkinson's disease. *Neurology.* 1999;53(2):438-439.

134. LeWitt PA, Bharucha A, Chitrit I, et al. Perceived exertion and muscle efficiency in Parkinson's disease: L-DOPA effects. *Clin Neuropharmacol.* 1994;17(5):454-459.

135. Goetz CG, Thelen JA, MacLeod CM, Carvey PM, Bartley EA, Stebbins GT. Blood levodopa levels and unified Parkinson's disease rating scale function: with and without exercise. *Neurology.* 1993;43(5):1040-1042.

136. Carter JH, Nutt JG, Woodward WR. The effect of exercise on levodopa absorption. *Neurology.* 1992;42(10):2042-2045.

137. Comella CL, Stebbins GT, Brown-Toms N, Goetz CG. Physical therapy and Parkinson's disease: a controlled clinical trial. *Neurology.* 1994;44(3, pt 1):376-378.

138. Inzelberg R, Peleg N, Nisipeanu P, Magadle R, Carasso RL, Weiner P. Inspiratory muscle training and the perception of dyspnea in Parkinson's disease. *Can J Neurol Sci.* 2005;32(2): 213-217.

139. Haas BM, Trew M, Castle PC. Effects of respiratory muscle weakness on daily living function, quality of life, activity levels, and exercise capacity in mild to moderate Parkinson's disease. *Am J Phys Med Rehabil.* 2004;83(8):601-607.

140. Reuter I, Engelhardt M, Freiwaldt J, Baas H. Exercise test in Parkinson's disease. *Clin Auton Res.* 1999;9(3):129-134.

141. Kuroda K, Tatara K, Takatorige T, Shinsho F. Effect of physical exercise on mortality in patients with Parkinson's disease. *Acta Neurol Scand.* 1992;86(1):55-59.

142. Sasco AJ, Paffenbarger RS Jr, Gendre I, Wing AL. The role of physical exercise in the occurrence of Parkinson's disease. *Arch Neurol.* 1992;49(4):360-365.

143. Schenkman M, Cutson TM, Kuchibhatla M, et al. Exercise to improve spinal flexibility and function for people with Parkinson's disease: a randomized, controlled trial. *J Am Geriatr Soc.* 1998; 46(10):1207-1216.

144. Rodrigues de Paula F, Teixeira-Salmela LF, Coelho de Morais Faria CD, Rocha de Brito P, Cardoso F. Impact of an exercise program on physical, emotional, and social aspects of quality of life of individuals with Parkinson's disease. *Mov Disord.* 2006;21(8):1073-1077.

145. Herman T, Giladi N, Gruendlinger L, Hausdorff JM. Six weeks of intensive treadmill training improves gait and quality of life in patients with Parkinson's disease: a pilot study. *Arch Phys Med Rehabil.* 2007;88(9):1154-1158.

146. Bassile C. Guillain-Barre syndrome. *Phys Ther Neurol Rep.* 1996; 20(2):31-36.

147. Ropper A. *Guillain-Barre Syndrome.* Philadelphia, PA: FA Davis Co; 1991.

148. Noonan V, Dean E. Submaximal exercise testing: clinical application and interpretation. *Phys Ther.* 2000;80(8):782-807.

149. Ropper AH, Wijdicks EF. Blood pressure fluctuations in the dysautonomia of Guillain-Barre syndrome. *Arch Neurol.* 1990;47(6):706-708.

150. Pitetti KH, Barrett PJ, Abbas D. Endurance exercise training in Guillain-Barre syndrome. *Arch Phys Med Rehabil.* 1993;74(7): 761-765.

151. Birk TJ. Poliomyelitis and the post-polio syndrome: exercise capacities and adaptation-current research, future directions, and widespread applicability. *Med Sci Sports Exerc.* 1993;25(4): 466-472.

152. Aston JW Jr. Post-polio syndrome. An emerging threat to polio survivors. *Postgrad Med.* 1992;92(1):249-256, 260.

153. Weinberg J, Borg J, Bevegard S, Sinderby C. Respiratory response to exercise in postpolio patients with severe inspiratory muscle dysfunction. *Arch Phys Med Rehabil.* 1999;80(9):1095-1100.

154. Willen C, Grimby G. Pain, physical activity, and disability in individuals with late effects of polio. *Arch Phys Med Rehabil.* 1998;79(8):915-919.

155. Stanghelle JK, Festvag L, Aksnes AK. Pulmonary function and symptom-limited exercise stress testing in subjects with late sequelae of poliomyelitis. *Scand J Rehabil Med.* 1993;25(3): 125-129.

156. Willen C, Cider A, Sunnerhagen KS. Physical performance in individuals with late effects of polio. *Scand J Rehabil Med.* 1999; 31(4):244-249.

157. Kriz JL, Jones DR, Speier JL, Canine JK, Owen RR, Serfass RC. Cardiorespiratory responses to upper extremity aerobic training by postpolio subjects. *Arch Phys Med Rehabil.* 1992;73(1): 49-54.

158. Wiesinger GF, Quittan M, Graninger M, et al. Benefit of 6 months long-term physical training in polymyositis/dermatomyositis patients. *Br J Rheumatol.* 1998;37(12):1338-1342.

159. Oncu J, Durmaz B, Karapolat H. Short-term effects of aerobic exercise on functional capacity, fatigue, and quality of life in patients with post-polio syndrome. *Clin Rehabil.* 2009;23(2): 155-163.

Physical Therapy Associated with Primary Prevention, Risk Reduction, and Deconditioning

Gary Brooks*

CHAPTER

15

INTRODUCTION

Physical therapists are often called on to treat patients/clients with one or more chronic medical conditions that are inherent causes of impairments, dysfunction, and disability and/or increase the risk of other pathologic conditions. Consider, for example, diabetes and coronary artery disease (CAD). Diabetes is, itself, a cause of considerable dysfunction and disability, and it is also a risk factor for CAD, which is the number one killer in the United States.[1] Both diabetes and CAD and other cardiopulmonary diseases are highly prevalent and may be present in medically complex patients/clients who are seen by physical therapists in a wide range of practice settings. CAD is also associated with other medical conditions (hypertension, hyperlipidemia, and obesity) and behaviors (cigarette smoking and physical inactivity) that are considered to be *risk factors*. These risk factors, too, are often encountered by physical therapists in clinical practice. Physical therapy (PT) interventions can help to prevent cardiopulmonary diseases from

developing, even among individuals with risk factors. This process is called *primary prevention,* and an individual referred to physical therapists for risk-factor management may be best referred to as a *client*. Physical therapists can also intervene in the presence of known, overt cardiopulmonary disease. These interventions are aimed at reducing symptoms and/or slowing the progression of the disease. This process is termed *secondary intervention* and these people are usually referred to as *patients*. Regardless of whether clients or patients seek physical therapy services, these individuals may be restricted in their activities due to deconditioning. Some have chronic medical conditions, including cardiopulmonary disease, and may restrict their activities because of symptoms, illness, or hospitalization. This deconditioning causes an impairment due to reduced aerobic capacity, which can lead to disability and dependency.

Both clients with risk factors and patients who are deconditioned may be treated in a variety of practice settings. They may be in hospital, recovering from surgery; they may be outpatients who visit the hospital several days a week for exercises and patient education, or they may receive services in the home. They may also be found in wellness centers for

weight-reduction programs and dietary counseling. Cardiopulmonary Practice Patterns A and B are intended to address both prevention of cardiopulmonary disease and the management of the deconditioning that often accompanies cardiopulmonary and other medical conditions.

Patterns A and B may be positioned on different points of the lifespan continuum. Pattern A is seen earlier, where the potential for cardiopulmonary disease is present, but not manifest. Pattern B represents progression such that cardiopulmonary disease may have occurred and has begun to affect not only physiology but also function. Many conditions that are "risk factors" for cardiopulmonary disease in Pattern A may also be present in pattern B. Moreover, Patterns A and B share common primary PT interventions—physical activity patient education—for which there is ample evidence of its effectiveness.

This chapter reviews the pathophysiology related to conditions and behaviors that underlie cardiopulmonary disease. We examine atherosclerosis, the fundamental disease process that leads not only to CAD but also to stroke, peripheral vascular disease, and kidney disease. The acute pathological processes associated with cigarette smoking, including how tobacco smoke damages the lungs, are also discussed. A case study of a prototypical high-risk individual, Joe Sixpack, will help us to understand the similarities and differences between Patterns A and B. The case study will serve as a springboard for a review of the medical conditions, behaviors, and traits that are risk factors for cardiovascular disease (CVD), including hypercholesterolemia (high blood cholesterol), hypertension, diabetes, obesity, cigarette smoking, physical inactivity, gender, family history, and psychosocial characteristics. To understand the rationale for intervention, the physiology of deconditioning and the benefits of physical activity and exercise are also discussed. We also describe appropriate PT examinations and interventions, highlighting the evidence for their effectiveness and considering extra- and intraindividual factors as described in the Disablement Model articulated by Verbrugge and Jette[2] (see Chapter 2).

RISK FACTORS: ATHEROSCLEROSIS AND SMOKING

A basic understanding of cardiopulmonary disease prevention requires knowledge of the underlying pathological process leading to cardiopulmonary disease. These topics have been the subject of extensive investigation in recent decades, resulting in voluminous literature. This chapter builds on material provided in earlier chapters—atherosclerosis (Chapter 6) and smoking (Chapter 7).

Atherosclerosis

Atherosclerosis, which is widespread in Western societies, is a major contributing factor to coronary heart disease, including angina pectoris and myocardial infarction. It is a complex disease process that evolves over a period of many years, in most cases decades, before clinical symptoms are apparent. The process is thought to begin with injury to the endothelium, the cells forming the inner layer of arteries, resulting in endothelial dysfunction. Sources of injury may be mechanical, as from

high blood pressure (BP); or biochemical, because of lipid accumulation, bacterial toxins, or viruses.[3]

The endothelium, rather than being merely a passive lining of the arterial lumen, is actually considered to be an organ with an active role in controlling vessel diameter, blood clotting (*thrombogenesis*), lipid metabolism, and blood vessel growth and repair.[4] Injury to endothelial cells initiates a cascading chain of events that eventually leads to formation of atherosclerotic plaque, causing obstruction of the lumen of the artery. These events are described in Chapter 6 (Figs. 6-1 and 6-2), which details the steps leading to plaque development.

Early in the progression, an inflammatory process attracts immune-related cells, including macrophages and T lymphocytes, which begin to undermine the endothelium. Macrophages engulf accumulated lipid molecules and become large, fatty *foam cells*. Smooth muscle cells, which comprise the layers of the arterial wall adjacent to the endothelium, migrate toward the developing lesion, further undermining the endothelium. Together with the foam cells and T lymphocytes, these cells form what is termed as the *fatty streak,* which is the earliest pathologically identifiable lesion in the atherosclerotic process.[3] These lesions have been found in children and adolescents[5,6] attesting to the early age at which this process begins.

The endothelium becomes disrupted and distorted and projects into the arterial lumen. Gaps develop between endothelial cells, attracting even more immune-related cells as well as platelets. Blood flow becomes turbulent, causing eddy currents with relatively static blood flow. All of these events set the stage for thrombus (blood clot) formation. Sites of arterial bifurcation are particularly vulnerable to this process. Lipids continue to accumulate within the lesion that becomes more fibrotic and often hardened by calcium deposits. Keep in mind that these events are ongoing and dynamic and result in space-occupying atheromas that progressively obstruct the arterial lumen over time. The good news is that there is a growing body of scientific evidence that indicates that the process is reversible through changes in lifestyle, including drugs.[3,7–12]

Cigarette Smoking

In addition to increasing CVD risk, cigarette smoking substantially increases the risk for other diseases, notably chronic obstructive pulmonary disease (COPD) and lung cancer. One out of every five deaths in the United States can be attributed to cigarette smoking. The death rate from COPD has been rising, in contrast to death rates from other major killers, including CVD and CAD, that have recently been falling. Lung cancer death rates rose dramatically throughout the previous century and are only now beginning to level off. Lung cancer is, for both men and women, the deadliest type of cancer.[13]

Nicotine, the primary ingredient in tobacco smoke, is a highly addictive compound, and cigarettes may be considered to be nicotine delivery devices. Most smokers say they would like to quit smoking, yet those who try to quit typically resume smoking. Physicians and other health care providers, including physical therapists, should discuss cigarette smoking and smoking cessation with their patients/clients, yet many health care providers miss the opportunities to do so. Recent data indicate that only approximately one-fifth of smokers' visits to physicians included any counseling on smoking cessation.[14]

In addition to nicotine, tobacco smoke also contains as many as 60 compounds that are or may be carcinogenic. A substance that is carcinogenic is one that damages cells, promoting rapid cell division leading to tumor growth. In addition to the airways of the lungs, many other tissues are exposed to tobacco-related carcinogens during the smoking of a cigarette, including the oral cavity, pharynx, and larynx. This explains why cancers of these tissues are also associated with tobacco use. Metabolites of tobacco smoke are also found in urine, which may explain the increased risk of bladder cancer among cigarette smokers.

Cigarette smoke and other toxic gases in inspired air injure cells within the lungs. This injury causes an inflammatory reaction in large and small airways and in the lung parenchyma that leads to the pathological changes in structure and function that are characteristic of COPD. This inflammatory reaction is part of a repair process that attempts to restore normal tissue where the injury has occurred. This process is illustrated in Fig. 15-1. Initially, toxic gases injure healthy epithelium, creating a *wound*. A provisional matrix is laid down over the wound that, along with chemoattractant signals from remaining cells within the wound, attracts epithelial cells and other agents involved in the inflammatory process. Epithelial cells adjacent to the wound become less differentiated and they begin to migrate in from the wound edges. These cells proliferate and eventually cover the wound and over the course of days to weeks, resume their normal structure and function.[15]

Unfortunately, because smoking tends to be an ongoing behavior, the inflammation typically becomes chronic and the damage irreversible. Bacteria that are ever present are drawn to the site, which presents an opportunity for colonization. This may be one reason that respiratory infections are commonly seen in smokers. Immune-related cells, including macrophages and neutrophils, are also attracted to the region. In the course of their efforts to clean up and repair the injury, these cells release enzymes that destroy healthy lung tissue. This ongoing injury, inflammation, and repair triggered by chronic cigarette smoking cause scarring and narrowing of small airways and disintegration of the lung parenchyma. The resulting obstruction of airflow and loss of elasticity are some of the hallmarks of COPD.[15,16]

CARDIOPULMONARY PRACTICE PATTERNS A AND B

Inclusion Criteria

A primary consideration in the decision to place a patient/client in a preferred practice pattern involves an assessment of

A. Normal epithelium

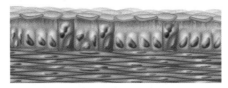

B.

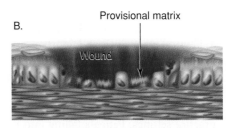

Provisional matrix

C.

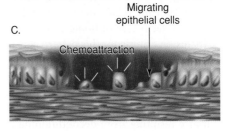

Migrating epithelial cells

D.

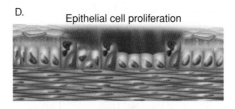

Epithelial cell proliferation

E. Restoration of normal epithelium

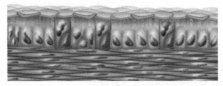

FIGURE 15-1 Injury and repair to airway epithelium. (**A**) Normal epithelium. (**B**) Wounding from toxic gases in cigarette smoke occurs. Provisional matrix is laid down. (**C**) Cells remaining in wound attract inflammatory agents. Epithelial cells begin to migrate in from wound edges. (**D**) Epithelial cells within wound proliferate. (**E**) Normal epithelium is restored. (Modified with permission from Rennard SI. Inflammation and repair processes in chronic obstructive pulmonary disease. *Am J Respir Crit Care Med.* 1999;160:S12.)

the medical diagnostic groups—the *includes* and *excludes*—for each pattern. For cardiopulmonary Practice Pattern A, *Primary Prevention/Risk Reduction for Cardiovascular/Pulmonary Disorders,* these include the risk factors for cardiopulmonary disease that were reviewed in the introduction. Because this is a primary prevention pattern, patients/clients with a current diagnosis of cardiopulmonary disease are excluded from Pattern A. Risk factors specifically listed for

Practice Pattern A in the 2nd edition of the *Guide* include diabetes, family history of heart disease, hypercholesterolemia, hypertension, obesity, sedentary lifestyle, and a history of smoking.[17] This list is not meant to be inclusive and other risk factors may also be considered.

One particular risk factor that has immediate relevance to physical therapists is sedentary lifestyle or a decrease in physical activity. This type of lifestyle will lead to a decrease in maximum aerobic capacity, which is listed as a functional limitation for Pattern A. Physical inactivity is an important risk factor for CVD because it leads to a host of pathological consequences, and it is a behavior that is a prime target for PT intervention.

Practice Pattern B, *Impaired Aerobic Capacity/Endurance Associated with Deconditioning,* has broad applications in diverse PT practice settings. Patients falling into this pattern may be seen in acute care, rehabilitation (including subacute rehabilitation), long-term care or home care, and other practice settings. Inclusion criteria for this pattern consist of a very wide range of medical conditions, including acquired immune deficiency syndrome (AIDS); cancer; chronic system failure, as well as cardiovascular, neuromuscular, and musculoskeletal disorders[17] (see p. S475 of the *Guide*). Impaired aerobic capacity and endurance resulting from deconditioning distinguish patients in this pattern. According to the *Guide,* aerobic capacity and endurance are impaired if dependency in activities of daily living (ADL) and/or instrumental activities of daily living (IADL) is present, or if the individual is symptomatic during activity, or unable to perform endurance conditioning. Typically, there is a period of substantially restricted activity or inactivity, such as bed rest, that precedes the diagnosis, which is caused by illness or medical treatment. This activity restriction frequently results from a systemic disorder, which then leads to deconditioning, rather than cardiovascular or respiratory pump dysfunction/failure, which would place the patient in a different practice pattern.

Similarities and Differences Between Practice Patterns A and B

Cardiopulmonary Practice Patterns A and B may be conceptually linked by physiologic, epidemiologic, and clinical elements. **A given patient/client may qualify for one or the other of these patterns at different points within the lifespan.** Pattern A applies when a sedentary individual, who is at risk for cardiopulmonary disease, is not yet impaired by deconditioning; that is, he or she does not have signs or symptoms during daily activities that are typical of deconditioning. Pattern B applies after the individual has developed impairment related to deconditioning as a result of either pathology or medical treatment, particularly if it involves prolonged bed rest. In contrast to Pattern A, impairment in Pattern B may be a result of diagnosed cardiopulmonary disease.

For both Patterns A and B, PT management should include interventions designed to increase physical activity. This may include physical activity counseling, exercise prescription, and/or training in ADL or IADL. The outcomes of PT intervention may differ, however, between Patterns A and B. For clients in Pattern A, the distinguishing outcome involves an understanding of the risk of continued physical inactivity and increasing their level of physical activity to appropriate levels. For patients in Pattern B, the outcomes are directed more toward improvement in the level of conditioning. Specific interventions as well as measurable outcomes for both Patterns A and B, and the evidence supporting them, are discussed later in this chapter.

Choosing Practice Pattern A or Pattern B

Figure 15-2 illustrates a decision algorithm for Patterns A and B that uses information from the PT examination and evaluation to arrive at a decision regarding the practice pattern to be applied to a patient/client. **Determining a practice pattern is, in effect, the equivalent of establishing a PT diagnosis.** At the apex of the algorithm is the determination of the individual's level of physical activity. Patients/clients who are physically active and who have no pathology, impairments, or disabilities, which are amenable to PT intervention, should not be treated. Patients who are physically active, but who may benefit from PT for reasons unrelated to physical activity, will be placed into other practice patterns. The decision to assign patients/clients, who are not physically active, to Pattern A or B or to another cardiopulmonary pattern is determined by the presence or absence of impaired aerobic capacity and endurance. Those who are physically inactive *without* aerobic impairment, which may be defined by the appearance of signs or symptoms of deconditioning during ADL or IADL, may be assigned to Pattern A. Those *with* aerobic impairment, who are symptomatic as a result of deconditioning, may be assigned to Pattern B, with the exception of those patients/clients who have cardiovascular pump dysfunction or failure or ventilatory pump failure who, therefore, belong in other cardiopulmonary patterns.

CASE EXAMPLE: MEET JOE SIXPACK

Joe Sixpack will show up in your clinic at some point, perhaps many times during your career (Fig. 15-3). He may be referred for any number of reasons, maybe not related to his cardiovascular risk status. You may encounter Joe in an outpatient clinic, where he wants you to cure his back pain. Perhaps you will meet him in a community setting, at a health fair, fitness clinic, or community exercise program. He saw on TV that he should have his BP checked or he wants to run in the 5-km race next month. When Joe gets sick or needs surgery or has an accident, you will encounter him in the bed at the acute hospital or rehabilitation facility. Joe is everywhere.

Joe is the embodiment of the CVD risk factors. He has hypertension, hypercholesterolemia, and for good measure, diabetes. He is also overweight, he smokes, and he is, of course, a "couch potato." We encounter Joe at two different times in his life. The first time that we meet him he qualifies for Pattern A, the primary prevention pattern. What can you offer Joe that

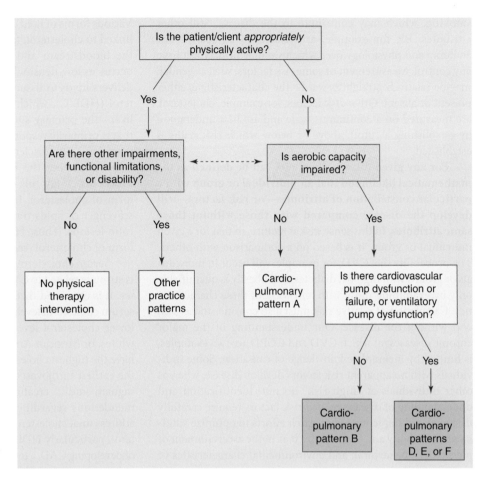

FIGURE 15-2 An algorithm for cardiopulmonary Practice Patterns A and B.

will help him to avoid, or postpone, the heart attack that seems inevitable? What are the clinical signs and symptoms and the physiologic responses that you need to monitor to safely help him to adopt a healthier lifestyle? These are the issues.

The next time you meet Joe he has been flat on his back for a while and you are going to help him get back on his feet—Pattern B applies here. You have treated lots of patients with his primary diagnosis, but Joe's medical history makes you a little nervous, and rightly so. He has a lot of hard work ahead of him and that is what worries you. What can you do to see him through his rehabilitation safely? The use of Joe as an example is going to show us how we can use cardiopulmonary Practice Patterns A and B. First, however, it is important to examine and understand the CVD risk factors he exhibits.

RISK FACTORS

Pattern A: Cardiovascular Risk Factors
Basis of Risk Determination
Before discussing specific conditions that are considered CVD risk factors, it may be helpful to review some of the concepts and the derivation of these risk factors that we so commonly associate with CVD. Health care professionals, as well as the concerned public, often wish an answer to the question: "What is the risk of developing a disease?" This concept of risk as it is applied to disease has been defined by studies of human populations. For any particular disease, there are typically numerous attributes that contribute, to varying degrees, to the pathogenesis of the disease. Some of these attributes are themselves diseases that may lead to, that is, increase the risk of the disease in question. An example of this in the context of CVD is diabetes. Other attributes are behaviors such as cigarette

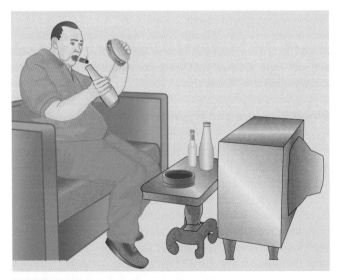

FIGURE 15-3 Meet Joe Sixpack.

smoking, which may contribute to the disease. Still other attributes, BP, for example, are related to aspects of our anatomy and physiology over which we may or may not have any control. Measurement of some risk factors, such as gender, may be relatively straightforward—the characteristic is either present or absent. Other risk factors, for example, cholesterol, are measured on a continuous scale and are best understood by establishing a cutoff, above or below which risk status is established.

For any given disease, then, *risk* can be defined as the mathematical likelihood that an individual or group with a particular constellation of attributes—or risk factors—will develop the disease compared with those without those same attributes. In this sense, risk is *relative,* in that for a given individual or group, it is based on a comparison with others. The probability that CVD, for example, will occur in individuals or groups with high BP, diabetes, and obesity is quantifiable only by examining those with and without these characteristics. Calculation of relative risk must also consider those with and without the disease. Our understanding of the major chronic diseases, of which CVD and COPD are two examples, is limited by incomplete knowledge of causation. Some individuals with no apparent risk factors develop disease, whereas other individuals at "high risk" do not. Identification and understanding of disease-related risk factors require carefully designed and implemented research efforts to optimize validity and reliability and to minimize bias in the ascertainment of physiologic, behavioral, and environmental characteristics of human populations.

One of the earliest and most important of the studies that established the basic risk factors for CVD is the Framingham study. Begun in 1948, the Framingham study has examined and reexamined over 5,000 residents of the town of Framingham, Massachusetts, and their offspring, looking for physiologic, psychosocial, and behavioral characteristics that may lead to CVD. This still-ongoing investigation has contributed enormously to the understanding of heart disease and stroke and has identified the chief risk factors for CVD.[18] Among the many benefits of this study, one that is applicable to cardiopulmonary Practice Pattern A includes a method for estimating cardiovascular risk, given the presence or absence of specific risk factors. This method makes use of tables derived from Framingham data that enable a clinician to calculate the approximate age- and gender-specific relative risk of heart disease in patients/clients without a documented history of CAD. Interested readers may study this method available at http://circ.ahajournals.org/cgi/content/full/100/13/1481.[19] This method is also used in this chapter to highlight the magnitude of risk for the individual risk factors identified by the Framingham study.

Cholesterol

Cholesterol is an essential compound that is used by the body for many important functions, including cell membrane structure and enzymatic activity. Its role as a risk factor for CVD stems from its function as a transporter of fatty acids or lipids.

Various forms of lipid-containing molecules (lipoproteins) are linked to cholesterol, forming complexes that circulate within the bloodstream and tissues. Most circulating cholesterol occurs as low-density lipoprotein cholesterol (LDL-C), which delivers lipids to tissues, and high-density lipoprotein cholesterol (HDL-C), which delivers lipids from the tissues to the liver—the primary site of lipid elimination. It is the LDL-C that is primarily responsible for the deposition of lipids within developing atherosclerotic lesions in arteries throughout the body, attracting the macrophages that eventually become foam cells.[3,20] For this reason, LDL-C is regarded as the "bad" form of cholesterol. In contrast, HDL-C is thought to be a scavenger of lipids transporting them away from atherosclerotic lesions. Thus, HDL-C is considered to be the "good" form of cholesterol (see Chapter 3).

Serum cholesterol, a common clinical laboratory measure, is strongly related to CVD in epidemiological and clinical studies. It is estimated that 19% of adult Americans have elevated serum cholesterol levels.[1] African American males tend to have lower cholesterol levels than do African American females, whites, or Mexican Americans, whereas white females tend to have the highest cholesterol levels. High cholesterol was one of the earliest cardiovascular risk factors identified by the Framingham study,[18] creating the basis for current clinical recommendations regarding cholesterol. These recommendations address total cholesterol (TC) as well as subfractions of cholesterol, particularly HDL-C and LDL-C. With regard to the risk of developing CAD, a total serum cholesterol level of <200 mg/dL is considered desirable, whereas serum cholesterol levels of 200 to 239 mg/dL and ≥240 mg/dL are considered to be borderline and high, respectively. A level of LDL-C <130 mg/dL is also considered desirable as is a level of HDL-C ≥45 mg/dL for men or ≥55 mg/dL for women.[19] Estimation of relative risk using Framingham risk tables[19] will give the reader a better sense of what is meant by the various risk levels. For example, a 40-year-old man with a TC of 250 (high) and a HDL-C level of 30 (also high) is approximately 2.5 times more likely to develop CAD than a 40-year-old man with desirable levels of TC and HDL-C. A 65-year-old woman with similar TC and HDL-C levels also has approximately 2.5 times the risk of CAD as does her counterpart with desirable levels. Men and women with very low TC (<160 mg/dL) and/or very high HDL-C (>60 mg/dL) actually have a *lower* CAD risk compared with those with merely "desirable" levels.

Blood Pressure and Hypertension

Blood pressure is the force exerted by blood on the arterial wall as it is pumped through the circulatory system. High BP causes mechanical damage to vascular endothelium resulting in areas that are stripped of normal endothelial cells. This facilitates the atherogenic processes discussed earlier, leading to increased thrombus and plaque formation. Furthermore, high BP also leads to intracerebral aneurisms and hemorrhage as well as left ventricular hypertrophy, a marker for severe CAD. Hypertension, defined as a systolic BP (SBP) of ≥140 mm Hg and/or a diastolic BP (DBP) ≥90 mm Hg,[21] is particularly insidious because, by itself, hypertension causes no symptoms, yet it can lead to a number of potentially fatal conditions.

Approximately 23% of adult Americans have hypertension. The prevalence of hypertension is higher among African Americans and among older Americans. A large majority of adults older than 65 years have hypertension.[1] Both SBP and DBP are positively related to atherosclerosis and CVD, that is, as resting BP rises so does the risk not only of CAD but also of stroke and all-cause mortality. Although persons with hypertension are particularly at risk, those with higher than optimal BP ($\geq$120/80 mm Hg) also face increasing risk.[19] According to Framingham tables, the risk of CAD for men is approximately 60% to 70% greater at a resting SBP of 140 to 150 mm Hg and 100% to 130% greater at $\geq$160 mm Hg. Women's risk is lower than that of men with regard to hypertension, yet they too have a 40% to 50% increased risk at a resting SBP of 160 mm Hg or more.[19] Systolic hypertension, without concomitant diastolic hypertension, is also an important risk factor. It has been estimated that a population-wide reduction of SBP of as little as 2 mm Hg would reduce CAD incidence by 6% and strokes by 13%.[22]

Cigarette Smoking

Unlike the other major CVD risk factors, cigarette smoking appears not to promote atherogenesis. Instead, the use of cigarettes enhances thrombus formation and affects vasomotor responses, interfering with coronary vasodilation. Keep in mind that cigarette use often coexists with other CVD risk factors, so these acute changes occur in the setting of atherosclerosis, further intensifying the danger of myocardial ischemia or infarction. In addition, cigarette use stimulates catecholamine release leading to hemodynamic responses that may be dangerous in the presence of CAD. Both heart rate (HR) and BP increase during cigarette smoking, causing elevated myocardial oxygen demand, which may induce ischemia if coronary circulation is inadequate to meet the increased demand. The acute nature of these physiologic alterations explains why cardiovascular risk associated with smoking is immediately reduced after quitting.[23]

Cigarette smoking is the nation's leading cause of mortality, responsible for approximately 430,000 deaths each year. Cigarette smoking is associated not only with CAD but also with stroke, COPD, and lung and other cancers. Women who smoke during pregnancy also have higher rates of low birth weight and subsequent illnesses in their children, including sudden infant death syndrome. Smokers also harm those around them through exposure to environmental tobacco smoke, which has been linked to CVD, lung cancer, and pediatric respiratory diseases in nonsmokers.[24]

Slightly less than one-fourth of adults in the United States are current smokers. The good news is that prevalence of smoking has declined since the 1960s, when over half of men and one-third of women smoked.[1] The bad news is that smoking rates are higher—more than one-third—among persons younger than 18 years, and they are rising.[24] On the basis of Framingham risk tables, cigarette smoking alone is responsi-

ble for a 50% to 70% increase in CAD risk for men and a 30% to 50% increase for women. These calculations are based on average consumption of one pack per day. Individuals who smoke more than this face dramatically greater risk.[19]

Diabetes

Diabetes mellitus is a disorder in which the body is unable to utilize glucose because of a disorder of insulin metabolism. The type of diabetes present in an individual determines the nature of this inability to metabolize glucose. Broadly, two types of diabetes are commonly seen in clinical practice: type 1 diabetes and type 2 diabetes, which is much more common. Type 1 diabetes includes persons who produce little or no insulin, typically because of autoimmune destruction of the pancreatic cells that secrete insulin. Onset of type 1 diabetes commonly occurs in childhood, though some adults develop the condition, and those with the disease generally require exogenous insulin administration for survival. Type 2 diabetes is characterized by insulin resistance, or the inability of target organs, particularly skeletal muscle to take in and utilize or store glucose. Adult onset of type 2 diabetes is common, and exogenous insulin dependency is uncommon. Obesity, especially central, or abdominal obesity is strongly associated with type 2 diabetes because it causes or exacerbates insulin resistance.[25]

Regardless of etiology, one of the central pathophysiologic features of untreated or inadequately managed diabetes is hyperglycemia—elevation of plasma glucose. This is a clinical laboratory value that is the most commonly used diagnostic measure for diabetes. A value of $\geq$126 mg/dL, drawn after an overnight fast, is the current criterion. Chronic hyperglycemia is associated with a number of microvascular (small-vessel) complications including retinopathy, a common cause of blindness in persons with diabetes, and with peripheral and autonomic neuropathy. The relationship of hyperglycemia with macrovascular (large-vessel) complications, such as accelerated atherosclerosis, in type 2 diabetes is less clear. It is now believed that type 2 diabetes is characterized by insulin resistance with compensatory hyperinsulinemia (elevated plasma insulin levels), which is etiologically related to atherosclerosis. Other powerful CVD risk factors such as dyslipidemia (high LDL-C and low HDL-C), hypertension, and as mentioned, obesity are also associated with this syndrome. **This complex mix of physiologic abnormalities accelerates the development of atherosclerosis and leads to many of the cardiovascular complications seen in diabetes.**[26]

Diabetes is highly prevalent in the United States, with type 2 diabetes being roughly 10 times more common than type 1 diabetes. Overall, approximately 5% of adults have diabetes; however, the prevalence rises to nearly 20% in adults older than 65 years. Many of those with diabetes—up to one-third of the total number of cases in older Americans—are unaware that they have the condition. Like many of the other CVD risk factors, diabetes prevalence varies by race and gender, with higher rates in women as well as in African Americans and Mexican Americans.[27] According to Framingham risk tables for men, diabetes confers an increased risk of CAD equal to that of cigarette smoking. However, women with diabetes lose the protective effect of their gender, so their CAD risk is essentially equal to that of men at any age.[19] Persons with diabetes often have asymptomatic CAD and tend to have more severe involvement at the time of diagnosis. They are also more likely to develop congestive heart failure due to cardiomyopathy.[28] Autonomic neuropathy, a common complication in diabetes, may cause abnormal physiologic changes during activity, such as postural hypotension or maladaptive HR and BP responses to exercise.[25] **For this reason it is particularly important to monitor vital signs during PT examination and intervention.**

Obesity

The role of obesity as an independent CVD risk factor is somewhat controversial because many of its effects appear to be mediated through other risk factors. Obesity, diabetes, and hypertension are often clustered together in what is known as the *metabolic syndrome.* Insulin resistance and dyslipidemia, characterized by low HDL-C and increased LDL-C, also appear as part of the metabolic syndrome, which greatly increases the risk of CVD.[26] It is hypothesized that abdominal obesity—fat deposition around the trunk rather than around the hips—is etiologically related to the abnormalities seen in the metabolic syndrome, contributing to insulin resistance and to the atherogenic lipid profile.[29] Cardiac abnormalities such as left ventricular hypertrophy and conduction disturbances are also more common in persons with obesity.[29]

There has been much recent concern about obesity in the United States. Approximately one-third of American adults may be considered overweight, a proportion that has increased from one-fourth since 1980. Higher rates of overweight are seen in African Americans and Mexican Americans, particularly among women in those ethnic groups. Among children, the proportion of those overweight has nearly doubled in the same time period, rising to more than 13% and 11% in children aged 6 to 11 years and 12 to 17 years, respectively.[1] See chapter 16.

Physical Inactivity

Among all the CVD risk factors, physical inactivity is perhaps the risk factor most relevant to PT because it is most clearly within our domain of practice. Physical therapists work to achieve desirable health outcomes by counseling patients/ clients to become more physically active or by prescribing exercise to improve fitness. As a CVD risk factor, physical inactivity like obesity may exert much of its influence through other risk factors.[30] Indeed, physical activity has been shown to improve lipid profile, improve insulin sensitivity and blood glucose control, and to reduce BP.[31] On the other hand, there is evidence that physical fitness is independently predictive of all-cause and CVD mortality.[32,33] Readers interested in a more comprehensive discussion of the risk-factor status of physical inactivity are invited to review the *Surgeon General's Report on Physical Activity.*[34] This seminal document is available at http://www.cdc.gov/nccdphp/sgr/sgr.htm.

Regardless of the "independence" of physical inactivity as a CVD risk factor, numerous public health and medical associations have identified physical inactivity as a significant risk factor for cardiovascular and other diseases.[30-32] The U.S. Surgeon General has determined that a majority of American adults do not participate in physical activity that is sufficient to achieve health or fitness benefits and that approximately one-fourth are completely inactive. Almost half of the nation's children are not active enough to ensure healthy futures.[34] Physical activity need not be vigorous to be beneficial. Men who are active enough to maintain a moderate level of physical fitness have *substantially* reduced mortality compared with men with low fitness.[33] Walking, a form of moderate physical activity, is associated with lower mortality and improved health outcomes in older men and women.[35,36] These, and many similar research findings, have led to the recommendation that all Americans should participate in at least 30 minutes of some form of moderate physical activity, such as brisk walking, on most if not all days in the week.[37-39] Exercise, which is a structured form of physical activity that is performed specifically to improve some aspect(s) of fitness and/or health,[40] is one way to achieve the desired outcomes. However, other "lifestyle" forms of activity, such as gardening, walking, or bicycling as transportation and occupational forms of physical activity, are also beneficial (see Chapter 3).

Gender

Although male gender has traditionally been listed as a CVD risk factor, this is a misleading characterization of the differences in risk between men and women. In fact, CAD is the number one killer of women, surpassing all forms of cancer, including breast cancer, combined. There are important differences, however, in CAD risk for women compared to men. There is, for example, an age differential, such that the risk of dying from CAD is roughly equal for a woman as compared to a man 10 years younger. Women also present somewhat more of a diagnostic challenge with regard to CAD. **This is because women are more likely to exhibit atypical symptoms, particularly variation or absence of chest pain, and because for women, the accuracy of many commonly used diagnostic tools is reduced. In addition, the prognosis following myocardial infarction is worse in women, with higher death rates compared to men.** This may be due to women's older age, more severe disease, and higher comorbidity rate at the time of the diagnosis. However, less aggressive treatment may also play a role. Differences in CAD occurrence are also seen among women in different ethnic groups. For example, CAD death rates among African American women are higher than those for white women, a difference that is considerably greater than the corresponding difference in mortality between African American and white men.[41]

At the onset of menopause, women's CAD risk begins to approach that of men. The hormone estrogen appears to have several physiologic effects that tend to protect women from CAD. Estrogen promotes fat deposition peripherally in thighs and buttocks, which is a more favorable pattern of fat deposition with regard to CAD. Estrogen increases HDL-C ("good cholesterol") levels and improves vasomotor reactivity, which promotes vasodilation and improved tissue perfusion. Estrogen and progestin, another female sex hormone, may also reduce the tendency to form clots, which may cause both strokes and heart attacks. **The protective effect of estrogen via hormone replacement therapy has become a common recommendation for some women who are past menopause to reduce the risk of CAD.** The protection against CAD conferred by estrogen is not universal. Obese women, especially those with abdominal adiposity, and women with diabetes lose the benefits conferred by their female status.

Family History

The Framingham study established family history of CAD as an important risk factor, one that is not subject to modification. **Family history is considered positive if myocardial infarction or sudden cardiac death occurred in a primary male relative, aged 55 years or less, or in a primary female relative, aged 65 years or less.** Because of family behavior patterns such as dietary and physical activity habits, the independence of family history as a risk factor is unclear. Recent investigations, however, have demonstrated that family history remains predictive for CAD even when other risk factors are accounted for.[42,43] Familial genetic characteristics appear to influence lipoprotein metabolism, providing a possible mechanism for the effect on atherosclerosis and CAD occurrence. Although family history is not, strictly speaking, a modifiable risk factor—one that an individual can do anything about—realization that many behaviors are culturally and therefore, familially derived can help to identify ways to effectively target those behaviors for CVD risk reduction efforts.

Psychosocial Factors

Researchers have long suspected that certain personality traits are associated with CAD. The term *type A personality* was coined to describe the driven, workaholic individual, usually male, who was more likely to succumb to heart disease because of chronic stress. It now appears that responses to stress that are characterized by hostility and impatience increase CAD risk. Other psychosocial factors have been linked to CAD. These include depression, social isolation, and yes, chronic stress, particularly the type of job-related stress that an individual feels unable to control. In addition, low socioeconomic status is related to CAD so that lower status predicts higher rates of disease. To be sure, psychosocial traits have a complex relationship with behaviors, such as smoking, and poor dietary habits that increase the risk of CAD, but there are plausible biologic mechanisms that explain why these characteristics may independently contribute to CAD. Many of the psychosocial traits linked to CAD are associated with arousal of the autonomic nervous system such that sympathetic stimulation is increased. This, in turn, results in higher HR and BP levels both at rest and in response to stressful events. These responses not only increase myocardial work but also promote endothelial dysfunction and atherosclerosis.

Furthermore, some characteristics also enhance blood clotting by way of increasing platelet activation.[44]

Co-occurrence of CVD Risk Factors and Clinical Implications

Most individuals at risk for CVD exhibit multiple risk factors, which accumulate to increase risk dramatically. For example, on the basis of the Framingham risk tables,[19] a 65-year-old man with high TC, say above 240, and a low HDL-C, below 35, faces 2.5 times the risk of CAD compared with a man of the same age with desirable TC and HDL-C levels. Add hypertension, for example, SBP >160 and the risk increases to 4.5 times. Add smoking and the risk is greater than 5.5 times that of a nonsmoking, normotensive man with desirable cholesterol levels. Risk continues to rise as additional risk factors are added. Risk factors may cluster, as is seen in the *metabolic syndrome*, in which obesity, especially central or abdominal obesity, diabetes, hypertension, and dyslipidemia coexist, often complicated by physical inactivity.

Clustering of risk factors has important clinical implications for the physical therapist treating patients like Joe Sixpack, particularly as a primary care provider. Clinicians must be aware of patient/client risk-factor status, especially in the absence of a documented history of CAD. Lack of a diagnosis of heart disease does not necessarily rule out the presence of the condition. It may be wise to refer back to the physician in cases where there is a suspicion of CAD and potential PT interventions will involve physical activity counseling or exercise prescription. A method for determining whether or not physician referral is indicated is presented later in this chapter. Box 15-1 summarizes the risk factors for Pattern A.

Pattern B: Deconditioning

The primary risk factor associated with Pattern B is deconditioning, a complex process that leads to significant changes in physiology, some of the consequences of which will be briefly summarized, particularly as they relate to clinical practice. Deconditioning may best be characterized by a decrease in maximal oxygen uptake ($\dot{V}O_{2max}$), which occurs relatively

---

BOX 15-1

Risk Factors Associated with Cardiopulmonary Practice Pattern A

Hypercholesterolemia
Hypertension
Cigarette smoking
Diabetes
Obesity
Physical inactivity
Family history
Hostile response to stress

quickly, within several days of the onset of maintained bed rest. **The rate of decrease in $\dot{V}O_{2max}$ is greatest in the first week of bedrest. There is a dose–response relationship between the duration of bedrest and the degree of deconditioning, meaning that the longer the bedrest continues, the greater will be the loss of $\dot{V}O_{2max}$. It is important to remember that deconditioning occurs even in the absence of concurrent disease processes.**[45]

Following bedrest or inactivity, loss of $\dot{V}O_{2max}$ uptake results from central and peripheral changes in physiology. Central changes appear to have the greatest effect on reduction in $\dot{V}O_{2max}$ and are primarily a result of a decrease in stroke volume during activity. This loss of stroke volume is due to a loss of plasma volume, and consequently of venous return, that occurs as a result of bedrest and/or inactivity, thus altering the Frank–Starling mechanism. To maintain cardiac output with the loss of stroke volume in the deconditioned state, there is an increased HR response, both at rest and during activity. This deconditioning-related physiologic change in HR is an important clinical indicator that is readily assessed during the PT examination and intervention.

CLINICAL CORRELATE

The clinician should be alert for higher-than-normal HR at rest and during activity and should consider the consequence of this response in regard to myocardial work.

Peripheral changes in physiology associated with bedrest or inactivity, which are characterized by reduced skeletal muscle blood flow and capillarization, also influence hemodynamic responses to activity.[45]

Clinically, these physiologic changes may become manifest as orthostatic intolerance, resulting from a tendency for venous pooling to occur when the individual assumes an upright posture and leg fatigue during activity. Furthermore, skeletal muscle mass and strength decreases and bone demineralization occurs.[45] Fortunately, the effects of deconditioning are readily reversed following bedrest. In one study, $\dot{V}O_{2max}$ returned to pre–bedrest levels within 30 days in subjects who participated in a post–bedrest reconditioning exercise program and subjects who merely resumed normal activities. The reconditioning exercise group, however, had a lower submaximal HR during a constant workload, an important potential benefit for subjects with CAD.[46] It should be kept in mind that the research on the physiologic effects of deconditioning has primarily involved healthy male subjects, necessitating caution in the generalization of the findings to patient populations. There are few studies that examine the effects of bedrest in patient populations. However, the consequences of physical inactivity on health in various patient populations may be inferred from results of epidemiologic studies.

Box 15-2 summarizes the effects of deconditioning.

BOX 15-2

Physiologic and Clinical Effects of Deconditioning

Decreased maximal oxygen uptake because of
  loss of plasma volume
    decreased venous return
    decreased stroke volume
    alteration in Frank–Starling mechanism
Orthostatic intolerance
Decreased skeletal muscle mass and strength
Bone demineralization

EXAMINATION TECHNIQUES

Use of the Guide and the Hypothesis Testing Process

The *Guide* characterizes the initial examination, which is performed when seeing the patient/client for the first time, as an "investigation"[17] (see p. S34) or a careful, systematic inquiry designed to provide data needed to formulate an appropriate plan of care.

CLINICAL CORRELATE

The examination, and subsequent evaluation, uses a form of *hypothesis testing*. In other words, the clinician tests a hypothesis, which may be thought of as an "educated guess," regarding a practice pattern. One's initial impression may be that a given patient/client fits a particular practice pattern. This "hypothesis" is then tested by evaluating the data gathered from the examination, and either the hypothesis is confirmed or another practice pattern is suggested. This new hypothesis is tested in light of the examination data and confirmed or refuted, and so on, until clinicians are satisfied that they have identified a tenable practice pattern.

Novice clinicians may be tempted to conclude that once they have completed the initial examination, and progressed to evaluation, diagnosis, prognosis, and intervention, the examination process is over. Certainly, one may foresee the need for a reexamination at some point, but in an important sense **the examination process is ongoing.** Perhaps we can best characterize this ongoing examination by another term, say *assessment* or *monitoring*. Indeed, when working with patients/clients with cardiopulmonary dysfunction, it is this ongoing assessment or monitoring of physiologic responses to activity that brings the full skill of the physical therapists to bear in a clinical encounter. The term *skill,* as used in the previous sentence, implies not only that the clinician has the technical ability to obtain measurements such as HR and BP during an examination or intervention but also that the clinician has the wisdom to interpret the information derived from clinical measurements to make appropriate decisions regarding continuation, modification, or termination of the procedure (see Chapter 12).

In the current health care environment, in which many clinicians are able to practice independently, without physician referral, the physical therapist may be acting as the primary provider of care. This adds to the responsibility of the clinicians who may be seeing Joe Sixpack in their clinic. It is incumbent on the primary care provider to gather as much information as possible regarding the health status of the patient or client. Referral to other health care provider(s) is indicated when additional information, which may be beyond the skill of the clinician or outside of the scope of PT practice, is needed. Furthermore, physician referral does not guarantee that all medically relevant information has been obtained or is provided or available to the physical therapist. Even in hospital settings, where there is typically an abundance of medical records, charts, and the like, information may be hard to come by. Charts can be misplaced, or in use by someone else, and sometimes they are inaccurate. Physicians and nurses (and yes, other physical therapists) are busy and may have neither the time nor the inclination to share information at a given point in time. The astute clinician in any setting must be prepared to gather information from as many sources as are available including the patient or client, family members and other associates, other health care providers, and the medical record.

Imagine that you are a therapist with a successful private practice who wishes to expand into a new territory by starting a "wellness" clinic. In walks Joe Sixpack. He saw a TV show, an infomercial perhaps, that featured young, slim, attractive men and women bouncing around some beach in the Caribbean doing aerobics in spandex and having lots of fun. Now Joe is no longer young (let's say he is "middle aged") nor is he slim and he (as you will soon discover) has lots of medical issues that put him "at risk" for cardiopulmonary disease. But he pictures himself on that beach someday. Fortunately, Joe had the good sense to come to you before embarking on his workout program and you eventually determine that he belongs to cardiopulmonary Practice Pattern A.

Now imagine that you are working in a busy hospital, or in a rehabilitation center, or may be doing home care, or even consulting in a nursing home. You receive a new PT referral—It is Joe. Only this time he is a little older, or maybe a lot older, and he has had _____. You can fill in the blank because his primary diagnosis is not the basis of your decision to place him in cardiopulmonary Practice Pattern B. Joe has been sick in bed for several weeks and he is quite deconditioned. For our purposes, let us say that Joe does not have a condition, like a stroke or a hip fracture or an amputation, that would place him in some other practice pattern. However, even if he did, much of the discussion about PT examination and intervention for Pattern B would still apply. This is because, regardless of his primary diagnosis, he is still deconditioned and he is what can be called a "complex medical patient," owing to the presence of multiple comorbidities[17] (*Guide,* see p. S475). This illustrates the extraordinary breadth of cardiopulmonary Pattern B. It encompasses a wide range of patients/clients that may include the presence of risk factors—those who have become deconditioned as a result of bed rest or inactivity due to medical illness.

History

The *Guide* lists a number of categories of data to be obtained when taking a history from the patient/client. All of the elements listed are important, but the clinician may elect to emphasize particular items in a given clinical scenario. This section discusses some of the more crucial factors to be obtained from Joe's history. A key area of inquiry involves his medical/surgical history. Whether one queries Joe himself, his family, or friends, or obtains the information from the medical record, the physical therapist will want to establish the presence or absence of medical comorbidities, particularly those that relate to cardiopulmonary disease. These include the Framingham risk factors—diabetes, hyperlipidemia, hypertension, and obesity—as well as other relevant conditions that impact on clinical decisions. The presence and nature of cardiopulmonary disease must be assessed. **A positive history of cardiopulmonary disease not only excludes a patient/client from Pattern A but also indicates heightened monitoring during intervention.** However, whether or not Joe has a *documented* history of CAD or other cardiopulmonary condition, the presence of multiple risk factors indicates *high-risk* status. In this case, the clinician is wise to proceed as though the patient/client *does* have cardiopulmonary disease and monitor accordingly during intervention.

More information about risk factors can be obtained when assessing Joe's past and current social habits, particularly with respect to cigarette smoking and physical activity, and his family history. Do not hesitate to discuss smoking with Joe: Ask him how many years he has smoked and how many packs per day he smokes. From this you can calculate his *pack-year smoking history,* a clinically useful measure of smoking status, simply by multiplying the number of packs per day smoked by the number of years of smoking. In Joe's case, he smoked two packs per day for approximately 30 years, so he has a 60-pack-year smoking history. If the patient/client is not currently smoking, you will also want to know about past smoking. Joe might tell you he does not smoke, and if you leave it at that you would not find out that he had "quit" smoking this morning. When assessing physical activity level, do not assume that lack of exercise during leisure time means patients/clients are inactive. They may have a physically active occupation, such as a letter carrier or homemaker/parent (think of all the work that goes into cleaning and vacuuming, etc, not to mention child care) or an active hobby like gardening. In Joe's case, however, we find that he is indeed a couch potato. When discussing family history, ask about primary relatives, parents, and siblings and whether there is a history of a heart attack before 55 years of age, for men, and 65 years, for women.

Also important are the medications that Joe is taking. It is imperative to get an accurate account of all drugs, including dosages and times and routes of administration. Not only will this information be crucial when assessing physiologic responses to activity, it can also provide valuable clues about risk factor and comorbidity status, particularly if the patient's/client's account or the medical record is lacking in detail regarding medications. If, for example, Joe is a bit fuzzy about his cholesterol levels, but he is taking medications you know to be drugs that lower cholesterol, it is a good bet that his cholesterol level is, or hopefully *was*, high. It is also important to assess the patient's/client's adherence with medication and, in some cases, the response to medication. Joe may well be taking antihypertensive medication; but if his resting BP is consistently high, say over 160/90 mm Hg, there is good reason to question him regarding adherence to his medication regime and if he is adherent, to discuss your concerns about the drug's effectiveness with his physician.

Laboratory and diagnostic tests provide important information regarding CVD risk factors, information that determines the course of medical therapy for individuals such as Joe. Joe's risk-factor history suggests that he may be classified as having the "metabolic syndrome," a common clustering of CVD risk factors that include diabetes, obesity, hypertension, and dyslipidemia. The physical therapist can learn much from laboratory test results for these conditions. For example, a lipid profile, from serum cholesterol measurement, provides information on TC, HDL-C, and LDL-C, which are all important indicators of CVD risk.

For diabetes, there are several useful, and sometimes necessary, laboratory tests including blood glucose, the amount of glucose within the plasma, and glycosylated hemoglobin (GHb), the fraction of hemoglobin bound with glucose. We have seen that hyperglycemia, or excessive blood glucose, is the primary diagnostic feature of diabetes, and it is a condition that has to be avoided to reduce the likelihood of the occurrence of diabetic complications. Fasting blood glucose (FBG), measured in blood drawn after at least 8 hours since eating, is used as a diagnostic indicator of diabetes. A FBG level of ≥126 mg/dL is considered to be diagnostic for diabetes. Blood glucose levels should also be monitored prior to, and sometimes during, exercise or sustained physical activity.

CLINICAL CORRELATE

If FBG is >250 mg/dL, exercise should be avoided until blood glucose levels are brought under better control. Exercise should also be avoided or stopped and a carbohydrate snack should be given, if blood glucose levels are <100 mg/dL at any time.[25]

Many individuals with diabetes, and many facilities that care for persons with diabetes, have blood glucose–monitoring kits available. These involve blood sampling by finger stick, rather than by venipuncture, and can be readily used for rapid determinations of blood glucose levels that are the basis for clinical decision making. Measurement of GHb is an indicator of overall blood glucose levels during the previous 2 to 3 months and as such, provides information on long-term diabetes control. As blood glucose levels rise, so do values of GHb. GHb values of 4% to 6% are considered normal, and values >8% are indicators of ongoing hyperglycemia and inadequate control. GHb is a particularly useful outcome measure for interventions designed to improve glycemic control and reduce diabetic complications.

Discussing the history of the current condition and health status presents an opportunity to learn why Joe has come to you, what his perceptions and concerns are about his health, and what his level of understanding is of his condition. A patient who when asked, "Why did you come here today?" answers with ". . . I dunno, the doctor told me I had to come here" has a very different understanding of his or her condition than one who answers with a 5-minute rendition of medical history, including details about drugs or surgery or other medical treatments. You want to know about functional status and activity level, paying particular attention to a recent decline in ADL and IADL. **Recent decline could be a key influence on the decision to place a patient/client in Pattern B rather than in Pattern A.**

Here you can get an idea of Joe's willingness to change behavior. Has he thought about his physical inactivity? Does he want to be more active? Has he tried to become more active in the past? Does he have a plan to increase his activity level by exercising or by some other activity? The answers to these questions help the clinician to design the most appropriate intervention, perhaps incorporating a behavior change theory such as the Transtheoretical Model.[47]

The Transtheoretical Model of behavior change provides a means to assess the patient's/client's willingness to change a behavior like physical activity. Using this approach, clinicians may tailor their intervention to optimize the chance of success in motivating the individual to progress to a higher stage toward behavior change. The model is based on a progression of stages of change that are listed in Table 15-1. For Pattern A, Joe is in the preparation stage, ready for action; he came to a physical therapist, looking for advice on how to become more physically active. Knowing this, the clinician can reasonably implement an exercise prescription or a specific plan to increase lifestyle physical activity. Had Joe been in an earlier stage, say precontemplation or contemplation, a specific action plan would be less likely to succeed. Provision of information about cardiovascular risk factors, or exposure to media campaigns, would be appropriate to help Joe progress toward the preparation or action stage. Once Joe adopts the desired behavior—he participates in regular exercise or lifestyle physical activity—the clinician may suggest strategies to encourage him to continue. These may include use of exercise groups for support or

TABLE 15-1   Five Stages of Change in the Transtheoretical Model of Behavior Change

Stage	Description
Precontemplation	Has no intention to take action within the next 6 months
Contemplation	Intends to take action within the next 6 months
Preparation	Intends to take action within the next 30 days and has taken some behavioral steps in this direction
Action	Has changed overt behavior for less than 6 months
Maintenance	Has changed overt behavior for more than 6 months

Adapted with permission from Prochaska JO, Redding CA, Evers K. The transtheoretical model and stages of change. In: Glanz K, Lewis FM, Rimer BK, eds. *Health Behavior and Health Education: Theory, Research, and Practice.* 3rd ed. San Francisco: Jossey-Bass Publishers; 1997.

reviewing contingency plans to exercise in different seasons or environments (indoors vs outdoors).

Systems Review

The *systems review* is where a scan of functions relating to the four primary domains of PT—musculoskeletal, neuromuscular, cardiopulmonary, and integumentary—is performed. In Joe's case, many of the assessments that fall under the cardiopulmonary domain will be emphasized as tests and measures during your examination. You will want, however, to quickly assess functional strength, range of motion, sensation, coordination, balance and equilibrium, and skin condition. A deficit in any of these areas indicates a need to assess the impairment in greater detail and will likely be a consideration in the type of physical activity you recommend or exercise you prescribe.

Tests and Measures

Placement of a patient/client in a particular practice pattern may require all the information that is gathered during the examination process before a final decision can be made. This can be said of many of the cardiopulmonary practice patterns, but for some patterns the decision is more apparent at the beginning of the episode of care. Pattern A may be one pattern in which the clinician senses at the outset that primary prevention is of interest. This determination needs to be confirmed by the examination, particularly by ruling out documented cardiopulmonary disease. If cardiopulmonary disease is present, Pattern A is excluded; however, the presence of one or more CVD risk factors should be established by reviewing the patient's/client's history. These risk factors are listed in the *Guide* under the Patient/Client Diagnostic Classification.[17] Note that many of the Framingham risk factors are listed.

Clinicians may wish to use structured screening tools that facilitate the assessment of CVD risk factors, such as that shown in the cardiac examination chapter *and* provide guidance regarding further referral and/or intervention. Formal cardiovascular risk screening procedures are desirable in settings where the clinician may be practicing without physician referral, or where the patient/client is referred for primary musculoskeletal or neuromuscular dysfunction and the physical therapist identifies physical activity or aerobic exercise as an appropriate intervention. Formal screening tools, like the Physical Activity Readiness Questionnaire (PAR-Q) or the American Heart Association/American College of Sports Medicine Health/Fitness Facility Preparticipation Screening Questionnaire are available at http://circ.ahajournals.org/cgi/content/full/97/22/2283.[48] However, the goal of screening is to identify patients who need additional medical assessment. In the absence of physician referral or evidence that the referring physician has sufficiently assessed CVD risk, additional consultation should be considered. Typically, this involves referral to a physician to rule out coronary or other heart disease, often by exercise testing, for patients/clients with multiple risk factors and/or symptoms. Some physical therapists may be qualified to conduct such assessments. Attributes that indicate the need for further medical evaluation include age (males >45 years and females >55 years) and/or the presence of two or more CVD risk factors.[48]

Utility of the Decision Algorithm

The decision algorithm (Fig. 15-2) is meant to facilitate the clinical decision process when considering the cardiopulmonary practice patterns, particularly Patterns A and B. According to the algorithm, once it has been established that the patients/clients are not physically active, the next step involves determining if they have aerobic impairment resulting from deconditioning. In some cases, this determination is fairly obvious. Most of us would have little difficulty choosing between Patterns A and B for a client who walks up to you at a health and fitness clinic in a shopping mall and for a patient who has been sick in an intensive care unit bed for several weeks. Clinical decisions are rarely that straightforward, however, and it is useful to consider the tests and measures that will help us to distinguish between Patterns A and B.

Impaired aerobic capacity, which is characteristic of Pattern B, is suggested by the impairments, functional limitations, and disabilities listed under the Patient/Client Diagnostic Classification. What are some of the tests and measures that correspond to these features? Table 15-2 lists impairments, functional limitations, or disabilities with some corresponding tests and measures. Ability to perform functional activities, including gait and locomotion, self-care, and other occupational activities, and to gain access to home, work, and community environments may be severely compromised by impaired aerobic capacity resulting from deconditioning. Unusual or abnormal responses, such as a high resting HR and an exaggerated HR response during activity or exercise, are hallmarks of deconditioning. In

TABLE 15-2   **Impairments, Functional Limitations, or Disabilities Associated with Impaired Aerobic Capacity in Pattern B with Corresponding Tests and Measures**

Impairments, Functional Limitations, or Disabilities	Tests and Measures
• Decreased endurance	Aerobic capacity and endurance • Aerobic capacity during functional activities • Aerobic capacity during standardized exercise test protocols • Cardiovascular symptoms in response to increased oxygen demand with exercise and activity • Pulmonary symptoms in response to increased oxygen demand with exercise and activity
• Increased cardiovascular response to low-level workloads	Assistive and adaptive devices • Safety during use of assistive or adaptive devices and equipment
• Increased perceived exertion with functional activities	Circulation (arterial, venous, and lymphatic) • Physiologic responses to position change, including autonomic responses, central and peripheral pressures (eg, sphygmomanometry), heart rate and rhythm, respiratory rate and rhythm, ventilatory pattern
• Increased pulmonary response to low level work loads	Gait, locomotion, and balance • Gait and locomotion during functional activities with or without the use of assistive, adaptive, orthotic, protective, supportive, or prosthetic devices and equipment • Safety during gait, locomotion, and balance
• Inability to perform routine work tasks due to shortness of breath	Self-care and home management (including ADL and IADL) • Ability to gain access to home environments • Ability to perform self-care and home management activities with or without the use of assistive, adaptive, orthotic, protective, supportive, or prosthetic devices and equipment • Safety in self-care and home management activities and environments • Ventilation and respiration/gas exchange • Pulmonary signs of respiration/gas exchange, including breath sounds • Pulmonary signs of ventilatory function, including airway protection, breath and voice sounds, respiratory rate, rhythm and pattern, ventilatory flow, forces and volumes Work (job/school/play), community, and leisure Integration or Reintegration (including IADL) • Ability to assume or resume work, community, and leisure activities with or without the use of assistive, adaptive, orthotic, protective, supportive, or prosthetic devices and equipment • Ability to gain access to work, community, and leisure environments • Safety in work, community, and leisure environments

Adapted from the American Physical Therapy Association. Guide to Physical Therapist Practice, 2nd ed. *Phys Ther.* 2001 Jan;81(1):9-746. Preferred Physical Therapist Practice Patterns[SM] is a service mark of the American Physical Therapy Association.

addition, ADL or IADL scales, which are available in some clinical databases (eg, the Minimum Data Sets (MDS) or Outcome and Assessment Information Set (OASIS)), are useful in that they provide valid and reliable quantitative measures of functional status. From a cardiovascular and pulmonary standpoint, safety during activity is measured by assessing physiologic responses to activity, including vital signs such as HR, BP, and RR, along with associated signs and symptoms. The Borg Perceived Exertion Scales are widely used and are valid and reliable measures of subjective responses to activity.[49]

Beyond assisting with practice pattern determination, the tests and measures performed during a PT examination also help to identify patient/client impairments that must be considered to provide the most appropriate intervention. Furthermore, **the tests and measures performed during an examination enable the clinician to assess the safety and effectiveness of interventions.** Selection of specific tests and measures by a clinician will depend not only on the practice pattern chosen but also on both the practice setting and the skill and experience of the therapist. We next review some tests and measures that might be used to assess Joe Sixpack for both Patterns A and B.

Tests and Measures for Pattern A

We first encounter Joe when he asks the physical therapist to advise him about physical activity. He realizes that his sedentary habits are not healthy and wants to change them. During the examination process, the clinician has determined that Joe has multiple CVD risk factors including diabetes, obesity, hypertension, and hyperlipidemia. Joe has discussed this with his primary care physician who has examined him and ruled out CAD. During the PT examination, the clinician collects information that suggests that Joe belongs to Practice Pattern A and that will help the physical therapist to provide a safe and effective intervention.

To assess Joe's aerobic capacity and endurance, the physical therapist performs a submaximal exercise test, using an established exercise protocol, to ascertain his physiologic responses to activity and to establish a safe level of activity. The protocol chosen is the modified Bruce protocol, which begins at a relatively low intensity. Because this was a submaximal exercise test, the clinician predetermined an endpoint based on HR, using 85% of Joe's age-related maximum HR as the primary termination criteria. Since Joe is 50 years old that

TABLE 15-3 Results of Submaximal Stress Test Using the Modified Bruce Protocol

Stage	Accrued Time (min)	Speed (mph)	Grade	METS	HR	BP	RPE
Rest	3	—	—	—	92	154/86	6
0	3	1.7	0%	3	106	162/84	9
1/2	6	1.7	5%	4	118	166/90	10
1	9	1.7	10%	5	134	170/86	13
2	12	2.5	12%	7	150	190/94	16
Recovery	5	—	—	—	126	164/84	8

RPE, rating of perceived exertion.

endpoint is approximately 173 beats per minute (bpm), using the revised formula:

$$ARMHR = 208 - 0.7 \times age.[50]$$

The stress test protocol and results are displayed in Table 15-3. Note that Joe's vital sign responses to the test were relatively normal, with the exception of elevated BP at rest with a hypertensive response to activity. Joe reached stage 2, where he just exceeded the termination criteria leading to cessation of the test. After 5 minutes of recovery, he had not attained resting values of HR and BP. At the highest metabolic equivalent (MET) level achieved on this test (7) Joe's perceived exertion level corresponded to "heavy." These findings indicate decreased aerobic capacity, an inclusion criterion for Practice Pattern A.

Measurement of height, weight, and girth will enable calculation of body mass index (BMI) and waist circumference, which are used to determine relative weight and body fat distribution (see Chapter 3). To calculate BMI using English measurements, divide the weight in pounds by the square of the height in inches and multiply the quotient by 703:

$$BMI = [body\ weight\ (lb)/height\ (in.)^2] \times 703.$$

In Joe's case, his weight is 240 lb and his height is 71 in. (5 ft 11 in.), yielding a BMI of 33.5 ($[240/(71)^2] \times 703 = 33.47$) that is well within the obese range (BMI $\geq$ 30 kg/m^2) according to National Institutes of Health criteria.[51] Joe's waist circumference is 43 in., which places him at "high risk" (>40 in.) for conditions associated with obesity.[51] Readers interested in online calculation of BMI and other information related to overweight and obesity may visit the National Heart, Lung, and Blood Institute Web site at http://www.nhlbi.nih.gov/guidelines/obesity/ob_home.htm.

For Pattern A, other tests and measures that are helpful to provide a safe and effective intervention may include performance of pulse oximetry and assessments of pulmonary function test results, ability to clear his airway, chest wall mobility, and cough assessment, particularly if there is a history of pulmonary disease or dysfunction. Questions about Joe's self-care and home management abilities, as well as work and leisure activities, will provide important information on ADL and IADL functioning. To assess potential neuromuscular or mus-

culoskeletal impairments that may necessitate modification of physical activity and/or exercise analysis of functional muscle strength, resting posture, and range of motion are useful. In Joe's case, no gross pulmonary, neuromuscular, or musculoskeletal abnormalities, other than generalized muscle tightness, are seen. To obtain more information about function and quality of life outcomes, a health-related quality-of-life instrument, the SF-12 (see Fig. 15-4), is administered.

Tests and Measures for Pattern B

The Pattern B scenario is quite different. This time we meet Joe when he is approximately 60 years old and has been hospitalized after surgery, resulting in a prolonged recovery period that required much bed rest. His primary medical comorbidities—hypertension, diabetes, and obesity—continue to be important clinical issues. Joe's level of conditioning, which was low to begin with, is now very poor. Just moving in bed causes him to be short of breath, and he feels woozy the first time you ask him to sit up at the side of the bed. He is barely able to perform active range-of-motion exercises and complains of excessive fatigue when asked to do so. Clearly, he meets the criteria for Pattern B.

Table 15-2 lists the tests and measures that can be used to qualify a patient/client for Pattern B. We now examine some other tests and measures that would assist the clinician in providing a safe and effective intervention. One of the more important categories of tests and measures, and one that relates directly to the primary impairment that characterizes this pattern, is appraisal of aerobic capacity and endurance. Assessment of performance during established exercise protocols can provide information that may be used to determine an appropriate intervention and to evaluate the effectiveness of the intervention. A good choice in this setting is the timed walk (6- or 12-minute walk). The procedure for this test is detailed in Chapter 9. The validity and reliability of this procedure have been established for patients/clients with COPD and other conditions,[52] and the test may be used as an outcome measure for patients/clients with chronic diseases. Joe's test results are presented in Table 15-4. Following a practice test, designed to wash out a learning effect, Joe is able to cover 385 ft in 6 minutes, stopping twice to rest during the procedure. During the procedure, Joe experienced shortness of breath and an elevated

---

Your Health and Well-Being

This survey asks for your views about your health. This information will help keep track of how you feel and how well you are able to do your usual activities. *Thank you for completing this survey!*

For each of the following questions, please mark an ☒ in the one box that best describes your answer.

1. In general, would you say your health is:

Excellent	Very good	Good	Fair	Poor
▼	▼	▼	▼	▼
□1	□2	☒3	□4	□5

2. The following questions are about activities you might do during a typical day. Does <u>your health now limit you</u> in these activities? If so, how much?

	Yes, limited a lot	Yes, limited a little	No, not limited at all
	▼	▼	▼
a <u>Moderate activities</u>, such as moving a table, pushing a vacuum cleaner, bowling, or playing golf...	□1	☒2	□3
b Climbing <u>several</u> flights of stairs...	□1	☒2	□3

3. During the <u>past 4 weeks</u>, have you had any of the following problems with your work or other regular daily activities <u>as a result of your physical health</u>?

	Yes	No
	▼	▼
a <u>Accomplished less</u> than you would like............................	□1	☒2
b Were limited in the <u>kind</u> of work or other activities..........	☒1	□2

4. During the past 4 weeks, have you had any of the following problems with your work or other regular daily activities <u>as a result of any emotional problems</u> (such as feeling depressed or anxious)?

	Yes	No
	▼	▼
a <u>Accomplished less</u> than you would like............................	□1	☒2
b Did work or other activities <u>less carefully than usual</u>........	□1	☒2

5. During <u>the past 4 weeks</u>, how much did <u>pain</u> interfere with your normal work (including both work outside the home and housework)?

Not at all	A little bit	Moderately	Quite a bit	Extremely
▼	▼	▼	▼	▼
☒1	□2	□3	□4	□5

6. These questions are about how you feel and how things have been with you <u>during the past 4 weeks</u>. For each question, please give the one answer that comes closest to the way you have been feeling. How much of the time during the <u>past 4 weeks</u>...

	All of the time	Most of the time	A good bit of the time	Some of the time	A little of the time	None of the time
	▼	▼	▼	▼	▼	▼
a Have you felt calm and peaceful?.................	□1	□2	☒3	□4	□5	□6
b Did you have a lot of energy?......................	□1	□2	□3	☒4	□5	□6
c Have you felt downhearted and blue...............	□1	□2	□3	□4	☒5	□6

7. During the <u>past 4 weeks</u>, how much of the time has your <u>physical health or emotional problems</u> interfered with your social activities (like visiting friends, relatives, etc.)?

All of the time	Most of the time	Some of the time	A little of the time	None of the time
▼	▼	▼	▼	▼
☒1	□2	□3	□4	☒5

Thank you for completing these questions!

FIGURE 15-4   SF-12(r) completed by Joe pre-PT. (Reprinted with permission from Ware JE Jr, Kosinski M, Turner-Bowker DM, et al. User's Manual for the SF-12v2™ Health Survey with a Supplement Documenting SF-12® Health Survey. Lincoln, RI: QualityMetric Incorporated, 2002.)

respiratory rate and rated his perceived exertion as 15 on the Borg scale.[49] Physiologic responses are mildly hypertensive but otherwise acceptable.

Other tests and measures appropriate here include assessments of orientation to time, place, person, and situation and screening for level of cognition. These assessments provide important information about Joe's safety awareness and his ability to follow your instructions. Joe has developed dependency in ADL such that the therapist elects to use assistive and/or adaptive devices during examination and intervention.

TABLE 15-4   Six-Minute Walk Performance

	HR	BP	RPE	O$_2$ Saturation (%)	Respiratory Rate
Rest	98	146/86	8	97	16
Peak	136	168/92	15	98	20
Recovery	102	150/82	9	98	16

A wheeled walker is less energy costly than a standard walker and is the assistive device of choice for this deconditioned patient. **Accordingly, the therapist should assess gait and locomotion during functional activities with or without the use of assistive, adaptive, orthotic, protective, supportive, or prosthetic devices and equipment**[17] (see p. S479 of the *Guide*). These analyses should indicate whether Joe is able to ambulate with fewer symptoms, less assistance, and reduced danger of falling when using the device. During the analysis of the wheeled walker, the therapist is also analyzing gait, locomotion and balance, and self-care and home management activities, specifically ambulation. **Other functional tests and measures include ability to gain access to home environments and safety in self-care and home management activities**[17] (see p. S479 of the *Guide*). These tests measure how well Joe is able to move about his hospital room and about the hospital floor and perform important ADL activities like using the toilet, washing up, and getting dressed. Analysis of *muscle strength, power, and endurance; functional range of motion;* and *postural alignment and position*[17] (see p. S479 of the *Guide*) provide evidence of other impairments that will need to be considered during intervention.

Among the most important function-related tests and measures are assessments of autonomic responses to position changes and of physiologic responses during self-care and home management activities, including, of course, transfers and ambulation. The significance of these assessments cannot be emphasized too strongly, for they are key elements of PT practice for patients such as Joe.

CLINICAL CORRELATE

All too often, the assessment of physiologic responses, such as HR and BP, *during* activity is ignored by practicing physical therapists. Not only is important information neglected—information that alerts the clinician to potentially unsafe responses—but also the therapist misses an opportunity to contribute in a meaningful way to the overall management of the patient.

Indeed, it is this type of assessment, performed during examinations and interventions, that many consider to be routine and mundane, which demonstrate the *skill* of the therapist. In the current health care environment, characterized by

cost-efficiency and competition, our profession must take every opportunity to demonstrate that the services we provide are unique and necessary and that we are the ones with the best skills to provide them. In most settings there may be other health care professionals, for example, nurses, who take vital signs; but it is the physical therapist who can and should monitor these responses before, *during*, and after activity.

A distinction may be made here between assessment of physiologic responses to activity as part of the PT examination and physiologic monitoring during intervention. During the examination, the therapist should perform an assessment of physiologic responses to activity for any patient/client who may qualify for Practice Patterns A or B as well as for any patient with two or more CVD risk factors or a documented history or CVD. Medical clearance may also be indicated in primary care settings. The choice to continue to monitor physiologic responses, including vital sign assessment, during intervention-related physical activities is based on the cardiovascular status and medical history of the individual. A proposed decision model for physiologic monitoring based on American Heart Association (AHA) risk stratification criteria is presented in Table 15-5.[48,52] This model is based on age, CVD risk factors, and known heart disease and includes patients/clients who may qualify for Pattern A or B. Although the AHA recommends a diagnostic exercise test performed by a physician, this information is typically not available in inpatient settings. A reasonable substitute for an exercise test, particularly when the primary PT intervention involves training in ADL (bed mobility, transfers, ambulation, etc) or aerobic exercise, is to assess physiologic responses during the examination.

CLINICAL CORRELATE

The decision to continue monitoring during intervention depends on the responses during examination as well as on the medical status of the patient.

This model proposes minimal criteria for physiologic monitoring and clinicians may, at their discretion, decide that physiologic monitoring is needed even though it may not be indicated here.

Monitoring for patients/clients with comorbid pulmonary disease (eg, COPD) should also include performance of pulse oximetry to assess oxygen saturation and assessment of dyspnea. Patients/clients with diabetes deserve special consideration when it comes to monitoring physiologic responses. Persons with diabetes may have unusual vital sign responses to activity, including changes in position. This is particularly important to remember when mobilizing someone like Joe out of bed after a prolonged period of bed rest. Assessment of orthostatic tolerance by monitoring vital signs and symptoms is essential (see Chapter 10).

TABLE 15-5   Criteria for Ongoing Physiologic Monitoring and Recommended Activity Intensity[48,52]

Criteria	GXT or Physician Examination Recommended	Monitoring During Exercise or Physical Activity	Activity Intensity Recommended
Apparently healthy individuals with no CVD risk factors and age <45 years (men) or <55 years (women)	No	None needed	Moderate and vigorous
Apparently healthy individuals with no CVD risk factors and age ≥45 years (men) or ≥55 years (women)	Yes	None, if GXT normal If no GXT available, on examination only unless activity responses are abnormal	Moderate without GXT Vigorous if GXT is negative for heart disease
Apparently healthy individuals with 2 or more CVD risk factors and age ≥45 years (men) or ≥55 years (women)	Yes	None, if GXT normal If no GXT available, on examination only unless activity responses are abnormal During intervention at the discretion of the therapist	Moderate without GXT Vigorous if GXT is negative for heart disease
Individuals with stable heart disease (no resting ischemia or angina) and normal exercise responses	Yes	On examination During intervention until safety demonstrated. Ongoing monitoring may be prudent when changing or increasing intensity of activity.	Medical examination and GXT recommended before either moderate or vigorous activity

GXT, graded exercise test.

Data from Balady GJ, Chaitman B, Driscoll D, et al. Recommendations for cardiovascular screening, staffing and emergency policies at health/fitness facilities. *Circulation.* 1998;97:2283.

Data from Fletcher GF, Balady GJ, Amsterdam EA, et al. Exercise standards for testing and training: a statement for healthcare professionals from the American Heart Association. *Circulation.* 2001;104:1694-1740.

INTERVENTION TECHNIQUES

The health care interventions for individuals like Joe Six-pack—individuals with multiple risk factors for cardiopulmonary disease—can be broadly classified into pharmacologic and lifestyle interventions. This section provides an overview of both categories of interventions that pertain to diabetes, hyperlipidemia, and hypertension—conditions we see in our case study. The key components of the health care management of all these are *weight loss* in those who are overweight or obese and adequate *physical activity* and/or exercise. Accordingly, this section also reviews health care interventions for patients/clients who are overweight and obese. Interventions for physical activity, a component of health care management that physical therapists are ideally suited to provide, are discussed separately. PT interventions emphasizing physical activity and/or exercise, as they pertain to Patterns A and B, are highlighted.

Interventions for Diabetes

The primary goal in management of both type 1 and type 2 diabetes is to achieve and maintain normal levels of blood glucose. Maintenance of euglycemia (normal blood glucose levels) will prevent the acute and chronic complications of diabetes. Among the most serious acute complications of diabetes are diabetic ketoacidosis, which occurs primarily in persons with type 1 diabetes, and hyperosmolar hyperglycemic nonketotic syndrome, which is seen mostly in those with type 2 diabetes.

Both conditions represent acute decompensation due to inadequate levels of insulin and/or uncontrolled hyperglycemia. These conditions, if untreated, may lead to coma and death. Hypoglycemia, which is also known as an insulin reaction, is an acute state characterized by an abnormally *low* level of blood glucose. This condition, which causes symptoms ranging from confusion, weakness, and irritability to unconsciousness, requires immediate intervention, typically in the form of rapidly absorbed carbohydrates. Chronic complications of diabetes become manifest in numerous ways ranging from accelerated CVD and its attendant pathologies to retinopathy and blindness to peripheral and autonomic neuropathies, which impair sensorimotor function and cardiovascular responses to activity.

Achievement of euglycemia involves both medical intervention, including pharmacologic intervention, and self-care on the part of persons with diabetes. Pharmacologic management differs according to whether or not endogenous insulin is present. In type 1 diabetes, little or no insulin is available and individuals must rely on exogenous insulin that is injected or supplied by an insulin pump. Ideally, the patient self-monitors blood glucose levels several times daily and adjusts insulin and food intake, as well as physical activity, accordingly. For those with type 2 diabetes, the problem typically is not inadequate insulin. In fact, hyperinsulinemia (too much insulin in the blood) is common; rather, the problem is resistance to insulin leading to poor glucose uptake by cells such as skeletal muscle cells. Pharmacologic management of type 2 diabetes often involves the use of oral medications (sulfonylureas) to lower blood glucose. In some cases, persons with type 2 diabetes require insulin, although typically an insulin schedule that is less complex is recommended in type 1 diabetes. On the basis of evidence that regular exercise or physical activity contributes to glycemic control in type 2 diabetes, and prevention of CVD in all persons with diabetes, **the American Diabetes Association recommends regular exercise as an important component of diabetes management.**[25]

Self-care in diabetes has taken on increased importance as the benefits of glycemic control have become evident. Self-care places more responsibility on the patient/client, but it enables the individual to maintain blood glucose within a much narrower range, potentially avoiding prolonged episodes of hypoglycemia or hyperglycemia. Cornerstones of self-care include monitoring of blood glucose and recognition of signs and symptoms associated with acute and chronic complications of diabetes as well as modifying diet and physical activity.

Home glucose monitoring kits are commonly used for self-monitoring of blood glucose. A drop of blood is obtained from a finger stick and tested in a small device that gives an immediate reading of blood glucose level. The results enable rapid adjustment of insulin and/or diet, if necessary, to normalize blood glucose. Patient/client use of home or ambulatory monitoring systems can be very helpful to the physical therapist in planning or adjusting physical activity and/or exercise, particularly if the patient/client is symptomatic or is known to have difficulty with glycemic control. The same types of devices may be used in inpatient settings for convenient blood glucose monitoring, avoiding costly and time-consuming laboratory work.

Patients are taught to recognize the signs and symptoms of acute decompensation and to monitor changes related to chronic complications. Foot care is particularly important for the person with diabetes because of the problems associated with sensory neuropathy, which affects distal extremities early in its course. Wearing well-fitting shoes that avoid friction or cramping, inspecting the feet daily for early signs of skin breakdown or infection, and taking care not to injure the feet during ADL are all important aspects of foot care. Many older people with diabetes have their toenails trimmed by a health care professional to avoid infection. Early skin problems can be quickly treated before they become catastrophes like amputation.

Dietary self-management is important for persons with both type 1 and type 2 diabetes. In type 1 diabetes, food intake should correspond with insulin administration to avoid hypoglycemia, which can result from inadequate food intake following insulin injection, and hyperglycemia, which may occur if food is eaten without exogenous insulin administration. In addition, persons with type 1 and type 2 diabetes are urged to maintain a healthy, balanced diet that is low in saturated fats and contains the recommended components from all food groups. Individuals with type 2 diabetes, most of whom are overweight or obese, should receive education in strategies to help them maintain a healthy weight. For sedentary individuals, increasing physical activity is a vital element in weight-loss efforts—one for which physical therapist referral may be indicated.

Interventions for High Blood Cholesterol

The health care management of hyperlipidemia is based on overall CVD risk as well as on cholesterol levels of the patient/client. For individuals with high blood cholesterol, the focus of management is on reducing LDL-C, a high level of which is recognized as a distinct CAD risk factor. The National Cholesterol Education Program (NCEP) recommends that persons with established CAD be treated more aggressively than those who are merely "at risk" due to other CAD risk factors as well as those who are otherwise at relatively low risk.[53] This risk stratification is reflected in the clinical management of different patient populations. For patients/clients with diagnosed CAD, nonpharmacologic intervention is initiated if LDL-C is >100 mg/dL, whereas pharmacologic intervention should be considered if LDL-C is >130 mg/dL. In the absence of CHD, but when multiple risk factors are present (the clinical scenario for Practice Pattern A), LDL-C values of ≥160 and ≥130 mg/dL are threshold levels for initiation of nonpharmacologic therapy and consideration of pharmacologic intervention, respectively.

Nonpharmacologic intervention for cholesterol management consists of lifestyle changes in diet and physical activity. Dietary modification follows a two-step plan based on progressively reducing intake of fats and cholesterol and on reducing weight in those who are overweight or obese. A recommendation for the step I diet is to limit fat intake to 30% of the total nutrients consumed, of which 8% to 10% should come from saturated fats. Consumption of less than 300 mg of cholesterol and of sufficient calories to maintain healthy weight are also components of the step I diet. For the step II diet, saturated fats should comprise less than 7% of total fat intake and less than 200 mg of cholesterol should be consumed. For those who are overweight or obese, adjustment of calorie intake to achieve weight loss is recommended.[54]

Pharmacologic intervention is reserved for those who are unable to lower LDL-C to desirable levels—desirability being based on risk-stratification thresholds—with dietary modification and physical activity. Several classes of drugs are currently used for their LDL-C–lowering characteristics, including bile acid sequestrants, "statins," and fibric acids. For postmenopausal women, estrogen replacement may be considered to help raise HDL-C levels and lower LDL-C levels.

Interventions for Hypertension

Risk stratification is also used to determine the medical treatment course for patients/clients with high BP. Risk is based not only on the magnitude of BP elevation but also on the presence or absence of other CVD risk factors and evidence of CVD. Diabetes is a particularly strong factor in clinical decisions, as is evidence of organ-related pathology, such as left ventricular hypertrophy or renal insufficiency. Patients with BP in the high-normal range (130–140 mm Hg systolic and 80–85 mm Hg diastolic) or who are hypertensive, with SBP ranging between 140 and 160 mm Hg and DBP ranging between 90 and 99 mm Hg, are urged to adopt lifestyle modification unless diabetes, CVD, or organ damage is present. Pharmacologic intervention is the recommended treatment for all individuals with BP higher than 160 mm Hg systolic or 100 mm Hg diastolic or who have elevated BP with diabetes, clinical CVD, or organ-related pathology.[21]

Recommended lifestyle modifications include dietary modification by reducing sodium and maintaining sufficient intake of potassium, calcium, and magnesium and limiting alcohol intake to no more than 1 oz of ethanol, which is roughly equal to 24 oz of beer, 10 oz of wine, or 2 oz of 100-proof liquor. Allowable amounts of alcohol are lower for women and other persons of smaller stature. Where appropriate, weight loss is strongly recommended, as is increasing physical activity. Other lifestyle modifications designed to reduce CVD, such as smoking cessation and limiting intake of saturated fats and cholesterol, are also recommended. Relaxation and biofeedback have been used as interventions for high BP; however, the benefit of these therapies is difficult to distinguish from that conferred by providing support or education. Clinical trials examining the efficacy of relaxation therapy and/or biofeedback have yielded mixed results.[21]

Pharmacologic management of hypertension is undertaken in a stepwise fashion. Initially, low-dose consumption of a drug that should be taken only once a day is tried. Dosages are increased, or other medications are added, if target BP ranges are not met. Many antihypertensive medications produce undesirable side effects, an important consideration in patient/client adherence. Dosages and combinations of medications are adjusted until sufficient reduction in BP is achieved with minimal side effects. Various classes of drugs are used in the management of hypertension, including diuretics, adrenergic inhibitors such as β-blockers, calcium antagonists, direct vasodialators, and ACE inhibitors. Combination medications are becoming more available.[21] Specifics regarding the classes of antihypertensive drugs are discussed in more detail in Chapter 8.

Interventions for Overweight and Obesity

Determination of treatment for the overweight and obese is based on several factors, including BMI, waist circumference, and other CVD risk factors. For adults who are obese (BMI $\geq$30 kg/m^2), intervention is recommended. Intervention is also recommended for adults who are overweight (BMI 25–29.9 kg/m^2) or who have increased waist circumference (males $\geq$40 in. and females $\geq$35 in.) *if* two or more CVD risk factors are present. Interventions that are effective for weight management include dietary modification, increased physical activity, drug therapy, and in some cases, surgery. The goals of intervention are highly dependent on the patient's/client's motivation to control weight. For some, an initial goal simply may be to prevent further weight gain. For more motivated individuals, weight loss is the goal and once weight loss has been achieved, maintenance of healthier weight becomes a long-term goal.[51]

Dietary modification involves reduction in the amount of calories as well as in the percentage of fats and saturated fats

consumed. Calorie reduction between 500 and 1,000 kcal/day from the patient's regular consumption is recommended. Crash diets are generally not effective in reducing and *maintaining* weight. Successful dietary modification programs consider individual food preferences as well as ethnic and cultural attitudes toward food and weight. Gradual weight loss, approximately 1 to 2 lb/wk, is preferred over more rapid, but difficult to maintain, weight-loss programs.[51]

Other interventions for weight loss and weight control include *behavior therapy* incorporating self-monitoring, *stimulus management* (recognizing and controlling the triggers that lead to overeating), *stress reduction* and management, and *cognitive retraining.* Consideration of pharmacotherapy is usually reserved for those in the obese range of BMI or for those who are overweight and who have multiple CVD risk factors. Drugs that have been used for weight loss are appetite suppressants, of which there are few available choices due to lack of the Food and Drug Administration approval and a history of abuse and addiction. One such drug, which combined phentermine and fenfluramine (phen/fen), was withdrawn from the market in the early 1990s after an unacceptably high number of patients taking this medication developed valvular heart disease. A new anorexiant, called sibutramine, has recently been approved. Another medication, orlistat, reduces weight by decreasing fat absorption and has also recently received approval. Patients/clients who are extremely obese (BMI $\geq$40 kg/m^2) may be offered surgical therapy, including gastric restriction by stapling or banding or gastric bypass.[51]

Finally, physical activity is considered to be an integral aspect of weight reduction and maintenance. See Chapter 16.

Intervention for Smoking Cessation

Every clinical interaction with a patient who smokes should include a discussion of smoking status and an offer of treatment for smoking cessation. This is the advice from the Agency for Health Care Research and Quality for primary care physicians, nurses, and respiratory therapists, and there is no reason why this advice should not pertain to physical therapists as well. Discussion and documentation of smoking status with patients is associated with higher rates of quitting.[55] As many readers may know from personal or family experience, quitting smoking is no easy matter. There are powerful environmental, social, and behavioral inducements to smoke, not to mention the highly addictive nature of nicotine. For example, fear of, or actually, gaining weight after quitting may reduce cessation prevalence. Cultural attitudes toward smoking and beliefs regarding the efficacy of personal behavior in disease prevention also affect quit rates.

An effective pharmacologic approach, particularly for heavy smokers, involves *nicotine replacement,* either with nicotine gum or with a nicotine skin patch. Programs using these interventions generally do not exceed 8 weeks in length. Relative precautions regarding the use of nicotine replacement include pregnancy and diagnosed CVD. For persons with these conditions, the risks of continued smoking may outweigh the risks of nicotine replacement. Individuals who find quitting especially difficult may benefit from specialized, intensive smoking cessation intervention. These interventions may include *counseling* and *behavior therapy*. Problem-solving skills and encouraging social support are two effective approaches.[55] Physical therapists can assist with smoking cessation efforts by avoiding cigarette smoking, themselves, by discussing smoking cessation with patients/clients and being knowledgeable about available smoking cessation programs in their communities.

Intervention to Promote Physical Activity

There is abundant evidence that increased physical activity and/or physical fitness confers substantial health benefits, including lower all-cause mortality and mortality from CHD.[32–34] Furthermore, regular physical activity is also associated with improvements in nearly all of the modifiable cardiovascular risk factors discussed in this chapter. For example, habitual physical activity helps to prevent hypertension, type 2 diabetes, and obesity.[34] Physical activity also contributes to an improvement in lipid profile, through an increase in HDL-C[20,34,56]; helps to lower BP[34]; and to improve glycemic control in type 2 diabetes.[25,34,57]

Virtually, all of the health care interventions for the conditions seen in Joe Sixpack include efforts to increase the individual's level of physical activity. Because increasing physical activity is a fundamental consideration in the management of CHD and its attendant risk factors, physical therapists have an outstanding opportunity to contribute to prevention of morbidity and mortality from the nation's number one killer. The remainder of this section is devoted to interventions designed to increase physical activity for individuals and for communities. Public health intervention strategies for physical activity promotion are briefly reviewed. A substantial portion of this section is also devoted to specific PT interventions as they relate to cardiopulmonary Practice Patterns A and B.

Public Health Approaches to Physical Activity Intervention

From the perspective of individual behavior change, there has been substantial interest in behavioral models of physical activity promotion. Many theories of behavior change, such as the Transtheoretical Model, described earlier in this chapter have been applied to physical activity intervention. Common strategies include education in the benefits of, and instruction in, physical activity, goal-setting, and self-monitoring; providing inducements and rewards; contests within and between groups; and development of skills to avoid resumption of inactivity. Mass-marketing strategies have also been used. Behavioral intervention trials have occurred in homes, schools, places of work and worship, as well as in whole communities or regions. Of primary importance to physical therapists, however, are potential interventions that may be applied in clinical settings.

Although physical therapists are primarily concerned with the level of physical fitness of their patients and clients, they may also have an interest in promoting physical activity within their communities as a public service to encourage wellness. Ecological approaches to physical activity promotion encompass *community-based* considerations and interventions. For example, the design of many of our communities, in which one must drive somewhere to shop, learn, or worship, actually discourages physical activity. Pedestrian and bicyclist safety is an issue in communities without sidewalks or bike paths or pedestrian traffic signals. Concerns about crime also prevent many individuals from walking outdoors. All of these factors increase dependence on automobile transportation and decrease community physical activity. Our lifestyles, too, have become impediments to physical activity. Human labor used to have a substantial physical component that is lacking in today's office-oriented environment. The ubiquity of television encourages physically inactive behavior, especially among youth.

Community- and worksite-based approaches to physical activity promotion involve a wide range of disciplines, including health care professionals who are knowledgeable about the benefits of physical activity and physical fitness. Advocates for physical activity can lobby for installation of sidewalks or pedestrian crossings and signals at intersections. By constructing bicycle paths, we can encourage bicycling to the workplace and to other locations. Communities can also preserve open spaces for recreation rather than industrial development. Playgrounds that are safe and pleasant places for children to play, with shade from the sun and water for drinking, can be built and/or maintained. Progressive physical education in our schools develops lifetime physical activity skills that are inclusive of all students, not just of those that are athletically inclined. Children, youths, and adults—all benefit from community athletic leagues and clubs such as soccer teams or Little League. Community institutions that install secure bicycle storage areas promote bicycle transportation to and from these locations. Workplaces can encourage physical activity by installing fitness facilities and encouraging their use through workplace policies. Shopping malls and schools can be opened during off-hours and used for indoor physical activity. These indoor facilities are especially important when very hot or cold weather, or air pollution, prohibits outdoor activities. Venues for physical activity should be accessible to persons with disabilities to encourage physical activity in this population.

Physical Therapy Interventions for Physical Activity

Physical therapists are ideally suited to play a vital role in disease and disability prevention, as well as wellness, through counseling in physical activity and exercise prescription—activities that are principal interventions for cardiopulmonary Practice Patterns A and B. Just as Patterns A and B may be distinguished by the presence or absence of pathology-related deconditioning so is the focus of intervention determined by the intent to reverse deconditioning or prevent pathology.

For Pattern A, the focus is on prevention of disease in the presence of multiple risk factors. We have seen what health care interventions may be applied to risk factors other than physical activity, and we have glimpsed some community- and

TABLE 15-6   Clinical Indicators of Activity/Exercise Intensity[52]

Intensity	Percent of Maximum HR	RPE (6–20)	MET Level[a]	
			Age ≤ 65 y	Age > 65 y
Light	40–59	<12	2.5–4.5	2–3.5
Moderate	60–75	12–13	4.5–6	3.5–5
Vigorous	≥75	>13	>6	>5

[a]MET levels are 1–2 points higher than listed for younger individuals (age 20–39 years) and 1–2 points lower for very old individuals (age ≥ 80 years), and for women in all age categories.

Data from Fletcher GF, Balady GJ, Amsterdam EA, et al. Exercise standards for testing and training: a statement for healthcare professionals from the American Heart Association. *Circulation*. 2001;104:1694-1740.

individual-based strategies. The task of the physical therapist is to safely increase the client's level of physical activity and to optimize the potential that the gains in physical activity will be maintained. To accomplish this, physical therapists may wish to familiarize themselves with a model of behavior change, such as the Transtheoretical Model,[47] that can help to focus the intervention in the most effective manner.

Pattern A may apply in primary care settings or in situations where CVD risk is not identified by the referring physician. Because of this, risk stratification can assist the physical therapist in determining the need for further referral and the level at which physical activity or exercise may be safely undertaken by the patient/client. Earlier in this chapter, a risk stratification model to identify individuals needing monitoring of physiologic responses during activity was proposed (see Table 15-5). The attributes identified in this table may also be used to determine safe intensity of physical activity or exercise. According to AHA guidelines,[48] all persons without diagnosed heart disease, including apparently healthy younger, older, and at-risk (two or more CVD risk factors) individuals, may participate in *moderate* physical activity or exercise without first having an exercise test or physician examination. Before participating in *vigorous* activity, however, apparently healthy older and at-risk individuals should have a physician examination. Individuals with stable heart disease should undergo a physician examination and diagnostic exercise test before participating in either moderate or vigorous activity.

Parameters that can be used to distinguish between moderate and vigorous activity include HR and RPE during activity, and the level of METs at which an individual is working during activity. Please refer to Chapter 3 for discussion of metabolic equivalents. Table 15-6 lists the approximate parameters that define activity or exercise intensity. For HR, the revised percentage of age-related maximum HR may be used. The RPE scale used is the 6- to 20-point Borg scale.[49]

Primary Prevention for Joe Sixpack

For Joe Sixpack in Pattern A, CHD has been ruled out by physician examination and he has undergone a submaximal exercise

test to assess physiologic responses to activity. This type of exercise test should not be confused with a diagnostic exercise test performed by a physician or other qualified health care professional. Such a test would include 12-lead electrocardiogram monitoring to detect myocardial ischemia during the procedure. Theoretically, he would be allowed to engage in vigorous activity; however, the therapist may choose to be more cautious given his risk-factor profile and in light of the evidence that substantial health benefits accrue from physical activity and exercise done at moderate intensities. In addition, a moderate exercise program is likely to result in better adherence than a vigorous program.

Specific Interventions: Physical Activity Prescription

Specific interventions from the *Guide* that will improve Joe's CVD risk status include aerobic endurance activities and conditioning and active strengthening exercises. Other intervention components that would promote overall health and fitness might include body mechanics education, breathing exercises, posture education, and stretching. A PT intervention program for Joe in Pattern A will include an aerobic exercise prescription. Joe states that walking is an activity that he might enjoy and that is feasible for him. In keeping with recommendations regarding frequency of physical activity, Joe should walk 4 to 5 d/wk, or more often if he is able to do so. His walking intensity is based on HR and RPE parameters, so Joe will also be instructed in self-monitoring of HR and RPE using the 6- to 20-point Borg scale. Because Joe is 50 years old, his target HR range during activity may be as low as 87 and as high as 121, which is approximately between 50% and 70% of his age-related maximum HR. RPE should be around 11 to 12 out of 20. There is certainly some "wiggle room" at the upper end of his target HR and RPE range, given that vigorous activity is not contraindicated in his case, and he could be allowed to achieve a higher HR, say 133, during exercise. Keep in mind, however, that physical activity should be enjoyable and that Joe may not perceive his exercise as such at higher intensities where perceived exertion is higher and symptoms such as shortness of breath may occur. Because Joe is sedentary, he has the most to gain simply from advancing to a moderate level of fitness,[33] which can be accomplished at moderate intensities of activity. **Duration of activity should be at least 30 minutes daily; however, at least initially, this need not occur all at once. The 30 minutes of daily activity may be accumulated throughout the day.** Sedentary individuals beginning a physical activity or exercise program may use shorter, but more frequent daily bouts of activity, for instance, 10 minutes, three times per day, to achieve the recommended dose of physical activity. Table 15-7 summarizes Joe's physical activity prescription.

Joe's program should include warm-up and cool-down periods before and after his walking. Three to 5 minutes of slower walking can suffice as warm-up and cool-down activities. Gentle stretching of major muscle groups will increase flexibility, whereas low-intensity, high-repetition resistance

TABLE 15-7 Joe Sixpack's Physical Activity Prescription for Pattern A

Intensity	Heart rate = 74–103 (50%–70% of age-adjusted maximum) Rating of perceived exertion = 9–12
Frequency	4–5 d/wk
Duration	30 min, may be accumulated throughout the day, eg, in three, 10-min bouts of activity.
Mode	Walking, bicycling, etc. Consider "lifestyle" activities, eg, gardening

training will improve lean muscle mass. Depending on Joe's level of motivation, the therapist may wish to observe caution in recommending too complex a regime. The main goal is to get Joe off the couch and get him to be more physically active on most days of the week. Of course, Joe can substitute other activities for walking such as bicycling or gardening. He should also be advised that incorporating activities into daily life, by walking to the corner store to pick up the newspaper or taking the stairs instead of the elevator at work, is a good way to increase overall physical activity.

As clinicians we might be tempted to treat Joe at our clinic 2 to 3 d/wk for as long as it takes for an improvement in conditioning to occur. This is neither feasible in the current health care environment nor necessary or desirable. In reality, we may have one shot to convince Joe of the necessity of becoming more physically active and to teach him what he needs to know to accomplish this safely. The upper limit of visits for Pattern A is six visits,[17(pS469)] so let us assume that we have several more visits. Following the examination, Joe receives an initial instruction session, covering the mode of activity, in his case walking; the frequency duration; and intensity. Because Joe seems to be fairly well motivated and ready to change his behavior, we also provide instruction in stretching and strengthening activities. Additional instruction in HR and RPE monitoring as well as symptom awareness is provided.

How should the remaining sessions be utilized? Joe may return once per week for the next week or two to check on his adherence, answer questions, and perhaps, assess his responses to an increase in intensity (ie, speed and/or grade on the treadmill). Following this, he may return once per month or every other month for an additional two to three visits to monitor adherence and progress and to troubleshoot. Joe will find, and the therapist will recommend, that he can walk a bit faster as he progresses, as long as he remains within his target HR and RPE levels. If he wishes, Joe may increase the intensity even further, into the vigorous range, but only if he does not exhibit any symptoms during activity that might suggest heart disease. If he began his program by accumulating shorter bouts of daily activity, he can try to exercise for longer periods, less frequently during the day. During the last session, the submaximal stress test should be repeated and we can assess his overall adherence with the recommendations. The goals of this intervention are to improve aerobic capacity, physical function, health status, and the physiologic response to activity. In addi-

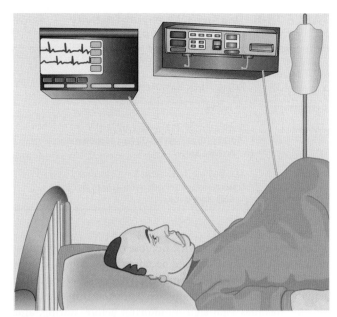

FIGURE 15-5 Joe Sixpack in the hospital.

tion, Joe should achieve a better understanding of personal and environmental factors that affect his health and adoption of health prevention strategies. Specifically, he becomes more physically active.

Joe Sixpack in the Hospital

When we encounter Joe in Pattern B, the clinical picture is very different. Now Joe is in the hospital and deconditioned; that is, he is short of breath during ADL such as moving in bed, transferring, and ambulating (Fig. 15-5). The focus of intervention will be to restore Joe to his previous level of function or at least to a functional level at which he is able to perform ADL and IADL without dyspnea. Interventions from the *Guide* that have the potential to remediate the primary impairment, deconditioning, include therapeutic exercise and functional training in self-care.

Specific Interventions: Physical Activity Prescription

Table 15-8 summarizes the physical activity prescription for Joe's PT intervention. The initial interventions will involve ADL training, including training in bed mobility, transfers, gait, and locomotion. These activities—moving in and arising from bed, sitting down in our favorite chair, and getting up and getting a cold drink from the kitchen—are activities that we tend to take for granted, and we no more think about the energy we expend doing these things than about breathing. For Joe, and many others like him who are recovering from or living with illness and are severely deconditioned, these tasks seem monumental. Simple daily activities represent a significant challenge to their cardiopulmonary system, causing them to work very hard indeed. The clinician must remember that performance of ADL in this setting may provide a more-than-adequate stimulus to reverse deconditioning and may be

TABLE 15-8   Joe Sixpack's Physical Activity Prescription for Pattern B

Intensity	Heart rate = 85–120 (50%–70% of age-adjusted maximum) Rating of perceived exertion = 9–12
Frequency	2–3 d/wk
Duration	Short bouts of 2–3 min, initially Progress to at least 15–20 min of continuous activity daily
Modes	ADL training, hallway walking, stationary bicycling Low-intensity strength training with elastic resistance bands

considered as *vigorous* activity. Because of the energy requirement associated with ADL and because of Joe's complex medical history, careful monitoring of physiologic responses to activity is indicated. As was discussed previously in this chapter, this includes vital sign monitoring before, during, and after activity and assessment of subjective responses including RPE, dyspnea, and other signs and symptoms.

As Joe improves—and with ADL training he improves quite quickly—aerobic conditioning and strengthening are added to his program. A stationary bicycle, which is often well tolerated by individuals who are deconditioned, is used for aerobic conditioning. Joe progresses from initially performing short bouts of 2 to 3 minutes, interspersed with 1- to 2-minute rest periods, to 15 to 20 minutes of continuous cycling. He also progresses from freewheeling, with no added resistance to cycling at 25 W. Other exercise modes are used as well, including hallway walking, which is part of an activity program that is carried out by nursing aides periodically during the day. Joe is also instructed in strengthening exercises using elastic resistance bands that are graded by resistance. Resistance is increased for each strengthening exercise pattern when Joe is able to perform 10 repetitions of a pattern without fatigue. An assistive device (wheeled walker) is prescribed, initially, to enhance his ambulatory safety. Over the course of time, as Joe's functional status improves he will be able to be weaned from this device.

For Pattern B, the course of treatment requires a longer period comprising a greater number of sessions that may span more than one practice setting. This particular episode of care begins in the acute hospital and culminates in an inpatient rehabilitation setting. In the acute hospital, the physical therapist sees Joe daily for four visits until he is transferred to the subacute rehabilitation unit. He resides there for 12 days where he is seen twice daily (once a day during the intervening weekend) and is discharged home. Before going home, Joe is instructed in a home walking program including self-monitoring of HR, RPE, and symptoms. A total of 26 PT treatment sessions were provided across two practice settings during this episode of care.

The goals for the interventions are to improve in performance of, and achieve independence in, ADL and IADL; to increase aerobic capacity and the ability to perform tasks related to self-care; and to improve the physiologic response to increased oxygen demand. Joe is able to perform ADL and IADL without the symptoms associated with deconditioning. The key outcomes associated with the course of treatment pertain to functional limitation and disability. Joe has returned to his former role function in his home environment where he safely and independently performs ADL and IADL. The risk of disability associated with acute and chronic illness is also prevented.

THRESHOLDS FOR INTERVENTION

This section summarizes the threshold parameters for health care interventions for the CVD risk factors seen in Joe Sixpack. Recall that a threshold behavior is one that triggers the inception of an intervention and identifies a minimum intensity, or higher, to realize the desired benefit (see Chapter 2). Tables 15-9 and 15-10 detail the thresholds, interventions, and potential benefits of treatment, according to risk-factor status, for obesity, hypertension, and high blood cholesterol. Health care interventions for these conditions are based on complex risk-stratification decisions that are somewhat simplified in this presentation. For high blood cholesterol, initial screening is based on TC, which, if elevated, triggers further laboratory analysis of the full lipid profile. Subsequent intervention decisions are based primarily on LDL-C. For high blood cholesterol, high BP/hypertension, and overweight/obesity, risk status is based on the presence and number of other CVD risk factors. For high BP/hypertension, an additional risk consideration is based on clinical evidence of organ damage such as renal insufficiency or left ventricular hypertrophy. Notice also that increased waist circumference qualifies as overweight status.[49,53,58]

Table 15-11 summarizes the clinical thresholds, interventions, and potential benefits for diabetes, stratified by type of diabetes. Regardless of type of diabetes, the clinical threshold for elevated blood glucose is 126 mg/dL, and the desired clinical response to intervention is a lowering of blood glucose to <120 mg/dL and of GHb to <7%. Interventions vary for type of diabetes based principally on use of exogenous insulin. Although some individuals with type 2 diabetes benefit from use of exogenous insulin, the decision to use insulin in type 2 diabetes usually occurs late in the course of the disease. Insulin use in type 1 diabetes is a fundamental component of management at the onset of the disease. Common elements of management in both type 1 and type 2 diabetes include dietary modification and physical activity. Because a high proportion of individuals with type 2 diabetes are also overweight or obese, weight loss is typically an additional consideration.[25]

Table 15-12 presents the thresholds that identify individuals as physically inactive, the desirable level of activity, and the potential benefits[34,35,38] of physical activity with regard to selected CVD risk factors and physiologic parameters measured during exercise. The benefits of increased physical activity and exercise extend to a wide range of conditions including CVD risk factors and physiologic parameters. A benefit of physical activity that may be especially

TABLE 15-9 Practice Pattern A: Threshold Values and Behaviors, Interventions, and Potential Improvement for Overweight and Obesity[51]

Type and Risk Profile	Threshold Value	Interventions	Potential Improvements
Overweight with <2 CVD risk factors	BMI 25–29 kg/m^2 or WC^a > 40 in males > 35 in females	Advise to lose weight and increase physical activity	10% reduction in body weight within 6 months
Overweight with ≥2 CVD risk factors	BMI 25–29 kg/m^2 or WC > 40 in males > 35 in females	Clinical intervention • Low-calorie diet • Increase physical activity • Behavior therapy • Consider pharmacologic therapy • if BMI ≥ 27 kg/m^2	10% reduction in body weight within 6 months
Obese	BMI ≥ 30 kg/m^2	Clinical intervention • Low-calorie diet • Increase physical activity • Behavior therapy • Consider pharmacologic therapy • Consider surgical therapy if BMI ≥ 40 kg/m^2	10% reduction in body weight within 6 months

^{a}WC, waist circumference.

Adapted from National Heart Lung and Blood Institute. *Clinical Guidelines on the Identification, Evaluation and Treatment of Overweight and Obesity in Adults: The Evidence Report.* Bethesda, MD: National Institutes of Health; 1998.

important to individuals with CHD is the reduced resting and submaximal HR and rate pressure product (RPP), which is seen following training. Lowering of these parameters reduces myocardial oxygen demand—the workload of the heart—at rest and during usual daily activities. Not listed in Table 15-12 is the potential benefit of increased physical activity and exercise with respect to weight loss and reduced incidence of CHD, hypertension, diabetes, osteoporosis,

some types of cancer, all-cause mortality, and overall physical functioning.[33,34]

It should be said that characterizing the benefits of physical activity and exercise is not a straightforward process. The issue is clouded by variation in measurement of physical activity and physical fitness, which are very different attributes. Further confusion results from studies in different populations, for example, healthy young subjects versus older

TABLE 15-10 Practice Pattern A: Threshold Values and Behaviors, Interventions, and Potential Improvement for High Blood Cholesterol and High Blood Pressure[21,54]

Risk Factor	Risk-Factor Profile	Threshold Value Nondrug Therapy	Threshold Value Pharmacologic Therapy	Interventions	Potential Improvement
High blood cholesterol	No CHD <2 risk factors	LDL-C ≥160	LDL-C ≥190	Nondrug interventions Dietary modification	Reduction of LDL-C to below threshold values:
(Unit values are mg/dL)	No CHD ≥2 risk factors	LDL-C ≥130	LDL-C ≥160	Increase physical activity Weight loss	<160 if no CHD and fewer than 2 risk factors
	CHD present	LDL-C ≥100	LDL-C ≥130	Pharmacologic interventions Statins Bile acid sequestrants Nicotinic acid (Fibrates)	<130 if no CHD and 2 or more risk factors <100 if CVD present
High blood pressure	One or more or no risk factors, no organ damage	130–160/ 85–99	>160/>100	Nondrug interventions Weight loss Increase physical activity	Reduction of blood pressure to below 140/90
(Unit values are mm Hg)	CVD and/or diabetes present	N/A	>130/>85	Pharmacologic interventions Stepwise management	

Data from National High Blood Pressure Education Program. The sixth report of the Joint National Committee on Prevention, Detection, Evaluation, and Treatment of High Blood Pressure. *Arch Intern Med.* 1997;157:2413.

Data from U.S. Department of Health and Human Services, National Cholesterol Education Program, National Heart, Lung, and Blood Institute, National Institutes of Health. *Third Report of the Expert Panel on Detection, Evaluation, and Treatment of High Blood Cholesterol in Adults (Adult Treatment Panel III).* NIH publication 01-3670, May 2001.

TABLE 15-11   Practice Pattern A: Threshold Values and Behaviors, Interventions, and Potential Improvement for Diabetes[25]

Type of Diabetes	Threshold Value	Interventions	Potential Improvements
Type 1	FPG[a] $\geq$ 126 mg/dL	Insulin injection Dietary modification Increase physical activity	Lower FBG to <120 mg/dL Lower GHb to <7%
Type 2	FPG $\geq$126 mg/dL	Dietary modification Increase physical activity Weight control Oral hypoglycemic medications May need insulin injection	Lower FBG to <120 mg/dL Lower GHb to <7%

[a]FPG, fasting plasma glucose.

Adapted from American Diabetes Association. Clinical practice recommendations, 2000. *Diabetes Care.* 2000;23(suppl 1).

patients with CAD or other pathology. The evidence that has accumulated regarding the benefits of physical activity and exercise is derived from various types of investigations, including epidemiologic studies and studies using an interventional approach. Therefore, the benefits of physical activity listed in Table 15-12 must be interpreted with caution. Just because an epidemiologic study shows that a particular parameter changes by x amount in a population does not necessarily mean that the same parameter will change by x amount in Joe Sixpack, the individual. Activity that fails to increase aerobic fitness may nevertheless result in improved health and decreased risk for disease. Taken as a whole, the evidence for the beneficial effects of an active lifestyle on disease incidence, risk factors, and physiologic parameters is strong and undeniable.

Intervention thresholds for Practice Pattern B are less clear in terms of measurable clinical and physiologic parameters. A decision method for physiologic monitoring based on age and the presence of CVD risk factors or CAD is proposed in Table 15-5. A maximal exercise capacity of 6 METs or less is considered to be a threshold for symptomatic deconditioning, which is the hallmark of Pattern B.[52] Maximal exercise capacity of 6 METs has also been associated with increased CAD and all-cause mortality.[33] Unfortunately, maximal exercise testing is not feasible in the typical clinical setting in which Pattern B is operative, so we are left with a more subjective assessment. The presence of any symptoms including dyspnea, dizziness, fatigue, or diaphoresis during ADL may be a reasonable threshold indicator for intervention in Pattern B. An additional threshold for consideration of immediate treatment modification or termination is a fall in SBP below resting value, particularly if the decrease is 20 mm Hg or more.

GOALS AND OUTCOMES

The *Guide to Physical Therapist Practice* was developed using the Disablement Model developed by Nagi and articulated by Verbrugge and Jette[2] to conceptualize the results of PT intervention. This model is discussed in Chapter 2. Briefly, goals and outcomes may be classified within the Disablement Model based on their impact on disability, functional limitation, and impairment and indirectly, on pathology pertaining to risk factors. Using the Disablement Model, Tables 15-13 and 15-14 summarize the results (ie, goals and outcomes) of PT intervention for Patterns A and B, respectively. Goals of PT intervention address impairments and at least one risk factor, physical inactivity, whereas outcomes of PT intervention address functional limitations and disabilities.

For Pattern A (Table 15-13) the episode of care spanned six visits over a 6-month period. Joe states that he now walks 4 to 5 d/wk, usually outdoors, but he uses the local shopping mall when weather prohibits outdoor activity. Performance on the repeat submaximal exercise test 6 months later improved by one stage to the 10-MET level. At this stage, peak HR was 146, BP was 184/90, and RPE was reported at 15—values that are essentially unchanged from his pretest performance. This indicates that his aerobic capacity has improved because he is able to achieve a higher workload without additional physiologic stress. Subjectively, Joe reports that ADL and IADL

TABLE 15-12   Threshold Parameters, Physical Activity (PA) Objectives and Benefits[34,37,38]

Threshold for Insufficient PA	Target PA Levels	Potential Benefits of PA
No moderate activity ($\leq$40% of HR_{max})	At least moderate PA (50%–65% of HR_{max})	Lipids: HDL-C increase 3–8 mg/dL
Activity <3 d/wk	At least 4–5 d/wk	BP: decrease 5–15 mm Hg in SBP and DBP
No sustained ($\geq$30 min) leisure or occupational PA	At least 30 min/d	Diabetes: 10%–20% improvement in GHb Resting HR decrease 10 bpm Decrease in resting and submaximal RPP

TABLE 15-13   Goals and Outcomes for Pattern B[17] (p S471) According to the Disablement Model

Pathology and Attendant Risk Factors[a]	Impairments[a]	Functional Limitations[a]	Disability (Including Quality of Life) [a]
• Physiologic response to increase oxygen demand is improved • Risk factors are reduced • Safety is improved • Walks 4–5 d/wk • Identifies risk behaviors, including weight loss, cigarette smoking and physical inactivity, and coping strategies that he is working to improve	• Endurance is increased • Energy expenditure per unit of work is decreased • Submaximal exercise test performance improved by one stage • Submaximal HR and BP are unchanged at higher workloads	• Ability to perform physical activities related to self-care, home management, work community and leisure is improved • Reports that it is "easier" to do yard work at home	• Ability to assume or resume required self-care, home management, work, community, and leisure roles is improved • Improved score on the SF-24 measure

HR, Heart rate; BP, Blood pressure.

[a]Joe's performance.

require less effort at home. The score on the SF-12 has improved, primarily because of increase in score in the physical functioning domain. Prior to PT intervention, Joe's SF-12 physical domain score was 42.00, which is below the national mean for the instrument. Following PT intervention, Joe achieved a physical domain score of 56.61, which is above the national mean (see Figs. 15-4 and 15-6). Joe now rates his overall health as "very good," is no longer "limited in the kind of work or other activities" he does, and now has "a lot of energy, most of the time." Finally, Joe relates how, in addition to acquiring the habit of walking on most days of the week, he has quit smoking and is eating a healthier diet, though he admits that he relies on snacks to help cope with cravings for cigarettes. Consequently, Joe has not lost as much weight as he had hoped—he has lost from 240 to 228 lb—although he appears trimmer, perhaps due to weight redistribution, and his waist circumference has decreased by 1.5 in.

Joe received a total of 26 visits from a physical therapist, 4 in the acute care setting and 22 in subacute inpatient rehabilitation. Table 15-14 presents the results of PT intervention for Pattern B. On admission to rehabilitation, the functional independence measure (FIM) and 6-minute walk were administered. Total score on the FIM also improved. End of program 6-minute walk distance was 625 ft, which is an improvement of 240 ft. Other changes noted during the exit test were a lower peak HR of 124 and a lower RR of 20, indicating an improvement in physiologic response to increased oxygen demand. On the stationary bicycle, Joe began his program by freewheeling—pedaling with no resistance—for several 2- to 3-minute bouts, with 1- to 2-minute rest periods each session. He has progressed to cycling

TABLE 15-14   Goals and Outcomes for Pattern B[17] (p S483) According to the Disablement Model

Pathology and Attendant Risk Factors[a]	Impairments[a]	Functional Limitations[a]	Disability, Including Quality of Life[a]
• Physiologic response to increase oxygen demand is improved • Symptoms associated with increased oxygen demand are decreased • Safety is improved • Able to move in bed, transfer and ambulate short distances without shortness of breath or dizziness • Demonstrates and discusses the importance of an independent walking program and accurate self-monitoring of HR, RPE, and symptoms prior to discharge	• Aerobic capacity is increased • Endurance is increased • Energy expenditure per unit of work is decreased • Muscle performance is increased • Improved 6-min walk performance • Progressed to 20 minutes of stationary cycling at 25 W with stable physiologic responses • Resistance of elastic strengthening bands increased by two grades	• Ability to perform physical activities related to self-care, home management, work community and leisure is improved • Level of supervision required for task performance is decreased • Performance of and independence in ADL and IADL are increased • Tolerance of positions and activities is increased • Able to move in bed, transfer and ambulate short distances independently • Improved score on the Functional Independence Measure	• Ability to assume or resume required self-care, home management, work, community, and leisure roles is improved • Discharged to home when independent in bed mobility, transfers and ambulation

ADL, Activities of daily living; IADL, Instrumental activities of daily living.

[a]Joe's performance.

Your Health and Well-Being

This survey asks for your views about your health. This information will help keep track of how you feel and how well you are able to do your usual activities. *Thank you for completing this survey!*

For each of the following questions, please mark an ⊠ in the one box that best describes your answer.

1. In general, would you say your health is:

Excellent	Very good	Good	Fair	Poor
▼	▼	▼	▼	▼
☐1	⊠2	☐3	☐4	☐5

2. The following questions are about activities you might do during a typical day. Does <u>your health now limit you</u> in these activities? If so, how much?

	Yes, limited a lot ▼	Yes, limited a little ▼	No, not limited at all ▼
a <u>Moderate activities</u>, such as moving a table, pushing a vacuum cleaner, bowling, or playing golf.	☐1	☐2	⊠3
b Climbing <u>several</u> flights of stairs	☐1	☐2	⊠3

3. During the <u>past 4 weeks</u>, have you had any of the following problems with your work or other regular daily activities <u>as a result of your physical health</u>?

	Yes ▼	No ▼
a <u>Accomplished less</u> than you would like	☐1	⊠2
b Were limited in the <u>kind</u> of work or other activities	☐1	⊠2

4. During the past 4 weeks, have you had any of the following problems with your work or other regular daily activities <u>as a result of any emotional problems</u> (such as feeling depressed or anxious)?

	Yes ▼	No ▼
a <u>Accomplished less</u> than you would like	☐1	⊠2
b Did work or other activities <u>less carefully than usual</u>	☐1	⊠2

5. During <u>the past 4 weeks</u>, how much did <u>pain</u> interfere with your normal work (including both work outside the home and housework)?

Not at all	A little bit	Moderately	Quite a bit	Extremely
▼	▼	▼	▼	▼
⊠1	☐2	☐3	☐4	☐5

6. These questions are about how you feel and how things have been with you <u>during the past 4 weeks</u>. For each question, please give the one answer that comes closest to the way you have been feeling. How much of the time during the <u>past 4 weeks</u>...

	All of the time ▼	Most of the time ▼	A good bit of the time ▼	Some of the time ▼	A little of the time ▼	None of the time ▼
a Have you felt calm and peaceful?	☐1	☐2	⊠3	☐4	☐5	☐6
b Did you have a lot of energy?	☐1	⊠2	☐3	☐4	☐5	☐6
c Have you felt downhearted and blue.	☐1	☐2	☐3	☐4	⊠5	☐6

7. During the <u>past 4 weeks</u>, how much of the time has your <u>physical health or emotional problems</u> interfered with your social activities (like visiting friends, relatives, etc.)?

All of the time	Most of the time	Some of the time	A little of the time	None of the time
▼	▼	▼	▼	▼
☐1	☐2	☐3	☐4	⊠5

Thank you for completing these questions!

FIGURE 15-6   SF-12(r) completed by Joe post-PT. (Reprinted with permission Ware JE Jr, Kosinski M, Turner-Bowker DM, et al. User's Manual for the SF-12v2™ Health Survey with a Supplement Documenting SF-12® Health Survey. Lincoln, RI: QualityMetric Incorporated, 2002.)

with resistance and revolutions per minute (rpm) set at 25 W for a total of 20 minutes. In his strengthening program, he progressed in grade of resistance bands by two grades throughout the episode of care. When Joe is discharged home he is independent in bed mobility and transfers and ambulates within and around his home. He understands the importance of maintaining his physical activity level and plans to continue with a walking program of moderate intensity. He is accurate in monitoring his own HR and uses HR and the RPE scale to maintain a safe level of independent activity while in the rehabilitation unit (Fig. 15-7).

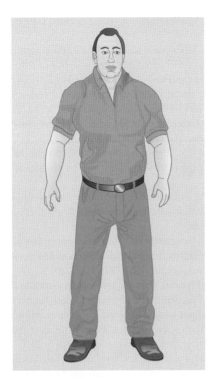

FIGURE 15-7   The new Joe Sixpack.

LIMITS OF KNOWLEDGE

The scientific evidence supporting the health care interventions discussed in this chapter is based on extensive clinical and epidemiologic research, which forms a large body of literature. However, much of the research that has informed us about the risk factors of CHD is based on studies of populations with relatively high socioeconomic status that has included few members of African American or Asian ethnic groups and many studies included only men. The generalizability of this research is limited by these considerations. There has been heightened interest, recently, in investigating CVD risk in women and in non-white ethnic groups, but the full impact of this research on clinical practice is yet to be seen. Research on the effects of deconditioning has similar limitations in that most of these studies, too, used young, healthy, predominantly male volunteers. Very little work has been done to investigate the effects of deconditioning on patient populations.

Other considerations regarding the literature on CVD risk factors are worth discussing. Risk factors, such as cholesterol, BP, BMI, and blood glucose, that are associated with CVD and related conditions are measured on continuous, numeric scales. For example, an SBP of 140 is 1 unit higher than an SBP of 139, 2 units higher than an SBP of 138, and 10 units higher than an SBP of 130, and so on. The epidemiologic research identifying these risk factors indicates that risk factors are associated with various disease outcomes, including CHD and mortality, in a continuous fashion. In other words, the risk of a developing CHD or of dying increases incrementally as, say, SBP increases. The risk for someone with an SBP of 130 is slightly higher than that for someone with an SBP of 120 or even 128, and it is higher still than that for someone with an SBP of 96. Yet, an SBP of 140 or higher is generally regarded as the point at which we decide that someone is hypertensive because of increased risk of undesirable outcomes such as CHD, stroke, or death. Indeed, virtually all clinical risk stratification guidelines identify risk-factor cut-points, above or below which the risk of disease is said to increase or decrease. Defining thresholds in this manner helps to translate scientific knowledge in ways that the public may better understand and use in personal decisions. Thresholds are also useful for clinical decision making, as is apparent in this chapter and textbook and in other works devoted to developing evidence-based clinical practice. Students, as well as practitioners at all levels of expertise, are wise to remember, however, that thresholds may not capture the true relationship between risk factor and disease occurrence or between clinical indicator and clinical outcome.

Another caveat regarding the setting of thresholds is that we may set them too high or too low. In so doing, we may misclassify individuals as being at high risk when they really are not or as being at low risk when they truly are at high risk. The former type of misclassification may needlessly stigmatize individuals and/or expose them to unnecessary diagnostic procedures or treatment interventions, with *their* inherent risks. The latter type of misclassification leads to withholding of potentially beneficial diagnostic procedures or interventions.

The recently updated BMI cut-points that define overweight and obesity, endorsed by the National Heart, Lung, and Blood Institute (NHLBI), provide an example of a controversial threshold. As Strawbridge and colleagues[57] point out in the *American Journal of Public Health,* the NHLBI threshold assigns a "disease" status to 55% of American adults. They argue that the evidence for increased risk of morbidity and mortality for those in the overweight range (BMI 25–29 kg/m^2) is weak and may not be equally valid for elders, women, and members of non-white ethnic groups. Furthermore, lowering the threshold for overweight and obesity may have the unintended consequence of promoting eating disorders such as anorexia and bulimia as people, particularly young women, strive to achieve an "acceptable" weight. The increased emphasis on overweight and obesity also tends to overlook the risk of underweight status (BMI < 18 kg/m^2), which is significantly related to mortality in women.[57]

This chapter emphasizes the interrelations between CHD risk factors and highlights how behaviors such as physical activity and exercise, cigarette smoking, and dietary modification are common elements in many interventions associated with reducing CHD risk. In the current health care environment in the United States, much emphasis is placed on an individual's behavior and the corresponding impact on health. We urge patients/clients to stop smoking, lose weight, and exercise more, and when they are unsuccessful in their efforts, as many are, we tend to hold the individual accountable and in effect, blame the victim. Individual behavior is subject to many powerful environmental influences from peers, culture, and the larger society. These influences can be very difficult to resist. Advertising, for example, portrays cigarette smoking as sociable, glamorous, and desirable. Tobacco companies have successfully marketed products to specific demographic groups, such as women and African Americans. Remember, too, that nicotine is highly addictive, making it difficult to quit once one has started smoking. Cultural preferences for high-fat foods may be difficult to overcome in prevention efforts. Healthy foods like fresh fruits and vegetables tend to be expensive and may not be available or accessible in low-income neighborhoods. The automobile culture and the design of our communities provide few opportunities for physical activity. The images of physical activity seen in broadcast and print media typically portray young, attractive, spandex-clad athletes engaging in sweaty and often painful appearing "workouts." Perhaps these images actually *discourage* physical activity when viewed by habitually sedentary, older individuals like Joe Six-pack. Remember that preventive health care interventions often must try to change the habits of a lifetime.

Heads Up!

This chapter contains a CD-ROM activity.

REFERENCES

1. Centers for Disease Control and Prevention, National Center for Health Statistics. *Fastats.* 1999. http://www.cdc.gov/nchs/fastats/fastats.htm. Accessed March 9, 2010.
2. Verbrugge L, Jette A. The disablement process. *Soc Sci Med.* 1994;38:1.
3. Ross R. The pathogenesis of atherosclerosis: a perspective for the 1990s. *Nature.* 1993;362:801.
4. Vogel R. Cholesterol lowering and endothelial function. *Am J Med.* 1999;107:479.
5. Tracy RE, Newman WP III, Wattigney WA, et al. Histologic features of atherosclerosis and hypertension from autopsies of young individuals in a defined geographic population: the Bogalusa Heart Study. *Atherosclerosis.* 1995;116:163.
6. Stary HC. Evolution and progression of atherosclerotic lesions in coronary arteries of children and young adults. *Arteriosclerosis.* 1989;9(1 suppl):I19.
7. Ornish D, Scherwitz LW, Billings JH, et al. Intensive lifestyle changes for reversal of coronary heart disease. *JAMA.* 1998;280:2001.
8. Baller D, Notohamiprodjo G, Gleichmann U, et al. Improvement in coronary flow reserve determined by positron emission tomography after 6 months of cholesterol-lowering therapy in patients with early stages of coronary atherosclerosis. *Circulation.* 1999;99(22):2871-2875.
9. Jukema J, Bruschke A, van Boven A, et al. Effects of lipid lowering by pravastatin on progression and regression of coronary artery disease in symptomatic men with normal to moderately elevated serum cholesterol levels. *Circulation.* 1995;91(10):2528-2540.
10. Mack W, Krauss R, Hodis H. Lipoprotein subclasses in the monitored atherosclerosis regression study (MARS). Treatment effects and relation to coronary angiographic progression. *Arterioscler Thromb Vasc Biol.* 1996;16(5):697-704.
11. deFaire U, Ericsson C, Grip L, Nilsson J, et al. Secondary preventive potential of lipid-lowering drugs: the bezafibrate coronary atherosclerosis intervention trial. *Eur Heart J.* 1996;17(suppl F):37-42.
12. Tamara A, Mikuriya Y, Nasu M. Effect of pravastatin (10 mg/day) on progression of coronary atherosclerosis in patients with serum total cholesterol levels from 160 to 220 mg/dL and angiographically documented coronary artery disease. *Am J Cardiol.* 1997;79(7):893-896.
13. American Cancer Society. *Statistics.* 1999. http://www.cancer.org/statistics.htm. Accessed March 9, 2010.
14. Thorndike AN, Rigotti NA, Stafford RS, Singer DE. National patterns in the treatment of smokers by physicians. *JAMA.* 1998;279:604.
15. Rennard SI. Inflammation and repair processes in chronic obstructive pulmonary disease. *Am J Respir Crit Care Med.* 1999;160:S12.
16. Cosio MG, Guerassimov A. Chronic obstructive pulmonary disease: inflammation of small airways and lung parenchyma. *Am J Respir Crit Care Med.* 1999;160:S21.
17. American Physical Therapy Association. Guide to Physical Therapist Practice, 2nd ed. *Phys Ther.* 2001 Jan;81(1):9-746.
18. National Heart Lung and Blood Institute. *Framingham Heart Study: 50 Years of Research Success.* 1998 (a). http://rover.nhlbi.nih.gov/about/framingham/. Accessed March 9, 2010.
19. Grundy SM, Pasternak R, Greenland P, et al. Assessment of cardiovascular risk by use of multiple-risk-factor assessment equations: a statement for healthcare professionals from the American Heart Association and the American College of Cardiology. *Circulation.* 1999;100:1481.
20. Hardman A. Interaction of physical activity and diet: implications for lipoprotein metabolism. *Public Health Nutr.* 1999;2:369.
21. National High Blood Pressure Education Program. The sixth report of the Joint National Committee on Prevention, Detection, Evaluation, and Treatment of High Blood Pressure. *Arch Intern Med.* 1997;157:2413.
22. Cook NR, Cohen J, Hebert PR, et al. Implications of small reductions in diastolic blood pressure for primary prevention. *Arch Intern Med.* 1995;155:701.
23. Bottcher M, Falk E. Pathology of the coronary arteries in smokers and non-smokers. *J Cardiovasc Risk.* 1999;6:299.
24. Centers for Disease Control and Prevention. *Targeting Tobacco Use: The Nation's Leading Cause of Death.* Atlanta, GA: U.S. Department of Health and Human Services; 2000.
25. American Diabetes Association. Clinical practice recommendations, 2000. *Diabetes Care.* 2000;23(suppl 1).
26. Hsueh WA, Law RE. Cardiovascular risk continuum: implications of insulin resistance and diabetes. *Am J Med.* 1998;105(1A):4S.
27. Harris MI, Flegal KM, Cowie CC, et al. Prevalence of diabetes, impaired fasting glucose and impaired glucose tolerance in US adults. The Third National Health and Nutrition and Examination Survey, 1988–1994. *Diabetes Care.* 1998;21(4):518-524.
28. Grundy SM, Benjamin IJ, Burke GL, et al. Diabetes and cardiovascular disease. A statement for healthcare professionals from the American Heart Association: *Circulation.* 1999;100:1134.
29. Abate N. Obesity as a risk factor for cardiovascular disease. *Am J Med.* 1999;107(2A):12S.
30. Grundy SM, Balady GJ, Criqui MH, et al. Primary Prevention of coronary heart disease: guidance from Framingham. A statement for healthcare professionals from the AHA Task Force on Risk Reduction: *Circulation.* 1998;97:1876.
31. Fletcher G. Physical inactivity as a risk factor for cardiovascular disease. *Am J Med.* 1999;107(2A):10S.

32. Blair SN, Kohl HW, Barlow CE, et al. Changes in physical fitness and all-cause mortality: a prospective study of healthy and unhealthy men. *JAMA.* 1995;273:1093.

33. Blair SN, Kohl HW, Paffenbarger RS, et al. Physical fitness and all-cause mortality: a prospective study of healthy men and women. *JAMA.* 1989;262:2395.

34. U.S. Department of Health and Human Services. *Physical Activity and Health: A Report of the Surgeon General.* Atlanta, GA: Centers for Disease Control and Prevention, National Center for Chronic Disease Prevention and Health Promotion; 1996.

35. Hakim AA, Petrovitch H, Burchfiel CM, et al. Effects of walking on mortality among nonsmoking retired men. *N Engl J Med.* 1998;338:94.

36. Pereira MA, Kriska AM, Day RD, et al. A randomized walking trial in postmenopausal women: effects on physical activity and health 10 years later. *Arch Intern Med.* 1998;158:1695.

37. Pollock ML, Gaesser GA, Butcher JD, et al. The recommended quantity and quality of exercise for developing and maintaining cardiorespiratory and muscular fitness, and flexibility in healthy adults. *Med Sci Sports Exerc.* 1998;30:975.

38. Fletcher GF, Balady G, Blair SN, et al. Statement on exercise: benefits and recommendations for physical activity programs for all Americans. A statement for health professionals by the Committee on Exercise and Cardiac Rehabilitation of the Council on Clinical Cardiology, American Heart Association. *Circulation.* 1996;94:857.

39. Pate RR, Pratt M, Blair SN, et al. Physical activity and public health: a recommendation from the Centers for Disease Control and Prevention and the American College of Sports Medicine. *JAMA.* 1995;273:402.

40. Caspersen CJ, Powell KE, Christenson GM. Physical activity, exercise, and physical fitness: definitions and distinctions for health-related research. *Public Health Rep.* 1985;100:126.

41. Mosca L, Manson JE, Sutherland SE, et al. Cardiovascular disease in women. A statement for healthcare professionals from the American Heart Association. *Circulation.* 1997;96:2468.

42. Friedlander Y, Siscovick DS, Weinmann S, et al. Family history as a risk factor for primary cardiac arrest. *Circulation.* 1998;97:155.

43. Schächinger V, Britten MB, Elsner M, et al. A positive family history of premature coronary artery disease is associated with impaired endothelium-dependent coronary blood flow regulation. *Circulation.* 1999;100:1502.

44. Rosanski A, Blumenthal JA, Kaplan J. Impact of psychological factors on the pathogenesis of cardiovascular disease and implications for therapy. *Circulation.* 1999;99:2192.

45. Convertino VA. Cardiovascular consequences of bed rest: effect on maximal oxygen uptake. *Med Sci Sports Exerc.* 1997;29:191.

46. DeBusk RF, Convertino VA, Hung J, Goldwater D. Exercise conditioning in middle-aged men after 10 days of bed rest. *Circulation.* 1983;68:245-250.

47. Prochaska JO, Redding CA, Evers K. The Transtheoretical Model and stages of change. In: Glanz K, Lewis FM, Rimer BK, eds. *Health Behavior and Health Education: Theory, Research, and Practice.* 3rd ed. San Francisco: Jossey-Bass Publishers; 1997.

48. Balady GJ, Chaitman B, Driscoll D, et al. Recommendations for cardiovascular screening, staffing and emergency policies at health/fitness facilities. *Circulation.* 1998;97:2283.

49. Borg G. Psychophysical bases of perceived exertion. *Med Sci Sports Exerc.* 1982;14:377.

50. Tanaka H, Monahan K, Seals D. Age-predicted maximal heart rate revisited. *J Am Coll Cardiol.* 2001;37:153-156.

51. National Heart Lung and Blood Institute. *Clinical Guidelines on the Identification, Evaluation and Treatment of Overweight and Obesity in Adults: The Evidence Report.* Bethesda, MD: National Institutes of Health; 1998.

52. Fletcher GF, Balady GJ, Amsterdam EA, et al. Exercise standards for testing and training: a statement for healthcare professionals from the American Heart Association. *Circulation.* 2001;104: 1694-1740.

53. National Cholesterol Education Program. Second report of the Expert Panel on detection, evaluation, and treatment of high cholesterol in adults (Adult Treatment Panel II). *Circulation.* 1994;89:1329.

54. U.S. Department of Health and Human Services, National Cholesterol Education Program, Bethesda, MD. National Heart, Lung, and Blood Institute, National Institutes of Health. *Third Report of the Expert Panel on Detection, Evaluation, and Treatment of High Blood Cholesterol in Adults (Adult Treatment Panel III).* May 2001. NIH publication 01–3670.

55. Fiore MC, Bailey WC, Cohen SJ, et al. *Treating Tobacco Use and Dependence. Clinical Practice Guideline.* Rockville, MD: U.S. Department of Health and Human Services, Public Health Service; 2000.

56. Leon AS. Effects of exercise conditioning on physiologic precursors of coronary heart disease. *J Cardiopulm Rehabil.* 1991;11:46.

57. Strawbridge WJ, Wallhagen MI, Shema SJ. New NHLBI clinical guidelines for obesity and overweight: will they promote health? *Am J Public Health.* 2000;90:340.

58. Steele B. Timed walking tests of exercise capacity in chronic cardiopulmonary illness. *J Cardiopulm Rehabil.* 1996;16:25.

C H A P T E R   15

An International Perspective: Canada

Elizabeth Dean

INTRODUCTION

As a backdrop to my commentary on the chapter by Dr. Brooks, I provide an overview of the status of contemporary physical therapy practice in Canada based on my observations as a practitioner and a scientist, and then on the practice of cardiovascular/cardiopulmonary physical therapy specifically. With respect to Dr. Brooks' chapter, in addition to reviewing aspects of the pathophysiology of cardiovascular disease and selected risk factors, Dr. Brooks has provided an overview of the process of decision making related to categorizing a given patient to either Practice Pattern A or B within the cardiovascular/pulmonary specialty. The purpose of my commentary on the chapter is twofold: first, to evaluate the application of practice patterns in the context of primary prevention, risk reduction, and deconditioning with respect to the patient described in the chapter; and second, to comment on the relevance of the model of practice patterns to Eastern cultures.

PHYSICAL THERAPY PRACTICE AND CARDIOVASCULAR/CARDIOPULMONARY PHYSICAL THERAPY IN CANADA

In my view, physical therapy practice in Canada, comparable to that in the United States, has advanced markedly in some notable domains over the past three decades, yet has remained relatively unchanged in others. With respect to areas of change, the majority of physical therapists in Canada can now practice without a physician referral. The trend with respect to scope of practice is away from doctor- and hospital-based care and toward community, home, and self-care. Despite this trend, as yet, there is less prominence of rehabilitation aides and assistants in Canada compared with the United States. I attribute this to a prevailing belief that assessment and treatment go hand in hand and that a physical therapist needs to perform ongoing assessment. In Canada, I anticipate that within the decade, physical therapy will be an outsourced service in the hospital sector, supporting the growing trend toward consultation services. This change has been paralleled by greater promotion of interdisciplinary team care in which patients are increasingly empowered to be active participants in preserving their health, self-healing, and long-term remediation of health problems. There has been exponential growth of not only scientific activity in the profession reflected by the growing number of doctoral qualified academic faculty members and numbers of graduate programs and students in the country but also recognition of the need to ensure scientific rigor and translate scientific findings into evidence-based practice. A growing number of studies are being published on the cost-effectiveness of treatments, which reflects demands on the profession to be increasingly accountable to the public and those paying the bills. These advances have all been very positive. But, I query whether these advances could be too much too late.

With respect to areas of relative stagnation within the profession in Canada and in the United States, in my view these include an inexplicable lag in physical therapists embracing their role foremost as clinical exercise physiologists and educators as integral components of their professional identity. Exercise is the hallmark of physical therapy and the physical therapist's principal "drug." We were strategically positioned to have been leaders in the clinical exercise physiology movement beginning in the 1970s; I believe this was a missed opportunity that has altered the course of the evolution of our profession. Exercise testing and training became integrated into "cardiac rehabilitation" and then "pulmonary rehabilitation" in the 1970s and 1980s. For many years it appeared that exercise testing and training were viewed by physical therapists as being unique to "cardiac and pulmonary rehabilitation" rather than principles and practices that were applicable across specialties. Only relatively recently have formal exercise testing and training become terms used in orthopedics and neurology, and even so this does not appear to be a consistent practice.

The cardiovascular/cardiopulmonary systems subserve every other system; therefore, physical therapists across specialties require assessment and treatment skills in this specialty. Conditions of these systems will invariably constitute comorbidities in patients being treated for orthopedic and neurologic conditions. Despite this, I have observed a deficiency in basic hemodynamic monitoring of patients with these conditions. Given the powerful combination of exercise and education tailored to both the needs and the wants of the patient, treatments require time. Appropriate treatment time is not reflected in most billing schedules. I would not find it surprising that physical therapy continues to be underfunded due to the lack of advocates supporting the need for the appropriate treatment frequency and course. PT will be shown to be ineffective because, like antibiotics, if the course of treatment is insufficient, so will the treatment be shown to be ineffective. The current structure and distribution of physical therapists across specialties (detailed further in reference to the cardiovascular/pulmonary specialty, in particular, later) have failed to expand and contract in the face of changing demographics. For example, in addition to cardiovascular/pulmonary physical therapy, other virtually invisible specialties are gerontology, oncology, and diabetes.

Despite the fact that patient education, a subspecialty in education, has also been a hallmark of physical therapy, in my view little of the scientific evidence supporting teaching principles is being integrated into contemporary physical therapy practice. This element of the patient–therapist relationship may determine whether a treatment succeeds or fails. Without question, most physical therapists would acknowledge that they advise their patients for prevention and instruct them in carrying out their treatment programs. I contend, however, that with the move toward greater empowerment and active participation in their care, patients require formalized education based on documented education principles including assessments of attitudes, learning style, and as required, readiness to adhere to treatment or change. This is particularly true considering that the leading causes of morbidity and mortality today in the more developed world are largely preventable according to the World Health Organization.

In my view, as a profession we have been slow in responding to the needs of those from other cultures. Immigration within Canada and the United States has enriched our respective societies with different attitudes, values, and beliefs. To maximize patient rapport, hence, treatment effectiveness, it behooves us to understand the values, attitudes, and beliefs of our patients regarding their health, ill health, and means of recovery and to incorporate this knowledge into our treatments. On the basis of my experience and observations in non-Western cultures, physical therapists from these cultures, who have qualified in Western-based programs either in the West or in their countries, are more adept than Western physical therapists treating individuals from non-Western countries, in ensuring that their treatments are culturally relevant and sensitive. Health care practitioners in the West, I believe, have a great deal to learn from our colleagues from other cultures—the success of our treatments depends on it.

The rapid change needed in these professional domains, during this period of shifting sands in the health care reform movement in Canada as well as in the United States, does not appear imminent to me. The slowness of change may give the impression that we are self-serving as a profession, rather than our priority being the public and societal need. In addition, it is clear that multiple other professions are encroaching on areas of practice in which the physical therapist, I believe, is the most qualified health care professional to provide such service.

Many of the areas of relative stagnation that I have identified in Canada as well as in the United States are particularly apparent in the cardiovascular/pulmonary specialty. Despite national and global indicators that the cardiovascular/pulmonary specialty should be one of the largest specialties, the conventional breakdown of specialty dominance is roughly 50%

orthopedics, 30% neurology, 15% cardiovascular/pulmonary, and 5% other. As therapists within the profession and within the specialty, we have fallen short in assuming prominent leadership roles in influential political, national, and provincial/state arenas including public health and health care policy. Further, I believe that the profession has failed in large part to update our health care colleagues and the public on changes in our practice. We seem bewildered when our expertise fails to be recognized and promoted by our health care colleagues. The profession needs articulate advocates to establish its rightful place in the health care delivery system as a primarily noninvasive health care service, whose benefits should be promoted as "primary" intervention before invasive care whenever possible and ethical to do so. It is clear that noninvasive care should be exploited primarily to support health ahead of invasive care, given the growth of iatrogenic conditions and their associated economic and societal costs. A prime example of the failure to exploit physical therapy is its diminishing presence in critical care—the most invasive and costly of health care settings; a trend widespread in the United States and increasingly in Canada. There is substantial lack of awareness, both within and outside the profession, of the essential role of physical therapy as a primarily noninvasive practice in this setting. The more high tech this setting becomes, the more noninvasive practices need to be exploited in my view for ethical and cost considerations as well as for minimizing the risk of iatrogenic effects. This area of practice provides an example of the lack of integration of the literature into practice. For several decades the literature has supported unequivocally the potent and direct effects of body positioning and exercise principles on gas exchange and that these potent interventions need prescription to achieve optimal results in critically ill patients. There appears to be an unsubstantiated belief that "routine" nonprescriptive body positioning and mobilizing performed by non–physical therapists achieves an equivalent result. The literature fails to support this view. Rather, body positioning and mobilization can be prescribed to enhance the steps of the oxygen transport pathway selectively, thereby impacting oxygen delivery directly. Considering the indications for a physical therapy presence in intensive care, how is our diminishing visibility explained?

APPLICATION OF PRACTICE PATTERNS IN THE CONTEXT OF PRIMARY PREVENTION, RISK REDUCTION, AND DECONDITIONING

The model of preferred practice patterns has emerged in the United States over the past decade, in response to the demand for physical therapist practice guidelines.[1] These guidelines were achieved through consensus. They describe the treatment options for each practice pattern that is recommended to affect an optimal outcome within an optimal number of treatments. Ten preferred practice patterns have been defined to encompass all possible physical therapy diagnoses within the cardiovascular/pulmonary specialty. The focus of this chapter is on primary prevention, risk reduction, and deconditioning; thus, my remarks will be confined to these. As a means of distinguishing the basis for selecting Practice Pattern A (*Primary Prevention/Risk Reduction for Cardiovascular/Pulmonary Disorders*) versus B (*Impaired Aerobic Capacity/Endurance Associated with Deconditioning*), Dr. Brooks describes two scenarios related to the case of Joe Sixpack.

The Case of Joe Sixpack

Joe's history included hypertension, hypercholesterolemia, and diabetes. In addition, he was overweight and sedentary, and he smoked. The first time we were introduced to Joe, he was seeking advice regarding preparation for a 5-km race in a month. He was categorized into Practice Pattern A, in that, this opportunity could be used to promote primary prevention and risk reduction related to cardiovascular or pulmonary disorders. At another time, Joe was described as having been "flat on his back for a while," presumably in an acute or rehabilitation setting following surgery or an accident. In this instance, Joe was categorized into Practice Pattern B, that is, consistent with *Impaired Aerobic Capacity/Endurance Associated with Deconditioning*.

Strengths and Limitations of Practice Patterns

The case of Joe Sixpack exemplifies the strengths and limitations of a model of practice based on practice patterns. With respect to strengths, practice patterns constitute the lowest common denominator of patient management. Practice patterns can increase the standards of physical therapy practice in situations or settings where practice standards are low. They aim to expand the level and scope of care by crossing specialty boundaries, promote safety standards, identify practice guidelines based on a consensus exercise of those in the specialty, and identify aspects of care that are outside as well as within the boundaries of physical therapist practice.

With respect to their limitations, practice patterns can promote a narrowness of focus in patient care because of the need to have the patient conform to one or more practice patterns within or outside the specialty. This limitation is particularly salient as health care delivery shifts toward holistic, integrative, patient-centered care. Joe Sixpack demonstrates this point.

On the basis of his risk-factor profile, Joe has both non-modifiable and modifiable risk factors for several "diseases of civilization" including lung disease, hypertension, stroke, cancer, and diabetes as well as atherosclerosis and coronary artery disease. With respect to the "number one killer" in the United States, namely, coronary artery disease, Joe's nonmodifiable risk factors include his gender and his age. His modifiable risk factors include cholesterol and saturated fat intake, smoking, sedentary lifestyle, and obesity. In the first instance, because he is currently asymptomatic for heart disease, Joe is classified

as Practice Pattern A (*Primary Prevention/Risk Reduction for Cardiovascular/Pulmonary Disorders*). Although hypertension, hypercholesterolemia, and diabetes are established risk factors for cardiovascular disease, these conditions are primarily life-threatening conditions that have been well documented to be amenable to diet, exercise, and education.[2-9] Joe has clinical signs of these conditions for which he is being medically managed. Noninvasive management in their primary management has yet to be exploited. There is substantial evidence supporting physical therapy intervention for these primary medical diagnoses[2-9] in the same way that there is for coronary artery disease[10] or for smoking-related pulmonary disease.[11] Potent noninvasive interventions need to be instituted as primary interventions for the management of these life-threatening conditions.

Joe Sixpack Falls Between the Practice Pattern Cracks

For optimal and safe management of Joe, he should be viewed as having multiple interrelated life-threatening conditions rather than as an individual with a collection of risk factors, ranging in degree of severity, for cardiovascular disease. He is a candidate for primary physical therapy to address his serious medical problems, namely, hypertension, hypercholesterolemia, and diabetes in addition to weight control, with the goal being to wean him from his medications, avoid surgery, and restore him to good health. Given this perspective, there is no ideal practice pattern for Joe.

On a general note, noninvasive interventions need to be promoted as the "primary" interventions in the absence of pharmacologic agents, coincident with pharmacologic agents until these can be weaned or in conjunction with these agents for a long term. As primarily a noninvasive practitioner, the physical therapist's principal goal is to eliminate the patient's need for medication and surgery and to promote lifelong self-responsibility for health and well-being. If medication is needed, then minimizing the potency of the medication and the dose in combination with noninvasive interventions is the priority. If the patient fails to adhere to a noninvasive program, in favor of invasive care only, then reasons for failure need to be addressed. The lack of appropriate practice patterns to identify the primary management of physical therapy for hypertension, hypercholesterolemia, and diabetes not only limits our professional "lens" in terms of our management of patients with these conditions but also conveys to others outside the profession an apparent lack of a primary role of physical therapy in the management of these conditions.

With respect to the second scenario, preferred Practice Pattern B (*Impaired Aerobic Capacity/Endurance Associated with Deconditioning*) fails to focus on Joe's more urgent problems. Deconditioning as a result of restricted activity would certainly be demonstrable; however, the severity of his other problems will contribute more significantly to reduced aerobic capacity and endurance. His other problems compound the complicating physiologic effects of recumbency and any further restriction in his physical activity. These factors should be the focus of the practice pattern in the context of his being hospitalized.

Both Practice Patterns A and B focus on functional capacity. This reflects, in part, the move away from the biomedical model to Nagi's Disablement Model and the levels problem definition, namely, impairment, action, and participation (or formerly impairment, disability, and handicap).[12,13] However, in the cardiovascular and pulmonary specialty, patients can have normal functional capacity in the presence of life-threatening impairments such as arrhythmias and conditions such as high blood pressure, hypercholesterolemia, and diabetes. Thus, in this specialty, impairment needs to be considered as a primary focus.

Noninvasive physical therapy practice needs to assume its rightful place in the health care delivery system. In the public's best interest, it is imperative that we within the profession do not marginalize the priority of physical therapy in the primary management of a range of cardiovascular/pulmonary conditions beyond primary cardiovascular and pulmonary disorders. The exploitation of noninvasive approaches needs to remain a priority and become an increasing and not less of a priority, commensurate with more costly, hi-tech, and invasive medical care that also constitutes greater risk. This is particularly evident in the management of chronic degenerative conditions whose management through traditional invasive care has been considerably less impressive than that through noninvasive management including diet, exercise, and education.

PRACTICE PATTERNS AND THEIR PSYCHOSOCIAL AND SOCIOCULTURAL RELEVANCE AND SENSITIVITY

At the psychosocial level, health care is shifting away from a patriarchal biomedical model to a patient-focused model that is reflected in the preferred practice patterns. Along with this trend has been a greater awareness of patients as individuals worthy of respect and having the opportunity to be active participants in their own care.

With respect to sociocultural considerations, the determinants of health and ill health reflect sociocultural as well as physical influences. At a global level, health care trends and rehabilitation, in particular, reflect Western culture, attitudes, values, and beliefs. Eastern-based medical philosophies have been largely ignored or minimized in importance yet have serviced well a large proportion of the world's population for several thousand years.[14] Even though there has been growing awareness and acceptance of Eastern-based health care practices, the prevailing attitude in the West is still one of these being "alternatives" or "complementary" rather than first-line interventions, implying that Western approaches remain those of choice. This is an interesting observation, given that Western-based medicine is in its

infancy compared to ancient Chinese medicine. Clearly, both approaches have strengths and limitations. Health care providers, educators, and researchers need to think beyond practice patterns based on Western values in order to be receptive to the merging of Eastern and Western philosophies to maximize interventions and health care outcomes by combining their strengths and minimizing the limitations of either philosophy individually.

SUMMARY AND CONCLUSION

Dr. Brooks's chapter describes a case that illustrates the decision-making process in assigning a client/patient to either Practice Pattern A or Practice Pattern B. The preferred practice patterns adopted by the American Physical Therapy Association have strengths and limitations and these are illustrated in relation to the patient featured in the chapter. In terms of strengths, preferred practice patterns maintain a standard for the lowest common denominator of practice with respect to both physical care and psychosocial considerations. In terms of limitations, difficulties can be anticipated when one attempts to pigeon-hole patients into restrictive practice patterns, which in turn, can lead to suboptimal care. In the case described, the patient has multiple life-threatening conditions such as hypertension, hypercholesterolemia, and diabetes that independently can be amenable to physical therapy care, in addition to being risk factors for cardiovascular disease. The present structure of the practice patterns tends to consider these primarily as modifiable risk factors, thereby minimizing the primary role of physical therapy in the management of each independently. Finally, psychosocial and sociocultural considerations are highlighted. Attention to these, and an appreciation of patients as individuals who should be treated with dignity, and that of other cultures and their perspectives on health and ill health will result in truly holistic, integrative health care in the years ahead. The integration of Eastern philosophies with Western philosophies will enhance approaches to wellness and health promotion, treatment interventions, and health outcomes, and overcome the limitations of either health care philosophy individually. By having adopted practice patterns within the profession, we need to ensure that our practice does not default to the lowest common denominator. Rather, we must be aware of their limitations and continually strive toward refining their application through a broad understanding of health and health care that cross the boundaries of both culture and practice patterns.

REFERENCES

1. American Physical Therapy Association. Guide to Physical Therapist Practice, 2nd ed. *Phys Ther.* 2001 Jan;81(1):9-746.
2. American Diabetes Association. Clinical practice recommendations, 2000. *Diabetes Care.* 2000;23(suppl 1).
3. Duncan J. The effects of an aerobic exercise program on sympathetic neural activity and blood pressure in mild hypertension. *Circulation.* 1983;68:285-288.

4. Hardman A. Interaction of physical activity and diet: implications for lipoprotein metabolism. *Public Health Nutr.* 1999;2:369.

5. Wood P. Increased exercise level and plasma lipoprotein concentrations: a one year, randomized, controlled study in sedentary, middle-aged men. *Metabolism.* 1983;32:31-39.

6. Richter E. Diabetes and exercise. *Am J Med.* 1984;70:201-209.

7. The Sixth Report of the Joint National Committee on Prevention, Detection, Evaluation, and Treatment of High Blood Pressure (JNC VI). *Arch Intern Med.* 1997;157:2413-2446.

8. American College of Sports Medicine. Physical activity, physical fitness, and hypertension. Position stand. *Med Sci Sports Exerc.* 1993;25:i-x.

9. Gordon NF. The exercise prescription. In: Derlin JT, Ruderman N, eds. *The Health Professional's Guide to Diabetes and Exercise.* Alexandria, VA: American Diabetes Association; 1995:70-82.

10. Wallace JP. Obesity. In: Durstine JL, ed. *ACSM's Exercise Management for Persons with Chronic Diseases and Disabilities.* Champagne, IL: Human Kinetics; 1997:106-111.

11. Hammond C. Smoking in relation to mortality and morbidity. Findings for mortality research. *J Natl Cancer Inst.* 65;5:1115-1124.

12. Nagi SZ. Some conceptual issues in disability and rehabilitation. In: Sussman MB, ed. *Sociology and Rehabilitation.* Washington, DC: American Sociological Association; 1965:100-113.

13. World Health Organization (WHO). *International Classification of Impairments, Disabilities, and Handicaps. A Manual of Classification Relating to the Consequences of Disease.* Geneva, Switzerland: World Health Organization; 1980.

14. *The Yellow Emperor's Classic of Medicine.* Boston: Shambhala Publications Inc; 1995.

Physical Therapy Associated with Obesity

Cheri L. Gostic & Dawn M. Blatt

INTRODUCTION

Obesity has grown into a major public health issue over the past several decades. Since 1980, the incidence of overweight adolescents and children has tripled, while the prevalence of obesity in adults has doubled in the United States.[1] The most recent data from the National Health and Nutrition Examination Survey (NHANES) from 2003 to 2004 reveal that 66% of adults in the United States are overweight with 32% of these individuals meeting the criteria for obesity.[2] Body mass index (BMI), defined as body weight (in kg) divided by height squared (in [meters]^2), has become the most commonly used indicator of overweight and obesity. Overweight is defined by a BMI between 25 and 29.9 kg/m^2. Adults with a BMI $\geq$30 kg/m^2 are classified as obese, and those with a BMI $\geq$40 kg/m^2 as morbidly obese (class III). Table 16-1 provides a chart that can be used to determine an adult's BMI and weight classification based on height and body weight. Children are at risk of being overweight if their BMI falls between the 85th to 95th percentile for their age and sex on standard growth charts, and considered obese at or above the 95th percentile.

CLINICAL MANIFESTATIONS

The National Center for Health Statistics reports that health risks become apparent at a BMI greater than 27 kg/m^2 (overweight). In adults, the adverse effects of obesity on health are well documented. Obesity increases the risks of cardiovascular disease, diabetes, stroke, arthritis, gall bladder disease, respiratory conditions, and certain cancers.[3] It is associated with an increased risk of morbidity and mortality as well as reduced life expectancy. Obesity is ranked second only to the use of tobacco as the leading preventable cause of death.[4]

Individuals who are overweight or obese are predisposed to coronary artery disease, heart failure, and sudden death due to changes in metabolism as well as a variety of alterations in cardiac structure and function that occur as adipose tissue accumulates in excess amounts throughout the body. Obesity also adversely affects the heart because of its association with hypertension, dyslipidemia, type 2 diabetes, inflammatory markers, obstructive sleep apnea, and a propensity for thrombosis.[5]

Obesity produces an increase in total blood volume and cardiac output that is caused by the high increased metabolic activity of excess adipose tissue. At any given level of activity, then, cardiac workload is greater for obese individuals than for individuals of normal weight. In moderate-to-severe cases of obesity, this increased workload can lead to left ventricular dilation, compensatory left ventricular hypertrophy, left ventricular diastolic dysfunction, and eventually heart failure.[6] Obese men and women have an increased risk of cardiac arrhythmias and sudden death that is about 40 times higher than the rate of unexplained cardiac arrest in individuals that are not obese.[7]

There are numerous respiratory complications associated with obesity, including hypoventilation and sleep apnea. Respiratory muscle expansion is restricted by the weight of the chest wall and pressure on the thoracic cavity from the large abdomen. Hypoventilation due to restrictive lung disease in individuals who are obese leads to an increase in $PaCO_2$ (hypercapnia) and chronic hypoxia. Studies reveal an increased demand for ventilation, an increased workload of breathing, respiratory muscle inefficiency, decreased functional reserve capacity and expiratory reserve volume, and atelectasis of peripheral alveoli in subjects who are obese.[5] Sleep apnea is characterized by multiple episodes of lengthy pauses in breathing during sleep that is associated with sleepiness and fatigue during the day. The airway narrows as a result of fat deposits in the upper airway and tongue. Sleep apnea and obesity hypoventilation place the patient at increased risk for respiratory failure, pneumonia, and dependence on mechanical ventilators.[8]

Children and adolescents who are overweight are at risk of developing type 2 diabetes, sleep apnea, and poor self-esteem, and have to deal with the social consequences of being overweight.[9] They are six times more likely to have at least one cardiovascular risk factor (ie, hypertension, hyperlipidemia, type 2 diabetes) as compared to children of healthy weight and are at increased risk for various chronic diseases such as osteoarthritis and sleep apnea as adults.[10]

TABLE 16-1　Adult BMI and Weight Classification Based on Height and Body Weight

	Normal Weight						Overweight					Obese: Class I					Obese: Class II					Obese: Class III				
BMI	19	20	21	22	23	24	25	26	27	28	29	30	31	32	33	34	35	36	37	38	39	40	41	42	43	44
Height (in.)												Body Weight (lb)														
58	91	96	100	105	110	115	120	124	129	134	139	144	148	153	158	163	167	172	177	182	187	191	196	201	206	211
59	94	99	104	109	114	119	124	129	134	139	144	149	153	158	163	168	173	178	183	188	193	198	203	208	213	218
60	97	102	108	113	118	123	128	133	138	143	148	154	159	164	169	174	179	184	189	195	200	205	210	215	220	225
61	101	106	111	116	122	127	132	138	143	148	153	159	164	169	175	180	185	191	196	201	206	212	217	222	228	233
62	104	109	115	120	126	131	137	142	147	153	158	164	169	175	181	186	191	197	202	208	213	219	224	230	235	241
63	107	113	119	124	130	135	141	147	152	158	164	169	175	181	186	192	198	203	209	215	220	226	231	237	243	248
64	111	117	122	128	134	140	146	151	157	163	169	175	180	186	192	198	204	210	216	221	227	233	239	245	251	256
65	114	120	126	132	138	144	150	156	162	168	174	180	186	192	198	204	210	216	222	228	234	240	246	252	258	264
66	118	124	130	136	142	149	155	161	167	173	180	186	192	198	204	211	216	223	229	235	242	248	254	260	266	273
67	121	128	134	140	147	153	160	166	172	179	185	192	198	204	211	217	223	230	236	243	249	255	262	268	275	281
68	125	132	138	145	151	158	164	171	178	184	191	197	204	210	217	224	230	237	243	250	256	263	270	276	283	289
69	129	135	142	149	156	163	169	176	183	190	196	203	210	217	223	230	237	244	251	258	264	271	278	284	291	298
70	132	139	146	153	160	167	174	181	188	195	202	209	216	223	230	237	244	251	258	265	272	279	286	293	300	307
71	136	143	151	158	165	172	179	186	194	201	208	215	222	229	237	244	251	258	265	272	280	287	294	301	308	315
72	140	147	155	162	170	177	184	192	199	206	214	221	229	236	243	251	258	265	273	280	288	295	302	310	317	324
73	144	152	159	167	174	182	189	197	205	212	220	227	235	243	250	258	265	273	280	288	296	303	311	318	326	333
74	148	156	164	171	179	187	195	203	210	218	226	234	241	249	257	265	273	280	288	296	304	312	319	327	335	343

TABLE 16-2   Metabolic Syndrome

Metabolic syndrome is defined by the presence of three or more of the following:
- **Elevated waist circumference:**
  - Men—equal to or greater than 40 in. (102 cm)
  - Women—equal to or greater than 35 in. (88 cm)
- **Elevated fasting glucose:** equal to or greater than 100 mg/dL or use of medication for hyperglycemia
- **Elevated triglycerides:** equal to or greater than 150 mg/dL
- **Elevated blood pressure:** equal to or greater than 130/85 mm Hg or use of medication for HTN
- **Reduced HDL** ("good" cholesterol):
  - Men—less than 40 mg/dL
  - Women—less than 50 mg/dL

Metabolic Syndrome

Metabolic syndrome is a cluster of conditions that have been found to directly promote the development of cardiovascular disease and type 2 diabetes. Abdominal or central obesity, fat deposition concentrated around the stomach rather than around the hips, and insulin resistance are considered the primary risk factors associated with metabolic syndrome.[11] Other medical findings associated with metabolic syndrome include elevated triglycerides and blood pressure and reduced HDLs. The presence of three or more of these five conditions constitute a diagnosis of metabolic syndrome (Table 16-2).

Research suggests that a measurement of waist circumference has a stronger correlation to health risks associated with metabolic syndrome than BMI or percent body fat and is an important adjunct in the clinical assessment of obesity[12] (Table 16-3).

ETIOLOGY

The problem of overweight and obesity results from an imbalance involving excessive caloric intake relative to energy expenditure and is influenced by genetic, metabolic, behavioral, and environmental factors. The World Health Organization Consultation on Obesity (2002) determined that overeating and physical inactivity were the factors primarily responsible for the obesity epidemic in the United States. Americans' devotion to television, video games, computers, remote controls, and other modern conveniences has contributed greatly to a more sedentary culture. Research has determined that there is a strong relationship between the amount of television an individual watches and the prevalence of obesity and diabetes.[13] The U.S. Department of Health and Human Services reports that 80% of overweight adults are completely sedentary and that 40% of adults in the United States engage in no leisure time physical activity.

INTERVENTION

Research consistently demonstrates that regular physical activity reduces many of the health risks associated with obesity. Individuals who are overweight or obese but are physically fit and active remarkably have lower morbidity and mortality than individuals of normal weight who are sedentary.[14] It is clear that regular exercise and physical activity result in improved fitness and health and need to be foundational elements in addressing obesity in the United States.

Despite national initiatives to reverse the growing problem of obesity in the United States, research shows that less than 43% of adults who are obese are advised to lose weight by their health care providers.[15] It is obvious that all health care professionals, including physical therapists, need to more consistently educate patients regarding the benefits of physical activity and weight loss if we are to effectively deal with this growing crisis.

The National Heart, Lung, and Blood Institute (NHLBI) recommends that all health care professionals address risk-factor reduction and weight management strategies with patients who are obese. The NHLBI also advocates the establishment of a modest target weight loss of 10% of body weight, at a rate of 1 to 2 lb/wk. Studies have demonstrated that even modest weight loss results in improvement in or prevention of hypertension, diabetes, and hyperlipidemia.[16] Goals related to weight management should focus on achieving and maintaining clinically meaningful weight loss that reduces the risk of obesity-related diseases. The promotion of long-term lifestyle changes in physical activity and diet in conjunction with the establishment of modest weight-loss goals provide a realistic chance of success in combating the obesity epidemic.

An approach to weight loss that combines a restriction of calories with an increase in physical activity and behavior modification has been shown to be the most effective regimen for

TABLE 16-3   Waist Circumference in Adults and Associated Risk of Cardiovascular Disease

Level of Risk	Males	Females
Very low	<31.5 in. (<80 cm)	<28.5 in. (<70 cm)
Low	31.5–39.0 in. (80–99 cm)	28.5–35.0 in. (70–89 cm)
High	39.5–47.0 in. (100–120 cm)	35.5–43.0 in. (90–109 cm)
Very high	>47.0 in. (>120 cm)	>43.5 in. (>110 cm)

Modified, with permission, from Bray GA. Don't throw the baby out with the bath water. *Am J Clin Nutr.* 2004;79:347.

TABLE 16-4   Indicators of Moderate-Intensity Exercise

55%–69% maximum heart rate[a]
Borg Rating of Perceived Exertion Scale 12–14 ("somewhat hard")[b]
3.0–6.0 METS[c]

[a]Parameters from Pollock ML, et al. The recommended quantity and quality of exercise for developing and maintaining cardiorespiratory and muscular fitness, and flexibility in healthy adults. *Med Sci Sports Exerc.* 1998;30:975.

[b]Parameters from Borg GA. Psychophysical bases of perceived exertion. *Med Sci Sports Exerc.* 1982;14:377.

[c]Haskell WL, Lee IM, Pate RR et al. Physical activity and public health: updated recommendations for adults from the American College of Sports Medicine and the American Heart Association. *Circulation.* 2007;116:1081-1093.

weight loss, weight maintenance, and improved quality of life.[16] Effective behavioral modification programs involve realistic goal-setting, stimulus control, problem-solving strategies, and contingency planning. Self-monitoring of diet and exercise using a journal and enlisting the support of friends and family can be useful in reinforcing positive changes in behavior. Time should be allocated for activities as trying to "squeeze" physical activity or exercise into the day is most often ineffective.

Daily Physical Activity

Daily physical activity plays a fundamental role in energy balance, weight control, and overall health. The National Academies Institute of Medicine issued new guidelines in 2002 on nutrition and exercise that recommend that children and adults get a minimum of 1 hour of physical activity daily, twice the previous public health recommendation.[17] The new guidelines reflect the need for 1 hour of moderate-intensity physical activity (see Table 16-4) to maintain healthy weight, but recognize that this activity can be accumulated in short periods (minimum of 10 minutes) of activity throughout the day. Research indicates that while significant health benefits can be obtained through participation in at least 2.5 hours of moderate-intensity physical activity or exercise per week, a gradual progression to 3.3 to 5 h/wk facilitates long-term maintenance of weight loss.[18] As long-term maintenance of weight loss is the goal for individuals who are overweight or obese, it is important that realistic goals be established and adequate time allotted to gradually progress to this higher recommended level of daily physical activity.

The incorporation of "lifestyle activity" to a weight-loss program can be an effective alternative or adjunct to more continuous, structured forms of exercise. Weight-loss programs of diet with moderate-intensity lifestyle activity have been shown to offer similar health and weight-loss benefits as those of diet with a structured aerobic exercise program.[14,19] Participation in moderate-intensity physical activities, such as those listed in Table 16-5, for at least 1 h/d in bouts of 10 minutes or more satisfies the National Academies Institute of Medicine guidelines. Individuals should be instructed to climb stairs instead of using elevators or escalators, perform

TABLE 16-5   Examples of Moderate-Intensity Physical Activity (3–6 METS)

Activity	METS
Swimming (leisurely)	6.0
General health club exercise	5.5
Tennis (doubles)	5.0
Walking 4 mph	5.0
Golf (walking and carrying clubs)	4.5
Mowing lawn (power mower)	4.5
Home repair (painting)	4.5
Washing windows	4.5
Gardening (weeding and cultivating)	4.5
Dancing (disco, folk, line, square, polka)	4.5
Golf (walking and pulling clubs)	4.3
Raking the lawn	4.0
Cycling (<10 mph)	4.0
Yoga, t'ai chi, stretching	4.0
Water aerobics	4.0
Fishing (standing in river bank)	3.5
Mopping floors	3.5
Childcare (bathing, feeding, dressing)	3.5
Vacuuming	3.5
Canoeing (rowing for pleasure)	3.5
Walking 3 mph	3.3
House cleaning	3.0
Loading/unloading a car	3.0
Carrying small children	3.0
Walking the dog	3.0

Data from Ainsworth BE, Haskell WL, White MC, et al. Compendium of physical activities: an update of activity codes and MET intensities. *Med Sci Sports Exerc.* 2000; 32(suppl 9):S498-S516.

their own household chores, park in distant parking spaces, get off the subway or bus a stop early and walk the remaining distance, walk during their lunch break, and participate in more physical leisure time activities on a regular basis. Research demonstrates that short bouts of moderate-intensity physical activity performed throughout the day provide an effective way to achieve the recommended quantity of daily physical activity. A comparison of the effects of performing multiple 10-minute bouts of exercise throughout the day with a single, longer bout in overweight subjects revealed greater adherence by those exercising in short bouts, with no negative impact on long-term weight loss or fitness.[20,21] Weight-loss programs that incorporate intermittent exercise or lifestyle activity will be more appealing to individuals under significant time constraints or to those that dislike structured exercise programs.

Exercise

Exercise is a critical component of a comprehensive weight-loss program. It not only increases energy expenditure, but has been shown to diminish the loss of lean body mass and associated decline in resting metabolic rate that is characteristic of dieting alone.[22] Exercise improves the body's ability to burn fat, enhancing the loss of adipose tissue.[23] In addition, it has been shown to improve dietary adherence while reducing anxiety, stress, and depression that can trigger overeating.[24] Research confirms that the combination of diet and exercise results in greater weight loss than diet or exercise alone.[25] Periods of severe caloric restriction can result in a significant decrease in metabolic rate that may persist after the dieting period ends, often promoting rapid weight regain. Research has repeatedly demonstrated that daily physical activity and exercise adherence are the greatest determinants of weight maintenance following weight loss.[19,20,26]

Exercise Prescription

Prior to prescribing an exercise program, medical history, risk factors, and medications should be assessed and when indicated, the patient should be referred to a physician for medical clearance. The Physical Activity Readiness Questionnaire (PAR-Q) has been recommended by the American College of Sports Medicine (ACSM) as a minimal standard for participation in a moderate-intensity exercise program.[27] The ACSM has developed risk stratification guidelines based on age, health status, and coronary artery disease risk factors and symptoms that can be utilized to determine the need for a medical examination and exercise testing prior to the initiation of an exercise program.[28] Patients who undergo an exercise stress test should have their heart rate parameters incorporated into the exercise prescription. Individuals at low risk can be instructed in self–heart rate monitoring and provided with patient education literature to guide them in progressing their exercise program. It is recommended that health care professionals monitor these individuals periodically to improve compliance and assess progress.

Physical therapists should question patients regarding their previous level of activity, exercise preferences, physical impairments, and time constraints. The type of exercise selected should be pain-free, convenient, and enjoyable to encourage long-term compliance. Whereas home-based exercise programs may improve compliance for some, exercise classes or group settings may provide valuable support and social benefits for others.

Physical therapists can play an integral role in prescribing an individualized exercise program for patients who are overweight or obese. The exercise prescription should include instruction in warm-up, training, and cool-down segments as well as guidelines for progression of intensity, duration, and frequency of exercise. The warm-up and cool-down portion should be designed to address deficits in strength, range of motion, and function that limit participation in activities of daily living, instrumental activities of daily living, and social and recreational activities while also serving to prevent injuries and sudden changes in heart rate and blood pressure. Warm-up and cool-down exercises can include flexibility, active, resistive or balance exercises tailored to address impairments in body structures or function. Flexibility exercises can enhance function, improve posture, and provide greater freedom of movement. Active and resistance exercises can be useful in improving strength and function. An increase in strength that results in an improved level of mobility can promote an increase in daily physical activity. Resistance exercises should target weak muscle groups involved in functional tasks. Balance exercises can be a valuable component of a warm-up or cool-down program and enhance function and safety during gait, reduce the risk of falls, and promote a more active lifestyle.

Individuals who are overweight or obese should be encouraged to gradually increase the intensity of their exercise from low to moderate over time when initiating an exercise program. Guidelines that can be shared with patients to promote an understanding of what constitutes moderate-intensity exercise are listed in Table 16-4. Duration and frequency of exercise should be gradually increased as well, based upon the individual's tolerance and prior activity level. The cumulative effect of exercise over time is substantial and research has demonstrated a clear, dose–response relationship between the amount of weekly exercise performed and the amount of weight lost in individuals who are overweight.[29] The most successful exercise programs for individuals who are obese are of moderate intensity, long duration, and are performed frequently.[18,30] Individuals should be encouraged to strive for a long-term goal of 60 minutes of moderate-intensity physical activity over the course of each day. An example of an aerobic exercise prescription is provided in Table 16-6.

Exercise Precautions and Contraindications

Diabetes and hypertension (HTN) are common comorbidities associated with obesity that require special consideration when prescribing exercise. Compliance with a regular exercise

TABLE 16-6 Example of an Aerobic Exercise Prescription for Weight Loss

	Duration (min)	Frequency (Times/wk)	Intensity	Time (Optional)
Initial phase: weeks 1–4	15–30	3–4	40%–55% HR$_{max}$	≥10-min bouts
Improvement phase: weeks 5–24	30–40	4–5	50%–69% HR$_{max}$	≥10-min bouts
Maintenance phase: weeks 25+	30–60	≥5	55%–69% HR$_{max}$	≥10-min bouts

program helps to diminish some of the health risks associated with these disease states. For individuals with diabetes, exercise is contraindicated when blood glucose is greater than 300 mg/dL or greater than 240 mg/dL with urinary ketone bodies. Blood glucose should be monitored before, during, and after activity at the initiation of an exercise program, if individuals are taking insulin or oral medications for diabetes. Exercise can lead to exercise-induced hypoglycemia when insulin is available in the bloodstream. A carbohydrate snack may be needed either before or during exercise. It is important to review the signs of hypoglycemia (shakiness, dizziness, hunger, headache, and diaphoresis) in individuals with diabetes. Exercise-induced hypoglycemia can occur up to 4 to 6 hours after the cessation of exercise. Evening exercise should be avoided because of an increased risk of nocturnal hypoglycemia. As the exercise program is progressed, insulin needs may change, so close monitoring and follow-up with a physician is important. People with diabetes are at risk for autonomic neuropathies associated with a blunted heart rate and blood pressure response to exercise and/or silent cardiac ischemia. It is important that heart rate monitoring be performed in conjunction with a rating of perceived exertion scale to determine a safe level of exercise intensity for individuals with diabetes.[31]

For individuals with hypertension, exercise is contraindicated if resting systolic blood pressure is greater than 200 mm Hg or diastolic is greater than 110 mm Hg. For persons on alpha-1, alpha-2, or calcium channel blockers or vasodilators, the risk of postexertion hypotension exists and the cool-down phase of the exercise program needs to be strictly adhered to.[31]

Aerobic Exercise

Aerobic exercise is the preferred type of exercise for individuals initiating a weight-loss program because of the volume of calories burned and its well-established cardiovascular benefits. Aerobic exercise options include swimming, rowing, upper-body cycles, stationary or recumbent cycles, bicycling, walking or the use of treadmills, exercise videos, or classes. The selection of an appropriate type of aerobic exercise should be based on an individual's preferences, access to equipment, time constraints, and physical factors. In a randomized controlled trial involving women who were overweight, having access to exercise equipment at home was associated with better exercise adherence and weight loss at 18 months when compared with women without home exercise equipment.[20]

Walking indoors can be accomplished at a local mall or on a treadmill when weather is a factor, or outdoors around a neighborhood or at a local track. Pedometers can be useful in improving compliance and quantifying activity and progress. On the basis of available evidence in the literature, it has been proposed that healthy individuals need to accrue 10,000 or more steps a day to be classified as "active."[32] Home cycle units, swimming, and aquatic therapy are excellent choices for individuals with arthritis as they impart minimal stress to the joints. Indoor pools can be found by contacting health clubs, school districts, Young Men's Christian Associations (YMCAs), or motels for information about pool membership and class availability.

Recumbent cycles provide a comfortable alternative to upright cycles. Exercise classes (aerobic, aquatic, yoga, t'ai chi) provide a structured environment with social support that may improve compliance for some individuals. Videotapes (dance, low-impact aerobics, t'ai chi, yoga) are an inexpensive and convenient choice for those who prefer to exercise at home. Health clubs are an option but individuals who are obese must be counseled that exercise equipment such as cycles, treadmills, and elliptical trainers manufactured for the general public tend to have weight limits of 300 to 350 lb. Individuals who are morbidly obese may require specialized equipment to facilitate an increase in physical activity.

Resistance Training

It is generally recommended that exercise programs for both weight loss and weight maintenance following weight loss consist primarily of aerobic exercise. There is not always a resistance exercise component. The benefits of resistance training include a reduction in cardiovascular disease risk factors, specifically diabetes, hypertension, and dyslipidemia. Resistance training may have an impact when addressing obesity, general physical inactivity, and predisposing risk factors in cardiovascular disease.[16] Resistance training can also assist an individual in leading an active lifestyle by increasing muscle strength and lean muscle mass. Studies that have examined the role of resistance training have demonstrated a reduction in body fat mass and an increase in resting metabolic rates in both men and women. This exercise approach has also been found to increase fat-free mass and resting metabolic rate despite weight loss in postmenopausal women.[33,34] Very low-calorie diets have been associated with a loss of lean muscle mass, resulting in a decrease in resting metabolic rate. The addition of resistance training, whether during the weight loss or weight maintenance phase of a program, can counteract these negative results. Overweight and obese persons may better tolerate this exercise modality since it involves slow, controlled movements and the positions can be tailored to the individual for comfort. It is common for obese patients to undertake walking programs, but this activity is sometimes poorly tolerated by weight-bearing joints. The above studies have examined resistance training, but not in combination with aerobic exercise. More research is needed to determine how to structure a weight loss and weight management program in regard to the mix of exercise options. The American Heart Association recommendations for resistance training for persons without cardiovascular disease are as follows[35]:

- Training at minimum of 2 d/wk, progressing to 3 d/wk
- Training of 8 to 10 major muscle groups including back, abdomen, thigh, lower legs, chest, shoulders, and arms
- Intensity of 30% to 40% of 1 repetition maximum for upper extremities and 50% to 60% for lower extremities; OR, determining a weight that can be lifted for 8 to 10 repetitions and progressing to 12 to 15 repetitions

A resistance training program can be developed in conjunction with an aerobic exercise program and can be progressed at a pace that will not be too overwhelming in regard to the time required for completion.

Patient Education

Health care providers are often reluctant to discuss weight loss with patients who are overweight or obese, but need to address this concern along with the patients' other medical issues. The topic of weight loss can be introduced into the conversation by discussing the benefits of healthy eating and physical activity. Physical therapists can refer patients to nutritionists or weight-loss centers for a dietary plan. If a patient is not ready to seek nutrition counseling, the individual should be provided with an accurate Web site or patient education pamphlet that can be reviewed independently. When raising the subject of weight loss with patients, be clear that the primary interest is in their health and current diagnosis/symptoms; it is not dependent on weight loss during the current episode of care. Patients who are in greatest need for a discussion of weight loss include those with a BMI $\geq$30 kg/m^2, those with a BMI between 25 and 30 kg/m^2 that demonstrate two or more weight-related issues (diabetes, personal or family history of cardiac disease, HTN, etc), and those with a waist measurement of $\geq$35 in. for women and $\geq$ 40 in. for men.[36] Patients need guidance with setting realistic goals for weight loss and a planned progression to increase physical activity without causing injury or exacerbating current musculoskeletal conditions. It is important for patients to gain an appreciation for the impact of small amounts of weight loss on their health. A weight loss of 5% to 10% of initial body weight can significantly lower blood pressure. A weight loss of 5% to 7% through diet and increased physical activity has been shown to delay or prevent the onset of type 2 diabetes in high-risk patients.[37]

Providing specific information regarding the benefits of weight loss will help make the discussion more concrete. Weight loss will assist in the following ways[16]:

- Decrease elevated blood pressure
- Decrease elevated blood glucose levels
- Decrease elevated total cholesterol, LDL, and triglycerides
- Increase low levels of HDL

As the plan for weight loss is developed, it needs to be tailored to the individual. There is no set of rules to guarantee success for each person. Including the patient's preferences in the plan will improve the chance of success. Consider cultural issues and other aspects of the patients' health care program that could impact the success of their weight-loss program.

The NHLBI recommends a three-step approach for discussing weight management with patients. The starting point sets the tone for communication. The conversation must be expressed in a nonjudgmental manner. Ask the patients if they are comfortable discussing their general health and include the topic of weight—weight history and the impact of excessive weight on their life. Step 2 is a discussion and assessment of their readiness to make changes in their life. What is their attitude toward exercise and physical activity, and what are potential barriers in this area? Have there been previous attempts to lose weight and increase activity and if so, what approach has been most successful/least successful? Listening to your patients will help you to determine if they are ready for this commitment. Ask specifically about their current perspective on losing weight and improving health on a 1 to 10 scale, 10 being 100% ready for a commitment. Responses between 1 and 4 reveal very little motivation or intention, between 5 and 7 ambivalence, and between 8 and 10 shows readiness to begin a program. The third step creates a partnership with the patients and establishes goals that are reasonable and achievable.[38]

Exclusions for Weight-Loss Therapy

There are certain patient populations to be excluded from weight-loss programs, and thus should not be counseled during physical therapy episodes of care. These include women who are pregnant or lactating, people with serious uncontrolled psychiatric illnesses such as major depression, those who have comorbidities that would be negatively impacted by a low-calorie diet, and persons having problems with substance abuse.[3]

SPECIAL CONSIDERATIONS IN BARIATRICS

Bariatrics is defined as the branch of medicine that deals with the causes, prevention, and treatment of obesity. This is a growing area of health care, in both the clinical environment and research arena because of the obesity epidemic in the United States. When treating the bariatric population in hospitals and rehabilitation settings, special considerations need to be addressed. Health care professionals are at high risk of musculoskeletal injuries when mobilizing patients who require assistance with bed mobility, transfers, and ambulation. Health care providers report fearing personal injury when moving heavy patients.[39] Facilities need to develop protocols when mobilizing patients who are morbidly obese, with consideration given to weight, body mass distribution, and clinical condition.

Mobilization of Patients

Suggestions for safer mobilization include placing a transfer sheet between the patient's body and the surface of the bed to avoid skin shear and the use of an overhead grab bar or trapeze to permit the patient to better participate in bed mobility and transfer activities. Refer to Table 16-7 for recommendations on mobilization of patients based on body type. Regular length gait belts should never be joined to accommodate a patient who is obese and caution should be taken to prevent gait belts from penetrating into skin folds.[40] Bariatric gait belts are available in lengths greater than 60 in. to accommodate patients who are morbidly obese. Before attempting to move a patient, include him/her in the plan. Ask questions such as "What works best for you?" or "How has this been done before?"

TABLE 16-7   Body Types and Suggested Methods of Mobility

Body Types	Definitions	Method of mobility
Apple ascites	Weight carried in abdominal region; abdomen may be rigid	Unable to tolerate supine or prone positions; supine to sitting position via supine on elbow perpendicular spin; push upper body to sitting while allowing legs to descend to floor
Apple pannus	Weight carried in abdominal region; abdomen mobile, hangs inferiorly	Supine tolerance is variable; too much weight in abdomen to roll sidelying to transition to sit Supine perpendicular flat spin with UE assist to sitting or prone flat spin with UE bench press to standing
Pear	Weight carried below waist: abducted—significant tissue bulk between knees adducted—significant tissue bulk on outside of thighs	Supine to long sit using bed controls to raise head of bed, may need to assist via draw sheet while patient weight shifts side to side and forward to transition to short sit at edge of bed; sit to stand by thrusting upper body forward

to solicit additional information that will assist in making the transfer successful. Facilitating patients' involvement protects their dignity and encourages them to be an active participant in their care.

Making the determination to stand and ambulate a patient who has morbid obesity can be a challenge for a physical therapist. It is difficult to provide more than guarding and verbal cueing without putting both the patient and PT at risk for injury. The Egress Test (described in Table 16-8), developed by Michael Dionne, PT, is a screening tool to determine if the patient is capable of ambulating with/without an assistive device or a mechanical lift device is needed. The tool is simple for a PT to remember as well as implement. The basis for the test is the patient's ability to perform repeated movements without assistance.

If all three steps of the Egress Test are completed without assistance from the PT, the patient is ready for the next step—ambulation. If they had difficulty with these basic movements, a mechanical lift is indicated until they can complete all three steps.[41]

Bariatric Equipment

When working with patients who are morbidly obese, it is important that physical therapists be familiar with and confident in the use of specialized bariatric equipment that is available.

TABLE 16-8   The Egress Test

The test comprises three steps:
- *Three repetitions of sit to stand:* The first repetition requires the patient to elevate from and clear the support surface by 1–2 in. The next two repetitions are performed to full standing position. The patient proves he can bear weight on his lower extremities and demonstrates lower extremity muscle strength.
- *Three repetitions of marching in place:* The patient demonstrates the ability to support body weight repeatedly in single leg stance.
- *Advance step and return each foot:* The patient is asked to step forward with one leg and bring it back to the start position, with each lower extremity. The advantage of this phase is that the patient has not left the safety of the bedside. It also confirms the ability of the patient to step backward.

All staff needs to be trained in the use, operation, and appropriateness of each piece of equipment and the special needs related to mobilization of bariatric patients. This training should also address body mechanics and the necessity for multiple person involvement in transfers, transitions, and repositioning of these patients.

Equipment with higher weight limits is available for rental or purchase, and there are many companies now supplying bariatric equipment. While typical hospital beds have weight limits of 300 lb, bariatric beds can accommodate patients weighing up to 1,000 lb and are wider in width to allow for the increased girth of this patient population. Some bariatric beds are designed to allow the patient to transition directly from supine to sitting position and permit egress from the foot of the bed (see Fig. 16-1). These beds allow the patient to stand and ambulate without expending additional energy to assume a seated position at the edge of the bed. Some bariatric chairs convert to stretchers to allow patients to be slid out of bed to the bariatric chair using a transfer sheet. The chair is then adjusted to the sitting position once the transfer has been completed (Fig. 16-2). For patients who are unable to be safely transferred out of bed with physical assistance, bariatric lifts should be used. These systems can be freestanding or mounted on track systems on the ceiling and may also be useful with extremity range-of-motion exercises (Figs. 16-3 and 16-4). Bariatric mobile lifts are available for this population as well. The patients are placed in a sling, which can assist the sit-to-stand transition and allow for safer ambulation and gait training. Patients can ambulate without the physical therapist's support, permitting the physical therapist to focus on gait training and patient technique (Fig. 16-5).

The bathroom is another area requiring consideration and planning. Toilets need to be floor mounted, as opposed to wall mounted, to handle the heavier weight. To assist in transfers on and off the commode, elevated bariatric toilet seats are also available. Appropriate shower chairs (higher weight ratings and larger widths) and shower nozzles with longer hoses may allow the patient more independence and dignity. For patients unable to get to the bathroom, bariatric size bedpans are available.

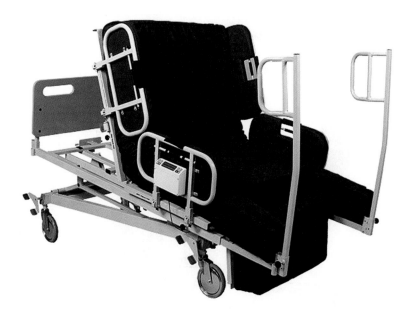

FIGURE 16-1 This specialized bariatric bed allows egress from the foot of the bed. (Courtesy of Convaquip—Extra Care Bariatric Bed Model 910EC.)

When working with the bariatric patient in an outpatient setting, consideration begins with the furniture in the waiting room. Sturdy wide chairs and sofas with firm, elevated seat surfaces that accommodate higher weight limits provide better patient comfort and ease in transfers. In the treatment area, a bariatric table that is wider and accommodates greater weight should be available. Extra large gowns will be helpful in making the patient less self-conscious at the start of treatment. Attention to these details will ensure safety of the patients as well as create a supportive environment that does not call attention to their difficulties due to size.

In the home setting, many of the same assistive devices and equipment are needed to ensure safety of the patient as well as the caretakers. Appropriate bariatric beds, lifting systems, commodes, and furniture, as discussed previously, will also improve the quality of life for the patient. This patient population may have difficulty reaching all areas of their body, making personal hygiene a challenge. Assistive devices can be purchased for the home: home scales, sponges on long handles for bathing, portable bidet systems, and toilet paper holders for toileting hygiene (see Fig. 16-6). More companies are increasing their product lines to include the bariatric population, and new companies are being introduced solely to meet the growing needs in our society. Specialized beds, wheelchairs, motorized scooters, and ambulation devices are available with varying weight limits of 600 to 1,000 lb. Architectural planning or revisions may be required in the home, including widening of doorways and extra wide ramps that can support heavier weights.

A checklist summarizing special considerations for treatment of bariatric patients can be found on Table 16-9.

Quality of Life

Morbid obesity, typically defined by BMI $\geq$40 kg/m^2, can also be defined as a condition in which body size limits health, mobility, and access to places and services that would otherwise be available. Morbid obesity has been recognized as a diagnosis protected by the Americans with Disabilities Act.[8] Patients with obesity have multiple health risks due to their weight and often experience a decreased quality of life. The patient–health care provider relationship should focus on

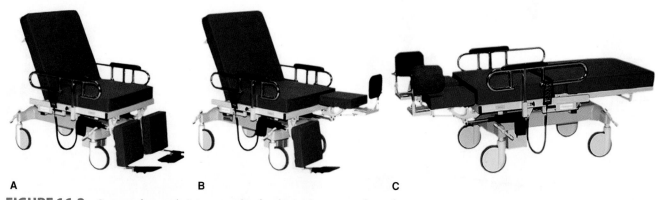

A **B** **C**

FIGURE 16-2 Converts from a chair to a stretcher for alternative means of transfers. (Courtesy of Convaquip—Model 900EC Bariatric Extra Care Chair.)

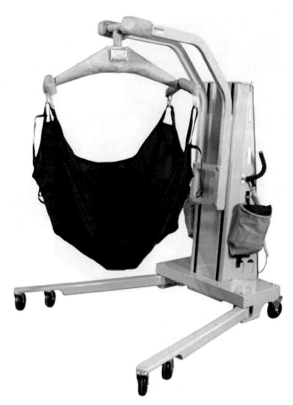

FIGURE 16-3   Electronic portable lift that includes a digital scale and can accommodate up to 1000 lb. (Courtesy of Convaquip—Model 9750.)

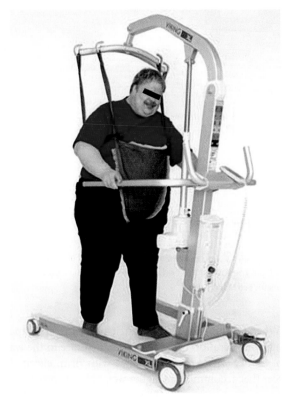

FIGURE 16-5   Gait training with Liko Lift Pants. (Courtesy of Liko North America.)

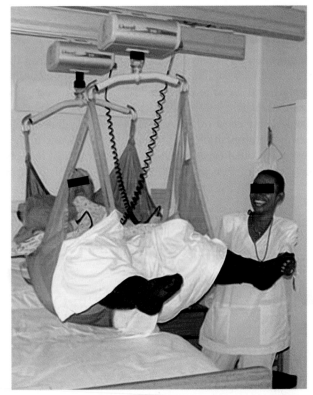

FIGURE 16-4   Liko Ultra twist, ceiling mounted lift system can accommodate up to 1100 lb. (Courtesy of Liko North America.)

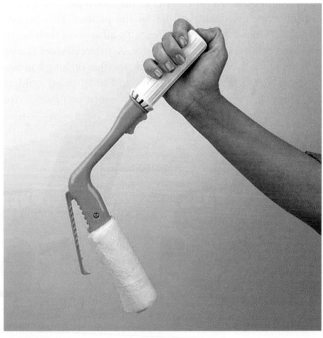

FIGURE 16-6   Self-wipe bathroom toilet aid. (Courtesy of Convaquip.)

TABLE 16-9   Bariatric Patient Checklist

Upon entering the room
❏ Transfer sheet for bed mobility
❏ Overhead grab bar or trapeze bar
❏ Question patients as to how they have successfully performed tasks previously

Performance of Egress Test
❏ Pass test—progress to ambulation
❏ Fail test—use bariatric lift device

Ambulation
❏ Gait belt, length greater than 60 in.
❏ Devices with adequate weight limit
❏ Gait training walker with sling (eg, see Fig. 16-5)

Durable medical equipment
❏ Ambulation device
❏ Bedside commode
❏ Chair

Bathroom
❏ Toilet mounted on the floor
❏ Elevated toilet seat
❏ Shower chair with higher weight limit and larger width

Assistive devices
❏ Sponges on long handles
❏ Shower head with a long hose
❏ Toileting devices
❏ Bariatric size bedpans

TABLE 16-10   Common Weight-Loss Medications[44]

Drug	Mechanism of Action	Possible Side Effects
Sibutramine	Appetite suppressant	Increased BP and HR
Phentermine	Appetite suppressant	Increased BP and HR, sleeplessness, nervousness
Orlistat	Lipase inhibitor	GI issues

(hypertension, dyslipidemia, congestive heart disease, type 2 diabetes, or sleep apnea) who have been unsuccessful achieving weight loss of 1 lb/wk while on a low-calorie diet and a program of increased physical activity.[16] Medication is intended to be part of a weight-loss program, not a singular approach. Weight-loss drugs work best with lifestyle changes such as diet and physical activity. The medications have different mechanisms of action and side effects that may impact exercise performance. Pharmacotherapy as part of a weight-loss plan is not a long-term solution. If a person is taking medication for 6 months and is not losing at least 1 lb/wk, it should be discontinued.[44] Commonly prescribed drugs, mechanism of action, and side effects are listed in Table 16-10.

Bariatric Surgery

Bariatric surgery is becoming the treatment of choice for severely obese patients, as it results in improvement in comorbidities and an overall decrease in mortality of 25% to 50%.[45] The number of bariatric surgeries performed in the United States has increased from 16,000 procedures in the early 1990s to 103,000 in 2003.[45] According to the National Institutes of Health, the surgical approach to weight loss is intended for persons with a BMI $\geq$40 kg/m^2 without comorbidities, or a BMI $\geq$35 kg/m^2 with serious obesity-related comorbidities. Candidates for surgery should have a history of unsuccessful attempts at weight-loss programs that included dietary changes, exercise, and behavioral changes. Prior to surgery, assessment of motivation and psychological stability for understanding the risks and benefits of surgery, the required lifestyle changes, and medical follow-up needed after undergoing a surgical approach to weight loss are necessary.[46]

Surgical Approaches

Three surgical approaches are commonly being performed: procedures that restrict the amount of food intake, procedures that limit absorption of nutrients, and one that combines the two. The most current restrictive surgical approach is the vertical banded gastroplasty (VBG) (Fig. 16-7). The capacity for food intake is greatly reduced through this procedure. A variation of this approach is the laparoscopic adjustable gastric banding (LAGB), which involves laparoscopic placement of a band around the upper stomach to create a smaller stomach pouch and a larger distal remaining stomach[47] (see Fig. 16-8). The second approach, biliopancreatic diversion

healthy behaviors and self-acceptance with less focus on weight loss. Having the proper sized equipment readily available (large blood pressure cuffs, weight scales with higher weight limits, and extra large gowns) assists in this relationship. Many patients who are overweight or obese report negative experiences during episodes of health care, making them reluctant to seek future treatment. There is fear of negative or inappropriate comments and/or of being judged for gaining weight or not losing weight since their last appointment. Health care providers need to examine their personal attitudes and barriers to intervention. Examples of possible barriers may include lack of appropriate medical equipment to assess and treat these patients, lack of training to accommodate their physical and emotional needs, perception that obesity is primarily due to a lack of willpower or that other health issues are not as important as weight loss, and difficulty performing a physical examination because of patient size.[42] The actual words that are used also have an impact on the patient–health care provider relationship. It is recommended that words such as "weight" and "excessive weight" be used, instead of terms like "obesity," "fat," and "excessive fat."[43]

Weight-Loss Medication

Numerous over-the-counter and prescription medications are available to individuals seeking this method for weight loss. Pharmacotherapy should be considered by physicians as an adjunct means of weight loss for patients with a BMI $\geq$30 kg/m^2 without risk factors or a BMI $\geq$27 kg/m^2 with risk factors

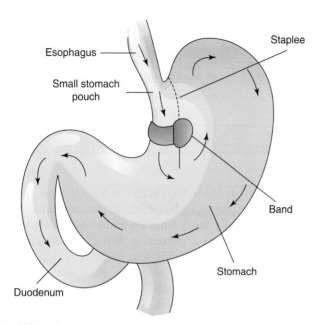

FIGURE 16-7   Diagram of vertical gastric banding surgery.

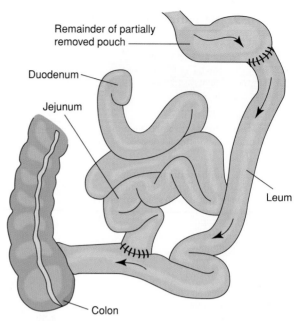

FIGURE 16-9   Diagram of biliopancreatic diversion surgery.

technique, works through malabsorption of nutrients. This surgical approach promotes weight loss by diverting pancreatic and biliary secretions to the distal portion of the ileum, causing lipid breakdown to be delayed in the digestive tract (see Fig. 16-9). The third surgical procedure, the Roux-en-Y gastric bypass (RYGB), combines both the restrictive and malabsorptive approaches. During this surgery, the stomach is partitioned into a 20-mL pouch, 5% of its normal volume, with an outlet to an anastomosed loop in the small intestine. Ninety-five percent of the stomach, the whole duodenum, and a small portion of the proximal jejunum are bypassed[47] (Fig. 16-10).

There has not been any research to determine which surgical approach is more successful with one exception. In the case of the superobese person, BMI $\geq$50 kg/m^2, the biliopancreatic diversion is the recommended procedure for surgical weight loss.[48] The long-term results of surgery show that persons undergoing restrictive surgical approach (VGB) demonstrate an average weight loss of 40% of excess weight, and persons undergoing RYGB and biliopancreatic diversion approaches experience an average weight loss of 60% of excess weight.[49]

A secondary benefit of weight-loss surgery that has been observed is the resolution of glucose intolerance in patients.

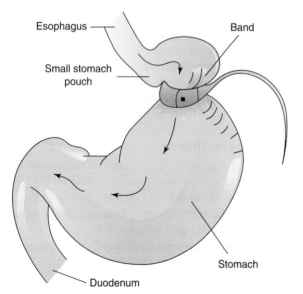

FIGURE 16-8   Diagram of laproscopic adjustable gastric banding surgery.

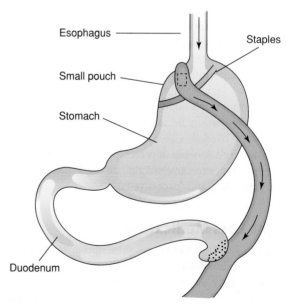

FIGURE 16-10   Diagram of Roux-en-Y gastric bypass surgery.

There are two theories proposed in the literature that can account for this metabolic change. First, it was noted that 73% of patients who underwent laparoscopic adjustable gastric banding had a complete remission of diabetes within 2 years following surgery. This was compared to 13% of patients who achieved weight loss through medical and behavioral interventions. The remission of diabetes was attributed to the amount of weight lost after the surgical procedure.[50] Another group of patients who underwent either RYGB or biliopancreatic diversion demonstrated an unexpected antidiabetic mechanism, more than expected with significant weight loss. These patients showed improved glucose metabolism within days to weeks following surgery, before any large amount of weight was lost.[50] A possible explanation for this positive response to surgery is the exclusion of the jejunum in the digestion process, perhaps eliminating the secretion of some unidentified hormone that affects insulin sensitivity.[51] More research in this area is needed to identify the mechanism responsible for this unexpected result of weight-loss surgery.

Exercise Recommendations

There is limited information available in the literature regarding preoperative and postoperative exercise recommendations. The American Society for Metabolic and Bariatric Surgery (ASBS) recommends mild exercise, 20 min/d, 3 to 4 d/wk, for the preoperative patient.[52] Specific recommendations by the ASBS include blowing up balloons to improve lung capacity, aerobic conditioning by walking, swimming, and biking, and use of light weights for strengthening. Northwest Kaiser Permanente includes a preoperative program for its bariatric surgical candidates, recommending a daily walking program, 60 to 90 minutes, in preparation for the postoperative aspect of care and to improve physical fitness. The goals of a preoperative exercise program include decreased surgical complications, facilitation of healing, and enhanced postoperative recovery. Patients should begin walking postoperative day 1. The distance or time can be increased each day as tolerated.[52] Postoperative patients are also at risk for blood clots and pneumonia; therefore, ankle pumps and deep breathing exercises should be encouraged.[53] Lifting should be restricted to no more than 15 to 20 lb for 6 weeks following invasive surgery and 3 weeks following laparoscopic approaches. Patients should be advised to progress their home walking program in both time and distance on a daily basis as tolerated. No specific exercise contraindications were found in the literature, with the exception of avoidance of "abdominal crunch" type machines in patients who had adjustable gastric banding surgeries because of one report of a port connection becoming dislodged after this type of exercise.[54] Aerobic exercise, light weight training, and abdominal exercises can be added as permitted by the surgeon.[53]

When working with the postoperative bariatric patient, potential changes in health status can impact participation in a physical therapy program. This population is at risk for poor nutritional status, potentially limiting exercise tolerance. Many patients take vitamins to supplement food intake. "Dumping syndrome," a common condition following gastric bypass surgery, is associated with food intake, usually after eating refined sugars, high glycemic carbohydrates, dairy products, and some fatty foods. The food quickly empties from the stomach into the small intestine, triggering a variety of symptoms. Early dumping syndrome occurs 30 to 60 minutes after eating and is characterized by symptoms of light-headedness, sweating, tachycardia, palpitations, nausea, diarrhea, and abdominal cramping. Late dumping syndrome occurs 1 to 3 hours after eating and is marked by signs and symptoms of hypoglycemia: sweating, shakiness, loss of concentration, hunger, and syncope. Individuals should be advised to speak with their physician if they experience symptoms associated with this syndrome, as this could be a signal to the patient for the need to more closely follow the required dietary recommendations.[53]

CASE STUDY

History of Present Illness

Millie is a 62-year-old female, admitted to the hospital on 11/14/08 complaining of worsening shortness of breath for 2 days and edema of the lower extremities. Her chest X-ray was consistent with pulmonary edema and mild cardiomegaly, but her lungs were free from infiltrates. Bilateral lower-extremity Doppler examination was negative for deep vein thrombosis. EKG showed sinus rhythm without any ST- or T-wave changes. Echocardiogram revealed LVEF = 50%, normal valves, and mild pulmonary hypertension.

Lab tests: serial CPK and troponins were within normal limits. Glucose was 271 mg/dL. Blood gas on admission: pH 7.3, P_{CO_2} = 53, P_{O_2} = 61, HCO_3 = 28.9, oxygen saturation = 89.1%, representing a partially compensated state of respiratory acidosis. Lipid profile: HDL = 38 mg/dL, LDL = 170 mg/dL, triglycerides = 187 mg/dL.

Admitting diagnosis was CHF. Patient was treated with Bi-PAP because of respiratory insufficiency, Lasix, insulin coverage for diabetes, and nebulizer treatments.

Past Medical History

Morbid obesity, OA, DJD of lumbar spine and bilateral knees, $L_{4/5}$ HNP with chronic LBP, type 2 DM since 1997, cataracts, history of TIA, S/P anterior wall MI 2006 with subsequent episodes of angina; patient underwent coronary angiography with placement of two cardiac stents to LAD and LM coronary arteries.

Medications at home: Nitro-patch, Percocet, β-blocker, insulin, aspirin, simvastatin, diuretic.

Social History

Millie lives with her spouse and has two adult children who do not live nearby. Equipment at home includes O_2 cylinders because of restrictive lung disease and hypoventilation, a rolling walker, and a bedside commode. She reports being overweight as a child and adolescent. She reports having been unable to lose all of the weight she had put on during her two pregnancies, with a slow, gradual gain in weight over the years to her current 230 lb. Millie attributes some of her recent weight gain to her chronic LBP and need for use of a walker to ambulate. Patient gave up cigarettes 5 years ago, but has a 20-pack-year history. Patient was referred to the physical therapy department of the hospital after being monitored and undergoing tests in ICU for 2 days, and then being transferred to the regular nursing floor.

Physical Examination

Patient is 5 ft 2 in. tall and weighs 230 lb with a BMI of 42. Her waist circumference is 124 cm, putting her at very high risk for cardiovascular disease. Body type identified as apple ascites.

Resting HR = 72, regular rhythm, no S_3, no murmur, RR = 22 on 2.5 L/min O_2 via nasal cannula with oxygen saturation of 92%, BP = 138/72. Breath sounds diminished bilaterally with minimal basilar crackles. No jugular venous distension noted; 1+ pedal edema noted bilaterally.

(+) Abdominal obesity

Mental status—alert and oriented × 3, cooperative

Sensation—intact to light touch (all dermatomes) and proprioception in all four extremities, but patient reports occasional paresthesias in left LE

Pain—reports 1/10 centralized chronic LBP at rest; (−) Homans sign bilateral LE

AROM—WNLs except shoulder flexion is limited to 130 degrees bilaterally with a springy end feel, ankle dorsiflexion to 0 degrees left and 2 degrees right because of decreased flexibility in gastrocsoleus, hip extension is 0 degrees bilaterally because of hip flexor tightness, hip flexion to 100 bilaterally secondary to abdominal girth

Bilateral UE strength is generally 4/5 except for shoulder flexors and abductors that are 4−/5 in the available ROM

Bilateral LE strength

  Ankle dorsiflexors: 3+/5 bilaterally in available ROM

  Ankle plantarflexors: 4/5

  Knee extensors: 4/5

  Knee flexors: 4−/5

  Hip flexors, adductors and abductors: 3+/5

  Hip extensors 4−/5

Neurological—normal muscle tone, 2+ reflexes, intermittent left LE paresthesias

Functional Assessment

Bed mobility: Patient utilized overhead bed trapeze to move upward in bed in a series of repeated attempts, after lowering the head of the bed to a flat position and following verbal cues to bend hip and knees to utilize LEs to push into extension. The overhead trapeze was moved sequentially toward the head of the bed along the support bar as the patient moved upward with each effort to provide her with adequate UE leverage.

Transfers: Patient transferred from long sitting to sitting at the edge of the bed using upper extremities to push up to sitting while allowing lower extremities to drop off the side of the bed to the floor. Patient did not report any dizziness in sitting. Vital signs were taken in sitting position: HR = 76, BP = 140/74, RR = 24 on oxygen with oxygen saturation = 93%. Pain was assessed and reported to be 2/10 in lumbar spine. Millie was encouraged to practice diaphragmatic breathing and rest before an attempt at standing was made.

Static and dynamic sitting balance: good.

Egress Test: A bariatric gait belt was applied to the patient. Patient was instructed that upon standing, if she felt she could not support her weight using the walker, she was to notify the PT and immediately sit back down on the bed. The patient was able to perform a sit-to-stand transition with the support of a bariatric walker three times under contact guard of two. Static standing balance with the use of the bariatric walker was assessed as good. Pain in standing was reported to be 3/10 in the lumbar region and 2/10 in bilateral knees. Patient was allowed to rest for 3 to 4 minutes. The patient then "marched in place" for 3 repetitions with the use of a bariatric walker and contact guard of two. Next, in standing, the patient was able to advance each foot and return it to the start position with support of the bariatric walker and contact guard of two individuals, thus successfully completing the Egress Test. It was determined that the patient was ready to ambulate. The patient practiced diaphragmatic breathing and was allowed to rest for 5 minutes.

Ambulation: A bariatric chair that had the capacity to convert to a stretcher was covered with a sheet and placed next to the patient's bed. This provided an alternate means for patient to be transferred back into bed if, after sitting up in the chair for an extended period of time, she did not feel she was capable of ambulating back to the bed safely. The patient transferred to stand under contact guard of two and following reassessment of her pain level and ability to bear weight on lower extremities, she ambulated with the rolling bariatric walker 5 ft to the chair under contact guard of two and transferred to sitting in the bariatric chair with verbal cueing. Dynamic standing balance with the use of the walker was fair.

Intervention

The nursing staff was informed of Millie's level of function and was instructed to assist the patient back to bed later that day using the walker or, if the patient felt unable to ambulate at that time, to convert the chair to a stretcher and utilize the sheet to assist the patient from the stretcher to her bed with the patient utilizing the overhead bed trapeze and her legs to shift sideways into bed. If the convertible bariatric chair is not available, a bariatric size hoyer sling could be placed on the chair to which the patient is to be transferred to provide an alternative means to return the patient to bed if it is deemed that she is unable to ambulate following sitting up for a period of time.

Patient Education

Millie was instructed in active exercises to be performed after a period of rest to strengthen her upper and lower extremities. The importance of independent exercise intermittently was stressed.

The PT brought up the topic of weight loss with Millie and asked her to assess her perception of her extra weight on her level of function. Millie expressed a readiness to lose weight and an understanding of how her weight impacted her respiratory status, level of pain, and activities at home and created severe restrictions in participation outside the home. Millie was asked if she had made any previous attempts at losing weight and what types of interventions had been successful. A referral was made to the hospital's dietician. The PT spoke with the patient's physician about medical clearance for an exercise program, and a stress test was ordered to provide cardiac clearance and provide heart rate parameters. Since Millie was prescribed a β-blocker to control HR, she was educated about other parameters that could be used to safely monitor her level of activity such as her respiratory rate or the Borg Scale of Perceived Exertion. The patient was educated on the benefits of physical activity and weight loss for her health: improved respiratory function, better glucose control, improved lipid profile, a reduction in risk factors of cardiovascular disease, and a potential decrease in pain associated with OA and her lumbar spine.

Millie was informed that weight loss would entail long-term lifestyle changes involving an increase in physical activity and a healthy diet. Personal factors that were perceived as barriers to exercise were discussed, primarily her dyspnea on exertion and chronic LBP and knee pain. Exercise options were discussed to minimize pain during exercise and promote long-term compliance. Millie saw potential options to include a recumbent cycle, aquatic therapy, and an upper-body ergometer. Since the patient was deemed high risk due to her previous cardiac history, it was determined that she would benefit from transfer to a subacute rehabilitation facility from the acute care hospital setting. This would provide her with the opportunity to improve her endurance and independence in activities of daily living in a monitored setting to assess exercise tolerance. It would also allow Millie the opportunity to evaluate the various types of exercise available to her to determine which best suited her lifestyle for long-term use.

Assessment

Millie presents with multiple factors associated with metabolic syndrome: an increased waist circumference, elevated triglycerides, reduced HDLs, and elevated blood glucose despite the use of medications for her type 2 DM. She reports a sedentary lifestyle due to her chronic LBP and OA as well as reports of dyspnea on exertion. She is at high risk for a cardiac event because of her history of an MI and CAD and will benefit from the initiation of an exercise program in a monitored setting such as a subacute rehabilitation center. This setting will also provide control over the patient's dietary intake as long as outside food is not brought into the center.

The patient has expressed a readiness to lose weight, and the recent hospital admission because of CHF provides motivation to decrease the health risks associated with obesity.

Plan of Care

A long-term target weight loss of 10% of body weight (23 lb) is established for this patient in compliance with NHLBI guidelines. She is instructed that her goal will be to lose 1 to 2 lb/wk through a gradual increase in physical activity and a low-fat diet. It is recommended that she utilize a diet and exercise journal to document her compliance. Problem-solving strategies are discussed to deal with her chronic pain, dyspnea on exertion, and food cravings. She is encouraged to speak with family and friends and instruct them to avoid bringing in food for her when they visit. Her exercise prescription will incorporate a target heart rate determined from the pending stress test as well as an alternative rate of perceived exertion score, "RPE," to guide intensity of the exercise. The patient will be taught self–heart rate monitoring if possible. The aerobic exercise prescription for Millie is outlined in Table 16-11.

In addition to her aerobic exercise program, Millie will be provided with a written exercise program that incorporates flexibility, strengthening, and standing balance exercises to address her deficits. Flexibility exercises will target limitations in shoulder flexion, ankle dorsiflexion, and hip extension. She will be instructed in theraband exercises to strengthen her ankle dorsiflexors and begin to use cuff weights to strengthen hamstrings and hip muscles. Millie's strengthening regimen can be progressed to include standing hip and hamstring strengthening exercises holding onto her walker using cuff

TABLE 16-11 **Millie's Aerobic Exercise Prescription**

	Total Duration (min)	Frequency (Times/wk)	Intensity	Time (Optional)
Initial phase: weeks 1–4 (subacute rehabilitation setting)	15–30	5 days a week while in rehabilitation	RPE: 9 (very light) 40%–55% HR$_{max}$	5- to 10-min bouts
Improvement phase: weeks 5–24 (following DC to home)	30–40	4–5	RPE: 11 (fairly light) 50%–69% HR$_{max}$	≥10-min bouts
Maintenance phase: weeks 25+	30–60	≥5	RPE: 13 (somewhat hard) 55%–69% HR$_{max}$	≥10-min bouts

weights, theraband, or a cable column weight machine to improve standing balance and core stability.

Because Millie is a type 2 diabetic patient who has become insulin dependent over time, blood glucose levels should be monitored before, during, and after activity for the first few months to prevent hypoglycemic episodes and to adjust medications in response to hyperglycemia. The signs of hypoglycemia should be reviewed with the patient and family. Exercise contraindications for this patient include glucose >300 mg/dL because of the risk of diabetic ketoacidosis.

PEDIATRIC OBESITY

The rate of overweight and obesity in children has continued to increase, with overweight children more likely to be obese as adults. Freedman et al. followed a group of children who were obese into adulthood and found that 77% of those with a BMI ≥95th percentile as a child had an adult BMI ≥30 kg/m^2.[55] The probability of obesity increases as the child ages. Obesity at 1 or 2 years of age is not associated with an increased risk of obesity as an adult. At 6 years of age, if the child is obese, there is a greater than 50% chance of being obese as an adult. In children and adolescents, the BMI of the parents has also been correlated with the weight of children as they reach adulthood. This is thought to relate to both genetic and environmental factors. Whitaker et al. looked at this relationship in a group of children and followed them into young adulthood (aged 21 to 29 years). If one parent is obese, there is greater risk for the child to be obese as an adult. If a child is younger than 6 years and both parents are obese, there is a substantially greater risk of becoming an overweight adult. As children get older, the parents' weight becomes less of a risk factor for adult obesity.[56]

Daily Physical Activity

The current activity recommendations for children from the U.S. Department of Health and Human Services is a *minimum of 60 minutes of moderate physical activity on most days of the week, daily if possible*.[57] As with adults, physical activity can be accumulated in short periods (minimum of 10 minutes) of activity over the course of the day. Children who are overweight or obese require more than 60 minutes of moderate physical activity to work toward a goal of weight loss or weight maintenance. Children can be guided toward activities that they enjoy, whether in a group or on an individual basis. Involvement in structured activities such as dance classes, martial arts, team sports, or swimming are appropriate options. The 60 minutes can also include recreational programs and unstructured free time, with a goal of developing interest in lifelong activities. The activities should provide them the opportunity to feel good about themselves. For older children, health club memberships (facilities generally allow children 12 years and older to join) can provide aerobic and resistance training. Resistance training should be carefully supervised by a competent instructor and performed 2 or 3 nonconsecutive days per week. Resistance should be set so that the child can

perform 8 to 15 repetitions per exercise, targeting 8 to 10 major muscle groups. The focus for this type of exercise should be on participation and proper technique, not the amount of resistance. If a child cannot perform 8 repetitions using good form, the amount of resistance should be decreased.[58]

Studies show that children who are obese are less active during the course of the day in comparison to children of normal weight.[59] While 90% of 9-year-olds get a couple of hours of exercise most days of the week, fewer than a third of American teenagers get the minimum recommended amount of activity per day according to a recent study that tracked approximately 1,000 U.S. children of various ages over a 6-year period.[37] A contributing factor to this sedentary lifestyle is television-viewing time. The NHANES survey in 2003–2004 found that the average television-viewing time for children aged 6 to 11 years is 2 h 13 min/d and those aged 12 to 17 years is 4 h/d.[2] Children are found to snack frequently while watching TV and are exposed to advertising related to candy, fast food, etc, contributing to the negative effect of television viewing.[60] Recommendations from the American Academy of Pediatrics include limiting "total screen time" to 1 to 2 h/d, including television, video games, computer games, and DVDs.[61]

It is important to have parental involvement when addressing weight issues in children. In addition to limiting sedentary activities, providing enjoyable active options for the children must be a goal. When giving children choices, they should include only active options such as "playing basketball *or* swimming in a pool." A 2-year study of a family-based behavioral weight program found that targeting a decrease in sedentary activities was as effective as targeting an increase in physical activity for children.[62] Participation in organized sports is one way to increase activity, but only if there is interest from the child. Other options such as jumping rope, dancing, shooting hoops in the driveway, and swimming are great alternatives. With the huge interest in video games, there are programs that promote exercise through the use of interactive dance mats available with video game systems. Children can set the mode of play (individual or competing with another person), time, and level of difficulty. A popular system at present is the Nintendo Wii, which includes games such as tennis and bowling to keep children from sitting on the couch. Nintendo also developed the Wii Fit accessory, which tracks the participants' BMI and weight over time. As users get on the device, it informs them of their current BMI and whether they are "normal, overweight, or obese" and allows them to set goals for weight loss if indicated. This system also has game modes, including strength, balance, yoga, and aerobics, that encourage users to be active. These games are appropriate for both children and adults and can be established as a regular family activity. Another option for the child with interest in video games is a stationary bicycle that plugs into a video game system, allowing the child to interact with the game. The Centers for Disease Control and Prevention (CDC) offers tips on making physical activity part of a child's life online.[63]

To address overweight and obesity in children, it is best to include both the family and school systems to obtain maximum benefit. A multifaceted intervention should target good nutritional habits, increased overall daily physical activity and exercise to increase energy expenditure, and optimization of physical fitness in the pediatric population. Schools are implementing nutrition and wellness policies to combat the rise in obesity rates. There is a trend, though, for less days and total time spent in physical education (PE) within the school day, a lost opportunity for children to be active. According to the National Center for Education Statistics, in 2005 public schools ranged in the number of days of PE programs were scheduled at the elementary level, with only 17% to 22% providing PE daily and 22% offering PE once per week. The time allotted for these classes was also low, with less than 30 minutes of PE time spent in 43% of first grade classes and 34% of fifth and sixth grade classes.[64]

The CDC published *The Youth Risk Behavior Surveillance Report* in 2006, stating that in high school only 54.2% of students were registered in PE classes and of those participating, only 20% were active for 20 minutes or more.[65] The CDC and the President's Council on Physical Fitness created Healthy People 2010 to improve Americans' health status, with one goal to increase the number of public and private schools requiring daily PE classes to 50%.[66] The school system is a key area to involve students in daily physical exercise and expose them to activities that may become lifelong interests. Recess within the school day is a second option for keeping children active during the school day. Schools should encourage children to go outdoors and participate in active play during recess. Health education is an additional venue for students to learn about the importance of an active lifestyle, providing the opportunity to develop healthy values and attitudes at young ages.

Bariatric Surgery in the Pediatric Population

Weight-loss surgery in adolescents is an area currently being studied to establish practice guidelines and ascertain the best surgical technique for this special population. Criteria for bariatric surgery have been offered by Inge et al. for severely overweight adolescents as follows:

- Failure ≥6 months in a behaviorally based weight-loss program
- Attainment of physiologic maturity (can be measured by X-ray, typically 13 years of age for girls and 15 years of age for boys)
- BMI ≥40 kg/m^2 with serious obesity-related comorbidities *or* BMI ≥50 kg/m^2 with less serious comorbidities
- Commitment to evaluation prior to surgery and close follow-up after surgery
- Willingness and capability to follow strict nutritional guidelines after surgery
- Avoidance of pregnancy for a minimum of 1 year postoperatively
- Demonstration of decisional capacity
- Parents/family supportive of the surgery and required follow-up care[67]

At this point in time, the only surgical approach approved by the FDA for patients under 18 years of age is gastric bypass.[67,68] Research needs to be conducted to determine the appropriateness, best surgical approach, and effectiveness of weight-loss surgery in the obese adolescent population.

In addition to the metabolic risks for children who are overweight and obese, overweight has been linked to orthopedic complications. A study involving the review of 355 children and adolescents' medical charts found a higher rate of documented skeletal fractures and complaints of musculoskeletal back and lower extremity pain in children who were overweight when compared with children of normal weight.[68] These children also scored higher in the mobility section on a self-reported written tool, The Impact of Weight on Quality of Life Questionnaire, when compared with children who were not overweight. The overweight group also had a higher level of lower extremity malalignment as measured on DEXA scans. The researchers suggest that the combination of overweight and lower extremity malalignment may be responsible for the musculoskeletal complaints. These complaints were likely to contribute to a decrease in physical activities, causing an increase in weight gain. Overweight children should be encouraged to choose activities that are of low impact to avoid musculoskeletal complaints.[69] If there is less discomfort experienced with activity, children may pursue a more active lifestyle.

PREVENTION

Three of the goals established by the NIH for Healthy People 2010, a statement of national health objectives developed at the turn of the century, are as follows:

- Increase the proportion of adults who are at a healthy weight
- Reduce the proportion of adults who are obese
- Reduce the proportion of children and adolescents who are overweight or obese

Unfortunately, despite our government's current efforts in combating obesity in the United States, the report of our nation's progress toward these goals, released in 2008, reveals a continued trend in the opposite direction. Data comparing statistics from 1988 to 1994 to that gathered between 2003 and 2006 reveal that the proportion of adults at a healthy weight has dropped from 42% to 32%, the proportion of adults who are obese has climbed from 24% to 33%, and the proportion of children and adolescents who are overweight or obese has increased from 11% to 17% in children and 18% in adolescents over this period of time. Clearly our efforts as a nation in this regard have so far been unsuccessful.[70]

Is it a wonder that obesity rates continue to rise when we consider our current cultural norms? Americans thrive on new technology and services that are developed to provide conveniences that reduce physical activity. Television, video games, and the generic use of computers have contributed greatly to our sedentary lifestyles. Take-out and fast foods are an inherent part of our daily routines. Education about the importance of good nutrition and benefits of physical activity is a necessity if future generations are to strive toward a healthy lifestyle and reverse the growing trend toward an obese population within our culture. Physical activity and exercise need to become a routine component of our lives.

A recent study found that people with a genetic variant that predisposes them to gain weight were no more likely to be overweight than those who did not possess this variant, as long as the individuals got 3 to 4 hours of moderate-intensity activity each day. These results strongly suggest that the increased risk of obesity due to genetic susceptibility can be curtailed with physical activity and emphasize the important role of physical activity in public health efforts to combat obesity.[71]

In order to make progress toward the objective of increasing the proportion of adults who are at a healthy weight, public health initiatives need to focus on prevention through education and the promotion of healthy lifestyles and behaviors, beginning in childhood. It is easier to maintain a healthy, active lifestyle into adulthood if the benefits of good nutrition and physical activity are valued and practiced at a young age than it is to improve dietary choices and incorporate physical activity into daily routines of sedentary adults.

It is important that children learn about proper nutrition and physical fitness not only at home but also in school as well. Cultivating an interest in physical activities at a young age should promote an active lifestyle as children enter adulthood. Parents should act as good role models for children at home. Parents should consistently strive to provide active choices to their children during leisure time. Health class, PE, recess, and extracurricular activities all provide wonderful opportunities to promote physical activity in the school environment. The food and drinks available to students in the schools should reflect healthy nutritional choices and reinforce information provided in classes about proper nutrition.

As previously noted, pediatric obesity is a predictor of adult obesity and therefore, it is especially important to address prevention in this population. On a national level, the "Child Nutrition and WIC Reauthorization Act of 2004" was signed into law to address the issue of childhood obesity through the public schools. Educational systems were charged with the task of developing a wellness policy to begin in 2006 to improve nutrition provided for lunch and snacks sold within the school, nutrition education, and physical activity. Each school district was required to develop a plan that incorporated both school faculty and community involvement.[72]

Prevention is key in combating the obesity epidemic in the United States. Research indicates that a small percentage of people who lose weight are successful in maintaining their weight loss. It is clear that changes in diet and physical activity that individuals make in order to lose weight must be maintained after the weight loss is achieved in order to sustain the weight loss. The concept that people can "go on a diet" temporarily to lose weight and expect that the weight loss is maintained when they revert to old eating habits is unreasonable. True weight management strategies in overweight patients need to promote long-term adherence to more healthy lifestyles.

It is critical that health care professionals consistently intervene when dealing with overweight individuals to prevent weight progression to the level of obesity and to prevent further weight gain in individuals who have demonstrated an increase in BMI from a healthy weight to one consistent with being overweight. In order to accomplish this, health care professionals, including physical therapists, should routinely include the determination of BMI and the measurement of waist circumference in initial examinations, introduce the topic of weight loss when warranted, provide patient information regarding the health risks associated with being overweight or obese, address risk-factor reduction, make referrals to nutritionists, and develop individualized weight-loss programs with these patients that includes an exercise prescription following medical clearance.

Weight gain seems to have a cyclical component to it. When an individual gains weight, the weight gain often makes physical activity more of an exertion, which can cause the individual to become less active and, in turn, leads to more weight gain. Physical activity can become more difficult due to pain, restrictive lung disease, the onset of diabetes, or the increased work of activity.

It is critical that an effort is made to break this cycle for individuals before long-term health issues develop or before the excessive weight makes exercise or physical activity too challenging to achieve (see Fig. 16-11).

It is apparent that there is a window of opportunity for patients to address the problem of excessive weight before the problem itself makes weight loss extremely difficult. When patients are overweight for many years, there is a greater risk of developing cardiovascular disease, restrictive pulmonary disease, and arthritis that make the initiation of an exercise program overwhelming. This is particularly true of patients with morbid obesity. Many of these individuals require assistive devices to ambulate and have difficulty accomplishing activities of daily living, let alone initiating an exercise program. Interventions in this population need to focus on proper eating habits, reducing impairments in body structures and function and enhancing daily activity and participation. Patients will benefit from adequate pain management, recommendations for appropriate assistive devices and equipment to enhance mobility and function, and an exercise program that addresses flexibility, balance, and strength deficits and permits pain-free physical activity. Successful long-term weight control requires that overweight or obese individuals develop an appreciation for physical activity and good nutrition as essential components of a healthy lifestyle.

In order to effectively address the obesity epidemic in the United States, an emphasis needs to be made to institute public policy that promotes education, prevention, and wellness for both adults and children. The lack of third-party payment for intervention or prevention of obesity continues to be a major obstacle in curtailing the continued trend toward obesity in our country. Cuts in state aid for our school systems make expansion of PE programs and extracurricular activities financially impossible. Strategies to address these problems

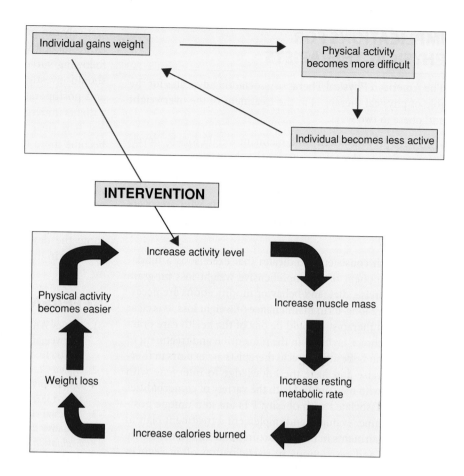

FIGURE 16-11   The cyclical components of weight gain and weight loss.

include government funding of such school programs and health insurance coverage or incentives for overweight individuals seeking a healthier lifestyle by joining a gym. Americans must begin to embrace physical activity as an essential component of their lives and improve their eating habits in order to reverse the growing trend toward obesity in our country.

LIMITS OF OUR KNOWLEDGE

Obesity is not a new diagnosis or comorbidity in health care, but has been identified as a growing epidemic in the United States. Physical therapists now need to address this issue with their patients as well as examining it from the perspective of prevention. Further research is needed to identify successful multifaceted approaches for adults and children who are overweight and obese in the areas of weight loss and weight management.

Some questions that need to be answered include the following:

• How can physical therapists impact society to develop healthy behaviors and attitudes to prevent the progression from healthy weight to overweight and obese?
• How can resistance training and aerobic training exercises best be combined to facilitate weight loss for long-term weight management/maintenance?

The second area for further exploration involves adults and adolescents who undergo bariatric surgery. There are no

research-based guidelines in the literature for postoperative exercise protocols following surgical intervention. As surgical approaches become more popular for weight loss in the obese, physical therapists should determine best practice for this population both pre- and postoperatively.

Questions for this population include the following:

• What activities/exercises demonstrate greatest benefits for patients undergoing bariatric surgery both pre- and postoperatively?
• Do patients benefit from physical therapist involvement pre- and postoperatively?

The third area for investigation involves prevention. The American Physical Therapy Association promotes health and wellness as an aspect of physical therapy practice. Preventative interventions are not typically covered by medical insurance plans but could have a significant impact on curbing the obesity epidemic in children and adults.

Questions to be addressed in the realm of prevention include the following:

• What is the impact of regular physical therapy examinations/evaluations in preventing weight gain in individuals who are overweight?
• Would physical therapy evaluations and interventions be cost-effective if overweight or obesity was a covered diagnosis?

IMPLICATIONS FOR PHYSICAL THERAPISTS

The American Physical Therapy Association advocates for the role of physical therapists in the treatment of the overweight and obese in two ways:

- To help prevent obesity and maintain weight loss by developing fitness plans that promote the ability to move, reduce pain, restore function, and prevent restrictions in participation for both children and adults
- To develop exercise programs for patients who are overweight or obese, taking into consideration safety and joint protection

Research consistently indicates that exercise is a fundamental component of a comprehensive weight-loss program and that exercise, diet, and behavior modifications are necessary to ensure long-term maintenance of weight loss. It is clear that physical therapists should be one of the health care practitioners of choice involved in the prevention and treatment of overweight and obesity. Physical therapists are experts in therapeutic exercise and have the knowledge to intervene with individuals who may present with the variety of comorbidities commonly associated with obesity. PTs are in a unique position to examine, evaluate, and implement a treatment plan to address impairments in body structures and function, activity limitations, and restrictions in participation often seen in patients who are obese. BMI and abdominal girth measurement should become a standard part of a physical therapy examination, and patient education should include a discussion of the health risks associated with being overweight or obese. All overweight individuals should be identified, evaluated, and counseled to begin a weight-reduction program even when only a modest weight gain is detected. Physical therapists are trained in prevention and wellness and are at an advantage in intervening to prevent weight progression to the level of obesity. An exercise prescription should be provided that takes into consideration the individual's previous level of activity, interests, time constraints, and impairments in body structures and function.

Pediatric physical therapists should network with pediatricians, nutritionists, and parents to inform them of how they can play a crucial role in preventing and treating obesity in children. Physical therapists possess the knowledge and skills necessary to work with children who are obese in prescribing and initiating an appropriate exercise program and to monitor their progress in achieving a healthy lifestyle. Physical therapists can also play a major role in research in the field of pediatric obesity.

As the field of bariatric surgery continues to grow, physical therapists should assume a role in the interdisciplinary team working with these patients. Many patients who are candidates for bariatric surgery present with muscular and joint problems that often limit their ability to exercise or walk long distances. Physical therapists are well trained to work with these patients to alleviate their impairments and improve their function and activity. Strength and endurance training preoperatively can prevent complications associated with immobility postoperatively and allow patients to recover more quickly following surgery. Research in the field of bariatric surgery should investigate the benefits of physical therapy both pre- and postoperatively in improving the health and fitness of patients undergoing bariatric surgery.

It is clear that physical therapists have an obligation to become more involved in combating the obesity epidemic in our country, through both prevention and intervention. Physical therapist education must include these topics to better prepare practitioners to intervene with these individuals. There are numerous niches that PTs can fill in the fields of pediatrics, bariatric surgery, prevention, and research to promote the development of healthier lifestyles in adults and children in the United States.

REFERENCES

1. Hedley AA, Ogden CL, Johnson CL, et al. Prevalence of overweight and obesity among US children, adolescents, and adults, 1999–2002. *JAMA*. 2004;291:2847-2850.
2. Ogden CL, Carroll MD, Curtin LR, et al. Prevalence of overweight and obesity in the United States, 1999–2004. *JAMA*. 2006;295:1549-1555.
3. National Heart, Lung, and Blood Institute, Obesity Education Initiative Expert Panel. *The Practical Guide: Identification, Evaluation and Treatment of Overweight and Obesity in Adults.* Rockville, MD: National Institutes of Health; 2000. NIH publication 00-4084.
4. Mokdad AH, Marks JS, Stroup DF, et al. Actual causes of death in the United States, 2000. *JAMA*. 2004;291:1238-1245.
5. Poirier P, Giles TD, Bray GA, et al. Obesity and cardiovascular disease: pathophysiology, evaluation, and effect of weight loss: an update of the 1997 American Heart Association scientific statement on obesity and heart disease from the obesity committee of the council on nutrition, physical activity and metabolism. *Circulation*. 2006;113:898-918.
6. Alpert MA. Obesity cardiomyopathy; pathophysiology and evolution of the clinical syndrome. *Am J Med Sci.* 2001;321:225-236.
7. Kannel WB, Plehn JF, Cupples LA. Cardiac failure and sudden death in the Framingham Study. *Am Heart J.* 1988;115:869-875.
8. Godell TT. The obese trauma patient: treatment strategies. *Adv Emerg Nurs J.* 2000;3:13-18.
9. Must A, Anderson SE. Effects of obesity on morbidity in children and adolescents. *Nutr Clin Care.* 2003;6:4-12.
10. Freedman DS, Dietz WH, Srinivasan SR, et al. The relation of overweight to cardiovascular risk factors among children and adolescents: The Bogalusa Heart Study. *Pediatrics*. 1999;103:1175-1182.
11. Grundy SM, Cleeman JI, Daniels RS, et al. Diagnosis and management of the metabolic syndrome: an American Heart Association/National Heart, Lung, and Blood Institute scientific statement. *Circulation*. 2005;112:2735-2752.
12. Shen W, Punyanitya M, Chen J, et al. Waist circumference correlates with metabolic syndrome indicators better than percentage fat. *Obesity*. 2006;4:727-736.
13. Hu FB, Li TY, Colditz GA, et al. Television watching and other sedentary behaviors in relation to risk of obesity and type 2 diabetes mellitus in women. *JAMA*. 2003;289:1785-1791.

14. Blair SN, Brodney S. Effects of physical inactivity and obesity on morbidity and mortality: current evidence and research issues. *Med Sci Sports Exerc.* 1999;31:S646-S662.

15. Mokdad AH, Bowman BA, Ford ES, et al. The continuing epidemics of obesity and diabetes in the United States. *JAMA.* 2001;286:1195-1200.

16. National Heart, Lung, and Blood Institute. Clinical Guidelines on the identification, evaluation, and treatment of overweight and obesity in adults—the evidence report. National Institutes of Health [published correction appears in *Obes Res.* 1998;6:464]. *Obes Res.* 1998;6(suppl 2):51S.

17. Food and Nutrition Board, Institute of Medicine. *Dietary Reference Intakes for Energy, Carbohydrate, Fiber, Fat, Protein, and Amino Acids (Macronutrients).* Washington, DC: National Academy Press; 2002.

18. Jakicic JM,Clark K, Coleman E, et al. Appropriate intervention strategies for weight loss and prevention of weight regain for adults. *Med Sci Sports Exerc.* 2001;33:2145-2156.

19. Anderson RE, Wadden TA, Bartlett SJ, et al. Effects of lifestyle activity versus structured aerobic exercise in obese women: a randomized trial. *JAMA.* 1999;281:335-340.

20. Jakicic JM, Winters C, Lang W, et al. Effects of intermittent exercise and use of home exercise equipment on adherence, weight loss, and fitness in overweight women: a randomized trial. *JAMA.* 1999;282:1554-1560.

21. Jakicic JM, Wing RR, Butler BA, et al. Prescribing exercise in multiple short bouts versus one continuous bout: effects on adherence, cardiorespiratory fitness, and weight loss in overweight women. *Int J Obes Relat Metab Disord.* 1995;19:893-901.

22. Svendsen OL, Hassager C, Christiansen C. Effect of an energy-restrictive diet, with or without exercise, on lean tissue mass, resting metabolic rate, cardiovascular risk factors, and bone in overweight postmenopausal women. *Am J Med.* 1993;95:131-140.

23. Racette SB, Schoeller DA, Kushner RF, et al. Effects of aerobic exercise and dietary carbohydrate on energy expenditure and body composition during weight reduction in obese women. *Am J Clin Nutr.* 1995;61:486-494.

24. Racette SB. Schoeller DA, Kushner RF, et al. Exercise enhances dietary compliance during moderate energy restriction in obese women. *Am J Clin Nutr.* 1995;62:345-349.

25. Orzano J, Scott JG. Diagnosis and treatment of obesity in adults: an applied evidence-based review. *J Am Board Fam Pract.* 2004;17:359-369.

26. Pronk NP, Wing RR. Physical activity and long-term maintenance of weight loss. *Obes Res.* 1994;2:287-299.

27. Adams R. Revised Physical Activity Readiness Questionnaire. *Can Fam Physician.* 1999;45:992, 995.

28. American College of Sports Medicine. *ACSM's Guidelines for Exercise Testing and Prescription.* 6th ed. Philadelphia, PA: Lippincott Williams & Wilkins; 2006:26-27.

29. Slentz CA, Duscha BD, Johnson JL, et al. Effects of the amount of exercise on body weight, body composition, and measures of central obesity. *Arch Intern Med.* 2004;164:31-39.

30. Jakicic JM, Marcus BH, Gallagher KI, et al. Effect of exercise duration and intensity on weight loss in overweight, sedentary women. *JAMA.* 2003;290:1323-1330.

31. American College of Sports Medicine. *ACSM's Guidelines for Exercise Testing and Prescription.* 6th ed. Philadelphia, PA: Lippincott Williams & Wilkins; 2006:207-215.

32. Tudor-Locke C, Bassett DR Jr. How many steps/day are enough? preliminary pedometer indices for public health. *Sports Med.* 2004;34:1-8.

33. Hunter GR, Bryan DR, Wetzstein CJ, et al. Resistance training and intra-abdominal adipose tissue in older men and women. *Med Sci Sports Exerc.* 2002;34:1023-1028.

34. Ryan AS, Pratley RE. Resistive training increases fat-free mass and maintains RMR despite weight loss in postmenopausal women. *J Appl Physiol.* 1995;79:818-823.

35. Braith RW, Stewart KJ. Resistance exercise training: its role in the prevention of cardiovascular disease. *Circulation.* 2006;113: 2642-2650.

36. U.S. Department of Health and Human Services, National Institutes of Health, Weight-control Network. *Understanding Adult Obesity.* Bethesda, MD: National Institutes of Health; October 2001. Updated March 2006. NIH publication 01-3680.

37. Nader PR, Bradley RH, Houts RM, et al. Moderate-to-vigorous physical activity from ages 9 to 15 years. *JAMA.* 2008;300:295-305.

38. U.S. Department of Health and Human Services, National Institutes of Health. *Three Steps to Initiate Discussion About Weight Management with Your Patients.* Bethesda, MD: National Institutes of Health; November 2002. NIH publication 02-5211.

39. Gallagher S, Arzouman J, Lacovara J, et al. Criteria-based protocols and the obese patient: pre-planning care for a high-risk population. *Ostomy Wound Manage.* 2004;50:32-44.

40. Dionne M. Ten tips for safe mobility in the bariatric population. *Rehab Manag.* 2002;15(8):28.

41. Dionne M. Stand and deliver. Physical therapy products, March 2005. http://www.ptproductsonline.com/issues/articles/2005-03_05.asp. Accessed January 27, 2009.

42. U.S. Department of Health and Human Services, National Institutes of Health, Weight-control Information Network. *Medical Care for Obese Patients.* Bethesda, MD: National Institutes of Health; February 2003. Updated January 2007. NIH publication 03-4159.

43. U.S. Department of Health and Human Services, National Institutes of Health, Weight-control Network. *Talking with Patients About Weight Loss: Tips for Primary Care Professionals.* Bethesda, MD: National Institutes of Health; November 2005. Updated December 2007. NIH publication 07-5634.

44. U.S. Department of Health and Human Services, National Institutes of Health, Weight-control Network. *Prescription Medications for the Treatment of Obesity.* Bethesda, MD: National Institutes of Health; November 2004. Updated December 2007. NIH publication 07-4191.

45. U.S. Department of Health and Human Services. *Longitudinal Assessment of Bariatric Surgery (LABS).* Bethesda, MD: National Institute of Diabetes and Digestive and Kidney Diseases; June 2005. Updated January 2007. NIH publication 04-5573.

46. U.S. Department of Health and Human Services, National Institutes of Health. *Bariatric Surgery for Severe Obesity.* Bethesda, MD: National Institutes of Health; December 2004. Updated March 2008. NIH publication 08-4006.

47. Manco M. Bariatric surgery in obesity and reversal of metabolic disorder. In: Bagchi D, Preuss H, eds. In: *Obesity: Epidemiology, Pathophysiology, and Prevention.* Boca Raton, FL: CRC Press; 2007:531-539.

48. Hainer V, Toplak H, Mitrakou A. Treatment modalities of Obesity. *Diabetes Care.* 2008;31:S269-S277.

49. Buchwald H, Avidor Y, Braunwald E, et al. Bariatric surgery: a systematic review and meta-analysis. *JAMA.* 2004;292:1724-1737.

50. Dixon JB, O'Brien PE, Playfair J, et al. Adjustable gastric banding and conventional therapy for type 2 diabetes. *JAMA.* 2008;299:316-323.

51. Manco M. Bariatric surgery in obesity and reversal of metabolic disorder. In: Bagchi D, Preuss H, eds. In: *Obesity: Epidemiology, Pathophysiology, and Prevention.* Boca Raton, FL: CRC Press; 2007:537.

52. *ASMBS Guidelines: Bariatric Surgery: Postoperative Concerns.* Public/Professional Education Committee notes—May 23, 2007. Revised February 7, 2008. http://www.asbs.org/html/pdf/asbs_bspc.pdf. Accessed March 3, 2009.

53. Bachman KH, Buck B, Hanna J, et al. Bariatric surgery in the KP northwest region: optimizing outcomes by using a multidisciplinary program. *Perm J.* 2005;9:52-57.

54. Felberbauer FX, Prager G, Wenzl E. The inflatable band and exercise machines. *Obes Surg.* 2001;11:532.

55. Freedman DS, Khan LK, Dietz WH, et al. Relationship of childhood obesity to coronary heart disease risk factors in adulthood: the Bogalusa Heart Study. *Pediatrics.* 2001;108:712-718.

56. Whitaker RC, Wright JA, Pepe MS, et al. Predicting obesity in young adulthood from childhood and parental obesity. *N Engl J Med.* 1997;869-873.

57. U.S. Department of Health and Human Services. *Overweight and Obesity: At a Glance Fact Sheet, 2007.* http://www.surgeongeneral.gov/topics/obesity/calltoaction/fact_glance.htm.

58. American College of Sports Medicine. *ACSM's Guidelines for Exercise Testing and Prescription.* 6th ed. Philadelphia, PA: Lippincott Williams & Wilkins; 2006:245.

59. Trost SG, Kerr LM, Pate RR. Physical activity and determinants of physical activity in obese and non-obese children. *Int J Obes.* 2001;25:822-829.

60. The Henry J. Kaiser Family Foundation. *The Role of Media in Childhood Obesity.* Washington, DC: Program for the Study of Media and Health. February 2004. Publication 7030.

61. American Academy of Pediatrics, Committee on Public Education. Children, adolescents, and television. *Pediatrics.* 2001;107:423-426.

62. Epstein LH, Paluch RA, Gordy CC, et al. Decreasing sedentary behaviors in treating pediatric obesity. *Arch Pediatr Adolesc Med.* 2000;154:220-226.

63. Centers for Disease Control and Prevention. Making physical activity a part of a child's life. http://www.cdc.gov/physicalactivity/everyone/getactive/children.html. Accessed January 7, 2010.

64. U.S. Department of Education. *Calories in, Calories Out: Food and Exercise in Public Elementary Schools 2005.* Washington, DC: National Center for Education Statistics; 2006. Publication NCES 2006057.

65. Centers for Disease Control and Prevention. Youth risk behavior surveillance—US June 2005. *MMWR CDC Surveill Summ.* 2006; 55(SS-5):24.

66. U.S. Department of Health and Human Services. *Healthy People 2010: Understanding and Improving Health.* 2nd ed. Washington, DC: U.S. Government Printing Office; 2000.

67. Spears BA, Barlow SE, Ervin C, et al. Recommendations for treatment of child and adolescent overweight and obesity. *Pediatrics.* 2007;120:S254-S288.

68. Inge TH, Krebs NF, Garcia VF, et al. Bariatric surgery for severely overweight adolescents: concerns and recommendations. *Pediatrics.* 2004;114:217-223.

69. Taylor ED, Theim KR, Mirch MC, et al. Orthopedic complications of overweight in children and adolescents. *Pediatrics.* 2006;117:2167-2174.

70. U.S. Department of Health & Human Services, Public Health Service. *Progress Review. Nutrition and Overweight.* http://www.healthypeople.gov/data/2010prog/focus19/default.htm. Accessed March 18, 2009.

71. Rampersaud E, Mitchell BD, Pollin TI, et al. Physical activity and the association of common FTO gene variants with body mass index and obesity. *Arch Intern Med.* 2008;168(16):1791-1797.

72. National Conference of State Legislators. PL 108–265. State issues in child nutrition: direct certification and local wellness policies. http://www.ncsl.org/statefed/humserv/summarys 2507.htm. Accessed March 3, 2009.

Physical Therapy Associated with Airway Clearance Dysfunction

Anne Mejia-Downs & Kathy Lee Bishop

INTRODUCTION

This chapter will address Practice Pattern 6C of the *Guide to Physical Therapist Practice*: *Impaired Ventilation, Respiration/Gas Exchange and Aerobic Capacity/Endurance Associated with Airway Clearance Dysfunction*. As you may recall from the oxygen transport pathway (see Chapter 5, Physiology of the Cardiovascular and Pulmonary Systems), the ability to exchange oxygen and carbon dioxide is dependent on an unobstructed path from the upper airways to the lungs. Normally, pulmonary secretions are easily removed from the airways by the mucociliary escalator, clearing the way for gas exchange to occur. When a dysfunction exists in the airway clearance mechanism, the inability to remove pulmonary secretions may result in decreased oxygen carried to the circulatory system, resulting in impaired muscle performance and aerobic endurance.

This chapter provides a review of the anatomy and physiology of the pulmonary system and describes the pathophysiology of cystic fibrosis (CF), an obstructive lung disease. The components of physical therapy (PT) management via Practice Pattern 6C will be illustrated, using a case study of a patient with CF. The management of airway clearance dysfunction is integral to this patient population and will demonstrate the effects of this dysfunction on impairments in physical function. Threshold levels or factors that affect ventilation, airway clearance, activity, and musculoskeletal function will be described and matched to appropriate interventions. The International Classification of Functioning, Disability and Health (ICF) will be used to demonstrate the body functions and structures evident in CF and their relation to activity and participation. Finally, though research efforts in this area are ongoing, there are limits to our knowledge about the disease of CF and the PT management that is currently used. Future directions for discovery in the realm of CF are discussed.

ANATOMY AND PHYSIOLOGY

Anatomy

The pulmonary system can be divided into two distinct categories: the musculoskeletal pump and a gas-exchanging organ.[1-3] These components act in synchrony to achieve both ventilation and respiration. Whereas the pump is made up of the thorax and attaching muscles, gas exchange is carried out by the upper and lower divisions of the airways and associated components.

There are 23 generations or divisions of airways.[2] The primary lobule or *acinus* consists of a transitional zone of bronchioles, alveolar ducts, and alveoli.[2,4] Capillaries surround the alveoli for ease of gas exchange. The lungs are supplied with blood from the bronchial circulation (airways) and the pulmonary artery (alveoli).[2,4] Gas exchange occurs by diffusion across the blood–gas barrier and follows the principles of Fick's law. Basically, the rate of gas transferred depends on the area of exchange, thickness of the area, and the partial pressure between the two sides.[2] If the lung tissue was spread out over the ground, the total size of the area would be similar to that of a tennis court.[2] The properties of the "gas" and tissue where the gas is being exchanged also affect the rate of diffusion.

Diseases such as CF may affect gas exchange in multiple ways: *distance for gas exchange* (clogged alveoli, chronically infected areas), *size of gas exchange area* (collapsed segments, shunted blood), and *alteration in the partial pressure gradient* (poor ventilation, poor distribution of air, elevation of arterial partial pressures). Chronic infected alveolar areas that are not cleared of secretions will result in shunting of the capillary blood away from the poorly oxygenated alveoli. This could result in a large portion of the pulmonary capillary blood being shunted that may lead to progression of right ventricular hypertrophy.[5,6] This shunting is due to poorly oxygenated alveoli and results in vasoconstriction of the pulmonary vascular bed.[7] In some cases, erosion into the capillary system can occur that causes bleeding.[5,7]

Surfactant is secreted in the alveoli to decrease surface tension and prevent alveolar collapse. Smoking, excessive secretion retention, exposure to general anesthesia, elimination of blood flow to an alveolar area (emboli), premature birth, and prolonged use of high concentrations of oxygen can lead to the elimination of the surfactant or a decrease in production.[2,8] Without the surfactant to lower the surface tension in the alveoli, there could be alveolar collapse, atelectasis, and possible infection.

The *pores of Kohn* connect adjacent alveoli and are in theory vital for collateral ventilation of blocked alveolar units.[2] They also participate in airway defense by allowing macrophages to move from one alveolus to another to engulf particles that are too small to be captured in the upper airway. This mechanism can also work against the lower airways, as in the case of exposure to tuberculosis: The bacilli are engulfed and cannot be digested but instead become part of the macrophage.[9] In the case of various airway clearance techniques, utilization of the collateral channels via the Lambert canals (respiratory bronchioles and alveoli) and the pores of Kohn promote equalization from one blocked alveolus to another blocked with secretions.[10] This allows movement of secretions from a blocked alveolus to the bronchiole and upward toward the carina (bifurcation of the right and left main stem bronchi) to be expectorated or swallowed.

Physiology

Mucociliary Escalator

Mucus is produced by the goblet cells, which line the tracheobronchial tree and acts as a medium to collect inhaled particles.[3,11] The mucus is primarily made up of water, glycoproteins, carbohydrates, and lipids. Dead cells, electrolytes, and foreign particles can also be found in the mucus.[1,11] More than 100 mL/d of mucus is produced by the respiratory tract.[11]

The lower airways act as a conduit for airflow and play a role in mucociliary transport.[1,2] Mucociliary transport refers to the action of the sol–gel layer and cilia, which trap and then sweep up the particles to be expectorated or swallowed (see Fig. 17-1).[1] This combination of a mucus layer and ciliary action is a major defense, protecting the lower airways from inhaled particles. Water, electrolytes, and several varieties of mucopolysaccharides account for the thickness of the mucus.[1] The cilia beat upward in a rhythmic fashion, moving the sol

layer and trapped particles upward and away from the lower airways. This layer is affected by smoking, anesthesia, dehydration, and various pathologies that lead to thick, tenacious secretions, and/or immotile cilia unable to sweep the mucus upward.[1,12,13] (See Chapter 5 for a detailed presentation of physiology.)

Cough

Exhalation is usually passive but can be forced with muscle contraction during a cough. Cough is an important protective reflex for the pulmonary system. An ineffective cough can lead to retained secretions, atelectasis, respiratory compromise, and in some cases respiratory failure.[10] A cough can be elicited consciously or by reflex stimulation.[2] A reflex cough occurs when irritants trigger impulses that are sent along the vagus nerve to the medulla. Mucus raised to the level of the carina stimulates a cough to expel the mucus.[3] The phases of the cough include a large inspiration of air; closing of the glottis; contraction of the abdominal and thoracic muscles to build up intrathoracic and intra-abdominal pressure; and sudden opening of the glottis, with explosive expulsion of air.[14] Forced exhalation or huffing may be used in place of or in addition to a cough to expectorate secretions. In order for forced exhalation to be effective, a large volume of air must be inhaled and the glottis must stay open.

Patients with CF or other obstructive lung diseases that are characterized by *air trapping* may have difficulty with effective forced exhalation or coughing because of premature closure of the smaller airways. A patient will often complain of the inability to catch their breath, but the problem is not on inhalation as might be assumed but rather on exhalation when the early collapse of the airways promotes air trapping. Over time, the respiratory muscles increase in length due to air trapping. This puts the respiratory muscles at a length–tension disadvantage. The poorly exhaled volumes combined with a dysfunctional musculoskeletal component and fatigue lead to poor timing of the cough sequence. The end result is a patient who is frustrated and fatigued and has been unable to effectively cough up the secretions that stimulated the cough.

The value of the cough as a defense mechanism is only effective down to the sixth and seventh generations of the bronchi.[14]

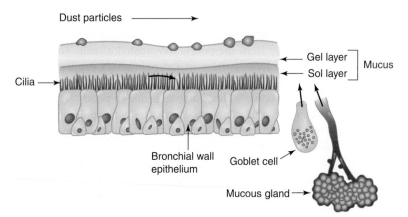

Dust particles ⟶

Gel layer ⎫
Sol layer ⎬ Mucus

Cilia ⟶

Bronchial wall epithelium

Goblet cell

Mucous gland ⟶

FIGURE 17-1   Mucociliary escalator.

The mucociliary blanket must work in synchrony with the cough as a defense mechanism. Constant irritation from persistent mucus may lead to bronchospasm, narrowing of the airway, and poor airflow, thereby lessening the benefit of the cough.[14] In chronic pulmonary diseases like CF, where coughing is a daily occurrence, supraclavicular retraction can be observed during paradoxical coughing, even in areas of the airway that have cartilage. Poor cough technique, excessive pressures generated during the coughs, and fatigue of the surrounding structures may lead to collapse in this area, adding to the ineffective and frustrating nonproductive cough.

PATHOPHYSIOLOGY OF CYSTIC FIBROSIS

Genetic Predisposition

CF is an inherited, autosomal recessive disease and the most common lethal genetic disease of the Caucasian population.[15] The altered gene is located on the long arm of chromosome 7.[15] The most common gene mutation is the delta F508.[15,16] There is a deletion of phenylalanine at position 508. This deletion leads to an altered production of the protein cystic fibrosis transmembrane conductance regulator (CFTR). The resulting defect affects chloride ion transmission across epithelial cells. Excessive sodium reabsorption is a consequence of CF transmembrane conductance regulator, which results in dehydration of surface fluids, abnormally salty sweat, and thick mucus that clogs up tubes, tubules, and ducts.[17]

Both parents must carry the genetic defect. The odds ratio of having a child with the disease is approximately 1 in 4 (see Fig. 17-2). The lungs are reported to be normal at birth, but changes in the mucus lining the airways rapidly occur. For this reason, newborn screening has been instituted in many states to identify individuals with CF as soon as possible.[18-20] In patients with CF, meconium ileus is a frequent occurrence at birth and has been considered one of the hallmarks for diagnosis. Essentially, meconium ileus is a bowel obstruction related to meconium (the substance found in newborn and fetal bowels), the change in the intestinal mucus, and pancreatic insufficiency.[15] In most cases, the diagnosis of CF will be made when stimulation from pilocarpine iontophoresis produces a positive sweat test, defined as >60 mEq/L of sodium.[15] Identification of the gene responsible for CF has made DNA testing to identify CF mutations possible as an additional diagnostic test.[21] *In individuals with a clinical picture of CF, identification of two known CF mutations by an accredited laboratory confirms the diagnosis.*[7,22] Although it is common for CF to be diagnosed at birth or in infancy, CF may not be suspected in patients until they are much older and symptoms have begun to interfere with their lifestyle. Presentation of exocrine pancreatic insufficiency, a family history, and chronic obstructive pulmonary changes confirm the CF diagnosis. In addition, problems with the reproductive system may lead to the diagnosis of CF; men are azoospermic and women have difficulty with fertilization as a result of thickening in the mucus lining of the uterus.[5]

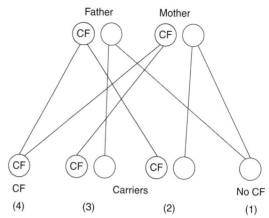

FIGURE 17-2   The inheritance of CF. Each parent of a child with CF has one abnormal CF gene (*blue circle*). The abnormal CF gene causes no problems if it is paired with a normal CF gene (*red circle*). When two parents each of whom carries an abnormal CF gene have children, each parent passes on either the normal or the abnormal CF gene. The figure shows the possible combinations of genes which children of carriers can have (1) a normal CF gene from both father and mother; (2) a normal CF gene from the mother and an abnormal gene from the father; (3) an abnormal CF gene from the mother and a normal gene from the father; and (4) an abnormal CF gene from each parent. Each of these four combinations is just as likely to occur as the others, meaning that the chances of two carrier parents having a child with CF is one in four each time they have a child. (Used with permission from D. M. Orenstein, Cystic Fibrosis: A Guide for Patient and Family, 2nd ed., Lippincott Williams & Wilkins, 1997.)

Clinical Manifestations of Cystic Fibrosis

The pathogenesis of CF is presented in Box 17-1. The pathologic changes in the lung occur at the bronchiole level. Inflammation and infection play active roles in destructive changes at this level. *Staphylococcus aureus* is one of the pathogens that can be seen early in the process, but *Pseudomonas aeruginosa* colonization is the primary culprit of infection. Initially, the organisms are nonmucoid, but a change occurs in which alginate, an exopolysaccharide, forms a gel-like substance incorporating the bacteria and protecting it from normal airway defenses.[5] Over time the larger and more central airways become involved. The glands that secrete the mucus become hypertrophied, and thick tenacious mucus is produced. This combination of hypertrophy and enhanced secretion adds to narrowing of the airways. The normal mucociliary clearance mechanism cannot function appropriately to mobilize the secretions upward and out of the lungs. The structural integrity of the airways is changed, and bronchiectatic reconstruction ensues.

Other clinical changes occur in patients with CF. *Clubbing*, a widening and flattening of the terminal portion of the digits, is a sign of hypoxemia that occurs because of the interruption of normal gas exchange. Progressive hypoxemia can lead to complications of pulmonary hypertension and right-sided heart failure or cor pulmonale. Pneumothorax (air in the chest cavity outside the lung) and *hemoptysis* (blood in the sputum or mucus) are two complications that can occur as a

BOX 17-1

Pathogenesis of Cystic Fibrosis

Pathogenesis of cystic fibrosis						
Genetic mutation Exocrine gland dysfunction						
Altered balance in electrolytes ⇓⇓	**Mucous abnormality**					
Sweat gland dysfunction ⇓⇓	**Intestines** ⇓⇓	**Liver** ⇓⇓	**Pancreas** ⇓⇓	**Reproductive tract** ⇓⇓	⇓⇓	**Airways/Lungs** ⇓⇓
			Pancreatic insufficiency in 50% of CF at birth			Normal at birth
						GI reflux, chronic airway infection
Heat intolerance and dehydration	Meconium ileus present in 10% at birth	Bile duct obstruction	Duct obstruction	Men ⇓⇓	Women ⇓⇓	Sticky, tenacious secretions
						Nasal polyps present in 25%
						Chronic infection
	Bowel obstructions	Cirrhosis ⇓⇓	Lack of pancreatic enzymes	Vas deferens blocked	Increased viscosity of cervical mucus	Air trapping
			Possible hyperglycemia and abnormal glucose tolerance tests			Poor ventilation
						Cor pulmonale
	20%–25% Later in life	**Liver Failure**	**Malnutrition**	**Sterility**		90% Morbidity/mortality
		Bone loss, decreased height, osteoporosis				**Respiratory Failure**

Adapted from Tucker DA. Normal and altered hepatobiliary and pancreatic exocrine function. In: Bullock BA, Henze RL, eds. *Pulmonary Rehabilitation: Focus on Physiology.* Philadelphia, PA: Lippincott–Raven Publishers; 2000, Orenstein DM, Noyes BE. Cystic fibrosis. In: Casaburi R, Petty TL, eds. *Principles and Practice of Pulmonary Rehabilitation.* Philadelphia, PA: WB Saunders; 1993, Yankaskas JR, Marshall BC, Sufian B, et al. Cystic fibrosis adult care. *Chest.* 2004;125:1S-39S.

result of the destruction of the integrity of the airways walls.[23,24] Recovery from these conditions is dependent on the extent of the damage and the ability to heal and compensate for the decreased function of the gas-exchanging organ.

Clinically, in patients with CF, one may observe increased accessory muscle use at rest when the work of breathing becomes greater. Additionally, development of a barrel chest related to air trapping, a need for supplemental oxygen for exercise with progression to continuous oxygen use, and a decline in activity may occur. An increase in the amount and viscosity of secretion production, a darkening in the color of secretions produced, and an elevated heart rate (HR) related to a chronically infected and hypoxic state may also be noted. In addition, patients with CF often exhibit a short stature and experience a decrease in body weight. Children with CF typically have voracious appetites yet fail to gain weight. Often, this phenomenon is what brings the child to the physician's office, where the diagnosis of CF is made. The inability to gain weight is caused by a high resting metabolic level and intestinal malabsorption. Malabsorption also plays a role in the development of osteopenia and premature osteoporosis. Decreased food intake is common in response to a sense of fullness from a barrel chest and flattened diaphragms compounded by a fear of vomiting with excessive, paradoxical coughs and traditional postural drainage with percussion for airway clearance.

TABLE 17-1   Clinical Signs and Symptoms of Cystic Fibrosis

Signs and Symptoms Impacting Lifestyle in Cystic Fibrosis				
Pancreas	**Liver**	**Lungs**	**Musculoskeletal**	**Reproductive**
Malnutrition: poor growth, cachexia; may need placement of feeding tube for night feedings; may require supplemental pancreatic enzymes with food, foul-smelling stools, foul breath, poor dentition (nutrition/vomiting); may need supplemental insulin; decreased energy, poor endurance, poor self-esteem	Cirrhosis/ascites: decreased energy, poor growth, cachexia, full feeling with even small meals, osteopenia, orthopnea, shortness of breath, risk of bleeding, hospitalization, liver transplant	Chronic infection: frequent airway clearance sessions; barrel chest; nasal polyps; clubbing of digits; cyanosis; shortness of breath; chronic productive cough; fatigue; dyspnea on exertion; accessory muscle use; pain; frequent exacerbations; hemoptysis; missed days or inability to do ADL,[a] school, or work without fatigue; orthopnea; poor appetite, nausea/vomiting with paroxysmal coughing; poor endurance; frequent hospitalizations; increased IV antibiotic use; placement of indwelling catheter; steroid usage resulting in side effects (facial and body changes); supplemental oxygen use; poor sleep, NIPPV[a]; lung transplant	Malnutrition: poor growth, increased fracture risk, osteoporosis, respiratory muscle fatigue, barrel chest, proximal muscle wasting, chronic pain, poor endurance, postural changes from muscle weakness and frequent flexion posture (for coughing, sleeping propped up on pillows, or in a hospital bed); pelvic floor weakness from chronic coughing	Infertility: impact on relationships in young to older adults, impact on child bearing, shortened life span to care for offspring

[a]ADL, activities of daily living; NIPPV, nasal intermittent positive pressure ventilation.

Data from Yankaskas JR, Marshall BC, Sufian B, et al. Cystic fibrosis adult care. *Chest.* 2004;125:1S-39S, Yankaskas JR, Knowles MR, eds. *Cystic Fibrosis in Adults.* Philadelphia, PA: Lippincott–Raven Publishers; 1999, The Thoracic Society of Australia and New Zealand. *Physiotherapy for Cystic Fibrosis in Australia: A Consensus Statement.* 2007. http://www.thoracic.org.au/physiotherapyforcf.pdf. Accessed February 26, 2009, and Dodds ME, Langman H. Urinary incontinence and cystic fibrosis. *J R Soc Med.* 2005;98(suppl 45):28-36.

In 2007, the mean survival according to the CF Foundation Registry was 37.4 years.[16] In more than 90% of patients with CF, the reason for mortality is respiratory failure.[25] Impending death is signaled by hypercarbia, hypoxemia, and acute exacerbations refractory to treatment.[25]

Table 17-1 provides a summary of the clinical presentation of a patient with CF.[23,25–28]

Case Study Patient/Client Diagnostic Classification

A key component of Pattern 6C of the cardiovascular and pulmonary preferred practice patterns in the *Guide* is airway clearance dysfunction.[29] The inability to mobilize pulmonary secretions from the tracheobronchial tree and/or expectorate them may result in decreased oxygen transport. This may, in turn, impair muscle performance and aerobic endurance. Patients/clients in this practice pattern are characterized by symptoms of shortness of breath, decline in pulmonary function, and decreased ability to perform activity.

This practice pattern includes patients with acute as well as chronic pulmonary disorders, oxygen dependency, and those patients who have undergone bone marrow and solid organ transplants, tracheostomy, and other cardiothoracic surgeries.[29] Patients who fall under these categories but have additional considerations may need to be managed through a different pattern or a combination of this pattern with another. Practice Pattern 6G covers patients aged 4 months or less, whereas older patients who may require mechanical ventilation are addressed in Practice Patterns 6E and 6F.[29] Patients with severe impairments or multiple complicating factors are not necessarily excluded from Pattern 6C; however, the frequency of visits and duration of care may require modification.

A patient with CF has been chosen to illustrate cardiopulmonary preferred Practice Pattern 6C: *Impaired Ventilation, Respiration/Gas Exchange, and Aerobic Capacity/Endurance*

Associated with Airway Clearance Dysfunction.[29] CF is included in the list of *ICD-9-CM* codes typically related to this pattern. It should be noted that CF falls under other cardiopulmonary practice patterns as well, namely, Patterns 6E and 6F.[29]

Description of the Case

Julia is a 35-year-old white female presently hospitalized with an acute exacerbation of CF. She was diagnosed with CF by a sweat test at 2 years of age when she failed to gain weight, even though she was eating a diet more than adequate for growth. This condition of "failure to thrive" is a clinical symptom of the gastrointestinal (GI) system, which should lead to further testing for CF.[30] Her younger brother has also been diagnosed with CF.

History of Present Illness

The patient is admitted with an increased weight loss and decreased exercise tolerance. Julia weighs 110 lb and is 5 ft 6 in. tall; her body mass index (BMI) is calculated at 17.8 (below normal). The patient uses 2 L of supplemental O_2 continuously and nasal intermittent positive-pressure ventilation (NIPPV) at night. Nocturnal NIPPV delivers positive-pressure ventilation through a tight-fitting mask (see Fig. 17-3). It is used to avoid endotracheal intubation and may prevent oxygen desaturation during sleep.[31]

Past Medical History

Julia was treated solely as an outpatient in the hospital's cystic fibrosis clinic; first in the pediatric clinic and after age 18 she was transitioned to the adult clinic. At the age of 24 years, when repeated lung infections from retained pulmonary secretions no longer responded to oral antibiotics, she was admitted to the hospital for intravenous (IV) antibiotics, which are able to be delivered in a more potent form. The following year, she had three hospital admissions and since that time has had an average of seven hospital admissions every year. Because of the severity of her disease, Julia was placed on the lung transplant list 1 year ago, at age 34. Her medical history includes sinusitis, otitis media, decreased bone mineral density (BMD), bronchospasm, pancreatic insufficiency, and hemoptysis.

Table 17-2 demonstrates the decline in Julia's lung function over time; there are 3 years between each of the test results.

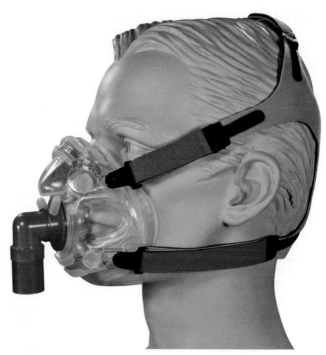

FIGURE 17-3   Nasal intermittent positive pressure ventilation (NIPPV) mask. (Reprinted with permission from Hans Rudolph, Inc., Kansas City, MO; 2009.)

Past Surgical History

At age 26, Julia had an indwelling venous catheter placed in the right anterior chest for ease of administering multiple courses of IV antibiotics. It is difficult to maintain patency in a peripheral IV line in patients with CF; peripherally inserted central catheters are also used for antibiotic treatments. A feeding gastric tube (G-tube) was placed, at age 30, to enhance weight gain with night-time feedings.

Social History

Julia earned a college degree and worked as a special education teacher until 2 years ago when she was placed on disability. She has no history of tobacco or alcohol abuse. Julia, who describes herself as very independent, lives alone and finds it increasingly difficult to carry out her treatment regime and activities of daily living (ADL) on her own.

TABLE 17-2   Julia's Pulmonary Function Tests[a]

	Forced Vital Capacity (FVC)		Forced Expiratory Volume in 1 Second (FEV$_1$)	
Test	Liters	Percentage of Predicted	Liters	Percentage of Predicted
1	2.52	89%	1.24	50%
2	1.67	67%	0.87	38%
3	1.10	32%	0.6	20%

[a]Note that there are 3 years between each of the test results.

Treatment History

Julia performs airway clearance (ie, techniques to mobilize and expectorate pulmonary secretions) three times a day, uses an exercise bicycle at home three times a week, inhales nebulized medication twice a day, uses a metered dose inhaler (MDI) for additional medications, takes pancreatic enzymes with food, and receives antibiotics by mouth and through her indwelling catheter.

Hospital Course

Julia demonstrates increased sputum production and decreased lung function upon admission. Her requirement for supplemental oxygen has also been increased—she currently requires 4 L of O_2 to maintain her oxygen saturation at 92% or greater. Julia reports pain with coughing, as a result of GI and musculoskeletal symptoms, and often has discomfort associated with treatment (eg, chest percussion, drawing arterial blood gases [ABGs]). Sputum cultures were performed to tailor the administration of antibiotics to cover the microorganisms present.

PT Examination

Julia's decline in pulmonary function tests (PFTs) on admission suggested the need for more aggressive airway clearance, which was addressed by increasing her airway clearance regimen from that performed at home. Julia was tachycardic at rest because of numerous factors including respiratory distress, deconditioning, and side effects of a prescribed bronchodilator. This increased HR affected her response to activity by limiting her ability for endurance exercise. Julia's exercise regimen was modified to consist of intermittent activity, which was well-tolerated. Additionally, the initial PT examination demonstrated a desaturation in Julia's oxygen levels with increased activity. This prompted a request for physician orders to allow titration of supplemental oxygen as needed during periods of activity.

Julia demonstrates impairments in pulmonary function, exercise tolerance, secretion clearance, posture, and muscle strength. The results of specific PT tests and measures will be described later. Julia's case demonstrates several components of Practice Pattern 6C, specifically an obstructive pulmonary disease with recurring pulmonary infections and chronic oxygen dependency. Julia falls within the appropriate age for this pattern, does not have respiratory failure, and does not require continuous mechanical ventilation, any of which might require classification in a different practice pattern or combination with another pattern.

EXAMINATION

Patient/Client History

The patient examination begins with a review of the patient's chart. This review is not meant to be a summary of the patient's entire medical history, but rather a distillation of information pertinent to the PT treatment including a review of medications. Medications may affect the response of the patient to a PT intervention, and conversely, an intervention by a physical therapist may require an adjustment of the medication regimen. The physical therapist should also be aware of the results of laboratory and medical tests that have been performed. Medical studies illuminate a patient's condition, giving clues to a patient's course of illness and indicate how an intervention by the physical therapist may need to be modified. Tracking Julia's PFT results informs the therapist of the possible need for a more aggressive regimen of airway clearance or a decrease in exercise intensity when the pulmonary flow rates show consistent decline.

Laboratory tests and medical studies document the progression of a patients' disease and identify appropriate interventions. These investigations include sputum culture, imaging studies, ABGs, and PFTs. Culture sensitivities are performed on sputum samples of patients with CF to treat the microorganisms present. BMD is measured in adults with CF, as it has been demonstrated that this population is at increased risk of osteoporosis.[23,32] Another routine medical test is chest radiography. A typical chest X-ray of a patient with CF demonstrates hyperinflation and flat diaphragms, usually accompanied by a kyphotic spine. X-ray changes initially occur in the upper lobes, especially on the right side for reasons unknown, and include increased interstitial markings in a cystic bronchiectatic pattern and atelectasis (see Fig. 17-4).[33] Bronchoscopy is performed by introducing a lighted bronchoscope down the airway, usually starting at the nasal cavity and steering into first one bronchus and then the other to visually inspect the upper branches of the tracheobronchial tree. Secretions can be suctioned and bronchial washings may be performed and sent for culture.

ABGs identify levels of oxygen and carbon dioxide in the blood. This will identify hypoxemia, which results in a decrease in oxygen available to be delivered to the tissues or a problem with retention of carbon dioxide. A blood sample is taken from an arterial site, usually the radial artery, and sent to the laboratory for analysis. If the patient requires close monitoring while in the hospital, an arterial line is placed for increased ease in obtaining repeated samples. Physical therapists, not having access to real time ABG values during treatment, use a pulse oximeter to determine the arterial oxygen saturation (SpO_2) level in the blood noninvasively. *The ABG value for the partial pressure of arterial oxygen (PaO_2) should be at least 60 mm Hg (corresponding to 90% oxygen saturation per pulse oximetry) without a substantial increase in the partial pressure of carbon dioxide ($PaCO_2$).*[34] On admission, Julia's ABG results showed a PaO_2 of 55 mm Hg on 2 L O_2 and a $PaCO_2$ of 45 mm Hg. Pulse oximetry revealed an SpO_2 of 86% at rest. These results indicated the need to increase Julia's level of supplemental oxygen.

PFTs provide information about the severity of pulmonary disease and treatment needed. PFTs assess flow rates and volume levels, diffusion, and airway compliance. These tests can assist with the diagnosis of restrictive or obstructive

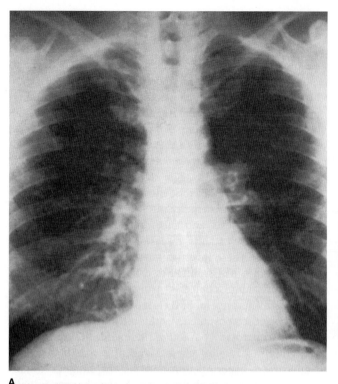

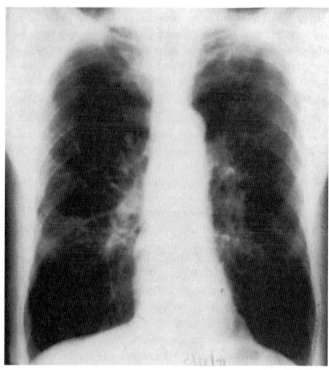

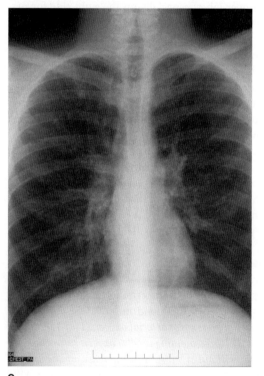

FIGURE 17-4   Chest radiograph of (**A**) a patient with healthy normal lungs and (**B**) a patient with emphysema, similar in pathophysiology to cystic fibrosis. Note the hyperinflation, flattened diaphragm, and narrow mediastinum. (**C**) Chest radiograph of a young patient with cystic fibrosis. (**A**) and (**B**) (Used with permission from West JB. *Pulmonary Pathophysiology: The Essentials.* 5th ed. Lippincott Williams & Wilkins; 1998.) (**C**) (Reprinted with permission from Michelle S. Howenstine, MD; Indiana University School of Medicine.)

components of lung disease; patients with CF exhibit an obstructive pattern.[23] PFTs are also used to document disease progression, since it has been shown that the forced expiratory volume in 1 second (FEV_1) in patients with CF is correlated with survival.[16,33] Normal test value predictions of lung function are based on a patient's sex, height, race, and age.

A patient with CF is likely to be exposed to a variety of antibiotics throughout life to combat the persistent infections that are common to the disease.[33] Although the choice of antibiotic is dominated by culture sensitivity, the growing resistance of microorganisms to antibiotics often causes the choice to be influenced by the experience of the clinician.[35] In

Julia's case, she was treated with azithromycin as an outpatient for pulmonary infections.[16] When her disease progressed and IV antibiotics were required, Julia was prescribed gentamicin or levofloxacin. The infusion was often initiated in the hospital and continued through her indwelling catheter at home after discharge. If the IV antibiotic was prescribed during a clinic visit, the necessary dosages were delivered to her home and a home health nurse initiated the therapy. Inhaled antibiotics, such as tobramycin (Tobi), are prescribed for a number of patients with CF,[16,23] more often for pulmonary exacerbations than prophylactically.[36]

Other categories of pulmonary medications with which patients with CF become all too familiar include bronchodilators, corticosteroids, and nebulized hypertonic saline.[13,16,36] There are different mechanisms and methods of delivering medication to dilate the airways; often more than one bronchodilator is prescribed. In Julia's case, she uses salmeterol in a nebulizer and levalbuterol in a metered dose inhaler. Corticosteroids and cromolyn are often used in patients with CF who have a component of bronchospasm or asthma.[36] Julia uses fluticasone, an inhaled corticosteroid (which has significantly fewer side effects than steroids delivered orally) to manage her bronchospasm. Hypertonic saline is used as a mucus therapy in CF.[13] This agent is used on a regular basis by more than one-third of patients over 6 years of age.[16] Dornase alfa is prescribed for patients with CF with the aim of thinning pulmonary secretions. Recombinant human deoxyribonuclease (DNase), marketed as *Pulmozyme*, actively digests DNA in the sputum to reduce the viscosity of pulmonary secretions.[13,35] Julia's use of DNase has resulted in a slight improvement in pulmonary function. See Chapter 8.

Oxygen should be included in the medication category as it requires a physician's prescription for administration. In the early stages of lung disease, supplemental oxygen is usually not required. It often becomes necessary in more advanced stages of pulmonary dysfunction and precipitates significant lifestyle change.[23,35] Supplemental oxygen is prescribed initially with sleep and increased activity and later may become necessary as a continuous therapy. NIPPV is used in patients with severe disease when increased levels of carbon dioxide become symptomatic.[31] Julia's case is representative of this pattern of supplemental oxygen use, starting with low levels of supplemental oxygen only for sleep and exercise sessions and progressing to continuous use of oxygen during the day and NIPPV for sleep.

Systems Review

The majority of the patient examination for this practice pattern focuses on the cardiovascular and pulmonary systems with attention to the musculoskeletal system, but a brief examination of the other systems should be included. *The integumentary system gives clues to the patient's state of hydration and nutrition.* Julia's skin is dry, suggesting dehydration, and she is pale in color upon admission. The integrity of her skin is interrupted by the indwelling catheter that is accessed in her right anterior chest. The neuromuscular assessment gives cues about locomotion and balance, especially with a change in position. No neuromuscular deficits were noted, as Julia presented no difficulty with any self-care tasks. Julia is well-coordinated in her efforts to move about her hospital room.

Another aspect of the systems review includes addressing the patient's communication skills and learning preferences. Julia is oriented × 4 and has no difficulty communicating with the medical team overseeing her care or the other health professionals with whom she comes into contact. Her sense of humor and ease in conversation with medical personnel reflect her extensive experience with hospitalizations in the past. Julia prefers to hear all of the information available to health care professionals about her course of treatment and wishes to be intimately involved with decisions about her care. Because of the chronic nature of her disease, Julia is often more informed about treatment options and their consequences than is some of the less experienced medical staff.

Physical Therapy Tests and Measures

After the patient history has been taken, the next step is to gather additional information from tests and measures to further describe the patient's status and to suggest appropriate interventions. Tests and measures that would be especially applicable to a patient with CF are described in the following section.

Aerobic Capacity and Endurance

Exercise capacity is reduced in this patient population so monitoring the response to activity is important.[23,27,37] This is done by measuring vital signs and response of the patient at rest and repeating the same measures during activity and again during recovery. *Some of the measurements to be recorded include heart rate (HR), blood pressure (BP), respiratory rate (RR), rating of perceived exertion (RPE) (be sure to document which scale is being used, 6–20 vs 1–10), dyspnea, and pulse oximetry. These measures should be recorded during an exercise test or the performance of functional activities.*

A test commonly used for patients with CF is the 6-minute walk (6MW) test in which a patient is asked to cover as much ground as possible by walking in 6 minutes while the distance is recorded.[23,27,37] The 6MW test is more accurate in patients with moderate to severe lung disease and is well-accepted at this stage because it is self-paced, unlike treadmill protocols. In patients with milder disease, a step test, shuttle test, or graded exercise test on a treadmill or bicycle would be appropriate.

CLINICAL CORRELATE

Evaluation of the exercise capacity of this patient population is vital because it is known that patients with CF who are physically fit survive longer than those who are less fit and that aerobic capacity is a marker for disease severity.[38,39]

Anthropometric Characteristics

The *Guide to Physical Therapist Practice* includes the measurement of body composition and edema in this practice pattern.[29] Monitoring the anthropometric components of height and weight of patients with CF is an important part of the PT management in this population. Patients with CF have decreased digestion and absorption of nutrients in their GI tract; therefore, they often have difficulty maintaining or gaining weight.[30] The energy expended in the performance of physical activity must be balanced with the intake of calories. A simple screening tool to document anthropometric status in patients with CF is the BMI, but skinfold thickness measurements and midarm circumference are also used.[30] Referring the patient to a dietitian may be beneficial for recommendations for a higher calorie diet to offset the energy expended with a recommended program of physical activity.

Circulation

The patient's circulation should be noted by observing the fingertips and lips for signs of cyanosis. Capillary refill can be assessed at the nail beds while observing the extent of finger clubbing present, a trait frequently possessed by patients with CF. Further discussion about cardiovascular symptoms and the response to activity is included under the section "Ventilation and Respiration."

Muscle Performance

Strength, power, and endurance of the musculoskeletal system are crucial to the accomplishment of daily activities, work or school performance, and exercise or physical activity. Range of motion, muscle strength, and endurance should be measured and tracked over time. It is known that patients with CF exhibit a decrease in maximal muscle force even in the absence of diminished pulmonary status.[40] Assessment and recommendation for a muscle strengthening program for patients with CF are therefore important. The primary and accessory muscles of respiration are forced to work overtime to compensate for the diseased state of the lungs.[41] These muscles warrant special examination for strength and endurance.

Another group of muscles that require specific attention are the muscles of the pelvic floor. Many patients with CF and COPD experience urinary stress incontinence during periods of increased abdominal pressure such as during coughing, laughing, and exercise.[27,28] A good rapport should be established with the patient before approaching this topic. It may be advisable to refer the patient to a physical therapist experienced in women's health issues to fully address this aspect of muscle strength.

Pain

The chronic nature of CF and its effect on many bodily systems predisposes patients to many years of treatment. Unfortunately, pain is frequently associated with the systems affected and the treatment involved. CF-related joint pain is frequently reported.[27] Chronic coughing and physical activity also contribute to musculoskeletal pain, and GI obstruction is often responsible for abdominal pain.[23] Pain associated with interventions includes ABG testing, placement of a G-tube or indwelling catheter, and even percussion and shaking for airway clearance. Pain should be inquired about regularly and can be reported during rest, activity, and procedures using a simple 1 to 10 pain scale.

Posture

The optimal alignment or musculoskeletal balance of good posture is altered in many patients with CF (Fig. 17-5). This is in part due to the forward position of the head and shoulders adopted during repeated bouts of coughing and periods of respiratory distress. The length–tension relationship of the respiratory muscles is altered, necessitating attention to the examination of posture and chest mobility.[27,41]

Self-care and Home Management

The daily routine of a patient with CF can be complicated and time-consuming. Daily treatments may include self-administering airway clearance and medications several times a day, regular exercise, and getting adequate sustenance in the face of decreased absorption of nutrients. Managing equipment needed for treatments such as the delivery of supplemental oxygen requires attention as well. In addition, the frequency of airway clearance and antibiotic treatments increase with the severity of the disease so that the most compromised patients

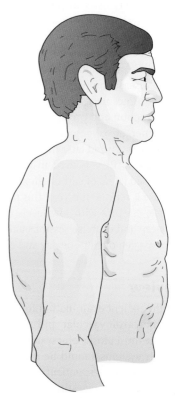

FIGURE 17-5   Typical posture of a patient with cystic fibrosis. Note the barrel chest, hypertrophied neck (accessory) muscles, and the forward head.

often find themselves saddled with the most exhausting treatments. Examination of the patient's ability to carry out a prescribed routine is important in recommending assistance for the patient to accomplish necessary tasks of disease management and self-care.

Ventilation and Respiration/Gas Exchange

This area is the crux of this practice pattern and will consume the greatest amount of examination time. This portion of the examination should include observation, auscultation, and examination of the components of the patient as well as the ventilatory response to activity.

The initial assessment should include observation of the patient's thoracoabdominal movements and breathing pattern; work of breathing; and use of the accessory muscles of ventilation, both at rest and in response to activity. The level and position of the diaphragms should also be assessed.

Auscultation of the lungs should be rendered before and after the patient performs airway clearance maneuvers to ascertain the effectiveness of these methods. In patients with moderate-to-severe CF, crackles are the norm, with the upper lobes being the most affected. Wheezing is indicative of bronchospasm, and its presence will necessitate the modification of an airway clearance regimen that prevents airway collapse. An additional component of the assessment involves listening to the patient's phonation, specifically, the strength of the voice and the ability to finish a complete sentence without breathlessness.

Palpation of the chest wall and assessment of chest mobility should be performed to identify any limitations in air exchange afforded by the mechanics of the chest wall. A simple measurement of chest wall excursion with a tape measure can be performed before and after a maximal inhalation. An additional assessment involves the performance of the ventilatory muscles. The primary and accessory muscles of ventilation are forced to work overtime to compensate for the diseased state of the lungs and warrant an examination of strength, muscle length, and endurance.

The techniques for airway clearance used by the patient should be thoroughly assessed. Many patients with CF are well-versed in a variety of methods and interchange them depending on the need for portability, the onset of an acute infection, or the stage of their disease.[42,43] In addition to the mobilization of the secretions from the airways, it is important to observe the effectiveness of their expectoration. The strength of the huff or cough effort is integral to the efficacy of secretion clearance. Many patients with CF exhibit severe and frequent coughing fits, which are extremely energy consuming and require an inordinate amount of recovery time. These patients may benefit from recommendations to stem the coughing impulse by breathing through the nose or taking sips of water and to use the coughing effort more effectively. Lastly, the sputum should be examined and quantified. If the sputum has increased in amount or thickness, or hemoptysis has occurred, it may be necessary to alter the performance of airway clearance techniques. As was discussed in the test of aerobic capacity and endurance, the patient's response at rest and with activity should be monitored. The HR, BP, RR, and SpO_2 are all indicative of the extent that the patient's ventilatory capacity affects the performance of activity. Subjective measures of RPE and dyspnea are important to consider as well, as these can be signals of limitations to the patient's activity irrespective of the vital sign values. Ventilatory muscle strength and endurance can be assessed by PFT results or use of a peak flow meter or handheld spirometer in the clinic. Response to activity is also a suitable measure of ventilatory muscle function.

Work, Community, and Leisure Integration or Reintegration

Before recent advances in CF treatment became available, many patients did not live long enough to make plans for employment or a career and advanced education was not emphasized. However, now that patients with CF survive into adulthood, integrating medical treatment into the patient's lifestyle to support continued employment and education is of greater importance. The tests of aerobic capacity will provide insight into the ability of the patient to carry out daily activities in these areas. Recommendations for modification of school or work schedules and daily activities are based on this information. In addition, modifications to the living environment or design of tasks related to community activities may be necessary.

APPLICATION OF THE GUIDE

Aerobic Capacity and Endurance

Julia's consistent use of her exercise bicycle was spurred on by the realization that exercise training on a regular basis allowed her to perform her ADL, treatment regimen, and work tasks more effectively. This regular activity enabled her to readily identify a decrease in her exercise tolerance. The 6MW is an appropriate test of endurance in Julia's disease state, and this test was performed on a regular basis to monitor this.

Julia's following 6MW results for consecutive years demonstrate a decline in exercise tolerance (Table 17-3).

Anthropometric Characteristics

In Julia's case, one of her symptoms on admission was weight loss, with a BMI of 17.8, well below normal. The issue of shoring up Julia's nutritional status needs to be addressed before her energy output is further increased with an exercise program. This is especially important at the time of an acute exacerbation.

Circulation

Julia was noted to have severe clubbing of the fingers and toes. Cyanosis was only present in the fingertips during occasional bouts of sustained coughing.

Posture

Julia's posture is typical of a patient with moderate-to-severe lung disease: forward head, rounded shoulders, shortened

TABLE 17-3   **Julia's 6-Minute Walk Results**[a]

Test	O₂ Required	Spo₂ (s)	HR (s)	RPE (6–20 scale)	Distance (ft)
1	Room air	90	140	13	1461
2a (On admission)	2 L O₂	88–90	150	15	1055
2b (At discharge)	Room air	90	140	13	1901
3	2–3 L O₂	85–90	150	14	1400
4	3–4 L O₂	90	160	17	1000

[a]Tests are yearly, from most recent years. Note that tests 2a and 2b were performed in the same year—on admission to the hospital and on discharge, 10 days later.

pectoral muscles, overstretched posterior thoracic muscles, and kyphotic spinal position. A postural exercise program using resistive tubing was prescribed the extensors, and cues to correct posture were provided.

Self-Care and Home Management

Julia's regimen at home consists of airway clearance three times during the day interspersed with nebulized, oral, and IV medications; pancreatic enzymes taken with high-calorie meals and snacks; maintaining oxygen equipment, regular exercise, and use of NIPPV and G-tube feedings each night. This routine would be taxing on even the most organized mind and well-tuned body. As Julia's disease has progressed, the topic of home assistance is regularly discussed and consultations with a social worker have been included in hospital visits.

Ventilation and Respiration

Examination of Julia revealed that, although accessory ventilatory muscle use was not marked at rest, she did exhibit extensive use of these muscles during exercise, leaning her forearms on the stationary bicycle handlebars to make optimal use of them. On auscultation of Julia's lungs, she was noted to have expiratory wheezes and crackles throughout both lung fields, most pronounced in the right upper lobe.

On admission, Julia had an increase in sputum production in recent days and that her sputum was streaked with blood, though without frank hemoptysis. Julia used autogenic drainage (AD) for airway clearance in the past, but this method became too energy consuming as her disease progressed, and she currently uses a combination of positive expiratory pressure (PEP) with inhaled albuterol and a manual percussor, which she uses in modified postural drainage positions. When admitted to the hospital, she prefers to continue her usual regimen, but this is increased to four times daily.

The following table is an excerpt of Julia's response to exercise sessions over time as her disease progresses (Table 17-4).

Work, Community, and Leisure Integration or Reintegration

As was mentioned earlier, Julia had completed a college degree and secured a professional position before her CF progressed to the point of requiring her to resign from her position as a special education teacher. Julia benefits from discussing her career accomplishments and how she enjoys using her precious free time to read. Discussion of energy conservation techniques is helpful to Julia as her disease progresses.

INTERVENTION

Multiple PT interventions may be used to improve ventilation, respiration, and aerobic capacity associated with airway clearance dysfunction. This section addresses patient and family education, therapeutic exercise, breathing strategies, and secretion clearance. Each of the subsections describes various techniques, which will promote achievement of anticipated goals and expected outcomes, and specific interventions to meet those goals will be proposed. Coordination of care and

TABLE 17-4   **Samples of Julia's Exercise Sessions as Her Disease Progresses**

Session	Treadmill Speed (mph)	Duration (min)	Oxygen Use	Heart Rate (bpm)	RPE (6–20 scale)	Spo₂
1	2.5–3.0	30	Room air	100	11	95%
2	2.5–3.0	30	2 L	102	12	91%
3	2.0–2.5	20	2 L	120	14	95%
4	1.5–2.0	25	4 L	132	16	93%
5	1.2–1.8	20	6 L	138	16	91%

communication to the patient, family, and care team as well as documentation are also reviewed throughout the section. Goals for the patient include the following: to enhance airway clearance, decrease energy expenditure, enhance physical tasks related to community and work integration with decreased pulmonary symptoms, improve functional capacity, promote independence in ADL, reduce risks of secondary impairments, promote safety to oneself and caregiver, promote self-management of symptoms, and improve sense of well-being. Establishing goals, documenting progress, and achieving measurable outcomes are the foundations of intervention.

Coordination, Communication, and Documentation

All the interventions addressed in the following sections require interaction with the patient and should include the family or support system. Basic understanding of the underlying disease pathology and physiology of why and how the interventions may affect the impairments will assist the patient in learning and adhering to the interventions. Allowing the patient and support personnel to participate in goal-setting and development of the plan of care reinforces that this is an individualized plan and the input of the patient is vital to its success.

Patient-/Client-Related Instruction

Education of the patient should be done according to need. Any impairment that would inhibit the ability to learn should be assessed. Visual and hearing impairments need to be incorporated in the delivery of the education, whether verbal, written, or via demonstration. Assessment of understanding should also be included once the education has been completed by having the patient repeat the information, demonstrate the technique, list or say precautions, and practice the technique until no verbal or tactile cues are required. The availability of return visits may determine how much material should be taught during the initial session. Videotaping the interventions is helpful for reinforcement once the patient leaves the clinic or hospital setting. The language in all handouts should be simple and straightforward to ensure comprehension by patients with all levels of literacy, and a phone number should be included with any written material. Having figures and drawings in addition to the written information and using a large font for easier readability are also important as is limiting the information on any one page.

Use simple steps to provide a straightforward and thorough approach to the intervention. For example, if an airway clearance technique is being taught, assess the patient by auscultation and clinical presentation. For Julia, a 35-year-old woman living alone with end-stage CF, it is important to choose a technique that is effective for the patient, nonfatiguing, can be performed independently, and allows freedom of performance anytime during the day. Julia, like many patients with CF, would benefit from a home exercise program using a safe method of exercise to improve posture, promote increased endurance, and improve airway clearance. In the clinic, the therapist should assess desaturation with the same exercise intervention being used at home and give exact parameters for HR, rating of perceived exertion, and frequency, duration, and intensity of the exercise. Instruct in proper use of medication to enhance bronchodilation and improve oxygen delivery and make sure the patient is aware of the need to modify or stop exercise if symptoms or clinical signs worsen. Each detail of this plan must be reviewed with the patient to make sure that there is a clear understanding of the parameters for hemodynamic response and benefits of the exercise. These steps will promote adherence and safety. Finally, include when the goals and intervention will be reexamined and what discharge outcomes will be.

Procedural Interventions
Therapeutic Exercise

Aerobic capacity/endurance conditioning—Aerobic or endurance exercise has multiple benefits. It enhances physical function and health status, improves physiologic response to increased oxygen demand, and may shorten recovery from infection.[3,15,17] Aerobic exercise is characterized by the use of large muscle groups, activated in a rhythmic fashion over time. Walking, bicycling, swimming, dancing, stair climbing, and jogging are examples of aerobic exercises.

Many systems of the body will be affected by aerobic training: cardiovascular, pulmonary, immune, metabolic, musculoskeletal, and neurologic.[15,44,45] The heart and lungs become more efficient at gas exchange and oxygen delivery to the tissues, the muscles become stronger and more effective at utilizing oxygen delivered to the tissues, there is a reduction in bone loss during weight-bearing exercises, skill and coordination are enhanced, and there is a sense of well-being. Metabolically, the processing of free fatty acids and glucose is enhanced along with utilization of insulin, the immune system is positively affected, motility of the GI system is improved, and in some cases, recovery from infections is enhanced.[45]

Julia's exercise prescription (Box 17-2) includes frequency of the aerobic exercise, intensity duration, and mode. In addition, strength training and flexibility exercises are included. The exercise prescription should also address precautions for implementing the exercise program. The prescription is developed once examination, systems review, and tests and measures are completed (see Chapter 3).

Nixon and colleagues found that higher aerobic fitness levels in patients with CF were related to improved survival.[38] In other words, the more fit and active a patient's lifestyle, obtained through regular aerobic exercise, the better the chance of living longer. Julia should stay as active as possible while awaiting her lung transplant for two primary reasons: her capacity to tolerate the surgery will improve and her recovery following lung transplantation may be shortened.

BOX 17-2

Julia's Exercise Prescription

Aerobic Intensity

70%–85% heart rate range from peak 6MW

Resting heart rate plus 10 (low level)

RPE scale 11–15/20 or 3–5/10 (see Box 14-2)

0–1 ventilatory scale (number of breaths to count to 15 in an 8-second period; highest level 4)

Resting respiratory rate plus 4–10 (depending on severity of illness)

Aerobic mode

Stationary cycle (home program)

Walking in the house or outside on level surface (could be at a mall)

Treadmill (when admitted to hospital)

Aerobic duration

Goal of 20–30 continuous minutes of exercise in target intensity range

Interval training for initial program: build up to 2–4 intervals of 5–10 min/d; progress to continuous level when time >10 min/interval

Aerobic frequency

If continuous program, 4–5 times per week

If unable to do continuous program, 6–7 times per week

With severe disease, 2–3 times per week

Flexibility and posture

Warm up—5 minutes of low-level cycling without resistance

Cool down—5 minutes of low-level cycling without resistance

ROM exercises: pick three exercises and rotate each session (can also be part of warm-up and/or cool-down; exercises to be combined with controlled breathing to incorporate chest wall mobility and relaxed breathing pattern)

Cervical extension (turtle necks) 3 × 5 sets

Bilateral shoulder flexion with elbows extended 3 × 5 sets

Standing against a wall: heels about 1 ft from wall, buttocks, head, and shoulders against wall, feet shoulder-width apart: elbows at 90 degrees and shoulders at 90 degrees for scapular retraction 3 × 5 sets

Knees bent slightly (stand clear of any objects), feet are shoulder-width apart; hold a towel or a dowel stick in hands with elbows extended; raise arms to shoulder height; slowly rotate arms with towel or dowel horizontal; hold count at each end of the rotation for at least 5–10 seconds; 3 × 5 sets

Calf stretches: stand on a step holding the rail; balls of the feet on the edge of the step; slowly lower 1 heel down and hold for 5–10 seconds; 2 × 2 sets on each leg

Hamstring stretch: stand or sit for comfort; back as straight as possible; place a bath towel around the ball of the foot; other leg should be bent; leg with towel should be fully extended; lean forward until pull is felt behind knee; do not hyperextend knee; 2 × 2 sets on each leg

Quadriceps stretch: hold onto couch back, chair, railing; keep your thighs parallel and stand as straight as possible; cradle your leg with a towel; now stand on one leg while raising the cradled leg to at least 90 degrees or more of knee flexion; keep your trunk as straight as possible so the pull is in the upper part of the thigh lifted by the towel; 2 × 2 sets on each leg

Strength Training

General instructions: do every other day or rotate muscle group (pick at least one exercise from each area of the body and rotate that exercise each time you do strength training; exercises to be combined with controlled breathing to incorporate chest wall mobility and relaxed breathing pattern)

Bicep curls (seated or standing) 3 × 10 with 1–5 lb weight

Triceps extension (seated or standing) 3 × 10 with 1–5 lb weight

Abduction (seated or standing; singles or bilateral depending on breathing) 3 × 10 with 1–5 lb weight

Shoulder flexion (seated or standing; singles or bilateral depending on breathing) 3 × 10 with 1–5 lb weight

Shoulder extension (seated or standing; singles or bilateral depending on breathing) 3 × 10 with 1–5 lb weight

Abdominal curls (supine, knees bent, and feet flat on floor): (1) progress from pelvic tilts to single leg lift to 4 in. holding pelvic tilt and then adding 1–3 lb leg weight as tolerated); (2) practice pelvic tilt and progress to abdominal curl with maintaining pelvic tilt; (3) progress to obliques/rotation when above levels tolerated with maintaining pelvic tilt (3 × 12 sets with each level of progression)

Standing lunges: start without weights and progress up to 5 lb weights after 15 on each leg without balance loss and maintaining upright trunk extension and appropriate pelvic tilt

Hip abduction/adduction (standing/supine/or sidelying): begin with 3 × 10 on each leg and maintain pelvic tilt and trunk extension for alignment; progress to add 1–5 lb weights for each leg

Hip extension (standing or prone): avoid any rotation and keep knee extended; lift the leg up approximately 4 in. off the surface-hold for 5 seconds; progress from 0 to 5 lb; 3 × 10 sets

Hip extension (standing or prone): avoid any rotation and keep knee flexed to 90 degrees; lift the leg up approximately 4 in off the surface-hold for 5 seconds; progress from 0 to 5 lb; 3 × 10 sets

Precautions

Evaluation prior to starting an exercise program (oxygen saturation at rest and with activity)

Use bronchodilator prior to exercise to prevent bronchospasm

Avoid strenuous exercise with an exacerbation/fever/hemoptysis/untreated pneumothorax

Precautions for osteopenia/osteoporosis

Proper hydration and calorie intake

Avoid poorly controlled climate conditions (hot, humid, freezing, high levels of pollution, windy, etc)

(continued)

BOX 17-2 (Continued)

Watch for signs of decompensation: color, breathing pattern, increase in dyspnea, etc.

Watch for sudden chest pain or any type of pain (musculoskeletal)

When indwelling venous catheter in place, avoid resistance exercise with affected upper extremity

Exercise with a buddy if possible; carry identification

Evaluate best time for airway clearance and timing of exercise

Be aware of any declines in activity level; keep a diary of exercise program/progression

Reevaluate exercise program in a timely manner (3–6 months depending on the level of illness and frequency of return visits to clinic)

Flexibility exercises—Flexibility is another important component of an exercise prescription. A commonly used phrase among physical therapists is "the position of comfort is a position of muscle shortening." Flexibility is key in preventing injury, enhancing chest wall expansion, and promoting healthy postures. Most patients with CF similar in age to Julia present with distinct shortening of the anterior chest muscles, overstretched posterior upper thoracic muscles, and shortening of the hip and knee flexors. Weakness in the lower abdominal region and pelvic floor is not uncommon as is weakness and loss of range of motion in the cervical and thoracic spine. Usually the lumbar spine assumes a flexed position.

Stretching of target areas is vital for ease of chest wall movement. Proximal muscles of the upper and lower extremities as well as trunk musculature play a role in inhibition of chest wall movement if muscle shortening has occurred from poor posture, weak muscles, and muscle imbalances.[46] It is important to stabilize the proximal segments to assess shortening of muscles, which cross two joints and influence movement of the chest wall. Instruction in corrective postures and integration of breathing strategies with flexibility exercises reinforce and encourage proper control of airflow while limiting discomfort and bronchospasm with exercise.

Strength, power, and endurance training for head and neck, limb, pelvic floor, trunk, and ventilatory muscles[27,28,47–53]—Strength Training is also an important component of a therapeutic exercise intervention. Strength training will improve muscle tone and BMD, and in some cases, pulmonary function.[15,46] Low weight and higher repetitions should be incorporated into a normal exercise routine. The exercises can be performed with dumbbells, soup cans, or resistance equipment. Breathing exercises should be utilized to decrease dyspnea and fear or anxiety that may occur with participation in this type of exercise. Exhalation on the "work" or "lift" part of the exercise will encourage good airflow, lessen the chance of a Valsalva maneuver, and improve strength and coordination of extremities and respiratory muscles. In addition, teaching patients to "brace" the pelvic floor by tightening the muscles before a lifting maneuver may prevent further stress on these muscles. Every other day, strength training in addition to rotation of targeted body segments is recommended to decrease the chance of musculoskeletal injury.

Relaxation—Breathing and movement strategies are important components of relaxation and energy conservation for patients with pulmonary disease. Although not intuitively included in the realm of relaxation, *energy conservation techniques* are probably best incorporated in this section, which includes breathing and movement strategies. Instruction in conservation techniques to promote a decrease in energy expenditure during daily activities will give the patient a sense of independence, decrease the fear of shortness of breath, and promote an increase in activity.

First pick simple activities like walking on level ground, getting out of a chair, or putting on a shirt before the patient/client is progressed to more energy-consuming and fearful activities like tying one's shoes, climbing stairs, or carrying objects while ascending stairs. Planning out the day or even just an hour at a time will help lessen the fear and anxiety of rushing to do a task. If the patient knows he or she will be spending the majority of the day on the first floor of the house and the bronchodilators are kept on the second floor by the bed, a mental note or an actual list should be made of what the patient needs to bring *before* he or she moves down to the first floor. Planning ahead for bathroom needs is also important. Rushing up a flight of stairs to get to the bathroom is a task that makes many patients feel short of breath and anxious. If the patient is on a diuretic, steps should be taken to plan when the medication is taken, limit the distance to the bathroom after the medication is taken, and eliminate obstacles on the way to the bathroom, all of which may decrease the energy cost of getting to the bathroom. A final area for improving the ease of ADL should be the process of showering. One suggestion is to bring a chair into the shower or have a chair just outside the shower so the patient/client can be sitting during the shower or immediately after the shower. In addition, if a terry-cloth robe is donned after a shower, the energy-consuming task of drying the patient's backside is eliminated. Pursed-lip breathing, planning ahead, and decreasing anxiety and fear are keys to conservation techniques and give the patient/client a sense of accomplishment. Relaxation techniques are very important for energy conservation, and are described elsewhere. They can be incorporated into daily activities or airway clearance techniques to decrease bronchospasm, control paroxysmal coughing, decrease metabolic demand or energy expenditure, enhance airflow, and promote a sense of well-being. The exercises or techniques can be performed in any position or location.

Functional training in self-care and home management— An evaluation of the home environment should include a review of daily activities. For example, on which level are bathrooms and bedrooms located, how many stairs are there in order to enter the house, are there handrails accompanying the stairs, where are the laundry facilities located, how accessible is the kitchen for demands on breathing, is there a gas stove versus electric (Julia uses oxygen), and how will she get her groceries? Julia presently functions independently at home, but she is finding it more difficult to carry out her day-to-day treatment regime and ADL. Education on ways to conserve energy (work of breathing), reduction of cough during ADL, and devices that may assist her to continue to live independently at home should be incorporated into the treatment (see sections on Breathing Strategies).

Functional training in work (job/school/play), community, and leisure integration or reintegration— Julia is no longer working and is on disability due to her illness. She does not have any hobbies besides reading and primarily focuses on her daily maintenance treatments. This topic should be examined in order to prepare Julia for discharge from the hospital. Julia may choose to visit with family and friends either at her home or away from her home. Evaluation of situations with which Julia may be presented during these times should be addressed by careful planning and assessment. A mockup of situations may be practiced in the hospital setting prior to discharge in order to evaluate hemodynamic responses and other challenges.

Once she receives the lung transplant, her functional training will have to be reassessed to see if she will be able to return to employment as a teacher. This evaluation should include examining the risk of infection, injury prevention and reduction, and safety awareness training during work, community, and leisure. Musculoskeletal components include assessment of osteoporotic changes, decreased activity, and falls from muscle weakness. Additional factors to consider are the ease of bruising, pain, and the physical side effects of the posttransplant medication including self-perception in the workplace as well as self-confidence related to these side effects. Finally, the evaluation should address the level of endurance related to work demands, hemodynamic challenges to the work area (stairs, inclines, uneven surfaces as on a playground), and other environmental considerations (smog, pollen, dust).

Manual therapy techniques— Techniques for mobilization of the rib cage, thorax, pelvic and shoulder girdle have been described to enhance ventilation and improve respiration. A working clinician can easily document the relationship between improvements in range of motion of the shoulder girdle, anterior chest wall, neck and upper thorax with improvements in relaxation, breathing pattern, perception of work of breathing (RPE), RR, level of anxiety, and in some cases, oxygen saturation. Applying the principles of proprioceptive neuromuscular techniques to the chest wall (musculoskeletal pump) can enhance relaxation, stimulate enhanced tidal volume or inspiratory capacity, and, as a result, may improve mucus mobilization and clearance.

Massage can be used to decrease muscle tension, anxiety, and work of breathing and enhance comfort. Massage of the upper posterior thorax and neck area may be beneficial following paradoxical coughing, vomiting initiated by coughing, or positioning, and to decrease musculoskeletal pain related to coughing and poor posture. Ventilation may be enhanced by utilizing massage in conjunction with manual techniques in order to provide relaxation of shortened accessory muscles.

Prescription application and, as appropriate, fabrication of devices and equipment— In the case of most individuals with CF, assistive or orthotic type devices are not indicated unless there is another superimposed pathology that would affect neuromuscular control. In the case of Julia, she had an indwelling venous catheter placed at age 26. If Julia and her care team decide that high-frequency chest wall oscillation (HFCWO) is the best form of airway clearance for her, fabrication of a device to offer relief around the catheter site may be necessary for comfort and safety reasons. The vest should be fit to Julia, and then the catheter area can be measured to have an appropriately sized padded device fabricated to prevent discomfort. This same type of device may also be utilized around gastric or jejunal tubes and chest tubes.[54-56]

Airway clearance techniques— When prescribing airway clearance techniques, many factors should be considered including the severity of disease, the patient's lifestyle, and factors affecting adherence (Table 17-5). Goals for airway clearance should be measurable and time oriented. Measuring sputum production, monitoring changes in color or viscosity, and measuring hemodynamic changes (SpO_2, HR, RR, and BP) allow appropriate goals to be set. Specific examples of goals included in this section are improvements in breath sounds, PFTs, chest radiography, subjective measurements, and treatment adherence. These goals may be obtained by performing the airway clearance interventions outlined in Box 17-3 and described in the following section.

TABLE 17-5   Decision Making for Airway Clearance Techniques

Considerations When Recommending Airway Clearance Techniques [5,27,42-44]	
History of esophageal reflux	Cost of device or technique
Osteopenia or osteoporosis	Lifestyle
Hemoptysis	Energy cost
Pulmonary function	Portability/space constraints
Severity of exacerbation	Energy source
Bronchospasm	Time constraints
Claustrophobia	Available assistance
Age	Comprehension (ease of learning, ease of teaching)
Patient preference	

BOX 17-3

Airway Clearance Techniques

Breathing strategies

Active cycle of breathing
Assisted cough/huff
Autogenic drainage
Paced breathing
Pursed-lips breathing
Techniques to maximize ventilation

Manual/mechanical techniques

Assistive Devices (positive expiratory pressure (PEP), including oscillatory PEP, high-frequency chest wall oscillation, intrapulmonary percussive ventilation)
Chest percussion, vibration, shaking
Chest wall manipulation
Suctioning
Ventilatory aids

Positioning

To alter the work of breathing
To maximize ventilation and perfusion
Pulmonary postural drainage

Exercise

Aerobic or endurance exercise

Breathing strategies: active cycle of breathing or forced expiratory technique[10,43,57-59]—The forced expiratory technique is based on optimal airflow and avoidance of a cough to prevent premature airway collapse to improve secretion mobilization and airway clearance. The technique can be done in any position. Quiet, tidal volume breathing is performed by the patient prior to a mid-to-large inhalation initiated from the lower rib cage. Then the glottis remains open and the air is then "huffed" out. The sound should be very breathy and the mouth should be in a shape of an "O." There should not be a high-pitched wheezing sound, as this would indicate too forceful of a maneuver, which would promote airway narrowing. The technique is easy to learn, can be performed independently, and can be taught to youngsters by using games that employ bubbles, cotton balls, handheld mirrors, and ping pong balls. The individual is taught to use huffs to loosen and then clear audible secretions until the huff sounds dry.

The active cycle of breathing technique (ACBT) combines the forced expiratory technique, bronchial drainage, and manual techniques. This technique is easy to learn, easy to teach, and can also be performed by the patient independently. The individual assumes a bronchial drainage position and focuses on a quiet breathing pattern using the lower rib cage area without upper chest movement. This is followed by a large inspiration again initiated in the region of the lower rib cage, a breath-hold for 3 to 4 seconds, and finally a sigh out through an open mouth. The theory of the inspiratory hold allows for air to equalize from an "open alveoli" to a "clogged one" to assist with secretion clearance from the blocked alveoli, thereby increasing the efficiency and effectiveness of the technique. This cycle can be repeated as dictated by the patient and then followed by one to two huffs to clear the secretions. The full cycle can then be repeated (see Fig. 17-6B). A caregiver or the patient may assist with manual techniques during expiration (such as vibration or shaking), but this is not necessary; rather, it is indicated if the patient feels it is beneficial.

Breathing strategies: assisted cough/huff techniques[5,10,14,43,57,59]—The *huff* or forced expiratory technique was explained previously. The assisted cough can be employed independently or with the help of an assistant. The technique can be as simple as placing a pillow over an incision to help splint the area or as vigorous as using a manual technique at the time of the cough. Massery describes four types of manual assistance: costophrenic (hand placement), abdominal thrust, anterior chest compression, and a counter-rotation assist.[14] Refer to Chapter 20 and the CD-ROM for explanations and demonstrations of these maneuvers. Pain, fullness of gastric contents, mental status, innervation, and expertise of the instructor or caregiver are a few factors to consider when determining whether an assisted cough is appropriate. After a surgical procedure, the simple act of coughing may be limited because of pain, which will inhibit a large inhalation and a forceful exhalation. Assisting a patient with splinting of the incision, along with assuring that adequate pain medication is provided, may improve the pain tolerance.

In Julia's case, she has pain with coughing from GI and musculoskeletal symptoms. During forced expiratory techniques, huffing, or controlled coughing, she may use hand placement to brace her lower rib cage, a towel wrapped around her lower rib cage, or a pillow to brace against the abdominal area and lower rib cage to lessen the complaint of pain and assist with a more effective cough. If the pain subsides with the bracing, Julia could be instructed to press inward on the lower rib cage and upward on the abdominal area to improve her cough.

The cough is best performed using a flexed posture. Another way of performing an assisted cough is to instruct the patient to assume certain postures to encourage flexion, such as sitting forward while in bed. Julia could be instructed that sidelying with hips and knees flexed may be an advantageous position to enhance her cough. Also while in bed, her head could be elevated on pillows (or by raising the head of the hospital bed) to increase flexion; Julia may already have her trunk and hips flexed. The disadvantage of elevating the head of the bed to place the patient in the flexed position is that the volume of air inhaled during the initial phase of the cough may be limited. If in a standing position, the patient could be taught to bend forcefully at the waist during the cough to assist with the movement of air. One disadvantage of this position is safety; if the patient is unstable or has near syncopal episodes with coughs, there is an opportunity for injury by bumping or falling against objects.[14]

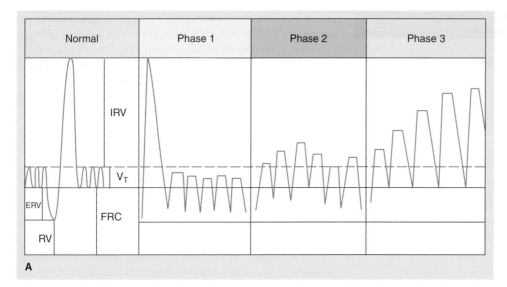

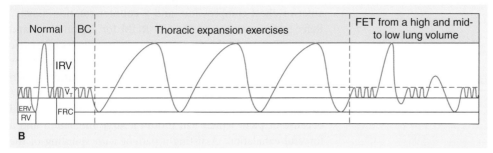

FIGURE 17-6   Autogenic drainage (AD) (**A**) versus active cycle of breathing (ACB) (**B**), both from spirograms of normal individuals. AD: phase 1 = peripheral loosening of mucus; phase 2 = collection of mucus in large airways; phase 3 = transport of mucus to the mouth. ACB: BC = breathing control, FET = forced expiration technique. (Republished with permission of Lippincott Williams & Wilkins, from Savci S, Ince DI, Arikan H. A comparison of autogenic drainage and the active cycle of breathing in patients with chronic obstructive pulmonary disorders. *J Cardiopulm Rehabil.* 2000;20(1); permission conveyed through Copyright Clearance Center, Inc.)

Breathing strategies: autogenic drainage[10,43,57,59–61]—AD is an airway clearance technique that can be used independent of assistance. This is a challenging technique to learn, requires a great amount of concentration, should only be instructed by experienced clinicians, and initially may be time consuming to use. However, these disadvantages are offset by the great freedom the technique offers to patients with pulmonary disease.

The technique can be done in sitting position and, once learned, can be performed nearly anywhere. Coughing is suppressed initially, and only lower chest wall movement is encouraged. Because the technique utilizes some of the same theories of active cycle of breathing (equalization of air across alveoli for mobilization of secretions), the bronchioles and alveoli should be fully developed to get the full benefit. This physiological consideration, plus the great level of concentration and patience required, makes this technique less suitable for patients younger than 12 years.

The patient is instructed to breathe out through an "o"-shaped mouth (or the nose) while learning the technique. The patient should be taught to listen during inhalation and exhalation for noises indicative of secretions such as high-pitched wheezes, gurgling, or popping sounds. The timing and pitch of these sounds give cues to where the secretions may be located. If the sounds are heard initially on inhalation and are lower in pitch, most likely the secretions are in the larger, upper airways. These airways must be cleared with huffs or coughs prior to continuation of the technique. If these larger airways

are not cleared, the patient will experience frustration from trying to continuously suppress the urge to cough. The patient should practice quiet breaths, using only the lower rib cage. A mirror is a good teaching tool to make sure the upper chest remains still during the technique.

Once the patient is comfortable with using only the lower rib cage, he or she is instructed to exhale down into expiratory reserve volume. This should be "sighing" out rather than a forceful exhalation. Once expiratory reserve volume is reached, the individual should inhale a "tidal volume" breath at this level. If the patient feels light-headed or dizzy at any time, he or she can resume a regular breathing pattern until the feeling subsides. The sounds described here should occur following multiple cycles at this low lung volume (a tidal volume breath just into expiratory reserve volume). Once the sounds are heard close to mid-exhalation, the patient then inhales to a slightly larger volume to move closer to a volume of breath where normal tidal volume would be performed. Again, if the patient feels light-headed or dizzy, he or she should resume normal tidal volume breaths or a couple of larger breaths until these symptoms pass. The patient is instructed to resume a "midlevel" of breathing and not to move to a higher level until the popping, wheezing, and gurgle sounds are heard midway through the exhalation phase. Once the sounds occur at this point in the breathing cycle, the patient can take a much deeper breath to reach the highest part of the pattern. Again, once the highest level of breathing is reached, only the amount of air in a tidal volume is used. If symptoms are experienced anytime during this phase of the cycle, instruct the patient to take a regular or larger breath until the symptoms pass and then resume the cycle where he or she left off. Once mobilized, the secretions are cleared through huffing or coughing.

The keys to this technique are airflow and volume control, suppression of cough until secretions are mobilized, inspiratory hold at the end of inhalation to equalize air across alveoli, and most importantly, patience. Because of the immense amount of concentration and the requirement of using audible and tactile cues, this technique is not appropriate for all patients with excessive production of sputum. See Figure 17-6 for a schematic of AD compared to active cycle of breathing.

Breathing strategies: techniques to maximize ventilation, pursed-lip breathing, paced breathing[4,15,62,63]—Although this category of breathing strategies is placed under the heading of Airway Clearance in the *Guide,* these techniques are also useful in other situations when secretion removal is not the primary goal. Many of these techniques may be incorporated into daily activities or exercise routines. This section also includes techniques useful for promotion of energy conservation or relaxation.

Techniques to maximize ventilation: The terms *diaphragmatic breathing* or *lower rib cage breathing* are both used to describe strategies to expand the lower chest in place of upper chest expansion. In order to teach lower rib cage breathing, the client should be in a comfortable position. The preferred position is one that enhances the movement of the diaphragm against gravity (side-lying or semifowlers). A tactile cue of a hand or a tissue box over the lower rib cage will help visualize how the lower rib cage should move on inhalation and exhalation. On inhalation, the hand on the lower rib cage or tissue box should rise, indicating air filling the lungs. When done correctly, the upper chest will have little movement because there should not be large volumes of air moved during a relaxation technique.

Stacking breaths is a useful technique to maximize ventilation when the volume of air a patient/client can inhale is limited. This may be due to a neuromuscular insult, postsurgical pain, trapped air, weak muscles, or large inspiratory airflow leading to bronchospasm. Breath stacking is accomplished by taking a small-to-moderate size breath and adding it to two or three additional breaths to increase inspiratory volume, thereby decreasing atelectasis, moving air behind the secretions, and increasing inspiratory volume to enhance a huff or cough. The patient is instructed to take in siplike volumes of air on top of one another without exhaling. After three to four breaths, an inspiratory hold should be done for 1 to 2 seconds followed by a huff or a controlled cough. It may be helpful for the patient/client to see a demonstration and use a mirror for visual cues. Any symptoms of dizziness or light-headedness are indications to stop the technique. The inhalation and inspiratory hold phases of breath stacking can be incorporated with many other airway clearance techniques such as the forced expiratory technique, AD, active cycle of breathing, PEP, oscillating positive pressure, and during bronchial drainage and manual techniques.

Segmental breathing combines manual cues and breathing control to improve ventilation to specific areas of the chest wall. If during evaluation of chest wall movement asymmetry is identified, this could coincide with the underlying pathology of pneumonia, an area with pleuritic chest wall pain or an area with poor air movement from retained secretions. Placing a hand on that area and coordinating chest wall movement with downward hand movement will enhance expansion in this area. Facilitation or inhibition of a segment can be controlled with proper timing, hand placement, and verbal cues for breathing coordination. Utilization of the principles of proprioceptive neuromuscular techniques will allow the therapist to increase chest wall movement, stimulate a productive cough in some cases, and improve overall ventilation and chest wall symmetry.

Combining *pursed-lip breathing* during exhalation with diaphragmatic breathing should enhance relaxation and promote a better overall breathing pattern with less accessory muscle use. Pursed-lip breathing is accomplished by breathing in through the nose to a count of "1, 2" and out via pursed lips to a count of "1, 2, 3, 4." This will prolong the expiratory phase, slow the RR, and delay small airway closure. It will also decrease dyspnea, improve airflow, and calm anxiety. Instruct the patient to sit in front of a mirror or use a handheld mirror for feedback. Repeat the previous sequence of taking a breath in through the nose and exhaling via the lips in a whistle-ready position. If the patient or client is very anxious, it is not as important how the breath is taken in, as how the air is exhaled through the pursed lips. If the patient or client has end-stage lung disease and the diaphragms are flattened from air trapping, diaphragmatic breathing may not be as beneficial as pursed-lip breathing.

Pursed-lip breathing and diaphragmatic breathing should be incorporated into functional activities like walking. This strategy is referred to as *paced breathing.* The patient is instructed to take a breath in through the nose and walk two steps to a count of "1, 2." The patient then exhales to a count of "1, 2, 3, 4" as they walk the next 4 steps. The inspiration-to-expiration ratio is 1:2, thus prolonging the expiratory phase and delaying small airway closure. Once the patient is able to use these strategies on level surfaces, they can advance to stair climbing. Instruct the patient to use a "step-to" strategy (ie, one foot meets the other on the same step), and avoid "step-over-step" (ie, one foot moves past the other to the next step above). Also make sure that his or her foot is placed fully on the step and not on the edge before going up to the next step. A handrail may allow the patient to use accessory muscles as needed. A handrail may also lessen the fear of falling, thereby reducing the anxiety that accompanies fear. Fear of falling promotes anxiety, which leads to shortness of breath and poor airflow.

Expiratory exercises that prolong the expiratory phase can be used as measurable outcomes as well as interventions.

Instructing the patient/client to read a phrase, sentence, or paragraph aloud promotes expiratory control. The number of words stated during exhalation can be measured by the patient/client for feedback and demonstration of progress. This same technique can incorporate singing for expiratory airflow control. The patient can place a hand on the abdominal area to palpate abdominal muscle activation during the technique. This exercise will promote endurance training of the expiratory muscles and can be used during ADL in combination with conservation techniques.

Manual/mechanical techniques: assistive devices[5,8,10,31,42,44,57,60,61,64–74]—PEP, oscillatory PEP (*Flutter* or *Acapella*), HFCWO, intrapulmonary percussive ventilation (IPPV), and the Frequencer are all mechanical devices used for airway clearance.

PEP can be produced using pursed lips, a mouthpiece, a mask, or various devices. For the purpose of airway clearance, only the devices used for PEP will be discussed in this section. The technique(s) are easy to learn, can be performed in the sitting position, done independently, taught to children, are very portable, and have been shown to be an effective method of airway clearance. There are many devices available in the market at a wide variety of prices. The devices used should include an exhalation port, a release-type valve, and be used for only a single individual. Ideally, they should also have a port for either oxygen or nebulized medication to be delivered during the technique. Pressures between 10 and 20 cm H_2O are optimal to build up back pressure and promote equalization of pressure across alveoli for mobilization of secretions. The back pressure is also theorized to promote airway stabilization to increase time for secretion mobilization.

The individual is instructed to sit upright with his or her elbows on a table, to exhale just greater than a normal tidal breath, and inhale into the mask or mouthpiece of the device. A manometer is placed in-line to measure pressure levels and give visual cues. A resistor is placed in the exhalation port to promote positive pressure in the range of 10 to 20 cm H_2O. When initially teaching an individual how to use the device, a larger resistor is used with progressively smaller ones put in place until the desired pressure range is reached. The manometer acts as biofeedback until the individual has learned the sequence. If a mouthpiece is used instead of a mask, a nose clip should be used to prevent air leakage. As with other devices used for airway clearance, secretions are expectorated by huffing or coughing.

Oscillating positive pressure is an alternative to a stable level of pressure in PEP devices. These pocket-sized devices (*Flutter* or *Acapella*) provide the benefits of a positive-pressure device plus the "interruptions" from the oscillations that promote changes in the viscosity of the secretions and enhance expiratory airflow. This category of PEP devices has been shown to be an effective mode of airway clearance. Pneumothoraces, claustrophobia, recent facial or nasal surgery, or injury are precautions that should be considered when weighing the benefits against the risks of using positive-pressure devices for airway clearance.

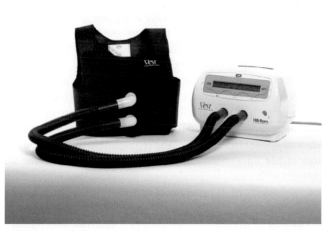

FIGURE 17-7   The *Vest* airway clearance system. (Courtesy of Advanced Respiratory, Inc, St Paul, MN.)

HFCWO (*the Vest Airway Clearance System* or the *SmartVest System*) is an individually sized chest wall jacket powered by a generator, which promotes secretion clearance of the entire lung fields while performed in the seated position (Fig. 17-7). HFCWO offers the advantage of independence and has been shown to be an effective airway clearance method. The device has been used in the home, acute and long-term care settings, and intensive care settings. The principal theory of the vest is that at various pressures and oscillations, airflow is enhanced and viscosity of secretions is altered, which promotes ease of secretion mobilization and clearance. The device requires an electrical source, comes with a prefitted vest, a compressor unit, a hand or foot pedal, and tubes to connect the vest to the compressor. Three frequency ranges are used to enhance secretion movement: 5 to 10 cycles/s, 10 to 15 cycles/s, and 15 to 20 cycles/s.

The individual is instructed to start at the lower settings to allow loosening of secretions from the periphery and then progress to the higher settings to move the secretions toward the upper airways for expectoration. More than 10 minutes should be spent at each level to promote the most efficient and effective airway clearance. A nebulizer can be used along with the vest. A properly fitted vest is imperative for comfort and to limit side effects such as nausea, abdominal discomfort, chest wall discomfort, and complaints of urinary urgency. If an indwelling venous catheter is in place, padding can be placed around the site to limit discomfort. These devices are expensive but are covered by most insurance companies.

The *IPPV* device works in a similar way to HFCWO. The device is based on theories of airflow and oscillation but is delivered internally via a mouthpiece compared to HFCWO, which is external. Cost and comfort are two key areas of patient concern, as a feeling of claustrophobia and chest fullness may be experienced during the application of the device. The changes in frequency and pressure delivered internally assist with airway stabilization, thereby decreasing secretion viscosity and enhancing secretion mobilization.

The Frequencer is a newly developed device for airway clearance. The electroacoustical device, which has recently received FDA approval in the United States, applies vibrations at a rate of 20 to 120 Hz to the chest wall to assist with the mobilization of mucus. A preliminary study demonstrated that the Frequencer was equal to conventional postural drainage and percussion in 22 patients with CF when used between 25 and 40 Hz. Although safety and efficacy of the Frequencer have been demonstrated, its use is not yet widespread enough to determine acceptance by the CF population.

Manual/mechanical techniques: chest percussion, vibration, and shaking[8–10,12,42,43,57,60,72,75]—Manual techniques have traditionally been used to enhance bronchial drainage. These techniques include *percussion, vibration,* and *shaking,* which are often collectively referred to as traditional *chest PT.* Treatments with these techniques can be performed with an assistant, independently via self-percussion/vibration, or with mechanical devices. The mechanical devices may be difficult to hold in the correct position to get the similar effect of manually delivered percussion or vibration. The mechanical devices can be expensive if not covered by insurance and could be unreliable at producing the correct rate and pressure required for optimal airway clearance. On the other hand, performing the technique manually can be fatiguing for the person performing the technique as well as for the person receiving the percussion, vibration, or shaking. Correct hand posture and position are needed to prevent injury to the performer and receiver of the percussion. The caregiver may be at risk for a repetitive-type injury at the wrist, elbow, or shoulder, and the individual receiving the technique may be at risk for bruising, soreness, and fractures of the ribs if too much pressure is applied and the patient does not communicate to the caregiver their tolerance to treatment.

The cupped-hand position is used for percussion to transmit energy through the chest wall to loosen thick secretions. The technique may be done concurrently with a drainage position to enhance secretion mobilization. Once the secretions are loosened with percussion, the techniques of vibration and shaking help to mobilize the secretions from the periphery and move them toward the trachea for expectoration and evaluation of the secretions. Vibration and shaking are done in a rhythmic pattern. The caregiver's shoulders should be positioned directly over the hands. As the patient exhales, a downward motion is made by the caregiver in a vibrating motion while maintaining full contact of the hands on the chest wall. Shaking results in an exaggeration of vibration and appears more like a plunging motion.

For each of the manual techniques, hand placement should avoid bony prominences such as the scapula, spinous processes, and clavicles. Ribs and breast tissue may be very sensitive and special care should be given in those areas. The patient receiving the manual techniques should be allowed to rest after three to four cycles. The caregiver should watch for fatigue and signs of decompensation: increased RR, reports of shortness of breath, a change in coloration or mental status, and a change from baseline breathing pattern. An individual may use self-percussion and vibration independent of a caregiver for certain drainage positions, but these exclude any of the posterior regions. Box 17-4 lists precautions for percussion and vibration.

Positioning for airway clearance[5,8,10,42,43,57,60–62,75]—*Bronchial drainage* or *postural drainage* has been utilized for treating pulmonary congestion for decades. The primary principle of the technique is to utilize the shape and direction of the lung segments and to place the individual in gravity-enhancing postures or positions that drain the uppermost segment of the lung once in that position. Ten positions are used to drain all the segments of the lung (see Fig. 17-8). It may not be necessary to use all 10 positions. The treatment should be based on the PT examination to focus on the areas most in need in addition to being tolerated by the patient. Elevated BP, anxiety, esophageal reflux, and decompensation of the cardiopulmonary system are precautions, which should always be observed if this technique is utilized. Bronchial drainage can be done independently and modified to reduce the aforementioned precautions; however, performing all 10 positions can be very time consuming. Precautions for postural drainage should be observed (Box 17-4).

BOX 17-4

Precautions for Postural Drainage and Manual Techniques

Precautions for Bronchial Drainage and Manual Techniques [5,42,44]

Esophageal reflux
Hemoptysis
Dyspnea
Orthopnea
Bruising/rib fractures/flail chest
Coagulopathy
Cardiac arrhythmias
Desaturation/hemodynamic decompensation
Large pleural effusion
Bronchospasm
Spinal instability
Recent burn graphs
Osteopenia/osteoporosis
Requires assistance
Pain
Level of alertness
Risk for injury to caregiver and/or recipient
Nausea and vomiting
Untreated pneumothorax
Increased intracranial pressure
Recent surgery
Appropriate light, loose clothing
Indwelling venous catheter
Feeding tubes (jejunal, gastric)
Timing of tube feeds prior to treatment
Mechanical percussor/vibrators need electrical source, rate may be inconsistent

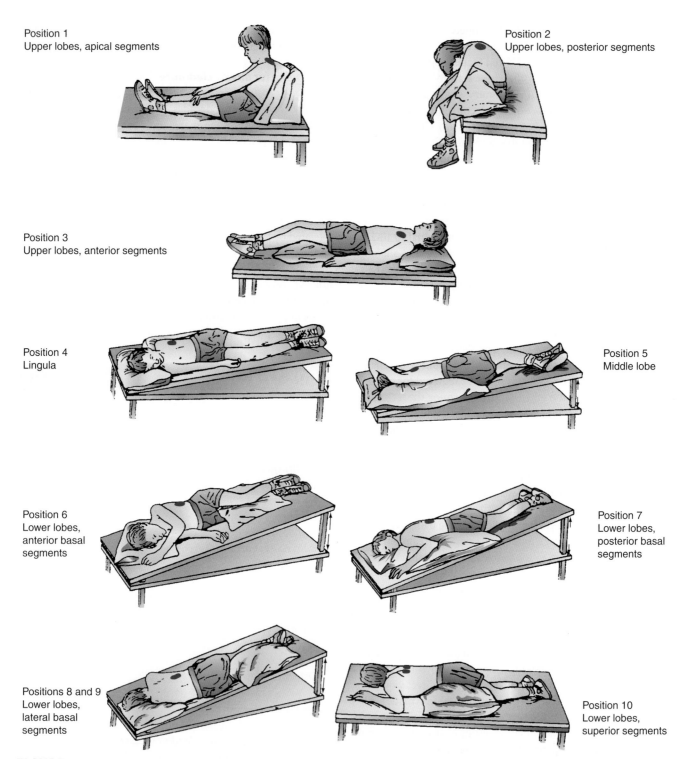

Position 1
Upper lobes, apical segments

Position 2
Upper lobes, posterior segments

Position 3
Upper lobes, anterior segments

Position 4
Lingula

Position 5
Middle lobe

Position 6
Lower lobes,
anterior basal
segments

Position 7
Lower lobes,
posterior basal
segments

Positions 8 and 9
Lower lobes,
lateral basal
segments

Position 10
Lower lobes,
superior segments

FIGURE 17-8   Postural drainage positions. Position 1 = patient leans back 30 degrees; position 2 = patient leans forward 30 degrees; position 3 = patient flatlying; positions 4 and 5 = patient with head down 15 degrees, rotated one-quarter turn backward; position 6 = patient with head down 30 degrees, sidelying; position 7 = patient with head down 30 degrees, prone; position 8 and 9 = patient with head down 30 degrees, rotated one-quarter turn forward; position 10 = patient prone with bed flat. (Reprinted with permission from the Cystic Fibrosis Foundation. *An Introduction to Chest Physical Therapy*. Bethesda, MD; 1997.)

TABLE 17-6   Threshold Behaviors: Impaired Ventilation and Respiration/Gas Exchange

Normal or baseline level	Minimal work of breathing at rest	Resting RR 12–16 breaths per minute	Temperature of 36–37.8°C	Paco₂ at 35–45 mm Hg	Absence of bronchoconstriction	Dyspnea rated as mild or absent at rest	Normal endurance of respiratory muscles
Abnormal or change in baseline	Increased work of breathing at rest	Increase in RR at rest	Elevated temperature indicative of infection	Elevated Paco₂ level	Increase in FEV₁ after bronchodilation[25]	Dyspnea rated as moderate or severe at rest	Excessive fatigue of respiratory muscles
Intervention	Techniques to maximize ventilation, relaxation techniques	Techniques to maximize ventilation, relaxation techniques, increased ACT[a]	More aggressive or increase frequency of ACT (antibiotics)	More aggressive or increase frequency of ACT	Use of bronchodilator or modify ACT	Techniques to maximize ventilation, relaxation techniques	Ventilatory muscle training, energy conservation, endurance conditioning

[a]ACT, airway clearance technique.

Exercise for airway clearance[15,17,43,60,75]—Although not listed in the *Guide* under Airway Clearance Techniques, *exercise* may be used to enhance clearance of secretions. Exercise promotes improvement in ventilation, airflow, air volume, chest wall movement, secretion movement, and functional capacity. Exercise has not been advocated as an independent method of airway clearance for patients with chronic pulmonary conditions and should be performed in conjunction with other techniques. Exercise to enhance airway clearance should involve large muscle groups, thereby promoting an increase in tidal volume and airflow and be done regularly for a training effect. Exercise should be age appropriate and enjoyable for the patient. Oxygen desaturation and hemodynamic decompensation should be a key concern when initiating any type of an exercise program with a patient with pulmonary disease and excessive secretion production. Monitoring pulse oximetry is a must for patient safety. Precaution for musculoskeletal injury should also be included in the plan. Substitut-ing one of the multiday airway clearance treatments with exercise will encourage independence and enjoyment and promote another component of health.

THRESHOLD BEHAVIORS

Threshold behaviors have been defined as measurable behaviors at the pathology, impairment, functional, disability, or quality of life level that triggers an intervention.[76] Identifying threshold behaviors in patients with CF may provide insight into which of these patients would benefit from the specific intervention techniques described. Many of the tests previously described measure levels of impairment and function in patients with CF. The following tables will identify numerous threshold behaviors for patients with CF and match them with appropriate interventions based on the level of impairment or function that has been identified (Tables 17-6 to 17-9).

TABLE 17-7   Threshold Behaviors: Airway Clearance Dysfunction

Normal or baseline level	Lungs clear to auscultation	FEV₁ and FVC[a] at standard for age, height, weight	Sputum produced is at patient's baseline	Hemoptysis is absent	Spo₂ 95% or > at rest	Adherence to ACTs as prescribed	Min to mod effort required to perform ACT
Abnormal or change in baseline	Increased crackles and wheezes from baseline	Decrease in baseline pulmonary function[25]	Increase in sputum produced[25]	Presence of hemoptysis	Spo₂ ≤ 90% or a in baseline at rest	Decreased adherence to prescribed ACTs	Excessive effort required to perform ACT
Intervention	More aggressive, or Δ in ACT, or increase frequency	More aggressive, or Δ in ACT, or increase frequency	More aggressive, or Δ in ACT, or increase frequency	Refer to physician and modify ACT	Δ PD position or increase frequency of ACT	Identify factors affecting adherence and Δ ACT	Modify or Δ ACT

[a]FVC, forced vital capacity; PD, postural drainage; Min to mod, minimal to moderate; Δ = change.

TABLE 17-8   Threshold Behaviors: Aerobic Capacity/Endurance

Normal or baseline level	Vital signs (HR, BP, RR) WNL[a] during activity	$SpO_2 \geq 95\%$ with activity	Dyspnea rated as mild or moderate with activity	RPE rated as 11–13 (6–20 scale) with activity	Normal exercise tolerance	Adherence to prescribed exercise program	Minimal to moderate effort required for self-care
Abnormal or change in baseline	Abnormal vital sign response to activity	$SpO_2 \geq 90\%$ or a Δ in baseline with activity	Dyspnea rated as severe with activity	RPE rated as 15 or higher (6–20 scale) with activity	Decrease in exercise tolerance or Δ in baseline	Decreased adherence to prescribed exercise or activity	Excessive effort required for self-care
Intervention	Prescribe intermittent activity, Δ mode, or decrease intensity	Obtain prescription for oxygen use and titration with activity	Decrease intensity of activity, use breathing strategies with activity	Prescribe intermittent activity, Δ mode, or decrease intensity	Prescribe intermittent activity, decrease intensity, endurance conditioning	Identify factors affecting adherence and Δ exercise	Energy conservation, endurance conditioning

[a]WNL, within normal limits; Δ = change.

INTERNATIONAL CLASSIFICATION OF FUNCTIONING, DISABILITY, AND HEALTH MODEL (ICF MODEL)

In the first edition of this chapter, the Nagi Disablement Model was used to describe the relationships among disease pathology, impairments, functional limitations, and disability. Included in the model were the risk factors for a particular pathology, factors that are specific to an individual patient's health status, and extraneous factors that impact a patient's treatment and lifestyle.[77] The components of the more recent ICF, a common language for function, disability, and health model[78] have been applied to the pathology of CF[79] using Julia's case to demonstrate a potential path to identify impairments, limitation, and disability (Table 17-10).

The ICF model "attempts to provide a coherent biopsychosocial view of health states from a biological, personal, and social perspective."[79] Three key levels of human function are identified to better describe the patient's limitations: body functions and structures and activity and participation. These levels are interconnected to the patient's health condition and contextual factors. In this model, health condition replaces the terms for diseases, injuries, or disorders.[79,80] Some examples of contextual factors would be environmental or personal factors that influence the patient's perception of how disablement is experienced.[79] Body functions and structures refer to physiological functions and anatomical parts of the body, and impairments are identified problems in those areas. Activity and activity limitations relate to tasks or actions by an individual and any difficulties encountered executing the activity.[79] Participation is the involvement of the individual in a specific life situation, while participation restrictions refer to problems experienced in a life situation.[79,80] Some examples of subdomains used in both activity and participation, which further identify patient limitations or restrictions, are communication,

TABLE 17-9   Threshold Behaviors: Posture, Muscle Performance

Normal or baseline level	Posture WNL,[a] absence of kyphosis	ROM in extremities WNL	Normal thoracic expansion	Bone density within 1 SD expected for age	5/5 on MMT for major muscle groups
Abnormal or change in baseline	Kyphotic or abnormal posture	Decreased ROM in upper or lower extremities	Limited thoracic expansion	Bone density greater than 1 SD below expected for age	Less than 5/5 on MMT for major muscle groups
Intervention	Strength training, flexibility exercises to improve posture and muscle balance	Flexibility exercises to improve ROM	Flexibility exercises to increase thoracic mobility breathing strategies	Patient education, modify exercise program, wt-bearing activity, strength training	Strength training, functional activities

[a]WNL, within normal limits; ROM, range of motion; wt, weight; MMT, manual muscle test.

TABLE 17-10 The International Classification of Function, Disability and Health (ICF)[78–82]

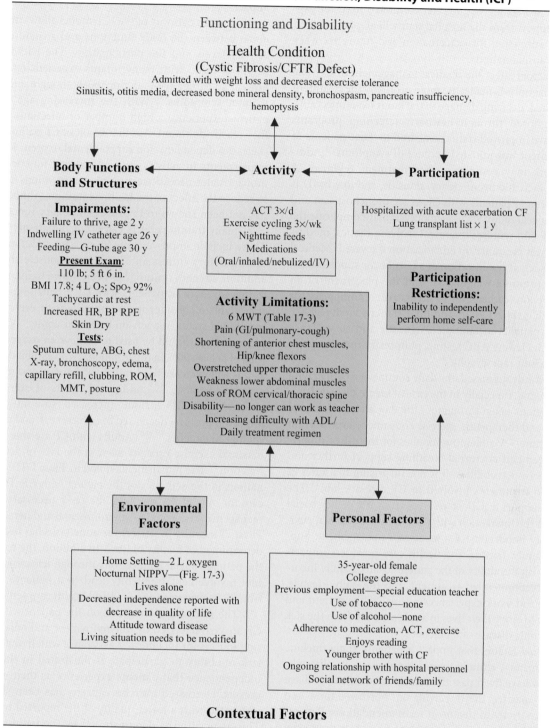

self-care, domestic life, and learning and applying knowledge.[79]

This newer classification emphasizes the components of health versus the consequences of disease.[81] From the clinician's perspective this shift in how disability and health are examined or classified focuses the patients' functioning and health away from merely the consequences of a disease or condition.[82] The ICF model takes into consideration how the patients' health and functioning are associated with their disease as well as the influence of personal and environmental factors. A full description and discussion of the qualifiers and scoring of the ICF is beyond the scope of this chapter. For

Julia, assessing factors such as her home setting, her inability to work, her worsening CF, and her continued need for psychosocial support from the hospital staff will all play a role in her present admission for exacerbation and future recovery from lung transplantation.

Many factors affect the medical management of CF. The earlier the diagnosis is made, the more promptly the treatment can be initiated, delaying damage to the lungs from infections. Infants diagnosed through newborn screening programs appear to have improved status compared to those patients in whom treatment was initiated because of symptoms.[33] Additional factors may complicate the treatment regimen. A history of pancreatic insufficiency, sinusitis, and low BMD is frequently seen in patients with CF, as are bronchospasm and gastroesophogeal reflux.[32,34,35] Hemoptysis may complicate the course of CF and requires treatment with antibiotics, modification of airway clearance, or embolization if severe.[34] Medical procedures such as the insertion of a G-tube for supplemental feedings to promote weight gain and the placement of an indwelling venous catheter for IV access are commonplace for patients with severe CF. In addition, the chronicity of CF predisposes patients to multiple diagnostic and surveillance procedures, including ABG testing, pulmonary function evaluation, and chest radiography.[34]

As previously discussed, the daily routine of a patient with CF can be taxing, especially in the case of severe disease. Multiple medications taken throughout the day, airway clearance techniques, and therapeutic exercise consume a large portion of patients' time.[26] Maintaining supplies for the use of supplemental oxygen and nocturnal breathing support further add to a patient's responsibilities. It is not surprising that rates of adherence to treatments involved in CF care are low.[35] The amount of support a patient receives from his or her social network and the interaction with the physical and social environment play important roles in disease management. Support from family, friends, and health care providers impacts significantly on the ability of the patient to successfully incorporate the recommended treatment into the daily lifestyle. Educational and work experiences normalize the patient and enable them to enjoy their lives in a role separate from the sick role that chronic disease often dictates.

Additional factors that impact a patient's status include age, family history, attitude toward the disease, and lifestyle. Patients who have lived past the current median survival age of 37 years[16] may feel they are living on "borrowed time" and adhere more strictly to treatment recommendations. Patients with genetic diseases may have grown up with parents who experienced guilt as a result of passing a disease to their children, and this may affect psychosocial interactions of family members in many different ways. A patient's attitude toward CF and the lifestyle they lead are important factors in the management of the disease. Regular use of tobacco would have negative consequences on disease progression, as would disregarding treatment recommendations or failing to take medications as directed. On the other hand, a positive attitude paired with the ability to accomplish airway clearance, exercise, and the taking of medications regularly would have a positive impact.

The main pathway of the ICF model allows linkages to be made between the body functions and structures of CF, to activity levels and the participation. The pathology of CF begins at birth, with many infants experiencing lung infections at an earlier age than previously thought and frequently without symptoms.[33] With the increasing age of survival, patients experience a high number of infections by the time they reach adulthood. Another result of CF pathology in later stages is a dependence on supplemental oxygen. The resulting impairments in activity, musculoskeletal function, and pulmonary status necessitate multiple interventions in an attempt to reduce the effect of the health condition. Although exercise has not been shown to improve pulmonary function specifically, many training effects can occur in patients with CF.[34,83] These include improvements in exercise endurance and cardiorespiratory fitness and inspiratory muscle strength.[83] In addition, strength training has been shown to improve skeletal muscle strength in patients with CF.[83] Nutritional therapy is important to consider in conjunction with exercise, as poor nutritional status impacts on muscular ability.[83] Oxygen supplementation should be used to achieve an oxygen saturation level of at least 90% in those patients who exhibit desaturation, as this will decrease the ventilatory demand and may improve exercise tolerance.[34,83] Additional effects of exercise seen in patients with CF include increased sputum production, improved posture, decreased breathlessness, and positive psychological benefits.[26,34,83] Adults with CF are able to maintain maximal exercise capacity even in the face of declining lung function.[83] The impairments noted in Table 17-10 lead to limitations in the activities of the patient with CF. The ability to care for oneself and perform the tasks necessary for disease management is related to environmental and personal factors. Physical inability to perform routine tasks has been cited as a determinant of quality of life.[83] In addition, the restrictions of the patient's social connections through leisure and community involvement frequently lead to a patient's withdrawal from the world outside home and health care settings.

The resulting restrictions on the patient with advanced CF are characterized by unemployment and reliance on outside sources for income and assistance with living needs. This lack of ability to participate is illustrated in the decreased independence that patients experience as their disease progresses. Decreased exercise capacity has been shown to be associated with a lower quality of life reported by patients.[83] This association is demonstrated by the pathway from the body structures and functions of CF to its resulting limitations in participation.

THE LIMITS OF OUR KNOWLEDGE

Manifestations of Cystic Fibrosis

There continue to be tremendous advances in the diagnosis and treatment of CF.[84] As genetic testing of CF is employed, the number of identified mutations has grown. Research continues into the correlation between genotype and clinical manifestations of lung disease.[21] As more states adopt newborn screening of CF, the identification of infants with the diagnosis allows earlier treatment.[19,20] Since the identification of the CF gene in 1989, research continues to play an important role in the development of new treatments available to patients with CF.[21] The trials and disappointments of gene therapy demonstrate that there are still many challenges to overcome.

With longer survival also comes an increased incidence of pulmonary complications of CF such as respiratory failure and hemoptysis and an increase in lung transplantation to treat end-stage disease.[23,24] Further research continues to search for optimal methods of managing this chronic disease to decrease the impact on disability and improve quality of life. Although the connection between the aforementioned structural changes and resulting functional limitations is apparent, the extent of the impact cannot be easily predicted.

Physical Therapy Interventions

The growing numbers of patients with CF surviving into adulthood depend on the expertise of the health care team to direct and support their treatment. The physical therapist plays an integral role on this team, with the ability to intervene in musculoskeletal, cardiovascular, and ventilatory impairments to improve the function of the patient. Although in the United States, we are historically more experienced in exercise interventions, we now have an increased variety of airway clearance techniques at our disposal. It has been demonstrated that many of the techniques are as effective as traditional postural drainage and percussion.[10,42] What is not proven, however, are the optimal strategies for patients at different stages of lifespan and disease. In addition, it is not known if there are certain patients who may in fact do well without any formal intervention, especially in light of the fact that there are now patients with the genetic diagnosis of CF, but without clinical signs and symptoms. We have yet to demonstrate that airway clearance prolongs life if done prophylactically, starting with infants.

Likewise with exercise interventions, we are challenged to discover which exercise training regimen is the most effective or appropriate for individual patients at different stages of their disease. For example, how long should we wait (if at all), before initiating exercise in a patient admitted to the hospital with an acute exacerbation, and what is the optimal balance between endurance and strength training in a patient with limited exercise tolerance, and finally, are there patients who will decompensate with exercise to the extent that it will prove harmful in the long term?

Finally, as the number of patients with CF increases because of augmented survival and new advances come to light in the treatment of CF, we are challenged to modify our PT interventions in order to optimize the benefits of these new therapies for our patients.

REFERENCES

1. Dean E, Hobson L. Cardiopulmonary anatomy. In: Frownfelter D, Dean E, eds. *Cardiovascular and Pulmonary Physical Therapy: Evidence and Practice.* 4th ed. St Louis, MO: Mosby–Elsevier; 2006.
2. West JB. *Respiratory Physiology—The Essentials.* 3rd ed. Baltimore, MD: Williams & Wilkins; 1985.
3. Cohen M, Michel TH. *Cardiopulmonary Symptoms in Physical Therpy Practice.* New York: Churchill Livingstone; 1988.
4. Mackin LA, Bullock BL. Altered pulmonary function. In: Bullock BA, Henze RL, eds. *Focus on Pathophysiology.* Philadelphia, PA: Lippincott–Raven Publishers; 2000.
5. Watchie J. *Cardiopulmonary Physical Therapy: A Clinical Manual.* Philadelphia, PA: WB Saunders; 1995.
6. Tucker DA. Normal and altered hepatobiliary and pancreatic exocrine function. In: Bullock BA, Henze RL, eds. *Pulmonary Rehabilitation: Focus on Physiology.* Philadelphia, PA: Lippincott–Raven Publishers; 2000.
7. Hillberg RE. Chronic obstructive pulmonary disease: causes and clinicopathologic considerations. In: Bach JR, ed. *Pulmonary Rehabilitation: The Obstructive and Paralytic Conditions.* Philadelphia, PA: Hanley & Belfus Inc; 1996.
8. Kigin CM. Chest physical therapy for the postoperative or traumatic injury patient. *Phys Ther.* 1981;61(12):1724-1736.
9. Dean E. Individuals with acute medical conditions. In: Frownfelter D, Dean E, eds. *Cardiovascular and Pulmonary Physical Therapy: Evidence and Practice.* 4th ed. St Louis, MO: Mosby–Elsevier; 2006.
10. Downs AM. Physiological basis for airway clearance techniques. In: Frownfelter D, Dean E, eds. *Cardiovascular and Pulmonary Physical Therapy: Evidence and Practice.* 4th ed. St Louis, MO: Mosby–Elsevier; 2006.
11. Mackin LA, Bullock BL. Normal pulmonary function. In: Bullock BA, Henze RL, eds. *Pulmonary Rehabilitation: Focus on Pathophysiology.* Philadelphia, PA: Lippincott–Raven Publishers; 2000.
12. Van der Schans CP. Bronchial mucus transport. *Respir Care.* 2007;52(9):1150-1156.
13. Rogers DF. Physiology of airway mucus secretion and pathophysiology of hypersecretion. *Respir Care.* 2007;52(9):1134-1146.
14. Massery M, Frownfelter D. Facilitating airway clearance with cough techniques. In: Frownfelter D, Dean E, eds. *Cardiovascular and Pulmonary Physical Therapy: Evidence and Practice.* 4th ed. St Louis, MO: Mosby–Elsevier; 2006.
15. Orenstein DM, Noyes BE. Cystic fibrosis. In: Casaburi R, Petty TL, eds. *Principles and Practice of Pulmonary Rehabilitation.* Philadelphia, PA: WB Saunders; 1993.
16. Cystic Fibrosis Foundation Patient Registry. *2007 Annual Data Report.* Bethesda, MD: Cystic Fibrosis Foundation; 2008.
17. Nixon PA. Cystic fibrosis. In: *ACSM's Exercise Management for Persons with Chronic Diseases and Disabilities.* 2nd ed: Champaign, IL: Human Kinetics; 2003.
18. Ratjen F. Update in cystic fibrosis. *Am J Respir Crit Care Med.* 2009;179:445-448.
19. Farrell PM, Lai HJ, Li Z, et al. Evidence on improved outcomes with early diagnosis of cystic fibrosis is through neonatal screening: enough is enough! *J Pediatr.* 2005;147(3 suppl):S30-S36.
20. Rock MJ. Newborn screening for cystic fibrosis. *Clin Chest Med.* 2007;28(2):297-305.

21. Knowles MR, Friedman KJ, Silverman LM. Genetics, diagnosis, and clinical phonotype. In: Yankaskas JR, Knowles MR, eds. *Cystic Fibrosis in Adults*. Philadelphia, PA: Lippincott–Raven Publishers; 1999:27-42.

22. Rosenstein BJ, Cutting GR. The diagnosis of cystic fibrosis: a consensus statement. *J Pediatr*. 1998;132:589-595.

23. Yankaskas JR, Marshall BC, Sufian B, et al. Cystic fibrosis adult care. *Chest*. 2004;125:1S-39S.

24. Stenbit A, Flume PA. Pulmonary complications in adult patients with cystic fibrosis. *Am J Med Sci*. 2008;335(1):55-59.

25. Yankaskas JR, Knowles MR, eds. *Cystic Fibrosis in Adults*. Philadelphia, PA: Lippincott–Raven Publishers; 1999.

26. Dean E, Frownfelter D. *Clinical Case Study Guide to Accompany Principles and Practice of Cardiopulmonary Physical Therapy*. 3rd ed. Philadelphia, PA: Mosby Year Book; 1996:144-151.

27. The Thoracic Society of Australia and New Zealand. *Physiotherapy for Cystic Fibrosis in Australia: A Consensus Statement*. Sydney, NSW: The Thoracic Society of Australia and New Zealand; 2007. http://www.thoracic.org.au/physiotherapyforcf.pdf. Accessed February 26, 2009.

28. Dodds ME, Langman H. Urinary incontinence and cystic fibrosis. *J R Soc Med*. 2005;98(suppl 45):28-36.

29. American Physical Therapy Association. *Interactive Guide to Physical Therapist Practice with Catalog of Tests and Measures, Version 1.0*. Alexandria, VA: American Physical Therapy Association; 2002.

30. Orenstein DM. *Cystic Fibrosis: A Guide for Patient and Family*. 3rd ed. Philadelphia, PA: Lippincott Williams & Wilkins; 2003.

31. Paradowski LJ, Egan TM. Lung transplantation for cystic fibrosis. In: Yankaskas JR, Knowles MR, eds. *Cystic Fibrosis in Adults*. Philadelphia, PA: Lippincott–Raven Publishers; 1999:195-219.

32. Robbins MK, Ontjes DA. Endocrine and renal disorders in cystic fibrosis. In: Yankaskas JR, Knowles MR, eds. *Cystic Fibrosis in Adults*. Philadelphia, PA: Lippincott–Raven Publishers; 1999: 383-418.

33. Davis PB. Clinical pathophysiology and manifestations of lung disease. In: Yankaskas JR, Knowles MR, eds. *Cystic Fibrosis in Adults*. Philadelphia, PA: Lippincott–Raven Publishers; 1999:145-173.

34. Noone PG, Knowles MR. Standard therapy of cystic fibrosis lung disease. In: Yankaskas JR, Knowles MR, eds. *Cystic Fibrosis in Adults*. Philadelphia, PA: Lippincott–Raven Publishers; 1999:145-173.

35. Elborn S. The management of young adults with cystic fibrosis: "genes, jeans and genies." *Disabil Rehabil*. 1998;20(6):217-225.

36. Konstan MW, Butler SM, Schidlow DV, et al. Patterns of medical practice in cystic fibrosis: part II. Use of therapies. *Pediatr Pulmonol*. 1999;28:248-254.

37. Ziegler B, Roveder PME, Lukrafka JL, et al. Submaximal exercise capacity in adolescent and adult patients with cystic fibrosis. *J Bras Pneumol*. 2007;33(3):263-269.

38. Nixon PA, Orenstein DM, Kelsey SF, et al. The prognostic value of exercise testing in patients with cystic fibrosis. *N Engl J Med*. 1992;327:1785-1788.

39. Selvadurai HC, Van Asperen PP, Mellis CM, et al. A comparison of fitness versus static lung function measurements as indicators of disease severity in children with cystic fibrosis [abstract]. *Pediatr Pulmonol*. 1998;26(S17):195.

40. de Meer K, Gulmans VAM, van der Laag J. Peripheral muscle weakness and exercise capacity in children with cystic fibrosis. *Am J Respir Crit Care Med*. 1999;159:748-754.

41. Massery M. Musculoskeletal and neuromuscular interventions: a physical approach to cystic fibrosis. *J R Soc Med*. 2005:98(suppl 45):55-66.

42. Downs AM. Clinical application of airway clearance techniques. In: Frownfelter D, Dean E, eds. *Cardiovascular and Pulmonary Physical Therapy: Evidence and Practice*. 4th ed. St Louis, MO: Mosby–Elsevier; 2006.

43. Hardy KA. A review of airway clearance: new techniques, indications, and recommendations. *Respir Care*. 1994;39(5):440-452.

44. Bishop-Lindsay KL, Lee GS. Rehabilitation for the pediatric patient with pulmonary disease. In: Hodgkin JE, Celli BR, Connors GL, eds. *Pulmonary Rehabilitation: Guidelines to Success*. 3rd ed. Philadelphia, PA: Lippincott Williams & Wilkins; 2000.

45. Dean E. Mobilization and exercise. In: Frownfelter D, Dean E, eds. *Cardiovascular and Pulmonary Physical Therapy: Evidence and Practice*. 4th ed. St Louis, MO: Mosby–Elsevier; 2006.

46. Resnick B, Henze R. Normal and altered functions of the musculoskeletal system. In: Bullock BA, Henze RL, eds. *Pulmonary Rehabilitation: Focus on Pathophysiology*. Philadelphia, PA: Lippincott–Raven Publishers; 2000.

47. Scherer S. The transplant patient. In: Frownfelter D, Dean E, eds. *Cardiovascular and Pulmonary Physical Therapy: Evidence and Practice*. 4th ed. St Louis, MO: Mosby–Elsevier; 2006.

48. Warren A. Mobilization of the chest wall. *Phys Ther*. 1968; 48(6):582-585.

49. Watts N. Improvement of breathing patterns. *Phys Ther*. 1968;48(6):563-576.

50. Dail CW. Respiratory aspects of rehabilitation in neuromuscular conditions. *Arch Phys Med Rehabil*. 1965;46(10):655-675.

51. Bishop KL. Pulmonary rehabilitation in the intensive care unit. In: Fishman AP, ed. *Pulmonary Rehabilitation*. New York: Marcel Dekker Inc; 1996:525–738.

52. Dean E, Frownfelter D. Individuals with chronic primary cardiopulmonary dysfunction, individuals with chronic secondary cardiopulmonary dysfunction. In: Frownfelter D, Dean E, eds. *Cardiovascular and Pulmonary Physical Therapy: Evidence and Practice*. 4th ed. St Louis, MO: Mosby–Elsevier; 2006.

53. Knott M, Voss DE. *Proprioceptive Neuromuscular Facilitation: Patterns and Techniques*. 2nd ed. Philadelphia, PA: Harper & Row Publishers; 1968.

54. *Advanced Respiratory Contract Trainer's Manual*. St Paul, MN: Advanced Respiratory, formerly American Biosystems Inc; 2001.

55. Anderson CA, Palmer CA, Ney AL, et al. Evaluation of the safety of high-frequency chest wall oscillation (HFCWO) therapy in blunt thoracic trauma patients. *J Trauma Manag Outcomes*. 2008;2:8.

56. Brierley S, Adams C, Suelter J, et al. Safety and tolerance of high-frequency chest wall oscillation (HFCWO) in hospitalized critical care patients. *Respir Care*. 2003;48(11):1112.

57. Mcllwaine M. *Physiotherapy in the Treatment of Cystic Fibrosis (CF)*. 4th ed. Canada: International Physiotherapy Group for Cystic Fibrosis (IPG/CF); 2009.

58. Phillips GE, Pike SE, Jaffe A, et al. Comparison of active cycle of breathing and high-frequency oscillation jacket in children with cystic fibrosis. *Pediatr Pulmonol*. 2004;37:71-75.

59. Fink JB. Forced expiratory technique, directed cough, and autogenic drainage. *Respir Care*. 2007;52(9):1210-1221.

60. Thomas J, Cook DJ, Brooks D. Chest physical therapy management of patients with cystic fibrosis. A meta-analysis. *Am J Respir Crit Care Med*. 1995;151(3, pt 1):846-850.

61. Miller S, Hall DO, Calyton CB, et al. Chest physiotherapy in cystic fibrosis: a comparative study of autogenic drainage and the active cycle of breathing techniques with postural drainage. *Thorax.* 1995;50:165-169.

62. Frownfelter D, Massery M. Facilitating ventilation patterns and breathing strategies. In: Frownfelter D, Dean E, eds. *Cardiovascular and Pulmonary Physical Therapy: Evidence and Practice.* 4th ed. St Louis, MO: Mosby–Elsevier; 2006.

63. Crouch R, Ryan K. Physical therapy and respiratory care: integration as a team in pulmonary rehabilitation. In: Hodgkin JE, Celli BR, Connors GL, eds. *Pulmonary Rehabilitation: Guidelines to Success.* 3rd ed. Philadelphia, PA: Lippincott Williams & Wilkins; 2000.

64. Murray JF. The ketchup-bottle method. *N Engl J Med.* 1979;300(20):1155-1157.

65. Konstan MW, Stern RC, Doershuk CF. Efficacy of the flutter device for airway mucus clearance in patients with cystic fibrosis. *J Pediatr.* 1994;124(5, pt 1):689-693.

66. Langenderfer B. Alternatives to percussion and postural drainage. A review of mucus clearance therapies: percussion and postural drainage, autogenic drainage, positive expiratory pressure, flutter valve, intrapulmonary percussive ventilation, and high-frequency chest compression with the ThAIRapy Vest. *J Cardiopulm Rehabil.* 1998;18(4):283-289.

67. Newhouse PA, White F, Marks JH, et al. The intrapulmonary percussive ventilator and flutter device compared to standard chest physiotherapy in patients with cystic fibrosis. *Clin Pediatr.* 1998;37:427-432.

68. Marks JH. Airway clearance devices in cystic fibrosis. *Paediatr Respir Rev.* 2007;8:17-23.

69. Darbee JC, Kanga JF, Ohtake PJ. Physiologic evidence for high-frequency chest wall oscillation and positive expiratory pressure breathing in hospitalized subjects with cystic fibrosis. *Phys Ther.* 2005;85(12):1278-1289.

70. Myers TR. Positive expiratory pressure and oscillatory positive expiratory pressure therapies. *Respir Care.* 2007;52(10):1308-1326.

71. Chatburn RL. High-frequency assisted airway clearance. *Respir Care.* 2007;52(9):1224-1235.

72. Scherer TA, Barandun J, Martinez E, Wanner A, Rubin EM. Effect of high-frequency oral airway and chest wall oscillation and conventional chest physical therapy on expectoration in patients with stable cystic fibrosis. *Chest.* 1998;113:1019-1027.

73. Dymedso, Inc. The Frequencer: Overview. http://www.dymedso.com/study.html. Accessed March 21, 2009.

74. Cantin AM, Bacon M, Berthiaume Y. Mechanical airway clearance using the frequencer electro-acoustical transducer in cystic fibrosis. *Clin Invest Med.* 2006;29(3):159-165.

75. Lannefors L, Wollmer P. Mucus clearance with three chest physiotherapy regimes in cystic fibrosis: a comparison between postural drainage, PEP and physical exercise. *Eur Respir J.* 1992;5:748-753.

76. Cahalin LP. Applying the cardiopulmonary practice patterns: heart failure. *Cardiopulm Phys Ther.* 1999;10(3):90-97.

77. Gordon J, Quinn L. Guide to physical therapy practice: a critical appraisal. *Neurol Rep.* 1999;23(3):122-128.

78. World Health Organization. *International Classification of Functioning, Disability, and Health (ICF).* Geneva, Switzerland: World Health Organization. http://www.who.int/classifications/icf/en/. Accessed March 31, 2009.

79. Jette AM. Toward a common language for function, disability, and health. *Phys Ther.* 2006:86:726-734.

80. Stucki G. International Classification of Functioning, Disability, and Health (ICF): a promising framework and classification for rehabilitation medicine. *Am J Phys Med Rehabil.* 2005;84: 733-740.

81. Perenboom RJM, Chorus AMJ. Measuring participation according to the International Classification of Functioning, Disability and Health (ICF). *Disabil Rehabil.* 2003;25(11-12):577-587.

82. Cieza A, Stucki G. Content comparison of health-related quality of life (HRQOL) instruments based on the International Classification of Functioning, Disability and Health (ICF). *Qual Life Res.* 2005;14:1225-1237.

83. Lands LC, Coates, AL. Cardiopulmonary and skeletal muscle function and their effects on exercise limitation. In: Yankaskas JR, Knowles MR, eds. *Cystic Fibrosis in Adults.* Philadelphia, PA: Lippincott–Raven Publishers; 1999:365-382.

84. Johnson LG, Knowles MR. New therapeutic strategies for cystic fibrosis lung disease. In: Yankaskas JR, Knowles MR, eds. *Cystic Fibrosis in Adults.* Philadelphia, PA: Lippincott–Raven Publishers; 1999:233-258.

Physical Therapy Associated with Cardiovascular Pump Dysfunction and Failure

Lawrence P. Cahalin & Lori A. Buck*

INTRODUCTION

Practice Pattern D represents a progression in heart disease beginning with cardiac pump dysfunction, which eventually may progress to cardiac pump failure. It is critically important that a physical therapist be able to distinguish between a person with cardiac pump dysfunction and a person with cardiac pump failure. The inclusion/exclusion criteria of Practice Pattern D list two specific pathologies that may distinguish between cardiac pump dysfunction from cardiac pump failure (ejection fraction <30% and exercise-induced myocardial ischemia) and two specific impairments that may distinguish between cardiac pump dysfunction from cardiac pump failure (hypoadaptive blood pressure response to exercise and achieved MET level during exercise testing).[1] These distinguishing characteristics are listed in Box 18-1.

Although these tests and measures are available from the patient's medical history, they may, in fact, be history and not represent current cardiac performance. Similarly, the only aforementioned test providing specific information to distinguish cardiac pump dysfunction from failure is the ejection fraction. Another simple measurement that can be performed by a physical therapist that may provide important information to distinguish cardiac pump dysfunction from failure is observing the blood pressure response during a controlled expiratory maneuver.[2-10] This simple test can provide important information about the disablement of heart disease and can provide a basis upon which the physical therapist can determine necessary outcomes, subsequent examinations, and specific treatment methods. The most relevant characteristics of cardiac pump dysfunction and cardiac pump failure will be presented in the following sections beginning with the microanatomy and physiology of both the dysfunctional and the failing cardiac pump, which will be followed by a brief review of the effects of cardiac pump dysfunction and failure on the pulmonary system and skeletal muscles.

MICROANATOMY AND PHYSIOLOGY

Cardiac Pump Dysfunction

The microanatomy and physiology of cardiac pump dysfunction are similar to cardiac pump failure. However, the pathological microanatomy and physiology are less extreme in cardiac pump dysfunction.[11] The primary characteristic of cardiac pump dysfunction is cardiac muscle dysfunction which produces a slight to modest cardiac impairment represented by slight to modest reductions in stroke volume, cardiac output, and ejection fraction.[11] These impairments often produce limitations in functional abilities which lead to some level of disability (Fig. 18-1). Functional abilities and disability are less marked in cardiac pump dysfunction compared to the significant reductions in function and greater levels of disability in cardiac pump failure.[11-15] In cardiac pump failure, the cardiac muscle fails to contract or relax adequately and results in marked reductions in stroke volume, cardiac output, and ejection fraction.[16,17]

The effects of cardiac muscle dysfunction or failure on the aforementioned areas of disablement are essentially due to changes in microanatomy and physiology from cardiac muscle damage or specific pathological processes which impair cardiac muscle performance. The specific pathological processes are listed in Box 18-2. Cardiac muscle damage from myocardial infarction is the most common cause of cardiac muscle dysfunction.[18] The predominant factors contributing to cardiac muscle dysfunction include myocardial cell death, myocardial scar formation, and subsequent physiologic changes associated with myocardial cell death such as impaired cardiac action potential propagation or cardiac arrhythmias which cause alterations in action potential movement in and around damaged myocardial cells[18] (see Chapter 6, Fig. 6-5).

BOX 18-1

Patients/Clients Diagnostic Group Characteristics for Practice Pattern D

Practice Pattern D: *Impaired Aerobic Capacity and Endurance Associated with Cardiovascular Pump* **Dysfunction**/*Failure*
Patients/clients who have impaired aerobic capacity associated with cardiovascular pump **dysfunction** and who may have one or a combination of the following:

Abnormal heart rate response to increased oxygen demand
Decreased ejection fraction (30%–50%)
Exercise-induced myocardial ischemia (1–2 mm ST-segment depression)
Functional capacity of less than or equal to 5–6 METS
Hypertensive blood pressure response to increased oxygen demand
Nonmalignant arrhythmias
Symptomatic response to increased oxygen demand
Angioplasty or atherectomy
Cardiomyopathy
Coronary artery bypass grafting
Coronary artery disease
Hypertensive heart disease
Uncomplicated myocardial infarction
Valvular heart disease
Excludes patients/clients with:
  Age <4 months
  Airway clearance impairment
  Mechanical ventilation
  Heart failure

Practice Pattern D: *Impaired Aerobic Capacity and Endurance Associated with Cardiovascular Pump Dysfunction/***Failure**
Patients/clients who have impaired aerobic capacity associated with cardiovascular pump **failure** and who may have one or a combination of the following:

Abnormal heart rate response to increased oxygen demand
Ejection fraction of less than 30%
Severe exercise-induced myocardial ischemia (>2 mm ST-segment depression)
Functional capacity of less than or equal to 4–5 METs
Flat or falling blood pressure response to increased oxygen demand
Complex ventricular arrhythmias
Symptomatic response to increased oxygen demand
Atrioventricular block
Cardiogenic shock
Cardiomyopathy
Complicated myocardial infarction

Age <4 months
Mechanical ventilation
Membrane oxygenator
Intra-aortic balloon pump
Ventricular assist device

Modified with permission from American Physical Therapy Association. Guide to Physical Therapist Practice. 2nd ed. *Phys Ther.* 2001 Jan;81(1):9-746.

Myocardial Cell Death

Myocardial cell death is initially characterized by interstitial edema, fatty deposits in muscle fibers, and infiltration of neutrophils and red blood cells. Over the 4 to 6 weeks following infarction, macrophages remove the necrotic muscle fibers until a scar has formed.[18]

Myocardial Scar Formation

Myocardial scar formation is characterized by a thin layer of connective tissue interspersed with muscle cells. Over time the scar gets stronger, initially in the periphery, and later progressing to its center.[18]

Pathophysiology of Myocardial Cell Death, Scar Formation, and Myocardial Dysfunction

The pathophysiology of myocardial cell death is associated with the aforementioned changes in myocardial cells and the resultant dysfunction as well as the consequences of cardiac muscle dysfunction.[18] The consequences of dysfunctional cardiac muscle include the aforementioned impairments of stroke volume, cardiac output, and ejection fraction as well as elevated pressures

within the cardiac chambers, pulmonary artery, and throughout the peripheral and pulmonary vasculature.[18] Elevation of the pressure in the pulmonary vasculature past 25 mm Hg often leads to pulmonary congestion, the hallmark of congestive heart failure and cardiac pump failure.[16,17] The pathophysiological consequences of cardiac pump failure are described in Table 18-1 and will be discussed further in the following section.

Cardiac Pump Failure

Cardiac failure is often described and defined as a syndrome of signs and symptoms due to the heart's inability to provide an adequate amount of blood flow to sustain normal organ and physiologic system function.[16,17] The signs and symptoms of cardiac failure are listed in Box 18-3; the two most common symptoms are dyspnea and fatigue. The dyspnea and fatigue resulting from cardiac failure are due to the inadequate delivery of blood to the lungs, organs, and periphery as well as to the accumulation of blood in the chambers of the heart. The accumulation of blood in the chambers of the heart increases the pressures within the cardiovascular system both centrally and peripherally. The increase in peripheral arterial pressure

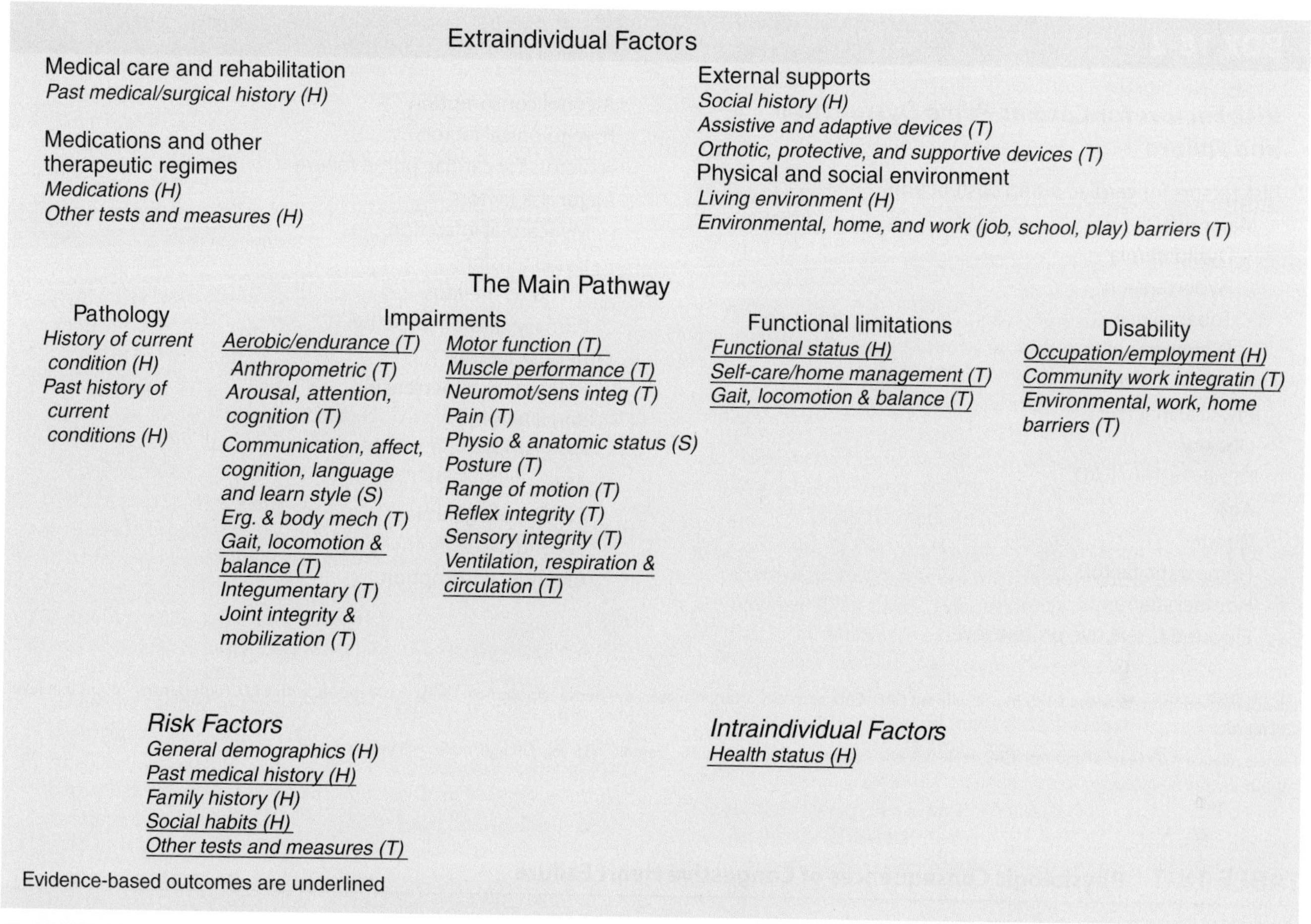

Extraindividual Factors

Medical care and rehabilitation
Past medical/surgical history (H)

Medications and other therapeutic regimes
Medications (H)
Other tests and measures (H)

External supports
Social history (H)
Assistive and adaptive devices (T)
Orthotic, protective, and supportive devices (T)
Physical and social environment
Living environment (H)
Environmental, home, and work (job, school, play) barriers (T)

The Main Pathway

Pathology
History of current condition (H)
Past history of current conditions (H)

Impairments
Aerobic/endurance (T)
Anthropometric (T)
Arousal, attention, cognition (T)
Communication, affect, cognition, language and learn style (S)
Erg. & body mech (T)
Gait, locomotion & balance (T)
Integumentary (T)
Joint integrity & mobilization (T)

Motor function (T)
Muscle performance (T)
Neuromot/sens integ (T)
Pain (T)
Physio & anatomic status (S)
Posture (T)
Range of motion (T)
Reflex integrity (T)
Sensory integrity (T)
Ventilation, respiration & circulation (T)

Functional limitations
Functional status (H)
Self-care/home management (T)
Gait, locomotion & balance (T)

Disability
Occupation/employment (H)
Community work integratin (T)
Environmental, work, home barriers (T)

Risk Factors
General demographics (H)
Past medical history (H)
Family history (H)
Social habits (H)
Other tests and measures (T)

Intraindividual Factors
Health status (H)

Evidence-based outcomes are underlined

FIGURE 18-1 The Nagi Disablement Model applied to the examination component of Practice Pattern D. Items from the *Guide* are listed underneath the major headings of the Disablement Model. Sections within the examination component of the *Guide* that each item is categorized are indicated in parentheses: H, History; S, Systems Review; T, Tests and Measures. Evidence-based outcomes are underlined. (Adapted with permission from Gordon J, Quinn L. Guide to Physical Therapist Practice: a critical appraisal. *Neurol Rep.* 1999;23(3):122-128.)

(eg, due to increases in the peripheral vascular resistance) further decreases cardiac performance because the blood ejected from the heart must overcome the increased peripheral vascular resistance. Ejecting blood from a failing left ventricle against increased resistance in the peripheral vasculature is difficult because the failing cardiac pump must contract with greater force. Frequently, the failing cardiac pump has no capacity to generate a greater force of contraction, and heart failure worsens.[16,17]

Centrally, the accumulation of blood in the chambers of the heart elevates the systolic and diastolic pressures within the (1) chambers of the heart and (2) vasculature within the thorax such as the pulmonary artery and veins, superior and inferior vena cava, and the jugular veins. This increase in pressure within the pulmonary vasculature often produces pulmonary edema.[16,17] The pressure within the pulmonary vasculature at which pulmonary edema begins is approximately 25 mm Hg. The aforementioned increase in pressure in the pulmonary vasculature, chambers of the heart, and peripheral vasculature leads to worsening cardiac performance, cardiac failure, and signs and symptoms of cardiac failure.[16,17] Therefore, treatment of cardiac failure is often

directed toward decreasing the elevated pressures in the aforementioned areas (eg, to unload the heart) and improving the pathophysiological events associated with heart failure. The pathophysiological processes at a microanatomical level will be presented in the following section.

Microanatomy and Pathophysiological Processes of Cardiac Failure

The microanatomical processes associated with cardiac failure are due to apoptosis. Apoptosis is the programmed death of cells, which is often extreme in persons with heart failure. Although heart failure may be due to a variety of causes, apoptosis appears to occur at a greater rate in all persons with heart failure despite the etiology of the heart failure. This suggests that a specific genetic predisposition which aggressively "turns on" myocardial cell death may be present in persons with heart failure.[19]

The causes of apoptosis are thought to be due to either genetic predisposition from birth (eg, some types of cardiomyopathy) or genetic reprogramming/mutation from specific types of heart disease including hypertension, coronary artery disease, or chronic valvular heart disease.[20]

BOX 18-2

Risk Factors for Cardiac Pump Dysfunction and Failure

Risk factors for cardiac pump dysfunction
- Major risk factors
    - Dyslipidemia*
    - Hypertension
    - Tobacco use
    - Diabetes mellitus
- Other risk factors
    - Physical inactivity
    - Obesity
    - Family history CAD[†]
    - Age[‡]
    - Gender[‡]
    - Hemostatic factors
    - Homocysteinemia
    - Elevated C-reactive protein levels

Alcohol consumption
Psychological factors
Risk factors for cardiac pump failure
- Major risk factors
    - Myocardial infarction
    - Hypertension
    - Diabetes mellitus
    - Primary cardiomyopathy
- Other risk factors
    - Pulmonary hypertension
    - Renal failure
    - Myocarditis
    - Age
    - Cardiac arrhythmias
    - Secondary cardiomyopathy
    - Alcohol consumption

*Low-density lipoprotein levels ≥130 mg/dL without CAD. CAD, coronary artery disease. Low-density lipoprotein levels >100 mg/dL with CAD. High-density lipoprotein levels <35 mg/dL.

[†]Female relative <65 years of age with CAD; male relative <55 years of age with CAD. [‡]Female >55 years of age; male >45 years of age.

TABLE 18-1　Physiologic Consequences of Congestive Heart Failure

Pathology	Effects
Cardiovascular	Decreased myocardial performance, with subsequent peripheral vascular constriction to increase venous return (attempting to increase stroke volume and cardiac output) ⇓
Pulmonary	Pulmonary edema because of elevated cardiac filling pressures due to poor cardiac performance and fluid overload ⇓
Renal	Water retention because of decreased cardiac output ⇓
Neurohumoral	Increased sympathetic stimulation that eventually desensitizes the heart to β_1-adrenergic receptor stimulation, thus decreasing the heart's inotropic effect ⇓
Musculoskeletal	Skeletal muscle wasting and possible skeletal muscle myopathies as well as osteoporosis from inactivity or other accompanying diseases ⇓
Hematologic	Possible polycythemia, anemia, and hemostatic abnormalities because of a reduction in oxygen transport, accompanying liver disease, or stagnant blood flow in the heart's chambers because of poor cardiac contraction ⇓
Hepatic	Possible cardiac cirrhosis from hypoperfusion due to an inadequate cardiac output or hepatic venous congestion ⇓
Pancreatic	Possible impaired insulin secretion and glucose tolerance as well as the source of a possible myocardial depressant factor ⇓
Nutritional/biochemical	Anorexia that leads to malnutrition (protein-calorie and vitamin deficiencies) and cachexia

Adapted with permission from Cahalin LP. Cardiac muscle dysfunction. In: Hillegas and Sadowsky, eds. *Essentials of Cardiopulmonary Physical Therapy*. Philadelphia, PA: WB Saunders; 1995.

BOX 18-3

Clinical Manifestations of Congestive Heart Failure

1. Dyspnea and fatigue
2. Tachypnea
3. Paroxysmal nocturnal dyspnea
4. Orthopnea
5. Peripheral edema
6. Cold, pale, and possibly cyanotic extremities
7. Weight gain
8. Hepatomegaly
9. Jugular venous distention
10. Crackles (rales)
11. Tubular breath sounds and consolidation
12. Presence of a third heart sound (S_3)
13. Sinus tachycardia
14. Decreased peripheral skeletal muscle strength and endurance
15. Decreased ventilatory muscle strength and endurance
16. Decreased exercise tolerance or physical work capacity
17. Functional limitations (eg, limited walking, stair climbing)
18. Disabilities (eg, difficulty doing things with family or friends and being a burden to family or friends)

BOX 18-4

The Three Stages of Pulmonary Edema

Stage 1 Difficult to detect: because of increased lymph flow without significant interstitial liquid in vessels and airways.

Stage 2 Detectable via auscultation of the lungs that will produce crackles (rales) and an absence of air movement in the lungs (no breath sounds due to consolidation): because of increased lymph flow with increased liquid in vessels and airways with potential for $\dot{V}/\dot{Q}$ mismatch.

Stage 3 Detectable via auscultation of the lungs that will produce greater crackles (rales) and a greater absence of air movement in the lungs (no breath sounds due to consolidation): because of increased lymph flow with increased liquid in vessels and airways with greater potential for $\dot{V}/\dot{Q}$ mismatch. As lymph flow increases, alveoli become flooded with potential for (1) filling of the large airways with blood-tinged foam, which can be expectorated; (2) reductions in most lung volumes (eg, vital capacity); (3) a right-to-left intrapulmonary shunt; and (4) hypercapnia with acute respiratory acidosis.

Apoptosis from either genetic predisposition or genetic reprogramming/mutation from heart disease will frequently produce a cardiomyopathy. Cardiomyopathy is a disease in which the contraction, relaxation, or both the contraction and the relaxation of myocardial muscle fibers are impaired. These are described in detail in Chapter 6.[21]

Pulmonary Function in Cardiac Pump Dysfunction and Failure

One of the hallmark signs of heart failure is pulmonary edema, and it is therefore the reason the word "congestive" is often added to heart failure.[16] The following review of the pulmonary pathophysiology associated with congestive heart failure (CHF) assists in the understanding of pulmonary edema and particular aspects of the examination of persons with CHF such as the presence of inspiratory rales, tachypnea, and dyspnea.

Pulmonary edema can be cardiogenic (hemodynamic) or noncardiogenic (caused by alterations in the pulmonary capillary membrane) in origin.[22] The differential diagnosis can be made by history, physical examination, and laboratory examination, as shown in Box 18-4. Despite the different origins of pulmonary edema, the "sequence of liquid accumulation" is similar for both and appears to consist of three distinct stages that are also described in Box 18-4.[22]

Perhaps the most important principle in treating pulmonary edema is that of "maintaining pulmonary capillary

pressures at the lowest possible levels," because it has been demonstrated that pulmonary edema can be decreased by more than 50% when pulmonary capillary wedge pressures are decreased from 12 to 6 mm Hg.[22]

The effect of repeated bouts of pulmonary edema (which is common in CHF) upon pulmonary function appears to be profound. In fact, it is believed that more advanced CHF may produce a "global respiratory impairment" that is associated with varying degrees of obstructive and restrictive lung disease.[23,24] In fact, several measures of pulmonary function have recently been found to be significantly related to the level of dyspnea of persons with advanced CHF (Table 18-2).[25]

Neurohumoral Consequences of Cardiac Pump Dysfunction and Failure

The neurohumoral system profoundly affects heart function in physiologic (eg, fight-or-flight mechanism) and pathologic states such as cardiac pump failure. In general, the neural effects are much more rapid, whereas humoral effects are slower. This is because the information sent by the autonomic nervous system via efferent nerves travels faster than the information traveling through the vascular system.[26]

Neurohumoral signals to the heart are perceived, interpreted, and augmented by the transmembrane signal transduction systems in myocardial cells. The primary signaling system in the heart appears to be the receptor-G protein-adenylate

TABLE 18-2   Relationship Between Pulmonary Function and Symptoms in CHF[a]

Dyspnea Variable	FEV$_1$ (%)	FVC (%)	FVC (L)	TLC (L)
Pre-IMT dyspnea at rest (N = 14)	−0.60	−0.59	—	—
Pre-IMT dyspnea during exercise (N = 14)	−0.57	−0.67	—	—
Post-IMT dyspnea at rest (N = 8)	—	—	−0.77	−0.82

Values are Pearson product–moment correlation coefficients between dyspnea and measurements of pulmonary function.

[a]FEV$_1$, forced expiratory volume in 1 second; FVC, forced vital capacity; IMT, inspiratory muscle trainer; TLC, total lung capacity.

cyclase (RGC) complex as it regulates myocardial contractility. Figure 18-2 illustrates the complexity of this system, which consists of (1) membrane receptors; (2) guanine nucleotide-binding regulatory proteins (the G proteins, which transmit stimulatory or inhibitory signals); and (3) adenylate cyclase, which converts adenosine triphosphate (ATP) to cyclic adenosine monophosphate (cAMP). Adenylate cyclase is an effector enzyme activated by a receptor agonist, thus enhancing cAMP synthesis. The lower portion of Figure 18-2 shows that increased cAMP synthesis ultimately increases the force of myocardial contraction (the inotropic effect).[26]

The top portion of Fig. 18-2 shows the receptor agonists responsible for the initial activation of the "receptor-G protein-adenylate cyclase complex." They include norepinephrine, epinephrine, histamine, vasoactive intestinal peptide, adenosine, and acetylcholine.

Figure 18-2 does not reveal the degree of influence each receptor agonist has on cardiac function. In general, the most influential receptor agonists are the sympathetic neurotransmitters norepinephrine and epinephrine, as they relay excitatory autonomic nervous system stimuli to both postsynaptic α- and β-adrenergic receptors in the myocardium. Inhibitory autonomic nervous system stimuli are transmitted by the parasympathetic nervous system via the vagus nerve and the neurotransmitter acetylcholine.[26]

β$_2$-receptor stimulation promotes vasodilation of the capillary beds and muscle relaxation in the bronchial tracts, whereas β$_1$-adrenergic receptor stimulation increases heart rate and myocardial force of contraction.[26] The stimulation of α$_1$-adrenergic receptors appears to activate the phosphoinositide transmembrane signaling system,[27,28] which increases phosphodiesterase and activates protein kinase, thus marginally increasing the inotropic effect.[29] Conversely, stimulation of α$_2$-adrenergic receptors activates the G-inhibitory protein and inhibits adenylate cyclase, which decreases the inotropic effect.[30]

The activation of adenylate cyclase (and subsequent increase in myocardial force of contraction) is, unfortunately, poorly understood but has been observed to be decreased in

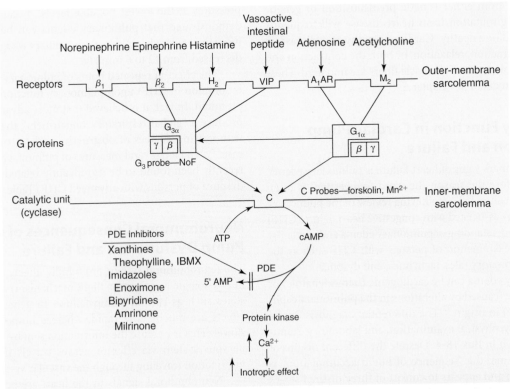

FIGURE 18-2   Neurohumoral system in CHF. The receptor G protein-adenylate cyclase complex and other important receptors, all of which affect the inotropic state of the heart. G$_s$, G-stimulatory protein; G$_1$, G-inhibitory protein; PDE, phosphodiesterase; IBMX, isobutylmethylxanthine; ATP, adenosine triphosphate; cAMP, cyclic adenosine monophosphate. (Adapted with permission from Cahalin LP. Cardiac muscle dysfunction. In: Hillegass EA, Sadowsky HS, eds. *Essentials of Cardiopulmonary Physical Therapy*. 2nd ed. Philadelphia, PA: WB Saunders; 2001:139.)

patients with CHF. This is the result of "a paradoxical diminution in the function of the RGC complex,"[26] which alters the receptor–effector coupling and "limits the ability of both endogenous and exogenous adrenergic agonists to augment cardiac contractility." The inability of endogenous (produced in the body) or exogenous (medications) adrenergic agonists to increase the force of myocardial contraction is frequently seen in patients with CHF.[26–32]

The abnormal RGC complex function in CHF appears to be associated with the insensitivity of the failing heart to β-adrenergic stimulation. This insensitivity to β-adrenergic stimulation is apparently the result of a decrease in $β_1$-adrenergic receptor density and is very important because the heart contains a ratio of 3.3 to 1.0 $β_1$- to $β_2$-adrenergic receptors.[26] In CHF, the ratio decreases to approximately 1.5 to 1.0, producing a 62% decrease in the $β_1$-adrenergic receptors. This marked decrease in $β_1$-adrenergic receptors decreases the ability of the heart to respond to increased β-adrenergic stimulation and results in a less than optimal increase in heart rate and myocardial force of contraction.[26]

Skeletal Muscle in Cardiac Pump Dysfunction and Failure

No specific skeletal muscle abnormalities have been observed in patients with cardiac pump dysfunction. However, inactivity due to coronary artery disease or inactivity alone is associated with skeletal muscle weakness, decreased endurance, and atrophy.[33]

The skeletal muscle of persons with heart failure appears to be markedly impaired in the areas of strength, endurance, mitochondrial function, and energy production.[34–45] These impairments of skeletal muscle have been hypothesized to be due to marked neurohumoral activation associated with heart failure, deconditioning associated with heart failure, or the presence of a myopathic process that is not limited to only cardiac muscle, but to all muscles. Studies of patients with CHF with and without cardiomyopathy have identified several important characteristics of skeletal muscles in CHF.

Skeletal Muscle Activity in CHF Without Cardiomyopathy

Results of a study by Shafiq et al. revealed no abnormalities in the skeletal muscles of normal subjects. In patients with CHF but without cardiomyopathy there was a decrease in the average diameters of the type I and type II fibers and in the patients with CHF and cardiomyopathy three distinct skeletal muscle abnormalities were observed including selective atrophy of type II fibers, pronounced nonselective myopathy and hypotrophy of type I fibers.[34]

Lipkin et al. studied nine patients with CHF of whom three had a dilated cardiomyopathy, five had coronary artery disease, and one had a previous aortic valve surgery for aortic regurgitation. The results of the study by Lipkin et al. revealed low maximal oxygen consumption (11.7 mL/kg/min) and isometric maximal voluntary contraction of the quadriceps (only 55% of the predicted value for weight), increased intracellular

acid phosphatase activity in six subjects, increased intracellular lipid accumulation in four subjects, and atrophy of type I and type II muscle fibers in four subjects.[35] In conclusion, the previous results and the results of a nuclear magnetic resonance spectroscopy study have shown that skeletal muscle fatigue in patients with CHF is associated with intracellular acidosis and phosphocreatinine depletion,[36] which if prolonged may predispose to myopathic processes.

CLINICAL CORRELATE

In view of this, physical therapists should utilize appropriate modes of exercise and exercise prescriptions that minimize intracellular acidosis and phosphocreatinine depletion. This can often be accomplished by beginning with low-level exercise and gradually progressing to higher levels of exercise based on objective signs and symptoms. Activation of the short-term energy system (glycolysis) should be minimized, and exercises utilizing the long-term aerobic energy system (citric acid cycle) will decrease the likelihood of this phenomenon (see Chapter 3).

Skeletal Muscle Activity in CHF with Cardiomyopathy

Skeletal muscle activity is apparently impaired by chronic CHF as well as cardiomyopathy. Skeletal muscle abnormalities due to dilated[37–39] and hypertrophic[40–44] cardiomyopathies have previously been reported and have consistently revealed type I and type II fiber atrophy.[37–44]

Caforio et al. studied 11 patients with dilated cardiomyopathy and eight patients with hypertrophic cardiomyopathy via neuromuscular and electromyographic analysis of the right biceps brachii muscle during a maximal voluntary contraction.[45] Six of the 19 patients underwent muscle biopsy of the right biceps brachii, and three underwent biopsy of the deltoid muscle with light and electron microscopy analysis.

Results of the neuromuscular assessment were relatively insignificant, except that (1) all symptomatic patients with dilated and one with hypertrophic cardiomyopathy demonstrated a slight hyposthenia in the girdles or proximal limbs, and (2) none of the patients had muscular hypotrophy. Electromyography revealed abnormalities typical of myogenic myopathy in nine patients (five dilated and four hypertrophic), but none showed signs of neurogenic alteration (ie, a reduction of nerve conduction velocities or increase in single motor unit potential duration).[45]

Muscle biopsies consistently detected pathologic changes (primarily mitochondrial abnormalities) in the type I (slow twitch) fibers in all nine patients from whom a biopsy was obtained, eight of which demonstrated increases of atrophy factors. No alteration of type II fibers was observed in any patient.[45]

Although echocardiographic and hemodynamic indices of ventricular function were similar in patients with and without EMG abnormalities, patients in functional class III were slightly, but not statistically, more likely to have EMG abnormalities.[45]

Caforio et al. believe the findings from this study support the hypothesis that skeletal myopathic changes, which are occasionally observed in patients with cardiomyopathy, are of a primary rather than a secondary nature.[45] It is likely that both chronic CHF and cardiomyopathy have profound effects on skeletal muscle activity that have been observed to reduce isometric muscle strength by nearly 50%. This reduction may be due to specific changes in skeletal muscle metabolism that produce fatigue at lower absolute workloads, hence limiting maximal exercise capacity in patients with chronic CHF.[35] The physical therapist must therefore examine and address many characteristics of the skeletal muscles of persons with CHF and determine how the pathologies and impairments of skeletal muscles impact upon functional abilities and disabilities.

CASE STUDY: A GUIDE AND EVIDENCE-BASED EXAMPLE

Inclusion and Exclusion Criteria for Practice Pattern D

Practice Pattern D describes the generally accepted elements of the management that physical therapists provide to patients who have impaired aerobic capacity associated with cardiovascular pump dysfunction or failure.[1] The specific characteristics of the patient/client diagnostic groups for each of the two subgroups of Practice Pattern D are listed in Box 18-1. The inclusion and exclusion criteria for each of the two subgroups in Practice Pattern D are also presented in Box 18-1.

The case chosen to illustrate the physical therapy management of a patient fitting the diagnostic classification of Practice Pattern D is George, a 41-year-old man who suffered a small uncomplicated myocardial infarction (MI) in 1995 at the age of 35 years. He subsequently underwent coronary artery bypass grafting (CABG) 2 months later for recurrent angina. He fit the broad diagnostic classification for Practice Pattern D, *Impaired Aerobic Capacity/Endurance Associated with Cardiovascular Pump Dysfunction or Failure*. More specifically, his examination findings of having suffered a small uncomplicated MI, having an ejection fraction (EF) of 50%, and having a mild impairment in aerobic capacity of six metabolic equivalents (METs) are common to patients/clients with cardiovascular pump dysfunction. Six years later, George suffered a second massive anterior wall myocardial infarction complicated by congestive heart failure. The progression of his disease resulted in severe impairments, functional limitations, and disabilities consistent with cardiovascular pump failure. He had an abnormal heart rate response to increased oxygen demand, a left ventricular ejection fraction of 25%, a functional capacity of far less than four METs, and a symptomatic response to increased oxygen demand. He also demonstrated an abnormal phase 2 arterial blood pressure response (eg, the blood pressure was

maintained) during a controlled expiratory maneuver, which prior to the massive anterior wall myocardial infarction was normal (eg, phase 2 arterial blood pressure decreasing during a controlled expiratory maneuver). This patient met the criteria for a patient/client with cardiovascular pump failure because of the (1) massive anterior wall myocardial infarction which reduced the ejection fraction and produced an abnormal heart rate, functional capacity, and symptoms during increased oxygen demand and (2) abnormal phase 2 arterial blood pressure response during a controlled expiratory maneuver.

The Disablement of Cardiac Pump Dysfunction and Cardiac Pump Failure

The disablement of the patient in this case involved both cardiac pump dysfunction and failure. The active pathology illustrated in the case study is coronary artery disease with subsequent myocardial infarction. The patient had impairments in aerobic capacity, muscle performance, ventilation, respiration and circulation. Functional limitations in self-care, bed mobility, transfers, and gait were noted. He was disabled in that he was unable to work or perform usual household chores/duties, and his family and social relationships were interrupted. These aspects of disablement are shown in Figure 18-1.

Risk Factors
Risk Factors for Developing Coronary Artery Disease

Coronary artery disease is the most common cause of cardiac pump dysfunction and failure (eg, CHF) and is true for this case study.[15] Risk factors associated with the development of coronary atherosclerosis[46,47] are listed in Box 18-2 and are discussed in detail in Chapters 6 and 15. Identifying risk factors is important in order to assign appropriate risk for recurrent events and therapeutic interventions. A patient at high risk for developing coronary artery disease will be more aggressively managed in those areas of greatest risk. Identifying key risk factors specific to the individual will help the health care professional select the most appropriate interventions. For example, a patient with a past MI and risk factor of inactivity alone can be best managed by prescribing physical exercise alone, whereas another patient with a past MI and risk factors of inactivity, hypertension, elevated lipids, and cigarette smoking is likely in need of an exercise prescription as well as management of lipids, hypertension, and cigarette smoking.

The major risk factors for developing coronary atherosclerosis are dyslipidemia, hypertension, diabetes mellitus, and tobacco use.[46] This patient's major risk factors were dyslipidemia (elevated low-density lipoproteins) and hypertension. He did not have diabetes mellitus nor did he use tobacco. His other risk factors included a family history of heart disease (mother, brother, and sister); age and gender (63-year-old man); and psychological factors (stressful job, history of anxiety for which he takes Xanax, rare bouts of intense anger). Though he did not participate in regular aerobic exercise, he had a physically active work environment (owner of a building supply company) and enjoyed yardwork during leisure time. He was overweight but not obese (height 5 ft 6 in., weight 75.2 kg, body mass index [BMI] 27.6 kg/m^2). Premorbid hemostatic factors and serum homocysteine and C-reactive protein levels were not available. He reported alcohol consumption of 2 beers/wk. In summary, this patient had multiple risk factors for developing coronary atherosclerosis, which put him at high risk for a recurrent event.

Risk Factors for Developing Cardiomyopathy and Cardiac Pump Failure

A multitude of inflammatory, metabolic, toxic, infiltrative, fibroplastic, hematological, hypersensitivity, genetic, miscellaneous acquired, and physical agent–related factors have been associated with the development of cardiomyopathy.[21] This patient did not have any of these conditions, confirming that coronary atherosclerosis with subsequent myocardial infarctions was the active pathology responsible for his cardiomyopathy and cardiac pump failure.

Examination Techniques

History

Through a careful review of the medical record, consultation with other members of the health care team, and interview of the patient and support system, the physical therapist obtained a detailed history of George's past and current health status. The information obtained indicated that the patient/client would benefit from physical therapy.

George was married for 18 years and had a 15-year-old daughter who was in highschool. He owned a building supply company. He lived with his family in a two-story private home.

His general health status had been relatively good since his coronary artery bypass graft (CABG) surgery and was limited only by rare episodes of angina, panic attacks, and bouts of anger. He did not smoke or use recreational drugs, and he only drank approximately 2 beers/wk. He worked full-time until this admission, and in his leisure time, he enjoyed yardwork and outings with family and friends. Prior to this admission, George was independent in both activities of daily living (ADL) and instrumental activities of daily living (IADL). His family history was positive for heart disease. The past medical history was significant only for the cardiac issues described in detail in the following section.

In July of 1995, George suffered an inferior MI. This was followed 2 months later by CABG of saphenous vein grafts to the left anterior descending artery, left circumflex artery, and right coronary artery because of recurrent angina. He subsequently returned to full activities including work. He was maintained on cardizem, a calcium channel blocker for its antianginal and antihypertensive properties; mevacor, a statin drug for its lipid-lowering effects; Xanax, a benzodiazepine used for the treatment of anxiety and panic attacks; and, sublingual nitroglycerin (SLNTG), a nitrate used for rare angina. At this time the patient entered a local outpatient multidisciplinary cardiac rehabilitation program. A complete examination including risk-factor analysis and a maximal exercise tolerance test was performed (see Chapter 10 and the CD-ROM for risk-factor analyses and exercise test methods). He also underwent arterial blood pressure measurement during a controlled expiratory maneuver and was found to have a normal response. The patient subsequently participated in an individually tailored rehabilitation program consisting of education, exercise training, and stress management.

Six years later on October 24, 2001, while working in his yard, George developed sudden onset of chest pain, nausea, and diaphoresis. It was the worst pain he had ever felt. He took two SLNTGs without relief and went to the emergency room of the local community hospital. He arrived in the emergency room within 1 hour of onset of chest pain.

Tests and Measures

The electrocardiogram showed ST-segment elevation in leads V$_2$ through V$_4$. He was given tissue plasminogen activator (tPA), a thrombolytic agent; heparin, an anticoagulant; lopressor, a β-blocker to decrease the demand for oxygen; and aspirin, a platelet inhibitor and anti-inflammatory agent. The creatine phosphokinase (CPK) peaked at 2,900 (reference range = 37–200) with a myocardial band fraction of 14%, which was diagnostic for a myocardial infarction. The following day the patient became progressively cold, clammy, and hypotensive. A chest radiograph showed moderate pulmonary vascular congestion and bilateral pleural effusions. He developed cardiogenic shock for which an intra-aortic balloon pump (IABP) was placed, and intravenous dobutamine, a positive inotropic medication, was started. The lopressor was held because it would lower the blood pressure further. The patient was then transferred to the university medical center for further management.

At the university medical center George underwent a cardiac catheterization, which showed occluded grafts to the left anterior descending artery and left circumflex artery. The graft to the right coronary artery was patent. An echocardiogram showed akinesis of the entire anterior wall, septum, and apex; basal and posterior areas were hypokinetic. The left ventricular ejection fraction (LVEF) was severely depressed at 25%. A 24-hour thallium scan was performed to search for areas of hibernating myocardium, which could have benefited from coronary revascularization. Unfortunately there was no viability in any of the infarcted areas. Therefore it was decided that CABG surgery would not yield therapeutic gain. Based on the LVEF of 25% his prognosis was poor with a 40% to 60% 1 year mortality rate.[48] Because of the poor prognosis, the patient was referred for a cardiac transplantation evaluation.

On October 30, 6 days after admission, the intra-aortic balloon pump was discontinued. He continued to undergo therapeutic diuresis with careful observation of hemodynamic measures through a Swan–Ganz catheter (see Chapter 19).

George was referred to physical therapy upon IABP removal. The physical therapy tests and measures are detailed at the end of this section and in Box 18-5. Although the patient had a Swan–Ganz catheter, he was still able to actively participate in formal exercise training, which was initiated with

BOX 18-5

George's Initial Examination, 10/31/2001

General demographics

41-Year-old, English-speaking, black man

Social history

Married 18 years with one 15-year-old daughter in high-school, strong family relationships

Occupation/work environment

Owner of building supply company, since 1993

Living environment

Lives with family in a private two-story home

General health status

In general, easy-going personality per family report

Occasional panic attacks since MI, *prescriptioned* (Rx'd) with Xanax

Successful at work; strong family relationships

Social/health habits

No tobacco use, no IVDA

Reports ~2 beers/wk

Worked full-time until 1 week ago

Enjoys yard work and family outings

Family history

Father died at 60 years of age from stroke

Mother died due to heart attack at 78 years

Brother died due to heart attack at 49 years

Sister died from liver cancer in her 60s

Sister alive at 65 though is s/p CABG

Past medical/surgical history

s/p MI 7/95

s/p CABG 9/95

Hypercholesterolemia

Hypertension

Had a blood transfusion following a nosebleed

History of current condition

7/95   Suffered inferior wall myocardial infarction

9/95   Underwent CABG × 3 (Sag's to LAD, LCX, RCA)

Patient returned to full activities with rare episodes of anginafor which he took sublingual nitroglycerin; additionally he was taking Cardizem, Mevacor, and Xanax.

10/24/2001 Patient developed sudden onset chest pain, nausea, and diaphoresis while performing heavy yard work. He took two tablets of sublingual nitroglycerin without relief and subsequently went to the local community hospital ER. He arrived at the ER within 1 hour of onset of chest pain. The EKG showed ST-segment elevation in leads V_2V_4. He was given TPA, Heparin, Lopressor, Nitroglycerin, and aspirin.

10/25/2001 An intra-aortic balloon pump was placed and IV dobutamine was started because of cardiogenic shock. The patient was transferred to the university medical center for further management.

10/26/2001 At the university medical center the patient underwent a cardiac catheterization, which showed occluded grafts to the LAD and LCX; the graft to the RCA was patent.

10/27/2001 An echocardiogram showed akinesis of the anterior wall, septum and apex. Other areas were hypokinetic. The left ventricular ejection fraction was 25%.

10/28/2001 A 24-hour thallium scan showed uptake only in areas of normal contractility. There was no viability in the anterior wall, septum, or apex. Therefore, it was decided that CABG would not yield therapeutic gain. Cardiac transplantation evaluation was begun.

10/30/2001 The intra-aortic balloon pump was weaned off. The patient continued to undergo diuresis with careful observation of hemodynamic measures through a Swan–Ganz catheter in the CCU. Cardiac rehabilitation was ordered.

Functional status and activity level

Independent in all ADLs and IADLs immediately prior to this admission

Medications

Dobutamine, dopamine, Heparin, Digoxin, Lasix, Vasotec, and Coreg

Other clinical tests

Peak CPK 2900, MB + (10/24/95)

BUN 36 Creat 1.5 Hgb 9.8 Hct 29.6

Chest radiograph:	Pulmonary vascular congestion, bilateral pleural effusions
Electrocardiogram:	Sinus tachycardia at 112 bpm, left atrial enlargement
	Old inferior infarction (Q waves, leads II, III, aVF)
	Evolving anterior infarction (ST-elevation leads V_2 through V_4)
2-D echocardiogram:	Anterior, septal, and apical akinesis, otherwise hypokinetic
	Mild-to-moderate MR, mild TR, LVEF 25%
Cardiac catheterization:	Occluded grafts to the LAD and LCX, patent graft to the PDA
24 hour thallium:	No viability in the anterior, septal, or apical regions

Systems review

Cardiopulmonary	BP 90/60 HR 110 R 20 SpO$_2$ 92%
Integumentary	Intact
Musculoskeletal	Normal
Neuromuscular	Normal

Arousal, attention, and cognition

Alert and oriented to person and place (date accurate to month/year)

Follows commands slowly, anxious, fearful

(continued)

BOX 18-5 *(Continued)*

Aerobic capacity and endurance/circulation

Observation: Patient was resting semifowlers in bed, +diaphoresis at rest

Cor: RRR, S_1, S_2, +S_3, S_4

Lungs: Bibasilar crackles

BP 90/60	HR110	SpO$_2$ 92%	Supine at rest on 5 L O$_2$ NC
80/60	118	93%	Sitting at edge of bed at rest on 5 L O$_2$ NC
84/60	120	93%	Sitting at edge of bed p 15 reps knee ext 5 L O$_2$ NC
78/60	124	92%	Standing at rest on 5 L O$_2$ Nasal Cannula
80/60	118	93%	Sitting in chair, recovery on 5 L O$_2$ NC

Symptoms: Initially a little dizzy upon sitting, resolved quickly

Dizzy and SOB when standing; there was no chest pain

HR and BP response: Resting tachycardia c/w pump failure and deconditioning

Mild postural hypotension c/w orthostasis

Appropriate increase in HR and BP with low-level exercise

Telemetry: Sinus tachycardia, no ectopy observed during session

Anthropometric characteristics

3+ Bipedal edema two-third the way up the lower leg

Assistive and adaptive devices

An occupational therapy consultation may be valuable to evaluate the patient for assistive devices, which would decrease his energy cost of performing simple ADLs. Because of the prolonged stay in intensive care, patient's fearfulness, and orthostatic responses; anticipate that he will eventually need an assistive device for ambulation

Gait, locomotion, and balance

Static standing balance required contact guard

Dynamic standing balance required minimal assistance

Gait was not assessed at this time because of hypotension in standing; and, because of the risk of dislodging the Swan–Ganz catheter

Integumentary integrity

Intact at occiput, sacrum, and heels

Muscle performance

≥3/5 throughout all extremities

Pain

Denies chest pain

Posture

Excessive thoracic kyphosis, perhaps related to monitors and/or fear

Range of motion

Within functional limits throughout except hamstrings, ~0 degree to −40 degrees bilaterally

Self care

Supine to sit transfer requires moderate assistance

Static sitting balance (at edge of bed) requires close supervision/contact guard

Stand pivot transfer requires minimal assistance

Bathing, grooming, toileting requires minimal assistance

Ventilation and respiration

Lungs with crackles bibasilar SpO$_2$ is 92% at rest on 5 L O$_2$ NC

Cough is effective at mobilizing sputum which is loose, white (~2 cc at this time)

Evaluation/diagnosis/prognosis

The patient is a 41-year-old male with primary impairments in aerobic capacity and endurance; and ventilation and respiration associated with cardiovascular pump failure. Additionally he has secondary impairments in range of motion, muscle strength, self-care, and gait and balance. Short-term goals to be achieved within two to three sessions include: (1) the patient will be independent in diaphragmatic breathing and cough; (2) the patient will require supervision and verbal cues for gentle active range of motion exercises; (3) the patient will move from supine to sit with minimal assistance; (4) the patient will require close supervision only for static sitting balance; and (5) the patient will require contact guarding/minimal assistance for stand pivot transfers. Goals to be achieved within 2 weeks include the following: (1) the patient will be independent in gentle active range of motion exercises; (2) the patient will move from supine to sit with close supervision; (3) the patient will be independent in static sitting balance; (4) the patient will require close supervision for stand pivot transfers; and (5) the patient will tolerate 5 minutes of cycle ergometry with no or minimal tension from a position seated in the bedside chair. Long-term goals to be achieved over 8 to 16 weeks include the following: (1) patient will be independent in self-care; (2) patient will be independent in ambulation on level surfaces and 1 to 2 flights of stairs; (3) patient will demonstrate maximal strength and aerobic capacity within the constraints of his disease, impairments, functional limitations, and disability. Frequency of intervention will be daily until he is an independent ambulator and then reduced progressively until all goals are achieved.

ADLs, activities of daily living.

breathing exercises and progressed to inspiratory, and expiratory muscle training and cycle ergometry. In fact, the Swan–Ganz catheter enabled more specific exercise to be provided with a better understanding of the effects of exercise on the cardiovascular system. Before, during, and after all breathing and cycling exercises the mean arterial pressure, pulmonary artery pressure, and occasionally the pulmonary artery wedge pressure could be examined with the information provided by the Swan–Ganz catheter. This information was combined and evaluated with the more traditional exercise measurements of electrocardiography and oxygen saturation. Appropriate changes were then made in the patient's exercise prescription.

On November 7, eight days after admission, the Swan–Ganz catheter was removed and the patient was transferred from the intensive care unit (ICU) to the cardiac telemetry floor. More aggressive cardiac rehabilitation was instituted upon transfer out of the ICU. His medications upon transfer included Dobutamine, for inotropic support; Dopamine, for increased renal perfusion; Digoxin, for inotropic support; Lasix, for diuresis; and, Vasotec, for afterload reduction. His laboratory values upon transfer to the floor include hemoglobin (Hgb) 10.2 g/dL, hematocrit (Hct) 30.1%, blood urea nitrogen (BUN) 30 g/dL, and creatine (Cr) 1.3 g/dL. On the floor the patient's activities were increased, but he consistently complained of increased dyspnea and fatigue. In addition, the patient's blood pressure continued to decrease with increasing exercise until the patient lost consciousness during hallway ambulation. At this time the patient was transferred back to the cardiac care unit (CCU) because of hypotension despite the addition of the inotropic drug Dobutamine, which was administered intravenously. Another inotropic agent, Milrinone, was added; however, he continued to be hemodynamically unstable despite a maximal medical regimen. Therefore the patient was evaluated for left ventricular assist device (LVAD) implantation. Because the patient remained hypotensive even at rest (despite maximal inotropic therapy) and had other specific indications for LVAD implantation (Table 18-3), an LVAD was implanted on December 7.

Physical therapy reexamination of the patient following LVAD implantation is outlined in Box 18-6. As suggested by the literature, this patient's initial physical therapy goals were directed toward preventing the ill effects of immobility while he required multiple vasopressive agents for hemodynamic stability.[49-52] Specific interventions included airway clearance techniques, upright positioning, active range of motion exercises and bedside functional training activities. When he consistently demonstrated appropriate responses to sitting out of bed and all prohibitive lines (Swan–Ganz catheter, femoral arterial line, or CVVHD) had been removed, the treatment was progressed to training in LVAD battery management and gait training. Methods for the early mobilization of a patient on LVAD support are suggested in Box 18-7.[50] Once the patient gained independence in ambulation on level surfaces, the treatment was advanced to aerobic conditioning on a treadmill in a gymnasium setting.[49-51] The physical therapist used the Borg Scale of Perceived Exertion (see Chapter 9) to *guide* the intensity of the exercise aiming for a grade of 11 to 13 on the 6 to 20 scale.[49-51] Selected treatment sessions following LVAD implantation are presented in Box 18-8. A cycle ergometer was also used by ensuring that the exit site for the LVAD drive line was not too low to inhibit the hip flexion necessary for cycling (Fig. 18-3). Resistive exercise for the upper extremities was purposefully omitted to ensure adequate sternal healing.

Systems Review

The systems review (limited examination) in this case study was normal except for the cardiopulmonary impairments in aerobic capacity, ventilation, and respiration as expected from the history.

Physical Therapy Tests and Measures

Arousal, attention, and cognition—Measures of arousal, attention, and cognition are important to evaluate in order to determine the patient's ability to participate in the plan of care and to adhere to safety precautions. This patient was alert and oriented to person and place. On questions relating to time, he was accurate to the month and year. He followed commands tentatively and appeared anxious and fearful.

Aerobic capacity and endurance—The initial examination of aerobic capacity and endurance began with observation of the patient. On observation the patient was found to be diaphoretic at rest, reclining in the bed. Cardiac auscultation

TABLE 18-3   Indications for LVAD Placement

FDA-Approved Inclusion Criteria for LVAD Implantation	This Patient's Specific Indications for LVAD Implantation
PCWP $\geq$ 20 mm Hg and	PCWP = 27 mm Hg
Dependence on IV Inotrope and	Dependent on IV Dobutamine, Milrinone
Systolic BP $\leq$ 80 mm Hg or	Systolic BP = 80 mm Hg
Cardiac index $\leq$ 2.0 L/min/m^2 and	Cardiac Index = 2.2 L/min/m^2
Candidate for cardiac transplantation	Listed for transplantation on 12/7/95

Medical Devices, Diagnostics and Instrumentation Reports. Chevy Chase, MD: F-D-C Reports, Inc; October 10, 1994.

BOX 18-6

12/11/2001 Reexamination Following LVAD Implantation

Hospital course update

12/01/2001 Patient was transferred to the CCU because of progressive SOB and hypotension. IV milrinone was added for its +inotropic effect. Diuresis was limited by hypotension. Right heart cath. = RA 14 RV 49/14 PA 49/25 PCWP 32 CO 3.86

12/07/2001 The medical team did not feel he would survive until a donor heart became available. Therefore, a left ventricular assist device was implanted as a bridge to transplantation. Arrived in recovery on Levophed, Dobutamine, Nitroglycerin, Primacor, and Pitressin.

12/09/2001 Extubated

12/10/2001 Cardiopulmonary physical therapy was ordered

Medications

Dobutamine, Dopamine, Milrinone, Vancomycin, Cefotaxime, Fluconazole, Percocet

Laboratory tests

WBC 10K Hct 26 Creat 1.8

Urine culture: *Klebsiella* and *Enterococcus*

Arousal, attention, and cognition

Alert and oriented ×3, follows all commands

Aerobic capacity and endurance/circulation

Observations: Supine in bed, Swan–Ganz catheter, arterial line, telemetry, foley,

35% O_2 via face tent and 6 L O_2 via nasal cannula; afebrile

Heartmate VE LVAD auto mode 62 bpm 66 mL 5.0 L/min

Cor: Obscured by LVAD

Lungs: Crackles halfway up on the right, 1/4 on left

Integumentary integrity

Sacral area a little red but intact, occiput and heels intact; incisions dressed

Muscle performance

≥3/5 throughout all extremities

Pain

Midsternal and LVAD pocket incisions 7/10 on a scale of 0 to 10

Posture

Marked thoracic kyphosis most likely self-protective due to the presence of the LVAD

Range of motion

Within functional limits except SLR ~0 degree to 30 degree, ankle dorsiflexion ~0 degree to 5 degrees

Self-care

Supine to sitting transfer requires moderate assistance

Stand pivot transfer bed to chair required minimal assistance

Bathing, grooming, and toilet needs require moderate assistance per patient and nurse

LVAD management requires maximal assistance

Ventilation and respiration

Lungs and SpO_2 as in previous

Cough is effective but difficult because of incisional pain.

Evaluation/diagnosis/prognosis

41-year-old man who suffered a massive AWMI with subsequent cardiogenic shock 10/24/2001 is now 2 days s/p *Heartmate* electric LVAD implantation as a bridge to cardiac transplantation. He has impairments in aerobic capacity and endurance; muscle performance; pain; posture; range of motion; gait; self-care; and ventilation and respiration. Short-term goals to be achieved within 2 to 3 sessions include the following: (1) patient will move

BP	HR	SpO_2	LVAD			
140/60	116	98%	62 bpm	66 mL	5.0 L/min	Supine at rest
135/60	118	98%	62	76	4.2	Sitting in chair

Symptoms: +mild DOE, resolves quickly with rest; +fatigue; denied dizziness

HR and BP Responses: very small (acceptable) drop in BP and LVAD flows in upright

Telemetry: sinus tachycardia without ectopy

Anthropometric characteristics

3+ Bipedal edema up to mid thigh

Assistive and adaptive equipment

May benefit from an OT consultation to evaluate the patient for assistive devices (ie, long-handled reacher, sock aide). Will likely benefit from rolling walker to initially assist ambulation

Gait, locomotion, and balance

Static standing balance required contact guard

Dynamic standing balance required minimal assistance gait was not tested from supine to sit with minimal assistance, (2) stand pivot transfers will require contact guard, (3) LVAD battery management will require moderate assistance, and (4) the patient will ambulate 25 ft × 2 with a rolling walker and contact guard/minimal assistance. Within 3 weeks he will be independent in ambulation on level surfaces with/without an assistive device, and, in self-care. Long-term goals to be achieved within 6 to 12 weeks include the following: (1) the patient will be independent in an aerobic/strength/flexibility exercise program; (2) the patient will be able to identify signs and symptoms of exercise intolerance, and (3) the patient will be independent in device management. Frequency of care will be daily until the patient is and independent ambulator and then reduced progressively until all goals are achieved. Medical/surgical complications (ie, bleeding, infection, etc) may prolong the duration of care or may cause a pause in the episode of care.

CCU, cardiac care unit; SOB, shortness of breath; RA, right atrium; RV, right ventricle; PA, pulmonary artery; PCWP, pulmonary capillary wedge pressure; CO, cardiac output; OT, occupational therapy; SLR, straight leg raise; DOE, dyspnea on exertion.

BOX 18-7

Mobilizing a Patient on LVAD Support

1. Note resting supine HR, BP, LVAD rate, flow, and volumes
2. Note all drips, lines, and tubes
3. In general, treatment would be held for:
   a. LVAD rate < 50 bpm
   b. LVAD volumes < 30 mL
   c. LVAD flows < 3.0 L/min
   d. Systolic BP < 80 mm Hg
   e. Heart rate > 150 bpm
   f. Sustained ventricular tachycardia or ventricular fibrillation
4. Assist patient supine to sitting, being certain not to kink or apply torque to the drive line
5. Dangle legs 3 to 5 minutes
6. Assess for orthostasis using parameters listed in number 1 and note any signs or symptoms of intolerance

7. Proceed to LE AROM exercises or;
8. Prepare to ambulate (*Heartmate* VE LVAD)
   Attach fully charged batteries one at a time. Apply holster and insert batteries. Clip controller to waist belt or holster (procedure must be reviewed with the LVAD coordinator)
9. Assist patient sitting to standing and begin ambulation as quickly as possible to prevent orthostasis. It is highly recommended to have the assistance of another health care worker when ambulating for the first time. There is a high incidence of orthostasis due to prolonged bed rest, and the sequelae of falling include LVAD dislodgement and hemorrhage.
10. Reassess: BP, LVAD rate, HR (if telemetry available), symptoms

Adapted with permission from Humphrey R, Buck L, Cahalin L, et al. Physical therapy assessment and intervention for patients with left ventricular assist devices. *Cardiopulmonary Phys Ther.* 1998;9(2):3-7.

revealed a normal first heart sound (S_1) and second heart sound (S_2) and presence of third heart sound (S_3) and fourth heart sound (S_4), frequently referred to as a summation gallop. The S_3 was heard because of a noncompliant left ventricle.[53–55] It is a classic sign of congestive heart failure.[56] The "(S_4) is heard when augmented atrial contraction generates presystolic ventricular distension."[57] Auscultation of the lungs revealed bibasilar crackles, a common finding in CHF due to pulmonary edema and fluid overload.

Changes in body position and exercise tolerance were initially assessed at the bedside. Heart rate, blood pressure, and oxygen saturation levels were measured with changes from supine to sitting and standing; and, with gentle active range of motion exercises. The results are listed in Box 18-5 and 18-6. Resting tachycardia consistent with cardiac pump failure and deconditioning was found. Mild orthostatic changes were noted. There was an appropriate increase in heart rate and blood pressure to low-level exercise.

The patient also underwent measurement of the arterial blood pressure during a controlled expiratory maneuver, which revealed an arterial blood pressure that remained elevated throughout the maneuver (Fig. 18-3). This abnormal response to the valsalva maneuver indicated that the cardiac pump was failing.

A 6-minute walk test was performed several days after cardiovascular stability was observed and revealed poor exercise tolerance and aerobic capacity/endurance. The results of the 6-minute walk test are shown in Table 18-4. The information obtained from the 6-minute walk test was used to establish a baseline from which to evaluate progress over time and to prescribe exercise and functional training.[58] More recently the 6-minute walk test has been shown to predict mortality in patients with heart failure and to predict aerobic capacity.[59,60] Aerobic capacity and endurance were measured to assess the patient's ability to tolerate increased activity and the subsequent increase in demand for oxygen.

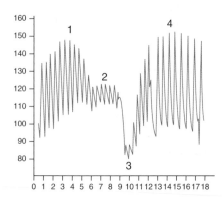

A

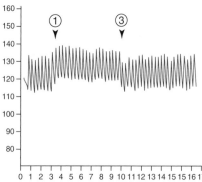

B

FIGURE 18-3 Arterial blood pressure response to the valsalva maneuver. (**A**) Normal response. (**B**) Abnormal response.

BOX 18-8

Selected Treatment Sessions for George Following LVAD Implantation

12/12/2001 POD 5

S: Patient c/o incisional pain

O: 4 L O$_2$ NC, telemetry, foley, IV Dobutamine, Dopamine, Milrinone

Afebrile Cor: obscured by LVAD Lungs: basilar crackles

Tx: Supine to sitting with contact guard

Diaphragmatic breathing and splinted cough

Don and doff LVAD batteries with maximal assistance

Sitting to standing with contact guard

Amb 25 ft with rolling walker and contact guard

BP 140/56	HR 80	SpO$_2$ 95%	LVAD 65 bpm	4.7 L/min	Supine
130/60	86	96%	62	4.3	Sitting
140/60	98	93%	66	4.6	Amb

A: + mild DOE, transient dizziness upon standing

Mild postural hypotension; appropriate responses to activity

Telem: Normal sinus rhythm

STGs: Mobilize and clear secretions

Don and doff batteries with mod assist

Supine to sitting with close supervision

Sitting to standing with close supervision

Amb 50 ft ×2 with rolling walker and close supervision

P: Airway clearance techniques

Education re: battery management of the LVAD

Bed mobility, transfer, and gait training

12/15/2001 POD 8

S: Fearful

O: He was transferred from the ICU to the cardiac floor yesterday.

IV Dobutamine is being weaned.

Afebrile Cor: LVAD Lungs: Bronchial breath sounds left base

Tx: Instruction in donning/doffing batteries, requires mod assist

Sitting to standing requires contact guard

Ambulation 200 ft × 1 with contact guard

Splinted coughing

BP 120/70	HR 108	LVAD 62 bpm	60 mL	4.3 L/min	Sitting
114/70	117	62	76	4.4	Standing
140/90	120	66	…	…	Amb

A: +fatigue, −SOB; VSS

STGs: Don/doff batteries with minimum assistance

Sitting to standing with close supervision

Amb 300 ft × 2 with close supervision

P: Education, transfer training, gait training

12/18/2001 POD 11

S: Very fearful of LVAD

O: Patient and wife instructed in battery management of LVAD

Sitting to standing with close supervision

Ambulate 500 ft × 1, 800 ft × 1 with close supervision

BP 120/60	LVAD Rate 72	Sitting at rest
120/60	96	Sitting after amb 500 ft
120/60	114	Sitting after amb 800 ft

A: Mild fatigue and slightly winded after session

STG: Increase confidence in himself in managing device

Sitting to standing independent

Amb level surfaces 1000 ft × 2 independently

(continued)

BOX 18-8 *(Continued)*

    P: Reassurance and education

       Transfer training, gait training

12/20/2001 POD 13

    S: Feels well, eager for P.T

    O: Afebrile lungs: decreased breath sounds left base

       Wearing batteries on my arrival

       Tx: sit to stand independent

       Amb level surfaces to/from gym (200 ft each way), independent

       Treadmill at 1.5 mph 0% grade for 10 minutes

BP 100/70	LVAD rate 78	Sitting at rest
120/80	96	Treadmill at 1.5 mph 0% × 5 min
120/80	102	Treadmill at 1.5 mph 0% × 5 min
120/80	72	Sitting—recovery

    A: Asymptomatic, vital signs stable.

       Good progress in function, endurance, and confidence

    STGs: Treadmill 15 minutes

           Independent in lower extremity stretching

    P: General conditioning, education

12/26/2001 POD 19

    S: Walked 8 laps around the nursing station this morning

    O: Tx: hamstring and calf stretching

       Treadmill ×20 minutes

	BP 118/60	LVAD Rate 90	Standing at rest
RPE 9/20	110/70	108	Treadmill at 1.6 mph 0%grade × 5 min
RPE 13/20	128/70	114	Treadmill at 2.0 mph 0%grade × 5 min
	120/70	114	Treadmill at 2.0 mph 0%grade × 5 min
	122/70	114	Treadmill at 1.6 mph 0%grade × 5 min
	130/70	78	Recovery

    A: Mild fatigue; no SOB; HR and BP responses acceptable

    STG's: Treadmill 20 minutes; 10/20 with small elevation

            Independent stretching program

    P: Aerobic exercise program, stretching; 3×/wk

01/03/2002 POD 27 s/p LVAD

    S: No complaints

    O: Afebrile, Lungs are clear

       Tx: Treadmill ×25 minutes

          Hamstring and calf stretching

BP 120/70	LVAD Rate 72	Resting
110/70	100	Treadmill at 2.2 mph 0% grade, 5 min
112/70	114	Treadmill at 2.4 mph 2% grade, 5 min
110/70	14	Treadmill at 2.4 mph 2% grade, 5 min
110/70	120	Treadmill at 2.4 mph 2% grade, 5 min
110/70	114	Treadmill at 2.2 mph 0% grade, 5 min
96/64	66	Recovery

    A: Asymptomatic throughout. Small drop in BP during exercise but pt. asymptomatic throughout and recovery BP did not rebound up; therefore, doubt ischemia or failure the reason. Could be somewhat volume depleted. Will discuss with MD.

    P: Continue 3×/wk. Encourage hallway amb on alternate days

01/11/2002 Suitable donor was identified; patient underwent heart transplant

01/26/2002 After a relatively uncomplicated course patient was discharged home

       In PT he was able to perform the treadmill ×25 minutes @ workloads of 01/03/2002

LVAD, left ventricular assist device; DOE, dyspnea on exertion; POD, post-operative day; STG, short-term goals; BP, blood pressure; re, regarding; Cor, heart; RPE, rating of perceived exertion; VSS, vital signs stable.

TABLE 18-4 Six-Minute Walk Test Results, 11/10/2001

Parameter Measured	Resting Value	Maximum Value from 6-Minute Walk Test
Distance ambulated, m		75
HR, bpm	110	132
BP, mm Hg	90/66	84/70
RPP,[a] $\times 10^3$	9.9	11.1
SpO$_2$,% while on room air	95	89
RPE,[a] 0–10	2	5

[a]RPE, rating of perceived exertion.

Anthropometric characteristics—An examination of the extremities showed 3+ bipedal edema. The fluid overload of congestive heart failure frequently accumulates in the extracellular spaces of the dependent parts of the body, usually the lower extremities. The pitting edema scale may help measurements to be more objective so that change can be followed over time (see Chapter 10).

Assistive and adaptive devices—An occupational therapy consultation was obtained in order to evaluate the patient for assistive devices which would decrease his energy cost of performing simple ADL. Because of the prolonged stay in intensive care, patient's fearfulness, and orthostatic responses; the therapist anticipated that the patient would eventually need an assistive device for ambulation. A rolling walker may require less energy than a standard walker and therefore would be helpful for the patient with heart failure.

Gait, locomotion, and balance—Static standing balance at the bedside required contact guard. Dynamic standing balance tested upon transfer to the chair required minimal assistance. Gait was not assessed at this time because of hypotension in standing; and, because of the risk of dislodging the Swan–Ganz catheter.

Integumentary integrity—The integumentary system was intact. The patient was at high risk for skin breakdown due to his impaired mobility and poor nutritional intake. Frequent reexamination was performed before and after each treatment session.

Muscle performance—A gross assessment of peripheral muscle strength was performed through observation of active limb movement against gravity. Manual resistance was not given because of his severely compromised pump function.

Range of motion—A standard physical therapy range of motion assessment was performed revealing significant limitation in hamstring length only with a straight leg test bilaterally of approximately 0 degree to 40 degrees.

Self-care—Moving from supine to sitting required moderate assistance. Static short sitting balance (at edge of bed) required

close supervision to contact guard. Stand pivot transfer from the bed to the chair required minimal assistance. Bathing, grooming, and toilet needs also required minimal assistance by patient and nursing report.

Ventilation and respiration—Many of the tests and measures presented earlier provided information about ventilation and respiration. An additional area worthy of examination was cough. The patient was observed to have a strong cough, which was sufficient to clear his airway. He produced 2 cc of pink frothy sputum, a classic finding in congestive heart failure.[61]

Evaluation, Diagnosis, and Prognosis

George is a 41-year-old man with primary impairments in aerobic capacity and endurance associated with cardiovascular pump failure. Additionally he has secondary impairments in range of motion, muscle strength, self-care, and gait and balance. Short-term goals to be achieved within two to three sessions include (1) the patient will be independent in diaphragmatic breathing and cough, (2) the patient will require supervision and verbal cues for gentle active range of motion exercises, (3) the patient will move from supine to sitting with minimal assistance, (4) the patient will require close supervision only for static sitting balance, and (5) the patient will require contact guarding/minimal assistance for stand pivot transfers. Long-term goals to be achieved over 8 to 16 weeks include the following: (1) patient will be independent in self-care; (2) patient will be independent in ambulation on level surfaces and one to two flights of stairs; (3) patient will demonstrate maximal strength and aerobic capacity within the constraints of his disease, impairments, functional limitations, and disability. Goals were progressed as they were achieved or as external constraints were removed allowing greater freedom of movement (ie, the Swan–Ganz catheter removal will allow ambulation). Goals remained unchanged or were decreased when signs or symptoms of intolerance to exercise or instability were observed. Medical instability occasionally increased the duration of care by causing a pause in the provision of physical therapy. The frequency of intervention was daily until the patient became independent in ambulation after which the frequency of intervention was progressively decreased until all goals were achieved.

Results of the initial and subsequent physical therapy examinations provided important diagnostic and prognostic information. The key examination findings in this case include the poor ejection fraction, maintenance of the blood pressure response during a controlled expiratory maneuver (rather than the normal decrease in blood pressure during the maneuver), poor 6-minute walk test distance ambulated, and abnormal cardiorespiratory responses during the 6-minute walk test and during attempts to increase exercises and activities of daily living. Specific characteristics of cardiac pump dysfunction and failure can be extremely useful in the diagnosis and prognosis of patients with cardiovascular disease. A complete description of the rationale and cause of many of the characteristic signs and symptoms of cardiac pump dysfunction and failure are presented in the following sections.

Characteristics of cardiac pump dysfunction—Cardiac pump dysfunction is commonly associated with several characteristic signs and symptoms which are thoroughly described in Chapters 6 and 10 and briefly described in the following:

- Ejection fraction greater than 30% to 40%
- Angina and anginal equivalents and myocardial ischemia
- Cardiac arrhythmias
- Myocardial infarction
- Hypertension
- Decrease in the systolic blood pressure during a controlled expiratory maneuver
- Mild-to-moderate decrease in exercise tolerance and functional abilities
- Disability
- Decreased quality of life

Laboratory findings of cardiac pump dysfunction—The laboratory finding of cardiac pump dysfunction is ventriculographic evidence (via radiologic or echocardiographic methods) of a cardiac ejection fraction above a threshold level of approximately 30% to 40%. It has been accepted that an ejection fraction greater than 40% is associated with adequate cardiac performance.[62]

Angina and anginal equivalents and myocardial ischemia—Angina is well described in Chapter 10 and can be summarized as the discomfort of myocardial ischemia which may occur in the chest, left arm, neck, back, jaw, teeth, or ears and is frequently described as a heaviness, pressure, or squeezing sensation brought on by exercise, eating a large meal, or emotional excitement or stress. An anginal equivalent is another symptom of myocardial ischemia that is frequently represented by dyspnea and fatigue. The myocardial ischemia producing angina may subsequently result in cardiac pump dysfunction due to inadequate oxygen supply to the heart (the demand for oxygen is greater than the supply). The lack of adequate oxygenation to the heart can also be observed in the electrocardiogram and is often associated with ST-segment depression and cardiac arrhythmias.[62]

Cardiac arrhythmias—Cardiac arrhythmias may produce cardiac pump dysfunction and are most likely due to myocardial ischemia, electrolyte imbalance, autonomic nervous system abnormalities. Though usually not life threatening, arrhythmias often need to be controlled with medication, and/or a pacemaker or pacemaker/defibrillator in order to optimize myocardial function through proper atrioventricular conduction.[62]

Myocardial infarction—Myocardial infarction is the most common cause of cardiac pump dysfunction. It is the result of a sustained inadequate supply of oxygen to meet the demands of the myocardium because of (1) coronary artery smooth muscle spasm, or (2) a sudden thrombotic occlusion at the site

of a previously atherosclerotic coronary artery culminating in regional myocardial cell necrosis and the associated impairment of cardiac pump dysfunction.[62]

Hypertension—Hypertension is thoroughly discussed in Chapters 6, 10, and 15 and can be summarized as an arterial blood pressure observed in repeated examinations to be greater than 140/90 mm Hg.[63] Chronic uncontrolled hypertension places excessive strain on the left ventricle. Initially the ventricle hypertrophies concentrically as a compensation to overcome the afterload. It also stiffens causing systolic and/or diastolic dysfunction. Eventually, the left ventricle will weaken and dilate resulting in CHF. Additionally, hypertension increases the likelihood of coronary atherosclerosis and myocardial infarction.

Mild-to-moderate decrease in exercise tolerance and functional abilities—The exercise tolerance and functional abilities of patients with cardiac pump dysfunction are mildly to moderately decreased compared to the more significant reduction in exercise tolerance and function of patients with cardiac pump failure. The reduction in exercise and functional abilities of patients with cardiac pump dysfunction are often due to limited cardiac performance from myocardial ischemia and associated angina, myocardial infarction, and cardiac arrhythmias. The patient with cardiac pump failure has greater limitations in cardiac performance yielding a much greater decrease in exercise tolerance and functional abilities.[62]

Disability and decreased quality of life—Disability and quality of life are mildly to modestly affected in patients with cardiac pump dysfunction. Numerous instruments have been used to measure disability and quality of life in patients with cardiac pump dysfunction and include both general and disease-specific instruments. Several examples of general instruments include the Medical Outcomes Study Short Form (SF-36), Sickness Impact Profile, and the DUKE Health Profiles. Several examples of disease-specific instruments include the Quality of Life After Myocardial Infarction, Outcomes Institute Angina Type Specification, and Ferrans and Powers Quality of Life Index-Cardiac Version.[64] Chapter 10 provides a brief summary of several of the aforementioned instruments.

Characteristics of cardiac pump failure—Cardiac pump failure is commonly associated with several characteristic signs and symptoms which are thoroughly described in Chapter 10 and briefly described here:

- Chest X-ray evidence of pulmonary edema
- Ejection fraction less than 30% to 40%
- Dyspnea and fatigue
- Tachypnea
- Paroxysmal nocturnal dyspnea
- Orthopnea
- Abnormal breathing patterns
- Peripheral edema
- Cold, pale, and possibly cyanotic extremities

- Weight gain
- Hepatomegaly
- Jugular venous distention
- Crackles (rales)
- Tubular breath sounds and consolidation
- Presence of an S_3 heart sound
- Sinus tachycardia
- Maintenance of the systolic blood pressure during a controlled expiratory maneuver
- Markedly decreased exercise tolerance (functional abilities) and peak oxygen consumption
- Decrease in systolic blood pressure and increase in diastolic blood pressure during incremental exercise
- Disability
- Markedly decreased quality of life

Laboratory findings of cardiac pump failure—Laboratory findings of cardiac pump failure include radiologic and ventriculographic evidence of pulmonary edema and a cardiac ejection fraction below a threshold level of 30% to 40%; elevated urine-specific gravity, blood urea nitrogen (BUN), and creatinine levels; decreased erythrocyte sedimentation rates (because of decreased fibrinogen concentrations resulting from impaired fibrinogen synthesis); and occasionally reduced partial pressure of oxygen, arterial (PaO_2), and oxygen saturation levels and elevated partial pressure of carbon dioxide, arterial ($PaCO_2$) and liver enzyme (eg, serum glutamic-oxaloacetic transaminase [SGOT], alkaline phosphatase) levels; and abnormal serum electrolytes during rigid sodium restriction and diuretic therapy.[16,17]

Radiologic evidence of CHF is dependent on the size and shape of the cardiac silhouette as well as on the presence of interstitial, perivascular, and alveolar edema (evaluating fluid in the lungs).[16] Interstitial, perivascular, and alveolar edemas are the radiologic hallmarks of CHF. The other traditional hallmark of cardiac pump failure is a cardiac ejection fraction below the threshold level of approximately 30% to 40%. It has been accepted that an ejection fraction (measured via radiography or echocardiography) less than 40% is associated with inadequate cardiac performance.[16,17,62]

Symptoms of cardiac pump failure—*Dyspnea*: It is often described as breathlessness or air hunger and is probably the most common finding associated with CHF. It is frequently the result of (1) poor gas transport because of acute and chronic pulmonary edema, (2) abdominal ascites from peripheral edema and the potential limitation in diaphragmatic descent, and (3) ventilatory muscle weakness all of which may contribute to an inadequate oxygen supply.[16,17,22–25] Inadequate oxygen supply either at rest or during exercise will increase the respiratory rate and tidal volume and frequently produces easily provoked dyspnea or, in severe cases of CHF, dyspnea at rest.[16]

Paroxysmal nocturnal dyspnea and orthopnea—Sudden shortness of breath awakening a patient with CHF from sleep

(eg, nocturnal) is often referred to as paroxysmal nocturnal dyspnea (PND).[16] The supine body position assumed during sleep increases venous return to an overloaded cardiac pump which worsens cardiac performance and increases pulmonary edema. In fact, patients with CHF who become dyspneic in the supine position are described as suffering from orthopnea, which can be improved by assuming a more upright body position. Often patients with CHF, PND, and orthopnea will use many pillows to attain a more upright position and sleep more comfortably. The severity of CHF and orthopnea (and essentially cardiac pump failure) can be roughly estimated by determining the number of pillows needed to improve orthopnea and sleep. Four-pillow orthopnea (or more) would suggest more severe pump failure than two-pillow orthopnea. Patients with frequent PND and orthopnea will often place the head of the bed on blocks or sleep in a reclining chair rather than on a bed.[16]

Signs associated with cardiac pump failure—*Abnormal breathing patterns*: Rapid and shallow breathing at rest which worsens with exercise is common in patients with CHF. A clinical finding observed in many patients with CHF is extreme dyspnea with quick and shallow breaths after a change in position, most frequently from sitting to standing. This response appears to be associated with orthostatic hypotension and tachycardia and is most profound in patients with more severe CHF. Measuring blood pressure and heart rate while timing the duration of dyspnea may be useful to document progress or deterioration in patient status. Cheyne–Stokes breathing is also frequently associated with CHF and is characterized by waxing and waning depths of respiration with recurring periods of apnea.[16]

Crackles (rales)—Pulmonary crackles are abnormal breath sounds that were formerly referred to as rales. Crackles are heard during inspiration due to alveolar opening in the presence of pulmonary edema and are considered a hallmark sign (although nonspecific) of CHF. The sound of crackles is identical to that of hair near the ears being rubbed between the thumb and index finger. Crackles are frequently heard at both lung bases in individuals with CHF but may extend upward depending on the patient's position, the severity of CHF, or both. The importance of the presence and magnitude of rales was first addressed in 1967 and provided data for the Killip and Kimball classification of patients with acute myocardial infarction.[65] Individuals with rales extending more than 50% of the lung fields have been observed to have a far poorer prognosis.[65]

Abnormal heart sounds—The normal heart sounds include the S_1 and S_2. S_1 represents closure of the mitral and tricuspid valves, and S_2 represents closure of the aortic and pulmonic valves (see Chapter 10 for a more complete description of examining heart sounds). The most common abnormal heart sounds are S_3 and S_4. S_3 occurs early in diastole (immediately after S_2) as blood begins to rapidly fill a stiff, noncompliant ventricle. S_4 occurs late in diastole (immediately before S_1) as the final filling of a ventricle is assisted by an exaggerated atrial kick to complete ventricular filling. Note that S_3 may be normal in children, young adults, and pregnancy. The presence of an S_3 is considered the hallmark of CHF.[56,57] An S_4 is commonly heard in patients with hypertension, left ventricular hypertrophy, increased left ventricular end-diastolic pressure, pulmonary hypertension, and pulmonic stenosis, all of whom need assistance (via an atrial "kick") with the final filling of the ventricles. Auscultation of the heart may also reveal adventitious (additional) sounds, most frequently murmurs. They not only are common in patients with cardiac pump failure but also appear to be of great clinical significance by identifying CHF patients most responsive to medical therapy or patients with papillary muscle ischemia.[56,57]

Peripheral edema—Peripheral edema frequently accompanies CHF, but may, in some clinical situations, be absent when, in fact, a patient has significant CHF.[16] **The failing pumping ability of the heart provides an inadequate amount of blood to peripheral tissues and central organs. As a result, the body senses a decreased volume of blood, which promotes a decrease in fluid excretion with subsequent fluid retention.**

Increased fluid retention further loads the heart and makes the work of the heart greater which further decreases its pumping ability. Retained fluid commonly accumulates bilaterally in the dependent extracellular spaces of the periphery such as the ankles, pretibial areas, as well as sacral and abdominal areas (see Chapter 10 for examination of peripheral edema).[16]

Jugular venous distention—Jugular venous distention (JVD) may also accompany CHF. It may occur as fluid is retained and the heart's ability to pump is further compromised; the retained fluid increases the filling pressures of the cardiac chambers and results in pulmonary edema and less forward venous flow. Slowed or stagnant venous flow will distend the jugular veins and produce the characteristic JVD of CHF (see Chapter 10 for the examination and a photo of JVD).[16]

Weight gain—As fluid is retained, total body fluid volume increases as does total body weight. Fluctuations of a few pounds from day to day are usually considered normal, but increases of several pounds per day (>3 lb) are suggestive of CHF.[16] Body weight should always be measured from the same scale at approximately the same time of day with similar clothing before exercise is started.

Maintenance of the systolic blood pressure during a controlled expiratory maneuver—The systolic blood pressure response during a controlled expiratory maneuver has an extensive evidence base indicating the important role it has in examining persons with heart disease.[2–10] It has been very useful in determining the presence or absence of heart failure. A systolic blood pressure that is well maintained is associated with cardiac pump failure, whereas a systolic blood that decreases during a controlled expiratory maneuver is associated with cardiac pump dysfunction or normal cardiac performance. Other tests and measures must be used to distinguish between cardiac pump dysfunction and normal cardiac performance including

the cardiac ejection fraction and exercise test results. See Chapter 10 and the CD-ROM for a complete description of the methods used to perform and interpret the blood pressure response to a controlled expiratory maneuver.

Cold, pale, and possible cyanotic extremities—The extremities of persons with cardiac pump failure may occasionally be cold, pale, and cyanotic. This abnormal sensation and appearance are due to the increased sympathetic nervous system activation of CHF which increases peripheral vascular vasoconstriction and decreases peripheral blood flow.[66,67]

Sinus tachycardia—Persons with cardiac pump failure may also experience sinus tachycardia or other tachyarrhythmias because of increased sympathetic nervous system stimulation.[16] The sinus tachycardia or tachyarrthymias attempt to improve physiologic function by increasing cardiac output. Unfortunately, this makes the work of the heart greater, which further impairs its ability to pump.

Decreased exercise tolerance, low peak oxygen consumption, and abnormal blood pressure responses to exercise—The exercise tolerance of patients with CHF is significantly less than that of normal subjects and patients with cardiac pump dysfunction.[68–74] The substantial decrease in exercise tolerance of persons with cardiac pump failure is due to the numerous pathophysiologies and subsequent signs and symptoms of CHF, as well as the constraints of the Fick equation (oxygen consumption per unit time [$\dot{V}O_2$] = cardiac output × arteriovenous oxygen difference). Oxygen supply is limited by a poor cardiac output and an inadequate arteriovenous oxygen difference because of poor delivery of blood to exercising muscle and the possible myopathic changes in the skeletal muscles of patients with CHF. During exercise, a poor cardiac output may be manifested by a decrease in systolic blood pressure and subsequent increase in diastolic blood pressure, whereas an inadequate arteriovenous oxygen difference is manifested by a narrow arteriovenous oxygen difference (limited capacity to widen) and low peak oxygen consumption (see Chapter 10). In fact, patients with CHF often have peak oxygen consumption levels in the range of 10 to 20 mL/kg/min (approximately 3–6 METs). Peak oxygen consumption less than 10 to 14 mL/kg/min is often used as a threshold level range to list patients for cardiac transplantation.[74]

Such a low level of peak oxygen consumption was apparent in the preexercise training exercise test results of the case study patient. Peak oxygen consumption was observed to be substantially greater after LVAD implantation and physical therapy. Measurement of the ventilatory threshold (VT) and the change in oxygen consumption to change in work rate above the anaerobic threshold also appear to be useful and relatively reliable when examining exercise tolerance in patients with CHF.[68–73] The effects of LVAD implantation and physical therapy on these parameters are also apparent in that the VT moved to the right, yielding increased aerobic capacity and improved cardiorespiratory function of the patient presented in the case. Finally, it is apparent that as individuals at rest become short of breath, retain fluid, develop peripheral and pulmonary edema, gain weight, and develop a faster resting heart rate, their ability to exercise is dramatically decreased.

Disability and decreased quality of life—In the past several years much research has been performed in the area of quality of life in CHF.[75–90] Early attempts to measure quality of life used instruments that were limited, such as dyspnea indices and exercise tolerance tests. More comprehensive instruments have been designed and consist primarily of questionnaires that measure specific attributes of life such as socioeconomic, psychologic, and physical functioning (see Chapter 10). Several such instruments include the Minnesota Living with Heart Failure Questionnaire, Chronic Heart Failure Questionnaire, and the Kansas City Heart Failure Questionnaire. These instruments have consistently found significantly greater disablement and poorer quality of life in patients with cardiac pump failure compared to patients with cardiac pump dysfunction and normal individuals.[75–90]

Intervention Techniques

Medical Interventions for Cardiac Pump Dysfunction

The medical interventions for cardiac pump dysfunction include several of the interventions presented for the acute treatment of a myocardial infarction presented in Chapter 6. The acute treatment of a myocardial infarction via PTCA with or without stenting is used not only for an acute myocardial infarction but also for patients with chronic coronary artery disease and coronary occlusion in need of reduction.[91] Although this is the current standard of care for coronary artery disease, increasing evidence suggests that pharmacologic treatment may be just as effective as these more invasive and costly interventions.[92] Many of the pharmacologic interventions that have the potential to manage coronary artery disease are listed in Table 18-5.

Table 18-5 also lists other medical interventions that all have the potential to (1) decrease the work of the heart, (2) decrease the amount of blockage in a coronary artery, or (3) provide new "plumbing" to the myocardium of a person with cardiac pump dysfunction. It is important to note that pharmacologic agents combined with optimal cardiac rehabilitation services have the potential to decrease the work of the heart and blockage in a coronary artery as well as improve myocardial blood flow.[93–95]

The first goals of medical treatment of persons with cardiac muscle dysfunction are to decrease the work of the heart and to decrease the amount of blockage in a coronary artery. Pharmacologic agents accomplish the aforementioned goals by decreasing the preload, afterload, and heart rate. In view of this, β-adrenergic blockers are a class of drugs frequently used to treat patients with coronary artery disease due to the reduction in both afterload and heart rate (see Chapter 8 for more information regarding β-adrenergic blockers). If this and other forms of medical treatment are ineffective in controlling the signs and symptoms of coronary artery disease, many

patients undergo PTCA with and without stenting and experience results that are somewhat inconclusive.[91,92] These results are shown in Table 18-6.[92]

Medical Interventions for Cardiac Pump Failure

The medical interventions for cardiac pump failure are also listed in Table 18-5 and have the potential to either (1) decrease venous return and decrease the work of the heart or (2) improve the work of the heart.[96] The methods to attain these goals are quite different from one intervention to another as is evident in Table 18-5. However, all of the medical interventions listed for the treatment of cardiac pump failure in Table 18-5 decrease the work of the heart and improve the work of the heart.

Utilization of Specific Tests and Measures to Direct Therapeutic Intervention

The medical treatment of patients with heart disease is based on the results of numerous tests and measures of which the preceding signs and symptoms of cardiac pump dysfunction and failure are instrumental in prescribing physical therapy.[57] Each of these tests and measures are thoroughly discussed in Chapter 10, but the method to use the results of these tests and measurements to direct and provide physical therapy will be discussed here.

CLINICAL CORRELATE

The most useful measurements to categorize patients with cardiac pump dysfunction or failure and provide physical therapy appear to be ejection fraction, electrocardiographic signs of myocardial ischemia, blood pressure monitoring during exercise, estimated or measured MET level achieved during an exercise test, and the blood pressure response to a controlled expiratory maneuver.[2–10,57]

The blood pressure response to a controlled expiratory maneuver (Fig. 18-3) may also be valuable when providing specific interventions to patients with cardiac pump dysfunction and failure. Recently, the medical treatment of persons with heart failure has been directed by evaluating the arterial blood pressure response during a controlled expiratory maneuver.[2–10] A patient with a blood pressure response like that in Figure 18-3 (indicating a failing cardiovascular pump) would receive medical treatments like digoxin, diuretics, and afterload reducers to improve the cardiac pump by (1) decreasing the venous return and fluid volume and (2) improving the force of myocardial contraction. These effects appear to improve cardiovascular and functional performance of patients with CHF and even improve the arterial blood pressure response

TABLE 18-5 Medical Interventions for Cardiac Pump Dysfunction and Failure

	Description	Outcome
Medical interventions for cardiac pump dysfunction		
Pharmacologic agents		
NTG	Venous dilation	Decrease venous return and work of heart
Calcium channel blockers	Reduce smooth mm contraction	Decrease smooth mm contraction in CA and PA
β-Blockers	Reduce HR and BP	Decrease work of the heart
ACE inhibitors	Afterload reduction	Decrease work of the heart
Cholesterol-lowering drugs	Decrease lipids	Decrease CA plaque
Aspirin	Platelet inhibition	Decrease CA thrombosis
Comprehensive cardiac rehabilitation	Ex., psych, social, dietary interventions	Risk factor reduction with decreased morbidity and mortality
PTCA with or without stenting	Inflation of a balloon at the end of a catheter to compress CA plaque against the wall of the CA with or without wire mesh compressed into the CA wall	Reduction in the size of the CA plaque, but often with residual stenosis or reocclusion of the CA
Atherectomy	Atherosclerotic plaque "shaved off" the wall of the CA much like a carpenters planer	Reduction in the size of the CA plaque, but often with residual stenosis or reocclusion of the CA
Rotobladder	"Roto-Rooter Unclogging" of CA blockage by boring through stenosis with an auger-like device attached to the tip of a catheter	Reduction in the size of the CA plaque, but often with residual stenosis or reocclusion of the CA
CABG, MID-CABG, or off-pump CABG	Saphenous vein, mammary artery, radial artery grafting around CA blockage	Improved blood flow to myocardium via "new plumbing," but occasionally with residual stenosis or reocclusion
Laser to coronary arteries or myocardial tissue	Laser beam directed at CA blockage or to areas of LV with reduced blood flow	Reduction in the size of the CA plaque or laser-induced injury to the LV which is believed to stimulate collateral artery growth and improve myocardial blood flow
Medical interventions for cardiac pump failure		
Pharmacologic agents		
NTG	Venous dilation	Decrease venous return and work of the heart Decrease work of the heart
β-Blockers	Reduce HR and BP	Decrease work of the heart
Diuretics	Increase urinary output	Decrease venous return and work of the heart
ACE inhibitors	Afterload reduction	Decrease work of the heart
Digoxin	Increase inotropy	Increase cardiac output
Intra-aortic balloon pump	Balloon in the descending aorta which deflates during systole and inflates during diastole	Deflation of balloon during systole "sucks" blood from the failing LV to improve cardiac output and inflation of the balloon during diastole improves myocardial blood flow reducing ischemic myocardium
LVAD/RVAD/BiVAD	Mechanical assistance with ventricular pumping	Improves cardiac output which improves the disablement of cardiac pump failure
Cardiac transplantation	Donor heart provided to a patient with end-stage heart failure	Improved morbidity, mortality, and disablement compared to cardiac pump failure, but with adverse effects of immunosuppressive therapy and rejection
Artificial heart	Mechanical heart replaces the failing heart	Improved cardiac performance for a limited period of time

NTG, nitroglycerin; CA, coronary artery; ACE, angiotensin-converting enzyme; PTCA, percutaneous transluminal coronary angioplasty; CABG, coronary artery bypass graft; LV, left ventricle; LVAD, left ventricular assist device; RVAD, right ventricular assist device; BiVAD, biventricular assist device; PA, pulmonary artery; HR, heart rate; BP, blood pressure.

during a controlled expiratory maneuver (yielding a more normal response similar to that in Figure 18-3A).[2-10]

Therefore, initial measurement of blood pressure during a controlled expiratory maneuver may be the most clinically efficacious method to categorize a patient with a failing cardiac pump or a dysfunctional cardiac pump (see Chapter 10 and Fig. 18-3) from which a hypothesis-oriented algorithm can be developed (Fig. 18-4). Maintenance of the systolic blood pressure during a controlled expiratory maneuver (Fig. 18-4)

indicates that the cardiac pump is failing and prefers to have less venous return. A decrease in systolic blood pressure during a controlled expiratory maneuver indicates that the cardiac pump is either normal or dysfunctional and prefers to have an increased venous return.

Other specific tests and measures that would categorize a patient with cardiac pump dysfunction include an ejection fraction between 30% and 50%, exercise-induced myocardial ischemia, a functional capacity of less than or equal to 5 or

TABLE 18-6   Invasive Versus Noninvasive Treatment of Stable CAD

Study Acronym	N	Severity of CAD	Study Design	Outcomes[a]
ACME	212	1-vessel CAD	Med. Rx vs PTCA	PTCA improved exercise tolerance and decreased need for antianginal medications, but without decrease in clinical events
ACME2	101	2-vessel CAD	Med. Rx vs PTCA	No benefit of PTCA over medical treatment
ACIP	558	Ischemia suitable for revascularization	Med. Rx vs CABG	CABG was associated with better event-free survival
MASS	214	Prox. LAD stenosis	Med. Rx vs PTCA vs. CABG	CABG was associated with better event-free survival
RITA2	1,018	1- to 2-vessel CAD	Med. Rx vs PTCA	PTCA was associated with fewer MIs
AVERT	341	1- to 2-vessel CAD	Med. Rx vs PTCA	Strong trend for fewer events in the patients receiving Med. Rx
COURAGE	3260	1- to 3-vessel CAD (mL/kg/min)	Med. Rx vs Med. Rx + PTCA	GET results—it just finished and an abstract should be in Circ Associated with greater potential for training
Belardinelli	94	Thallium uptake score index	<2.0	Normal thallium uptake to a moderate reduction in uptake with a score index <2.0 indicating less myocardial ischemia and the possible likelihood for greater safety and training
Belardinelli	94	$\dot{V}o_2$ @ VT (mL/kg/min)	>10 mL/kg/min	Less cardiac events if VT >10 mL/kg/min possibly due to a healthier cardiorespiratory system

CAD, coronary artery disease; Med. Rx, medical treatment; PTCA, percutaneous transluminal coronary angioplasty; LAD, left anterior descending coronary artery; MIs, myocardial infarctions; VT, ventilatory threshold; $\dot{V}o_2$, oxygen consumption.

[a]Success, improvement in disablement (cardiovascular or pulmonary function, exercise tolerance, aerobic capacity, functional performance, disability), completion of cardiac rehabilitation program, and absence of complications.

6 METs with a history of heart disease, a hypertensive blood pressure response, nonmalignant arrhythmias, and dyspnea and fatigue with a history of heart disease.[57]

Other tests and measures that would categorize a patient as having cardiac pump failure include an ejection fraction of less than 30%, complex ventricular arrhythmias, falling systolic blood pressure response to increased oxygen demand, functional capacity of less than or equal to 4 or 5 METs, marked exercise-induced myocardial ischemia, and marked dyspnea and fatigue in a person with evidence of a failing cardiac pump.[57]

Physical therapy intervention should incorporate methods of treatment that mimic the traditional medical therapy for persons with cardiac pump failure and dysfunction while increasing strength, endurance, and functional abilities. Utilization of body positions that decrease venous return and maximize ventilatory strategies are keys to improving the impairments, functional limitations, and disabilities associated with cardiac pump failure (associated with a well-maintained blood pressure during a controlled expiratory maneuver). Likewise, breathing exercises and possibly noninvasive positive-pressure ventilation at rest and during exercise may improve the disablement of cardiac pump failure.[25,97–103] Conversely, a decrease in blood pressure during a controlled expiratory maneuver indicates that the heart can very likely tolerate substantial increases in venous return from supine body positions, physical exercise, and other modalities or physical therapy treatments

that may increase venous return (eg, aquatic physical therapy in cold or lukewarm water).

The interventions for the patient with cardiac pump dysfunction are very similar to those for the patient with cardiac pump failure, but subtle differences in the application and progression of treatments exist (Fig. 18-4). The examination and treatment differences between these patients are shown in the decision tree for a patient categorized with a dysfunctional or failing cardiovascular pump.

CLINICAL CORRELATE

Patients with cardiac pump failure have been observed to train more effectively with one-legged cycling than with two-legged cycling (indicating that the patient with cardiac pump failure prefers to have a limited venous return).[104]

Conversely, patients with cardiac pump dysfunction or clients who have been identified as healthy with normal cardiac pump performance favor an increase in venous return which could be accomplished via two-legged cycling or a variety of other modes of exercise at higher exercise intensities.[79,105,106]

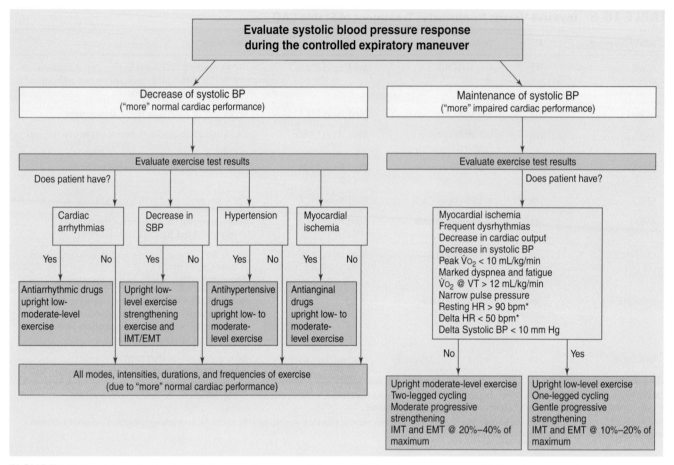

FIGURE 18-4   A hypothesis-oriented algorithm for the use of the controlled expiratory maneuver. IMT, inspiratory muscle trainer; EMT, expiratory muscle trainer.

Although patients with cardiac pump dysfunction can tolerate daily, high-intensity exercise reasonably well, the patient with cardiac pump failure is likely to train most effectively at lower exercise intensities, less often.[107–109]

CLINICAL CORRELATE

The frequency of exercise for a patient with cardiac pump failure may be best if prescribed every second or third day based on observations that patients with cardiac pump failure experience diastolic cardiac dysfunction for 24 hours or more after a single symptom-limited exercise test.[109]

However, there is little consensus regarding the intensity or duration of rehabilitative treatment for a person with a failing or dysfunctional cardiac pump.[108]

Although the medical management of persons with cardiovascular pump dysfunction and failure is similar with respect to the fundamental basis of treatment (eg, to decrease

the workload imposed on the heart often by decreasing venous return) particular results of different tests and measures can more clearly direct physical therapy. Some of the additional tests and measures include the observation of a decrease in the cardiac output and systolic blood pressure during exercise, an elevated resting heart rate, electrocardiographic evidence of myocardial ischemia or cardiac arrhythmias, and a low level of peak oxygen consumption (Table 18-7).[75,88,90,106,110–115] Utilization of the test results in Table 18-7 can better direct the specific intervention, frequency of intervention, and outcomes for a patient with cardiovascular pump dysfunction and failure.

The specific interventions for patients with specific threshold behaviors suffering from cardiovascular pump dysfunction and failure outlined in the branching diagram of Fig. 18-4 are based on peer-reviewed published research.[2–10,75,88,90,106,110–166] The initial branching is dependent on the arterial blood pressure response to a controlled expiratory maneuver and the remaining branches are dependent on many of the threshold behaviors listed in Box 18-1 and Table 18-7.[2–10,75,88,90,106,110–166] Subtle adjustments in the exercise prescription of patients with cardiac pump dysfunction and failure may improve the outcomes of patients in both subgroups. The methods to provide these subtle adjustments in the exercise prescription will be discussed in the following sections.

TABLE 18-7 Possible Predictors of Success or Failure of Patients with Cardiac Pump Dysfunction in Cardiac Rehabilitation[a]

Author	N	Baseline Study Predictor	Possible Threshold for Success	Rationale
Arvan[111]	65	Ejection fraction and myocardial ischemia	Ejection fraction > 40% with and without myocardial ischemia	Patients with an ejection fraction >40% appear to better tolerate episodes of myocardial ischemia and develop training adaptations, whereas patients with an ejection fraction <40% with myocardial ischemia (MI) developed fewer training adaptations
Digenio et al.[112]	171	Systolic and diastolic myocardial function and myocardial ischemia	None—patients with varying degrees of systolic and diastolic function and myocardial ischemia were all successful in cardiac rehabilitation	Because patients with varying degrees of systolic and diastolic function and myocardial ischemia developed training adaptations, the authors were unable to identify one of more predictors of success in cardiac rehabilitation
Vanhees et al.[115]	417	$\dot{V}_{O_{2peak}}$[b]	A 2% decrease in cardiovascular mortality was associated with every 1% increase in $\dot{V}_{O_{2peak}}$	Improved fitness and cardiovascular health via exercise training improved cardiovascular mortality
Vanhees et al.[115]	527	$\dot{V}_{O_{2peak}}$ expressed in METs	Attainment of 7 METs was associated with lower all-cause and cardiovascular mortality	Greater fitness was associated with improved all-cause and cardiovascular mortality in patients with MI and/or CABG
Vanhees et al.[115]	63	Atrial fibrillation	Presence or absence of atrial fibrillation	Cardiac patients with and without atrial fibrillation developed training adaptations
Wilson[90]	32	Cardiac output	Maintenance during exercise	Improved peripheral and central blood flow
Wilson[90]	32	Heart rate (HR) and mean arterial pressure (MAP)	Greater difference between rest and peak exercise HR and MAP (>50 bpm and 5 mm Hg, respectively)	A greater difference between rest and peak exercise HR and mean arterial pressure may be suggestive of a less impaired cardiovascular system which may be more likely to improve
Wielenga et al.[88]	80	Modified Naughton exercise test	Exercise test duration >7 min	Better conditioned which may be associated with greater potential for training
Meyer et al.[110]	18	$\dot{V}_{O_2}$/kg @ VT (% predicted maximum)	<30% predicted maximum	Marked deconditioning which may be more likely to improve
Meyer et al.[110]	18	$\dot{V}_{O_{2peak}}$ (mL/kg/min)	<12 mL/kg/min	Marked deconditioning which may be more likely to improve
Belardinelli et al.[133,134]	94	$\dot{V}_{O_{2peak}}$ (mL/kg/min)	>11.3 mL/kg/min	Better conditioned which may be associated with greater potential for training
Belardinelli et al.[133,134]	94	Thallium uptake score index	<2.0	Normal thallium uptake to a moderate reduction in uptake with a score index <2.0 indicating less myocardial ischemia and the possible likelihood for greater safety and training
Belardinelli et al.[133,134]	94	$\dot{V}_{O_2}$ at VT (mL/kg/min)	>10 mL/kg/min	Less cardiac events if VT >10 mL/kg/min possibly due to a healthier cardiorespiratory system

[a]Success, improvement in disablement (cardiovascular or pulmonary function, exercise tolerance, aerobic capacity, functional performance, disability), completion of cardiac rehabilitation program, and absence of complications.

[b]$\dot{V}_{O_{2peak}}$, peak oxygen consumption; VT, ventilatory threshold.

Exercise Training: Management of Pathology, Impairments, Functional Abilities, Disability, and Quality of Life in Persons with Cardiac Pump Dysfunction

The results of numerous studies of persons with cardiac pump dysfunction reveal the important role of exercise training in improving the pathology, impairments, functional abilities, disability, and quality of life. Perhaps the most important evidence documenting the role of exercise training and cardiac rehabilitation for patients with cardiac pump dysfunction are the results of several meta-analyses of exercise training in patients with coronary artery disease and the United States Cardiac Rehabilitation Guidelines (USCRG) document.[93,116–118] The USCRG outlined and categorized the strength of the evidence for cardiac rehabilitation on the disablement of patients with cardiac pump dysfunction. The

BOX 18-9

Effects of Cardiac Rehabilitation on Disablement

Effects of exercise training on improving	Strength of evidence
1. Exercise tolerance—increases ex.* ability safely	A
2. Strength training—increases strength safely	B
3. Exercise habits—promotes short-term ex. Participation	B
4. Symptoms—decreases angina and CHF symptoms	B
5. Smoking cessation—little to no effect	B
6. Lipids—inconsistent effect on lipid management	B
7. Body weight—not recommended as sole intervention	C
8. Blood Pressure—inconsistent effect on hypertension	B
9. Psychological well-being—enhances physiological functioning	B
10. Social adjustment and functioning—improves both areas	B
11. Return to work—not recommended as sole intervention	A
12. Morbidity and safety—safe and no effect on morbidity	A
13. Mortality and safety—safe and reduced mortality	B
14. Regression/limit of CAD—not recommended as sole intervention	A and B†
15. Coronary collateralization—does not promote collateralization	B
16. Myocardial perfusion/ischemia—decreases myocardial ischemia	B
17. Myocardial contractility—very little effect on contractility	B

	Strength of evidence
18. Cardiac arrhythmias—inconsistent effects on arrhythmias	B
19. Congestive heart failure—improves function and symptoms	A
20. Cardiac transplantation—improves ex. Tolerance	B
21. Elderly patients—develops training adaptations safely	B

Effects of education, counseling, and behavioral Interventions on improving	Strength of evidence
1. Smoking cessation—combined interventions recommended	B
2. Lipids—combined interventions improve lipids	B
3. Body weight—combined interventions reduce body weight	B
4. Blood pressure—not recommended as sole intervention	B
5. Exercise tolerance—not recommended as sole intervention	C
6. Symptoms—alone or combined reduces angina	B
7. Return to work—does not improve rates of return to work	C
8. Stress and psychological well-being—alone or combined improves both	A
9. Morbidity—ineffective in altering morbidity as sole intervention	B
10. Mortality—reduces mortality and recommended as a combined intervention	B

Effects of organizational issues on improving	Strength of evidence
1. Patient participation via alternate approaches—safe and effective	A
2. Patient adherence—may improve adherence	C
3. Medical costs—cardiac rehabilitation is cost-effective	B

*ex., exercise; CAD, coronary artery disease.
†Strength of evidence: A, for exercise training alone; B, for multifactorial intervention.

strength of the evidence for many domains of disablement was determined from the available literature and was based on the lettering criteria cited in the following and is shown in Box 18-9.[93]

- A = Scientific evidence provided by well-designed, well-conducted, controlled trials (randomized and nonrandomized) with statistically significant results that consistently support the guideline recommendation.
- B = Scientific evidence provided by observational studies or by controlled trials with less consistent results to support the guideline recommendation.

- C = Expert opinion that supports the guideline recommendation because the available scientific evidence did not present consistent results, or controlled trials were lacking.

Exercise Training: Management of Pathology, Impairments, Functional Abilities, Disability, and Quality of life in Persons with Cardiac Pump Failure

Historically, physical activity was restricted in persons with CHF. Patients were commonly confined to their homes and were restricted from cardiac rehabilitation. Even today, cardiac

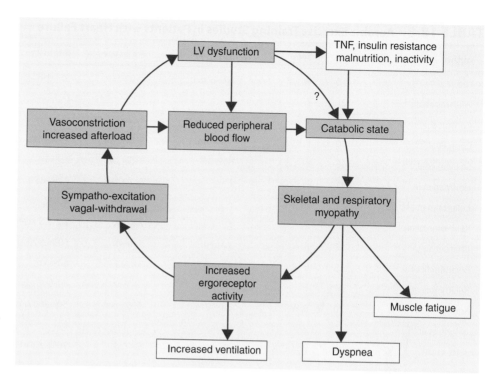

FIGURE 18-5 The muscle hypothesis of chronic heart failure. (Used with permission from Piepoli M, Clark A, Volterrani M, et al. Contribution of muscle afferents to the hemodynamic, autonomic, and ventilatory responses to exercise in patients with chronic heart failure. *Circulation.* 1996;93: 940-952.)

rehabilitation for patients with CHF is not reimbursed, yet it is these patients who may benefit the most from cardiac rehabilitation.[93] The following section will provide evidence of the important role exercise training and physical therapy have for patients with CHF.

A significant literature exists regarding the efficacy of cardiac rehabilitation in patients with NYHA class II–III heart failure.[75–90,119–152] The major areas which will be discussed in this section include the muscle hypothesis of chronic heart failure, aerobic exercise training (inpatient exercise, home exercise, and rehabilitation center exercise programs), strength training, breathing exercises, left ventricular assist device care, and heart failure clinic care for patients with heart failure. Tables 18-8 through 18-12 show the studies that have been performed in each of the previously cited areas.

The muscle hypothesis of chronic heart failure—is shown in Figure 18-5 and presents the interrelated manifestations of chronic heart failure.[153–156] Central to this conceptual model is the role of skeletal muscle. It is hypothesized that a reduction in peripheral blood flow to skeletal muscle contributes substantially to the vicious cycle of heart failure resulting in skeletal muscle catabolism, myopathy, increased ventilation, increased dyspnea and fatigue, sympathetic nervous system activation, vagal nervous system withdrawal, vascular constriction, and poorer left ventricular function.[153–156] It is important to note that vascular constriction (and the resultant increase in afterload) not only produces poorer left ventricular function, but also further diminishes peripheral blood flow to skeletal muscle. In fact, each of the above manifestations is intimately interrelated with the capacity to substantially worsen cardiovascular pump function if not managed and or treated. Properly pre-

scribed exercise is a key modality that has been suggested to manage and improve many of the manifestations of chronic heart failure shown in Figure 18-5.[153–156] The following sections will provide the rationale and methods that support the favorable role of exercise in addressing almost all of the manifestations of chronic heart failure.

Inpatient care—Several inpatient studies of aerobic exercise have been performed and have affirmed the safety of inpatient aerobic exercise training and significant improvements in many areas of disablement including symptoms, heart rate, exercise tolerance via exercise test or 6-minute walk test, and peak oxygen consumption.[80,119–122] **The exercise training programs in these studies consisted of flexibility exercises, cycle ergometry, and treadmill ambulation for an average of 30 minutes total, 3 to 5 days/wk for 2 to 4 weeks duration at 50% to 70% of peak cycle ergometry work rate and a mean of 2.4 mph on the treadmill.**

Home care—Aerobic exercise training in the home of heart failure patients has been performed safely in seven separate studies in which significant improvements have been observed in many areas of disablement including symptoms, heart rate, blood pressure, exercise tolerance via exercise test, and peak oxygen consumption.[75,77,89,121–124] One recent study demonstrated improved quality of life in patients with heart failure who exercised at home.[75] **The exercise training programs in these studies consisted of cycle ergometry or walking for an average of 20 to 60 minutes, 3 to 7 days/wk for 2 to 6 months duration at 50% to 80% of peak heart rate or oxygen consumption.**

Rehabilitation center care—The majority of studies investigating aerobic exercise training have been performed in

TABLE 18-8   Aerobic Exercise Training Studies in Patients with Heart Failure

Author	N	Type[a]	Duration	Frequency	Intensity	Period	Effect
Lee et al.[125]	18	W, J, B	20–45 min	2–6×/wk	85% HR_{max}	12–42 mo	Positive
Williams et al.[126]	121	?	?	?	?	2–57 mo	Positive
Cody et al.[127]	32	?	?	4×/wk	?	12 mo	Positive
Conn et al.[128]	10	B, W/J	35–45 min	3–5×/wk	70%–80%	4–37 mo	Positive
Sullivan et al.[129]	16	W, J, B	60 min	3–5×/wk	75% $\dot{V}O_{2max}$	4–6 mo	Positive
Hoffman et al.[130]	41	?	?	3–7×/wk	70%–85%	4 mo	Positive
Kellerman et al.[131,132]	11	AE	?	2×/wk	90%	36 mo	Positive
Kellerman et al.[131,132]	11	C	?	2×/wk	2.2–7.5 kcal/min	12 mo	Positive
Coats et al.[71]	17	B	20 min	5×/wk	60%–80% HR_{max}	2 mo	Positive
Belardinelli et al.[133,134b]	55	B	40 min	3×/wk	60% $\dot{V}O_{2max}$	2 mo	Positive
Belardinelli et al.[133,134]	27	B	30 min	3×/wk	40% $\dot{V}O_{2max}$	2 mo	Positive
Squires et al.[135]	20	B, W	30–40 min	4–6×/wk	50%–60% $\dot{V}O_{2max}$	2 mo	Positive
Baigrie et al.[136]	17	W	16 min	?	?	4 mo	Positive
Jette et al.[120]	39	W, J, C, B	30–60 min 2×/d	5×/wk	70%–80% HR_{max}	1 mo	Positive
Meyer et al.[119]	15	B	20–25 min	5×/wk	70%–80% HR_{max}	1.5 mo	Positive
Hambrecht et al.[121]	22	B	10 min 6×/d for 3 wk; then 40–60 min	7×/wk	70% $\dot{V}O_{2max}$	6 mo	Positive
Kulavuori et al.[139]	20	B	30 min	3×/wk	50%–60% $\dot{V}O_{2max}$	3 mo	Positive
Davey et al.[140]	22	B	20 min	5×/wk	70%–80% HR_{max}	2 mo	Positive
Koch et al.[141]	25	K	90 min	3×/wk	?	3 mo	Positive
Kostis et al.[76]	20	W, B, RW, SC	60 min	3–5×/wk	40%–60% functioning capacity	3 mo	Positive
Meyer et al.[81c]	18	B, W	15 min[c]	3–5×/wk	50% WORKmax[c]	3 wk	Positive
Kavanagh et al.[78c,d]	30	W	26–48 min	5×/wk	50%–60% $\dot{V}O_{2max}$	12 mo	Positive
Tyni-Lenne et al.[79c,d]	21	B	15 min	3×/wk	I:35%WORKmax II:70%WORKmax	2 mo	Positive Positive[c]
Flynn et al.[152]	2331	Multiple modes	30 min	3×/wk	75–85% $\dot{V}O_{2max}$	3 mo	Positive

The question mark in the table indicates unknown or data not reported.

[a]Type of exercise codes: IT, interval training; W, walking; J, jogging; B, bicycling; R, running; SR, stationary running; K, Koch device (strength and endurance cycling); RW, rowing; G, gymnastics; W/J, walking/jogging; SC, stair climbing; AE, arm ergometry; C, calisthenics.

[b]First study to evaluate the effects of exercise training in patients with diastolic dysfunction.

[c]Bicycling exercise was performed 5×/wk for 15 minutes in an interval manner with work phases of 30 seconds at 50% of the maximal work rate achieved and active recovery phases of 60 seconds during which patients pedaled at 15 W. Walking exercise was performed 3×/wk for 10 minutes in an interval manner with work phases of 60 seconds (mean treadmill speed = 2.4 mph) and 60 seconds of active recovery (mean treadmill speed = 0.9 mph).

[d]First studies to evaluate the quality of life of persons with heart failure before and after exercise training. Improvements in quality of life and beneficial training effects were observed in both studies.

Adapted with permission from Cahalin LP. Cardiac muscle dysfunction. In: Hillegass E, Sadowsky HS, eds. *Essentials of Cardiopulmonary Physical Therapy*. Philadelphia, PA: WB Saunders; 2001:153.

supervised rehabilitation centers. These studies have consistently shown that aerobic exercise training can be performed safely with significant improvements in many areas of disablement including symptoms, heart rate, blood pressure, exercise tolerance via exercise test or 6-minute walk test, peak oxygen consumption, and recently, quality of life.[75,76,78–88,90,106,110–122,125–152] **The exercise training programs in these studies consisted of a variety of modes of exercise (however, cycling was the most frequent mode) for 20 to 60 minutes, 3 to 7 days/wk for 1 to 57 months duration at 40% to 90% of peak heart rate or oxygen consumption.**

The results of the multicenter HF-Action trial of cardiac rehabilitation in persons with heart failure demonstrated nonsignificant effects of cardiac rehabilitation on all-cause mortality,

TABLE 18-9 Strength Training Studies in Patients with Heart Failure

Study	Sample Size and Characteristics	Design	Intervention	Clinically Significant or Statistically Significant Outcomes	Area Affected in Muscle Hypothesis
Koch et al.[141]	Exercise group $N = 25$ (19 men, 6 women) Age: 55 ± 10 y Ejection fraction: 26 ± 11% $\dot{V}O_{2peak}$: 19 ± 6.5 mL/kg/min NYHA: 2.4 ± .5 Control group ($N = 13$): details were not reported	RT	*Exercise protocol:* RT[a] (via KOCH bench; Genin Medical) for 90 min over a 12-wk study period; the frequency and intensity of RT/wk was not reported	Significant improvement in exercise duration and quality of life with an increase in skeletal muscle strength, but it was not reported if the increase from 77 ± 20 kg to 112 ± 24 kg was statistically significant; there was no change in myocardial function nor complications from RT	• Skeletal muscle • Catabolic state • Possible increase in activity which may decrease deconditioning
Pu et al.[162]	Sample size: 16 (all women) Age: 76.6 ± 2 y Ejection fraction: 36.3 ± 2.7% $\dot{V}O_{2peak}$: 15.46 ± 1.04 mL/kg/min NYHA: 2.2 ± 0.1	RT	**RT group ($N = 9$):** *Exercise protocol:* 80% of 1-RM for 10 wk (3×/wk for 60 min each session) *Exercises:* pneumatic-resistance using seated leg press, chest press, knee extension, triceps, and knee flexion **Control group ($N = 7$):** 60 min of low-intensity stretching exercises to the neck, trunk, and extremities	Significant improvement in muscle strength and endurance as well as 6-minute walk test distance ambulated in the RT group Near significant improvement in the treadmill time to exhaustion (80% of each subject's habitual gait speed for 2 min at 0% grade followed by 2% increase in treadmill grade every minute) and type I muscle fiber cross-sectional area in the RT group ($p = 0.06$ and $p = 0.08$, respectively)	• Skeletal muscle • Catabolic state • Possible increase in activity which may decrease deconditioning • Possible Ergoreflex due to near significant improvement in type I muscle fiber cross-sectional area
Maiorana et al.[159]	Sample size: 13 (all men) Age: 60 ± 2 y EF: 26 ± 3% $\dot{V}O_{2peak}$: approximately 20.0 mL/kg/min NYHA: 1–3	RT with ST AE	**RT Period ($N = 12,13$)[11,12]:** *Exercise protocol:* 55%–65% of 1-RM for 8 wk (3×/wk for 60 min each session); progression based on retesting of strength during first 2–3 wk; 1–3 sets of 15 reps *Exercises:* dual seated leg press, left and right hip extension, seated abdominal flexion, dual leg flexion, dual pectoral flexion, and dual shoulder extension; the methods used to determine 1-RM were not reported *Endurance training:* 45 s of cycling at 70%–85% of peak heart rate; treadmill walking for 5 min at 70%–85% of the peak heart rate **Control period ($N = 12, 13$)[11,12]:** crossover design during which subjects did no formal exercise	Significant improvement in peak reactive hyperemic blood flow, forearm vascular resistance, forearm blood flow, forearm blood flow ratio, and peak oxygen consumption during the RT period	• Skeletal muscle • Vasodilation and decreased afterload • Increase peripheral blood flow • Possible increase in activity, which may decrease deconditioning • Possible catabolic state due to improved peripheral blood flow • Possible Ergoreflex due to improved $\dot{V}O_{2peak}$ and forearm blood flow

(continued)

TABLE 18-9 **Strength Training Studies in Patients with Heart Failure (Continued)**

Study	Sample Size and Characteristics	Design	Intervention	Clinically Significant or Statistically Significant Outcomes	Area Affected in Muscle Hypothesis
Selig et al.	Sample size: 39 (33 men, 6 women) Age: 65 ± 11 y EF: 28 ± 7% $\dot{V}o_{2peak}$: not reported NYHA: 2.4 ± .5	RT with ST AE	**RT group (N = 19):** *Exercise protocol:* 12 wk (3×/wk) 3 hydraulic resistance exercises were each performed for 30 seconds; the methods used to determine maximal muscle strength were not thoroughly reported *Exercises:* elbow extension/flexion, knee extension/flexion, and shoulder press/pull *Endurance training:* either leg cycling, stair climbing, or arm cycling performed at moderate intensity via heart rate, but no specific intensity was reported; 5-min warm-up and cool-down periods consisting of gentle aerobic exercise and stretching were performed **Control group (N = 20):** usual care without change in activity level	Significant improvement in strength (however, no report of the shoulder press/pull was provided) and endurance, oxygen consumption, forearm blood flow, and heart rate variability in the RT group	• Peripheral blood flow • Skeletal muscle • Catabolic state • Possible Ergoreflex due to improved $\dot{V}o_{2peak}$ and forearm blood flow • Possible LV dysfunction due to improved heart rate variability
Hare et al.[157]	Sample size: 9 (all men) Age: 63 ± 11 y EF: 26 ± 6% $\dot{V}o_2$: 17.6 ± 1.6 mL/kg/min NYHA: 2.4	RT with ST AE	**RT & AE group (N = 9):** *Exercise protocol:* 11-wk circuit training program using a hydraulic resistance system[b] with 3 activities done for a 30–60 s duration *Exercises:* chest push-pull, knee extension/flexion; shoulder push-pull *Endurance:* RT was interspersed with 1–2 min of stair climbing, stationary cycling, arm cycling **Control group** This was a prospective, uncontrolled observational study	Significant improvement in basal forearm blood flow, skeletal muscle strength and endurance with an increase in total work for chest pull, chest push, and knee extension	• Peripheral blood flow • Skeletal muscle • Catabolic state • Possible Ergoreflex due to improved forearm blood flow
Magnusson et al.[161]	Sample size: 11 (9 men, 2 women; gender makeup of groups not reported) Age = 56 ± 9 y EF = 19.8 ± 11.3% $\dot{V}o_{2peak}$ = 15.1 ± 2.9 mL/kg/min NYHA = 2.6 ± 0.7	RT with ST AE	**RT group (N = 5):** *Exercise protocol:* 3 days/wk for 8 wk. 4 sets/6–10 reps/80% of 1-RM for 45 min[c] *Exercise:* leg extension **AE group (N = 6):** aerobic exercise consisted of cycling at 65%–75% of absolute one-legged peak workload for 45 min **Control group:** this was a novel study which employed one leg of one group of individuals to perform no exercise while the other leg performed RT; the other group of individuals performed AE with one leg while the other leg performed AE and RT	Significant improvement in exercise intensity, dynamic and isometric strength, and cross-sectional area of biceps femoris after RT; significant increases in the oxidative enzyme activity in m. vastus lateralis (above 50%), capillary per fiber ratio of m. vastus lateralis, and peak dynamic knee extensor work after endurance training	• Skeletal muscle • Vasculature • Catabolic state • Dyspnea due to improved oxidative enzyme activity • Possible Ergoreflex due to improved oxidative enzyme activity

Cider et al.	RT with ST AE	Sample size: 24 (16 men, 8 women) Age = 63 + 7.5 y EF = not reported $\dot{V}O_{2peak}$ = 14.3 + 6.3 mL/kg/min NYHA = 2.5 ± 0.5	**RT group (N = 12):** *Exercise protocol:* 60% 1-RM, 30 RT rep/min for 60 min; $3\times$/wk; muscle strength and endurance were measured isokinetically at 60 and 180 degrees/s, respectively, with subjects seated. Endurance was measured at 180 degrees/s with patients performing 50 repeated muscle contractions[d] *Exercises:* shoulder flexion, abduction, elbow flexion; knee flexion and extension *Circuit:* stretching exercises and functional tasks (heel raises, sit to stand, etc) **Control group (N = 12):** nontraining group	Significant improvement in the anaerobic threshold, the patients' ability to lift weights and performance of heel-lift	• Skeletal muscle • Catabolic state • Function/exercise tolerance • Possible increase in activity, which may decrease deconditioning • Possible Ergoreflex due to improvement in the anaerobic threshold
Levinger et al.	RT	Sample size: 15 (all men) Age = 57 ± 10 y EF = 34.7 ± 7.2% $\dot{V}O_{2peak}$ = 14.6 ± 2.3 mL/kg/min NYHA = 2.5 ± 0.5	**RT group (N = 8):** *Exercise Protocol:* 50 min of RT at 40%–60% of maximal strength (with one set of 15–20 repetitions) initially which was progressed to 80%–90% of maximal strength (with three sets of 8–12 repetitions); $3\times$/wk for 8 wk.[e] *Exercises:* chest press, leg press, lateral pull-down, triceps extension, knee extension, upright row, sitting row, and biceps curl, and abdominal curl **Control group (N = 7):** nontraining group	Significant improvement in skeletal muscle strength, walking time, peak oxygen consumption, quality of life, left ventricular fractional shortening, and left ventricular ejection fraction in the RT group.	• Skeletal muscle • Catabolic state • Function/exercise tolerance • Possible increase in activity, which may decrease deconditioning • Possible Ergoreflex due to improved $\dot{V}O_{2peak}$
Grosse et al.	RT	Sample size: 27 (22 men, 5 women) Age = 57 ± 8 y EF = 27 ± 10.5% $\dot{V}O_{2peak}$ = 12.6 ± 3.6 mL/kg/min NYHA = 3.0 ± 0.5	**RT group (N = 14):** *Exercise protocol:* wrist and ankle weights used $2\times$/wk (2–3 sets of 15 reps with a 2-min rest) for 12 wk to strengthen the biceps brachealis, quadriceps femoris, triceps, and biceps femoris Measurement of maximal strength did not appear to be performed, but wrist and ankle weights were provided to patients at an intensity that made it difficult for the patients to do 2–3 sets of 15 reps with the weights being increased to maintain difficulty *Exercises:* elbow flexion and extension and knee flexion and extension **Control group (N = 13):** nontraining group	Significant improvement in skeletal muscle strength, peak oxygen consumption, NYHA class, ergometric efficiency, and resting heart rate without complication or adverse event	• Skeletal muscle • Catabolic state • Function/exercise tolerance • Possible increase in activity, which may decrease deconditioning • Possible Ergoreflex due to improved $\dot{V}O_{2peak}$

(continued)

TABLE 18-9 Strength Training Studies in Patients with Heart Failure (*Continued*)

Study	Sample Size and Characteristics	Design	Intervention	Clinically Significant or Statistically Significant Outcomes	Area Affected in Muscle Hypothesis
Witham et al.	Sample size: 82 (45 men, 37 women) Age = 80 ± 5 y EF = not reported, but LV systolic function was reported as mild, moderate, or severe with each representing 35%, 30%, and 35% of the study population $\dot{V}O_{2peak}$ = not measured NYHA = class 2 = 46 subjects, class 3 = 36 subjects	RT	**RT group (N = 41; 26 men, 15 women):** *Exercise protocol:* 6-month study of 20-min of a supervised and home RT exercise program during weeks 1–12 (23×/wk) and weeks 13–24 (2–3×/wk), respectively, performed at an intensity of 11–13 using the Borg RPE scale during which a poorly described RT program was provided that consisted of upper and lower limb exercises as well as slow and fast whole body aerobic movements were performed with 500-g wrist and 1.1-kg ankle weights; RT was followed with 10 min of breathing exercises and relaxation[f] **Control group (N = 41; 19 men, 22 women):** nontraining usual care group	Significant improvement in daily activity measured via accelerometry, but no significant improvement in 6-minute walk test or quality of life	• Function/exercise tolerance • Increase in activity, which may decrease deconditioning
Feiereisen et al.	Sample size: 8 (number of men and women unreported) Age = not reported EF = 22.25 ± 6.5% $\dot{V}O_{2peak}$ = 14.3 ± 1.9 mL/kg/min NYHA = not reported	RT	**RT group (N = 8):** RT program not reported except that it was performed 3×/wk for 3 m Knee extensor strength and endurance were measured isokinetically at 60 and 180 degrees/s, respectively **Control group:** this was a prospective, uncontrolled observational study	Significant improvement in skeletal muscle strength and volume, left ventricular ejection fraction, peak oxygen consumption, and quality of life	• Skeletal muscle • Catabolic state • Function/exercise tolerance • Possible INCREASE in activity, which may decrease deconditioning • Possible Ergoreflex due to improved $\dot{V}O_{2peak}$
Resistance training combined with long-duration aerobic exercise Barnard et al.	Sample size: 21 (all male) Age: 58 ± 12 y Ejection fraction: 24 ± 9% $\dot{V}O_{2peak}$: 19 ± 9 mL/kg/min NYHA: not reported	RT with LT AE	**RT + AE group (N = 14):** *Exercise protocol:* 8-wk program: Strength training 2×/wk, Weeks 1–2: 60% 1-RM, 2 sets/12 reps; Weeks 3–4: 80% 1-RM 2 sets/8 reps; Weeks 5–8: max weight ensuring a max of 8 repetitions occurred. *RT exercises:* isokinetic RT using seated shoulder press, leg extension, lat pull-down, 2 arm biceps curl, and the horizontal squat.[9] AE: 30 minutes(15 min of cycling and 15 min of treadmill exercise) 3×/wk **AE group (N = 7):** Aerobic training only performed for 30 min (15 min of Schwinn Air Dyne cycling and 15 min of treadmill exercise) 3/wk at 60%–80% of maximum heart rate reserve and increased by 0.5 METs/wk	Significant improvement in strength in all RT exercises in only the RT+AE group. After the study period only the AE group was observed to have a significantly greater heart rate and rate pressure product during the 1-RM horizontal squat while that of the RT group was relatively unchanged (yielding less cardiac work). Also, no significant muscle soreness was reported in either group	• Skeletal muscle • Catabolic state • Possible increase in activity/function • Improvement in LV dysfunction in the RT + AE group

| Conradds et al. | RT with LT AE | Sample size: 41 (28 men, 13 women; the 23 patients in the training group consisted of 12 with CAD and 11 with IDCM)
Age: approximately 63 y
Ejection fraction: 27.5%
$\dot{V}o_{2peak}$: 18.7 ml/kg/min
NYHA: classes 1–2 = 11 subjects, classes 3–4 = 12 subjects; data for control group not reported | **RT & AE group (N = 23):**
Exercise protocol: 30 min of RT @ 50% of 1-RM, 2 sets of 10 reps/set, 3×/wk for 16 wk; the form of RT was not reported and the methods used to determine 1-RM were not reported
RT exercises: 9 RT exercises to muscle groups of lower and upper limbs and torso
AE: 20 min of cycling and/or jogging @ target HR of 90% of ventilatory threshold. RT and AE training modalities were alternated
Control group (N = 18):
Age and sex matched patients attending outpatient heart failure clinic served as untrained heart failure control group | Significant decrease in inflammatory cytokines (TNFR1 and TNFR2) in the CAD patients performing RT+AE. Significant increase in NYHA functional class and an improvement in submaximal and maximal work performance (greater peak Watts, $\dot{V}o_{2peak}$ and W/$\dot{V}o_2$) for the entire RT + AE group; however, only the CAD group was observed to have a significant increase in $\dot{V}o_{2peak}$ and $\dot{V}o_2$ @ the anaerobic threshold; skeletal muscle strength gains were not reported | • Skeletal muscle
• Catabolic state
• Function/exercise tolerance
• Possible increase in activity, which may decrease deconditioning
• TNFR levels
• Vasoconstriction (decreased TNFR leads to reversal of peripheral vascular endothelial dysfunction)
• Dyspnea and fatigue (higher $\dot{V}o_{2peak}$ levels and workrates at anaerobic threshold and peak exercise)
• Possible Ergoreflex due to improved $\dot{V}o_{2peak}$ |
| Sabelis et al. | RT with LT AE | Sample size: 61 (45 men, 16 women)
Age: 60±9 y
Ejection fraction: 26.9±8.1%
$\dot{V}o_{2peak}$: 19±4.8 mL/kg/min
NYHA: classes 2–3 | **RT & AE group (N = 36; 25 men, 11 women):**
Exercise protocol: 26 wk; four times per week, two times supervised and two times at home performed for 11 min each session
RT exercises[h]: poorly described strength training program (5BX of the Royal Canadian Air Force) for the abdominal, gluteal, posterior leg, and arm muscles that were performed continuously at home and during supervised sessions each of the exercises were performed for 1 min and were separated by 30 s of rest yielding 11 min of RT exercise; skeletal muscle strength did not appear to be tested
AE[h]: AE consisted of interval training via cycle ergometer at 50% of the maximum exercise capacity (obtained from a steep ramp exercise test, which was repeated every 4 wk) for 30 s of cycling and 60 seconds of rest which was repeated 10 times[h]
Control group (N = 25; 20 men, 5 women):
Patients were randomly assigned to a control group in which individuals were untrained | Significant increase in peak workload and oxygen consumption and a trend towards significance in increasing insulin sensitivity; 16 patients dropped out of the study (8 from each group) due to numerous reasons that the investigators stated were unrelated to the study (6 patients died, 3 patients could not be reassessed due to medical reasons, and 7 patients chose to not participate for personal reasons); skeletal muscle strength was not reported | • Skeletal muscle
• Catabolic state
• Function/exercise tolerance
• Possible increase in activity, which may decrease deconditioning
• Possible insulin resistance
• Possible Ergoreflex due to improved $\dot{V}o_{2peak}$ |

(continued)

TABLE 18-9 Strength Training Studies in Patients with Heart Failure (Continued)

Study	Sample Size and Characteristics	Design	Intervention	Clinically Significant or Statistically Significant Outcomes	Area Affected in Muscle Hypothesis
Stolen et al.	Sample size: 15 (13 men, 2 women) Age: 56 ± 6.5 y Ejection fraction: 34 ± 8% $\dot{V}o_{2peak}$: 20 ± 4.2 mL/kg/min NYHA: 1.3 ± 0.4	RT with LT AE	**RT & AE group (N = 8; 6 men, 2 women):** *Exercise protocol:* 5-month AE endurance and strength training program with 3 supervised and 2 home exercise sessions per week performed at a goal intensity and duration of 70% of $\dot{V}o_{2peak}$ and 45 min, respectively; RT was added 4 wk after the commencement of AE and consisted of 9 exercises/2 sets/15 reps for each muscle group; intensity was determined by RPE; measurement of skeletal muscle strength did not appear to occur *Exercises:* not reported **Control group (N = 7; all men)** 7 randomized untrained patients from original sample group	Significant improvement in peak oxygen consumption, body composition, insulin-stimulated myocardial fractional uptake and glucose uptake, whole-body insulin-stimulated glucose uptake, and serum free fatty acid levels	• Skeletal muscle • Catabolic state • Function/exercise tolerance • Possible increase in activity, which may decrease deconditioning • Insulin resistance • LV dysfunction • Possible Ergoreflex (from decreased fatty acid levels and improved $\dot{V}o_{2peak}$)
Delagardelle et al.[158]	Sample size: 14 (11 men, 3 women) Age: 57 ± 8 y Ejection fraction: 29 ± 2.7% $\dot{V}o_{2peak}$: 17.2 ± 1.04 mL/kg/min NYHA: 2.7 ± 0.1	RT with LT AE	**RT & AE group (N = 14):** *RT exercise protocol:* 6 mo of RT+ET performed 3×/wk for 60 min with 3 sets of 15 reps/set using 6 exercises (leg extensors and flexors, shoulder muscles, and abdominal muscles) performed at 60%–80% of 10-RM; skeletal muscle strength was measured via isokinetic testing; the specific methods used to determine 10-RM were not reported *RT exercises:* leg extensors and flexors were exercised via pulley weight system, shoulder muscles were exercised via shoulder abduction using dumb bells, and abdominal muscles were exercised via curl-up exercises; three sets of stair-climbing and throwing a medicine ball at a wall were also performed using 15 to 20 repetitions *AE:* 10 min of endurance cycling during first session that was replaced with walking at 60% to 75% of $\dot{V}o_{2peak}$ followed by 18 min of interval cycling from 50% to 75% of $\dot{V}o_{2peak}$ **Control group** This was a prospective, uncontrolled observational study	Significant improvement in knee flexor and extensor endurance, NYHA class, work capacity, and $\dot{V}o_{2peak}$; maximal exercise lactate production was observed to increase significantly; the increase of peak torque, total work, and average power reached statistical significance only for the knee extensors	• Skeletal muscle • Catabolic state • Function/exercise tolerance • Possible increase in activity, which may decrease deconditioning • Possibly Ergoreflex (via alteration of H+[lactate] and improved $\dot{V}o_{2peak}$)

Study	Intervention	Sample	Protocol	Results	Outcomes
Delagardelle et al.[158]	RT with LT AE	Sample size: 20 (all men) Age: approximately 58 y Ejection fraction: Approx. 28% $\dot{V}o_{2peak}$: approximately 18 mL/kg/min NYHA: approximately 2.6	**RT & AE group (N = 10):** *RT exercise protocol:* 12 wk of 20 min of RT (via 3 sets of 10 repetitions at 6 exercise stations performed at 60% of 1-RM) combined with 20 min of interval cycling 3×/wk; one repetition lasted 6 seconds with a 3-s concentric phase and 3 s eccentric phase resulting in a set being completed in 1 min (followed by a 1-min rest period between sets); strength was measured via 1-RM and reassessed after 6 wk; the specific methods used to determine 1-RM were not reported *RT exercises:* undefined type of weight machines used to exercise the quadriceps and biceps femoris, pectoral muscles (seated arm press), latissimus dorsi (pull down), rhomboids (rowing), and deltoids (lateral arm abduction using dumbbells) *AE:* 20 min of interval cycling performed 3×/wk at 50% of $\dot{V}o_{2peak}$ for 2 min followed by 2 min at 75% of $\dot{V}o_{2peak}$ **AE group (N = 10):** 40 min of interval cycling performed 3×/wk at 50% of $\dot{V}o_{2peak}$ for 2 min followed by 2 min at 75% of $\dot{V}o_{2peak}$	The combined RT & AE group was observed to have a significant improvement in NYHA class, peak work capacity, $\dot{V}o_{2peak}$, peak lactate production, peak skeletal muscle torque and endurance, LVEF, FS, and LVED	• LV dysfunction • Skeletal muscle • Catabolic state • Function/exercise tolerance • Possible increase in activity, which may decrease deconditioning • Possibly Ergoreflex (via alteration of H+[lactate] and improved $\dot{V}o_{2peak}$)
Oka et al.[203]	RT with LT AE	Sample size: 40 (31 men, 9 women) Age: not reported, but range = 30–76 y Ejection fraction: 23 ± 7% $\dot{V}o_{2peak}$: 18.6 ± 3.8 mL/kg/min NYHA = class 2 = 15 subjects, class 3 = 25 subjects	**RT & AE group (17 men, 3 women):** *RT exercise protocol:* poorly described 12-wk home-based RT program via an unreported mode of unilateral total body RT performed at 75% 1-RM, 2×/wk; the methods used to determine the 1-RM were not reported *AE:* home-based walking program at 70% of peak heart rate for 40–60 min, 3×/wk **Control Group (14 men, 6 women):** Subjects randomly assigned to usual care who met study criteria.	Significantly improved quality of life, level of fatigue, emotional function, and mastery/perceived control over symptoms. Improvement in dyspnea was near significance ($p = 0.08$); higher levels of adherence to AE vs RT was observed and no complications were observed during the study. No report of change in skeletal muscle strength, method of 1-RM testing, or progression of the RT program	• Fatigue • Possible increase in activity, which may decrease deconditioning • Dyspnea (trending towards significance) • Possible Ergoreflex due to near significant improvement in dyspnea

(continued)

TABLE 18-9 Strength Training Studies in Patients with Heart Failure (*Continued*)

Study	Sample Size and Characteristics	Design	Intervention	Clinically Significant or Statistically Significant Outcomes	Area Affected in Muscle Hypothesis
Haykowsky et al.	Sample size: 20 (all women) Age: 72 ± 8 y Ejection fraction: approximately 36 ± 20% $\dot{V}o_{2peak}$: approximately 12 ± 3 mL/kg/min NYHA: Class 1 = 1, Class 2 = 17 subjects, Class 3 = 2 subjects	RT with LT AE	**RT & AE group (N = 10):** *RT exercise protocol:* 24-wk program (supervised weeks 1–12 and unsupervised weeks 13–24) of AE vs AE + RT; supervised RT: consisted of 1–2 sets of vertical row, chest press, shoulder press, triceps pushdown, biceps curl, and leg press via unreported resistance or machine at 50%–70% of maximal strength (which was assessed via repetitive lifts with progressively heavier weights until a lift with smooth, full ROM was no longer possible using unreported commercially available equipment), 2×/wk **Unsupervised RT:** home RT consisting of 1–2 sets of upper and lower extremity RT exercises using light hand weights (2.5–4.5 kg) or leg weights (2.5 kg). 2×/wk AE:[l] **Supervised AE:** cycle ergometry 2×/wk at 60%–70% of heart rate reserve for 15–28 min **Unsupervised AE:** home cycle ergometry or walking 2×/wk at Borg RPE of 12–14 for 20–40 min	A comprehensive comparison between the RT+AE vs AE alone groups was not performed, but after the supervised portion of the study the combined RT+AE and AE groups were found to have a significant improvement in leg press strength and vertical rowing (although the one reported comparison between the RT+AE and AE groups found that only the vertical row of the RT+AE group was significantly greater) and $\dot{V}o_{2peak}$; no significant change in quality of life was observed After the unsupervised portion of the study the strength gains and improvements in $\dot{V}o_{2peak}$ returned to baseline except for the vertical row strength of the RT + AE group, which remained significantly greater than at baseline; one patient did not complete the study due to worsening CHF	• Skeletal muscle • Catabolic state • Function/exercise tolerance • Possible increase in activity, which may decrease deconditioning • Possible Ergoreflex due to improved $\dot{V}o_{2peak}$
Jonsdottir et al.	Sample size: 43 (34 men, 9 women) Age: 68 ± 6 y Ejection fraction: 41 ± 13.6% $\dot{V}o_{2peak}$: 15.6 ± 3 mL/kg/min NYHA: class 2 and 3, but the number of patients in each class was not reported	RT with LT AE	**RT & AE group (16 men, 5 women):** *RT + AE protocol:* 20 wk supervised RT + AE program which consisted of 10 min of warm-up exercises (breathing exercises and nonresistance arm and leg movements), 15 min of cycling at 50% of peak workload (which was progressed, but the specific method was not reported), and 20 min of circuit RT via Evient sequence equipment (from of RT not reported), free weights, and elastic rubber-bands (Thera-bands) at 20%–40% of 1-RM followed by 5 min of cool-down (stretching of exercised muscles), 2×/wk; the method used to determine 1-RM was "the heaviest weight lifted once through a full range of motion was the patient's 1-RM", but the process/methods used to achieve this weight was not reported **Control group (18 men, 4 women):** Subjects randomly assigned to usual care who met study criteria	Significant improvements in quadriceps muscle strength, 6-min walk test distance, peak cycle ergometry work load and cycling duration, and quality of life; no complications were observed during the study	• Skeletal muscle • Catabolic state • Function/exercise tolerance • Possible increase in activity, which may decrease deconditioning

Study			
Smith et al.[40]	Sample size: 1 woman Age: 54 y Ejection fraction: 19% $\dot{V}o_{2peak}$: 15.7 mL/kg/min NYHA: not reported	RT with LT AE	*RT+AE Protocol:* 12 wk (36 sessions) of AE and RT consisting of 15 min of treadmill ambulation and 15 min of Schwinn Air-Dyne exercise 3×/wk at 60%–80% of heart rate reserve with an increase of 0.5 METs/wk and progressive RT of 6 muscle groups at 50%–80% of 1-RM,[h] 2×/wk, respectively *RT exercises:* isokinetic RT (Trotter-Cybex Int, Inc) exercises via leg press, shoulder press, leg extension, lat pulldown, cable biceps curl, and horizontal squat. The number of repetitions and sets was not reported; the method of progressing the 2×/wk RT program is outlined below: Weeks 1–2: 60% of 1-RM[h] Week 3: 70% of 1-RM[h] Weeks 4–12: 80% of 1-RM[h] [h]1-RM was determined with a warm-up set of resistance at 50% of the pre-determined 1-RM followed by 3 sets at 70% of 1-RM (the number of repetitions was not reported)	28%–90% increase in strength in all muscle groups/exercises except for the shoulder press which was unchanged. 14% increase in METs, $\dot{V}o_{2peak}$ 35% increase in METs, and an increase in peak workload; no change in psychosocial or personality measurements the EF was unchanged with RT + AE, but examination of the EF via echocardiography during the leg press revealed a consistent increase from a baseline of 19% to 33%–39% during pre- and poststudy measurements • Skeletal muscle • Catabolic state • Function/exercise tolerance • Possible increase in activity, which may decrease deconditioning • Possible Ergoreflex due to improved $\dot{V}o_{2peak}$
Radzewitz et al.	Sample size: 88 (67 men, 21 women) Age: 65.8±8.2 y Ejection fraction: 31±8% $\dot{V}o_{2peak}$: 13.9±4.6 mL/kg/min NYHA: not reported	RT with LT AE	*RT + AE protocol:* 4 wk RT + AE program; moderate strength training via shuttle exercising device (semifowlers position leg press with resistance provided by rubber bands yielding specific units of measure [kg/path and muscle strength units; MST]) performed 2–3×/wk without information about repetitions, sets, or duration of the RT exercise; AE consisted of cycle ergometry at 60%–80% of $\dot{V}o_{2peak}$ for 15–20 min, 3×/wk and the 6-minute walk performed 2×/wk **Control group** This was a prospective, uncontrolled observational study	Significant improvement in skeletal muscle strength, LVEF, LVEDD, and quality of life, but without change in anxiety and depression; near significant improvement in $\dot{V}o_{2peak}$ ($p = 0.05$); decrease in the peak exercise RPP, but not statistically significant • LV dysfunction • Skeletal muscle • Catabolic state • Function/exercise tolerance • Possible increase in activity, which may decrease deconditioning

[a]The description of RT exercises was "they consisted of the building up of a small number of muscle groups at a time and simultaneously so as to avoid too much pressure on the heart. The load of each patient was chosen according to the results of the exercise test and the measurement of maximum muscular strength (MMS) which was measured by a dynamometer for each muscle group on position on the training bench." The MMS was measured four times during the study (after each patient completed 10 RT sessions) after which the RT program was progressed, but the progression nor the number of repetitions of RT were not reported.

[b]Muscle strength and endurance were measured isokinetically at 60 and 120/180 degrees/s, respectively, using three consecutive maximal repetitions (lower extremity endurance was measured at 180 degrees/s). The intensity of RT was not reported.

[c]Maximal concentric muscle strength was measured with free weights and was defined as the maximal weight that could be lifted not more than twice. Maximal isometric strength was measured with the knee angle at 60 degrees and was defined as the maximal weight that could be held for 4 seconds.

[d]Isometric endurance was defined as the duration of time that 40% or greater of the maximal isometric strength with the knee at a 60 degree angle could be maintained.

[e]Maximal strength was described as the heaviest weight a patient could lift with 1–4 repetitions with proper lifting and breathing (beginning with one set of 10 reps followed by a gradual increase in weight until failure).

[f]Muscle strength did not appear to be tested.

[g]1-RM was determined using the methods described by Kraemer and Fry before and after the RT program, but the specific method used was not reported.

[h]Supervised AE: RT was performed at a target heart rate >70% of peak heart rate obtained from the steep ramp exercise test and was performed for 60 minutes.

[i]Aerobic Exercise Alone Group (N = 10): Supervised AE: Cycle ergometry 2×/wk at 60%–70% of heart rate reserve for 15–28 minutes. Unsupervised AE: Home cycle ergometry or walking 2×/wk at Borg RPE of 12–14 for 20–40 minutes.

Adapted with permission from Cahalin LP, Ferreira DC, Yamada S, Canavan PK. Review of the effects of resistance training in patients with chronic heart failure: potential effects upon the muscle hypothesis. *Cardiopulm Phys Ther J.* 2006;17(1):16–29.

TABLE 18-10   Breathing Exercise Studies in Patients with Heart Failure

Author	N	Type of Breathing Exercise	Study Measurements	Study Outcomes
Mancini et al.[165]	8	Extensive ventilatory muscle training program[a]	Ventilatory muscle strength and endurance; exercise tolerance; cardiorespiratory function; dyspnea	Improved ventilatory muscle strength and endurance, exercise tolerance, and dyspnea
Cahalin et al.[25]	8	Threshold IMT	Ventilatory muscle strength and dyspnea	Improved ventilatory muscle strength and dyspnea
Johnson et al.[166]	16	Threshold IMT	Ventilatory muscle strength, exercise tolerance, dyspnea, and QOL	Improved ventilatory muscle strength, but no change in other Measures
Weiner et al.[167]	20	Threshold IMT	Ventilatory muscle strength, and endurance; PFTs; exercise tolerance; and dyspnea	Improved ventilatory muscle strength and endurance, exercise tolerance, PFTs, and dyspnea
Bernardi et al.[168]	50 + 15[b]	Complete yoga breathing[c]	Sao_2, exercise tolerance, cardiorespiratory function; dyspnea	Improved Sao_2, exercise tolerance, cardiorespiratory function, and dyspnea
Martinez et al.[169]	20	Threshold IMT	Ventilatory muscle strength and endurance; peak oxygen uptake; 6-min walk; dyspnea	Improved ventilatory muscle strength and endurance, peak oxygen uptake, 6-min walk, and dyspnea
Dall'Ago et al.[170]	32	Threshold IMT	Ventilatory muscle strength and endurance; peak oxygen uptake; 6-min walk; dyspnea	Improved ventilatory muscle strength and endurance, peak oxygen uptake, 6-min walk, and dyspnea
Chiappa et al.[171]	18	Threshold IMT	Ventilatory muscle strength; diaphragm thickness; resting and exercise calf and forearm blood flow.	Improved ventilatory muscle strength, diaphragm thickness, and resting and exercise blood flow to the calf and forearm

[a]Extensive ventilatory muscle training included isocapnic hyperpnea, threshold IMT, strength training, and breathing calisthenics.

[b]Fifteen additional patients underwent 1 month of complete yoga breathing.

[c]Complete yoga breathing was performed at a rate of 15, 6, and 3 breaths/min. Threshold IMT, inspiratory muscle training with a portable handheld device through which a patient can breathe only when they overcome the threshold resistance (provided via a calibrated spring) of the device.

TABLE 18-11   Aerobic Exercise and Strength Training Studies in Patients with Heart Failure and Left Ventricular Assist Device

Author	N	LVAD Type[a]	Study Measurements	Study Outcomes
Morrone et al.[49]	34	TCI HeartMate 1000 IP and 1205 VE	Ambulatory status, METs, functional status, and complications	IA by 14 days in 55% of subjects; TA was tolerated by 82% of subjects; greatest improvement observed by 6–8 wk; only four minor incidents (2.9/1000 patient hours) of a transient decrease in pump flow
Humphrey et al.[50]	1	?	Exercise tolerance, cardiorespiratory function, and complications	Improvement in $\dot{V}o_{2peak}$, $\dot{V}o_2$ @ VT, and RPP without complication
Buck et al.[173]	6	5 TCI HeartMate 1000 IP and One 1205 VE	Exercise tolerance, cardiorespiratory function, and complications	No substantial change in $\dot{V}o_{2peak}$, but approximately 10% increase in peak ex. dur., VE, and LVAD flow rate and a 21% increase in $\dot{V}o_2$ at VT without complication
Buck et al.[174]	3	1 HeartMate 1000 IP and two 1205 VE	Ambulatory status, METs, functional status, and complications	Improvement in ambulatory status, METs, and functional status with relatively few minor complications
Arena et al.[175]	1	1205 VE	PFT, exercise tolerance, cardiorespiratory function, and complications	PFT and ex. test results suggestive of a restrictive defect possibly due to abdominal LVAD implantation restricting diaphragmatic descent, but without major complication

[a]IA, independent ambulation; TA, treadmill ambulation; $\dot{V}o_2$, oxygen consumption; $\dot{V}o_{2peak}$, peak oxygen consumption; VT, ventilatory threshold; RPP, rate pressure product; VE, ventilation; METs, metabolic equivalents; PFT, pulmonary function test; ex, exercise; dur., duration.

TABLE 18-12 Studies of Structured Heart Failure Clinics

Author	N	Provider	Outcomes
Cintron et al.[176]	15	NP and MD	Fewer admissions (61%) and hospital days (85%); lower cost ($8000.00/patient/y)
Kornowski et al.[177]	42	MD and health care team	Fewer admissions (62%) and hospital days (77%); improved ADLs
Lasater[178]	80	RN and MD	Fewer admissions (14%) and hospital days (22%); lower hospital costs ($500.00/patient)
West et al.[179]	51	RN and MD	Fewer admissions (74%) and CHF admissions (87%); improved symptoms, QOL, and ex. Tolerance
Fonarow et al.[180]	214	CHF/heart transplant team	Fewer admissions (44%) and improved NYHA class and ex. tolerance; lower cost ($9800.00/patient)
Hanumanthu et al.[181]	134	CHF/heart transplant team	Fewer CHF admissions (69%) and improved peak oxygen consumption (23%)
Smith et al.[182]	21	NP and MD	Fewer CHF admissions (87%) and improved NYHA class, QOL, and ex. tolerance
Shah et al.[183]	27	RN and MD	Fewer admissions (50%) and hospital days (92%)
Dennis et al.[184]	24	Home care RN	Fewer readmissions with greater frequency and intensity of visits
Martens and Mellor[185]	924	Home care RN	Fewer readmissions (36%) with home care
Rich[186]	98	RN and multidisciplined health care team	Fewer admissions (27%) and hospital days (25%)
Schneider[187]	54	RN	Fewer admissions (73%)
Kostis[76]	20	Multidisciplined team	Improved ex. tolerance, anxiety, and depression
Rich et al.[188]	282	RN and multidisciplined health care team	Fewer admissions (44%) and CHF admissions (56%); improved QOL and lower cost ($460.00/patient)
Stewart[189]	97	Home-based RN and pharmacist team	Fewer admissions (42%) and hospital days (43%); lower hospital costs (41%)
Serxner[190]	109	Educational mailings	Fewer admissions (52%) and improved health status and compliance; lower costs

cardiovascular mortality, cardiovascular hospitalization, or heart failure hospitalization. However, analyses adjusted for baseline characteristics found that patients with heart failure undergoing cardiac rehabilitation had significantly improved all-cause mortality or hospitalization, cardiovascular mortality or cardiovascular hospitalization, and cardiovascular mortality or heart failure hospitalization.[151] Additional analyses demonstrated that heart failure patients undergoing cardiac rehabilitation had significantly greater self-reported health status that persisted after the rehabilitation program.[152]

Strength training—A number of studies have been published investigating the clinical efficacy of strength training in patients with heart failure (Table 18-9).[157-164] This literature suggests that strength training may be an important mode of exercise training that is safe and effective in patients with heart failure. Circuit strength training combined with aerobic exercise appears to improve peripheral muscle strength and endurance, exercise tolerance, cardiorespiratory function, and symptoms. **The strength training performed in these studies was administered to major muscle groups at 60% to 80% of maximum voluntary contraction or of the 10-repetition method (10-RM) for 2 to 6 months.**

The number of repetitions and strength training session durations were slowly progressed and varied among studies. No major complications were observed in the studies.

The manner by which the above strength training studies are related to the muscle hypothesis of chronic heart failure is also shown in Table 18-9. It is important to note that almost every domain of the muscle hypothesis of chronic heart failure was favorably affected by resistance training or a combination of resistance training and aerobic exercise.[164]

Breathing exercises—An increasing number of studies have investigated the effects of breathing exercises on the clinical manifestations of heart failure (Table 18-10).[25,165-171] Five of the six studies utilized a *threshold* inspiratory muscle training device which consisted of a portable handheld device through which a patient would inspire only when they overcame the threshold resistance (provided via a calibrated spring) of the device. Such a *Threshold* inspiratory muscle trainer is shown in Figure 18-6. **Inspiratory muscle training was performed daily for an average of 15 to 30 minutes at 15% to 60% of maximal inspiratory mouth pressure for 2 to 3 months.**[167-171]

One additional study investigated the acute and chronic effects of slowing the respiratory rate via yoga breathing. *Threshold* inspiratory muscle training appears to consistently improve ventilatory muscle strength and endurance and dyspnea. Yoga breathing appears to have both acute and chronic benefits including improved oxygen saturation, exercise tolerance, cardiorespiratory function, and dyspnea.

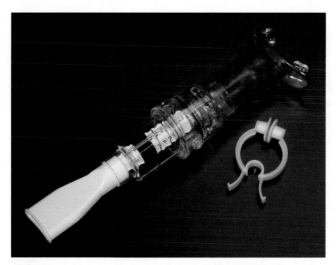

FIGURE 18-6   A *Threshold* inspiratory muscle trainer.

Left ventricular assist devices—Left ventricular assist devices are becoming more commonplace, yet have received very little clinical rehabilitative investigation (Table 18-11).[49,50,172–175] Exercise training of patients with LVADs appears to be safe, but requires gradual progressive mobilization which can lead to treadmill or cycling exercise. Treadmill or cycle ergometry exercise often begins after patients become independent with hallway ambulation. Specific criteria for mobilization and progression of a patient with heart failure and LVAD will be provided in the following section. Mobilization and progression of such patients has been observed to improve functional status and exercise tolerance and to optimize recovery before heart transplantation.

Heart failure clinics—Table 18-12 also includes a number of studies that have investigated the usefulness of heart failure clinics.[76,176–190] Heart failure clinics provide comprehensive heart failure management, frequently through a physician and nurse team. The team often follows specific patient care pathways, which ensure timely performance of specific tests and measures as well as allocation of a variety of services. Heart failure clinics are becoming more popular due to favorable economic and patient outcomes including a reduction in hospital admissions, readmissions, days, and costs as well as an improvement in quality of life and morbidity.

Specific Methods of Exercise Training for Patients with Cardiac Pump Dysfunction and Failure

Boxes 18-10 and 18-11 provide an overview of several important aspects of exercise training in patients with cardiac pump dysfunction and failure. As previously mentioned, **patients with cardiac pump dysfunction can tolerate an increase in**

BOX 18-10

Exercise Training Methods for Patients with Cardiac Pump Dysfunction

1. Perform an exercise test or utilize recent exercise test results.
2. Determine whether the cardiovascular and pulmonary responses during the exercise test are adaptive.
3. If exercise test results are adaptive without signs or symptoms of myocardial ischemia or cardiac arrhythmias, the exercise prescription should be developed via one of several methods including:
   a. Karvonen method
   b. 60% to 85% of peak heart rate or peak oxygen consumption
   c. Rate of perceived exertion corresponding to optimal training heart rate or level of oxygen consumption
   d. Heart rate or rate of perceived exertion just below the ventilatory threshold/anaerobic threshold
4. If exercise test results are not adaptive and show signs or symptoms of myocardial ischemia or cardiac arrhythmias, the exercise prescription should be developed via one of several methods including:
   a. Ischemic threshold via heart rate
   b. Ischemic threshold via rate pressure product (double product)
   c. Ischemic threshold via electrocardiographic evidence of myocardial ischemia or cardiac arrhythmias

d. Heart rate or rate of perceived exertion just below the threshold for maladaptive cardiovascular or pulmonary exercise test results
5. Perform physical exercise using the most appropriate mode, duration, frequency, and duration based on exercise test results, the blood pressure response during a controlled expiratory maneuver, and patient goals/enjoyment.
6. Begin with gentle stretching and aerobic exercise and progress to a greater exercise duration and intensity as exercise training is continued.
7. Set realistic goals for exercise with a range of 20 to 45 minutes of exercise duration, at a frequency of 3–5 ×/wk, and at an appropriate training intensity based on numbers 3 and 4.
8. Monitor patient during exercise using the methods described in chapter 10 and determine the frequency of monitoring during an exercise training session based on the exercise test results, blood pressure response during a controlled expiratory maneuver, and patient signs/symptoms.
9. Reexamine the patient during each exercise session using the methods described in Chapter 10.
10. Perform a second exercise test after 1 to 3 months of exercise training to establish safety of progressive exercise training and develop a new exercise prescription.

Criteria for the Initiation and Progression of Exercise Training in Patients with Cardiac Pump Failure

I. Relative criteria necessary for the initiation of an aerobic exercise training program—**Compensated heart failure:**
   1. Ability to speak without signs or symptoms of dyspnea (able to speak comfortably with an RR <30 breaths/min)
   2. Moderate fatigue
   3. Crackles present in <1/2 of the lungs
   4. Resting heart rate <120 bpm
   5. Cardiac index ≥2.0 L/min/m^2 (for invasively monitored patients)
   6. Central venous pressure <12 mm Hg (for invasively monitored patients)

II. Relative criteria indicating a need to modify or terminate exercise training
   (a) Marked dyspnea or fatigue (eg, Borg rating > 3/10)
   (b) Respiratory rate >40 breaths/min during exercise
   (c) Development of S$_3$ or pulmonary crackles
   (d) Increase in pulmonary crackles
   (e) Significant increase in the intensity of the second component of the second heart sound (P$_2$)
   (f) Poor pulse pressure (<10 mm Hg difference between the systolic and diastolic blood pressures)
   (g) Decrease in heart rate or blood pressure of >10 bpm or mm Hg, respectively, during continuous (steady-state) or progressive (increasing workloads) exercise
   (h) Increased supraventricular or ventricular ectopy
   (i) Increase of >10 mm Hg in the mean pulmonary artery pressure (for invasively monitored patients)
   (j) Increase or decrease of >6 mm Hg in the central venous pressure (for invasively monitored patients)
   (k) Diaphoresis, pallor, or confusion

Adapted with permission from Cahalin LP. Heart failure. *Phys Ther.* 1996;76:529.

venous return relatively well and can exercise at a greater intensity, duration, and frequency while utilizing a greater number of modalities and body positions than can the patient with cardiac pump failure. The exercise prescription for a patient with cardiac pump dysfunction should be developed from exercise test results when available and should likely follow the methods outlined in Box 18-10.[64,93]

In contrast to the patient with cardiac pump dysfunction, the patient with cardiac pump failure cannot tolerate a substantial increase in venous return. Therefore, the exercise prescription should be developed with this in mind (Box 18-11) and should be provided at a lesser intensity, duration, and frequency with a thorough appreciation for body position (and the effect of body position on venous return) and patient signs

and symptoms (requiring more thorough monitoring). Of primary concern for the patient with cardiac pump failure is the degree of heart failure and whether it is compensated or decompensated.[16,191] Several clinical findings appear to be suggestive of decompensated heart failure (Box 18-11), and identification of one or more of these findings may be sufficient to terminate exercise training until heart failure has become compensated.[16,191] Clinical findings suggesting modification or termination of exercise training are also listed in Box 18-11 and include marked dyspnea and fatigue, a fall in systolic blood pressure response during progressive exercise, and development of a S$_3$ or crackles in a patient who did not demonstrate these signs prior to exercise.[16,191]

Table 18-13 provides a structured approach to the rehabilitation of patients with heart failure in a variety of settings such as those who are hospitalized, seen in the home, or attending a rehabilitation center.[182] Patients who are debilitated may require a more gradual exercise progression (gradual activity protocol), whereas patients who are less debilitated may progress more rapidly through a rehabilitation program (standard activity protocol). The progression of the patient through either activity protocol or in any setting is based on the initial patient status and subsequent responses to exercise and other components of the cardiac rehabilitation program that have been identified as necessary.[191]

For most patients, ambulation may be the most effective and functional mode of exercise to administer and prescribe, beginning with frequent short walks and progressing to less frequent, longer bouts of exercise. Occasionally, patients may be so deconditioned that gentle strengthening exercises, restorator cycling, or ventilatory muscle training is the preferred mode of exercise conditioning. As strength and endurance improve, patients can be progressed to upright cycle ergometry or ambulating with a rolling walker.

Because dyspnea is the most common complaint of patients with CHF, the level of dyspnea or Borg rating of perceived exertion appears to be an acceptable method to prescribe an exercise program.[182] This is supported by the observation that these subjective indices correlate well with training heart rate ranges in this patient population. Therefore, a basic guideline of increasing the exercise intensity to a level that produces a moderate degree of dyspnea (conversing with modest difficulty, ability to count to 5 without taking a breath, or a Borg rating of 3/10) may be the simplest and most effective method to prescribe exercise for patients with CHF. It also appears to be the most effective method to progress a patient's exercise prescription. The exercise prescription can be progressed when (1) the cardiopulmonary response to exercise is adaptive and (2) workloads which previously produced moderate dyspnea (eg, Borg rating of 3/10) produce mild dyspnea (eg, Borg rating of ≤2/10).[191]

Ventricular Assist Devices

Patients with end-stage heart failure who are refractory to maximal inotropic therapy may benefit from a ventricular assist device. Currently there are two intracorporeal devices

TABLE 18-13   Two Different Methods of Activity Progression in Patients with Heart Failure[a]

Day	Standard Activity Regimen	Gradual Activity Regimen
1	Commode/chair	Bed rest
2	Room ambulation	Bed rest/gentle active strengthening exercises
3	Hallway ambulation and cycle ergometry ×2 (1–10 min); MET-level goal = 2.0–3.0	Commode/chair/bathroom/restorator cycling/room ambulation/gentle strengthening exercises
4	Independent hallway ambulation ×3 (1–15 min); MET-level goal = 3.0–4.0; patient adequately ascends/descends 2 flights of stairs and is showering independently; adequate understanding of home exercise prescription; outpatient cardiac rehabilitation appointment scheduled; patient discharged	Hallway ambulation/restorator or cycle ergometry ×2 exercise duration (1–5 min); MET-level goal = 1.0–2.0 strengthening exercises
5		Hallway ambulation/restorator or cycle ergometry ×2, exercise duration (1–8 min); MET-level goal = 1.5–2.5 strengthening exercises
6		Hallway ambulation/restorator or cycle ergometry ×2, exercise duration (1–10 min); MET-level goal = 2.0–3.0 strengthening exercises
7		Hallway ambulation ×2, exercise duration (1–15 min); MET-level goal = 2.0–4.0; strengthening exercises; patient adequately ascends/descends 2 flights of stairs and is showering independently; adequate understanding of home exercise prescription; outpatient cardiac rehabilitation appointment scheduled; patient discharged.

[a]Activity protocol is based on risk stratification of patients (eg, degree of ventricular dysfunction and signs/symptoms) and on the cardiopulmonary response (heart rate not >20–30 bpm above resting heart rate without hypoadaptive BP response (not >10–20 mm Hg decrease) and without significant arrhythmias or dyspnea). (Adapted with permission from Cahalin LP. Heart failure. *Phys Ther*. 1996;76:530).

operated by battery packs, which are approved by the United States Food and Drug Administration (USFDA) for use as a bridge to transplantation and/or a bridge to recovery of function. Thoratec, Inc. (Heartmate VE, Fig. 18-7A) and Novacor (Oakland, CA) have developed these portable devices allowing the patient mobility not afforded by earlier generations of assist devices with the potential for discharge home.[192–195] Additionally, the USFDA has recently approved the Heartmate VE LVAD as a destination therapy in those patients who are not candidates for heart transplantation following successful outcomes in a multicenter study.[186] Physical therapy has been shown to be safe and effective at helping these patients to regain independence in ADL and gait; and to maximize strength, flexibility, and endurance while awaiting transplantation.[49] The reexamination of the case study following LVAD implantation is presented in Box 18-6. Clinical trials are currently in progress to evaluate the Novacor LVAD as a destination therapy.

As more and more patients are being discharged home following LVAD implantation to wait until a donor heart becomes available, more attention needs to be given to discharge planning. Adequate social support and home environment must be considered. It is the LVAD nurse coordinator's responsibility to perform the final safety check-out of the patient and family in performing LVAD emergency procedures. It is the physical therapist's responsibility to provide the patient and family with verbal and written instructions for a home exercise program. Those who have had a complicated hospital course and who are very weak and debilitated may benefit from transfer to an inpatient rehabilitation center prior

to discharge home. In the rare case in which the patient is not independent in their ADL or in ambulation prior to discharge home but has the potential to make progress, home physical therapy would be warranted. Finally, contact information regarding local outpatient cardiac rehabilitation facilities should be provided to the patient prior to discharge home. A nurse coordinator may provide on-site training (device management and emergency procedures) to staff at a local cardiac rehabilitation facility prior to their accepting this type of patient.[51]

The right ventricular assist device (RVAD) and biventricular assist device (BiVAD) have been utilized clinically, but minimal research has investigated the best methods to provide exercise to patients provided an RVAD or BiVAD. The available data suggest that the LVAD provides better hemodynamic support and exercise tolerance than the BiVAD. However, more research in this area is needed. Nonetheless, the rehabilitation of patients with an RVAD or BiVAD appears to be similar to that provided to patients with an LVAD.

Allocation of Services in Cardiac Rehabilitation for Persons with Cardiac Pump Dysfunction and Failure

The allocation of appropriate services for patients with cardiac pump dysfunction and failure participating in cardiac rehabilitation can be performed via a detailed history, results of medical and psychological tests, and results from disease specific and general health status questionnaires.[16,106,111–118,196] Exercise test results often provide important information about the severity of heart failure, safety of exercise training, and exercise prescription. Patients with a peak oxygen consumption

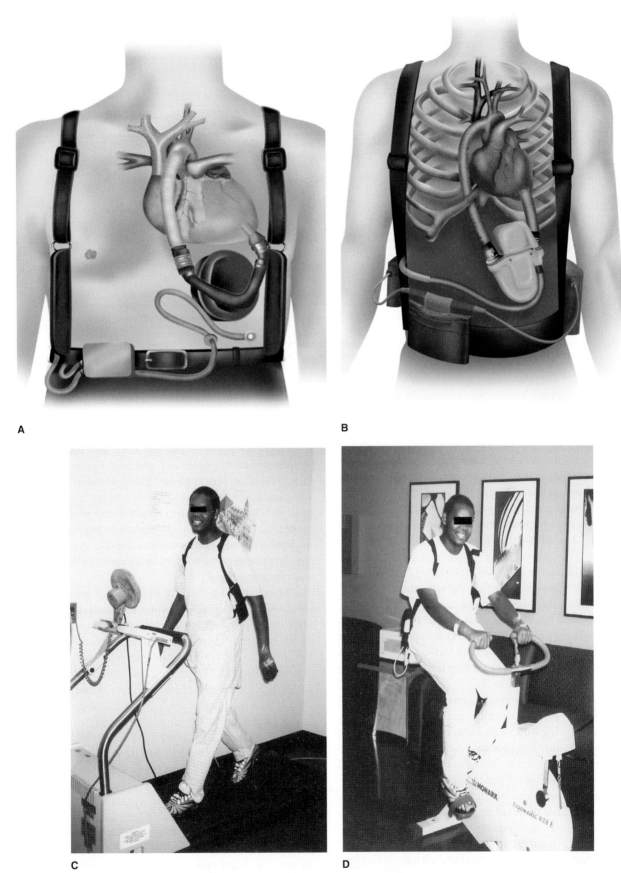

A

B

C

D

FIGURE 18-7 Diagram of LVAD types with photo of treadmill and cycle exercise. (**A**) Schematic representation of the *HeartMate* VE LVAD; (**B**) schematic representation of the *Novacor* N100PC LVAS; (**C**) photo of George with *HeartMate* VE LVAD performing treadmill exercise; (**D**) Photo of George with *HeartMate* VE LVAD performing bicycle exercise.

TABLE 18-14   **Allocation of Cardiac Rehabilitation Based on Risk Stratification**

Risk Factor	Low Risk	Moderate Risk	High Risk
Smoking	None	Recent smoking cessation	Current smoker
Diet	<20% fat <7% saturated fat <150 mg cholesterol	20%–29% fat 7%–10% saturated fat 150–300 mg cholesterol	>29% fat >10% saturated fat >300 mg cholesterol
LDL			
Cholesterol	LDL < 100 mg/dL	LDL = 100–129 mg/dL	LDL > 130 mg/dL
Diabetes	FBG < 120 mg/dL	FBG = 120–180 mg/dL	FBG > 180 mg/dL
Mellitus	or Hb A_{1c} < 7%	or Hb A_{1c} = 7%–9%	or Hb A_{1c} > 9%
Weight	BMI < 25	BMI = 25–29	BMI > 30
Hypertension	SBP < 130 mm Hg DBP < 85 mm Hg	SBP = 130–159 mm Hg DBP = 85–99 mm Hg	SBP ≥ 160 mm Hg DBP ≥ 100 mm Hg
Depression	No clinical depression	moderate clinical depression	Significant clinical depression
Exercise	>6300 kJ/wk	2940–6300 kJ/wk	<2940 kJ/wk

LDL, low-density lipoprotein; FBG, fasting blood glucose; Hb A1c, glycosylated hemoglobin; BMI, body mass index; SBP, systolic blood pressure; DBP, diastolic blood pressure.

Adapted with permission from Roitman JL, LaFontaine T, Drimmer AM. A new model for risk stratification and delivery of cardiovascular rehabilitation services in the long-term clinical management of patients with coronary artery disease. *J Cardiopulm Rehabil*. 1998;18:113-123.

of less than 10 to 14 mL/kg/min appear to have a poorer prognosis and are often considered candidates for cardiac transplantation. However, these same patients may benefit from closely monitored and gradually progressed cardiac rehabilitation. Exercise test results can also provide (1) some indication of the potential for complications during exercise training based on the comprehensive examination of the cardiorespiratory response (eg, peak oxygen consumption, heart rate and blood pressure response, electrocardiogram, and symptoms) and (2) patient-specific exercise training parameters.[16,106,111–118,196]

Additional data may be helpful in allocating cardiac rehabilitation as recently presented for the long-term clinical management of patients with coronary artery disease (Table 18-14).[196] As shown in Table 18-14, important patient data and critical threshold levels may help to stratify and subsequently allocate cardiac rehabilitation. The patient data include traditional risk factors as well as other factors that may influence the risk for the progression of atherosclerosis.

Examination of the results of a general health status questionnaire (eg, SF-36) or a disease-specific questionnaire like the Minnesota Living with Heart Failure Questionnaire or the Chronic Heart Failure Questionnaire can also provide important information about the domain of disablement most affected by heart disease for patients with cardiac pump dysfunction and failure. These instruments can also address the specific areas in need of direct medical, physical, educational, psychological, social, occupational, and nutritional interventions.[64] Cardiac rehabilitation provided in this manner will likely address the specific disablement of each patient and provide cost-effective and comprehensive care.

Monitoring and Reexamination

Monitoring persons with cardiac pump dysfunction and failure is dependent on the past history as well as on the findings from specific physical therapy tests and measures. These include symptoms, heart rate and blood pressure at rest and during exercise, heart rate and blood pressure during the valsalva maneuver, and exercise test results (eg, exercise duration, peak workload, peak oxygen consumption, and electrocardiographic findings such as ST-segment depression). Specific medical tests and measurements (eg, ejection fraction) can also provide important information about patient monitoring and reexamination.[16,64,106,111–118]

Monitoring of persons with cardiac pump failure and LVAD support requires constant monitoring of the patient's response to physical therapy intervention in order to ensure safety and to evaluate effectiveness of the intervention. Heart rate and rhythm (via telemetry), blood pressure, oxygen saturation, LVAD rate (pulse), stroke volume, and flow, and the patient's symptoms are monitored with position change and with exercise.[49–52] Once the patient is transferred from alternating current to battery operation of the LVAD, the power base display of device rate, volume, and flow is no longer available. The rate of the device can still be ascertained by counting the pulse. Rhythm would be monitored in patients with known or suspected arrhythmia. Blood pressure and symptoms would continue to be watched. Treatment would be terminated for LVAD rate <50 bpm, LVAD volume <30 mL, LVAD flows <3.0 L/min, symptomatic drop in blood pressure of more than 10 mm Hg, heart rate >150 bpm, or sustained ventricular tachycardia or ventricular fibrillation.[49–51]

TABLE 18-15 Possible Outcomes After Cardiac Transplantion

Possible Adverse Outcomes	Possible Favorable Outcomes
1. Allograft rejection and cardiac dysfunction/failure	1. Improved cardiac and multisystem Function
2. Immunosuppressive issues (eg, infection, malignancies, myopathy)	2. Ability to exercise and increase functional tasks
3. Deconditioning and muscle weakness	3. Improvement in psychological function
4. Significantly blunted heart rate to exercise	4. Exercise training adaptations
5. Greater dependency on anaerobic metabolism	a. Improved skeletal and cardiac muscle function
6. Obesity	b. Lower resting heart rate and blood pressure
7. Hypertension	c. Lower rate pressure product
8. Hyperlipidemia	d. Increased peak oxygen consumption
9. Diabetes	e. Increased lean muscle mass
10. Accelerated Coronary Artery Disease	f. Decreased body weight and body fat
11. Osteoporosis	g. Greater heart rate responsiveness during exercise
12. Psychological dysfunction	h. Improved lipid and blood sugar profiles
	i. Decreased bone mineral loss

Adapted from Cahalin LP. Cardiac transplantation and acute care outcomes. *Acute Care Perspect*. 2005;14(3):1-8.

Allocation of Services for Persons After Cardiac Transplantation

The care provided to persons before cardiac transplantation is identical to that provided to persons with cardiac pump failure. However, after cardiac transplantation several important issues must be considered including the effects of cardiac denervation on heart rate, immunosuppression on skeletal muscle, and marked deconditioning on the progression of therapeutic exercise.[197-199]

Table 18-15 provides an overview of the possible outcomes after cardiac transplantation. Cardiac denervation produces a blunted heart rate during exercise and a slower decrease in heart rate after exercise, which reinforces the importance of a proper warm-up and cool-down period after exercise for patients after a cardiac transplant. Immunosuppressive drugs are provided to patients after a cardiac transplant to prevent the body from rejecting the transplanted heart. However, immunosuppressive drugs weaken the immune system making infection and the development of malignancies a potential problem. Furthermore, immunosuppressive drugs have been associated with the development of skeletal muscle myopathies making the rehabilitation of cardiac transplant recipients challenging. Finally, almost all cardiac transplant recipients have suffered from chronic heart failure and the marked deconditioning associated with chronic heart failure. Despite these issues, favorable outcomes are associated with

TABLE 18-16 The Primary Domains of Disablement in Cardiac Pump Dysfunction and Failure

	Cardiac Rehabilitation Interventions
Key impairments	
Dyspnea	Supplemental oxygen, pursed-lip breathing, breathing exercises, ventilatory muscle training
Fatigue	Supplemental oxygen, rest, proper diet and nutrition, pharmacologic agents, individualized gradual progressive exercise training program, patient education
Decreased exercise tolerance	Supplemental oxygen, rest, proper diet and nutrition, pharmacologic agents, individualized gradual progressive exercise training program, pursed-lip breathing, patient education
Key functional limitations	
Walking	Gait training, strength and aerobic exercise training, balance training
Climbing stairs	Gentle stair stepper exercise, functional exercise training (stair climbing)
Housework and yardwork	Functional activity training
Lifting boxes	Functional activity training
Recreational pastimes and hobbies	Recreational/hobby training
Key disabilities	
Unable to do things with family or friends	Patient and family/friend education, functional exercise and activity training
Being a burden to family or friends	Patient and family/friend education, functional exercise and activity training
Traveling away from home	Patient and family/friend education, functional exercise and activity training
Working to earn a living	Occupational therapy, social services, patient and family/friend education, functional exercise and activity training
Paying for the costs of medical care	Social services, patient and family education

TABLE 18-17   **Differences in the Physiologic Profile of Cardiac Transplant Recipients Compared to Healthy Subjects**

Higher	Lower
Resting heart rate	Lean body mass
Resting systolic and diastolic blood pressure	Peak exercise heart rate
Peak ventilatory equivalent	Peak exercise systolic blood pressure
Resting cardiac output	Peak double product Peak power output (watts) Peak oxygen consumption Absolute anaerobic threshold

Differences in the cardiovascular and cardiorespiratory response of cardiac transplant recipients compared to age matched healthy subjects

Adapted from Kavanagh T et al. *Circulation.* 1988;77(1):162-171.

TABLE 18-18   **Training Adaptations in Cardiac Transplant Recipients**

Variables	Before	After	% Change
Body mass (kg)	69.9	73.9	+6
Lean body mass (kg)	56.2	58.2	+4
Resting heart rate (bpm)	104	100	−4
Peak heart rate (bpm)	135	148	+10
Resting systolic blood pressure (mm Hg)	138	125	−9
Resting diastolic blood pressure (mm Hg)	95	86	−9
Peak diastolic blood pressure (mm Hg)[a]	100	92	−8
Peak ventilation (1-min^{-1} btps)[a]	70	91	+30
Peak oxygen consumption (mL/kg/min)	22	26	+18
Peak power (W)	101	150	±49

[a]Significant reductions in submaximal exercise at equivalent workloads was observed in the above variables and in the patients ratings of perceived exertion.

Training effects in cardiac transplant recipients adapted from Kavanagh T et al. *Circulation.* 1988;77(1):162-171.

cardiac transplantation and it has been shown that properly prescribed exercise can facilitate the favorable outcomes.[197–199]

Because of the above possible adverse outcomes after cardiac transplantation, cardiac transplant recipients demonstrate a very different physiologic profile from age- and gender-matched healthy subjects which is shown in Table 18-17. The major differences include the higher resting heart rate and lower peak exercise heart rate, higher resting systolic and diastolic blood pressure, higher resting cardiac output, and lower lean body mass, peak power, and peak oxygen consumption.[197–199]

However, properly prescribed exercise can improve many of the less than favorable outcomes after cardiac transplantation and make the cardiac transplant recipient more physiologically similar to healthy individuals. The potential for change is shown in Table 18-18 with substantial improvement likely in peak power, peak ventilation, and peak oxygen consumption.[197–199]

Finally, the methods to develop the favorable exercise training adaptations shown in Table 18-18 can be appreciated by examining the exercise training methods outlined in Table 18-19. Gradual increases in strengthening as well as functional and exercise training before and after transplantation are likely to safely promote training adaptations. Breathing exercises may also be of benefit and prescription of exercise using rating of perceived exertion as opposed to heart rate is preferred because of the blunted heart rate from cardiac denervation.[197–199]

Outcomes—Utilization of Threshold Behaviors for Improvements in Exercise and Functional Abilities as a Result of Aerobic Exercise Training

A review of the outcomes listed in the *Guide* for patients with cardiovascular pump dysfunction and failure in Practice Pattern D reveals a lack of specificity.[1] Despite the fact that the medical management of persons with cardiovascular pump dysfunction

and failure is similar (eg, the fundamental basis of treatment which is to decrease the workload imposed on the heart and to decrease venous return) the specific outcomes are likely to be different and should be based on the results of specific tests and measures. Several such results of specific tests and measures include the observation of a decrease in cardiac output during exercise, an elevated resting heart rate, and low level of peak

TABLE 18-19   **Exercise Training Before and After Cardiac Transplantation[a]**

Before TX in Hospital	Before TX at Home	After TX
		Airway clearance
Breathing exercises	Breathing exercises	Breathing exercises
Gentle strengthening	Gentle strengthening	LE strength < 6 wk Add UE strength > 6wk
Progressive amb	Progressive amb	Progressive amb
Treadmill/cycle	Treadmill/cycle	Treadmill/cycle
RPE < 13	RPE < 13	RPE 11–13 < 6 wk RPE 13–14 ≥ 6 wk

TX, transplant; RPE, rating of perceived exertion.

[a]LVAD patients exercising in the hospital or at home before transplantation can exercise at a slightly greater intensity (Borg RPE of 13–14) and are usually more stable than CHF patients exercising without an LVAD. However, specific procedures should likely be followed for LVAD patients to exercise safely at home or in the hospital.

Data from Matsuo Y, Cahalin LP, Buck L. Cardiac transplantation. *Japanese Phys Ther J.* 2005;39(9):785-793.

oxygen consumption. Identification of particular responses of key tests and measures can provide important prognostic information regarding the likelihood of success or failure of aerobic exercise training. Understanding the likelihood for success or failure during specific therapeutic interventions can better direct specific patient outcomes. The specific signs and symptoms of cardiac pump dysfunction and failure listed in Table 18-7 provide important outcome and prognostic information. The results of these tests and measures can provide an evidence base for goal-setting and patient outcomes.[16,106,111–118,196]

Important outcomes for physical therapy and potential goals for patients with cardiac pump dysfunction and failure are listed in Table 18-16. The key areas of disablement in cardiac pump dysfunction and failure are listed in this table, from which the specific results of tests and measures of persons with cardiac pump dysfunction and failure can be compared. The list of key disablements are supported by a substantial literature which has identified important patient characteristics associated with heart disease and successful outcomes.[200–205] The results of these specific tests and measures within their respective domains of disablement are described in the following sections.

Pathology concept—etiology of heart failure—The etiology of CHF is often due to either an ischemic cardiomyopathy or an idiopathic cardiomyopathy. Persons with CHF due to an ischemic cardiomyopathy have a poorer prognosis and exercise tolerance than do patients with an idiopathic cardiomyopathy.[206] The presence of myocardial ischemia in a patient with depressed myocardial performance appears to predispose a patient to poorer exercise tolerance and prognosis.[111] **Poor prognosis and exercise intolerance (a health outcome and impairment measure, respectively) are therefore negative outcomes that may be expected in patients with CHF due to an ischemic cardiomyopathy. The use of pathological information such as this may alert a therapist to provide more frequent monitoring and a more gradual progression in exercise for a patient with an ischemic cardiomyopathy.**

Impairment concept—peak oxygen consumption and oxygen consumption at the ventilatory threshold—A great deal of investigation has been done on measuring exercise tolerance, functional capacity, and survival in persons with heart disease.[68,69,71–75,207–212] Peak oxygen consumption measurements have traditionally been used to categorize persons with heart disease, and numerous studies have shown that persons with lower levels of peak oxygen consumption have poorer exercise tolerance, functional capacity, and survival than persons with greater levels of peak oxygen consumption.[68,69,71–73,207–212]

It has been observed that a peak oxygen consumption and oxygen consumption at the ventilatory threshold have been identified as important threshold behaviors.[73–75,106]

These values likely represent a moderate degree of CHF (patients who are not severely deconditioned or suffering from decompensated CHF). If patients had more severe CHF they would have lower levels of peak oxygen consumption (less than 10 mL/kg/min) and higher levels of oxygen consumption at the ventilatory threshold (greater than 12 mL/kg/min).

Similar findings have recently been observed by Belardinelli et al.[75]

Impairment concept—reduced cardiac output during exercise—A reduction in the cardiac output during exercise is indicative of poor myocardial function that will unlikely improve with chronic aerobic exercise training.[107,116]

Impairment concept—resting heart rate and heart rate change during exercise—**A resting heart rate of less than 90 bpm and a change in heart rate during exercise testing that is greater than 50 bpm appear to be associated with successful rehabilitation of persons with CHF.**[106,110,116,118] These findings are likely due to a healthier person with CHF and a better preserved stroke volume which would provide an adequate cardiac output at rest and during exercise with lower heart rates. Patients with a resting heart rate greater than 90 bpm and a change in heart rate during exercise testing that is less than 50 bpm will have less cardiac reserve for aerobic exercise training and therefore may predispose such patients to less exercise tolerance and earlier dyspnea, fatigue, and myocardial ischemia if coronary artery disease exists. Similar findings have recently been observed by Belardinelli et al.[75] These patients may benefit from the same interventions that were described previously for patients with a reduction in cardiac output during exercise.

Impairment concept—peak systolic blood pressure—A peak exercise systolic blood pressure that is greater than 10 mm Hg from the resting blood pressure appears to be associated with successful rehabilitation.[116] A peak systolic blood pressure which is unable to increase greater than 10 mm Hg likely identifies a poor level of myocardial performance. Systolic blood pressure characteristically rises with progressive incremental exercise, but in a patient with a poor cardiac pump, the rise may be less than 10 mm Hg from the resting level or the systolic blood pressure may rise, but precipitously fall to a level that is less than 10 mm Hg above the resting systolic blood pressure at peak exercise. Patients presenting with a peak systolic blood pressure that is less than 10 mm Hg above the resting systolic blood pressure may benefit from the same interventions listed previously for patients with a reduction in cardiac output during exercise.

Impairment concept—pulse pressure—A pulse pressure (the difference between the systolic and diastolic blood pressures) greater than 10 mm Hg is likely to be associated with successful rehabilitation.[110,116] The greater the pulse pressure, the greater will be the perfusion pressure to vital organs and to peripheral musculature and tissues. Improved perfusion to organs and peripheral tissues and musculature will likely yield greater exercise tolerance and an improved exercise response due to maintenance of organ function (including the heart), adequate blood flow to exercising muscles, and cooling of the body during exercise. A smaller pulse pressure reflects not only poorer myocardial performance and an inability to increase the systolic blood pressure but also increased peripheral vascular constriction that may be associated with an increase in diastolic blood pressure. Thus, a narrowing of the pulse pressure may ensue in a person with CHF who has poor myocardial performance and increased peripheral vascular resistance because of worsening blood flow to the periphery and to vital organs. Patients presenting with a narrow pulse pressure less than 10 mm Hg during exercise testing should likely be prescribed very low-level strength training to the peripheral musculature and the muscles of breathing as well as energy conservation techniques and patient education.

Functional abilities/disability/quality-of-life concepts— 6-minute walk test distance ambulated—Results of the 6-minute walk test (a functional performance measure) have recently been shown to be helpful in estimating peak oxygen consumption (an impairment measure) and survival (an important measurement of health outcome) in persons with heart failure.[60] The distance ambulated during the 6-minute walk test was significantly related to the measured peak oxygen consumption during cycle ergometry exercise testing. The distance ambulated during the 6-minute walk test can be used to estimate peak oxygen consumption via a number of prediction equations (see Chapter 10).[60]

Another important finding from the results of the 6-minute walk test is that patients walking less than 300 m (approximately 1,000 ft) appear to have a poorer survival.[60] This has been observed in a relatively large number of studies of persons with heart failure. Observation of such poor exercise tolerance and functional ability provides a threshold behavior level which may be useful for the medical management of patients with heart failure and in directing physical therapy intervention. Heart failure patients ambulating less than 300 m are frequently provided more extensive and structured physical therapy interventions than patients ambulating greater than 300 m.

Overall disablement—Minnesota Living With Heart Failure Questionnaire (MLWHFQ)—A total score of 50 or greater on the MLWHFQ appears to be associated with greater potential for successful rehabilitation.[116] The greater the score on the MLWHFQ, the greater the functional limitation and disability and the poorer the quality of life (see Chapter 10). A total score of 50 or greater may be a threshold level below which disablement is less likely to change, but above which (because of greater disability and functional limitation) disablement may be more prone to improve.

Outcomes—utilization of threshold behaviors for improvements of symptoms and ventilatory muscle strength as a result of ventilatory muscle training— *Impairment Concept—Ventilatory Muscle Strength and Dyspnea:* A previous study investigating the effects of inspiratory muscle training on ventilatory muscle strength and symptoms of persons with heart failure can be used to show a more specific application of a threshold behavior to direct physical therapy intervention.[25,213,214] It was observed that ventilatory muscle strength and symptoms (eg, dyspnea) improved significantly after an 8-week period of inspiratory muscle training.[25,213,214] Univariate and multivariate regression analyses revealed that the percent change in dyspnea at rest and during exercise was significantly related to the pulmonary artery pressure, right ventricular ejection fraction, and left ventricular end-diastolic volume of the heart failure patients.[214]

It appears that patients with heart failure will benefit from inspiratory muscle training when they have (1) a poor right ventricular ejection fraction (less than 45% = a threshold behavior level), (2) elevated pulmonary artery pressure (greater than 20 mm Hg = a threshold behavior level), and (3) elevated left ventricular end-diastolic volume (greater than 150 mL = a threshold behavior level).

Patients with one or more of these particular threshold behaviors are likely to succeed with inspiratory muscle training performed in the manner described in this research study.[213,214] In fact, from these preliminary data, it may even be possible to predict the degree of improvement in dyspnea from inspiratory muscle training. The use of such threshold behaviors, therefore, may enable the prediction of physical therapy intervention outcomes in much the same way that the degree of success with medical intervention is predicted.

Outcomes—utilization of threshold behaviors for improvements in exercise and functional abilities as a result of aerobic and strength training in patients with cardiac pump failure and left ventricular assist devices—
Extraindividual concept: Many extraindividual concepts appear to be related to the improvements in exercise and functional abilities of persons with LVAD and include the possible constraints of the LVAD, the possible contribution of the native heart to cardiac output during exercise, the duration post-LVAD implantation when exercise training is performed, and whether or not exercise training was performed as well as the potential role training adaptations may have on cardiorespiratory performance after LVAD implantation.[215] $\dot{V}O_{2peak}$ and $\dot{V}E$ have been observed to be significantly greater in LVAD patients than in patients with CHF, and a trend for greater $\dot{V}E/\dot{V}O_2$ has been observed in LVAD patients. The available literature of exercise for LVAD patients is limited, but the results of a recent research synthesis reveal that (1) many issues involving the possible constraints and benefits of the LVAD need further investigation, (2) persons with LVAD have greater $\dot{V}O_{2peak}$ and $\dot{V}E$ than persons with end-stage CHF, (3) LVAD patients appear to have greater levels of $\dot{V}O_{2peak}$, $\dot{V}E$, and $\dot{V}E/\dot{V}O_2$ when exercise is performed, and (4) more substantial improvements in $\dot{V}O_{2peak}$, $\dot{V}E$, and $\dot{V}E/\dot{V}O_2$ appear to occur later, rather than earlier, after LVAD implantation.[215] These are important issues, because an improvement in $\dot{V}O_{2peak}$ and $\dot{V}E$ due to LVAD implantation will likely yield greater functional abilities in persons with end-stage CHF. Knowledge of the expected timeline of these improvements can help to develop realistic and comprehensive patient goals, exercise prescriptions, and discharge plans. Physical therapists examining and treating patients with end-stage CHF should appreciate and further examine the safety and possible role of LVAD combined with exercise to improve the disablement of end-stage CHF.

It is presumed that all acute LVAD patients will benefit from airway clearance techniques, deep breathing, splinted coughing, positioning (+/- splinting), and range-of-motion exercises until they are able to be mobilized as dictated by their hemodynamic stability and by their external supports (ie, CVVHD). Instruction in LVAD management, bed mobility, transfers, and gait is indicated until the patient is independent in these activities or until it is determined that they have reached a plateau in their progress toward these goals. It seems logical that all LVAD patients would benefit from specific and individualized strengthening and aerobic training until they are independent in their training program or in their physiologic and functional adaptations to training plateau. A plateau in exercise duration, symptom relief, 6-minute walk distance, or $\dot{V}O_{2peak}$ is examples whichever comes first. It is likely that the same threshold behaviors that have been established in patients/clients with cardiovascular pump dysfunction/failure (distance walked in 6 minutes and MIP) may hold true in patients/clients following LVAD implantation and warrant clinical investigation. Additional behaviors, which may prove to be valuable markers, include peripheral muscle strength, vital capacity, and maximal or submaximal $\dot{V}O_2$ as well as LVAD type and the period of time since LVAD implantation. Further research may validate these threshold behaviors.[215]

Criteria for Discharge

The criteria for discharge of persons with cardiac pump dysfunction, cardiac pump failure, and cardiac pump failure with LVAD have not been established. The criteria for discharge are dependent on the attainment of the anticipated goals and outcomes. Anticipated goals and outcomes will be based on the initial and subsequent results of specific tests and measures such as exercise testing, functional activities, questionnaires, and patient symptoms. Further investigation of the specific tests and measures and the level of improvement needed to ensure safe and optimal function after discharge from physical therapy is needed. Medical deterioration from compensated to uncompensated CHF would also warrant discharge from physical therapy until the patient is stabilized.

NAGI MODEL

Gordon and Quinn suggest organizing the physical therapy examination according to the expanded version of the Nagi model of disablement as described by Verbrugge and Jette.[216,217] Figure 18-1 demonstrates how this model can be applied to the examination component of a patient with cardiac pump dysfunction and failure (Practice Pattern D). The evidence-based outcomes to date for physical therapy interventions in these practice patterns are underlined.

THE LIMITS OF OUR KNOWLEDGE

Cardiac Pump Dysfunction and Failure

The rehabilitation of persons with cardiac pump dysfunction and failure has evolved tremendously. Substantial evidence exists for the rehabilitation of persons with cardiac pump dysfunction, and more evidence is becoming available for the rehabilitation of persons with cardiac pump failure. Although the knowledge of rehabilitation of persons with cardiac pump dysfunction is extensive, much is unknown about the rehabilitation of persons with cardiac pump failure.

The future rehabilitation of persons with heart failure will likely utilize the results of exercise training trials to develop prediction equations to determine the degree of success or failure with specific modes of exercise. Specific patient populations with CHF will likely be observed to improve a specific amount in particular areas of disablement from physical therapy and other rehabilitation interventions. The percentage of improvement in aerobic exercise capacity and other areas of disablement will likely be accurately predicted once specific baseline threshold behaviors are identified. Such an evolution in the rehabilitative care of persons with CHF is in keeping with the medical management of many diseases.

Patients with CHF not presenting with particular threshold behaviors of success may still be successful with rehabilitation efforts, and patients presenting with particular evidence-based threshold behaviors may not necessarily respond favorably to rehabilitation. Threshold behaviors can only provide us with some degree of likelihood for success or failure during rehabilitative care. In fact, a recent European multicenter study of exercise training in CHF found no significant correlations between baseline patient characteristics and successful rehabilitation.[88] Threshold behaviors may better direct our treatment and allow us to treat the most important concept of disablement that will most likely improve a patient's functional abilities and quality of life. They may provide physical therapists with very specific evidence-based practice.

The specific intervention provided to a patient with CHF will be based on the patient's primary need and will likely result in very specific educational and therapeutic programs aimed at the area of disablement most affected. Methods to identify the areas of disablement most affected by CHF should include specific tests and measures such as the 6-minute walk test or other functional tests and measures. General and specific questionnaires of a patient's perceived health status such as the Medical Outcomes Study SF-36 and the MLWHFQ, respectively, may also be helpful in identifying the areas of disablement in need of intervention.[218] Provision of therapeutic exercise will likely be much more specific using not only aerobic exercise training but also strength training to peripheral skeletal muscles. Improving the strength and endurance of the breathing muscles via inspiratory muscle training may also prove to be helpful for patients with CHF by directing intervention at the two main complaints of persons with CHF—dyspnea and fatigue.[25] Aerobic exercise will likely continue to be prescribed using symptom scores of dyspnea and fatigue (Borg rating of perceived exertion score of 3–4/10 or 12–14/20), but may include other objective indices (in combination with symptom scores or separate) such as heart rate, systolic and diastolic blood pressures at rest and during exercise, pulse pressures, rate–pressure product, ventilatory threshold, oxygen consumption, or even lactate levels. However, much more research is needed to identify the specific exercise prescription most effective for patients with cardiac pump failure. Such specific allocation of an exercise prescription directed at the primary areas of disablement and utilizing specific threshold behaviors will likely result in optimal physical therapy. However, future investigation is needed in all of the aforementioned areas to expand our knowledge base and improve the care provided to patients with cardiac pump dysfunction and failure.

Left Ventricular Assist Devices

Exercise training following LVAD implantation is safe and increases the duration and intensity of submaximal exercise.[49] Patients following LVAD implantation have an improved $\dot{V}O_{2peak}$.[219]

We do not know which impairments keep these patients from regaining normal exercise capacity. It has been suggested that persistent right ventricular failure and chronic peripheral changes may be the limiting factors.[220] Can specific exercise conditioning in patients following LVAD placement reverse the peripheral skeletal muscle and vascular changes that occur in congestive heart failure, thus further improving their exercise capacity? It has also been hypothesized that the presence of the rather large LVAD pump in the abdomen below the left hemidiaphragm may cause a restrictive lung dysfunction preventing the LVAD patient from achieving a greater exercise capacity.[173–175] Further defining the causes for peak exercise deficits may help to develop more specific interventions that will in turn improve exercise performance and thereby reverse the functional limitations and disability imposed by the device and the underlying pathology.

We also have not established threshold behaviors for determining which LVAD patient will benefit most from a specific intervention. Furthermore, investigation of right ventricular and biventricular assist devices is needed to facilitate the rehabilitation of this increasing patient population.[221] This information would enable us to quickly identify patients at risk for a poor outcome and respond by delivering the appropriate therapy. Additionally, these threshold behaviors could be used to justify insurance reimbursement. Administratively these markers may help us to ensure that physical therapy services are being utilized in an appropriate and efficient manner.

Heads Up!

This chapter contains a CD-ROM activity.

REFERENCES

1. American Physical Therapy Association. *Guide to Physical Therapist Practice*. 2nd ed. *Phys Ther*. 2001 Jan;81(1):9-746.

2. Knowles JH, Gorlin R, Storey CF. Clinical test for pulmonary congestion with use of the Valsalva maneuver. *JAMA*. 1956;160:44.

3. Zema MJ, Restivo B, Sos T, et al. Left ventricular dysfunction: bedside Valsalva maneuver revisited. *Br Heart J*. 1980;44:560.

4. Marantz PR, Kaplan MC, Alderman MH. Clinical diagnosis of congestive heart failure in patients with acute dyspnea. *Chest*. 1990;97:776.

5. Zema MJ. Diagnosing heart failure by the Valsalva maneuver: isn't it finally time? *Chest*. 1999;116(4):851.

6. Rocca HP, Weilenmann D, Rickli H, Follath F, Kiowski W. Is blood pressure response to the Valsalva maneuver related to neurohormones, exercise capacity, and clinical findings in heart failure? *Chest*. 1999;116(4):861.

7. van Kraaij DJ, Jansen RW, Bouwels LH, et al. Use of Valsalva's maneuver to detect early recurrence of congestive heart failure in a randomized trial of furosemide withdrawal in older patients. *J Am Geriatr Soc*. 1999;47(11):1384.

8. van Kraaij DJ, Schuurmans MM, Jansen RW, Hoefnagels WH, Go RI. Use of the Valsalva manoeuvre to identify haemodialysis patients at risk of congestive heart failure. *Nephrol Dial Transplant*. 1998;13(6):1518.

9. Rostagno C, Galanti G, Felici M, et al. Prognostic value of baroreflex sensitivity assessed by phase IV of Valsalva manoeuvre in patients with mild to moderate heart failure. *Eur J*. 2000;2(1):41.

10. Cahalin LP, Zema MJ. Expansion of the clinical practice guideline decision tree for cardiac rehabilitation: a theoretical application of the Valsalva maneuver and exercise test results for optimal exercise training. *J Cardiopul Rehabil*. 22(5):368, 2002.

11. McKee PA, Castelli WP, McNamara PM, et al. The natural history of congestive heart failure: the Framingham Study. *N Engl J Med*. 1971;26:1441.

12. Kannel WB: Epidemiological aspects of heart failure. *Cardiol Clin*. 1989;7:1.

13. Yancy CW, Firth BG. Congestive heart failure. *Dis Mon*. 1988;34:467.

14. Kannel WB, Ho K, Thom T. Changing epidemiological features of cardiac failure. *Br Heart J*. 1994;72:S3-S9.

15. Kannel WB, Belanger AJ. Epidemiology of heart failure. *Am Heart J*. 1991;121:951.

16. Braunwald E. Clinical manifestations of heart failure. In: Braunwald E, ed. *Heart Disease—A Textbook of Cardiovascular Medicine*. Vol 1. Philadelphia, PA: WB Saunders; 1988:chap 16.

17. Braunwald E. Pathophysiology of heart failure. In: Braunwald E, ed. *Heart Disease—A Textbook of Cardiovascular Medicine*. Vol 1. Philadelphia, PA: WB Saunders; 1988:chap 14.

18. Antman EM, Braunwald E. Acute myocardial infarction. In: Braunwald E, ed. *Heart Disease—A Textbook of Cardiovascular Medicine*. Vol 2. 5th ed. Philadelphia, PA: WB Saunders; 1997: chap 37.

19. Abbate A, Biondi-Zoccai GG. Baldi: myocardiocyte loss due to apoptosis. *Eur Heart J*. 2002;23(23):1889-1890.

20. Tomei LD, Umansky SR. Apoptosis and the heart: a brief review. *Ann NY Acad Sci*. 2001;946:160-168.

21. Wynne J, Braunwald E. The cardiomyopathies and myocarditides. In: Braunwald E, ed. *Heart Disease—A Textbook of Cardiovascular Medicine*. Vol. 2. Philadelphia, PA: WB Saunders; 1988:chap 42.

22. Ingram RH Jr, Braunwald E. pulmonary edema: cardiogenic and noncardiogenic. In: Braunwald E, ed. *Heart Disease—A Textbook of Cardiovascular Medicine*. Vol 1. Philadelphia, PA: WB Saunders; 1988:chap 18.

23. Light RW, George RB. Serial pulmonary function in patients with acute heart failure. *Arch Intern Med*. 1983;143:429.

24. Wright RS, Levine MS, Bellamy PE, et al. Ventilatory and diffusion abnormalities in potential heart transplant recipients. *Chest*. 1990;98:816.

25. Cahalin LP, Semigran MJ, Dec GW. Inspiratory muscle training in patients with chronic heart failure awaiting cardiac transplantation: results of a pilot clinical trial. *Phys Ther*. 1997; 77:830.

26. Feldman AM, Bristow MR. The beta-adrenergic pathway in the failing human heart: implications for inotropic theraopy. *Cardiology*. 1990;77(suppl D):1.

27. Lefkowitz RJ, Caron MG. Adrenergic receptors: models for the study of receptors coupled to guanine nucleiotide regulatory proteins. *J Biol Chem*. 1988;263:4993.

28. Exton JH. Molecular mechanisms involved in alpha-adrenergic responses. *Mol Cell Endocrinol*. 1981;23:233.

29. Scholz A, Schaefer B, Schmitz W, et al. Alpha1-mediated positive inotropic effect and inositol triphosphate increase in mammalian heart. *J Pharamaccol Exp Ther*. 1988;245:327.

30. Gilman AG. G proteins: transducers of receptor-generated signals. *Annu Rev Biochem*. 1987;56:615.

31. Bristow MR. The beta-adrenergic receptor. Configuration, regulataion, mechanism of action. *Postrad Med*. 1988;29:19.

32. Bristow MR, Ginsburg R, Umans V, et al. Alpha1-adrenergic receptors in the non-failing and failing human heart. *J Pharmaccol Exp Ther*. 1989;247:1039.

33. Weisfeldt ML, Lakatta EG, Gerstenblith G. Aging and cardiac disease. In: Braunwald E, ed. *Heart Disease—A Textbook of Cardiovascular Medicine*. Vol 2. Philadelphia, PA: WB Saunders; 1988:chap 50.

34. Shafiq SA, Sande MA, Carruthers RR, et al. Skeletal muscle in idiopathic cardiomyopathy. *J Neurol Sci*. 1972;15:303.

35. Lipkin DP, Jones DA, Round JM, Poole-Wilson PA. Abnormalities of skeletal muscle in patients with chronic heart failure. *Int J Cardiol*. 1988;18:187.

36. Wilson JR, Fink L, Maris J, et al. Evaluation of energy metabolism in skeletal muscle of patients with heart failure with gated phosphorus-31 nuclear magnetic resonance. *Circulation*. 1985; 71:57.

37. Isaacs H, Muncke G. Idiopathic cardiomyopathy and skeletal muscle abnormality. *Am Heart J*. 1975;90:767.

38. Dunnigan A, Pierpont ME, Smith SA, et al. Cardiac and skeletal myopathy associated with cardiac arrhythmias. *Am J Cardiol*. 1984;53:731.

39. Dunnigan A, Staley NA, Smith SA, et al. Cardiac and skeletal muscle abnormalities in cardiomyopathy: comparison of patients with ventricular tachycardia or congestive heart failure. *J Am Coll Cardiol*. 1987;10:608.

40. Smith ER, Heffernan LP, Sangalang VE, et al. Voluntary muscle involvement in hypertrophic cardiomyopathy: a study of 11 patients. *Ann Intern Med*. 1976;85:566.

41. Hootsmans WJM, Meerschwam IS. Electromyography in patients with hypertrophic obstructive cardiomyopathy. *Neurology*. 1971; 21:810.

42. Meerschwam IS, Hootsmans WJM. An electromyographic study in hypertrophic obstructive cardiomyopathy. In: Wolsterholme GEW, O'Connor M, London J, Churchill A, eds. *Hypertrophic Obstructive Cardiomyopathy*. Ciba Foundation Study Group No. 37. New York: Wiley; 1971.

43. Przybosewki JZ, Hoffman HD, Graff AS, et al. A study of family with inherited disease of cardiac and skeletal muscle. Part 1: clinical electrocardiographic, echocardiographic, hemodynamic, electrophysiological and electron microscopic studies. *S Afr Med J*. 1981;59:363.

44. Lochner A, Hewlett RH, O'Kennedy A, et al. A study of a family with inherited disease of cardiac and skeletal muscle. Part 2: skeletal muscle morphology and mitochondrial oxidative phosphorilation. *S Afr Med J*. 1981;59:453.

45. Caforio ALP, Rossi B, Risaliti R, et al. Type 1 fiber abnormalities in skeletal muscle of patients with hypertrophic and dilated cardiomyopathy: evidence of subclinical myogenic myopathy. *J Am Coll Cardiol*. 1989;14:1464.

46. Farmer JA, Gotto AM. Dyslipidemia and other risk factors for coronary artery disease. In: Braunwald E, ed. *Heart Disease: A Textbook of Cardiovascular Medicine*. 5th ed. Philadelphia, PA: WB Saunders; 1997:1126.

47. Expert Panel on Detection, Evaluation, and Treatment of High Blood Cholesterol in Adults: Summary of the second report of the National Cholesterol Education Program (NCEP) Expert Panel on Detection, Evaluation, and Treatment of High Blood Cholesterol in Adults (Adult Treatment Panel II). *JAMA*. 1993;269:3015.

48. Dargie HJ, McMurray JJ, McDonough TA. Heart failure: implications of the true size of the problem. *J Int Med*. 1996;239(4): 309-315.

49. Morrone TM, Buck LA, Catanese KA, et al. Early progressive mobilization for patients with left ventricular assist devices is safe and optimizes recovery before heart transplantation. *J Heart Lung Transplant*. 1996;15:423-429.

50. Humphrey R, Buck L, Cahalin L, et al. Physical therapy assessment and intervention for patients with left ventricular assist devices. *Cardiopulm Phys Ther*. 1998;9(2):3-7.

51. Morrone TM, Buck LA. Rehabilitation of the ventricular assist device recipient. In: Goldstein DJ, Oz MC, eds. *Cardiac Assist Devices*. Armonk, NY: Futura Publishing Co; 2000:167-176.

52. Dean E. Bedrest and deconditioning. *Neurol Rep*. 1993;17(1):6-9.

53. Ozawa Y, Smith D, Craige E. Origin of the third heart sound. II. Studies in human subjects. *Circulation*. 1983;67:399.

54. Drzewiecki GM, Wasicko MJ, Li JK. Diastolic mechanics and the origin of the third heart sound. *Ann Biomed Engin*. 1991; 19:651.

55. Downes TR, Dunson W, Stewart K. Mechanisms of physiologic and pathologic S_3 gallop sounds. *Am Soc Echocardiol*. 1992;5:211.

56. Chizner MA. Cardiac auscultation: heart sounds. *Cardiol Pract*. 1984;Sept/Oct:141.

57. Perloff JK, Braunwald E. Physical examination of the heart and circulation. In: Braunwald E, ed. *Heart Disease: A Textbook of Cardiovascular Medicine*. 5th ed. Philadelphia, PA: WB Saunders; 1997:35.

58. Guyatt GH, Sullivan MJ, Thompson PJ, et al. The 6-minute walk: a new measure of exercise capacity in patients with chronic heart failure. *Can Med Assoc J*. 1985;132:919-923.

59. Bittner V, Weiner DH, Yusuf S, et al. Prediction of mortality and morbidity with a 6-minute walk test in patients with left ventricular dysfunction. *JAMA*. 1993;270:1702-1707.

60. Cahalin LP, Mathier MM, Semigran MJ, et al. The six-minute walk test predicts peak oxygen uptake and survival in advanced heart failure. *Chest*. 1996;110:325-332.

61. Fishman AP. Approach to the patient with respiratory symptoms. In: Fishman AP, ed. *Fishman's Pulmonary Diseases and Disorders*. 3rd ed. New York: McGraw-Hill; 1997:chap 28, 361-394.

62. Braunwald E. Assessment of cardiac function. In: Braunwald E, ed. *Heart Disease—A Textbook of Cardiovascular Medicine*. Vol 1. Philadelphia, PA: WB Saunders; 1988:chap 15.

63. Joint National Committee on Detection, Evaluation, and Treatment of High Blood Pressure. The fifth report of the Joint National Committee on Detection, Evaluation, and Treatment of High Blood Pressure (JNC-V). *Arch Intern Med*. 1993;153:154.

64. American Association of Cardiovascular and Pulmonary Rehabilitation. *Guidelines for Cardiac Rehabilitation*. 2nd ed. Chicago, IL: Human Kinetics Books; 1994.

65. Killip T, Kimball JT. Treatment of myocardial infarction in a coronary care unit. A two-year experience with 250 patients. *Am J Cardiol*. 1967;20:457.

66. Constant J. *Bedside Cardiology*. Boston, MA: Little, Brown and Company; 1985.

67. Guyton AC. The relationship of cardiac output and atrial pressure control. *Circulation*. 1981;64:1079.

68. Sullivan MJ, Cobb FR. The anaerobic threshold in chronic heart failure. Relation to blood lactate, ventilatory basis, reproducibility, and response to exercise training. *Circulation*. 1990;81 (suppl II):II47-II58.

69. Tavazzi L, Gattone M, Corra U, De Vito F. The anaerobic index: uses and limitations in the assessment of heart failure. *Cardiology*. 1989;76:357-367.

70. Wasserman K, Beaver WL, Whipp BJ. Gas exchange theory and the lactic acidosis (anaerobic) threshold. *Circulation*. 1990; 81(suppl II):14.

71. Koike A, Itoh H, Taniguchi K, Marumo F. Relationship of anaerobic threshold (AT) to AVO$_2$/WR in patients with heart disease [abstract]. *Circulation*. 1988;78(suppl II):624.

72. Griffin BP, Shah PK, Ferguson J, Rubin SA. Incremental prognostic value of exercise hemodynamic variables in chronic congestive heart failure secondary to coronary artery disease or to dilated cardiomyopathy. *Am J Cardiol*. 1991;67:848-853.

73. Pilote L, Silberberg J, Lisbona R, Snideman A. Prognosis in patients with low left ventricular ejection fraction after myocardial infarction: importance of exercise capacity. *Circulation*. 1989;80:1636-1641.

74. Mancini DM, Eisen H, Kussmaul W, Mull R, Edmunds LH Jr, Wilson JR. Value of peak exercise oxygen consumption for optimal timing of cardiac transplantation in ambulatory patients with heart failure. *Circulation*. 1991;83:778.

75. Belardinelli R et al. Randomized, controlled trial of long-term moderate exercise training in chronic heart failure: effects on functional capacity, quality of life, and clinical outcome. *Circulation*. 1999;99:1173-1182.

76. Kostis JB, Rosen RC, Cosgrove NM, Shindler DM, Wilson AC. Nonpharmacologic therapy improves functional and emotional status in congestive heart failure. *Chest*. 1994;106:996-1001.

77. Coats AJS, Adamoupoulos S, Radaelli A, et al. Controlled trial of physical training in chronic heart failure: exercise performance, hemodynamics, ventilation, and autonomic function. *Circulation*. 1992;85:2119-2131.

78. Kavanagh T, Myers MG, Baigrie RS, Mertens DJ, Sawyer P, Shephard RJ. Quality of life and cardiorespiratory function in

chronic heart failure: effects of 12 months' aerobic training. *Heart.* 1996;76:42-49.

79. Tyni-Lenne R, Gordon A, Sylven C. Improved quality of life in chronic heart failure patients following local endurance training with leg muscles. *J Cardiac Failure.* 1996;2(2):111-117.

80. Tyni-Lenne R, Gordon A, Jansson E, Bermann G, Sylven C. Skeletal muscle endurance training improves peripheral oxidative capacity, exercise tolerance, and health-related quality of life in women with chronic congestive heart failure secondary to either ischemic cardiomyopathy or idiopathic dilated cardiomyopathy. *Am J Cardiol.* 1997;80:1025-1029.

81. Meyer K, Schwaibold M, Westbrook S, et al. Effects of exercise training and activity restriction on 6-minute walking test performance in patients with chronic heart failure. *Am Heart J.* 1997;133:447-453.

82. Willenheimer R, Erhardt L, Cline C, Rydberg E, Israelsson B. Exercise training in heart failure improves quality of life and exercise capacity. *Eur Heart J.* 1998;19:774-781.

83. McKelvie RS, Teo KK, Roberts R, et al. Effects of exercise training in patients with heart failure: the exercise rehabilitation trial (EXERT). *Am Heart J.* 2002;144(1):23-30.

84. Tokmakova M, Dobreva B, Kostianev S. Effects of short-term exercise training in patients with heart failure. *Folia Medica.* 1999;41(1):68-71.

85. Keteyian SJ, Brawner CA, Schairer JR, et al. Effects of exercise training on chronotropic incompetence in patients with heart failure. *Am Heart J.* 1999;138:233-240.

86. Gottlieb SS, Fisher ML, Freudenberger R, et al. Effects of exercise training on peak performance and quality of life in congestive heart failure patients. *J Cardiac Failure.* 1999;5(3):188-194.

87. Quittan M, Sturm B, Wiesinger GF, Pacher R, Fialka-Moser V. Quality of life in patients with chronic heart failure: a randomized controlled trial of changes induced by a regular exercise program. *Scand J Rehab Med.* 1999;31:223-228.

88. Wielenga RP, Huisveld IA, Bol E, et al. Safety and effects of physical training in chronic heart failure. Results of the chronic heart failure and graded exercise study (CHANGE). *Eur Heart J.* 1999;20(12):872-879.

89. Oka RK, DeMarco T, Haskell WL, et al. Impact of a home-based walking and resistance training program on quality of life in patients with heart failure. *Am J Cardiol.* 2000;85(3):365-369.

90. Wilson JR, Groves J, Rayos G. Circulatory status and response to cardiac rehabilitation in patients with heart failure. *Circulation.* 1996;94:1567-1572.

91. Gersh BJ, Braunwald E, Rutherford JD. Chronic coronary artery disease. In: Braunwald E, ed. *Heart Disease: A Textbook of Cardiovascular Medicine.* 5th ed. Philadelphia, PA: WB Saunders; 1997:1299-1313.

92. Blumenthal RS, Cohn G, Schulman SP. Medical therapy versus coronary angioplasty in stable coronary artery disease: a review of the literature. *J Am Coll Cardiol.* 2000;36:668.

93. U.S. Department of Health and Human Services. *Clinical Practice Guideline Number 17: Cardiac Rehabilitation.* AHCPR Publication No. 96-0672, October 1995.

94. Ornish D, Scherwitz LW, Billings JH, et al. Intense lifestyle changes for reversal of coronary heart disease. *JAMA.* 1998;280(23):2001-2007.

95. Ornish D. Avoiding revascularization with lifestyle changes: the multicenter lifestyle demonstration project. *Am J Cardiol.* 1998;82(10B):72T-76T.

96. Smith TW, Kelly RA, Stevenson LW, et al. Management of heart failure. In: Braunwald E, ed. *Heart Disease: A Textbook of Cardiovascular Medicine.* 5th ed. Philadelphia, PA: WB Saunders; 1997:492-514.

97. Cahalin L, Zambernardi L, Dec G. Multiple systems assessment during inpatient cardiopulmonary rehabilitation [abstract]. *J Cardiopulm Rehab.* 1993;13:344.

98. Baratz DM, Westbrooke PR, Shah PK, Mohsenifar Z. Effect of nasal continuous positive airway pressure on cardiac output and oxygen delivery in patients with congestive heart failure. *Chest.* 1992;102:1397-1401.

99. Bradley TD, Holloway RM, McLaughlin PR, Ross BL, Walters J, Liu PP. Cardiac output responses to continuous positive airway pressure in congestive heart failure. *Am Rev Respir Dis.* 1992;145:377.

100. Naughton MT, Rahman MA, Hara K, Floras JS, Bradley TD. Effect of continuous positive airway pressure on intrathoracic and left ventricular transmural pressures in patients with congestive heart failure. *Circulation.* 1995;91:1725.

101. Malone S, Liu PP, Hollway R, Rutherford R, Xie A, Bradley TD. Obstructive sleep apnea in patients with dilated cardiomyopathy: effects of continuous positive airway pressure. *Lancet.* 1991;338:1480.

102. Takasaki Y, Orr D, Popkin J, Rutherford R, Liu P, Bradley TD. Effect of nasal continuous positive airway pressure on sleep apnea in congestive heart failure. *Am Rev Respir Dis.* 1989;140:1578.

103. Acosta B, DiBenedetto R, Rahimi A, et al. Hemodynamic effects of noninvasive bilevel positive airway pressure on patients with chronic congestive heart failure with systolic dysfunction. *Chest.* 2000;118:1004.

104. Gordon A, Tyni-Lenne R, Jansson E, et al. Beneficial effects of exercise training in heart failure patients with low cardiac output response to exercise—a comparison of two training models. *J Intern Med.* 1999;246(2):175.

105. Foster C, Dymond DS, Anholm JD, et al. Effect of exercise protocol on the left ventricular response to exercise. *Am J Cardiol.* 1983;51:859.

106. Meyer K, Samek L, Schwaibold M, et al. Interval training in patients with severe chronic heart failure: analysis and recommendations for exercise procedures. *Med Sci Sports Exerc.* 1997;29:306.

107. Strzelczyk TA, Quigg RJ, Pfeifer PB, et al. Accuracy of estimating exercise prescription intensity in patients with left ventricular systolic dysfunction. *J Cardiopulm Rehabil.* 2001;21:158.

108. Keteyian SJ. How hard should we exercise the failing human heart? *J Cardiopulm Rehabil.* 2001;21:164.

109. Morikawa M, Sato H, Sato H, et al. Sustained left ventricular diastolic dysfunction after exercise in patients with dilated cardiomyopathy. *Heart.* 1998;80:263.

110. Meyer K, Gornandt L, Schwaibold M, et al. Predictors of response to exercise training in severe chronic congestive heart failure. *Am J Cardiol.* 1997;80(1):56.

111. Arvan S. Exercise performance of the high risk acute myocardial infarction patient after cardiac rehabilitaton. *Am J Cardiol.* 1988;62:197.

112. Digenio AG, Noakes TD, Cantor A, et al. Predictors of exercise capacity and adaptability to training in patients with coronary artery disease. *J Cardiopulm Rehabil.* 1997;17:110.

113. Vanhees L, Fagard R, Thijs L, Amery A. Prognostic value of training-induced change in peak exercise capacity in patients with myocardial infarcts and patients with coronary bypass surgery. *Am J Cardiol.* 1995;76(14):1014.

114. Vanhees L, Schepers D, Fagard R. Comparison of maximum versus submaximum exercise testing in providing prognostic information after acute myocardial infarction and/or coronary artery bypass grafting. *Am J Cardiol.* 1997;80(3):257.

115. Vanhees L, Schepers D, Defoor J, et al. Exercise performance and training in cardiac patients with atrial fibrillation. *J Cardiopulm Rehabil.* 2000;20(6):346.

116. Oldridge NB et al. Cardiac rehabilitation after myocardial infarction. *JAMA.* 1988;260:945.

117. Greenland P, Chu JS. Efficacy of cardiac rehabilitation services with emphasis on patients after myocardial infarction. *Ann Intern Med.* 1988;109:650.

118. Greenland P, Chu JS. Cardiac rehabilitation services. *Ann Intern Med.* 1988;109:671.

119. Meyer K, Schwaibold M, Westbrook S, et al. Effects of short-term exercise training and activity restriction on functional capacity in patients with severe chronic congestive heart failure. *Am J Cardiol.* 1996;78:1017.

120. Jette M, Heller R, Landrey F, Blumchen G. Randomized 4-week exercise program in patients with impaired left ventricular function. *Circulation.* 1991;84:1561-1567.

121. Hambrecht R, Gielen S, Linke A, et al. Effects of exercise training on left ventricular function and peripheral resistance in patients with chronic heart failure. *JAMA.* 2000;283(23):3095.

122. Kiilavuori K, Sovijarvi A, Naveri H, et al. Effect of physical training on exercise capacity and gas exchange in patients with chronic heart failure. *Chest.* 1996;110:985.

123. Barlow CW, Qayyum MS, Davey PP, et al. Effect of heart failure and physical training on the acute ventilatory response to hypoxia at rest and during exercise. *Respiration.* 1997;64:131.

124. European Heart Failure Training Group. Experience from controlled trials of physical training in chronic heart failure. *Eur Heart J.* 1998;19:466.

125. Lee AP, Ice R, Blessey R, et al. Long-term effects of physical training on coronary patients with impaired ventricular function. *Circulation.* 1979;60:1519-1526.

126. Williams RS, Conn EH, Wallace AG. Enhanced exercise performance following physical training in coronary patients stratified by left ventricular ejection fraction (abstract). *Circulation.* 1981;64:IV-186.

127. Cody DV, Denniss AR, Ross DA, et al. Early exercise testing, physical training and mortality in patients with severe left ventricular dysfunction (abstract). *J Am Coll Cardiol.* 1983;1(2):718.

128. Conn EH, Williams RS, Wallace AG. Exercise responses before and after physical conditioning in patients with severely depressed left ventricular function. *Am J Cardiol.* 1982;49:296-300.

129. Sullivan MJ, Higginbotham MB, Cobb FR. Exercise training in patients with severe left ventricular dysfunction: hemodynamic and metabolic effects. *Circulation.* 1988;78:506-515.

130. Hoffman A. The effects of training on the physical working capacity of MI patients with left ventricular dysfunction. *Eur Heart J.* 1987;8(suppl G):43-53.

131. Kellerman JJ, Shemesh J, Fisman E, et al. Arm exercise training in the rehabilitation of patients with impaired ventricular function and heart failure. *Cardiology.* 1990;77:130-138.

132. Kellerman JJ, Shemesh J. Exercise training of patients with severe heart failure. *J Cardiovasc Pharm.* 1987;10(6):S172-S183.

133. Belardinelli R, Georgiou D, Cianci G, et al. Exercise training improves left ventricular diastolic filling in patients with dilated cardiomyopathy: clinical and prognostic implications. *Circulation.* 1995;91:2775-2784.

134. Belardinelli R, Georgiou D, Scocco V, et al. Low intensity exercise training in patients with chronic heart failure. *J Am Coll Cardiol.* 1995;26:975-982.

135. Squires RW, Lavie CJ, Brandt TR, et al. Cardiac rehabilitation in patients with severe ischemic left ventricular dysfunction. *Mayo Clin Proc.* 1987;62:997-1002.

136. Baigre RS, Myers MG, Kavanagh T, et al. Benefits of physical training in patients with heart failure [abstract]. *Can J Cardiol.* 1992;8(suppl B):107B.

137. Meyer TE, Casadei B, Coats AJS, et al. Angiotensin-converting enzyme inhibition and physical training in heart failure. *J Intern Med.* 1991;230:407-413.

138. Hambrecht R, Niebauer J, Fiehn E, et al. Physical training in patients with stable chronic heart failure: effects on cardiorespiratory fitness and ultrastructural abnormalities of leg muscles. *J Am Coll Cardiol.* 1995;25:1239-1249.

139. Kulavuori K, Toivonen L, Naveri H, Leinonen H. Reversal of autonomic derangements by physical training in chronic heart failure. *Eur Heart J.* 1995;16:490-495.

140. Davey P, Meyer TE, Coats AJS, et al. Ventilation in chronic heart failure: effects of physical training. *Br Heart J.* 1992;68: 474-477.

141. Koch M, Douard H, Broustet JP. The benefit of graded physical exercise in chronic heart failure. *Chest.* 1992;101:231S-235S.

142. Demopoulos L, Bijou R, Fergus I, Jones M, Strom J, LeJemtel TH. Exercise training in patients with severe congestive heart failure: enhancing peak aerobic capacity while minimizing the increase in ventricular wall stress. *J Am Coll Cardiol.* 1997;29: 597-603.

143. Barlow CW, Quayyum MS, Davey PP, Conway J, Paterson DJ, Robbins P. Effect of physical training on exercise-induced hyperkalemia in chronic heart failure. Relation with ventilation and catecholamines. *Circulation.* 1994;89:1144-1152.

144. Kayanakis JG, Page E, Aros F, Borau F. Readaptation des malades en insuffisance cardiaque chronique. Effets immediats et a moyen terme. *Presse Med.* 1994;23:121-126.

145. Scalvini S, Marangoni S, Volterrani M, et al. Physical rehabilitation in coronary patients who have suffered from episodes of cardiac failure. *Cardiology.* 1992;80:417-423.

146. Hornig B, Maier V, Drexler H. Physical training improves endothelial function in patients with chronic heart failure. *Circulation.* 1996;93:210-214.

147. Piepoli M, Volterrani M, Clark AL, Adamopoulos S, Sleight P, Coats AJS. Contribution of muscle afferents to the hemodynamic, autonomic, and ventilatory responses to exercise in patients with chronic heart failure. Effects of physical training. *Circulation.* 1996;93:940-952.

148. Jugdutt BI, Bogdon L, Michorowski BL, Kappagoda CT. Exercise training after anterior Q wave myocardial infarction: importance of regional left ventricular function and topography. *J Am Coll Cardiol.* 1988;12:362.

149. Ennezat PV, Malendowicz SL, Testa M, et al. Physical training in patients with chronic heart failure enhances the expression of genes encoding antioxidative enzymes. *J Am Coll Cardiol.* 2001;38(1):194.

150. Curnier D, Galinier M, Pathak A, et al. Rehabilitation of patients with congestive heart failure with or without beta-blockade therapy. *J Card Fail.* 2001;7(3):241.

151. O'Connor CM, Whellan DJ, Lee KL, et al. Efficacy and safety of exercise training in patients with chronic heart failure: HF-ACTION randomized controlled trial. *JAMA*. 2009;301(14):1439-1450.

152. Flynn KE, Pina IL, Whellan DJ, et al. Effects of exercise training on health status in patients with chronic heart failure: HF-ACTION randomized controlled trial. *JAMA*. 2009;301(14):1451-1459.

153. Coats A. The 'muscle hypothesis' of chronic heart failure. *J Mol Cell Cardiol*. 1996;28(11):2255-2262.

154. Clark A, Poole-Wilson P, Coats A. Exercise limitation in chronic heart failure: central role of the periphery. *J Am Coll Cardiol*. 1996;28(5):1092-1102.

155. Coats A, Clark A, Piepoli M, et al. Symptoms and quality of life in heart failure: the muscle hypothesis. *Br Heart J*. 1994;72:S36-S39.

156. Piepoli M, Clark A, Volterrani M, et al. Contribution of muscle afferents to the hemodynamic, autonomic, and ventilatory responses to exercise in patients with chronic heart failure. *Circulation*. 1996;93:940-952.

157. Hare DL, Ryan TM, Selig SE, et al. Resistance exercise training increases muscle strength, endurance, and blood flow in patients with chronic heart failure. *Am J Cardiol*. 1999;83:1674.

158. Delagardelle C, Feiereisen P, Krecke R, Essamri B, Beissel J. Objective effects of a 6 months' endurance and strength training program in outpatients with congestive heart failure. *Med Sci Sports Exerc*. 1999;31(8):1102.

159. Maiorana A, O'Driscoll G, Cheetham C, et al. Combined aerobic and resistance exercise training improves functional capacity and strength in CHF. *J Appl Physiol*. 2000;88(5):1565.

160. Meyer K, Hajric R, Westbrook S, et al. Hemodynamic responses during leg press exercise in patients with chronic congestive heart failure. *Am J Cardiol*. 1999;83(11):1537.

161. Magnusson G, Gordon A, Kaijser L, et al. High intensity knee extensor training in patients with chronic heart failure: major skeletal muscle improvement. *Eur Heart J*. 1996;17(7):1048.

162. Pu CT, Johnson MT, Forman DE, et al. Randomized trial of progressive resistance training to counteract the myopathy of chronic heart failure. *J Appl Physiol*. 2001;90(6):2341.

163. Quittan M, Sochor A, Wiesinger GF, et al. Strength improvement of knee extensor muscles in patients with chronic heart failure by neuromuscular electrical stimulation. *Artif Organs*. 1999;23(5):432.

164. Cahalin LP, Ferreira DC, Yamada S, Canavan PK. Review of the effects of resistance training in patients with chronic heart failure: potential effects upon the muscle hypothesis. *Cardiopulm Phys Ther J*. 2006;17(1):16-29.

165. Mancini DM, Henson D, La Manca J, Donchez L, Levine S. Benefit of selective respiratory muscle training on exercise capacity in patients with chronic congestive heart failure. *Circulaton*. 1995;91:320.

166. Johnson PH, Cowley AJ, Kinnear WJM. A randomized controlled trial of inspiratory muscle training in stable chronic heart failure. *Eur Heart J*. 1998;19:1249.

167. Weiner P, Waizman J, Magadle R, Berar-Yanay N, Pelled B. The effect of specific inspiratory muscle training on the sensation of dyspnea and exercise tolerance in patients with congestive heart failure. *Clin Cardiol*. 1999;22:727.

168. Bernardi L, Spadacini G, Bellwon J, et al. Effect of breathing rate on oxygen saturation and exercise performance in chronic heart failure. *Lancet*. 1998;351:1308.

169. Martinez A, Lisboa C, Jalil J, et al. Selective training of respiratory muscles in patients with chronic heart failure. *Rev Med Chil*. 2001;129(2):133.

170. Dall'Ago P, Chiappa GRS, Guths H, et al. Inspiratory muscle training in patients with heart failure and inspiratory muscle weakness—a randomized trial. *J Am Coll Cardiol*. 2006;47:757-763.

171. Chiappa GR, Roseguini BT, Vieira PJC, et al. Inspiratory muscle training improves blood flow to resting and exercising limbs in patients with chronic heart failure. *J Am Coll Cardiol*. 2008;51:1663-1671.

172. Humphrey R. LVAD (abstract). Exercise physiology in patients with left ventricular assist devices. *J Cardiopulm Rehabil*. 1997:17(2):73-75.

173. Buck L, Morrone T, Goldsmith R, et al. Exercise training of patients with left ventricular assist devices: a pilot study of physiologic adaptations [abstract]. *J Cardiopulm Rehabil*. 1997:18:86.

174. Buck L. Physical therapy management of three patients following left ventricular assist device implantation: a case report. *Cardiopulm Phys Ther*. 1998;9:8-14.

175. Arena R, Humphrey R, McCall R. Altered exercise pulmonary function after left ventricular assist device implantation. *J Cardiopulm Rehabil*. 1999;19:344-346.

176. Cintron G, Bigas C, Linares E, et al. Nurse practitioner role in a chronic congestive heart failure clinic: in-hospital time, costs, and patient satisfaction. *Heart Lung*. 1983;12:237.

177. Kornowski R, Seeli D, Averbuch M, et al. Intensive home care surveillance prevents hospitalization and improves morbidity rates among elderly patients with severe congestive heart failure. *Am Heart J*. 1995;129:762.

178. Lasater M. The effect of a nurse-managed CHF clinic on patient readmission and length of stay. *Home Healthcare Nurse*. 1996;14:351.

179. West JA, Miller NH, Parker KM, et al. A comprehensive management system for heart failure improves clinical outcomes and reduces medical resource utilization. *Am J Cardiol*. 1997;79:58.

180. Fonarow GC, Stevenson LW, Walden JA, et al. Impact of a comprehensive heart failure management program on hospital readmission and functional status of patients with advanced heart failure. *J Am Coll Cardiol*. 1997;30:725.

181. Hanumanthu S, Butler J, Chomsky D, et al. Effect of a heart failure program on hospitalization frequency and exercise tolerance. *Circulation*. 1997;96:2842.

182. Smith LE, Fabbri SA, Pai R, et al. Symptomatic improvement and reduced hospitalization for patients attending a cardiomyopathy clinic. *Clin Cardiol*. 1997;20:949.

183. Shah NB, Der E, Ruggerio C, et al. Prevention of hospitalizations for heart failure with an interactive home monitoring program. *Am Heart J*. 1998;135:373.

184. Dennis LI, Blue CL, Stahl SM, Benge ME, Carol CJ. The relationship between hospital readmission of Medicare beneficiaries with chronic illness and home care nursing interventions. *Home Healthc Nurse*. 1996;14:303.

185. Martens KH, Mellor SD. A study of the relationship between home care services and hospital readmission of patients with congestive heart failure. *Home Healthc Nurse*. 1997;15:123.

186. Rich MW, Vinson JM, Sperry JC, et al. Prevention of readmission in elderly patients with congestive heart failure: results of a prospective, randomized pilot study. *J Gen Intern Med*. 1993;8:585.

187. Schneider JK, Hornberger S, Booker J, et al. A medication discharge planning program: measuring the effect on readmissions. *Clin Nurs Res.* 1993;2:41.

188. Rich MW, Beckham V, Wittenberg C, et al. A multidisciplinary intervention to prevent the readmission of elderly patients with congestive heart failure. *N Engl J Med.* 1995;333:1190.

189. Stewart S, Pearson S, Horrowitz JD. Effects of a home-based intervention among patients with congestive heart failure discharged from acute hospital care. *Arch Intern Med.* 1988;158:1067.

190. Serxner S, Miyaji M, Jeffords J. Congestive heart failure disease management study: a patient education intervention. *Congestive Heart Fail.* 1998;4:23.

191. Cahalin LP. Heart failure. *Phys Ther.* 1996;76:516.

192. Goldstein DJ. Intracorporeal support: thermo cardiosystems ventricular assist devices. In: Goldstein DJ, Oz MC, eds. *Cardiac Assist Devices.* Armonk, NY: Futura Publishing Co; 2000:307-321.

193. Ramasamy N, Vargo RL, Kormos RL, et al. Intracorporeal support: the novacor left ventricular assist system. In: Goldstein DJ, Oz MC, eds. *Cardiac Assist Devices.* Armonk, NY: Futura Publishing Co; 2000:323-339.

194. de Jonge N, Kirkels H, Lahpor JR, et al. Exercise performance in patients with end-stage heart failure after implantation of a left ventricular assist device and after heart transplantation: an outlook for permanent assisting? *J Am Coll Cardiol.* 2001;37(7):1794.

195. Rose EA, Moskowitz AJ, Packer M, et al. The REMATCH trial: rationale, design, and endpoints. *Ann Thorac Surg.* 1999;67:723-730.

196. Roitman JL, LaFontaine T, Drimmer AM. A new model for risk stratification and delivery of cardiovascular rehabilitation services in the long-term clinical management of patients with coronary artery disease. *J Cardiopulm Rehabil.* 1998;18:113.

197. Matsuo Y, Cahalin LP, Buck L. Cardiac transplantation. *Jpn Phys Ther J.* 2005;39(9):785-793.

198. Cahalin LP. Cardiac transplantation and acute care outcomes. *Acute Care Perspect.* 2005;14(3):1-8.

199. Kavanagh T, Yacoub MH, Mertens DJ, et al. Cardiorespiratory responses to exercise training after orthotopic cardiac transplantation. *Circulation.* 1988;77:162-171.

200. Feinstein AR, Fisher MB, Pigeon JG. Changes in dyspnea-fatigue ratings as indicators of quality of life in the treatment of congestive heart failure. *Am J Cardiol.* 1989;64:50.

201. Guyatt GH, Thompson PJ, Berman LB, et al. How should we measure function in patients with chronic heart and lung disease? *J Chron Dis.* 1985;38:517-524.

202. Rector TS, Kubo SH, Cohn JN. Patients' self-assessment of their congestive heart failure. Part 2: content, reliability and valifity of a new measure, The Minnesota Living with Heart Failure Questionnaire. *Heart Fail.* 1987;3:198-209.

203. Oka RK, Stotts NA, Dae MW, Haskell WL, Gortner SR. Daily physical activity levels in congestive heart failure. *Am J Cardiol.* 1993;71:921.

204. Guccione AA, Felson DT, Anderson JJ, et al. The effects of specific medical conditions on the functional limitations of elders in the Framingham study. *Am J Public Health.* 1994;84:351-358.

205. Cahalin LP. Physiotherapy for the disablement of heart failure—Part II. *Physiotherap Singapore.* 2000;3(1):31.

206. Clark AL, Harrington D, Chua TP, Coats AJS. Exercise capacity in chronic heart failure is related to the aetiology of heart disease. *Heart.* 1997;78:569.

207. Cohn JN, Rector TS. Prognosis of congestive heart failure and predictors of mortality. *Am J Cardiol.* 1988;62:25A-30A.

208. Szlachcic J, Massie BM, Kramer BL, Topic N, Tubau J. Correlates and prognostic implication of exercise capacity in chronic congestive heart failure. *Am J Cardiol.* 1985;55:1037-1042.

209. Likoff MJ, Chandler SL, Kay HR. Clinical determinants of mortality in chronic congestive heart failure secondary to idiopathic dilated or to ischemic cardiomyopathy. *Am J Cardiol.* 1987;59:634-638.

210. Cohn JN, Johnson GR, Shabetai R, et al. Ejection fraction, peak exercise oxygen consumption, cardiothoracic ratio, ventricular arrhythmias, and plasma norepinephrine as determinants of prognosis in heart failure. *Circulation.* 1993;87(VI):VI5-VI16.

211. Aaronson KD, Mancini DM. Is percentage of predicted maximal exercise oxygen consumption a better predictor of survival than peak exercise oxygen consumption for patients with severe heart failure? *J Heart Lung Transplant.* 1995;14:981-989.

212. Cohen-Solal A, Barnier P, Pessione F, et al. Comparison of the long term prognostic value of peak oxygen pulse and peak oxygen uptake in patients with chronic heart failure. *Heart.* 1997;78:572-576.

213. Cahalin LP, Semigran MJ, Dec GW. Inspiratory muscle training in advanced heart failure: Reflections on a pilot study. *Phys Ther.* 1997;77:1764.

214. Cahalin LP, Semigran MJ, Dec GW. Inspiratory muscle training in patients with chronic heart failure awaiting cardiac transplantation: reexamination of pilot data. *World Confederation of Physical Therapy Proceedings.* 1999;302.

215. Higgens T, Cahalin L. A meta-analysis comparing cardiorespiratory performance in persons with left ventricular assist device and end-stage heart failure [abstract]. *Cardiopulm Phys Ther J.* 2001;12(4):147-148.

216. Gordon J, Quinn L. Guide to physical therapist practice: a critical appraisal. *Neurol Rep.* 1999;23:122-128.

217. Verbrugge L, Jette A. The disablement process. *Soc Sci Med.* 1994;38:1-14.

218. Stewart AL, Hays RD, Ware JE. The MOS Short-Form General Health Survey—reliability and validity in a patient population. *Med Care.* 1988;26:724.

219. Mancini D, Goldsmith R, Levin H, et al. Comparison of exercise performance in patients with severe heart failure versus left ventricular assist devices. *Circulation.* 1998;98:1178-1183.

220. Mancini D, Beniaminovitz A. Exercise performance in patients with left ventricular assist devices. In: Goldstein DJ, Oz MC, eds. *Cardiac Assist Devices.* Armonk, NY: Futura Publishing Co; 2000:137-152.

221. Simon MA, Kormos RL, Gorcsan J, et al. Differential exercise performance on ventricular assist device support. *J Heart Lung Transplant.* 2005;24(10):1506-1512.

Physical Therapy Associated with Respiratory Failure

CHAPTER

19

Nancy D. Ciesla & Jill D. Kuramoto

INTRODUCTION

Recent literature supports the need for early mobility in the intensive care unit (ICU), and that patients can be safely mobilized.[1-6] Acute respiratory distress syndrome (ARDS) survivors report significant impairments in quality of life, including physical functioning, which may be more impaired than respiratory function.[7,8] One year following mechanical ventilation for at least 48 hours more than half of the survivors required caregiver support at home.[9]

New evidence suggests 7 day per week physical therapy as part of a protocol-driven mobility team is associated with earlier mobilization out of bed, ambulation, and decreased ICU and hospital length of stay.[4,5] Therefore, support and demand for physical therapy interventions are increasing in the ICU, particularly with mechanically ventilated patients.

Mechanically ventilated patients are often acutely ill, hospitalized in an ICU, and connected to a plethora of lines, tubes, and monitors to sustain life. Examining medically and surgically complex patients with all of this paraphernalia can be quite intimidating for both the novice and experienced physical therapist with little training in the critical care setting. This chapter provides a basic understanding of the physiological aspects of pulmonary function related to mechanical ventilation. Respiratory failure is defined, and the student is introduced to the criteria used to initiate and discontinue mechanical ventilatory support. Commonly utilized modes of mechanical ventilation are described to enable the entry-level therapist to examine and safely treat patients requiring artificial ventilation. This knowledge can be utilized not only in the acute care setting but also in rehabilitation, subacute, and home care settings, where greater numbers of patients are being discharged with a continued need for mechanical ventilation. Physical therapy examination and interventions are described in detail using a case demonstration of a monitored and mechanically ventilated tetraplegic patient with a complete lesion at the C5 level on the American Spinal Injury Association impairment scale, the standard neurological classification of spinal cord injury. Physical therapy interventions such as secretion clearance techniques, breathing exercises, therapeutic exercises, and functional mobility training may assist the patient in being weaned from a ventilator and improve functional outcomes. The risks of mechanical ventilation, ICU interventions, and immobility are discussed throughout this chapter, with an introduction to evidence-based practice and the future for physical therapists working with mechanically ventilated patients.

DESCRIPTION OF PATTERN 6F

A practice pattern has been developed by the American Physical Therapy Association for patients who are in respiratory failure. This Practice Pattern, Pattern 6F, *Impaired Ventilation and Respiration/Gas Exchange Associated with Respiratory Failure,* is the basis for this chapter (Fig. 19-1).[10] Mechanical ventilation is frequently required until the cause of respiratory failure is improved, removed, or reversed. This chapter addresses patients who require mechanical ventilation 24 hours per day and who may require weaning to be liberated from mechanical ventilatory support. A description of the modes of mechanical ventilation, including continuous positive airway pressure and bilevel ventilation, is included.

RESPIRATORY PHYSIOLOGY: APPLICATION TO THE MECHANICALLY VENTILATED PATIENT

During normal breathing, inspired air passes from the mouth through the trachea and bronchial tree to the alveoli where most gas exchange takes place. Oxygen diffuses across the alveolar capillary membrane into the circulating blood where it binds with hemoglobin. Oxygen is then carried from the lungs to the capillary beds that are present in all metabolically active tissues. Oxygen then dissociates from hemoglobin and diffuses into the cells. (Refer to Chapter 5 for a description of oxyhemoglobin dissociation.) For adequate oxygenation, there must

585

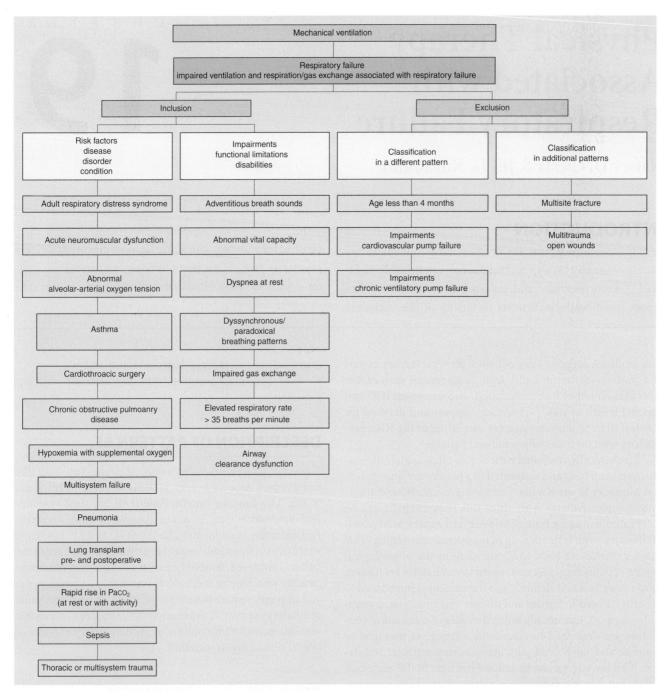

FIGURE 19-1   Patient/client diagnostic classification adapted from Practice Pattern 6F. (Reproduced with permission from American Physical Therapy Association. Guide to Physical Therapist Practice, 2nd ed. *Phys Ther.* 2001 Jan;81:539–553.)

be sufficient oxygen carried in the blood, or oxygen-carrying capacity. The total oxygen concentration of a sample of blood (dissociated oxygen and the oxygen combined with hemoglobin) is determined using the formula[11]:

$$Ca_{O_2} = (1.39 \times Hb \times Sat/100) + 0.003\ P_{O_2}$$

Hb refers to hemoglobin concentration in grams per 100 mL; Sat is the arterial hemoglobin saturation as a percentage; and P_{O_2} is the partial pressure of oxygen dissolved in the blood.[11,12] With this simple equation, note that nearly all the oxygen carried in the blood is bound to hemoglobin, and only a small clinically insignificant amount is transported and dissolved in the plasma (approximately 1%–2%). Hypoxemia results when either the lungs are unable to diffuse sufficient oxygen to saturate hemoglobin or the red blood cell count is insufficient.

Normally, a healthy person breathing room air has a hemoglobin concentration of 15 g/100 mL of blood, an arterial saturation of 97.5%, and a P_{O_2} of 100 mm Hg. Therefore, a normal arterial oxygen concentration is approximately 20.8 mL of

O_2/100 mL of blood.[11] Venous blood contains less saturated hemoglobin, about 15 mL of O_2/100 mL of blood. When patient oxygen-carrying content is low due to low hemoglobin, a blood transfusion may be necessary, yet the patient may have normal lung function and normal oxygen saturation. However, if the oxygen-carrying content is low due to a low oxygen saturation and P_{O_2}, the appropriate treatment may be to deliver supplemental oxygen. *Supplemental oxygen* is defined as a percentage of oxygen greater than 21% (room air contains 21% oxygen). A patient may receive supplemental oxygen through a face mask, tracheostomy collar, or nasal prongs, which require the patient to breathe independently, or oxygen may be delivered via positive pressure using a mechanical ventilator. After administering supplemental oxygen, the medical team must determine the cause of the hypoxemia. The cause of hypoxemia may be either pulmonary (lung injury or disease) or nonpulmonary (respiratory muscle or metabolic) dysfunction. A patient with severe chronic obstructive pulmonary disease (COPD) or a lung contusion may be hypoxemic as a result of secretion retention, lung injury, lung disease, or an obstruction in the tracheobronchial tree, all pulmonary causes of hypoxemia. A patient who has a chest radiograph that denotes a severe hemothorax compressing the lung would have a nonpulmonary cause of hypoxemia. Once a chest tube is inserted and blood is drained from the pleural cavity, the patient's Pa_{O_2} and Sa_{O_2} are likely to improve. A patient in respiratory failure as a result of septic shock would have a metabolic, nonpulmonary indication for mechanical ventilation (Table 19-1).

The matching of ventilation to perfusion ($\dot{V}/\dot{Q}$) is the principal determinant of Pa_{O_2}. $\dot{V}/\dot{Q}$ is the matching of ventilation (respiratory gases) to perfusion (pulmonary blood). Shunt refers to the amount of blood entering the left heart without passing through ventilated areas of the lung.[11,13] Ninety-five percent of the blood entering the pulmonary circulation passes through the alveoli and equilibrates with inspired respiratory gases. A shunt greater than 20% may indicate the need for mechanical ventilation.[12] Arterial oxygen saturation and Pa_{O_2} may be decreased because of $\dot{V}/\dot{Q}$ mismatching, alveolar hypoventilation, anatomic right to left shunt, decreased ambient oxygen, and a limitation in diffusion.[11] Physical therapists working with mechanically ventilated patients should review the most recent arterial blood gases or oxygen saturation prior to physical therapy interventions. For example, a patient breathing room air with a $\dot{V}/\dot{Q}$ mismatch exceeding 20% may have a Pa_{O_2} of only 50 mm Hg. Mechanical ventilation may be necessary if increasing the Fi_{O_2} with spontaneous breathing is unsuccessful. Physical therapy may be indicated once the patient is adequately oxygenated.

Minute Ventilation

Normally, an adult patient's minute ventilation is about 7.5 L/min. Total minute ventilation is the sum of alveolar ventilation ($\dot{V}A$) and dead space ventilation ($\dot{V}D$). Alveolar ventilation represents the volume of gas that reaches the respiratory zone, and is therefore available for gas exchange, and accounts for approximately two-thirds of normal minute ventilation. Dead space ventilation may be considered in two different ways, either anatomic or physiologic. Anatomic dead space represents the volume of the conducting airways, whereas physiologic dead space represents the volume of the lung that does not exchange carbon dioxide (CO_2). Normally, anatomic and physiologic dead space are virtually the same, but in the patient with pulmonary dysfunction, physiologic dead space may be greater due to $\dot{V}/\dot{Q}$ mismatch.[11] The ventilator usually supplies a calculated minute ventilation, or the therapist may be able calculate it by multiplying the respiratory rate by the tidal volume if tidal volume has been set on the ventilator. For a patient receiving mechanical ventilation, the expired minute volume is a combination of mandatory machine breaths and patient-initiated breaths. During physical therapy interventions, the physical therapist should note any significant changes in respiratory rate, tidal volume, or minute ventilation.

Carbon dioxide (CO_2) is a by-product of cellular aerobic metabolism and diffuses from the tissues into venous capillary blood. The pulmonary capillary network surrounds the alveoli, and CO_2 diffuses into the alveoli and is exhaled through the mouth and nose after passing through the tracheobronchial tree. The partial pressure of carbon dioxide (Pa_{CO_2}) is determined by the balance between carbon dioxide production that occurs during cellular metabolism and the amount removed by the lungs during ventilation. Carbon dioxide is highly soluble and is not usually affected clinically by changes in $\dot{V}/\dot{Q}$. When a patient is at rest we can assume that CO_2 tension is constant. Changes in Pa_{CO_2} can be attributed to changes in $\dot{V}A$. Increases in Pa_{CO_2} occur when changes in carbon dioxide production are not accompanied by a proportional change in minute ventilation. Exercise, fever, and an increase in dead space ventilation are conditions that may cause an increase in Pa_{CO_2}.[12] High levels of Pa_{CO_2} may not be as detrimental as originally thought.[14] Therapists working in the intensive care unit may see mechanically ventilated patients with Pa_{CO_2} levels exceeding 80 mm Hg without known deleterious side effects. An intentional mechanical ventilation strategy which incorporates an elevated Pa_{CO_2} is referred to as *permissive hypercapnia*.[15]

TABLE 19-1 Common Causes of Hypoxemia/Hypoxia

Pulmonary	Non Pulmonary
Pneumonia	Respiratory muscle weakness/fatigue
Lung injury (eg, contusion)	Congestive heart failure
Acute respiratory distress syndrome	Anemia
Lung diseases (eg, chronic obstructive lung disease)	Metabolic (eg, septic shock)
Secretion retention	Pneumothorax
Airway obstruction	Hemothorax

Work of Breathing

Work of breathing is defined as energy a patient must expend to move gases into and out of the lung. During normal ventilation, inspiration involves the contraction of the respiratory muscles, and expiration occurs passively, using the elastic recoil of the lung and chest wall. The normal work of breathing is around 3 mL/min or less than 2% of the total metabolic rate. Only 10% of the energy consumed during respiration is a result of contraction of the respiratory muscles to move gases against the resistance and compliance factors of the airways and lung tissues; 90% of the energy consumed during ventilation is wasted and used to generate heat. However, the respiratory work of breathing is also the result of both the airway pressures required to overcome airway resistance and the elastic forces of the lung and thorax. Therefore respiratory work increases during periods of high airway resistance and rapid respiratory rates, or with large lung volumes and low lung–thorax compliance. Asthmatic patients and patients with a tracheostomy or endotracheal tube may have increased airway resistance and breathe optimally with a slower respiratory rate at higher tidal volumes. Conversely, patients with low lung compliance, such as those with severe ARDS, pulmonary edema, pulmonary fibrosis, atelectasis, and pulmonary contusion, breathe more efficiently at faster respiratory rates using smaller tidal volumes.[16,17] The ventilator can be adjusted to minimize the patient's work of breathing. This will be explained later in this chapter in the section on *Modes of Mechanical Ventilation*. The optimal respiratory frequency is a balance between the resistive and the elastic forces of the lung. See Chapter 5 for more details regarding respiratory physiology.

RESPIRATORY FAILURE

Respiratory failure occurs when the exchange of gases (oxygen and carbon dioxide) is inadequate to meet the patient's metabolic needs. *Acute respiratory failure* is a life-threatening condition, diagnosed clinically, and the primary indication for mechanical ventilation. Breathing requires integration of the respiratory centers in the brainstem, the respiratory muscles, and connecting nerves. Injury or disease negatively impacting this integration, or the lung parenchyma, may lead to respiratory failure. Patients in respiratory failure usually require mechanical ventilation and therefore fall into physical therapy Practice Pattern 6F. A patient may present with hypoxemia, hypercarbia, acidosis, or a combination of these three conditions. This clinical presentation may result from the lung not being efficient as a gas-exchange membrane, from inadequate gas exchange, or from the patient being unable to support respiratory function because it requires too much work. Common clinical indications for intubation and mechanical ventilation that the physical therapist may encounter are listed in Table 19-2. The exact criteria used to intubate and mechanically ventilate a patient may vary depending on patient diagnosis, physician preference and training, and institutional guidelines.

TABLE 19-2   Indications for Endotracheal Intubation

Couple patient to ventilator
Acute hypoxemia respiratory failure
Ventilatory failure
Periodic respiratory failure
Circulatory instability or shock
Maintain patent airway
Neurologic impairment
Sleep apnea
Oropharyngeal edema or hematoma
Laryngospasm
Glottic edema or stenosis
Aid pulmonary toilet
Massive hemoptysis
Excessive secretions
Minimize aspiration of oropharyngeal or gastric contents

Reprinted with permission from Schmidt G, Hall J, Wood L. Management of the ventilated patient. In: Murray JF, Nadel JA, eds. *Textbook of Respiratory Medicine.* 2nd ed. Philadelphia, PA: WB Saunders; 1994:2637.

MECHANICAL VENTILATION

The critical care physical therapist may be challenged by the variety of ventilators and ventilator settings they encounter while treating ICU patients. Ventilator preferences vary between facilities based on physician preference, patient population, funding, and staff knowledge. This section will describe frequently used types and modes of ventilators for adult patients receiving physical therapy interventions. Most are positive-pressure ventilators with a multitude of dials, digital readouts, lines, tubes, and alarms. Although there are many theories in practice about the pros and cons of each ventilator type and the modes of ventilation, it is vital to remember the most important factor related to the duration and success of mechanical ventilation: treatment of the patient's underlying condition causing respiratory failure. This is far more important in influencing patient morbidity and mortality than the type of ventilator. Although ventilators from different manufacturers may have controls, dials, and digital readouts that appear very different, the principles and functions of most ventilators are similar.

While mechanical ventilation is a common medical intervention, 80% of patients are weaned without difficulty after only a short duration of mechanical ventilation.[18] For the 20% of mechanically ventilated requiring more complex weaning, the newer more sophisticated ventilators may hold advantages for patients with resolving severe respiratory failure.

The first positive pressure ventilators were developed in the early part of the 20th century by anesthesiologists to deliver anesthetic agents via an endotracheal tube to patients having surgery, and to support breathing during thoracic surgery. In 1952, positive pressure ventilation was brought to the bedside, when medical students in Copenhagen were scheduled by Dr. Isben, an anesthetist, to manually inflate the lungs of patients with poliomyelitis using *manual resuscitator bags,* 24 hours per day.[19] Manual resuscitator bags, often referred to as *ambu*

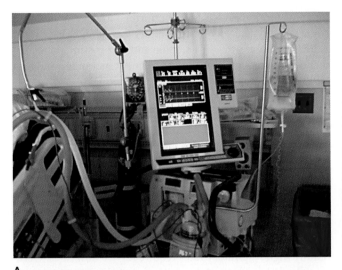

A

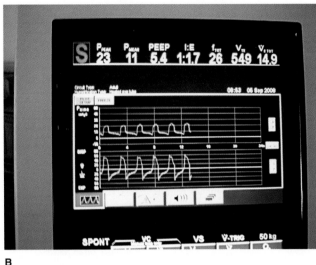

B

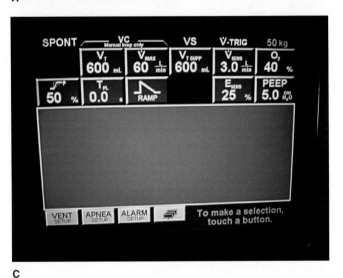

C

FIGURE 19-2 Mechanical ventilator. (**A**) Ventilator and humidifier at the patient's bedside. (**B**) Patient's actual ventilation: note airway pressure (mean airway pressure 11), Peep, inspiratory—expiratory time, respiratory rate (f$_{tot}$), and tidal volume. (**C**) Ventilator settings: note tidal volume, 600 mL, Fio$_2$ 40%, Peep 5. The patient is spontaneously breathing; there is no preset respiratory rate.

bags, delivered a concentration of oxygen greater than 21% (oxygenation) and a larger than resting tidal volume (ventilation); the respiratory rate (work of breathing) was controlled by the medical student. The same goals, for example, improving oxygenation, ventilation, and the work of breathing, are the basis for mechanical ventilation today. In addition, recent technological advances allow some ventilators to automatically adjust parameters to the patient's physiological response to the disease process and the demands associated with medical and physical therapy interventions. Figure 19-2 shows the common features of a mechanical ventilator.

Oxygenation

Oxygenation is primarily controlled by the concentration (percentage) of oxygen in the inspired gas and the positive end-expiratory pressure (PEEP). The concentration of oxygen is referred to as the Fio$_2$, the percentage or fraction of inspired oxygen. Additional oxygen is usually delivered by a ventilator after other methods of supplemental oxygen delivery have failed

to achieve adequate oxygenation. In addition to increasing the Fio$_2$, PEEP may be added. PEEP retards small airway and alveoli closure, thus preventing derecruitment of alveoli. Derecruited alveoli do not participate in gas exchange.[20] Therefore, PEEP prevents early airway and alveolar collapse at the end of expiration by increasing functional residual capacity, increasing end-expiratory lung volumes, and improving the matching of ventilation to perfusion by decreasing intrapulmonary shunt (Table 19-3).[21]

Oxygenation may also be enhanced by increasing tidal volume or increasing inspiratory versus expiratory (inverse I:E ratio) ventilation, providing increased time for gas exchange to occur in ventilated alveoli. Some advocate transient use of high levels of PEEP in conjunction with recruitment maneuvers to facilitate recruitment or reopening of collapsed alveoli. More recently, facilitation of spontaneous breathing has also been shown to improve oxygenation[22] (see Table 19-3).

Functional residual capacity (FRC) may be negatively impacted in the sick lung and in patients lying in the supine or near supine position. A means of increasing FRC is to add

TABLE 19-3   Interventions to Increase PaO$_2$

Increase FiO$_2$—fraction (%) of inspired oxygen
Increase tidal volume
Increase inspiratory: expiratory ratio
Facilitate spontaneous breathing
Add positive end expiratory pressure (PEEP)

Mechanisms of increased PaO$_2$ with PEEP
Increase in end-expiratory lung volume
   Distension of patent lung units
   Prevent derecruitment of collapsed lung units
   Redistribution of fluid within the lung

Decrease in intrapulmonary shunt (Arterial blood not passing
   through normal ventilated lung)
   Increase in end-expiratory lung volume
   Decrease in cardiac output

Adapted from Tobin M. Mechanical ventilation: conventional modes and settings. In: Fishman A, ed. *Fishman's Pulmonary Diseases and Disorders*. 3rd ed. New York: McGraw-Hill; 1998:2691-2699. West JB. Respiratory physiology: Ventilation, blood flow, and gas exchange. In: Murray JF, Nadel JA, eds. *Textbook of Respiratory Medicine*. 2nd ed. Philadelphia, PA: WB Saunders; 1994:75. Putensen C, Muders T, Varelmann D, Wrigge H. The impact of spontaneous breathing during mechanical ventilation. *Curr Opin Crit Care*. 2006;12(1):13-18.

PEEP or continuous positive airway pressure (CPAP). Some believe physiological PEEP, defined as positive pressure within the alveoli in the presence of a closed glottis, is lost with the presence of a tracheal tube. This is because the tracheal tube either passes through the glottis, which remains open, or the tube is placed below the glottis and vocal cords. However, evidence is lacking as to whether physiological PEEP actually exists.[23]

To restore FRC, 5 cm H$_2$O of PEEP is usually applied during mechanical ventilation. A fixed resistance is applied to the expiratory limb of the ventilator circuit to maintain a positive pressure at the end of expiration. PEEP is increased by the physician as clinically indicated; levels as high as 15 to 20 cm H$_2$O may be necessary with ARDS, severe pulmonary edema, and severe bilateral pneumonia when distal airways may be edematous and prone to collapse. PEEP is increased cautiously as it may decrease cardiac output and adversely affect blood pressure. Patients who require frequent adjustments of FiO$_2$ and PEEP usually have continuous blood pressure monitoring via an arterial line and may have pulmonary artery catheters to measure pulmonary artery pressures and cardiac output as the level of PEEP is titrated. PEEP may be contraindicated for patients with untreated pneumothorax, or bronchopleural fistulas.[24]

As a general rule those patients requiring PEEP greater than 10 cm H$_2$O pressure should not be routinely disconnected from the ventilator for turning, suctioning, and transfer activities. Disconnection, either intentional or inadvertent, may result in alveolar derecruitment with ensuing complications. High levels of PEEP alone usually do not preclude a patient from tolerating secretion clearance techniques and mobilization, including ambulation with a portable ventilator. It is important to maximally mobilize the patient and perform secretion clearance techniques, as immobility and secretion retention may be contributing to the hypoxemia for which high levels of PEEP are required. Functional mobility and range-of-motion exercises are performed to patient tolerance, while the physical therapist monitors the patient's vital signs. A PEEP adapter or in-line suction catheter is strongly recommended for patients who require frequent suctioning and have a PEEP of 10 cm H$_2$O or greater (see CD-ROM).

Ventilation

There are several controls or dials on the ventilator that regulate ventilation. These include controls for respiratory rate, tidal volume, inspiratory flow rate, and inspiratory/expiratory (I:E) ratio. Tidal volume and respiratory rate regulate PaCO$_2$. In volume targeted modes of ventilation the inspiratory flow rate is the speed with which inspired gas is delivered to the lungs and may be adjusted to meet the patient's demand. Patients who require high respiratory rates require higher flow rates. Occasionally, during physical therapy interventions the patient may seem to be "bucking" or dyssynchronous with the ventilator due to higher minute ventilation requirements. This may be due to a flow rate that is not adequate and the patient subsequently breathes against a fixed resistance. The result is an increased work of breathing for the patient and increased inspiratory effort. In pressure targeted and dual targeting modes of ventilation, the inspiratory flow is variable and may be advantageous to meet varying patient demands. Critically ill patients may also have an increase in dead space ventilation as high as 70% of minute ventilation, secondary to increased $\dot{V}/\dot{Q}$ mismatch or shunt related to their disease process.[25] Thus, mechanically ventilated patients routinely require a higher than normal minute ventilation to meet their metabolic demand.

Work of Breathing

Work of breathing will be influenced by the mode of ventilation used. A mode of ventilation is defined by the interaction between machine and patient. How the breath is delivered and how the patient participates or interacts with that delivery defines the mode.[26] It is essential that the physical therapist understand the concepts of the different modes of mechanical ventilation if they are to independently deliver care. For example, a patient may have a resting respiratory rate of 21 breaths/min, with 8 mandatory breaths and 13 spontaneous breaths. During physical therapy treatment, without any ventilator adjustments, the respiratory rate may temporarily increase to 35 breaths/min. The therapist will note that the spontaneous respiratory rate is now 27 breaths/min and there is an increased work of breathing. The patient may need to rest before additional physical therapy interventions. Temporary changes in respiratory rate are normal and should not interfere with physical therapy interventions if they quickly return to baseline. However, the number of breaths per minute delivered by the ventilator can be increased (with a physician order) to allow a patient to tolerate more physical therapy and nursing interventions such as side-to-side turning, therapeutic exercises, and bed-to-chair transfers.

Physical therapists usually do not adjust ventilator settings. After consultation with the critical care personnel: physician, respiratory therapist and/or nurse, orders may be written that permit adjustments by appropriate staff to support physical therapy interventions.

CLINICAL CORRELATE

Mechanical ventilation should be a dynamic process, similar to changes in spontaneous breathing during changes in activity levels. It therefore may be necessary to change the mode of ventilation or increase the flow rate, respiratory rate, or FiO_2 during all or part of a patient's physical therapy treatment. Collaboration between the physical therapist and the ICU clinicians trained in the complexities of mechanical ventilation is recommended to determine the best ventilator settings during physical therapy interventions.

VENTILATOR ALARMS

Prior to treating ventilated patients, the physical therapist must have a basic understanding of the alarms generic to all ventilators. The therapist should be able to discriminate between those requiring emergent nursing or medical interventions and alarms which may be the result of normal changes in respiratory parameters/mechanics in response to the treatment intervention. The parameters for each alarm are selected by the bedside clinician and are typically set for the patient in a resting state. Therefore normal physiological responses to position changes, activity, coughing, suctioning, and therapeutic exercise may activate an alarm.

Alarms may be divided into three categories: those alarms resulting from oxygenation/system failure, pressure changes, and volume changes.

Oxygen/System Failure Alarms

Though infrequent, the alarm associated with one of the most serious consequences notifies the clinician of system failure or a low or nonexistent oxygen supply. This alarm usually has a piercing sound that calls immediate attention to the situation. Most hospitals have a backup generator system that will immediately take over in cases of electrical failure. When a ventilator becomes nonoperational, the therapist should immediately turn the wall oxygen flow rate up as high as possible (usually around 15 L/min) and begin ventilating the patient with a manual resuscitator bag, while calling for assistance. Whenever the therapist is treating a ventilated patient outside the ICU setting, he or she should check that an oxygen supply is readily available from either a portable tank or a wall oxygen supply. Manual resuscitator bags, oxygen tubing, an oxygen supply, and tracheal suction equipment and supplies should be in the work area and checked daily according to hospital/departmental standards.

Pressure Alarms

Pressure alarms notify the clinician that the ventilator is operating outside preset pressure ranges, either high or low. These alarms require that the clinician determine the cause of the alarm and whether any additional interventions are necessary.

High-pressure alarms indicate that higher than expected pressures are necessary to deliver the desired tidal volume. High-pressure alarms may be triggered by either an increase in airway resistance or a decrease in lung compliance. Increase in airway resistance occurs because of an obstruction in the tracheal tube, coughing, or agitation causing the patient to breathe in a way that is not in synchrony with the ventilator settings. The tracheal tube may be obstructed by a mucus plug, blood clot, or by a patient biting the endotracheal tube. When a mucus plug or blood clot is suspected, the therapist should immediately suction the patient. While suctioning, the therapist should note whether the catheter could reach the carina. Noting the distance from the opening of the tracheal tube to the carina will help the therapist determine whether there is still an obstruction in the airway after suctioning. The therapist should also auscultate the chest and note any changes in breath sounds since the beginning of the physical therapy intervention. If it is suspected that the patient is biting the endotracheal tube, or that the tube is kinked, the nurse should be notified and a bite block may be placed in the patient's mouth or sedation administered. If the alarm persists after suctioning, placing a bite block, and sedation, medical attention may be necessary. The physician evaluates the situation and may need to change the tracheal tube.

High-pressure alarms may also be activated when a patient's lungs are becoming less compliant due to a worsening medical condition such as ARDS or pneumothorax. In this situation, the ventilator must generate higher pressures in order to maintain the same tidal volume. The physician or respiratory therapist may change the mode of ventilation, targeted tidal volume, or increase the upper limit of the pressure alarm setting in order to resolve the situation. Changes in patient position may also decrease thoracic compliance, care should be taken with upper extremity positioning to facilitate versus inhibit chest wall expansion, particularly in the side-lying position.

Low-pressure alarms are the result of some type of leak in the respiratory circuit. This occurs when the endotracheal tube is disconnected, there is a break in the integrity of the tubing circuit, or there is an air leak around the tracheal tube. The nurse, patient, or therapist may inadvertently disconnect the ventilator tubing from the tracheal tube, or open an access port within the ventilator circuit. If consistent with institutional policies, therapists may briefly disconnect the tracheal tube from the ventilator tube for suctioning, when mobilizing a patient, or to remove excess water from condensation in the tubing. As disconnection will eliminate PEEP, the frequency and duration of disconnection will depend upon the level of PEEP the patient requires. Once the tube is reconnected, the alarm will no longer sound. While working with a patient who disconnects him or herself from the ventilator, the therapist should not hesitate to reattach the ventilator tubing to the tracheal tube and report this behavior to the bedside nurse. Such circumstances may make it appropriate to apply protective devices that restrain movement, for which a physician order is usually required. If a patient pulls out the tracheal tube (self-extubates), the therapist should immediately begin bagging the patient with a manual resuscitator bag, supplemental oxygen and a face mask while summoning help.

Volume Alarms

Volume alarms signal that the ventilator is operating outside the expected volume ranges set by the operator. These alarms may be set to monitor minute ventilation and/or tidal volume. It is expected that the inhaled and exhaled lung volumes of a mechanically ventilated patient are close. When the cuff on the tracheostomy or endotracheal tube ruptures, leaks, or is deflated, there will be a marked difference in inhaled and exhaled volumes causing the low-volume alarm to sound. The therapist should notify the nurse, physician, or respiratory therapist when this is suspected.

High-volume alarms alert the clinician that the patient is getting a higher than preset minute ventilation. This may occur with an increase in respiratory rate in response to agitation or to a change in the patient's mental status. The high-volume alarm frequently sounds while turning a patient or moving a patient to sit on the edge of the bed or transfer. Once the activity is completed, the patient usually returns to the baseline ventilatory pattern, and the alarm stops. This is a normal response to physical therapy and does not require any special intervention. However, if the patient becomes agitated, and does not respond to activity or the therapist trying to calm the patient, the nurse should be notified. There may be a better time of day to see the patient, or the nurse may need to administer medication to enhance participation. It is recommended that the therapist anticipate the need for additional medication and speak with the nurse prior to physical therapy interventions.

It is notable that an increase in respiratory rate is a normal response to activity. Therefore, a marked increase in respiratory rate with an exercise program may necessitate a change in the ventilator settings, not medication.

CLINICAL CORRELATE

The decision to use sedation or antianxiety medication to facilitate therapy interventions must always take into account the detrimental effects the medication may have on the patient's ability to interact and actively participate in the therapeutic intervention as well as potential detrimental long-term effects of the medication.

Low-exhaled-volume alarms are usually the result of the patient becoming disconnected from the ventilator or from a leak in the cuff of the tracheal tube or ventilator circuit, as previously discussed. However, a low-volume alarm may also sound when a spontaneously breathing patient receiving ventilatory support is given a narcotic, sedative, or paralytic medication, decreasing their respiratory drive or ability. Patients who require ventilatory support may benefit from a short-acting drug for some physical therapy interventions. For example, patients with abnormal muscle tone may require pharmacological intervention to optimize joint positioning prior to serial casting. Close monitoring is required. Ventilatory support may need to be increased for the procedure; yet, once the patient's spontaneous respirations return, the ventilator is adjusted back to the original baseline settings.

MODES OF MECHANICAL VENTILATION

A mode of ventilation is a means to deliver a breath to a patient and is defined by the interaction between patient and machine. There are many different modes with specific characteristics. At times, these differences may appear subtle, but are sufficient to warrant distinction. Modes may be considered on a continuum, from the ventilator assuming all or the vast majority of the patient's breathing, to the patient primarily breathing on his own.

There are numerous modes of ventilation utilized in clinical practice that are designed to improve oxygenation and subsequently support oxygen consumption. Oxygen consumption ($\dot{V}O_2$) of the respiratory muscles depends on the patient's clinical condition and ranges from 2% to 3% of total body $\dot{V}O_2$ in healthy spontaneously breathing subjects, 5% to 10% in patients breathing on a ventilator during assisted modes, and up to 50% in patients with severe respiratory failure on mechanical ventilation.[27,28] Patients with high oxygen consumption may require the more complex and sophisticated modes of ventilation, whereas patients with lower oxygen demands may only require continuous positive airway pressure (CPAP). Although medical centers and physicians have distinct preferences for the mode of ventilation used, research is limited regarding mortality, length of stay, and functional outcome. Most studies examine physiological variables during the time of mechanical ventilation. The most cost-effective modes that provide the best outcomes have yet to be substantiated. Recent studies advocate low tidal volumes and higher levels of PEEP for the management of acute respiratory failure.[29,30] High tidal volumes and progressive ventilator-free breathing are advocated for weaning the tetraplegic patient when conventional weaning techniques have failed.[31] Figure 19-3 demonstrates pressure waveforms with spontaneous breathing and various forms of mechanical ventilation.

Ventilatory Support
Control Modes

Critically ill patients who are unable to maintain adequate oxygenation and/or carbon dioxide removal without support require a mode of ventilation that relieves the patient of the majority of the work of breathing while ensuring ventilation

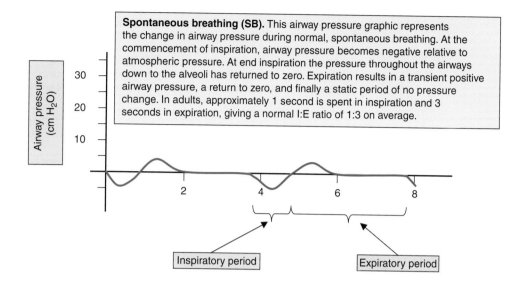

Spontaneous breathing (SB). This airway pressure graphic represents the change in airway pressure during normal, spontaneous breathing. At the commencement of inspiration, airway pressure becomes negative relative to atmospheric pressure. At end inspiration the pressure throughout the airways down to the alveoli has returned to zero. Expiration results in a transient positive airway pressure, a return to zero, and finally a static period of no pressure change. In adults, approximately 1 second is spent in inspiration and 3 seconds in expiration, giving a normal I:E ratio of 1:3 on average.

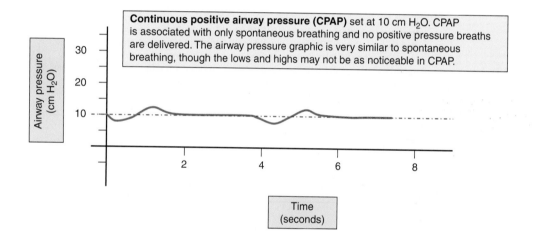

Continuous positive airway pressure (CPAP) set at 10 cm H_2O. CPAP is associated with only spontaneous breathing and no positive pressure breaths are delivered. The airway pressure graphic is very similar to spontaneous breathing, though the lows and highs may not be as noticeable in CPAP.

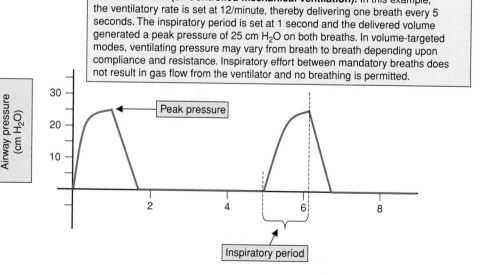

Volume control (or Controlled mechanical ventilation). In this example, the ventilatory rate is set at 12/minute, thereby delivering one breath every 5 seconds. The inspiratory period is set at 1 second and the delivered volume generated a peak pressure of 25 cm H_2O on both breaths. In volume-targeted modes, ventilating pressure may vary from breath to breath depending upon compliance and resistance. Inspiratory effort between mandatory breaths does not result in gas flow from the ventilator and no breathing is permitted.

FIGURE 19-3 Pressure waveforms with spontaneous breathing and various forms of mechanical ventilation. (This article was published in Trauma nursing: from resuscitation through rehabilitation, 4th edition, McQuillan KA, Makic MB, Whalen E, eds. Thoracic Trauma, pp 614-677, Copyright Saunders Elsevier (2009).) *(continued)*

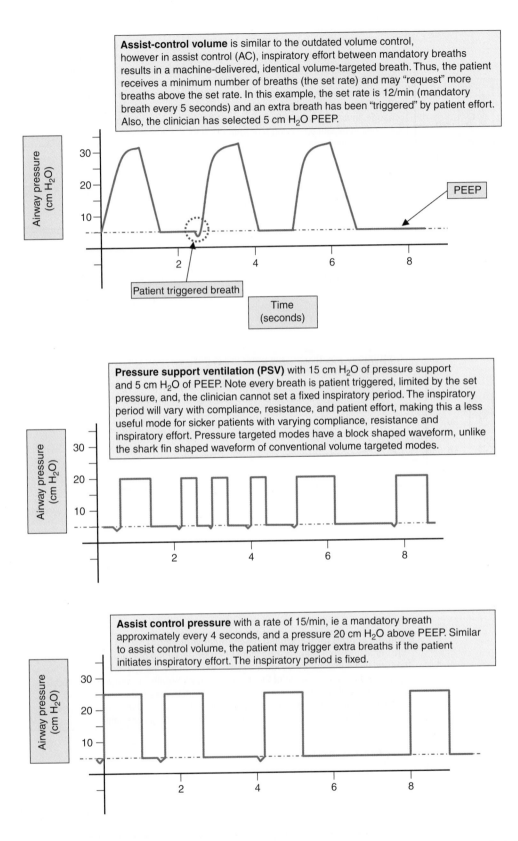

Assist-control volume is similar to the outdated volume control, however in assist control (AC), inspiratory effort between mandatory breaths results in a machine-delivered, identical volume-targeted breath. Thus, the patient receives a minimum number of breaths (the set rate) and may "request" more breaths above the set rate. In this example, the set rate is 12/min (mandatory breath every 5 seconds) and an extra breath has been "triggered" by patient effort. Also, the clinician has selected 5 cm H_2O PEEP.

Airway pressure (cm H_2O)

PEEP

Patient triggered breath

Time (seconds)

Pressure support ventilation (PSV) with 15 cm H_2O of pressure support and 5 cm H_2O of PEEP. Note every breath is patient triggered, limited by the set pressure, and, the clinician cannot set a fixed inspiratory period. The inspiratory period will vary with compliance, resistance, and patient effort, making this a less useful mode for sicker patients with varying compliance, resistance and inspiratory effort. Pressure targeted modes have a block shaped waveform, unlike the shark fin shaped waveform of conventional volume targeted modes.

Airway pressure (cm H_2O)

Assist control pressure with a rate of 15/min, ie a mandatory breath approximately every 4 seconds, and a pressure 20 cm H_2O above PEEP. Similar to assist control volume, the patient may trigger extra breaths if the patient initiates inspiratory effort. The inspiratory period is fixed.

Airway pressure (cm H_2O)

FIGURE 19-3   *(Continued)*

and oxygenation. Depending upon the mode selected and level of sedation utilized, the patient may initiate some breaths, and/or breathe spontaneously. Thus, even for the critically ill, there is a continuum of ventilatory support from maximal to minimal support.[26] Historically, the disadvantages to maximum ventilatory support included the need for frequent sedation and possibly neuromuscular blockade. In turn, this led to decreased spontaneous respiratory efforts, muscle atrophy, increased atelectasis, and inspissated secretions. These disadvantages were reluctantly accepted as necessary to sustain life.

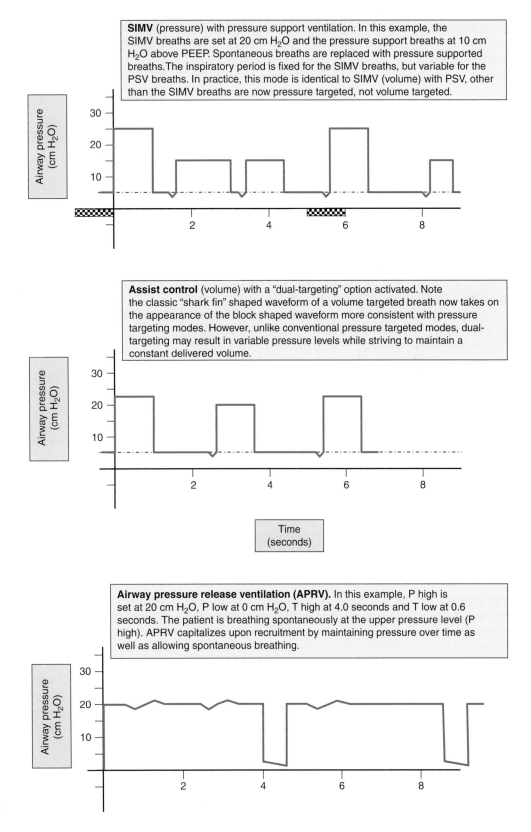

SIMV (pressure) with pressure support ventilation. In this example, the SIMV breaths are set at 20 cm H_2O and the pressure support breaths at 10 cm H_2O above PEEP. Spontaneous breaths are replaced with pressure supported breaths. The inspiratory period is fixed for the SIMV breaths, but variable for the PSV breaths. In practice, this mode is identical to SIMV (volume) with PSV, other than the SIMV breaths are now pressure targeted, not volume targeted.

Assist control (volume) with a "dual-targeting" option activated. Note the classic "shark fin" shaped waveform of a volume targeted breath now takes on the appearance of the block shaped waveform more consistent with pressure targeting modes. However, unlike conventional pressure targeted modes, dual-targeting may result in variable pressure levels while striving to maintain a constant delivered volume.

Airway pressure release ventilation (APRV). In this example, P high is set at 20 cm H_2O, P low at 0 cm H_2O, T high at 4.0 seconds and T low at 0.6 seconds. The patient is breathing spontaneously at the upper pressure level (P high). APRV capitalizes upon recruitment by maintaining pressure over time as well as allowing spontaneous breathing.

FIGURE 19-3   *(Continued)*

However, technological advances in mechanical ventilation now offer options that allow more limited use of sedation, and particularly paralytics.

For many years, modes of ventilation were broadly categorized into either volume targeted or pressure targeted modes.

The volume targeted modes required the clinician to select a tidal volume for the ventilator to deliver (or target) with each mandatory breath, while pressure targeted modes required selection of a fixed ventilating pressure for each mandatory breath. The incorporation of computer technology into the ventilator has allowed increasing sophistication in the delivery of breaths. Computer science, along with evolving clinical knowledge, has paved the way for a third classification of modes known as dual-targeting. In the 1990s, dual-targeting modes permitted the clinician to deliver a breath that combined features from both volume and pressure targeting ventilation.[26]

***Volume-controlled ventilation*—**Volume-controlled ventilation is probably the simplest and earliest method of positive pressure ventilation. Developed in the 1950s, adults were the primary patient group. In this mode the patient is not allowed, nor required, to initiate a breath, and the work of breathing is primarily provided by the ventilator, as long as the patient's respiratory cycle is synchronized with the mechanically delivered breaths. All breaths are initiated by the ventilator at the rate that has been set by the clinician. The tidal volume is preset for each breath, and the minute ventilation becomes the product of the set rate and the tidal volume. Respiratory muscle efforts and their contribution to oxygen consumption may be eliminated if the patient is chemically paralyzed. Some also believe that subsequent relaxation of the chest wall muscles may enhance recruitment of lung tissue.[32] Eliminating patient effort may also relieve patient dyssynchrony, although anxiety can be high. Lung thorax compliance, airway resistance, and auto-PEEP are easily calculated for pressure and flow measurements. The generation of high tidal volumes from volume-controlled ventilation may increase the risk of volutrauma, a major facet of ventilator induced lung injury (VILI)[33] (see page 612). It is recommended that tidal volumes and airway pressures be closely monitored to minimize the risk of alveolar over distension and VILI.

***Pressure-controlled ventilation*—**Pressure-controlled ventilation applies a pressure that is preset by the clinician, as is the ventilatory rate. The clinician also sets a fixed inspiratory time. In pure control modes, the patient cannot trigger or initiate a breath. Inspiratory effort may appear as dyssynchrony between the patient and the machine, as the patient attempts to draw gas into their lungs, but the machine does not respond. Controlled breaths are delivered at a predictable interval, ie, a rate of 12/min results in a breath every 5 seconds. The inspiratory flow from the ventilator is high initially, the flow decelerates as the alveolar pressure rises with lung inflation. The delivered tidal volume varies depending on the inspiratory time, patient effort, as well as the patient's lung compliance and airway resistance. Minute ventilation is not predetermined.[34]

Patients receiving ventilatory support frequently require postural drainage with or without manual techniques and suctioning for secretion retention. The physical therapist should be careful not to dislodge or pull on the tracheal tube when turning the patient. With careful positioning, manual techniques and most postural drainage positions, including the prone position, are possible (Fig. 19-4). Obstacles to the prone position include severe kyphosis or a pelvic external fixator. It is possible to place a patient prone while wearing a brace to stabilize spinal fractures, if the patient requires manual techniques, braces such as thoracolumbosacral orthoses (TLSOs)

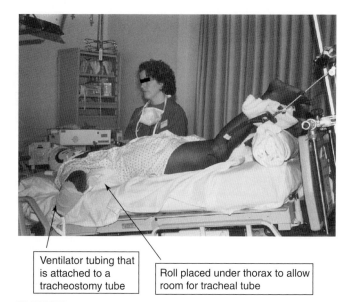

Ventilator tubing that is attached to a tracheostomy tube

Roll placed under thorax to allow room for tracheal tube

FIGURE 19-4   Prone positioning.

can often be opened once the patient is securely positioned. For patients with cervical bracing such as Halo vests or Yale braces, full prone positioning may be problematic. In these instances, the therapist should try to position the patient as close to one-fourth turn to prone from side-lying as possible. If a patient does not have adequate cervical rotation to lie prone, a towel roll can be placed both under the forehead and under the upper thorax. For patients with a tracheostomy a blanket roll, a sheet roll or wedge is carefully placed under the upper thorax to allow room for the tracheostomy tube and airway suctioning. A roll under the pelvis may also be helpful to allow for a shift in abdominal contents, particularly for patients with a large abdominal girth.

In summary, the disadvantages of control modes of mechanical ventilation include the need for heavy sedation and possibly neuromuscular blockade, decreased spontaneous respiratory efforts, respiratory alkalosis, and progressive atelectasis. Progressive infiltrates and atelectasis develop in dependent lung zones as a result of the gravitational redistribution of fluid, impaired secretion clearance, and poor inflation. The positive pressure breaths of mechanical ventilation result in ventilation along the path of least resistance, hence upper/anterior lung regions (when the patient is supine) are more readily ventilated than the posterior lung, while perfusion is primarily gravity dependent and greater in dependent/posterior regions, creating a $\dot{V}/\dot{Q}$ mismatch.[11] The decrease in spontaneous respiratory effort associated with control modes of ventilation is unfortunate, as it has potential to mitigate negative effects of positive pressure ventilation. Spontaneous breathing has been shown to decrease the development of atelectasis and reduce $\dot{V}/\dot{Q}$ mismatch, as it improves ventilation of posterior/dependent lung regions based on diaphragmatic mechanics.[35-38] Mechanically ventilated patients in the ICU frequently experience atelectasis and consolidation in the dorsal dependent lung regions. Therefore strategies which enhance ventilation and recruitment of these lung regions, such as facilitation of spontaneous breathing, are valuable. Recent studies, primarily in the animal model, have also shown significant decrement in diaphragmatic muscle force[39,40] and diaphragm atrophy[41] as a result of mechanical ventilation.

Controlled mechanical ventilation results in a greater decrease in diaphragmatic force than assist control ventilation.[42] If paralytic agents are required to maintain compliance with a controlled mode of ventilation, inadvertent disconnection from the ventilator can be life-threatening. Despite these disadvantages, controlled mechanical ventilation with low tidal volumes and PEEP remains an option for ventilation of patients with severe respiratory failure and elevated intracranial pressure. Arguably, the simplicity, and immediate responsiveness, makes it an attractive choice for clinicians with less expertise in other modes.

Assist-Control Modes

Assist-control (AC) modes may be either volume or pressure targeted, and while similar to their precursors, the control modes, the AC modes are far more commonly used.[26] The difference between control and assist-control is the ability of the patient to trigger or request breaths above the set ventilatory rate. All breaths continue to be of the same size and type as the mandatory breaths. The rate set by the clinician becomes the minimum number of breaths a patient will receive, however if the patient initiates additional breaths, the ventilator will reward the patient with a machine breath.

The goals of assist control modes are to allow and improve synchrony between the patient and the ventilator, reduce patient effort, and optimize comfort. However, how a particular mode of ventilation is used may be equally as important as the chosen mode of ventilation. Physical therapists should be familiar with the terms and general principles of AC, synchronized intermittent mandatory ventilation (SIMV), pressure support ventilation (PSV), pressure regulated volume control ventilation (PRVC), airway pressure release ventilation (APRV), and proportional assist ventilation (PAV) when working with mechanically ventilated patients.

Synchronized intermittent mandatory ventilation—

Synchronized intermittent mandatory ventilation (SIMV) appears the same as AC ventilation when the patient is receiving only ventilator-assisted breaths (not taking any spontaneous breaths). The patient receives periodic positive-pressure breaths from the ventilator at a preset volume or pressure and rate. With SIMV, the patient can inhale with unassisted spontaneous breaths between mechanically assisted breaths. When a patient is able to breathe spontaneously, spontaneous efforts will be synchronized with the timing of the mandatory ventilator breaths. If spontaneous breaths are taken within the preset triggering period that a mechanical breath is scheduled to be delivered (usually about a 1-second zone), the ventilator will deliver the mandatory breath while synchronizing with the patient's inspiratory effort.[19] If the patient makes no effort during the triggering period, the ventilator waits until the end of the triggering period and delivers the targeted volume or

pressure. The precursor to SIMV was intermittent mandatory ventilation (IMV), which was developed to facilitate weaning.[43,44] SIMV evolved with the goal to avoid problems with dyssynchrony when weaning patients from the ventilator and to gradually decrease the number of mechanically assisted breaths to decrease the duration of mechanical ventilation. However, the use of SIMV to decrease weaning time has not been substantiated in clinical studies (see page 603). SIMV may actually contribute to respiratory muscle fatigue when the patient has a high respiratory rate and increased work of breathing.[45,46] SIMV was historically a volume targeted mode until the 1990s with the mainstream introduction of SIMV as a pressure targeted mode as well. In clinical practice SIMV, whether volume or pressure targeted, is routinely used with pressure-support ventilation.

Pressure regulated volume control—Pressure regulated volume control (PRVC) is a combination of volume control and pressure regulation. In this mode, the ventilator initially delivers a volume-controlled breath, while measuring the plateau pressure. The next breath is delivered using the measured pressure of the previous breath. If subsequent breaths increase above the preset volume, the pressure level is incrementally decreased until the preset tidal volume is delivered. If measured tidal volumes fall below the preset volumes, pressure is increased incrementally to reach the preset volume, up to a preset maximum upper pressure limit. In this mode, the ventilator is set to deliver a guaranteed respiratory rate, however breaths may be either ventilator or patient initiated. An alarm sounds if the ventilator is unable to deliver the preset volume within the preset pressure limit. It has been theorized that PRVC may decrease work of breathing while being used in a lung protective strategy, however this has not yet been established.[47]

Pressure-support ventilation—Pressure-support ventilation (PSV) is a pressure targeted mode requiring the patient to trigger every breath. The clinician does not set a machine rate, so in the absence of patient effort, the ventilator will not deliver a breath. This, probably more than any other mode, gives the patient more freedom with breathing. With PSV the main setting is the pressure target. When the ventilator senses an inspiratory effort (dependent on the trigger sensitivity that has been set) it responds by delivering a decelerating gas flow which raises the pressure in the airways to the targeted pressure level and holds the pressure constant. Decelerating gas flow is a consistent feature of pressure-targeted modes, as compared to a fixed or constant gas flow, which is a consistent feature of volume targeted modes.[26] The pressure is maintained throughout inspiration. The inspiratory period terminates when the gas flow rate decreases to a preset value (typically 5%–25% of the peak inspiratory flow rate). Alternate measures to terminate the inspiratory period are available but are either uncommon or included as a safety feature.[48] The patient indirectly controls rate, tidal volume, minute ventilation, and I/E ratio. The two most notable features of PSV are that the patient must trigger every breath, and the clinician does not set a fixed inspiratory period (one of the only modes having this distinction).

In the stable lung, as pressure support increases, respiratory rate decreases and tidal volume increases. In most cases, minute ventilation is not significantly modified. Alveolar ventilation is increased and $PaCO_2$ decreases. Conversely, when pressure support is decreased the tidal volume decreases, PSV assists respiratory muscle activity by improving the efficacy of spontaneously initiated breaths, reducing the demand on the inspiratory muscles, and increasing tidal volume, therefore reducing the workload on the respiratory muscles. PSV has been shown to reduce the work of breathing and oxygen consumption of the inspiratory muscles.[28,49] Lower levels of PSV counteract the element of work of breathing incurred by the ventilator circuitry and, particularly, the endotracheal tube. However, resistance changes throughout inspiration, being greatest at the beginning of the breath and least at the end of the breath, but the pressure level remains fixed. Therefore, the support to overcome resistance initially under compensates and later overcompensates. Nonetheless, PSV has become a highly useful adjunct particularly in the stable ventilated patient and in the patient being weaned from ventilatory support.[26]

CLINICAL CORRELATE

Physical therapists should be aware that some physicians will use a pressure support of 5 cm of water pressure and a resting respiratory rate of <35 breaths/min as criteria for extubation.[50–52]

Airway-pressure-release ventilation—Airway-pressure-release ventilation (APRV) (also referred to as BiVent, BIPAP, DuoPAPBiLevel or Biphasic ventilation, depending upon the manufacturer) is simply a modified form of CPAP (continuous positive airway pressure) which uses two different levels of pressure.[53] As the name CPAP suggests, CPAP utilizes a continuous positive airway pressure while the patient breathes spontaneously. APRV is CPAP with a periodic release in the airway pressure to a lower level. Typically, the release is very short (less than 1 second) and the release level is to zero $cm\,H_2O$. The higher CPAP level of APRV allows the patient to breathe spontaneously, facilitating recruitment, and improving oxygenation. The release phase aids in the removal of CO_2. Conceptually, lowering the airway pressure to zero may seem like a bad idea. However, as the release phase is quite short, not all the gas empties from the lungs before the higher airway pressure is reinstituted, thus alveoli tend not to derecruit[54–56] (Fig. 19-3). APRV works well with ARDS where lung compliance is low and the respiratory muscles are intact. Proposed advantages of APRV include reducing the risk of VILI (see risks of mechanical ventilation) by limiting peak airway pressures, and a reduction in repetitive recruitment/derecruitment of alveoli, which results in atelectrauma. Studies have also shown a decreased need for patient sedation and neuromuscular

blockade,[22,57] as well as benefits associated with spontaneous breathing.[58] It should be noted that with critically ill patients who are unable to initiate spontaneous breathing, APRV can be used essentially as a "Full Support" mode of ventilation until the patient is able to initiate spontaneous breaths. APRV's standout feature is allowing patients to spontaneously breathe; therefore practices inhibiting breathing, such as heavy sedation and or paralytic use, limit the usefulness of this mode.

Proportional-assist ventilation—Proportional-assist ventilation (PAV) may have promise and replace other ventilatory modes though it has yet to gain widespread acceptance. PAV offers maximal patient autonomy; every breath is initiated and terminated by the patient. The ventilator essentially acts as an accessory muscle imposing no volume or pressure targets; the patient has total control over all aspects of breathing. The operator selects which portion of the work will be performed by the machine. Pressure assistance by the machine is proportional to a variable combination of the inspired volume (elastic assist) and the inspiratory flow rate (the resistive assist). Tidal volume and flow are totally controlled by the patient. When the patient pulls harder, the machine boosts its output, and as the patient relaxes, the machine cuts back.[49,59–61] This is different from the patient ventilator interaction observed in conventional modes, where the ventilator-generated pressure is either constant or inversely related to effort. The advantage of PAV is that it yields to the patient's own neuromuscular control mechanisms and is guided by motion of the respiratory system synchronizing the ventilator's output with the patient's continuously changing needs. Because tidal volume and flow rates are controlled by natural breathing with PAV they vary continuously; therefore, PAV requires backup in the event that the patient's ventilatory effort ceases. PAV has the potential for providing appropriate ventilatory support in a variety of clinical settings, ranging from acute lung injury, to weaning from mechanical ventilation, to increasing exercise tolerance in patients with COPD for pulmonary rehabilitation when used noninvasively.[62] PAV theoretically improves the physiological relationship between inspiratory effort and ventilatory return that often characterizes respiratory failure. PAV may require lower peak airway pressures than standard volume-targeted modes, improve patient comfort,[63] and provide a better synchrony of breathing[64], however, the clinical benefit has yet to be clearly established.

Dual-Targeting

In the 1990s, ventilator technology began incorporating a combination of both volume- and pressure-targeted features. In these new "modes", the clinician sets a volume target for each breath, but unlike historical volume targeting modes, the ventilator utilizes a decelerating gas flow to deliver the breath. This requires the ventilator to initially do a series of test breaths to gauge lung compliance. The ventilator is then able to calculate how to deliver the breath with the lowest possible pressure. Calculations are performed on every breath. As lung compliance improves, the ventilator requires less pressure, as lung compliance worsens, the ventilator will increase pressure. Pressure changes are incremental, usually no more than 3 cms H_2O at a time. The clinician sets a pressure limit not to be exceeded and the ventilator alarms as the pressure alarm level are reached. At that time, pressure will not increase, but volume will decrease until the clinician intervenes. Some ventilators have dual targeting designed modes, for example, PRVC, while other ventilators apply the feature of dual targeting to conventional volume modes, for example, SIMV with AutoFlow. It has been theorized that this technology may decrease work of breathing while being used in a lung protective strategy, however this has not yet been established.[47]

Noninvasive Ventilation

Noninvasive ventilation (NIV) is a term used to describe ventilatory support supplied via nasal prongs or some type of face mask to provide CPAP, BiPap or positive pressure ventilation to the nonintubated patient. Thus, NIV is not a mode of ventilation, rather a technique of delivering a mode. The machine used may be either a standard ventilator or a single purpose unit. Noninvasive positive pressure ventilation has been shown to have particular benefit for patients with COPD in avoiding intubation and failure of extubation, as well as facilitating weaning.[65] Noninvasive ventilation may also be used to increase exercise tolerance for patients with COPD[62] or for sleep apnea.

Continuous positive airway pressure—Continuous positive airway pressure (CPAP) is a form of ventilatory support that is simply PEEP delivered to a patient who is spontaneously breathing. No machine breaths, that is, positive pressure breaths, are delivered. CPAP is the terminology reserved for patients who are only spontaneously breathing, while PEEP is terminology used when patients are receiving some form of positive pressure breaths. Both CPAP and PEEP increase FRC and help prevent derecruitment of alveoli. In normal subjects, CPAP increases tidal volume by 25% and lowers respiratory rate by over 30%.[66] In intubated patients CPAP may decrease the work of breathing by 50%. CPAP is frequently used as a method of weaning the patient from the previously described modes of ventilatory support. CPAP can also prevent the flail action of a paralyzed hemidiaphragm, thereby improving the efficiency of the remaining innervated respiratory muscles, and may also prevent atelectasis.

CPAP can be delivered with a mechanical ventilator or a separate device via a tracheal tube, nasal prongs, or face mask. Nasal CPAP has been shown to reduce the number of apneic episodes, arrhythmias, and hypoxic episodes during sleep and to reduce daytime sleepiness and improve neuropsychiatric function in patients with obstructive sleep apnea, which affects 2% to 4% of the population.[67,68] Nasal CPAP provides a pneumatic splint for the airway, preventing airway collapse during sleep (when upper airway dilator muscle activity is low), and increases the airway caliber in the retropalatal and retroglossal regions. Nasal CPAP also increases the lateral dimensions of the airway and thins the lateral pharyngeal walls. Typical settings are 5 to 20 cm of H_2O pressure. Poor patient compliance is noted with nasal prongs and face masks, which may be related to facial and skin discomfort, rhinitis, nasal irritation and dryness, difficulty exhaling, and claustrophobia. Full-face face masks have been associated with increased aspiration and are typically reserved for patients with persistent mouth leaks.[68]

Because CPAP can increase functional residual capacity and shorten inspiratory muscles placing them at a mechanical disadvantage, there is the potential to worsen inspiratory muscle weakness. However, patients with preexisting shortened inspiratory muscles because of COPD may benefit from the ventilatory assistance of CPAP.[66–69] Some patients may require CPAP at night or while in bed to maintain adequate oxygenation, yet have adequate oxygenation while they are mobile. After consulting with the physician, the physical therapist can evaluate whether CPAP is required during mobility activities. CPAP can frequently be disconnected for short periods of time during ambulation and wheelchair mobility activities, or extension cords and battery packs can be used to provide adjunctive CPAP during functional tasks. Likewise, CPAP during physical therapy interventions such as aerobic exercise training or functional training may enhance patient tolerance, comfort, and compliance.

Bilevel positive airway pressure—Bilevel positive airway pressure (often referred to as BiPap) may be used with noninvasive ventilation for ventilatory support. As with CPAP, intubation is not required. Sleep apnea is a common indication, along with exacerbations of COPD, congestive heart failure, and cystic fibrosis. BiPap is sometimes referred to as bilevel CPAP because it adds the advantage of an inspiratory positive airway pressure to CPAP. As with CPAP, BiPap may be used exclusively at night or intermittently throughout the day depending on the patient's condition. Successful treatment can be predicted by improvement in pH, $PaCO_2$, PaO_2, and functional status.[18,69]

CLINICAL CORRELATE

Physical therapy interventions are used to assist in strengthening the respiratory muscles and provide general conditioning to assist in weaning the patient from the ventilator. The physical therapist should closely monitor oxygen saturation, respiratory rate, and the patient's tolerance to activity. The physical therapist should notify the physician when a patient has markedly abnormal signs and symptoms during treatment. It may be necessary to add invasive or noninvasive mechanical ventilation to allow the patient to tolerate physical therapy and nursing interventions.

IMPROVING OXYGENATION FOR THE DIFFICULT TO VENTILATE PATIENT

Patients with acute lung injury (ALI), ARDS, or other disease processes may reach a point in their management when they cannot be adequately oxygenated despite optimal traditional ventilation strategies. The physician may have tried several different modes of mechanical ventilation, and is now faced with a dilemma of how to best oxygenate the patient. The use of prone positioning, extracorporeal membrane oxygenation, nitric oxide, and independent lung ventilation are all options to improve oxygenation in patients with severe respiratory failure.[70-73]

Prone Positioning

Prone positioning has been used since the 1970s to improve oxygenation of patients with acute respiratory failure. The mechanism of action appears to be a reduction of compressed lung segments by the heart, recruitment of collapsed lung tissue by reexpansion of dependent consolidation as it shifts from dependent to nondependent positions, and improved gravity-related drainage from previously dependent consolidated lung tissue, all resulting in improved matching of ventilation to perfusion.[70,73] Turning a patient into the prone position for 7 to 20 hours per day has been shown to improve oxygenation within 2 hours to 10 days of implementing the procedure. It is also thought to decrease the incidence of ventilator-associated pneumonia.[70,74,75] In one study, 30 minutes of prone positioning recruited more edematous lung than adjusting ventilator settings to optimize PEEP, as noted by computed tomography. The results were most pronounced in patients with lobar ALI.[76] Turning a patient prone is considered safe without an increased incidence of displacement of the tracheal tube or accidental extubation, however; an increase in pressure sores without significant sequelae has been noted.[75,77] Introducing prone positioning earlier in a patient's care may prevent the need for 100% inspired oxygen.

Physical therapists may be consulted to assist the nursing staff in turning a patient with neuromuscular or musculoskeletal impairments into the prone position, or for airway clearance of the most involved dependent lung segments (Fig. 19-4). A good rule of thumb is to turn the patient from supine, onto the least involved side, and then prone. Range-of-motion exercises can also be performed. Nurses may look to physical therapists for guidance and instruction on how best to provide range of motion exercises and move limbs while in the prone position, as well as positioning of limbs during turning.

Extracorporeal Life Support

Extracorporeal life support (ECLS), also commonly referred to as: extracorporeal membrane oxygenation (ECMO), extracorporeal carbon dioxide removal (ECCO$_2$R), or extracorporeal lung assist (ECLA), is a supportive therapy that may be used in patients with severe, but reversible cardiorespiratory failure. Studies regarding the efficacy of ECLS in adults with respiratory failure are not conclusive, though its use in neonates and pediatric patients is well established.[78,79] Its use with adults continues in primarily large, academic centers of excellence, where clinical experience has supported its efficacy. ECLS, when used for respiratory failure in adults, most commonly utilizes a venovenous circuit. A common femoral venous cannula drains large volumes of deoxygenated blood, which is pumped through an oxygenating device and a heat exchanger prior to being infused back into the patient through a right internal jugular cannula.[80] The extracorporeal blood flow is titrated according to the patient's required level of support, generally beginning with full support, with flow rates of approximately 100 mL/kg/min.[81] Gas exchange takes place in the extracorporeal support system, allowing ventilator management to focus on lung protection, while aggressive measures to treat the underlying disease process continue. Patients on ECLS are often sedated (the degree of sedation may be minimal depending on institutional practice).

ECLS is an invasive and often intimidating form of life support, particularly for clinicians who have not been exposed to this modality. Although the cannulas are large, and the extracorporeal blood volume quite significant, these patients frequently require physical therapy interventions including airway clearance techniques, contracture prevention, and positioning. Patients requiring ECLS may also be positioned prone as an adjunctive therapy. As with most invasive monitoring lines, the cannulas are sutured, reducing the risk of dislodgement. They are also wire reinforced, significantly reducing the risk of kinking. Blood flow through the system is also closely monitored and tracked, another safeguard which allows judicious patient care. While studies examining the limits of ROM are lacking, it is the personal experience of these authors that hip flexion to 90 degrees, abduction to 45 degrees, internal and external rotation to 30 degrees, full shoulder flexion and abduction, and three-fourth prone positioning toward and away from the cannulated side can be performed without complications.

Inhaled Nitric Oxide

Inhaled nitric oxide (INO) is another adjunctive therapy for patients with ARDS/ALI and life-threatening hypoxemia, who have failed conventional lung protective ventilation. NO improves hypoxemia by causing vasodilation to areas of well-ventilated lung while diverting blood away from poorly ventilated lung, thus improving ventilation/perfusion matching.[70,71] Significant improvement in PaO$_2$/FiO$_2$ ratios, while decreasing pulmonary vascular resistance occurs with low doses of INO.[82]

NO appears to be a safe, yet expensive intervention; however, its effect on mortality, ICU stay and functional outcomes is not yet known. The precautions are the same as with all mechanically ventilated ICU patients; physical therapists should be careful not to displace any of the NO equipment when working with these patients and discuss any concerns with the nurse or physician. (See Chapters 6 and 8 for further discussion of NO.)

Synchronous Independent Lung Ventilation

Synchronous independent lung ventilation (SILV) may be required for patients who have failed conventional methods of full ventilatory support, because the injury or disease to one lung is so severe that it prevents both lungs from being adequately ventilated. Independent lung ventilation may be necessary with unilateral, or asymmetrical lung disease as a result of severe pulmonary trauma (blunt or penetrating), aspiration pneumonitis, or bronchopleural fistula. These patients usually do not tolerate position changes with conventional ventilation and ultimately may require resection of part or all of one lung (see Chapter 7). Pulmonary congestion and the loss or inactivation of surfactant in the diseased lung may lead to a decrease in tissue elasticity and decreased lung compliance. Therefore, the gases delivered to the lung follow the path of least resistance and the "healthy" or "better" lung receives the majority of the tidal volume delivered by the ventilator. Higher inspiratory pressures are required in attempts to ventilate the more diseased lung, which may have detrimental effects on the lung tissue and potentially a greater potential for VILI (see potential risks associated with mechanical ventilation section). Hyperinflation of the healthy lung may also occur, diverting blood flow to the affected lung, which results in a large dead space. Furthermore, overdistension of healthy alveoli may often result in volutrauma leading to ALI. Ventilation to the healthy lung continues, but pulmonary perfusion is either decreased or absent, resulting in poor gas exchange (Table 19-4).

The advantage of independent lung ventilation is that each lung can be ventilated separately; overdistension of the good lung can be prevented while adequately ventilating the "sick lung." Two ventilators are required. The patient is intubated with a double-lumen endotracheal tube. Intrapulmonary cross-contamination is prevented by the presence of a distal second cuff on the endotracheal tube, which is inflated in the mainstem bronchus, usually the left. The end of the tube has an attachment for each ventilator.[83] Computerized assessment techniques allow synchronous mechanical ventilation to each lung with a different FiO_2, different tidal volumes, and PEEP levels. Different modes of mechanical ventilation, tailored to the pathophysiology of each lung may be required.[73,83] Typically, oxygenation improves within hours after SILV is initiated.

TABLE 19-4 Effects of Conventional Mechanical Ventilation on Alveoli in Unilateral Lung Disease

	Healthy Lung	Diseased Lung
Tidal volume	↑	↓
Ventilation	↑	↓
Perfusion	↓	↑
V̇/Q̇ ratio	High *dead space*	Low *shunt*
Pao₂	↓	↓

TABLE 19-5 Recommended Suction Catheter Sizes with Tracheal Tube Sizes

Tracheal Tube Size (mm)	Suction Catheter Size (French)
5	8
6	8
7	10
8	12
9	14

Adapted from Vanner R, Bick E. Tracheal pressures during open suctioning. *Anaesthesia*. 2008;63(3):313-315.

Patients on SILV are typically on bed rest. Standard postural drainage positions and manual techniques can be administered. Because the patient is intubated with a double-lumen tube (which prevents transbronchial aspiration), each lung can be suctioned separately, as clinically indicated. The suction catheter is changed between passes to each lumen to prevent contamination from one lung to the other. Ideally, an in-line catheter is in use. The therapist should also note the size of the internal diameter of each port of the endotracheal tube because smaller suction catheters are usually necessary. The suction catheter should not exceed half the diameter of the airway (Table 19-5).

When deciding which intervention or combination of interventions is optimal to improve oxygenation for a specific patient, resource availability, physician preference, and the expertise of health care practitioners must be taken into consideration. The effect of these four interventions on long-term outcomes, including mortality, is unknown. Improvement in oxygenation may lead to a decrease in inflation pressures and could be associated with improved outcomes. However the mortality for patients with ventilator-associated lung injury and severe ARDS/ALI remains high.

LIBERATING THE PATIENT FROM MECHANICAL VENTILATION

1. Weaning is the term used when trying to liberate a patient from mechanical ventilation. Discontinuation from mechanical ventilation is easily achieved in the majority (70%–80%) of patients.[18] Weaning should not be initiated until the patient can maintain alveolar ventilation with less ventilator support without causing excessive stress, which may lead to respiratory muscle fatigue. It is advised that weaning not be initiated until the pathophysiology for weaning failure and any imbalance between energy supply and demand for the respiratory muscles is corrected.[52] Metabolic disturbances and circulatory disturbances are easier for the physician to correct than neuromuscular incompetence, where a program of exercise interspersed with rest may be necessary. The decision of how to wean depends partly on the type of ventilator and

TABLE 19-6A   Clinical Considerations (Adult) "Weaning" from Mechanical Ventilation

Parameter	Consider Weaning	Normal Value
Is the cause for respiratory failure resolving?	Yes/No	N/A
Is the patient hemodynamically stable?	Yes/No	Yes
Able to initiate inspiratory effort	Yes	Yes
Fio_2 (percentage of inspired oxygen concentration)	≤0.4–0.5	0.21 (room air)
Pao_2/Fio_2 ratio	≥150–300	≥380
PEEP (cm H_2O pressure)	≤5–10	Approximately 5
Respiratory rate	<30–38/min	12–20/min
Tidal volume[a]	325–408 (4–6 mL/kg)	500 mL(10–15 mL/kg)
Rapid shallow breathing index[a] (Respiratory rate/tidal volume)	60–105/L	50/L
Pi_{max}	−15 to −30 cm H_2O	M (−65 to −120) F (−46 to −79)

M = male; F = Female.

[a]Data while spontaneously breathing.

Adapted from Kondili E, Xirouchaki N, Vaporidi K, Klimathianaki M, Georgopoulos D. Short-term cardiorespiratory effects of proportional assist and pressure-support ventilation in patients with acute lung injury/acute respiratory distress syndrome. *Anesthesiology.* 2006;105(4):703-708. MacIntyre NR, Cook DJ, Ely EW Jr, et al. Evidence-based guidelines for weaning and discontinuing ventilatory support: a collective task force facilitated by the American College of Chest Physicians; the American Association for Respiratory Care; and the American College of Critical Care Medicine. *Chest.* 2001;120(suppl 6):375S-395S.

primarily on the physiologic response of the patient to the weaning process. To wean, a patient may be changed from assist-controlled ventilation to SIMV with pressure support, or from APRV to CPAP. In addition, the degree of pressure support, Fio_2, and PEEP may be lowered as the patient's condition improves. Once the PEEP and Fio_2 have been reduced, there are several methods to further reduce ventilatory support and assess the patient for extubation. Recent research strongly supports the use of daily spontaneous weaning trials (SBTs) to aid in determining a patient's readiness for ventilator discontinuance.[52,84] SBTs are recommended for patients who demonstrate reversal of the underlying cause of respiratory failure, adequate oxygenation, hemodynamic stability, and the ability to initiate an inspiratory effort[52] (Table 19-6A). SBTs are typically performed on low levels of pressure support, CPAP or a T-piece and lead to liberating the patient from the ventilator (Table 19-6B). Failure of a SBT requires that the medical team reevaluate the cause of respiratory failure, and attempt to rectify any reversible causes, after returning the patient to a stable, nonfatiguing mode of ventilation.[52] The physical therapist should be aware of the physician's or ICU's weaning protocol and different weaning modes to appropriately modify treatment interventions. The three most commonly used techniques are T-piece weaning, synchronized intermittent mandatory ventilation with pressure support, and pressure-support ventilation. All of these methods lead to removal of the mechanical ventilator and independent patient breathing. Daily physical therapy interventions may need to be timed to accommodate SBTs.

T-Piece Weaning

T-Piece weaning refers to removing the patient from the ventilator and placing a plastic adapter shaped like a T on the patient's tracheostomy or endotracheal tube. The patient is still intubated yet able to breathe on his or her own with humidified supplemental oxygen. If the patient maintains good vital signs,

TABLE 19-6B   Criteria for a Spontaneous Breathing Trial

Gas exchange acceptability	Spo_2 ≥ 85%–90% Po_2 ≥ 50–60 mm Hg pH ≥ 7.32 Increase in $Paco_2$ ≤ 10 mm Hg
Hemodynamic stability	HR < 120–140 beats/min (not changed >20%) Systolic BP <180–200 and >90 (not changed >20%, no vasopressors required)
Stable ventilatory pattern	RR 30–35 breaths/min (not changed >50%) No increased use of accessory respiratory muscles or paradoxical breathing
Mental status	No decline (eg, somnolence, agitation, anxiety, coma)
Other	No diaphoresis, other worsening/onset of discomfort

Adapted from MacIntyre NR, Cook DJ, Ely EW Jr, et al. Evidence-based guidelines for weaning and discontinuing ventilatory support: a collective task force facilitated by the American College of Chest Physicians; the American Association for Respiratory Care; and the American College of Critical Care Medicine. *Chest.* 2001;120(suppl 6): 375S-395S.

blood gases, oxygen saturation, and an appropriate breathing pattern, extubation usually occurs within hours. Supplemental oxygen is usually still required and is delivered through a face mask or nasal cannula. This is the oldest method of weaning and is associated with outcomes similar to other methods. Patients may receive airway secretion clearance techniques during T-piece weaning. This may enable them to better tolerate extubation. If a patient fails a T-piece trial, they will be put back on their previous mode of mechanical ventilation and physical therapy interventions can be continued. This decision is usually made within a few hours.

Synchronized Intermittent Mandatory Ventilation and Pressure Support

Synchronized intermittent mandatory ventilation can be used as a weaning mode by gradually reducing the number of breaths per minute delivered by the ventilator over several days or weeks. SIMV weaning was initially thought to be a weaning mode that would decrease the duration of mechanical ventilation. However, there is some evidence that this mode of ventilation increases weaning time rather than decreasing the time necessary for mechanical ventilatory support.[59,85] When mechanical breaths are decreased, there is a gradual increase in the mean inspiratory effort. When weaning with pressure support ventilation unloading of the respiratory muscles is more gradual. Pressure support can also be added to spontaneous breaths to reduce the additional work of breathing during SIMV weaning.

MacIntyre suggests that patients who remain mechanically ventilated for greater than 21 days "should not be considered permanently ventilator dependent until three months of weaning attempts have failed."[52] Ventilator support should be gradually reduced, and self-breathing trials of gradually increasing duration be employed.[52] Upper arm strength was a predictor of weaning time in the chronically ventilated patients, giving support to the role of physical therapy in this population.[86]

CLINICAL CORRELATE

When a patient is being weaned and does not tolerate physical therapy interventions during weaning trials, the physical therapist should confer with the physician to determine if the ventilator can be adjusted back to preweaning settings which may facilitate the provision of physical therapy interventions. As a general guideline, physical therapy treatments should be performed when the patient is not being weaned.

PNEUMONIA AND ATELECTASIS

Pneumonia is an inflammatory response of the bronchioles and alveolar spaces to an infective agent.[87] These infections may be bacterial, fungal, or viral. Exudates lead to lung consolidation, dyspnea, tachypnea, and adventitious breath sounds on clinical examination of the involved lung lobe or segment. Pneumonia is the leading cause of death in patients with spinal cord injury (SCI).[88]

Ventilator-associated pneumonia (VAP), the most frequent type of nosocomial infection in the ICU, occurs in up to 30% of intubated patients.[89] VAP consists of a pulmonary inflammatory reaction and sepsis in patients who are mechanically ventilated for a minimum of 48 hours. It is difficult to accurately diagnose, and because the underlying illness of critically ill patients often has a high mortality rate, it is difficult to differentiate to what extent mechanical ventilation contributes to the risk of nosocomial pneumonia.[90] Historically, clinical findings have been used to diagnose pneumonia yet have not been shown to have sufficient accuracy, leading to the overuse of antimicrobial therapy (Table 19-7). Quantitative cultures are recommended to determine the bacterial load in a tracheal sample to differentiate colonization from infection and avoid overutilization of antibiotics. Clinicians may also see the use of biomarkers to assist in the diagnosis of VAP in the future.[89]

Placing mechanically ventilated patients in a semirecumbent position of 45 degrees has been demonstrated to reduce the incidence of VAP. Physical therapists can assist the nursing staff in moving patients with abnormal muscle tone or orthopedic injuries, which make positioning supine, side-lying, and sitting a challenge. VAP has a documented mortality rate from 20% to as high as 70% with multi resistant pathogens, despite treatment with antibiotics.[91] Consequently, the treatment of pneumonia with antibiotics is controversial for the mechanically ventilated patient.[92-94] Antibiotic usage has its own adverse effects: allergic reactions, acute renal failure, development of antimicrobial resistance, superinfections, and death. Therefore antibiotics should be prescribed cautiously with consideration as to the cost and adverse effects. Pneumonia in patients who have received previous antibiotic therapies is associated with a higher mortality.[92] Antibiotics are given to

TABLE 19-7   Criteria for the Diagnosis of Pneumonia

Clinical
    Adventitious breath sounds
        Crackles, rhonchi, bronchial
    Fever greater than 38°C
    Cough
    Purulent sputum
    Consolidation on physical examination

Radiological
    Evidence of a new or worsening pulmonary infiltrate

Laboratory findings
    Sputum gram stain (polymorphonuclear cells and a single
        morphologically distinct organism, leukocytosis)
    Positive blood, sputum, pleural fluid cultures

Adapted from Weber DJ, Rutala WA, Mayhall GC. Nosocomial respiratory tract infections and gram-negative pneumonia. In: Fishman A, ed. *Fishman's Pulmonary Diseases and Disorders.* 3rd ed. New York: McGraw-Hill; 1998:2219.

patients who do not need them as much as 77% of the time, with some evidence that mortality is greater in those patients receiving antibiotics.[90]

Although a placebo-controlled trial for antibiotic treatment of VAP has not been conducted, there is some evidence that chest physical therapy may be utilized to help in the diagnosis of pneumonia prior to administering antibiotics. Joshi and colleagues studied 39 trauma patients, 32 of whom were intubated, mechanically ventilated, and diagnosed with pneumonia. Chest physical therapy was initiated within 72 hours. Thirty-one of the 39 patients showed complete or partial clearing of the pulmonary infiltrate without antimicrobial therapy.[95] Patients who present with the traditional signs of pneumonia may have atelectasis rather than a true infection of the bronchioles and alveoli. *Atelectasis* is defined as an incomplete expansion, or collapse, of the lung and can result from secretion retention for which airway clearance techniques are beneficial, even when the chest radiograph shows an infiltrate. Atelectasis without secretion retention may be the result of compression of the lung (eg, pneumothorax, hemothorax, pleural effusion, or lung tumor) and would therefore not be responsive to secretion removal techniques. When an infiltrate noted on the chest radiograph improves within 24 to 48 hours, it is not indicative of pneumonia. Therefore, chest physical therapy interventions that clear an infiltrate within hours or days may assist the physician in determining whether the patient truly has pneumonia and needs antibiotics. This is an example of an intervention that also aids in a diagnosis.

Newer techniques such as bronchoalveolar lavage and quantitative cultures of protected sputum brushings are reported to have better sensitivity and specificity in the diagnosis of pneumonia, yet there is controversy as to which technique is most effective. It is suggested that consideration be given to these examinations to better diagnose pneumonia and potential pathogens for immunocompromised patients who present with a broad range of potential pathogens (eg heart or lung transplant patients, critically ill patients with severe VAP) and when the patient's condition is not improving with empiric antimicrobial therapy. Invasive diagnostic testing may lower mortality and provides more antibiotic free days.[94]

TRACHEAL, BRONCHIAL, AND PULMONARY SECRETION REMOVAL

Tracheal Suctioning

Physical therapy interventions frequently mobilize pulmonary secretions. Tracheal suctioning may, therefore, be necessary to remove secretions from the upper airway. If a patient is unable to either cough or huff secretions to the proximal portion of the tracheal tube, deep suctioning is indicated. Suctioning is a sterile procedure. Eye protection, a mask, and sterile gloves should be worn when not using an inline catheter, as the physical therapist is at risk for exposure to blood and body fluids. Deep suctioning is required for many mechanically ventilated patients

TABLE 19-8   Recommended Procedure—Tracheal Suctioning

1. Check baseline vital signs (eg heart rate, blood pressure, SpO_2) and arterial blood gases.
2. Check equipment to make sure it is operational (vacuum pressure <120 mm Hg).
3. Note ventilator settings, increase FiO_2 if baseline SpO_2 < 92% to 95%.
4. Check with medical staff regarding need for a PEEP adapter if PEEP ≥10 cmH_2O pressure, if not using an inline catheter.
5. Explain procedure to patient.
6. Don mask, eye protection, gloves.
7. Attach suction catheter to suction tubing.
8. Discontinue patient from oxygen source.
9. Increase ventilation by giving 3–5 breaths with a manual resuscitator bag if the patient is breathing spontaneously.
10. Insert suction catheter into the airway until resistance is felt. Apply suction after withdrawing the catheter a few centimeters. Suction should be continuous, and catheter rotated while withdrawing. Assess vital signs during the procedure.
11. Ventilate with 3–5 breaths from a manual resuscitator bag if indicated. Reattach the patient to the oxygen source, recheck vital signs, if SpO_2 has dropped wait until it returns to baseline. Increase FiO_2 if indicated.
12. Repeat steps 9–11 as indicated for 2–4 suction catheter passes. Change suction catheter if the patient requires more than 3–4 passes of the suction catheter.
13. Suction the mouth.
14. Return FiO_2 to baseline setting and reassess vital signs.
15. Dispose of suction supplies.

and requires that the catheter be inserted until an obstruction is felt (usually the carina or wall of the right mainstem bronchus), then slightly withdrawn, suction is continuously applied while the catheter is withdrawn from the airway (Table 19-8).

The recommended features of tracheal suction catheters and complications of tracheal suctioning are listed in Tables 19-5 and 19-9. One of the complications of tracheal suctioning that contributes to tracheolaryngeal ciliary dysfunction is irritation of the airway mucosa. The greatest mucosal damage has been noted with vacuum pressures greater than 120 mm Hg, although pressures as high as 170 mm Hg are used. Clinicians should use the lowest pressure that is effective.[96] Inline tracheal suction catheters were initially thought to be more beneficial than using a port adapter with a standard catheter to maintain PEEP during the suctioning procedure. Currently, there is no evidence to support a reduction in ventilator-associated pneumonia, decrease in hospital stay, or a decrease in mortality with the inline devices. The inline devices have been shown to have more colonization of the respiratory tract and should be changed every 24 to 48 hours to minimize pulmonary infection.[97-100] The physical therapist may observe a clinician instilling saline in the tracheal tube to "loosen" secretions. However, saline does not reach the peripheral airways or change the rheological properties of the

TABLE 19-9 Tracheal Suctioning: Catheter Features and Complications

Recommended Features of Suction Catheters	
Size: <1/2 the internal diameter of the artificial airway	12–14 French for adults with a 7–9-mm endotracheal tube *Proper size reduces airway occlusion and suction-induced hypoxemia*
Material	Polyvinyl chloride *Reduces mechanical trauma associated with insertion of the catheter* *Allows visualization of color and quantity of secretions suctioned*
Tip design	Straight—routine use *Coude—to increase likelihood of intubating left mainstem bronchus*
Sideholes, endhole	Two or more sideholes and an endhole *Optimize secretion removal* *Reduce trauma to the tracheal mucosa*

Adapted from Vanner R, Bick E. Tracheal pressures during open suctioning. *Anaesthesia.* 2008;63(3):313-315. Shah S, Fung K, Brim S, Rubin BK. An in vitro evaluation of the effectiveness of endotracheal suction catheters. *Chest.* 2005;128(5): 3699-3704. O'Malley P, Zankofski MA. Nursing 79 product survey: Disposable suction catheters. *Nursing.* 1979;5:70-75.

mucus. Saline instillation may also cause nosocomial infection, and the fluid instilled is not all retrieved.[101–103] No studies have found that instillation of saline is beneficial, current recommendations are that instillation of normal saline should not be performed as a routine step with endotracheal suctioning.[104] Patients should receive adequate hydration and airway humidification rather than resort to instillation of saline.

Prior to decannulation (removal of the tracheal tube), some physicians prefer to insert a fenestrated tracheostomy tube. The fenestrated tube can be plugged and requires that the patient breathe though the oropharynx (Fig. 19-5A). If the tracheostomy tube has a cuff, the cuff is deflated, and inspired gases pass through the fenestration and around the tube. Patients with fenestrated tubes who are in need of suctioning should have the plug and inner cannula of the fenestrated tube removed and replaced with a nonfenestrated cannula to minimize the chances of irritating or puncturing the posterior tracheal wall (Fig. 19-5A). When the patient cannot take deep enough breaths to maintain adequate oxygenation during the suctioning procedure, a manual resuscitator bag (MRB) is used to provide greater lung volumes, or for preoxygenation. Use of an MRB requires inflation of the tracheal cuff.

In summary, suctioning through an artificial airway of a patient with adequate oxygenation and stable vital signs has relatively few contraindications. Suctioning should not be performed routinely, only when clinical indications for suctioning exist (rhonchi, increased airway pressure, decreased lung volumes, increased work of breathing, visible secretions) and with close monitoring of vital signs and vacuum pressures. Based upon the current literature, it is up to the clinician's discretion whether to use an open or closed suction technique.

To Suction or Not to Suction— That Is the Question!

Prior to suctioning a patient with unstable vital signs or a low SpO$_2$, the therapist should discuss the benefit of suction-ing versus the risk of causing additional arrhythmias or desaturation with the medical and nursing staff. However, suctioning should not be withheld when indicated because retained secretions may result in airway occlusion and hypoxemia.

Nasotracheal suctioning (suctioning through a catheter inserted from the nose to the trachea without an artificial airway) is recommended only when vigorous airway clearance techniques, including prolonged postural drainage, cough stimulation techniques, and suctioning the oropharynx, are ineffective and the medical team does not plan to intubate the patient. See Table 19-10 for the complications associated with nasotracheal suctioning.

Refer to the CD-ROM for a detailed description of tracheal suctioning including a patient demonstration.

CLINICAL CORRELATE

The therapist should note the type of tracheal tube the patient has in place (endotracheal vs tracheostomy) and if the tracheostomy tube has a fenestration. The length of the tracheal tube will give the therapist a gross assessment of how far the catheter may be inserted into the airway. Suctioning is recommended only when cough instruction and breathing exercises are ineffective. Deep suctioning is reserved for patients who cannot mobilize secretions into the tracheal tube. Vital signs and airway pressures are monitored throughout the procedure. Following suctioning, the therapist may note an improvement in breath sounds and lower airway pressures or increased volumes on the ventilator.

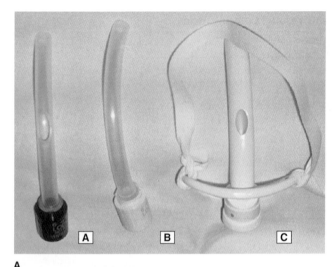

A

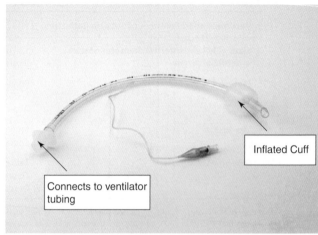

B

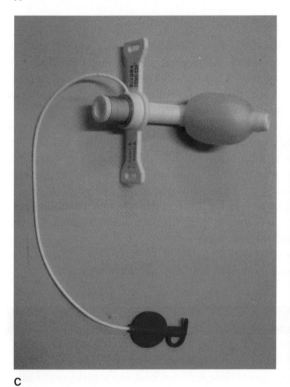

C

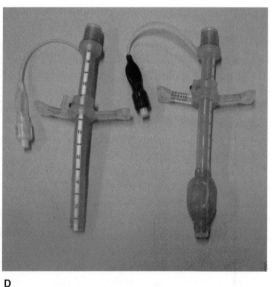

D

FIGURE 19-5   (**A**) Fenestrated tracheostomy tubes. (**B**) Standard endotracheal tube. (**C**) Bivona tracheostomy tube. (**D**) Variable length Bivona tracheostomy tubes.

Therapeutic Bronchoscopy Versus Chest Physical Therapy

Therapeutic Bronchoscopy

A *bronchoscope* is a multipurpose instrument that is inserted into the upper airway to perform diagnostic and therapeutic procedures. The procedure is performed by a physician and referred to as a *bronchoscopy,* a common therapeutic modality in the management of critically ill patients. Flexible bronchoscopes are used in conjunction with a swivel adaptor and rubber diaphragm to allow mechanical ventilation throughout the procedure.[105] Because of the associated risk of hypoxemia, the

FiO_2 is increased to 100% during the procedure. The diagnostic indications for bronchoscopy include visualization of the airway for tracheal or bronchial tears, burns, foreign bodies, tumors, and placement of airway stents. Qualitative cultures obtained via bronchoscopy may assist in the diagnosis of pneumonia and prescription of an appropriate antimicrobial agent (see Chapter 8). Bronchoscopic needle aspiration is used to stage lung cancer. The therapeutic indications include aspiration, lung contusion, lung abscess, atelectasis from secretion retention, and the removal of foreign bodies. These are the same therapeutic indications for airway clearance

TABLE 19-10 Complications Associated with Tracheal Suctioning

Complication	Recommended Intervention
Hypoxemia, death	Increase Fio_2 if baseline Spo_2 is less than 92% Use a port adapter with PEEP $>10\,cm\,H_2O$ to preserve PEEP and functional residual capacity Preoxygenate or add port adapter when there is a significant drop in Spo_2 or heart rate Limit procedure to 15–20 seconds Use inline suction catheter
Vasovagal response (may cause cardiac dysrhythmias)	Closely monitor cardiac function Notify medical staff
Elevated intracranial pressure (ICP)	Closely observe monitor, repeat suctioning after ICP has returned to baseline
Bacterial contamination	Sterile technique Change suction catheter every 2–4 passes
Atelectasis	Lung inflation prior to and following the procedure Minimize use of 100% oxygen
Mechanical trauma	Minimize the number of suction catheter passes Use continuous suction Use appropriate catheters Nasotracheal suctioning only after vigorous cough stimulation techniques, breathing exercises, mobilization, and postural drainage are unsuccessful
Nasotracheal suctioning	Only recommended when other airway clearance interventions have failed, and there is no plan to intubate. Consider: *Contraindications*: stridor, basilar skull fracture, facial fractures, known or suspected cerebrospinal fluid leak; *Complications*: apnea, laryngospasm, bronchospasm, severe cardiac arrhythmias, mechanical trauma to an edematous airway that may cause stridor

Adapted from Pedersen CM, Rosendahl-Nielsen M, Hjermind J, Egerod I. Endotracheal suctioning of the adult intubated patient-what is the evidence? *Intensive Crit Care Nurs.* 2009;25:21-30. Rauen CA, Chulay M, Bridges E, Vollman KM, Arbour R. Seven evidence-based practice habits: putting some sacred cows out to pasture. *Crit Care Nurse.* 2008;28(2):98-124. Fiorentini A. Potential hazards of tracheobronchial suctioning. *Intensive Crit Care Nurs.* 1992;8(4):217-226. Petersen GM, Pierson DJ, Hunter PM. Arterial oxygen saturation during nasotracheal suctioning. *Chest.* 1979;76(3):283-287.

techniques performed by physical therapists, nurses, and respiratory therapists.

The mechanically ventilated patient usually presents with borderline cardiopulmonary function where even small changes in ventilation and hemodynamics during bronchoscopy can have critical effects. Therefore, this procedure should be scrutinized, performed with caution, and utilized therapeutically when chest physical therapy treatment is unsuccessful.[105,106] The complications of therapeutic bronchoscopy with a comparison to chest physical therapy interventions are listed in Table 19-11. Although research comparing the advantages and disadvantages of chest physical therapy to therapeutic bronchoscopy is limited, there is some evidence that one chest physical therapy treatment is equally or more effective than therapeutic bronchoscopy in the treatment of lobar collapse from secretion retention.[107–112]

Chest Physical Therapy

Several case studies have demonstrated improved oxygenation and a decrease in the Fio_2 after one chest physical therapy intervention.[107,110,113] In these studies patients had a clear indication for chest physical therapy treatment.

TABLE 19-11 Complications of Bronchoscopy

Hypoxemia (requires 100% O_2 during procedure)
Pulmonary hemorrhage
Anesthesia/sedation-related risks (one-half of major complications)
Respiratory failure, hypoxia, hypotension, syncope, seizure, arrythmia
Pneumothorax/mediastinal emphysema
Bronchospasm, laryngospasm
Vasovagal reactions
Increased intra-cranial pressure
Pneumonia
Hemoptysis
Increased myocardial oxygen demand

Disadvantages of Therapeutic Bronchoscopy Compared to Chest Physical Therapy[a]

Requires 100% Fio_2 due to risk of hypoxemia
Risk of cross-contamination from equipment
May be limited by tracheal tube size,
  Bronchoscope occupies 51%–66% of the endotracheal tube (has a smaller orifice than standard suction catheter)
Limited to removing secretions from the lobar bronchus, not peripheral airways
Physician participation is necessary
Cost
Additional sedation is required

Adapted from Borchers SD, Beamis JF. Flexible bronchoscopy. *Chest Surg ClinN Am.* 1996;6:169-191. [a]Imle PC. Adjuncts to chest physiotherapy. In: Mackenzie CF, ed. *Chest Physiotherapy in the Intensive Care Unit.* 2nd ed. Baltimore, MD: Williams & Wilkins; 1989:308.

Jelic S, Cunningham JA, Factor P. Clinical review: airway hygiene in the intensive care unit. *Crit Care.* 2008;12(2):209.

CLINICAL CORRELATE

The indications for chest physical therapy include radiological evidence of atelectasis or infiltrate associated with secretion retention, adventitious breath sounds coupled with secretion retention, poor cough, and a decrease in arterial oxygenation thought to be a result of secretion retention.

Chest physical therapy consisted of postural drainage positioning to the areas of radiological involvement, manual percussion, manual vibration, airway suctioning and breathing exercises with assistive cough techniques for spontaneously breathing patients. Treatment duration was not predetermined. Patients were treated as long as they were productive of secretions; and breath sounds were improving, suggesting that pulmonary secretions were being mobilized.[107,110,114] Patients who are mobile and able to expectorate secretions would not require these airway clearance interventions. Patients with lobar collapse who are unable to be mobilized or optimally positioned for postural drainage to an area of radiologically proven pathology may be responsive to bronchoscopy if they remain symptomatic after 24 hours of aggressive chest physical therapy.[106] The primary problem for secretion retention should be resolved and not considered an indication for repeated invasive intervention of the airways.[106]

CLINICAL CORRELATE

With optimal positioning for postural drainage, percussion, and vibration, it may take 20 to 30 minutes to mobilize secretions from the lung parenchyma and alveolar areas. Evidence of successful secretion mobilization via positioning and manual techniques is typically characterized by diminished or absent breath sounds prior to positioning which become crackles, rhonchi, or vesicular during treatment.

POTENTIAL RISKS ASSOCIATED WITH MECHANICAL VENTILATION

Risk Factors Associated with Intubation

Patients requiring prolonged mechanical ventilation usually require tracheal intubation. A tube is placed in the trachea through the nose (nasotracheal tube), mouth (orotracheal tube), or an incision in the trachea (tracheostomy tube) (Fig. 19-5). The proximal/external end of the tracheal tube is connected to tubing and attached to the mechanical ventilator. In adults, tubes with an inflated cuff are used. Indications for tracheal intubation are included in Table 19-2. With a tracheal tube, the normal cough mechanism, which includes glottic closure, is interrupted and the inflated cuff inhibits mucociliary function. Complications of intubation include translocation of organisms from the oropharynx to the lung, intubation of the right mainstem bronchus, laryngeal or tracheal injury (perforation of the trachea is rare), and aspiration. After the patient is intubated by the physician (or in some institutions the respiratory therapist) the position of the tube is confirmed by a chest radiograph (distal end 2–3 cm above the carina) before the initial physical therapy intervention.[21] Airway clearance techniques may be indicated shortly after intubation if aspiration is suspected. Physical therapists working with intubated patients should check that the tube is secured in place and that the patient is appropriately restrained if at high risk for self-extubation. During treatment interventions the physical therapist should note if there is a marked difference in inhaled and exhaled tidal volumes, which may denote an air leak around the tracheal tube, or a cuff that is not properly inflated or may be damaged. This finding should be reported immediately to the nurse or physician. If inflating the cuff does not resolve the problem, the tracheal tube may need to be changed by the physician prior to any further physical therapy interventions.

It has been reported that the majority of patients intubated for greater than 3 days have some type of tracheal or laryngeal injury ranging from mild mucosal erythema to ulceration, granuloma formation, or vocal cord immobility.[115] Laryngotracheal injury or edema narrow the upper airway, predisposing the patient to *stridor* (a high pitched inspiratory wheeze located in the trachea or larynx) once the tube is removed. Stridor is a serious complication, which may require that the patient be reintubated because of upper airway occlusion when the lungs themselves are functioning normally. The highest risk of stridor is when a patient extubates himself or herself without the cuff being deflated, causing the inflated cuff to be pulled through the vocal cords. Stridor does not appear to be related to the number of intubations and usually occurs within the first few hours after extubation.[116,117]

The initial treatment for stridor is inhalation of racemic epinephrine and intravenous corticosteroids, or inhalation of a helium–oxygen gas mixture (heliox). Inhaling heliox reduces the large pressure drop associated with turbulent flow across the obstruction.[118,119] Secretion removal techniques, including head-down positioning, may be necessary to assist in the removal of pulmonary secretions.

Head-down positioning with close monitoring of vital signs is less invasive in assisting secretions to drain to the oropharynx than is nasotracheal suctioning. Nasotracheal suctioning is contraindicated with stridor due to the mechanical injury it may cause to the soft tissues. Reintubation is necessary if stridor does not respond to the treatment interventions previously described. Physical therapists should closely monitor patients postextubation and report any suspicion of stridor to the nurse or physician.

Endotracheal or tracheal tube cuffs may also cause pressure necrosis of the trachea resulting in tracheal stenosis and tracheal malacia. Using tracheal tubes with high-volume, low-pressure cuffs and monitoring cuff pressures reduces the complication of tracheal ischemia. Cuff pressures should be maintained below the pressure that occludes capillary blood flow to the tracheal tissues that are compressed by the cuff. Cuff pressures between 20 and 30 cm H_2O pressure are recommended.[120] Mean tracheal capillary perfusion pressure is approximately 30 mm Hg. The lowest pressure that prevents leakage around the cuff is used. A minimal air leak at the moment in the ventilatory cycle when the tracheal diameter is greatest will also act to minimize tracheal ischemia. Patients who have developed tracheal injury related to the cuff may require a tracheal tube with a foam cuff (Fig. 19-5C).[121]

Nursing, speech–language pathology, and respiratory therapy personnel are usually capable of inflating and deflating the cuff on the tracheal tube. However, it has been shown that periodic cuff deflation is not beneficial. Deflating the cuff 5 minutes each hour does not restore blood flow to the tracheal mucosa and can create periods of inadequate ventilation, potential cardiovascular instability, and potential aspiration. Erosion of the trachea may also result in a fistula forming between the trachea and the esophagus (tracheal-esophageal fistula) or into the innominate artery (tracheal-innominate fistula). These complications are rare yet life threatening when they occur, requiring immediate surgical repair.

Impaired Mucociliary Function and Lack of Humidification

The presence of an endotracheal tube bypasses the naso-, oro-, laryngo-pharynx that humidifies inspired gases to 100% relative humidity and protects the lung from particulate, chemical and microbiologic matter.[122] Inhalation of dry respiratory gases that bypass the normal mechanisms of warming and humidification can irritate the respiratory mucosa, reduce mucociliary transport, and cause drying and retention of lung

secretions. Therefore, mechanically ventilated patients require some type of airway humidification.

The most common methods of airway humidification for mechanically ventilated patients are use of a heated humidifier or a heat and moisture exchanger.[123] The humidifier allows gas to pass over a water reservoir and water is evaporated into the gas, increasing the humidity level of the gas delivered to the patient (Fig. 19-6A). The humidified gas then passes through a delivery tube to the patient. Most systems can deliver near 100% humidity at 37°C.[123] Water temperature is closely monitored to minimize condensation and prevent burning of the airway. Because condensation is often present in the tubing, humidifiers and ventilator tubing should be positioned lower than the patient to prevent the water from spilling back into the patient's airway. When turning or mobilizing a patient, the physical therapist may need to maneuver the tubing to prevent backflow of water into the patient's airway.

Heat and moisture exchangers (HME) are placed on the distal end of the tracheal tube to minimize the loss of heat and humidity from the upper respiratory tract. They are commonly referred to as an *artificial nose* (Fig. 19-6B). This device recovers part of the heat and moisture contained in the expired air. Humidified expired gases pass through a sponge or similar material with low thermal conductivity, which conserves heat and causes condensation of moisture and heat retention. The retained heat and moisture are added to the inspired gases. The humidifying process is possible because of the condensation of water vapor during expiration and its subsequent evaporation during inspiration.[123] HMEs are thought to require less maintenance than a heated humidifier.

HMEs may be sufficient for patients ventilated for a short duration, and patient transport, however for patients with long-term mechanical ventilation, haemoptysis, tenacious secretions, increased airway resistance and hypothermia, a heated humidifier is recommended.[124,125] In the ICU setting, an increased viscosity of bronchial secretions has been noted during prolonged mechanical ventilation with an HME. Thick secretions can increase airway resistance due to clogging of the endotracheal tube or HME and may lead to increased respiratory effort by the patient, air trapping, airway obstruction, and pulmonary infection. The physical therapist working in the ICU should evaluate the consistency of the patient's secretions and be aware of both the type and presence of humidification. Institutional protocols will determine which type of humidification is routinely used. Patients with bloody, copious, or viscous secretions with a HME may require increased systemic hydration or another type of humidification. The therapist should discuss this with the patient's physician who may decide to increase the patient's fluid intake or change the method of humidification.

Respiratory Muscle Weakness and Fatigue

It is generally accepted that patients requiring prolonged mechanical ventilation are subject to respiratory muscle

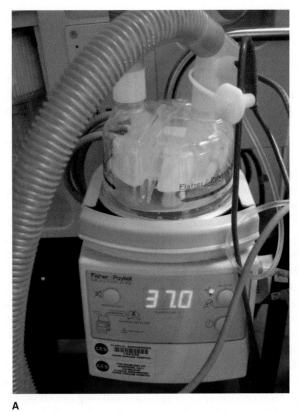

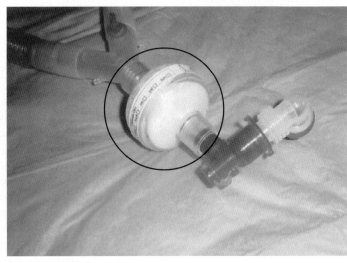

A

B

FIGURE 19-6   (**A**) Heated humidifier. (**B**) Heat and moisture exchanger—"artificial nose."

weakness. This may be the result of inadequate neuromuscular function, atrophy of the respiratory muscles, paralysis due to administration of a neuromuscular blockade, electrolyte imbalance, inadequate nutritional support, fibers remodeling, oxidative stress, and/or steroid myopathy.[60,126] Future research may assist physical therapists to determine the type and timing of inspiratory, and expiratory (including diaphragmatic) muscle strength training, which may assist the weaning process. There is also interest in the potential for newer modes of mechanical ventilation, which allow unassisted spontaneous breathing, for example, APRV, which may limit development of diaphragmatic weakness.

The degree of support offered to the respiratory muscles will vary with the chosen mode of mechanical ventilation. When pharmacological paralysis of the respiratory muscles is necessary to sustain life (see Chapter 8), and where a higher incidence of respiratory muscle atrophy is suspected, modes of ventilation such as volume control or pressure control are used. However, it is difficult to precisely determine the volume or pressure required. Offering more support than is necessary may contribute to respiratory muscle atrophy, whereas not providing enough support may lead to respiratory muscle fatigue. Modes utilized for weaning, such as PSV and SIMV, as well as APRV or similar modes of ventilation allow for greater activity of the respiratory muscles. If muscles fatigue, the recommended treatment is rest, which is usually accomplished by either increasing the number of breaths offered by the ventilator per minute or increasing the pressure associated with each

breath or cycle. For example, increasing inspiratory pressure support increases tidal volume, decreases respiratory rate, decreases $PaCO_2$, and decreases oxygen consumption and the work of the inspiratory muscles.[49] Reducing PSV, a shorter inflation time and lower tidal volumes may decrease the work of breathing with patients requiring long-term ventilation.[127] Pressure support ventilation is therefore a mode of ventilation commonly used to assist weaning and prevent respiratory muscle fatigue. Unfortunately, the precise intensity and duration of mechanical ventilation needed to rest the inspiratory muscles without causing fatigue is unknown and probably varies from patient to patient.

Weaning is not attempted until the cause of respiratory muscle fatigue is reversed. Further research will determine the optimal modes of ventilation required to minimize respiratory muscle weakness and fatigue and enhance the patient's chances of successful liberation from a ventilator. Evidence suggesting that inspiratory muscle training (IMT) improves the strength and/or endurance of the respiratory muscles and enhances weaning from mechanical ventilation is limited to small sample sizes and case reports.[128–131] Although the mechanism for rapid increases in maximal inspiratory pressure (MIP) with training is unknown, it is speculated that neural adaptations rather than muscle hypertrophy occur because the duration of training is probably insufficient to elicit microscopic changes in muscle fibers.[132] Physical therapists usually do not provide inspiratory muscle training exercises to assist weaning unless the patient has a

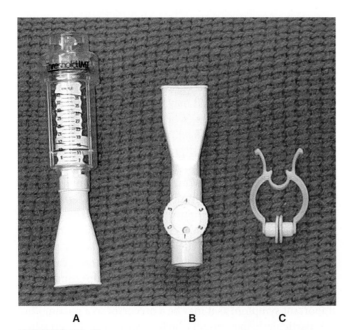

FIGURE 19-7 Inspiratory muscle trainers. (**A**) Resistive, linear device (**B**) Pressure, nonlinear device (**C**) Noseclip (Courtesy of Mary Massery, PT, DPT).

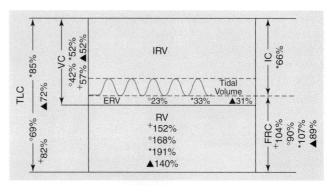

Percentage of Normal Lung Volumes in Tetraplegia Patients

[+] Bodin P, Kreuter M, Bake B, Olsen MF. Breathing patterns during breathing exercises in persons with tetraplegia. *Spinal?Cord.* 2003;41(5):290-295.

[°] Fugl-Meyer AR. Effects of respiratory muscle paralysis in tetraplegic and paraplegic patients. *Scand?J?Rehabil?Med.* 1971;3(4):141-150.

[*] Haas A, Lowman EW, Bergofsky EH. Impairment of respiration after spinal cord injury. *Arch?Phys?Med?Rehabil.* 1965;46:399-405.

[▲] Estenne M, De Troyer A. Mechanism of the postural dependence of vital capacity in tetraplegic subjects. *Am?Rev?Respir?Dis.* 1987;135(2):367-371.

FIGURE 19-8 Lung volumes.

neuromuscular injury or disease affecting the inspiratory muscles, or the patient has not responded to prior attempts to discontinue mechanical ventilation.

Inspiratory muscle training devices are usually either pressure (nonlinear) or resistive (linear) threshold devices with an adapter to attach the device to the tracheal tube (Fig. 19-7). A nose clip is not required when the cuff on the tracheal tube is inflated. The patient is trained once to twice daily in a position that optimizes vital capacity (sitting for nontetraplegic patients with the head of bed elevated to at least 30 degrees) for up to 30 minutes.[133] Mechanically ventilated patients may better tolerate morning training sessions.

With pressure threshold devices the patient breathes though a set of adjustable orifices and the resistance is increased as the size of the orifice is decreased, however the resistance is dependent upon airflow which can be modulated by the patient adjusting their tidal volume and respiratory rate. Resistive threshold devices are preferred as they can be adjusted to a specific workload to provide a constant pressure through the entire inspiration, independent of airflow. Depending upon the device used, the resistance is adjusted by assessing the rate of perceived exertion (RPE) or MIP (linear devices) or the patient's tolerance to the size of the orifice of the device (nonlinear devices). Based upon the limited evidence of the efficacy of inspiratory muscle training, it should be implemented on a case-by-case basis, when the physician has determined the patient is unable to wean by conventional methods, including maximal mobilization (page 601). Vital capacity, inspiratory mouth pressures, tidal volume, ventilator settings, resistance, training time, oxygen saturation, and heart rate should be monitored and recorded by the physical therapist during each training session and the resistance adjusted based upon the patient's response to treatment.

Tetraplegic patients are notoriously difficult to wean due to a reduction in lung volumes and inability to cough effectively due to the loss of abdominal muscle strength[133] (Fig. 19-8). Lesions above C5 result in impairment or loss of diaphragmatic muscle strength. Respiratory muscle strengthening exercises are therefore advocated. Inspiratory muscle training is often used however current evidence is inconclusive and primarily restricted to patients who have been weaned from the ventilator.[134–138] Training is initiated in the supine position during CPAP or during interruptions from mechanical ventilation twice daily 5 to 7 days per week.

A second type of respiratory muscle strengthening, abdominal weight training has been used with tetraplegic patients during periods of spontaneous breathing both with and without CPAP.[136,139] Theoretically, abdominal weight training, where cuff or dish weights are placed on the abdomen, would appear to provide more strength training than endurance training of the inspiratory muscles. During abdominal weight training the patient lies supine and the therapist determines a training load (Fig. 19-9). The inspiratory load can be determined by choosing the maximum weight with which a subject can breathe for 6 minutes, or by adding weights until the inspiratory capacity (grossly assessed using an incentive spirometer) decreases. Training protocols include a rate of 6 to 40 breaths per session or abdominal weight training for a predetermined time.

It is advisable to reevaluate the inspiratory mouth pressures and the training load at least weekly during either IMT or abdominal weight training. Literature is scant regarding which training method is optimal during weaning from mechanical ventilation. Some tetraplegic patients prefer abdominal weight training over inspiratory muscle training stating it is easier to learn. Pulmonary secretions may clog the diaphragm of the IMT device and require frequent cleaning. Conversely, IMT is easily performed in the sitting position once the patient's respiratory condition improves and can be performed more independently than abdominal weight training.

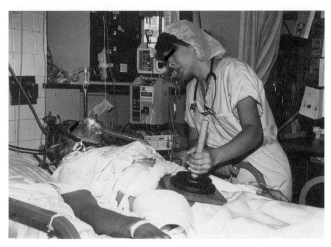

FIGURE 19-9 Abdominal weight training—tetraplegic patient.

Other respiratory interventions advocated for the tetraplegic patient include strengthening the latissimus dorsi and the clavicular portion of the pectoralis major, glossopharyngeal breathing, summed breathing, incentive spirometry, and strengthening the cervical accessory muscles of respiration. Strengthening the clavicular portion of the pectorals major, the latissimus dorsi, and cervical accessory muscles should be included in the physical therapy regimen starting while the patient is mechanically ventilated, as these muscles have been shown to increase peak expiratory flow rates and thus are likely to enhance cough efficacy.[140–142] Studies evaluating breathing exercises and glossopharyngeal breathing when the patient with tetraplegia is free from mechanical ventilation are covered in detail in Chapter 20. Objective assessment of the efficacy of breathing exercises requires electromyography and the insertion of gastric and esophageal balloons to measure gastric and subdiaphragmatic pressures and is therefore impractical in the ICU setting. However, examination of mouth pressures via manometers is simple and clinically useful, and can be taken when a patient has a tracheal tube (see Chapter 9).

Ventilator-Induced Lung Injury

Experimental studies have shown that excessive mechanical stresses associated with mechanical ventilation inflict injury on normal and acutely injured lungs. Repetitive application of excessive stress or strain to the lung by mechanical ventilation leads to diffuse alveolar damage, referred to as ventilator induced lung injury (VILI).[143] VILI may result from one of four different mechanisms—Barotrauma, volutrauma, atelectrauma, biotrauma[144,145]—and is thought to result in the release of inflammatory mediators and proteinaceous edema entering the alveolar space. This is very similar to the macroscopic and microscopic lung injury observed in ARDS.

Barotrauma is induced by high ventilating pressures and can describe alveolar rupture and extra-alveolar air present in abnormal locations. Risk factors thought to predispose a patient to ventilator-associated barotrauma include diminished lung integrity from necrotizing pneumonia, aspiration,

alveolar distension from high tidal volumes, high airway pressures, and possibly PEEP. Extra-alveolar air can be present in many locations including the pleural space, soft tissue, abdominal cavity, and pericardium. Extra-alveolar air occurs after alveolar rupture as air dissects along the vascular sheaths back to the mediastinum. It may then dissect the pleural space and cause a pneumothorax. When the air diffuses into the soft tissues, it is known as *subcutaneous emphysema*. Air in the abdominal cavity is termed *pneumoperitoneum*, while *pneumopericardium* refers to air in the pericardial space.

Subcutaneous emphysema is a frequent complication of barotrauma that has implications for physical therapy interventions. Subcutaneous emphysema is diagnosed by palpating crepitation in the neck, face, chest, axilla, or abdomen. The crepitus of subcutaneous emphysema feels like crisped rice cereal. The physical therapist may be the first health care practitioner to pick up this clinical sign during an examination or treatment intervention. Subcutaneous emphysema can be an important symptom as it may be a precursor to a pneumothorax, particularly in a patient who has elevated airway pressures and diminished or absent breath sounds in one lung. If the patient has not had a recent chest radiograph and been evaluated for pneumothoraces the physician will usually order a chest radiograph. Once a pneumothorax has been ruled out or treated, physical therapy interventions including mobility, manual techniques for secretion clearance and cough assistance techniques can be performed if clinically indicated. A sudden elevation in airway pressures and/or drop in tidal volume and decreased breath sounds in the absence of subcutaneous emphysema should also be brought to the physician's attention, as they may be indicative of a pneumothorax.

Volutrauma describes damage caused by overdistension of the alveoli occurring as a result of high volume ventilation. Overdistension of the alveoli results in diffuse alveolar damage, pulmonary edema, increased fluid filtration, epithelial permeability, and microvascular permeability and mostly affects healthy or highly compliant alveoli.[144] *Atelectrauma* is lung injury related to repetitive opening and closing of alveoli, and is theoretically prevented by the use of PEEP to prevent derecruitment or collapsing of alveoli.[33] *Biotrauma* describes inflammatory injury to the alveoli due to cytokine release in response to mechanical injury.[144] Ventilation at high tidal volumes, high pressures, or without peep can exacerbate VILI, and recent studies have demonstrated a reduced mortality with mechanical ventilation using low tidal volumes.[29,146,147] Plateau pressures should be monitored and ideally not exceed 30 cm H_2O pressure. The literature is inconclusive as to whether the tidal volume or plateau pressure is the best target for therapeutic interventions.[148] It is recommended that plateau pressure should be monitored during mechanical ventilation. Plateau pressure is a more accurate indicator of lung compliance than peak inspiratory pressure. As lung compliance falls, plateau pressure rises. Peak inspiratory pressures are influenced by decreasing lung compliance, but also influenced by any increase in airway resistance. Plateau pressures in the first 48 hours of ALI may reflect the severity of disease and mortality.[149]

Physical therapists should be aware that ventilatory management that emphasizes lower alveolar pressures and avoids hyperinflation may result in an intentional elevation of $PaCO_2$, which is usually well tolerated in critically ill patients, as long as the increases are gradual.[150]

COMPLICATIONS OF IMMOBILITY AND ICU INTERVENTIONS

The following quotation made by Dr. Henry Bendixon in 1974 remains true today and is worth reiterating.[151]

The importance of immobilization has been part of medicine's body of knowledge for many, many, years and can be accepted as fact. As with any fact, if not restated from time to time it tends to be forgotten. Our advanced knowledge and technology by themselves cannot save the patient. Instead, something so simple as turning the patient . . . at least hourly, may make the difference between living and dying for the intensive care patient.

Patients receiving mechanical ventilation are at risk for all the complications associated with immobility. The hazards of immobility alter the normal physiological function of most, if not all body systems. Interventions to prevent these complications are often overlooked, due to medical prioritization of the life-saving aspects of the patient's plan of care. Physical therapists working in the critical care unit often bring this necessary perspective of patient management to the ICU team. Once aware of the principles of mechanical ventilation, and the life-sustaining equipment these patients require, the physical therapist can develop a treatment plan to enhance respiratory, cardiovascular, neurological, and musculoskeletal function. Attention to respiratory function and mobility may decrease the risk of integumentary complications. The medical team is usually receptive to the physical therapist attending rounds and taking an active role as part of the interdisciplinary team.

EFFECTS OF BODY POSITION AND THE USE OF ABDOMINAL BINDERS FOR PATIENTS WITH TETRAPLEGIA

Changes in respiratory function occur during the initial period of adjustment from the sitting to the supine position. In normal subjects, total lung capacity, vital capacity, functional residual capacity, residual volume, and forced expiratory volume may all be reduced simply by lying down.[152-154] A reduction in rib cage compliance, decreased anterio-posterior diameter, and increased lateral diameter of the rib cage are also noted in the supine compared to the sitting position. Alveolar size decreases, and small airway closure increases in dependent lung zones with a decrease in PaO_2.[153] The normal subject may have a 7.5% decrease in vital capacity when assuming the supine position.[155,156] Similarly, a reduction in the FRC occurs consistently in changing from the sitting to supine position.[157] Therefore, patients with normal innervation of the respiratory muscles

usually tolerate weaning and functional activities better while sitting out of bed or in bed with the head of the bed elevated.

The tetraplegic patient may also have dramatic changes in respiratory function when moving from the upright or sitting position to the supine position. However, these changes are quite different from those noted in patients who have normal innervation of the respiratory muscles (Fig. 19-8). With tetraplegia, inspiratory muscle weakness results in a 15% to 31% reduction in total lung capacity, 48% to 58% loss of vital capacity, and a 34% loss of inspiratory capacity. Up to a 77% reduction in expiratory reserve volume and a 50% increase in residual volume are attributed to a lack of expiratory muscle function.[158-161]

The tetraplegic patient has a decreased tidal volume, vital capacity, inspiratory capacity, and decreased ventilation in the lung bases when assuming the sitting position from the supine position.[156,160] With tetraplegia an increase in vital capacity has also been noted in the 20-degree head-down position with supine positioning.[162] Therefore, the tetraplegic patient may better tolerate weaning trials, respiratory muscle strengthening exercises, and early rehabilitative interventions, while supine. Vital capacity may be greater during postural drainage positioning for the lower and middle lobes than in the upright position.

Abdominal binders are advocated for the spontaneously breathing or weaning tetraplegic patient in order to align the abdominal contents under the diaphragm, thus improving the length–tension relationship of the diaphragm. The effect of an abdominal binder is most evident in the seated position. Increases in inspiratory capacity, vital capacity, tidal volume, total lung capacity, and decreases in functional residual capacity have been documented.[163-165] These improved lung volumes assist the tetraplegic patient's ability to cough. Maximum expiratory airflow increases with an abdominal binder when manual lung inflation and chest compressions are utilized as an assistive cough maneuver.[166]

Physical therapists working with mechanically ventilated tetraplegic patients should recommend the use of an abdominal binder once the patient is spontaneously breathing during part of the ventilatory cycle, and prior to raising the head of the bed to initiate sitting. Elastic binders are recommended and can usually be obtained from the hospital medical supply department. Elastic binders usually come with 3 to 4 circumferential elastic panels (Fig. 19-10). The therapist should measure the distance from a few inches below the xiphoid process to the level of the anterior superior iliac spine (ASIS). Clinically, it has been noted that skin breakdown is greater when the binder extends below the ASIS. If the elastic binder is too wide, one or two panels can be cut away. Binders that are too tight or extend too high on the thorax may hinder inspiration. Although binders are recommended as a standard of care in acute rehabilitation the overall benefits are not known. A decrease in functional residual capacity with the use of a binder has the potential to impair gas exchange and abdominal strapping alone is unlikely to improve expiratory flow rates sufficient to improve the efficiency of cough in tetraplegic patients 6 to 200 months after injury.[167,168] However, abdominal binders appear to improve vital capacity and enhance the

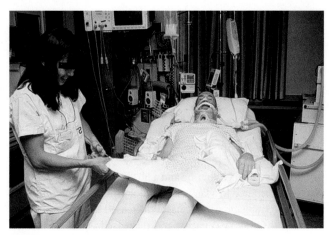

FIGURE 19-10   Abdominal binder.

patient's ability to cough by providing abdominal pressure, which may be assisted by the clinician during expiration.

CLINICAL CORRELATE

If the therapist is in doubt as to whether a binder is beneficial for a particular patient, vital capacity measurements can be taken with a respirometer both with and without the binder to determine if the binder is advantageous.

Some advocate that abdominal binders be worn until a plateau in pulmonary function or cough effectiveness/assistance is observed. When patients are observed to be stable and no further improvement in pulmonary function or cough is noted, abdominal binders are frequently removed. However, chronic abdominal binder use after spinal cord injury has been suggested to maintain and possibly improve pulmonary function, cardiovascular status, and posture. This will be presented in the following chapter where the patient in the case study of this chapter is progressed to a subacute facility and the physical therapist must consider the chronic ramifications of spinal cord injury.

Central Nervous System
Cognitive Impairment

Cognitive function can be dramatically altered by bedrest and particularly in mechanically ventilated ICU patients. Seventy-eight percent of ICU survivors of ARDS may have cognitive impairment at one year, which is severely underestimated by rehabilitation professionals.[169,170] College students placed on bedrest were noted to have slowing of electroencephalogram activity, emotional and behavioral changes, decreased psychomotor performance, and changes in sleep patterns.[171,172]

Decreased psychomotor performance in areas of intellect, perception, and coordination accompanied by visual and auditory changes have also been noted.[173]

Once mechanically ventilated, a patient is at a high risk for delirium due to acute multisystem illness, comorbidities, and medications.[174] *Delirium* is defined as an acute onset of impaired cognitive functioning which impacts the patient's ability to receive, process, store, and recall information.[174] Delirium can result in increased morbidity, including more time to liberate the patient from mechanical ventilation, higher rates of nosocomial pneumonia, delayed functional recovery, and a prolonged hospital stay.[175] ICU patients also experience a loss of circadian light patterns, electrolyte imbalances, fever, and hypoxia, and are subjected to monitoring alarms and numerous caregivers approaching the bedside to provide interventions around the clock, all of which disrupt their cognitive function.

It is not uncommon for mechanically ventilated patients to receive various forms of analgesia, sedation, and even neuromuscular blockade for surgical procedures and management while in the ICU. Sedation and delirium can have a dramatic impact on the ability of the patient to participate with physical therapy interventions. Recent literature recommends at least daily monitoring of sedation and delirium by nursing and other health care providers.[176] The Richmond Agitation—Sedation Scale (RAAS) assists physicians and nurses in determining appropriate doses of sedative and analgesic medications.[177] The Confusion Assessment Method for ICU patients (CAM-ICU) alerts the clinician to disorganized thinking, inattention, and altered level of consciousness, and is used to determine delirium.[174]

Most physical therapists are familiar with and can utilize the Glasgow Coma Scale (GCS), a 3- to 15-point scale rating eye opening, verbal, and motor responses to determine level of consciousness.[178] Despite its widespread use for neurological assessment in the ICU setting, it was developed for assessment of level of consciousness after head injury, and its use has not been validated in the general ICU population. Unfortunately, few physical therapists are aware of the RAAS and ICU–CAM, two highly reliable and valid tools for ICU patients that take 1 to 2 minutes to administer and are used to assess the patient's level of sedation and delerium.[174,176,179] It is therefore recommended that physical therapists working in the ICU learn the meaning of the scores and how to administer these tools to enhance communication with the medical team. Improved teamwork may lead to a change in sedation or analgesia and the physical therapist may gain a better understanding of the patient's mental status, therefore optimizing the patient's ability to participate in therapy.

The RAAS is a 10-point scale with four positive levels for agitation and five negative levels. The RAAS separates the patient's responses to verbal and physical stimulation. The ICU–CAM is recommended when a patient's RAAS score indicates the patient has some response to voice. Each visit the therapist should also orient the patient to place and time, work with the nursing staff to display pictures of family members, and procure audiotapes to assist with cognitive orientation. A calendar noting the day displayed within the patient's line of vision is helpful. The therapist should speak to the patient throughout the treatment session and never underestimate the patient's ability to understand the activity and environment around him or her. Upright positioning out of bed is recommended to enhance the patient's orientation to, and interaction with, their environment, as well as minimize the other associated complications of immobility.

Many clinicians (physicians, nurses, and therapists) currently defer getting out of bed for patients with a low level of consciousness, due to a perceived lack of ability to participate or benefit. Sitting in a chair out of bed, the patient may be stimulated to an increased level of consciousness, and demonstrate greater than expected participation, when attempts are made to begin mobility within days of admission to the ICU. It is the clinical experience of the authors that patients often demonstrate automatic responses to rolling, moving from supine to sitting, sitting to standing and transferring, despite the inability to follow commands or effectively participate in activities while supine in bed. Activities out of bed should not be discounted solely due to a patient's perceived inability to participate with physical therapy interventions.

Cardiovascular

Cardiac

While mechanically ventilated, most patients spend the majority of their day in bed. It is therefore assumed that the same risks associated with immobility that occur within the cardiovascular system with bedrest occur with mechanically ventilated patients. Decreased blood volume, decreased plasma and red blood cell mass, decreased hemoglobin concentration, increased basal and maximal heart rate, decreased maximum oxygen uptake, and a decreased transverse diameter of the heart have all been reported.[180,181] Critically ill patients without previous cardiac disease may also be susceptible to reversible myocardial dysfunction including systolic dysfunction, segmental contractility disturbances, and electrocardiographic changes.[182] Immobilized patients develop a decreased ability to perform aerobic work. Oxygen uptake during exercise decreases, whereas oxygen debt and blood lactate concentrations increase. Pharmacological agents are frequently required to maximize cardiac output. Detailed descriptions of the cardiac risks of immobility are described in Chapter 14.

Orthostatic or *postural hypotension* is the term used to describe a decrease in blood pressure upon assuming the erect position accompanied by symptoms of dizziness or syncope. Circulating blood volume is reduced with bed rest and vascular tone is decreased. Medical management will attempt to maximize circulating blood volume; however, sitting the patient up may result in decreased cardiac filling pressures and decreased cardiac output because of vasodilation of the lower extremity blood vessels. The resulting decreased blood flow to the brain may result in mild cerebral hypoxemia. The alert, oriented, and spontaneously breathing patient can report to the caretaker that they are feeling "lightheaded" or "dizzy" after sitting up. The mechanically ventilated patient usually cannot speak because of intubation and may have cognitive impairment, muscular weakness, or lines and tubes making it difficult to display discomfort with body language.

The therapist should be aware of whether the patient is taking any medications such as β-blockers that blunt the body's normal response to activity (see Chapter 8). The most common response to upright positioning is a drop in blood pressure with a compensatory increase in heart rate. Oxygen saturation may drop and may prompt the physician to increase the FiO_2 delivered by the ventilator.

The patient with an acute cervical spinal cord injury presents an additional challenge for the physical therapist. Rapid changes in body position for the acute tetraplegic patient in spinal shock may have a more dramatic adverse affect on cardiac function. Head elevation of greater than 20 degrees may cause a sudden decrease in cardiac filling pressures, resulting in a decrease in cardiac output, and even cardiac arrest. Similarly, sudden head-down positioning, as is necessary for postural drainage of the middle and lower lobes, may cause a rise in cardiac filling pressures. Because of the loss of sympathetic cardiac innervation associated with lesions above T1, the steep head-down position may precipitate acute myocardial failure with pulmonary edema. Therefore, in the early stages of acute tetraplegia, head elevation and head-down positioning should be performed with careful monitoring of arterial and venous pressures. Most mechanically ventilated tetraplegic patients tolerate head-down positioning when experienced personnel move the patient cautiously.

The lower extremities of a patient with acute tetraplegia should be wrapped with elastic bandages or elastic stockings that cover the entire lower extremity prior to sitting the patient upright, particularly after prolonged bedrest. Compression of the lower extremity veins will assist the return of venous blood to the heart. The benefits of using elastic bandages versus compression stockings are not known. However, some clinicians have noted that patients who do not tolerate upright position changes with elastic stockings are better able to tolerate these position changes with elastic bandages. Bandages are more time-consuming to don and require special training of the personnel who apply them. They should be wrapped in a spiral or figure-eight fashion. The greatest tension is applied distally over the foot and gradually reduced as the extremity is wrapped to the groin. If applied incorrectly circumferential pressure may impair blood flow and increase edema below the circumferential wrap. An abdominal binder is also recommended for patients with acute tetraplegia to prevent pooling of blood in the abdominal cavity.

Venous Thromboembolic Disease

Medical and surgical patients have a 10% to 30% incidence of deep venous thrombosis (DVT) within the first week of ICU admission.[183] The risk of DVT with acute spinal cord injury is extremely high at 60% to 80%.[184]

Venous thrombi are intravascular deposits composed mainly of fibrin and red blood cells with a variable platelet and leukocyte component, usually located in the deep veins. It is important that they are recognized early and treated effectively. DVTs occur in regions of slow or disturbed blood flow (vascular stasis) in the lower extremity, or with loss of vessel wall integrity as a result of trauma or disease. The majority are confined to the calf and are asymptomatic, small, and not associated with major complications.[185] However, venous thrombi, particularly in the proximal veins (popliteal, femoral, iliofemoral), may break off and form a pulmonary embolus (PE) which is life threatening.

Mechanical ventilation and the associated immobility causing venous stasis put the patient at high risk for DVT and subsequent PE. Cancer, autoimmune disorders, lower extremity fractures, trauma or surgery to the veins, congestive heart failure, neurological disorders, lack of skeletal muscle activity, and postoperative sepsis all increase the risk of DVT and PE. Patients on bedrest have impaired venous return from the lower extremities and abnormal coagulation factors. It is thought that the decreased circulating blood volume that occurs with immobility is due more to the loss of plasma than to a decrease in red blood cell mass. With loss of endothelial lining cells along a vein, platelets attach to the underlying collagen and release factors that cause more platelets to adhere and aggregate to underlying collagen. A fibrin mesh attaches to the platelets and eventually traps erythrocytes and leucocytes. The result is an intravascular clot or thrombus.[185]

Patients with a decreased level of consciousness and sensory deficits may not perceive pain or tenderness along the track of the deep venous system, making DVT even more difficult to diagnose. More than 50% of DVTs occur without signs or symptoms.[185] When a physical therapist suspects a patient may have a DVT due to the presence of new clinical signs, the physician should be notified and further diagnostic testing may be necessary. Scoring for probability of deep vein thrombosis may be accomplished by use of the scoring method as described by Anand et al.[186] Ultrasonography and venography are most commonly used to diagnose DVT in critically ill patients. Once a diagnosis is made the therapist should be aware of whether the DVT is from the calf, which is most common, or from a more proximal vein such as the popliteal, femoral, iliac, or inferior vena cava where there is a higher incidence of complications including pulmonary embolus.

Anticoagulation therapy is effective in the prevention of extension, embolization, and recurrence of DVT. However, although anticoagulation therapy prevents enlargement of the thrombus and allows for further attachment of the thrombus to the vessel wall to prevent a pulmonary embolus, it does not dissolve the DVT.[187] The treatment of choice for acute DVT, PE, or while awaiting the results of diagnostic tests when the clinician has a high index of suspicion for thromboembolitic disease is anticoagulation therapy. Options include subcutaneous low-molecular-weight heparin (Lovenox, Fragmin), monitored IV or subcutaneous unfractionated heparin (Heparin Sodium), or fondaparinux (Arixtra) a Factor Xa inhibitor in the coagulation cascade.[187] A treatment regimen is recommended for most ICU patients at risk of DVT, and for most major trauma and spinal cord injury patients.[184,188,189] The efficacy of unfractionated heparin is measured by clotting times such as the activated partial thromboplastin time (APTT or PTT). Because of the mechanism of action for the low-molecular-weight heparins and fondaparinux, monitoring bleeding times is not required. The International Normalized Ratio for Prothrombin time (PT INR) is used to monitor warfarin (Coumadin) (Table 19-12).

When anticoagulation is contraindicated because of a high risk of bleeding, elastic compression stockings (CS) with a pressure gradient of 30 to 40 mm Hg and/or intermittent pneumatic compression (IPC) is recommended until pharmacologic thromboprophylaxis can be started. The advantages of IPC and CS are that they do not increase the risk of bleeding, may reduce leg swelling, and may enhance the effectiveness of anticoagulant thromboprophylaxis. They also have a greater effect in reducing distal versus proximal DVT. However, they

TABLE 19-12   Laboratory Tests to Monitor Anticoagulant Therapy

Anticoagulant	Laboratory Test	Reference Range
Coumadin/Warfarin	INR	2.0–3.0 desired range 2.5–3.5 heart valve in place >4.0 risk of hemorrhage
Heparin	APTT	1.5–2.5 × the mean of Labs normal PTT range
	[a]anti-Xa	0.3–0.7 U/mL of anti-Xa
Low molecular weight heparin	anti-Xa	0.6–1.1 U/mL of anti-Xa

INR, international normalized ratio; APTT, activated partial thromboplastin time.

[a]anti Factor Xa is used to determine the therapeutic dose of heparin. The reagents are antithrombin and Factor Xa. The heparin in patient plasma binds with excess antithrombin and inhibits excess Xa. Factor Xa is measured and is inversely proportional to the amount of heparin in patient plasma.

Table courtesy of Betty Ciesla, MS, MT, (ASCP)SH.

are generally less efficacious than anticoagulation as a prophylactic measure, staff compliance is low and there are no standards for size, pressure, or physiologic features.[184,190] Studies have shown that CS may reduce postthrombotic sequelae by 50%, and therefore should be worn for at least 2 years in patients who have had a symptomatic proximal DVT.[191-193]

Placing a filter in the inferior vena cava is a treatment modality for DVT and PE and is used for PE prophylaxis. Currently vena cava filters are not recommended except when a patient has a PE or acute proximal DVT and anticoagulant therapy is not indicated because of the risk of bleeding.[191,194] Anticoagulant therapy is recommended once the risk of bleeding subsides.[191] Physical therapists working in the ICU may see filters being placed at the bedside or in the interventional radiology department.[195] The physical therapist should be aware of any postprocedure precautions, such as immobilization of the hip for several hours (filters are usually placed via the femoral vein). However, by the day following the procedure routine physical therapy interventions such as range-of-motion exercises and bed-chair transfers can usually be resumed. Once the filter is in place there is no contraindication to range-of-motion exercises to the limb with the DVT.

The medical recommendations for mobilizing patients with a DVT have dramatically changed over the past several years. Historically, bed rest was advocated. It is now generally accepted that bed rest is associated with a slower resolution of leg pain and swelling from a DVT, and does not lower the risk of PE.[187] Early ambulation and CS are recommended for patients with acute DVT and may provide even faster improvement with less pain, swelling, and minimize the extension of a DVT.[187,189,196-199] The physical therapist should treat the mechanically ventilated patient with a DVT, the same as a nonmechanically ventilated patient with a DVT or suspected DVT. If the clinical examination and chart review reveal that the patient can be mobilized and transferred out of bed, the therapist removes the IPC device, applies elastic stockings or elastic bandages to the lower extremities if the patient is having symptoms of orthostatic hypotension, and begins mobility training activities. For patients in whom an IPC device is prescribed the device is reapplied after transfer training or ambulation. A patient with an untreated DVT in one extremity can receive secretion removal techniques and range-of-motion exercises to the noninvolved extremities.

A patient with a DVT who develops unexplained breathlessness, desaturation, hemoptysis, pleuritic pain, arrhythmia, or fever is suspected of having developed a PE.[200] However, the mechanically ventilated patient may not demonstrate breathlessness, may have hemoptysis from tracheal irritation with suctioning or a lung contusion, and may have arrhythmias or fever unrelated to a PE. Therefore, the diagnosis of PE is more difficult. The nurse, physical therapist, or respiratory therapist may note a critical drop in PaO_2 or oxygen saturation that leads the physician to suspect a PE. The most frequent diagnostic testing for PE is serial computed tomography, followed by ventilation/perfusion scans, or pulmonary angiography.[201] A PE usually does not preclude airway clearance interventions

with manual techniques. To date there are no documented cases of PE dislodgement, with manual chest physical therapy techniques, coughing, or suctioning. Should an embolus be dislodged, it would move peripherally into the pulmonary vasculature, where there is less rather than more occlusion of pulmonary blood flow. Anatomically it is impossible for a pulmonary embolus to cause a cerebral vascular accident or occlusion of an extremity vessel; yet this is a common concern of many practicing physical therapists.

The patient with acute tetraplegia has both a high risk of pulmonary embolus and a high risk for hypoxemia due to pulmonary secretion retention. Figure 19-11 demonstrates a ventilation perfusion scan of a patient with tetraplegia suspected of having developed a pulmonary embolus accompanied by a drop of PaO_2 to 50 torr. Following the scan, intensive chest physical therapy was instituted and the patient's oxygenation status significantly improved. In this case the patient was ruled out for a PE and was diagnosed with a ventilation versus a perfusion abnormality for which physical therapy was indicated for secretion clearance. When in doubt as to the appropriateness of secretion clearance interventions for a suspected or confirmed PE, the therapist should discuss their concerns with the referral source.

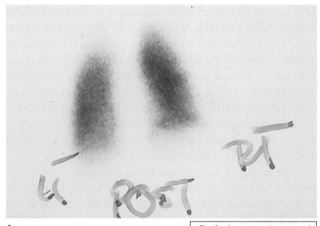

A   Perfusion scan is normal.

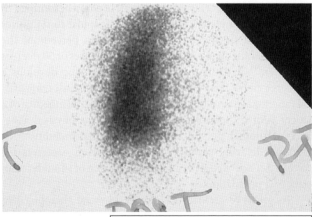

B   Ventilation scan—Note loss of ventilation to the right lung.

FIGURE 19-11   Ventilation–perfusion scans.

Neuro-musculoskeletal

The mechanically ventilated patient is subject to the same risks of contractures, muscle atrophy, and weakness as any immobilized, malnourished, or deconditioned patient. Because of the ventilator and the plethora of lines and tubes required for physiological monitoring, there may be an even greater risk of muscle wasting and limitations to joint mobility. Fourteen days of bedrest alone results in a 4.1% decrease in lean thigh mass, with a 15% to 30% decrease in quadriceps strength after 6 weeks.[202,203] Significant decrements in bone mineral density occur which may not be fully reversed after 6 months of normal weightbearing activities.[204] Heterotopic ossification, which increases the risk of contracture formation, has been documented in a variety of ICU populations, including patients with traumatic brain and/or spinal cord injuries, thermal burns, multitrauma without head trauma or simply long-term sedation.[205-209] Sedation and medical paralysis may be necessary to manage respiratory failure, placing some patients at an even higher risk of neuromusculoskeletal dysfunction.

Contractures

While research looking specifically at the relationship between contractures and mechanical ventilation is limited, there is some evidence that 34% of patients with ICU stays of greater than 14 days develop a functionally significant contracture in at least one joint at the time of ICU discharge, with 23% of the contractures present at the time of discharge to home.[210] In addition, clinical experience has noted contractures in the cervical spine, most likely due to the limitation of spontaneous cervical rotation by the ventilator tubing, and cervical extension contractures leading to a forward head from prolonged supine positioning with the head on pillows.

The incidence of contractures has been more clearly documented with acute SCI patients (who are usually admitted to an ICU) and may require mechanical ventilation. A study of 181 SCI patients demonstrated that those who are not admitted to an SCI center with early physical therapy developed more contractures.[211] Fifty-one percent of elbows examined in patients with complete C5 or C6 traumatic spinal cord injuries demonstrated flexion contractures. Sixteen percent of the upper extremities had elbow flexion contractures of 50 degrees or greater.[212] A patient with C6 tetraplegia who develops a 25-degree elbow flexion contracture frequently loses one critical functional neurological level, resulting in the mobility of a patient with C5 tetraplegia, who requires the physical assistance of another person for most functional mobility.[213] In addition, delaying shoulder range-of-motion exercises for 2 weeks is associated with a higher incidence of shoulder pain in the SCI population.

To preserve cervical ROM, the physical therapist can show the nursing staff how to position and maintain the head in the neutral position while the patient is supine. Outdated IV bags or rolled up towels placed on either side of the face will help to maintain the head in the neutral position. Active, active-assistive, and passive cervical ROM exercises (supine,

side-lying, and prone as indicated) are also recommended. The physical therapist and nursing staff may move the ventilator and ventilator tubing to provide enough slack for the patient to actively rotate the cervical spine. The alert patient should be periodically reminded to actively turn their head both toward and away from the ventilator while staff stabilizes the tubing. Alert and oriented patients who watch television may benefit from having the television placed on the side of the bed opposite the ventilator tubing. In rare cases, when a severe limitation of cervical motion rotation has developed, the ventilator can be moved to the other side of the bed (space permitting) to encourage spontaneous motion toward the most involved side.

The ICU physical therapist has a major role in preventing extremity contractures. Hip and knee flexion contractures, limited hip internal rotation, loss of ankle dorsiflexion; and limitations in scapular abduction, shoulder flexion, abduction, and external rotation are frequently noted in mechanically ventilated patients. ICU patients are at risk for losing motion in joints adjacent to lines and tubes due to discomfort and reluctance to spontaneously move the joint/extremity. No accidental removals or adverse effects have been found with physical therapy interventions for patients with arterial catheters.[4,5]

Many mechanically ventilated patients in acute respiratory failure present with subclavian and femoral lines. Central lines inserted in the subclavian vein with tubing extending perpendicular to the thorax contribute to decreased scapular mobility and limited shoulder motion. While some institutions advocate limiting shoulder ROM in the presence of subclavian lines, it should be noted that full-shoulder ROM can usually be accomplished without compromising the line. These lines are sutured in place and confirmed radiologically. The therapist carefully monitors the line for patency as the shoulder is moved to determine limitations in specific joint motions. When a central line is limiting shoulder motion, the therapist can speak with the physician and request that it be repositioned so that it does not cross the shoulder joint at the time of the next line change. If the line cannot be repositioned, side-to-side turning may pose greater challenges, requiring time-consuming positioning utilizing towels or outdated IV bags under the axilla to minimize the risk of occluding the line.

Therapists are sometimes fearful of moving the hip joint of a patient who has a femoral line. However, when therapists are working closely with the medical team this is usually not a problem, and the risks and benefits of hip flexion exercises and functional activities which incorporate hip flexion can be discussed on a case-by-case basis. Hip-extension contractures are rare; therefore, aggressive hip flexion exercises are usually not necessary. The presence of a femoral line does not preclude hip extension, abduction, adduction, and internal and external rotation unless the patient has an unusual acute condition where ROM exercises may increase bleeding at the site or the line is not sutured in properly. Transfers out of bed and even ambulation should not be aborted solely because a patient has a femoral line if it is adequately sutured in place. Early

TABLE 19-13 Physical Therapy Interventions That May Be Utilized During Mechanical Ventilation to Prevent Contractures

Side-to-side turning to 90 degrees or greater (Place a roll or foam wedge behind the patient's back, or turn patient onto the roll, so anterior trunk rests on the roll)
Dependent hip in neutral position
Uppermost shoulder flexed, scapula protracted

Move TV or ventilator side to side (increase rotation of the cervical spine)

Maintain cervical spine in neutral position while supine (place small towel rolls or expired IV bags on either side of the patient's neck)

Bed mobility exercises

Extremity therapeutic exercises

Splinting, serial casting

Sitting balance activities on edge of bed

Transfer patient to upright sitting position out of bed

Wheelchair propulsion or ambulation using a manual resuscitator bag or portable ventilator

---

mobility including ambulation has not been shown to adversely affect or dislodge arterial lines.

Many mechanically ventilated patients have chest tubes. These tubes are also sutured in place, and full shoulder ROM is not contraindicated, though care should be taken to assess the chest tube for drainage and possible air leaks both prior to and after intervention. Any change may indicate that the tube is not securely placed, and may need evaluation. Chest tubes placed for hemothorax or pneumothorax may well be accompanied by rib fractures, and early intervention to encourage full shoulder mobility and encourage deep breathing will reduce the risk of complications.

When possible, prone positioning is an ideal intervention to prevent hip flexion and shoulder internal rotation contractures. The prone or side-lying position facilitates hip extension and knee flexion exercises (Fig. 19-4).

In summary, contracture prevention for the mechanically ventilated patient should include the following: side-to-side turning to at least 90 degrees (a foam wedge or roll of several sheets or blankets is effective in keeping patients turned), ROM exercises, mobilization from supine to sit, bed to chair, and sitting the patient on the edge of the bed as soon as tolerated (Table 19-13). Early ambulation is also recommended (Fig. 19-12).

Splinting or serial casting (for patients who demonstrate increased muscle tone) can be applied to prevent contractures while patients are receiving mechanical ventilation. Short-acting pharmacological agents may be necessary to temporarily reduce spasticity for optimal joint positioning prior to serial casting (see Chapter 8). These drugs may temporarily decrease the patient's respiratory function necessitating an increase in ventilator support just prior to, during, and for a short time following the casting procedure.

CLINICAL CORRELATE

Early motion is recommended for most mechanically ventilated patients, particularly those with SCI or orthopedic injuries stabilized with internal and external fixation devices. The therapist should consult with the orthopedic or neurosurgeon for clarification of any precautions or restrictions to range-of-motion exercises, sitting upright, or weight bearing and instruct the nursing staff and family in ROM exercises that may enhance physical therapy sessions.

Critical Illness Neuromyopathy

Muscle weakness and atrophy are also significant complications for patients who require mechanical ventilation and ICU care. This weakness may be attributed to a variety of factors, including critical illness neuropathy and/or myopathy, corticosteroid use, hyperglycemia, immobility and deconditioning.[214,215] *Critical illness neuromyopathy (CINM)* has been defined as an illness that develops during a patient's ICU stay, involving peripheral nerves, muscles or the neuromuscular junction. Several risk factors have been identified, including sepsis, multiple organ failure and hyperglycemia.[216] While corticosteroid use has been suspected of increasing the risk of CINM, limited evidence suggests that corticosteroid use is not an independent risk factor for development of CINM.[217] Use of neuromuscular blockers has long been associated with muscle weakness, especially after prolonged use.[218,219] However, a clear causative role has not been established, as other known risk factors such as sepsis and hyperglycemia were not excluded. The typical patient with CINM presents with grossly symmetrical weakness without a known neuromuscular disease process predating ICU admission. Reflexes are typically depressed, yet may be normal, and muscle atrophy is often present. Facial musculature and sensation are generally spared.[215,220]

Quantification of muscle weakness is often difficult in the ICU patient who is sedated or delirious. Decreased motor response to noxious stimulus in the presence of facial grimacing may suggest CINM. Manual muscle testing is advocated for patients who can follow simple commands. For the critically ill patient who is unable to be turned 90 degrees side-lying, the therapist can raise the head of the bed as high as possible and with simple adaptations test the major muscle groups of the shoulder, wrist and hand as well as hip flexion, knee extension and ankle dorsiflexion and assign a 1-to 5- muscle grade.

Asymmetrical weakness, particularly in the peroneal or ulnar nerve distributions, should prompt consideration of compressive neuropathy, which is also common in the ICU patient population.[221] Respiratory muscles are also affected, and likely contribute to prolonged weaning from mechanical ventilation, based on studies which compared duration of mechanical ventilation between patients with and without CINM.[222-224]

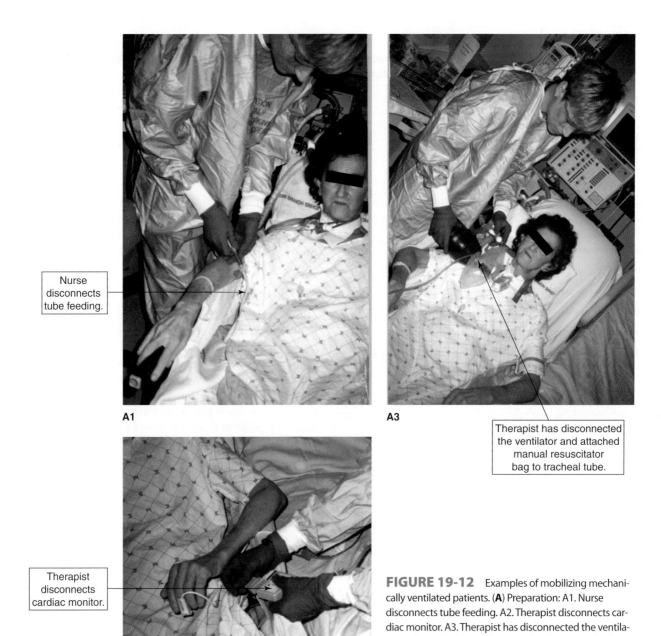

Nurse disconnects tube feeding.

A1

Therapist disconnects cardiac monitor.

A2

Therapist has disconnected the ventilator and attached manual resuscitator bag to tracheal tube.

A3

FIGURE 19-12 Examples of mobilizing mechanically ventilated patients. (**A**) Preparation: A1. Nurse disconnects tube feeding. A2. Therapist disconnects cardiac monitor. A3. Therapist has disconnected the ventilator and attached manual resuscitator bag to tracheal tube. *(continued)*

In clinical practice, diagnosis is typically made based on suggestive presentation, in the presence of known risk factors. Electroneuromyogram testing and neuroimaging may be used to confirm or rule out the CINM in the presence of other possible diagnoses.[220] Electroneuromyogram testing typically shows a reduced compound muscle action potential with normal conduction velocity, and spontaneous electrical activity on muscle needle recording.[220] To date, the only established preventative measure for CINM is intensive insulin control to prevent hyperglycemia. Intensive insulin therapy has been shown to decrease the incidence of CINM, and reduce prolonged mechanical ventilation in medical ICU patients.[216] An increasing attention to minimizing the use of sedation and analgesia in the ICU setting, while not initiated with this goal in mind, may aid in earlier diagnosis of CINM. Decreased use of sedation also has the potential to reduce drug-induced immobility. The value of early exercise and mobility in treating

CINM has yet to be established, although these interventions are safe for patients with respiratory failure.[2,4,6]

Disconnecting the patient from the ventilator and ambulating the patient using a manual resuscitator bag (MRB), or ambulation using a portable ventilator (many of the ventilators found in standard use in the ICU have this capability) are also recommended for difficult-to-wean patients (Fig. 19-12). If a patient is unable to ambulate due to injury or disease affecting the lower extremity, yet is having difficulty being weaned from the ventilator, the therapist can use an MRB or portable ventilator to assist with ventilation while the patient is trained in wheelchair transfers and propulsion. Research regarding this type of early intervention including mobilization and exercise in the ICU patient population is extremely limited. In a study of 103 patients admitted to a respiratory ICU, Bailey and colleagues demonstrated that early activity including transfers and ambulation was both safe and feasible, with a less than 1%

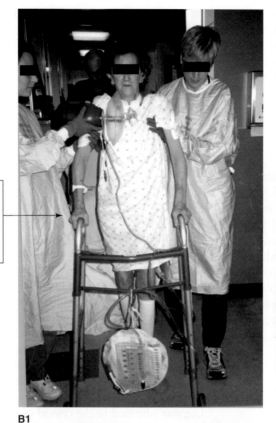

Nurse ventilating patient during ambulation (this can also be done by a second physical therapist).

B1

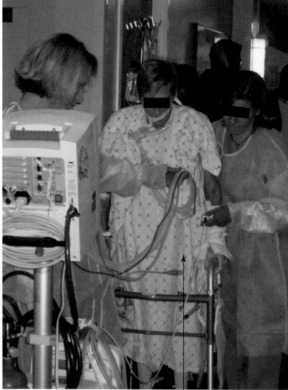

COPD patient ambulating while ventilated with a portable ventilator.

B2

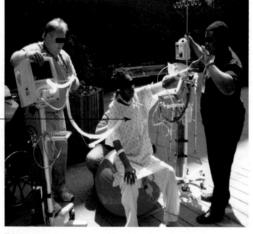

Patient receiving balancing activities as part of his physical therapy treatment while outdoors and on a portable ventilator.

B3

FIGURE 19-12 *(Continued)* (**B**) Mobility: B1. Nurse ventilating patient during ambulation (this can also be done by a second physical therapist). B2. COPD patient ambulating while ventilated with a portable ventilator. (Photo courtesy of Dale Needham, MD, PhD) B3. Patient receiving balancing activities as part of his physical therapy treatment while outdoors and on a portable ventilator. Pressure support ventilation 12, PEEP 5 cm H_2O, FiO_2 40%, Respiratory rate 20, tidal volume 438 ml, Fio_2 was increased by 20 % for patient mobilization. (Courtesy of Janette Scardillo, DPT)

adverse event rate. Additionally, 69% of their patients were able to ambulate >100 feet at the time of discharge from the RICU.[6]

Integumentary

The details of integumentary complications are discussed in Chapter 13. Rotating beds, bariatric beds, low-air-loss beds, air-fluidized beds, and mattresses that inflate at specified times to turn the patient 20 to 30 degrees to either side all assist in relieving capillary pressure on the skin to prevent pressure sores. Placing a patient in a bed that minimizes skin capillary pressure may prevent a pressure sore but does not prevent the other cardiopulmonary, musculoskeletal, and neurological hazards of immobility. Therapists should learn how to operate these beds and utilize any features that will assist

with mobility such as deflating the mattress to achieve a firm surface for bed mobility and transfer activities.

When a patient is in a specialty bed, part of the therapists' assessment should include whether the bed is optimal for patient mobility and pulmonary care. If it is suspected that a standard bed will enhance mobility and pulmonary care, this information should be relayed to the medical and nursing staff as a recommendation to change the bed. Newer standard beds allow mechanically ventilated patients to be positioned in the sitting position and begin sitting balance and standing activities without transferring to a chair.

In summary, patients who are mechanically ventilated and subsequently immobile benefit from the same interventions of cognitive orientation, positioning, therapeutic exercise, functional mobility, splinting, and serial casting as the patient who is not in respiratory failure. The same orthopedic precautions are followed regardless of whether the patient is mechanically ventilated. Special attention is paid to joints adjacent to intravascular lines and cervical ROM that may be limited because of bulky ventilator tubing.

Summary of Potential Risks Associated with Mechanical Ventilation

One may wonder why patients are intubated and mechanically ventilated after reviewing all of the associated risks. However, it is important to remember that the primary clinical concern is to provide adequate oxygenation for recovery from the underlying cause of respiratory failure. Given the inevitability of having patients who require mechanical ventilation, clear understanding of the potential risks will aid in their prevention. Therapists working with mechanically ventilated patients should always be cautious and aware of the modes and complications of mechanical ventilation. This will enable them to appropriately perform secretion clearance techniques and mobilize patients despite minute-by-minute changes in ventilatory and hemodynamic status.

CASE STUDY

Patient with C5 Tetraplegia

The intent of this case example is to familiarize the physical therapist with the medical, and physical therapy interventions pertinent to treating an ICU patient with tetraplegia. This multitrauma patient sustained a spinal cord injury following a motor vehicle collision (MVC). The patient fits the following inclusion criteria for Practice Pattern 6F. The patient has acute neuromuscular dysfunction, abnormal alveolar-arterial oxygen tension, and multisystem trauma. The patient also has adventitious breath sounds, abnormal vital capacity, elevated respiratory rate, dyspnea at rest and dyssynchronous (paradoxical) breathing patterns (without mechanical ventilation), and impaired gas exchange (Fig. 19-1).

The case presented is a 38-year-old Caucasian postal worker named Lee who sustained a C4-5 fracture dislocation in a motor vehicle crash, resulting in C5 motor complete tetraplegia. The case presentation follows the *Guide to Physical Therapist Practice* as applicable to the utilization of physical therapy in an ICU/trauma center. This case study is written as a physical therapist would realistically collect relevant data from the medical record, examine the patient, evaluate data, and determine a prognosis and intervention strategy within 24 hours of the patient's admission. Intervention strategies are modified as the patient's clinical condition changes. For the ICU patient the medical status can change hourly. Therefore, the physical therapist must continually modify the treatment plan and intervention strategies based on the patient's examination at each treatment session.

Initial Examination

When entering the ICU to examine a patient, the physical therapist must efficiently extract the most pertinent and relevant

information from the medical record and team members. It is most important to obtain general demographic information, a detailed history of the patient's current condition, medications pertinent to physical therapy interventions, a pertinent past medical history including social habits, and the patient's functional status at the time of the initial examination. Some centers utilize a paper form or computerized database to assure consistency of data collection at the initial and subsequent visits. Details regarding social history, employment, growth and development, living environments, family history, and the patient's general health status are frequently not available at the time of the first visit. This information can be obtained later in the hospitalization through discussion with team members and the patient's family, friends, and/or a significant other. Patients who are intubated have difficulty communicating and may be receiving medications or have injuries that make it difficult and sometimes impossible to obtain a complete history. Augmentative communication devices may be recommended by a speech–language pathologist, which enhance the physical therapist's ability to communicate with the patient. The patient history (Table 19-14) was obtained within Lee's first 10 days of hospitalization after attending rounds; meeting with the family in a family conference; reviewing the medical record daily prior to each visit; and speaking with the patient's nurse, physician, social worker, and occupational therapist.

Lee was admitted to the critical care unit 12 hours after reaching the trauma center. The physical therapy service had standing orders to evaluate and treat any patient admitted with suspected or diagnosed spinal cord injury. The physical therapist provided an initial examination 18 hours after the patient's hospital admission.

A chest radiograph was taken when Lee was admitted to the ICU. The report noted right rib fractures, clear lung fields, correct placement of the pulmonary artery catheter in the pulmonary artery, and the presence of electrocardiogram electrodes. Chest tubes and a feeding tube that passed through the stomach to the small intestine were also seen in proper position on the chest and abdominal radiographs. It was too early for an infiltrate from a pulmonary contusion to appear on the chest film.

Tests and Measures

Upon entering Lee's cubicle, the therapist noted that the patient was connected to numerous lines and tubes and mechanically ventilated via a tracheostomy tube. Table 19-15 shows the ventilator settings and arterial blood gas results. Humidification was delivered through a heated humidifier (Fig. 19-6A). The therapist also noted that the patient had a pulmonary artery catheter to measure central venous and pulmonary artery pressures. Pulmonary artery (PA) catheters can be inserted through the jugular, subclavian, brachial, or femoral veins. This patient's PA line was inserted through the subclavian vein, the most common insertion site. Figure 19-13 shows a quadruple lumen PA line and the waveforms associated with the line passing though the different chambers of the heart and into the pulmonary artery. The normal values for pulmonary artery pressures and other monitoring devices are noted in Table 19-16. Lee had chest leads connected to the cardiac monitor with a

TABLE 19-14 Lee's Patient History

General demographics	38-year-old Caucasian male Married × 16 y no children
Social history	Likes to travel Two sisters will take patient home following rehabilitation Resources available to modify apartment and acquire environmental control devices
Employment/work (job/school/play)	Postal worker × 15 y Prior to admission physically fit, independent in all ADL High school varsity wrestler
Growth and development	Right-hand dominant Nonsignificant developmental history
Living environment	Fourth floor apartment Elevator access Would like to return to work following rehabilitation
General health status	Excellent prior to admission
Social/health habits	No smoking history No alcohol history Occasional marijuana
Family history	Nonsignificant
Medical/surgical history	Left proximal humeral fracture 2 years ago, open reduction internal fixation, physical therapy × 4 wk, ROM WNL MVC, front-seat passenger with shoulder strap, No air bags, hit head-on by a tractor trailer truck Bronchitis × past 3 winters
Condition at scene	Conscious, lethargic EMS arrival: respiratory rate: 18 breaths/min Witnessed unconscious at scene Extrication: 20 min Med-evaced to trauma center Extremity motor and sensory function: not obtained, 2 IVs, LLE traction splint applied
Initial paramedic treatment	Patient placed on backboard Oxygen 15 L/min, nonrebreather face mask Spontaneous RR 40 bpm, rapid and shallow LOC
Trauma center admission	Suspected CHI Pulmonary secretions bloody—possible lung contusion Subcutaneous emphysema right anterior chest Edematous left thigh GCS 8/15 (eye 3, verbal 4, motor 1) Neurological examination C5 motor complete ABG's high flow aerosol mask at 10 L/min Pao_2 50 mm Hg, Ph 7.5, $Paco_2$ 30 mm Hg Hct 35%
Clinical tests	Chest radiograph—fx rib R 4–10, R pneumothorax, L hemothorax (R apical and L basilar chest tubes inserted and placed on wall suction) Cervical spine radiograph—Fx dislocation C4/C5 CAT scan—liver lac, ? cerebral contusion, L leg radiograph—midshaft L femur fracture
Admission medical/surgical interventions	Operative repair of liver lacerations Open reduction internal fixation of L midshaft femur fx by orthopedics Tracheostomy, mechanical ventilation initiated Blood and fluid resuscitation Neurosurgical stabilization of spinal fracture, patient placed on a turning frame with traction—Halo vest later applied
Functional status and activity level	Mechanically ventilated on bed rest dependent in all activities of daily living
Medications	Dulcolax suppository Pericolase Heparin Tylenol Morphine Levophed

ADL, activities of daily living; EMS, emergency medical system; IV, intravascular line; LLE, left lower extremity; CHI, closed head injury; L, left; MVC, motor vehicle collision.

TABLE 19-15 **Ventilator Settings and Arterial Blood Gas Measurements**

Ventilator settings	
Oxygenation	Fio_2 .50
	PEEP 8 cmH_2O pressure
Ventilation—	
Pressure Control Mode	35 cmH_2O pressure
Work of Breathing—minimal	Respiratory rate set by ventilator— 20 breaths/min
Arterial blood gases	
Pao_2	95 torr
$Paco_2$	35 torr
Ph	7.46
Spo_2	97%

continuous readout of heart rate and rhythm, a pulse oximeter probe on the right index finger, a peripheral IV for fluid administration, and a catheter inserted in the bladder to facilitate and monitor urine output. The patient's blood pressure was monitored through a peripheral radial arterial line.

Arterial pressure monitoring via an indwelling peripheral catheter (arterial line) is the most common mode of invasive hemodynamic monitoring. It is used to draw blood samples, and to monitor arterial blood pressure when rapid fluctuations are expected. The radial artery is the most common site for placement of a peripheral artery catheter. Radial arterial lines have the least discomfort and do not require total joint immobilization. They are associated with a low risk of ischemic injury to the hand, as there is usually adequate collateral circulation through the ulnar artery. Other sites for monitoring arterial pressures include the dorsalis pedis, femoral, and brachial arteries. The femoral artery is the preferred site for emergency cannulation and is easily catheterized with a low risk of thrombosis. Care should be taken not to dislodge an arterial line, and not to kink or disconnect the tubing. The transducer is positioned at the level of the right atrium when blood pressure measurements are taken.

The patient also had an oral feeding tube that passed through the stomach and terminated in the small intestine, an incision on the left proximal lateral thigh from insertion of an intramedullary rod to stabilize the femur fracture, and an abdominal incision from the surgical repair of liver lacerations. The patient was wearing sequential pneumatic compression devices for prevention of venous thromboembolism. Skin was intact. There was some bruising on the anterior chest from the seatbelt.

The therapist completed a neurological assessment of the patient's level of function at the initial visit. Lee's Glasgow Coma Scale was 11T (eye 4, motor 6, verbal 1T) and he was following simple commands (Table 19-17). "T" indicates that the patient was intubated and could not speak. Richmond agitation scale was 0 and CAM-ICU was administered by having the patient stick out his tongue as he did not have adequate hand function to use hand gestures. It was determined that Lee was not delirious at this time and would most likely be able to participate in the initial physical therapy examination. Lee luckily did not have a severe brain injury and therefore did not require intracranial pressure monitoring. However, concomitant brain injury with cervical spine injury is as high as 60%, 43% of these patients having severe brain injuries.[225] Had he sustained a severe brain injury in addition to his other injuries, he would most likely have had an intracranial pressure monitor inserted. Intracranial pressure monitoring alone is not a contraindication to physical therapy. Severe brain injury increases the risk of contractures, pulmonary infection, and hypoxemia and is therefore a strong indicator for physical therapy interventions. The therapist is responsible for monitoring the intracranial pressure and cerebral perfusion pressure during physical therapy interventions following institutional guidelines (see Table 19-16).

The therapist evaluated the patient's range of motion (ROM) (Table 19-17). Passive ROM in both lower extremities (LEs) was WNL except for some limitations in left hip and knee motions. Because of early fracture fixation, complete assessment of the left hip and knee was possible after consulting with the orthopedic surgeon. ROM was within normal limits in both upper extremities, and no pain was noted with any ROM exercises. The spine had been stabilized with the

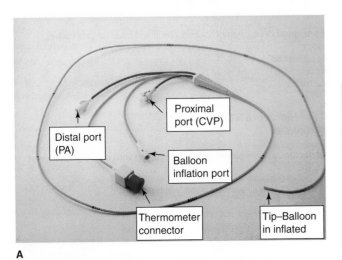

A

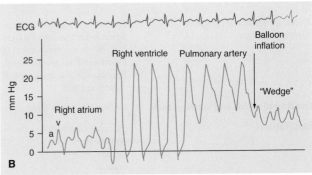

B

FIGURE 19-13 (**A**) Pulmonary artery line. (**B**) Waveforms seen on cardiac monitor as a pulmonary artery catheter passes through the chambers of the heart.

TABLE 19-16   Lines, Tubes, and Catheters: Summary of Precautions and Physical Therapy Implications

Device	Precautions	Physical Therapy Implications
Tracheal tube	If the therapist suspects the endotracheal tube is malpositioned (ie, cannulation of the right mainstem bronchus) this should be discussed with the nurse or physician prior to physical therapy interventions. Assure cuff is inflated during mechanical ventilation, when using a manual resuscitator bag, and during suctioning. Orotracheal and endotracheal tubes should be secured; tracheostomy tubes are secured by tying the string around the neck—avoid tension on carotid and jugular vessels.	Usually does not interfere with physical therapy interventions. Endotracheal tubes cannulating the right mainstem bronchus should be pulled back and placement confirmed radiologically prior to physical therapy interventions. Cervical ROM[a] exercises should be performed cautiously
Fenestrated	Insert inner cannula prior to mechanical ventilation, bagging, and suctioning. Never inflate cuff with fenestration occluded and tube plugged.	Same as tracheal tubes.
Chest tube	Avoid tipping drainage container; kinking and tension on tubes. Check for any new or increased air leaks prior to, during, or after physical therapy interventions. Maintain drainage collection container below level of insertion, prevent backflow of drainage into chest cavity.	Pneumothorax—consult with physician prior to discontinuing suction. May ambulate with portable suction or extended tubing. Hemothorax—usually can discontinue suction for mobility after consulting with physician. Shoulder ROM exercises, manual percussion and vibration to patient tolerance. Usually does not limit prone positioning.

Device	Normal Value	Precautions	Physical Therapy Implications
Pulse oximeter	$SpO_2 > 97\%$	Avoid motion artifact. Low values—nail polish, low tissue perfusion, vasoconstriction, improper probe placement. High values—heavy skin pigmentation, anemia. Doesn't differentiate oxyhemoglobin from carboxyhemoglobin, methemoglobin.	Move probe to another digit, extremity, or ear to verify low values. Warm cool extremities. Administer supplemental oxygen if $SpO_2 < 90\%$ or decline from baseline >5% when baseline is in the 80s. Notify nurse or physician per institutional guidelines. With normal oxyhemoglobin dissociation curve SpO_2 90% approximates PaO_2 60 mm Hg.
Hemodynamic monitoring devices general considerations		Assure lines are sutured in place; equipment is calibrated and transducer is at the level of the right atrium. Assure normal waveform prior to interpreting values. Notify nurse if air bubbles or blood are noted in the line. Avoid kinking or dislodging lines.	Patient movement and electrical interference may compromise the waveform.
Peripheral arterial	Systolic 100–130 mm Hg End diastolic 60–90 mm Hg Mean 70–90 mm Hg		Interferes little with physical therapy treatment. Move transducer to IV pole if not disconnected prior to ambulation. Femoral lines—observe waveform while exercising hip or when patient is sitting out of bed. Avoid severe hip flexion. Note changes in blood pressure from baseline.

(continued)

TABLE 19-16   Lines, Tubes, and Catheters: Summary of Precautions and Physical Therapy Implications *(Continued)*

Device	Normal Value	Precautions	Physical Therapy Implications
Central venous pressure	Mean 0–8 mm Hg	Waveform fluctuates with respiration.	Cautious range of motion to joints near insertion. For subclavian insertion may need to use towel rolls to avoid kinking of the catheter when turning patient to side or prone.
Pulmonary artery	Systolic 15–21 mm Hg End diastolic 4–13 mm Hg Mean 9–19 mm Hg		Same as central venous pressure.
Pulmonary artery wedge pressure	4–12 mm Hg	Waveform noting catheter in the wedged position.	Physical therapy is contraindicated if catheter is in the wedged position—Notify nurse or physician who will deflate the balloon and pull catheter back, then proceed with treatment.
ICP Monitors *Epidural Subdural/ subarachnoid Intraparenchymal*	ICP = 0–15 mm Hg at rest with head of bed elevated Cerebral perfusion pressure (CPP) = driving pressure of blood to the brain. Normal > 60 mm Hg	Assure proper waveform prior to interpreting values. CPP < 40 mm Hg—unable to sustain brain function. Increase in ICP to 20–25 mm Hg may result in decompensation and secondary brain injury from tissue compression, decreased cerebral blood flow, and decreased tissue perfusion. Intervention will be dictated by relationship of ICP to mean arterial blood pressure (within institutional guidelines).	May use to calculate CPP = MABP—ICP. Some institutions use CPP > 55 mm Hg for patients with craniectomies and > 60 mm Hg for other brain injury patients and ICP < 25 mm Hg for secretion removal techniques, including head-down positioning. Head-down positioning may be limited to 15 minutes at a time. Monitor waveform and pressure throughout intervention.
ICP Monitors Intraventricular	ICP = 0–15 mm Hg at rest with head of bed elevated. Most accurate monitoring device, highest risk of infection.	Same as ICP. Cerebral spinal fluid may be drained continuously or intermittently as prescribed by the physician.	Same as ICP. Note status of the drainage system. Accurate ICP measurements are only obtained when the system is turned off to drainage. Request nurse to close drainage system unless otherwise ordered by the physician. Consistency in the level of the drainage system is necessary for accurate interpretation of pressure readings.

[a]Key: ROM, range of motion; Spo$_2$, saturation of arterial oxygen by pulse oximetry; Pao$_2$, partial pressure of arterial oxygen; ICP, intracranial pressure; CPP, cerebral perfusion pressure.

Adapted from Ciesla N, Murdock K. Lines, tubes, catheters, and physiologic monitoring in the ICU. *Cardiopulm Phys Ther.* 1999;11:16-25. Darovic GO. *Hemodynamic Monitoring: Invasive and Noninvasive Clinical Application.* 2nd ed. Philadelphia, PA: WB Saunders; 1995:165-167, 253-274. *Manual of Bedside Monitoring.* Springhouse, PA: Springhouse Corporation; 1994:76, 95-111.

Halo vest, and therefore there were no restrictions to assessing shoulder strength and providing shoulder ROM exercises to the patient's tolerance.

The therapist then auscultated the patient's chest and noted upper-airway secretions (rhonchi). Lee was unable to effectively cough or mobilize his secretions, so the therapist suctioned the patient through the tracheostomy tube with a 14 French suction catheter (the patient had a size 9 tracheostomy tube) and reexamined the chest. Decreased breath sounds were noted over the right lower lobe (adventitious breath sounds may precede a change in chest radiograph). While pal-pating the right anterior thorax, the therapist also noticed that the patient had subcutaneous emphysema. The therapist checked the chest tubes for an air leak (there was none) and discussed this finding with the nurse. The nurse reported that both chest tubes had been functioning to this point without an air leak. The nurse and therapist checked the patient's airway pressures on the ventilator. They had not changed within the last few hours. After discussion and assessment, the therapist determined that the subcutaneous emphysema was likely residual from his admission pneumothorax, as resolution can sometimes take hours to several days.

TABLE 19-17 Lee's Physical Therapy Initial and Discharge Examinations

	Initial Examination *(18 h Following Admission)*	Discharge Examination (Day 17)
Monitoring **Hemodynamic**	BP 100/75 Sao$_2$ 97% (pressure control mechanical ventilation 50% Fio$_2$)	110/80 99% (spontaneous breathing, trach collar 40% Fio$_2$)
Cardiac	Electrocardiogram Normal sinus rhythm 100 bpm	Electrocardiogram Normal sinus rhythm 70 bpm
Glasgow Coma Scale	11 T/15 (eye 4, motor 6, verbal 1T)	11T/15
RAAS	0	Negative
CAM — ICU	Negative for dementia (although fluctuated throughout hospital course with changes in medical status)	
Breath sounds	Rhonchi, decreased RLL following suctioning	Vesicular after cough-assistive techniques
Range of motion (degrees) (involved joints) Left hip		
Flexion	70	100
Extension	−15	5
Abduction	5	35
Adduction	10	20
Internal rotation	0	30
Left knee		
Flexion	85	130
Extension	−20	0
Straight-leg raises		
Right	100	110
Left	70	95
Neurological examination	ASIA C5 complete	Unchanged
Functional mobility	On bed rest Dependent in all activities, unable to assume upright position	Sitting out of bed BID—90 minutes Assisting nurse/therapist with abdominal pressure for cough assistive techniques Side to side rolling—moderate assistance Sitting balance—10 min with BUE support

Evaluation

Following the examination, the therapist determined that Lee was at high risk for additional pulmonary complications and musculoskeletal impairments due to his injury. Table 19-18 outlines the physical therapy tests and measures that were appropriate to administer during this patient's hospital stay. The examination at each physical therapy visit determined which test was administered. Table 19-19 outlines the critical components of a physical therapy examination and evaluation for the mechanically ventilated patient.

Diagnosis

The therapist determined that Lee had impairments in airway clearance, ROM, muscle strength, sensation, and mobility that would benefit from physical therapy interventions.

Prognosis

The therapist estimated Lee's prognosis and outcome at the initial visit. The therapist expected the patient would leave the trauma center and enter a spinal cord injury rehabilitation center within 10 to 15 days, timing dependent upon the patient's medical complications such as developing an infection, DVT, PE or skin breakdown. The patient would be spontaneously breathing through a tracheostomy tube while receiving supplemental oxygen and have functional passive range of motion of all four extremities. The patient would also have an understanding of how to assist himself with deep breathing and coughing exercises and instruct a caretaker in pressure relief. It was anticipated that the patient would tolerate sitting on the edge of the bed with moderate assistance of one individual and sitting in a wheelchair with the legs dependent for 2 to 4 hours per day. It was hoped that the patient would not develop any skin breakdown or thromboemboli.

Physical Therapy Interventions During Mechanical Ventilation

The first physical therapy priority was to clear Lee's airway secretions, as a right lower lobe atelectasis due to secretion retention was suspected. The therapist and nurse positioned the patient in the left side-lying position, one-fourth turn from prone. They noted that there was no excessive drainage from

TABLE 19-18   **Lee's Physical Therapy Tests and Measures**

Aerobic capacity and endurance	Review ventilator settings and flowsheets. Determine mode and parameters of mechanical ventilation. Note number of spontaneous and ventilator-assisted breaths at baseline, during and following interventions. Monitor standard vital signs (heart rate and blood pressure) at baseline, during, and following interventions. Monitor oxygen saturation. Auscultate the lungs.
Anthropometric characteristics	Note subcutaneous emphysema, crackling from rib fractures. Note and report any increased extremity girth measurements.
Arousal, attention, and cognition	Assess level of consciousness, agitation, and delerium during each examination and intervention. Assess orientation to time, person, place, and situation (using eye blinking).
Assistive and adaptive devices	Handsplints, abdominal binder, footsplints (when ROM exercises and bed positioning do not maintain ankle dorsiflexion).
Cranial nerve integrity	Review neurosurgical assessment, determine whether physical therapy cranial nerve assessment is indicated.
Gait, locomotion, and balance	Assess static and dynamic sitting balance on edge of bed and in wheelchair, with upper extremity support. Note number of health care providers necessary to assist patient with balance in supported and unsupported sitting postures and transfers.
Integumentary integrity	Assess skin integrity at each visit while turning patient for each postural drainage or mobility intervention—particularly bony prominences, the back of the head, areas where brace touches skin, heels. Inspect skin each time binder, splints, and elastic stockings are donned and doffed.
Orthotic, protective, and supportive devices	Assess alignment, fit, and movement while patient wears the resting hand splints and abdominal binder.
Pain	Assess pain using a 1–10 Visual Analog Scale (note and rate pain at rest or during activity). Note changes on pain scale resulting from interventions.
Posture	Assess resting posture in wheelchair and static and dynamic postures while sitting on the edge of the bed with assistance.
Range of motion	Assess functional ROM and joint passive movements using a goniometer. Note hamstring length, and measure straight leg raises.
Muscle strength and sensation	Determine neurological level using ASIA standards of neurological classification.

either chest tube. There was also no air bubbling in the waterseal chamber of either chest tube, so it was unlikely that the patient had developed a bronchopleural fistula. The therapist and nurse monitored the patient's vital signs, lines, and tubes and positioned the bed in the head-down position. Aspiration was less of a concern, because the feeding tube passed through the stomach and extended to the small intestine; however, the tube feeding was turned off prior to head-down positioning. The uppermost lateral strap of the vest was opened and taped to the bedrails to allow the therapist access to the patient's chest for percussion and vibration. The therapist noted and marked which hole in the strap was used to secure the vest. The therapist manually percussed the right lateral chest below the axilla and posterior chest wall from thoracic vertebrae T3 to T10 (Fig. 19-14). Although the patient had right rib fractures, which were noted as a precaution, it was necessary to administer manual techniques to assist in secretion clearance on the right side because the patient could not be mobilized or cough sufficiently to clear retained pulmonary secretions. It should be noted that manual percussion may be performed judiciously over rib fractures without any known complications. When properly performed, there is no

known increased risk in the development of extrapleural hematomas, hemo- and/or pneumothorax.[226,227] Properly performed, percussion should cause less pressure over the thorax and ribs than coughing or lying on the involved side. A gentle form of vibration is used over rib fractures by some physical therapists.

After 10 minutes of percussion to the right lower lobe, the therapist noted crackles with auscultation, which was indicative of secretions loosened in the small airways. The therapist suctioned the trachea. A cough was stimulated with the suction catheter, but no secretions were suctioned. This is most likely because the secretions remained in the lower airways as the cough was ineffective, and secretions were unable to be suctioned into the suction catheter that most likely was at the carina (level of the second rib), or upper level of the right mainstem bronchus. The therapist continued with percussion over the right lower lobe for another 10 minutes. Subsequent auscultation of breath sounds revealed diffuse rhonchi and the patient was suctioned again. After three passes of the suction catheter 5 cc of bloody sputum was obtained. Bloody secretions are to be expected after a lung contusion. Upon auscultation, the therapist noted the breath

TABLE 19-19   **Mechanically Ventilated and Monitored Patient Components of Physical Therapist Examination and Evaluation During Physical Therapy Sessions**[a]

Initial screening of level of conscious (GCS, RASS, CAM–ICU as indicated)
Arterial oxygen saturation via pulse oximeter (SpO$_2$)
Recent arterial blood gases
Blood pressure—note waveform on bedside monitor
Heart rate and EKG—note waveform on bedside monitor
Mode of ventilation
   Volume controlled, PRVC, assist control, SIMV, pressure support, pressure control, APRV, CPAP
   Other _____
Fraction of inspired oxygen concentration (FiO$_2$)
Positive end-expiratory pressure (PEEP)
Tidal volume or minute ventilation (Inhaled and exhaled volumes)
Rate and depth of respiration (Ventilator vs patient's spontaneous breaths)
Airway pressures
Most recent chest X-ray report and/or view chest X-ray
Breath sounds
Sputum quantity and color, viscosity
Pain/discomfort associated with interventions
Integumentary inspection
Significant change in joint tightness/stiffness or patient's level of mobility

[a]Significant changes are noted in the medical record.

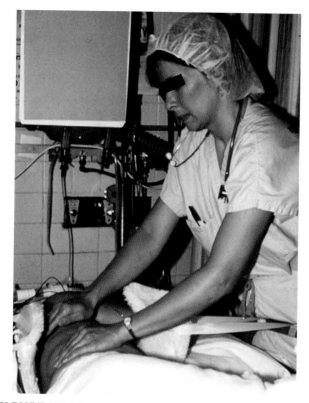

FIGURE 19-14   Physical therapist performing chest physical therapy to the right lower lobe of a patient with tetraplegia.

sounds had improved; there was increased air entry in the right lung base with some crackles. The therapist continued the treatment for 15 minutes with percussion, vibration, and suctioning after which vesicular or normal breath sounds were heard. The therapist closed the vest, placed the bed flat, and with the nurse turned the patient to the supine position. The therapist once again auscultated the chest and discovered that the breath sounds were normal in all lung zones, indicating that transbronchial aspiration of secretions was unlikely. It was therefore not necessary to turn the patient and treat the lung lobes and segments that were dependent during this portion of the treatment.

While Lee was supine, the therapist performed passive ROM exercises to both lower extremities with emphasis on straight-leg raises, ankle dorsiflexion, and the limited motion in the left hip and knee. The therapist was cautious while performing ROM exercises to the left hip and knee. Because of the patient's neurological injury, he was unable to perceive pain in the lower extremities. The therapist was cautious not to overstretch the lumbosacral musculature that would impair the patient's stability in sitting as he progressed through rehabilitation. To stretch the hamstrings, the therapist extended the knee while the hip was flexed to 90 degrees. The patient became exhausted and did not participate in any active or active-assistive ROM exercises of the innervated upper extremity muscles; therefore, passive ROM exercises were given. Emphasis was placed on achieving full wrist extension with elbow extension and shoulder external rotation to facilitate sitting at the edge of the bed. Care was taken

not to stretch the finger flexors during wrist extension to allow a tenodesis grip to develop, given the level of Lee's injury. Finger flexors were only stretched with the wrist in a neutral position. The therapist documented the physical therapy examination and interventions in the medical record. It was noted that the patient's vital signs were stable during each intervention and that breath sounds improved over the right lower lobe; 5 cc of blood-tinged secretions was suctioned, and the patient tolerated 65 minutes of physical therapy examination and treatment.

The therapist returned in the afternoon for a second assessment of the need for airway clearance techniques. Upon auscultation, the therapist noted that the patient had crackles over the lingula (comparable to the right middle lobe). Treatment was given as in the morning in the postural drainage position for the lingula: Lee was positioned one-fourth turn to the right in the head-down position. The vest was opened again after Lee was placed and stabilized in the head-down position, and closed prior to moving him. The therapist added vibration to the patient's tolerance. There were no documented rib fractures on the left side; therefore, vibration was added to mobilize secretions in the larger bronchi. During bronchoscopy, vibration has been shown to mobilize secretions into the upper airway, which in theory will decrease the duration of postural drainage.[228] A moderate quantity of clear secretions were suctioned. (Precise measurements of sputum volume are obtained only when a sputum trap is attached to the suction catheter.)

TABLE 19-20   Lee's Physical Therapy Interventions

Coordination, communication, documentation	Referrals to occupational therapy and speech–language pathology Attend patient care rounds Communication and coordination of care with health care team members, family Discharge planning

Patient/client/nursing staff-related instruction	Demonstrate proper positioning for opening the vest, postural drainage and
	    pressure relief, passive ROM exercises, sitting in high-back wheelchair
	Take digital photographs of binder and compression stocking placement, seating
	    and side-lying positioning and display at bedside for family and staff

Airway clearance techniques	Manual chest percussion Manual chest vibration Segmental postural drainage positioning Assistive cough techniques Tracheal suctioning
Therapeutic exercise	Diaphragmatic weight training Inspiratory muscle training Pectoralis and serratus anterior strengthening Active, active-assistive and resistive ROM exercises Hamstring stretching—avoid stretching low back Balance training
Prescription, application, and fabrication of devices and equipment	Resting hand splints Abdominal binder Lower extremity compression wraps Air splints or knee immobilizers Reclining high-back wheelchair with elevating leg rests Foot splints not required if full PROM maintained
Manual therapy techniques	Passive range of motion

The therapist continued the same treatment regimen for the next 2 days. During each treatment session the therapist noted the patient's breath sounds and determined which lung/lobes or segments required intervention. Table 19-20 lists the treatment interventions that were administered throughout the patient's hospital stay. Active, active-assistive, and passive ROM exercises were carried out to patient tolerance. The nursing staff supplemented physical therapy sessions with PROM exercises. Hip and shoulder extension exercises were administered in the side-lying position. Shoulder extension, shoulder external rotation, elbow extension, and wrist extension exercises with the fingers in a position of tenodesis were emphasized to enhance sitting balance. Strengthening of the pectoralis muscles was added and emphasized to further assist the patient with coughing.[140] Strengthening of serratus anterior was also included, to promote scapular stability, and facilitate functional use of the upper extremity. Occupational therapy made resting hand splints for the patient. The patient maintained ankle dorsiflexion with passive ROM exercises, had no increased plantarflexor muscle tone. Therefore, it was decided that ankle splints were not indicated.

The fourth day following admission, secretion clearance and early rehabilitative interventions continued as previously described. The therapist noted that the humidifier had been changed to a heat and moisture exchanger. Secretions were viscid and dry with suctioning. The therapist spoke with the physician and respiratory therapist, the heated humidifier was placed back on the ventilator, and the HME was removed. The physi-

cian also decided to increase the patient's fluid intake through the IV. Secretions were noted to be less viscid during suctioning throughout the day.

In addition, the therapist and nurse decided to transfer Lee from bed to chair, as the standing orders included progressing the patient's activity as tolerated. The patient's respiratory status had improved and he was no longer on pressure-controlled ventilation. However, pressure-controlled ventilation is not a contraindication for getting patients out of bed. Lee was on an SIMV of 12 breaths/min, pressure support of 15 cm H_2O pressure, $FiO_2 = 0.45$, and remained on a PEEP of 8 cm H_2O pressure. He was taking 10 spontaneous breaths per minute and therefore had a respiratory rate of 22 breaths/min. An abdominal binder was applied to aide in venous return and improve the biomechanics of breathing. The IPCs were removed from the patient's legs, and groin high compression stockings were applied to enhance venous return. The therapist examined the monitor and noted that the patient's blood pressure was 100/60 mm Hg while supine, and the heart rate was 90 bpm with a regular rhythm. The head of the bed was elevated 30 degrees for 15 minutes, and the patient's blood pressure was noted to be 110/95 mm Hg. The head of the bed was raised to 70 degrees, and the patient became diaphoretic, with a spontaneous respiratory rate of 21 breaths/min, and when questioned, he confirmed feeling dizzy. At this time, the patient's blood pressure was 80/60 mm Hg and the heart rate was 120 bpm. The patient's head was lowered to 50 degrees. Lee no longer felt dizzy and the blood pressure had returned to baseline. Because of the increase in heart rate, decrease in blood pressure, and the patient's complaints of dizziness the nurse increased his vasopressors (often used in the first 7 days to maintain mean arterial pressure and promote spinal cord perfusion), which allowed him to sit upright in bed and transfer out of bed that day. Because of numerous monitoring and therapeutic lines as well as to the patient's inability to assist, three caregivers were needed to transfer Lee out of bed. Each caregiver was careful not to dislodge the IV or any of the central monitoring lines. The ventilator was disconnected from the tracheostomy tube during the transfer and reconnected as soon as the patient was in the wheelchair. The patient sat out of bed for 30 minutes with pressure relief every 15 minutes. The hips were flexed to 90 degrees, and the leg rests were kept elevated to aide in venous return. Two pictures were taken and placed at the patient's bedside for the nursing staff. One picture showed the patient sitting in the high-back wheelchair, the other demonstrated the staff providing pressure relief. The nursing staff began getting the patient out of bed daily using the photographs to assure continuity in positioning, and inspecting the skin after each sitting intervention.

In a situation where the nurse does not have the ability to immediately titrate vasopressors the therapist would develop a plan with the nurse to monitor blood pressure and gradually increase the patient's sitting position in bed at least two times daily, time permitting. The nurse would inspect the skin and document the time the patient tolerated sitting up in bed with each session. Once the patient could tolerate sitting up in bed for 30 minutes transfers out of bed would be initiated.

Over the next 48 hours, Lee's physical therapy interventions included secretion removal techniques, active and active-assistive ROM exercises to the pectoralis and innervated cervical and upper extremity muscle groups, and passive ROM to the lower extremities. Patient education regarding the rationale as well as specific ROM exercises was incorporated in the treatment plan. He continued sitting out of bed in a highback reclining wheelchair with a pressure distributing cushion and a full sheet for rapid return to bed if necessary. Vital signs remained stable with a blood pressure of 100/80 mm Hg and heart rate of 85 bpm while wearing elastic bandages and an abdominal binder, with his legs dependent on the footrests of the wheelchair. On day 7, the therapist decided to attempt sitting balancing activities on the side of the bed with a therapy aide. Lee continued to improve and was now mechanically ventilated with an FiO_2 of 0.40, pressure support 12 cm of H_2O pressure, SIMV 8, and PEEP of 5 cm H_2O pressure. His respiratory rate was 18 breaths/min. Lee required maximal assistance to assume the sitting position, yet was able to tolerate sitting upright with the binder, leg wraps, and moderate assistance from the therapist (Fig. 19-15). During the treatment session Lee used his upper extremities for support for 10 minutes. The ankles were supported in a neutral position on a footstool. This treatment was continued throughout Lee's hospital stay with the goal of getting the

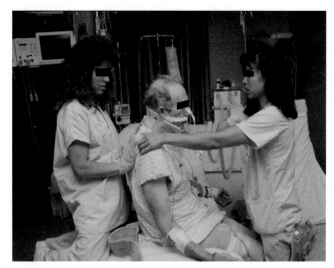

FIGURE 19-15 Patient with C5 tetraplegia—initiating sitting balancing activities.

patient to support his upper body with shoulders externally rotated and elbows and wrists extended, while the fingers remained flexed. After ensuring adequate scapular stability, the therapist also encouraged Lee to assist as much as possible with rolling in bed, and transfers from the side-lying to sitting position. Small knee immobilizers (air splints may also be used) were placed over the elbows during deltoid and serratus anterior strengthening exercises to give the patient a longer lever arm by maintaining the elbows in extension (Fig. 19-16).

On day 9, Lee developed a fever of 104°F (40.5°C) and was noted to have positive blood cultures. The source was thought to be pulmonary; yet this was never confirmed. Lee could no longer tolerate getting out of bed, and refused to turn onto his left side because of left shoulder pain. Although it is a routine procedure to turn a tetraplegic patient side to side every 2 hours and position them as comfortably as possible, this patient had a new nurse who felt badly about having to impose discomfort on the patient. Therefore, he was not turned onto his left side for 12 hours. Lee's oxygen saturation decreased to 85%, and upon clinical examination, the physician noted no air entry into the right lung. A chest radiograph was ordered and is shown in Figure 19-17. The physician decided a therapeutic bronchoscopy was indicated because of the significant right middle and lower lobe collapse noted on the chest radiograph. The FiO_2 was increased to 1.00, as is standard procedure during a bronchoscopy. Following the bronchoscopy the patient's chest radiograph was only minimally improved as seen in Figure 19-18. Physical therapy was immediately paged and asked to treat the patient. Immediate chest physical therapy treatment was given to the right lower and middle lobes for 35 minutes. Fifteen cc of whitish sputum was obtained, and breath sounds became audible over the right lower and middle lobes. During the treatment the breath sounds progressed from barely audible to rhonchi and slightly

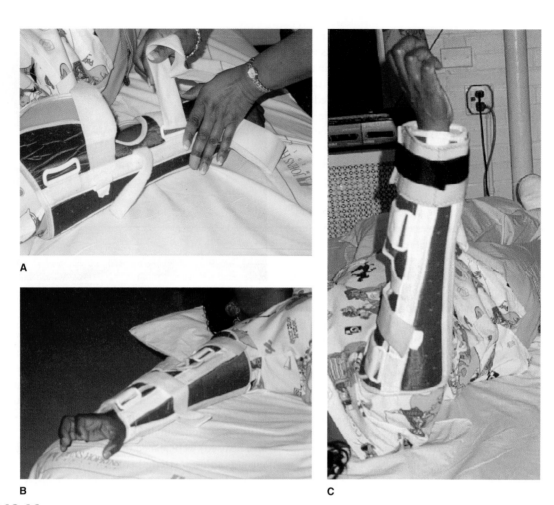

FIGURE 19-16   Use of small knee immobilizers to maintain elbow extension with deltoid exercises.

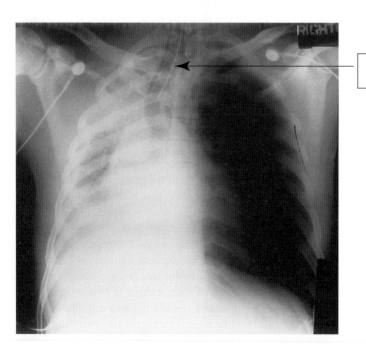

Endotracheal tube

FIGURE 19-17   Chest radiograph before therapeutic bronchoscopy.

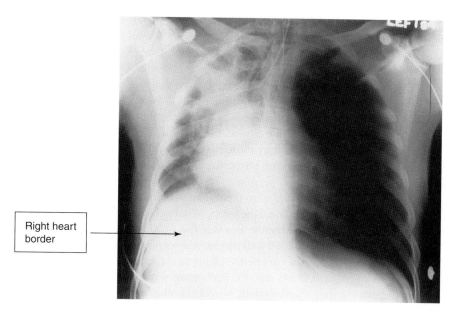

Right heart border →

FIGURE 19-18   Chest radiograph following therapeutic bronchoscopy.

diminished with a few crackles. Following the treatment, the therapist auscultated both sides of the patient's chest. After returning the patient to the supine position, the right lower lobe sounded clear and crackles were noted over the left lower lobe. Chest physical therapy was then provided to the left lower lobe for 25 minutes as it was suspected that the patient had aspirated secretions from the right to the left lung. A repeat chest X-ray was taken, and the right lower lobe atelectasis was markedly improved as shown in Figure 19-19. Lee tolerated having his FiO_2 decreased to 45% with a SpO_2 of 93% 30 minutes after physical therapy treatment.

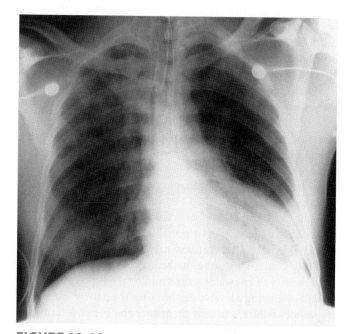

FIGURE 19-19   Chest radiograph following chest physical therapy.

Physical Therapy Interventions with Liberating the Patient from Mechanical Ventilation

On day 11, Lee's blood cultures were available and found to be negative. It was therefore believed that the patient was free of systemic infection. The physician decided to begin liberating Lee from the ventilator. Lee's temperature was 99°F, 37.2°C. The weaning procedure consisted of pressure support and SIMV ventilation for the majority of the day interspersed with periods CPAP. During CPAP the physical therapist was asked to provide respiratory muscle strengthening exercises and instruct the patient in how to assist with "quad coughing" (see Chapter 20). The therapist had two available options for respiratory muscle strengthening exercises—either abdominal weight training or inspiratory muscle training (IMT). The therapist chose to use abdominal weight training because the patient had difficulty understanding how to use the inspiratory muscle trainer, and each time the trainer was attached to the tracheostomy tube a cough was stimulated and secretions occluded the trainer. Greater patient education in IMT and frequent cleaning of the IMT device were needed to enhance the effectiveness of IMT in this patient, which was difficult during this acute period. Inspiratory muscle training was used later during the patient's hospital stay (see Chapter 20).

The therapist therefore used the method of diaphragmatic strength training described by Derrickson et al.[139] With the patient supine, the maximal inhaled volume without weights was recorded using an incentive spirometer. This was a gross assessment of the patient's inspiratory capacity (IC). Standard dish weights were placed on the patient's upper abdomen, just below the xiphoid process in 1/2- to 5-lb increments (Fig. 19-9).

The patient's baseline inspiratory capacity was 800 mL, and 1,000 mL after adding 15 lb. With 20 lb, the inspiratory capacity was 759 mL. The therapist decided to begin training with 20 lb twice per day. During each training session, the patient was disconnected from mechanical ventilation and performed 10 maximal inspirations, holding each breath for several seconds. This sequence was repeated three times for a total of 40 breaths per session. The patient continued with abdominal weight training twice daily for 5 days in conjunction with weaning. Initially therapeutic exercises, functional mobility activities, and postural drainage with manual techniques were continued while the patient was mechanically ventilated. During weaning it is important to prevent respiratory muscle fatigue; therefore, initially it was necessary to perform physical therapy interventions (with the exception of abdominal weight training) during periods of mechanical ventilation when the respiratory muscles were rested. The therapist monitored the patient's vital signs and used clinical judgment to determine whether the treatment interventions were best performed with mechanical ventilation or CPAP. The patient was able to tolerate all physical therapy interventions during CPAP on day 15. Suctioning was frequently necessary during diaphragmatic weight training, postural drainage, and functional mobility sessions because the patient mobilized secretions but could not adequately expectorate (cough) on his own. The patients need for postural drainage with manual techniques decreased as breathing exercises and functional mobility activities were better tolerated. (When adventitious breath sounds were improved by breathing exercises and mobility activities.)

On day 16, the patient's CPAP time had increased to 18 hours per day, with only 6 hours of mechanical ventilation during sleep. The physicians decided to monitor the patient during the night while on a CPAP of $8 \, cm \, H_2O$ pressure. The patient tolerated this final step in weaning through the next 48 hours and the patient was liberated from mechanical ventilation (Table 19-21).

TABLE 19-21   **Respiratory Parameters, Day 16 Clinical Considerations (Adult)— "Weaning" from Mechanical Ventilation**

Parameter	Consider Weaning
Is the cause for respiratory failure resolving?	Yes Chest X-ray clear Free of infection, afebrile Remains tetraplegic
Is the patient hemodynamically stable?	Yes
Able to initiate inspiratory effort	Yes
Fio_2 (percentage of inspired oxygen concentration)	0.35
Pao_2/Fio_2 ratio	271 (Pao_2 95)
PEEP (cm H_2O pressure)	8
Respiratory rate	25
Tidal Volume	500 mL
Rapid shallow breathing index (respiratory rate/tidal volume)	50
PI_{max}	−20

When Lee was weaned from the ventilator, he was tolerating CPAP sitting out of bed in a wheelchair twice daily with his legs dependent for 90-minute sessions, wearing the abdominal binder and elastic bandages. The nursing and physical therapy staff assisted the patient with forward and side bending for pressure relief every 15 to 30 minutes while sitting. He was participating in active and active-assistive ROM exercises to the upper extremities and able to sit on the edge of the bed supported by his upper extremities for 10 minutes. He was able to assist the nurses and therapists while they applied abdominal pressure to enable him to have a productive cough. Although he lacked independence in bed mobility, he could roll side to side and transfer from supine to sitting with moderate assistance from a caregiver. The patient was discontinued from this practice pattern because of successful separation from the mechanical ventilator. The patient's physical therapy program while spontaneously breathing is described in Chapter 20 where he was assigned to Practice Pattern E.

At the time of the initial physical therapy examination, Lee was dependent in all mobility and required mechanical ventilation 24 hours per day. After receiving physical therapy for 16 days, Lee demonstrated improvement in bed mobility, sitting balance, tolerance to the upright position, the ability to participate in active ROM exercises, and an improved cough. Nursing and physical therapy interventions prevented pressure sores and ROM was either maintained or improved in all extremity joints.

DISABLEMENT MODEL

The Disablement Model is described in detail in Chapter 2. The domain of physical therapy practice is primarily at the impairment and functional limitation levels. However, physical therapy airway clearance techniques for the mechanically ventilated patient with pulmonary secretion retention may also impact the pathology and pathophysiology of pneumonia and atelectasis. When performing secretion clearance techniques, an atelectasis can be completely reversed as noted in the case study. Treatment interventions that prevent pulmonary infection may reverse the pathophysiology of a developing pneumonia. Physical therapy interventions are also provided at the impairment level (to prevent or improve limitations in ROM or muscle strength, deconditioning); and at the level of functional limitation (when bed mobility activities, transfer training, and ambulation or wheelchair propulsion using a manual resuscitator bag or portable ventilator may be indicated). Medical interventions may take priority, yet early mobility can enhance the medical interventions. With our current level of knowledge, determining a long-term prognosis and predicting a level of disability for the patient with acute respiratory failure is usually premature and better determined in the rehabilitation or home setting after the patient's medical condition has plateaued. The patient's social situation, including family support and educational and vocational interests and aptitudes, can be better assessed outside the acute hospital setting. The patient's level of disability will vary depending on how the patient utilizes his or her inherent abilities.

The Limits of Our Knowledge

Despite physical therapists' role in mobilizing and providing airway clearance interventions to mechanically ventilated patients for the past 35 years, there is only scant evidence supporting the benefit of these interventions.[2,4–6,114,229–233] However, the need for compelling evidence to support physical therapy interventions is great since 57% of ARDS/ALI patients are unable to return to normal activity 12 months after hospitalization, and physical domains of survivors' quality of life are more adversely affected than mental health domains.[234,235] Moreover, after only 1 week of mechanical ventilation, 25% of conscious patients develop muscle weakness, and the risk of critical illness neuromuscular abnormalities is nearly 50% in ICU patients with sepsis, prolonged mechanical ventilation or multiorgan failure.[215,236,237] ICU-acquired weakness is also associated with a longer duration of mechanical ventilation.[214,215,220,237,238] Many believe that physical therapy interventions can have a positive effect on ventilator-associated pneumonia, muscle strength, functional mobility, and long-term functional outcomes. However, strong evidence to support these beliefs is lacking. One recent study demonstrated the safety and feasibility of physical therapy 48 hours after initiating mechanical ventilation with an associated decrease in hospital stay and cost for survivors.[4] More are needed.

Patient outcomes vary depending upon patient comorbidities, the nature of their critical illness and the associated ICU management. The use of corticosteroids and neuromuscular blocking agents, glycemic control, and sedation all may impact the duration of the ICU stay and functional outcomes.[214,215,236] Further research is necessary to establish the optimal type, timing, duration, and frequency of physical therapy services for patients who require mechanical ventilation. The most beneficial and cost-effective physical therapy interventions with the best outcome are also yet to be determined.

The Future

With advances in the management of critically ill patients, more patients may survive critical illness emphasizing the importance of optimizing ICU care to minimize patients' long-term sequelae. As the population ages, the frail elderly may have even greater representation within ICU patient populations. In this population, even a small decrement in physical function may move the patient from independent living to requiring care in a nursing facility. Although heavy sedation and immobility have been commonly associated with mechanical ventilation, this paradigm of ICU care is changing. The need for physical therapists to be comfortable with providing interventions to mechanically ventilated patients may grow. Thus, the need for airway clearance techniques, ROM exercises, and functional mobility training may expand within the intensive care setting and beyond, as patients move on to lower levels of care while continuing to require mechanical ventilation.

Support for physical therapists to work closely with the ICU clinicians and researchers is vital for developing evidence-based assessment tools and protocols regarding the utilization of rehabilitative care in the ICU. Physical therapy education needs to provide more time and clinical experience in caring for mechanically ventilated patients. All too often, patient care in the ICU is deprioritized in favor of less acutely ill patients, when in fact, theses patients may have the greatest need for physical therapy interventions. More training in assessing cognitive function is also needed.[169] Tapping into the resources of experienced, enthusiastic ICU physical therapists, and utilizing these experts when placing students at clinical education sites is essential. Training should emphasize the need for therapists to directly interact with ICU nurses and physicians in evaluating and encouraging safe and appropriate physical therapy interventions for critically ill patients.

Thoughts for the Future

What are the best type, timing, and duration, of physical therapy interventions?

How can physical therapy best be administered in an ICU when patients are frequently sedated and undergoing medical and nursing procedures?

Are outcomes better and costs reduced when therapists are assigned specifically to the ICU as an integral part of the ICU healthcare team?

Does inspiratory muscle training enhance weaning for patients who are optimally mobilized versus those who are unable to gain independence in functional mobility?

Do patients with pneumonia or atelectasis respond better to chest physical therapy interventions including directed postural drainage, percussion, and vibration than breathing exercises and mobilization?

What is the best timing for physical therapy interventions in conjunction with evidence-based daily spontaneous breathing trials to evaluate liberation from mechanical ventilation?

How can physical therapy interventions be best coordinated with evidence-based daily interruptions of continuous sedation?

What are optimal changes, if any, in mechanical ventilator settings for physical therapy interventions versus bed rest?

ACKNOWLEDGMENT

The authors would like to thank the following for their critical review and assistance with this chapter: Roy Brower, MD, for his review and expertise with mechanical ventilation; P Milo Frawley, RN, MS, ACNP, CCNS, for his critical review and assistance with the modes of mechanical ventilation; and Dale Needham, MD, PhD, for his review, photographs, references, and never-ending availability.

Heads Up!

This chapter contains a CD-ROM activity.

REFERENCES

1. Morris PE. Moving our critically ill patients: mobility barriers and benefits. *Crit Care Clin.* 2007;23(1):1-20.
2. Stiller K. Safety issues that should be considered when mobilizing critically ill patients. *Crit Care Clin.* 2007;23(1):35-53.
3. Perme CS, Southard RE, Joyce DL, Noon GP, Loebe M. Early mobilization of LVAD recipients who require prolonged mechanical ventilation. *Tex Heart Inst J.* 2006;33(2):130-133.
4. Morris PE, Goad A, Thompson C, et al. Early intensive care unit mobility therapy in the treatment of acute respiratory failure. *Crit Care Med.* 2008;36(8):2238-2243.
5. Thomsen GE, Snow GL, Rodriguez L, Hopkins RO. Patients with respiratory failure increase ambulation after transfer to an intensive care unit where early activity is a priority. *Crit Care Med.* 2008;36(4):1119-1124.
6. Bailey P, Thomsen GE, Spuhler VJ, et al. Early activity is feasible and safe in respiratory failure patients. *Crit Care Med.* 2007; 35(1):139-145.
7. Dowdy DW, Needham DM, Mendez-Tellez PA, Herridge MS, Pronovost PJ. Studying outcomes of intensive care unit survivors: the role of the cohort study. *Intensive Care Med.* 2005;31(7): 914-921.
8. Herridge M, Cheung AM, Tansey CM, Martyn AM, Diaz-Granados N. One-year outcomes in survivors of the acute respiratory distress syndrome. *N Engl J Med.* 2003;348(8): 683-693.
9. Chelluri L, Im KA, Belle SH, et al. Long-term mortality and quality of life after prolonged mechanical ventilation. *Crit Care Med.* 2004;32(1):61-69.
10. American Physical Therapy Association. Guide to Physical Therapist Practice, 2nd ed. *Phys Ther.* 2001 Jan;81:539-553.
11. West JB. *Respiratory Physiology—The Essentials.* 7th ed. Philadelphia, PA: Lippincott Williams & Wilkins; 2005:186.
12. Gerold K, Nussbaum E. Understanding mechanical ventilation. *Phys Ther Pract.* 1994;3:81-91.
13. Shaffer T, Wolfson M, Gault JH. Respiratory physiology. In: Shaffer T, Wolfson M, Gault JH, eds. *Cardiopulmonary Physical Therapy.* 3rd ed. Baltimore, MD: Mosby; 1995:260.
14. Kacmarek R, Hickling K. Permissive hypercapnia. *Respir Care.* 1993;38:373-386.
15. Hickling KG, Henderson SJ, Jackson R. Low mortality associated with low volume pressure limited ventilation with permissive hypercapnia in severe adult respiratory distress syndrome. *Intensive Care Med.* 1990;16(6):372-377.
16. Wolthuis EK, Choi G, Dessing MC, et al. Mechanical ventilation with lower tidal volumes and positive end-expiratory pressure prevents pulmonary inflammation in patients without preexisting lung injury. *Anesthesiology.* 2008;108(1):46-54.
17. Marini JJ, Brower RG. Auto-peep with low tidal volume. *Am J Respir Crit Care Med.* 2003;167(8):1150-1151; author reply 1151.
18. Rossi A, De Ninno G, Mergoni M. Respiratory muscles in intensive care medicine. *Monaldi Arch Chest Dis.* 1999;54(6): 532-538.
19. Tobin M. Mechanical ventilation: conventional modes and settings. In: Fishman A, ed. *Fishman's Pulmonary Diseases and Disorders.* 3rd ed. New York: McGraw-Hill; 1998: 2691-2699.
20. Kumar A, Falke KJ, Geffin B, et al. Continuous positive-pressure ventilation in acute respiratory failure. *N Engl J Med.* 1970; 283(26):1430-1436.
21. Levitzky M, Cairo J, Hall S. *Introduction to Respiratory Care.* Philadelphia, PA: WB Saunders; 1990:525-527,534.
22. Putensen C, Zech S, Wrigge H, et al. Long-term effects of spontaneous breathing during ventilatory support in patients with acute lung injury. *Am J Respir Crit Care Med.* 2001;164(1):43-49.
23. Deem S, Bishop MJ. Physiological consequences of intubation. In: Marini JJ, Slutsky AS, eds. *Physiologic Basis of Ventilatory Support.* New York: Marcel Dekker Inc; 1998:623-654.
24. Acosta P, Santisbon E. The use of positive end-expiratory pressure in mechanical ventilation. *Crit Care Clin.* 2007;23(2): 251-261.
25. Adams AB, Lim S. Monitoring and management of the patient in the intensive care unit. In: Wilkins RL, Stoller JK, Scanlan CL, eds. *Egan's Fundamentals of Respiratory Care.* 8th ed. St Louis, MO: Mosby; 2003:1081-1119.
26. Frawley PM. Thoracic trauma. In: McQuillan KA, Makic MB, Whalen E, eds. *Trauma Nursing: from Resuscitation Through Rehabilitation.* 4th ed. St Louis, MO: Saunders Elsevier; 2009:614-677.
27. Staudinger T, Kordova H, Roggla M, et al. Comparison of oxygen cost of breathing with pressure-support ventilation and biphasic intermittent positive airway pressure ventilation. *Crit Care Med.* 1998;26(9):1518-1522.
28. Brochard L, Harf A, Lorino H, Lemaire F. Inspiratory pressure support prevents diaphragmatic fatigue during weaning from mechanical ventilation. *Am Rev Respir Dis.* 1989;139(2):513-521.
29. Oba Y, Salzman GA. Ventilation with lower tidal volumes as compared with traditional tidal volumes for acute lung injury and the acute respiratory distress syndrome. *N Engl J Med.* 2000;343(11):812-814.
30. Brower RG, Ware LB, Berthiaume Y, Matthay MA. Treatment of ARDS. *Chest.* 2001;120(4):1347-1367.
31. Peterson WP, Barbalata L, Brooks CA, Gerhart KA, Mellick DC, Whiteneck GG. The effect of tidal volumes on the time to wean persons with high tetraplegia from ventilators. *Spinal Cord.* 1999;37(4):284-288.
32. Marcy T. Full ventilatory support. In: Marini J, Slutsky A, eds. *Physiological Basis of Ventilatory Support.* New York: Dekker; 1998:783-792,807.
33. Pinhu L, Whitehead T, Evans T, Griffiths M. Ventilator-associated lung injury. *Lancet.* 2003;361(9354):332-340.
34. Pocket Guide: Servo i modes of ventilation. Maquet – Products – Servo-i Adult Web site. http://www.maquet.com/productPage.aspx?m1=112599774495&m2=112808545902&m3=105584076919& productGroupID=112808545902&productConfigID=105584076919&productConfigViewID=3&imageViewCategoryID=112799157632&languageID=1&subID=Sales%20 Flyer. Published 2003. Accessed July 26, 2008.
35. Wrigge H, Zinserling J, Neumann P, et al. Spontaneous breathing improves lung aeration in oleic acid-induced lung injury. *Anesthesiology.* 2003;99(2):376-384.
36. Froese AB, Bryan AC. Effects of anesthesia and paralysis on diaphragmatic mechanics in man. *Anesthesiology.* 1974;41(3): 242-255.
37. Putensen C, Muders T, Varelmann D, Wrigge H. The impact of spontaneous breathing during mechanical ventilation. *Curr Opin Crit Care.* 2006;12(1):13-18.
38. Putensen C, Hering R, Muders T, Wrigge H. Assisted breathing is better in acute respiratory failure. *Curr Opin Crit Care.* 2005; 11(1):63-68.

39. Le Bourdelles G, Viires N, Boczkowski J, Seta N, Pavlovic D, Aubier M. Effects of mechanical ventilation on diaphragmatic contractile properties in rats. *Am J Respir Crit Care Med*. 1994; 149(6):1539-1544.

40. Powers SK, Shanely RA, Coombes JS, et al. Mechanical ventilation results in progressive contractile dysfunction in the diaphragm. *J Appl Physiol*. 2002;92(5):1851-1858.

41. Shanely RA, Zergeroglu MA, Lennon SL, et al. Mechanical ventilation-induced diaphragmatic atrophy is associated with oxidative injury and increased proteolytic activity. *Am J Respir Crit Care Med*. 2002;166(10):1369-1374.

42. Sassoon CS, Zhu E, Caiozzo VJ. Assist-control mechanical ventilation attenuates ventilator-induced diaphragmatic dysfunction. *Am J Respir Crit Care Med*. 2004;170(6):626-632.

43. Downs JB, Perkins HM, Modell JH. Intermittent mandatory ventilation. An evaluation. *Arch Surg*. 1974;109(4):519-523.

44. Downs JB, Klein EFJ, Desautels D, Modell JH, Kirby RR. Intermittent mandatory ventilation: a new approach to weaning patients from mechanical ventilators. *Chest*. 1973;64(3): 331-335.

45. Marini JJ, Smith TC, Lamb VJ. External work output and force generation during synchronized intermittent mechanical ventilation. Effect of machine assistance on breathing effort. *Am Rev Respir Dis*. 1988;138(5):1169-1179.

46. Imsand C, Feihl F, Perret C, Fitting JW. Regulation of inspiratory neuromuscular output during synchronized intermittent mechanical ventilation. *Anesthesiology*. 1994;80(1):13-22.

47. Kallet RH, Campbell AR, Dicker RA, Katz JA, Mackersie RC. Work of breathing during lung-protective ventilation in patients with acute lung injury and acute respiratory distress syndrome: a comparison between volume and pressure-regulated breathing modes. *Respir Care*. 2005;50(12):1623-1631.

48. Shelledy DC, Peters JI. Initiating and adjusting ventilatory support. In: Wilkins RL, Stoller JK, Scanlan CL, eds. *Egan's Fundamentals of Respiratory Care*. 8th ed. St Louis, MO: Mosby; 2003:1026.

49. Brochard L, Pluskwa F, Lemaire F. Improved efficacy of spontaneous breathing with inspiratory pressure support. *Am Rev Respir Dis*. 1987;136(2):411-415.

50. Esteban A, Alia I, Tobin MJ, et al. Effect of spontaneous breathing trial duration on outcome of attempts to discontinue mechanical ventilation. Spanish Lung Failure Collaborative Group. *Am J Respir Crit Care Med*. 1999;159(2):512-518.

51. Kollef MH, Shapiro SD, Silver P, et al. A randomized, controlled trial of protocol-directed versus physician-directed weaning from mechanical ventilation. *Crit Care Med*. 1997;25(4):567-574.

52. MacIntyre NR, Cook DJ, Ely EW Jr, et al. Evidence-based guidelines for weaning and discontinuing ventilatory support: a collective task force facilitated by the American College of Chest Physicians; the American Association for Respiratory Care; and the American College of Critical Care Medicine. *Chest*. 2001;120(suppl 6):375S-395S.

53. Rose L, Hawkins M. Airway pressure release ventilation and biphasic positive airway pressure: a systematic review of definitional criteria. *Intensive Care Med*. 2008;34(10): 1766-1773.

54. Frawley PM, Habashi NM. Airway pressure release ventilation: theory and practice. *AACN Clin Issues*. 2001;12(2):234-246.

55. Frawley PM, Habashi NM. Airway pressure release ventilation and pediatrics: theory and practice. *Crit Care Nurs Clin North Am*. 2004;16(3):337-348.

56. Habashi NM. Other approaches to open-lung ventilation: airway pressure release ventilation. *Crit Care Med*. 2005;33(suppl 3): S228-S240.

57. Rathgeber J, Schorn B, Falk V, Kazmaier S, Spiegel T, Burchardi H. The influence of controlled mandatory ventilation (CMV), intermittent mandatory ventilation (IMV) and biphasic intermittent positive airway pressure (BIPAP) on duration of intubation and consumption of analgesics and sedatives. A prospective analysis in 596 patients following adult cardiac surgery. *Eur J Anaesthesiol*. 1997;14(6):576-582.

58. Putensen C, Mutz NJ, Putensen-Himmer G, Zinserling J. Spontaneous breathing during ventilatory support improves ventilation-perfusion distributions in patients with acute respiratory distress syndrome. *Am J Respir Crit Care Med*. 1999; 159(4, pt 1):1241-1248.

59. Esteban A, Frutos F, Tobin MJ, et al. A comparison of four methods of weaning patients from mechanical ventilation. Spanish Lung Failure Collaborative Group. *N Engl J Med*. 1995; 332(6):345-350.

60. Hendra KP, Celli BR. Weaning from mechanical ventilation. *Int Anesthesiol Clin*. 1999;37(3):127-143.

61. Marini J. Mechanical ventilation: physiological considerations and newer ventilatory techniques. In: Fishman A, ed. *Fishman's pulmonary diseases and disorders*. 3rd ed. New York: McGraw-Hill; 1998:2714.

62. Bianchi L, Foglio K, Pagani M, Vitacca M, Rossi A, Ambrosino N. Effects of proportional assist ventilation on exercise tolerance in COPD patients with chronic hypercapnia. *Eur Respir J*. 1998; 11(2):422-427.

63. Grasso S, Puntillo F, Mascia L, et al. Compensation for increase in respiratory workload during mechanical ventilation. Pressure-support versus proportional-assist ventilation. *Am J Respir Crit Care Med*. 2000;161(3, pt 1):819-826.

64. Giannouli E, Webster K, Roberts D, Younes M. Response of ventilator-dependent patients to different levels of pressure support and proportional assist. *Am J Respir Crit Care Med*. 1999;159(6):1716-1725.

65. Liesching T, Kwok H, Hill NS. Acute applications of noninvasive positive pressure ventilation. *Chest*. 2003;124(2): 699-713.

66. Aldrich T, Rochester D. The lungs and neuromuscular diseases. In: Murray J, Nadel J, eds. *Textbook of Respiratory Medicine*. 2nd ed. Philadelphia: WB Saunders; 1994:2648.

67. Kotloff R. Acute respiratory failure in the surgical patient. In: Fishman A, ed. *Fishman's Pulmonary Diseases and Disorders*. 3rd ed. New York: McGraw-Hill; 1998:2603.

68. Schwab R, Goldberg A, Poack A. Sleep apnea syndromes. In: Fishman A, ed. *Fishman's Pulmonary Diseases and Disorders*. 3rd ed. New York: Mc Graw-Hill; 1998:1627.

69. Criner GJ, Brennan K, Travaline JM, Kreimer D. Efficacy and compliance with noninvasive positive pressure ventilation in patients with chronic respiratory failure. *Chest*. 1999;116(3): 667-675.

70. Dellinger RP. Inhaled nitric oxide versus prone positioning in acute respiratory distress syndrome. *Crit Care Med*. 2000;28(2): 572-574.

71. Dupont H, Mentec H, Cheval C, Moine P, Fierobe L, Timsit JF. Short-term effect of inhaled nitric oxide and prone positioning on gas exchange in patients with severe acute respiratory distress syndrome. *Crit Care Med*. 2000;28(2): 304-308.

72. Deja M, Hommel M, Weber-Carstens S, et al. Evidence-based therapy of severe acute respiratory distress syndrome: an algorithm-guided approach. *J Int Med Res.* 2008;36(2):211-221.

73. Rico FR, Cheng JD, Gestring ML, Piotrowski ES. Mechanical ventilation strategies in massive chest trauma. *Crit Care Clin.* 2007;23(2):299-315, xi.

74. Alsaghir AH, Martin CM. Effect of prone positioning in patients with acute respiratory distress syndrome: a meta-analysis. *Crit Care Med.* 2008;36(2):603-609.

75. Abroug F, Ouanes-Besbes L, Elatrous S, Brochard L. The effect of prone positioning in acute respiratory distress syndrome or acute lung injury: a meta-analysis. Areas of uncertainty and recommendations for research. *Intensive Care Med.* 2008;34(6):1002-1011.

76. Galiatsou E, Kostanti E, Svarna E, et al. Prone position augments recruitment and prevents alveolar overinflation in acute lung injury. *Am J Respir Crit Care Med.* 2006;174(2):187-197.

77. Fernandez R, Trenchs X, Klamburg J, et al. Prone positioning in acute respiratory distress syndrome: a multicenter randomized clinical trial. *Intensive Care Med.* 2008;:34(8):1487-1491.

78. Morris AH, Wallace CJ, Menlove RL, et al. Randomized clinical trial of pressure-controlled inverse ratio ventilation and extracorporeal CO_2 removal for adult respiratory distress syndrome. *Am J Respir Crit Care Med.* 1994;149(2, Pt 1):295-305.

79. Zapol WM, Snider MT, Hill JD, et al. Extracorporeal membrane oxygenation in severe acute respiratory failure. A randomized prospective study. *JAMA.* 1979;242(20):2193-2196.

80. Rich PB, Awad SS, Crotti S, Hirschl RB, Bartlett RH, Schreiner RJ. A prospective comparison of atrio-femoral and femoro-atrial flow in adult venovenous extracorporeal life support. *J Thorac Cardiovasc Surg.* 1998;116(4):628-632.

81. Rich PB, Rock P. Extracorporeal life suppport for severe adult respiratory failure. *Curr Opin Anaesthesiol.* 2003;16:105-111.

82. Hsu CW, Lee DL, Lin SL, Sun SF, Chang HW. The initial response to inhaled nitric oxide treatment for intensive care unit patients with acute respiratory distress syndrome. *Respiration.* 2008;75(3):288-295.

83. Mays LC, Eckert S. Synchronous independent lung ventilation. *Dimens Crit Care Nurs.* 1994;13(5):249-255.

84. Ely EW, Baker AM, Evans GW, Haponik EF. The prognostic significance of passing a daily screen of weaning parameters. *Intensive Care Med.* 1999;25(6):581-587.

85. Brochard L, Rauss A, Benito S, et al. Comparison of three methods of gradual withdrawal from ventilatory support during weaning from mechanical ventilation. *Am J Respir Crit Care Med.* 1994;150(4):896-903.

86. Martin UJ, Hincapie L, Nimchuk M, Gaughan J, Criner GJ. Impact of whole-body rehabilitation in patients receiving chronic mechanical ventilation. *Crit Care Med.* 2005;33(10):2259-2265.

87. Seidel H, Ball J, Dains J, Bendeict G. *Mosby's Guide to Physical Examination.* 3rd ed. Baltimore, MD: Mosby; 1995:358.

88. DeVivo MJ, Black KJ, Stover SL. Causes of death during the first 12 years after spinal cord injury. *Arch Phys Med Rehabil.* 1993;74(3):248-254.

89. Lisboa T, Rello J. Diagnosis of ventilator-associated pneumonia: is there a gold standard and a simple approach? *Curr Opin Infect Dis.* 2008;21:174-178.

90. Wunderink RG. Mortality and the diagnosis of ventilator-associated pneumonia: a new direction. *Am J Respir Crit Care Med.* 1998;157(2):349-350.

91. Sterling T, Ho E, Brehm W. Diagnosis and treatment of ventilator-associated pneumonia—Impact on survival. *Chest.* 1996;110:1025-1034.

92. Rello J, Ausina V, Ricart M, Castella J, Prats G. Impact of previous antimicrobial therapy on the etiology and outcome of ventilator-associated pneumonia. *Chest.* 1993;104(4):1230-1235.

93. Rello J, Quintana E, Ausina V, et al. Incidence, etiology, and outcome of nosocomial pneumonia in mechanically ventilated patients. *Chest.* 1991;100(2):439-444.

94. Fagon J, Chastre J, Hance A. Nosocomial pneumonia in ventilated patients: a cohort study evaluating attributable mortality and hospital stay. *Am J Med.* 1993;94:281.

95. Joshi M, Ciesla N, Caplan E. Diagnosis of pneumonia in critically ill patients. *Chest.* 1988;94:4s.

96. Donald KJ, Robertson VL, Tsebelis K. Setting safe and effective suction pressure: the effect of using a manometer in the suction circuit. *Intensive Care Med.* 2000;26(1):15.

97. Subirana M, Sola I. Closed tracheal suction systems versus open tracheal suction systems for mechanically ventilated adult patients. *Cochrane Datanbase Syst Rev.* 2007: Oct 17;(4): CD004581. Review

98. Siempos II, Vardakas KZ, Falagas ME. Closed tracheal suction systems for prevention of ventilator-associated pneumonia. *Br J Anaesth.* 2008;100(3):299-306.

99. Subirana M, Sola I, Benito S. Closed tracheal suction systems versus open tracheal suction systems for mechanically ventilated adult patients. *Anesth Analg.* 2008;106(4):1326.

100. Darvas JA, Leesa G Hawkins LG. The closed tracheal suction catheter: 24 hour or 48 hour change? *Aust Crit Care.* 2003: 86-92.

101. Celik SA, Kanan N. A current conflict: use of isotonic sodium chloride solution on endotracheal suctioning in critically ill patients. *Dimens Crit Care Nurs.* 2006:11-14.

102. Raymond J. Normal saline instillation before suctioning: helpful or harmful? A review of the literature. *Am J Crit Care.* 1995;4(4):267-271.

103. Akqui S, Akyolcu N. Effects of normal saline on endotracheal suctioning. *J Clin Nurs.* 2002;11(1):826-830.

104. Rauen CA, Chulay M, Bridges E, Vollman KM, Arbour R. Seven evidence-based practice habits: putting some sacred cows out to pasture. *Crit Care Nurse.* 2008;28(2):98-124.

105. Golden J, Wank K, Keith F. Bronchoscopy, lung biopsy, and other diagnostic procedures. In: Murray J, Nadel J, eds. *Textbook of Respiratory Medicine.* 2nd ed. Philadelphia, PA: WB Saunders; 1994:738-739.

106. Jelic S, Cunningham JA, Factor P. Clinical review: airway hygiene in the intensive care unit. *Crit Care.* 2008;12(2):209.

107. Ciesla N. Chest physical therapy for the adult intensive care unit trauma patient. *Phys Ther Pract.* 1994;3:102-105.

108. Ciesla N, Klemic N, Imle PC. Chest physical therapy to the patient with multiple trauma. Two case studies. *Phys Ther.* 1981;61(2):202-205.

109. Ciesla ND. Chest physical therapy for patients in the intensive care unit. *Phys Ther.* 1996;76(6):609-625.

110. Mars M, Ciesla N. Chest physical therapy may have prevented bronchoscopy and exploratory laparotomy: a case report. *Cardiopulm Phys Ther.* 1993;4:4-5.

111. Marini J, Pierson D, Hudson L. Comparison of fiberoptic bronchoscopy and respiratory therapy [letter]. *Am Rev Respir Dis.* 1984;126:368.

112. Marini JJ, Pierson DJ, Hudson LD. Acute lobar atelectasis: a prospective comparison of fiberoptic bronchoscopy and respiratory therapy. *Am Rev Respir Dis.* 1979;119(6):971-978.

113. Mackenzie CF, Shin B, McAslan TC. Chest physiotherapy: the effect on arterial oxygenation. *Anesth Analg.* 1978;57(1):28-30.

114. Mackenzie CF, Imle PC, Ciesla N. *Chest Physiotherapy in the Intensive Care Unit.* 2nd ed. Baltimore, MD: Williams & Wilkins; 1989.

115. Santos PM, Afrassiabi A, Weymuller EA Jr. Risk factors associated with prolonged intubation and laryngeal injury. *Otolaryngol Head Neck Surg.* 1994;111(4):453-459.

116. Maury E, Guglielminotti J, Alzieu M, Qureshi T, Guidet B, Offenstadt G. How to identify patients with no risk for postextubation stridor? *J Crit Care.* 2004;19(1):23-28.

117. Miller RL, Cole RP. Association between reduced cuff leak volume and postextubation stridor. *Chest.* 1996;110(4):1035-1040.

118. Houck JR, Keamy MF III, McDonough JM. Effect of helium concentration on experimental upper airway obstruction. *Ann Otol Rhinol Laryngol.* 1990;99(7, Pt 1):556-561.

119. Schmidt G, Hall J, Wood L. Management of the ventilated patient. In: Murray J, Nadel J, eds. *Textbook of Respiratory Medicine.* 2nd ed. Philadelphia, PA: WB Saunders; 1994:2640-2644, 2648.

120. Sengupta P, Sessler DI, Maglinger P, et al. Endotracheal tube cuff pressure in three hospitals, and the volume required to produce an appropriate cuff pressure. *BMC Anesthesiol.* 2004; 4(1):8.

121. Hess DR. Tracheostomy tubes and related appliances. *Respir Care.* 2005;50(4):497-510.

122. Shelly MP. The humidification and filtration functions of the airways. *Respir Care Clin N Am.* 2006;12(2):139-148.

123. Rathgeber J. Devices used to humidify respired gases. *Respir Care Clin N Am.* 2006;12(2):165-182.

124. Kola A, Eckmanns T, Gastmeier P. Efficacy of heat and moisture exchangers in preventing ventilator-associated pneumonia: meta-analysis of randomized controlled trials. *Intensive Care Med.* 2005;31(1):5-11.

125. Lorente L, Lecuona M, Jimenez A, Mora ML, Sierra A. Ventilator-associated pneumonia using a heated humidifier or a heat and moisture exchanger: a randomized controlled trial [ISRCTN88724583]. *Crit Care.* 2006;10(4):R116.

126. Jubran A. Critical illness and mechanical ventilation: effects on the diaphragm. *Respir Care.* 2006;51(9):1054-1061; discussion 1062-1064.

127. Thille AW, Cabello B, Galia F, Lyazidi A, Brochard L. Reduction of patient-ventilator asynchrony by reducing tidal volume during pressure-support ventilation. *Intensive Care Med.* 2008;34 (8):1477-1486.

128. Bissett B, Leditschke IA. Inspiratory muscle training to enhance weaning from mechanical ventilation. *Anaesth Intensive Care.* 2007;35(5):776-779.

129. Sprague SS, Hopkins PD. Use of inspiratory strength training to wean six patients who were ventilator-dependent. *Phys Ther.* 2003;83(2):171-181.

130. Martin AD, Davenport PD, Franceschi AC, Harman E. Use of inspiratory muscle strength training to facilitate ventilator weaning: a series of 10 consecutive patients. *Chest.* 2002; 122(1):192-196.

131. Abelson H, Brewer, K. Inspiratory muscle training in the mechanically ventilated patient. *Physiother Can.* 1987;39: 305-307.

132. Caruso P, Denari SD, Ruiz SA, et al. Inspiratory muscle training is ineffective in mechanically ventilated critically ill patients. *Clinics.* 2005;60(6):479-484.

133. Lin KH, Lai YL, Wu HD, Wang TQ, Wang YH. Cough threshold in people with spinal cord injuries. *Phys Ther.* 1999;79(11): 1026-1031.

134. Liaw MY, Lin MC, Cheng PT, Wong MK, Tang FT. Resistive inspiratory muscle training: its effectiveness in patients with acute complete cervical cord injury. *Arch Phys Med Rehabil.* 2000;81(6):752-756.

135. Brooks D, O'Brien K, Geddes EL, Crowe J, Reid WD. Is inspiratory muscle training effective for individuals with cervical spinal cord injury? A qualitative systematic review. *Clin Rehabil.* 2005;19(3):237-246.

136. Lin KH, Chuang CC, Wu HD, Chang CW, Kou YR. Abdominal weight and inspiratory resistance: their immediate effects on inspiratory muscle functions during maximal voluntary breathing in chronic tetraplegic patients. *Arch Phys Med Rehabil.* 1999;80(7):741-745.

137. Rutchik A, Weissman AR, Almenoff PL, Spungen AM, Bauman WA, Grimm DR. Resistive inspiratory muscle training in subjects with chronic cervical spinal cord injury. *Arch Phys Med Rehabil.* 1998;79(3):293-297.

138. Mueller G, Perret C, Spengler CM. Optimal intensity for respiratory muscle endurance training in patients with spinal cord injury. *J Rehabil Med.* 2006;38(6):381-386.

139. Derrickson J, Ciesla N, Simpson N, Imle PC. A comparison of two breathing exercise programs for patients with quadriplegia. *Phys Ther.* 1992;72(11):763-769.

140. Estenne M, Knoop C, Vanvaerenbergh J, Heilporn A, De Troyer A. The effect of pectoralis muscle training in tetraplegic subjects. *Am Rev Respir Dis.* 1989;139(5):1218-1222.

141. Fujiwara T, Hara Y, Chino N. Expiratory function in complete tetraplegics: study of spirometry, maximal expiratory pressure, and muscle activity of pectoralis major and latissimus dorsi muscles. *Am J Phys Med Rehabil.* 1999;78(5): 464-469.

142. Kang SW, Shin JC, Park CI, Moon JH, Rha DW, Cho DH. Relationship between inspiratory muscle strength and cough capacity in cervical spinal cord injured patients. *Spinal Cord.* 2006;44(4):242-248.

143. Marini JJ, Gattinoni L. Ventilatory management of acute respiratory distress syndrome: a consensus of two. *Crit Care Med.* 2004;32:250-255.

144. Slutsky AS. Lung injury caused by mechanical ventilation. *Chest.* 1999;116(suppl 1):9S-15S.

145. Carney D, DiRocco J, Nieman G. Dynamic alveolar mechanics and ventilator-induced lung injury. *Crit Care Med.* 2005;33 (suppl 3):S122-S128.

146. Halter JM, Steinberg JM, Gatto LA, et al. Effect of positive end-expiratory pressure and tidal volume on lung injury induced by alveolar instability. *Crit Care.* 2007;11(1):R20.

147. Yilmaz M, Gajic O. Optimal ventilator settings in acute lung injury and acute respiratory distress syndrome. *Eur J Anaesthesiol.* 2008;25(2):89-96.

148. Steinberg KP, Kacmarek RM. Respiratory controversies in the critical care setting. Should tidal volume be 6 mL/kg predicted body weight in virtually all patients with acute respiratory failure? *Respir Care.* 2007;52(5):556-564; discussion 565-567.

149. Checkley W, Brower R, Korpak A, Thompson BT; Acute Respiratory Distress Syndrome Network Investigators. Effects of a clinical trial on mechanical ventilation practices in patients with acute lung injury. *Am J Respir Crit Care Med.* 2008;177(11):1215-1222.

150. Hickling KG, Walsh J, Henderson S, Jackson R. Low mortality rate in adult respiratory distress syndrome using low-volume, pressure-limited ventilation with permissive hypercapnia: a prospective study. *Crit Care Med.* 1994;22(10):1568-1578.

151. Bendixen H. Editorial comment. *Arch Surg.* 1974:541.

152. Vilke GM, Chan TC, Neuman T, Clausen JL. Spirometry in normal subjects in sitting, prone, and supine positions. *Respir Care.* 2000;45(4):407-410.

153. Behrakis PK, Baydur A, Jaeger MJ, Milic-Emili J. Lung mechanics in sitting and horizontal body positions. *Chest.* 1983;83(4):643-646.

154. Vellody VP, Nassery M, Druz WS, Sharp JT. Effects of body position change on thoracoabdominal motion. *J Appl Physiol.* 1978;45(4):581-589.

155. Allen SM, Hunt B, Green M. Fall in vital capacity with posture. *Br J Dis Chest.* 1985;79(3):267-271.

156. Loveridge BM, Dubo HI. Breathing pattern in chronic quadriplegia. *Arch Phys Med Rehabil.* 1990;71(7):495-499.

157. Ibanez J, Raurich JM. Normal values of functional residual capacity in the sitting and supine positions. *Intensive Care Med.* 1982;8(4):173-177.

158. Anke A, Aksnes AK, Stanghelle JK, Hjeltnes N. Lung volumes in tetraplegic patients according to cervical spinal cord injury level. *Scand J Rehabil Med.* 1993;25(2):73-77.

159. Haas A, Lowman EW, Bergofsky EH. Impairment of respiration after spinal cord injury. *Arch Phys Med Rehabil.* 1965;46:399-405.

160. Estenne M, De Troyer A. Mechanism of the postural dependence of vital capacity in tetraplegic subjects. *Am Rev Respir Dis.* 1987;135(2):367-371.

161. Fugl-Meyer AR. Effects of respiratory muscle paralysis in tetraplegic and paraplegic patients. *Scand J Rehabil Med.* 1971;3(4):141-150.

162. Cameron GS, Scott JW, Jousse AT, Botterell EH. Diaphragmatic respiration in the quadriplegic patient and the effect of position on his vital capacity. *Ann Surg.* 1955;141(4):451-456.

163. Maloney FP. Pulmonary function in quadriplegia: effects of a corset. *Arch Phys Med Rehabil.* 1979;60(6):261-265.

164. McCool FD, Pichurko BM, Slutsky AS, Sarkarati M, Rossier A, Brown R. Changes in lung volume and rib cage configuration with abdominal binding in quadriplegia. *J Appl Physiol.* 1986;60(4):1198-1202.

165. Goldman JM, Rose LS, Williams SJ, Silver JR, Denison DM. Effect of abdominal binders on breathing in tetraplegic patients. *Thorax.* 1986;41(12):940-945.

166. MacLean D, Drummond G, Macpherson C, McLaren G, Prescott R. Maximum expiratory airflow during chest physiotherapy on ventilated patients before and after the application of an abdominal binder. *Intensive Care Med.* 1989;15(6):396-399.

167. Bodin P, Fagevik Olsen M, Bake B, Kreuter M. Effects of abdominal binding on breathing patterns during breathing exercises in persons with tetraplegia. *Spinal Cord.* 2005;43(2):117-122.

168. Estenne M, Pinet C, De Troyer A. Abdominal muscle strength in patients with tetraplegia. *Am J Respir Crit Care Med.* 2000;161(3, Pt 1):707-712.

169. Hopkins RO, Jackson JC. Long-term neurocognitive function after critical illness. *Chest.* 2006;130(3):869-878.

170. Hopkins RO, Weaver LK, Pope D, Orme JF, Bigler ED, Larson-LOHR V. Neuropsychological sequelae and impaired health status in survivors of severe acute respiratory distress syndrome. *Am J Respir Crit Care Med.* 1999;160(1):50-56.

171. Zubeck J, Wilgosh L. Prolonged immobilization of the body: changes in performance and in the electroencephalogram. *Science.* 1963;140:306.

172. Hammer R, Kenan E. The psychological aspects of immobilization. In: Steinberg F, ed. *The immobilized Patient: Functional Pathology and Management.* New York: Plenum Medical Company; 1980:123-149.

173. Greenleaf J, Kozlowski S. Psychological consequences of reduced physical activity during bedrest. *Exerc Sport Sci Rev.* 1982;10:84.

174. Ely EW, Inouye SK, Bernard GR, et al. Delirium in mechanically ventilated patients: validity and reliability of the confusion assessment method for the intensive care unit (CAM-ICU). *JAMA.* 2001;286(21):2703-2710.

175. Plaschke K, von Haken R, Scholz M, et al. Comparison of the confusion assessment method for the intensive care unit (CAM-ICU) with the Intensive Care Delirium Screening Checklist (ICDSC) for delirium in critical care patients gives high agreement rate(s). *Intensive Care Med.* 2008;34(3):431-436.

176. Soja SL, Pandharipande PP, Fleming SB, et al. Implementation, reliability testing, and compliance monitoring of the Confusion Assessment Method for the intensive care unit in trauma patients. *Intensive Care Med.* 2008;34(7):1263-1268.

177. Ely EW, Truman B, Shintani A, et al. Monitoring sedation status over time in ICU patients: reliability and validity of the Richmond Agitation-Sedation Scale (RASS). *JAMA.* 2003;289(22):2983-2991.

178. Teasdale G, Jennette B. Assessment of coma and impaired consciousness. A practical scale. *Lancet.* 1974;2:81-83.

179. Sessler CN, Jo Grap M, Ramsay MA. Evaluating and monitoring analgesia and sedation in the intensive care unit. *Crit Care.* 2008;12(suppl 3):S2.

180. Friman G. Effect of clinical bed rest for seven days on physical performance. *Acta Med Scand.* 1979;205(5):389-393.

181. Bassey EJ, Fentem PH. Extent of deterioration in physical condition during postoperative bed rest and its reversal by rehabilitation. *Br Med J.* 1974;4(5938):194-196.

182. Ruiz Bailen M, Aguayo de Hoyos E, Lopez Martnez A, et al. Reversible myocardial dysfunction, a possible complication in critically ill patients without heart disease. *J Crit Care.* 2003;18(4):245-252.

183. Attia J, Ray JG, Cook DJ, Douketis J, Ginsberg JS, Geerts WH. Deep vein thrombosis and its prevention in critically ill adults. *Arch Intern Med.* 2001;161(10):1268-1279.

184. Geerts WH, Bergqvisr D, Pineo GF, et al. Prevention of deep venous thromboembolism: ACCP evidence-based clinical practice guidelines. *Chest.* 2008;133(6):381s-453s.

185. Tepper S, McKeough D. Deep vein thrombosis: risks, diagnosis, treatment interventions and prevention. *Acute Care Perspect.* 2000;9-11.

186. Anand S, Wells P, Hunt D, et al. Does this patient have deep vein thrombosis? *JAMA.* 1998;279:1094-1099.

187. Kearon C, Kahn SR, Giancardo A, Goldhaber S, Raskob GE, Comerota AJ. Antithrombotic therapy for venous thromboboloc disease: ACCP evidence-based clinical practice guidelines. *Chest.* 2008;133:454S-545S.

188. Junger M, Diehm C, Storiko H, et al. Mobilization versus immobilization in the treatment of acute proximal deep venous thrombosis: a prospective, randomized, open, multicentre trial. *Curr Med Res Opin.* 2006;22(3):593-602.

189. Partsch H. Immediate ambulation and leg compression in the treatment of deep vein thrombosis. *Dis Mon.* 2005;51(2–3): 135-140.

190. Stannard JP, Lopez-Ben RR, Volgas DA, et al. Prophylaxis against deep-vein thrombosis following trauma: a prospective, randomized comparison of mechanical and pharmacologic prophylaxis. *J Bone Joint Surg Am.* 2006;88(2):261-266.

191. Hirsh J, Guyatt G, Albers G, Harrington R, Schunemann HJ. Executive summary: ACCP evidence-based clinical practice guidelines. *Chest.* 2008;133(6):71S.

192. Prandoni P, Lensing AW, Prins MH, et al. Below-knee elastic compression stockings to prevent the post-thrombotic syndrome: a randomized, controlled trial. *Ann Intern Med.* 2004;141(4):249-256.

193. Segal JB, Streiff MB, Hofmann LV, Thornton K, Bass EB. Management of venous thromboembolism: a systematic review for a practice guideline. *Ann Intern Med.* 2007;146(3):211-222.

194. Giannoudis PV, Pountos I, Pape HC, Patel JV. Safety and efficacy of vena cava filters in trauma patients. *Injury.* 2007;38(1):7-18.

195. Paton BL, Jacobs DG, Heniford BT, Kercher KW, Zerey M, Sing RF. Nine-year experience with insertion of vena cava filters in the intensive care unit. *Am J Surg.* 2006;192(6):795-800.

196. Aschwanden M, Labs KH, Engel H, et al. Acute deep vein thrombosis: early mobilization does not increase the frequency of pulmonary embolism. *Thromb Haemost.* 2001;85(1):42-46.

197. Kahn SR, Shrier I, Kearon C. Physical activity in patients with deep venous thrombosis: a systematic review. *Thromb Res.* 2008:122(6):763-73.

198. Trujillo-Santos J, Perea-Milla E, Jimenez-Puente A, et al. Bed rest or ambulation in the initial treatment of patients with acute deep vein thrombosis or pulmonary embolism: findings from the RIETE registry. *Chest.* 2005;127(5):1631-1636.

199. Phillips SM, Gallagher M, Buchan H. Use graduated compression stockings postoperatively to prevent deep vein thrombosis. *BMJ.* 2008;336(7650):943-944.

200. Palevsky H, Kelley M, Fishman A. Pulmonary thromboembolic disease. In: Fishman A, ed. *Fishmans Pulmonary Diseases and Disorders.* 3rd ed. New York: McGraw-Hill; 1998:1310-1325.

201. Cook D, McMullin J, Hodder R, et al. Prevention and diagnosis of venous thromboembolism in critically ill patients: a Canadian survey. *Crit Care.* 2001;5(6):336-342.

202. Ferrando AA, Lane HW, Stuart CA, Davis-Street J, Wolfe RR. Prolonged bed rest decreases skeletal muscle and whole body protein synthesis. *Am J Physiol.* 1996;270(4, Pt 1):E627-E633.

203. Berg HE, Larsson L, Tesch PA. Lower limb skeletal muscle function after 6 wk of bed rest. *J Appl Physiol.* 1997;82(1):182-188.

204. Bloomfield SA. Changes in musculoskeletal structure and function with prolonged bed rest. *Med Sci Sports Exerc.* 1997;29(2):197-206.

205. Dellestable F, Voltz C, Mariot J, Perrier JF, Gaucher A. Heterotopic ossification complicating long-term sedation. *Br J Rheumatol.* 1996;35(7):700-701.

206. Evans EB. Heterotopic bone formation in thermal burns. *Clin Orthop Relat Res.* 1991(263):94-101.

207. Garland DE. Clinical observations on fractures and heterotopic ossification in the spinal cord and traumatic brain injured populations. *Clin Orthop Relat Res.* 1988(233):86-101.

208. Pape HC, Lehmann U, van Griensven M, Gansslen A, von Glinski S, Krettek C. Heterotopic ossifications in patients after severe blunt trauma with and without head trauma: incidence and patterns of distribution. *J Orthop Trauma.* 2001;15(4): 229-237.

209. Sugita A, Hashimoto J, Maeda A, et al. Heterotopic ossification in bilateral knee and hip joints after long-term sedation. *J Bone Miner Metab.* 2005;23(4):329-332.

210. Clavet H, Hebert PC, Fergusson D, Doucette S, Trudel G. Joint contracture following prolonged stay in the intensive care unit. *CMAJ.* 2008;178(6):691-697.

211. Yarkony GM, Bass LM, Keenan V III, Meyer PR Jr. Contractures complicating spinal cord injury: incidence and comparison between spinal cord centre and general hospital acute care. *Paraplegia.* 1985;23(5):265-271.

212. Bryden AM, Kilgore KL, Lind BB, Yu DT. Triceps denervation as a predictor of elbow flexion contractures in C5 and C6 tetraplegia. *Arch Phys Med Rehabil.* 2004;85(11):1880-1885.

213. Grover J, Gellman H, Waters RL. The effect of a flexion contracture of the elbow on the ability to transfer in patients who have quadriplegia at the sixth cervical level. *J Bone Joint Surg Am.* 1996;78(9):1397-1400.

214. De Jonghe B, Sharshar T, Lefaucheur JP, et al. Paresis acquired in the intensive care unit: a prospective multicenter study. *JAMA.* 2002;288(22):2859-2867.

215. Schweickert WD, Hall J. ICU-acquired weakness. *Chest.* 2007; 131(5):1541-1549.

216. Hermans G, Wilmer A, Meersseman W, et al. Impact of intensive insulin therapy on neuromuscular complications and ventilator dependency in the medical intensive care unit. *Am J Respir Crit Care Med.* 2007;175(5):480-489.

217. Hermans G, De Jonghe B, Bruyninckx F, Van den Berghe G. Interventions for preventing critical illness polyneuropathy and critical illness myopathy. *Cochrane Database Syst Rev.* 2009;1:CD006832. 10.1002/14651858.CD006832.pub2.

218. Leatherman JW, Fluegel WL, David WS, Davies SF, Iber C. Muscle weakness in mechanically ventilated patients with severe asthma. *Am J Respir Crit Care Med.* 1996;153(5):1686-1690.

219. Segredo V, Caldwell JE, Matthay MA, Sharma ML, Gruenke LD, Miller RD. Persistent paralysis in critically ill patients after long-term administration of vecuronium. *N Engl J Med.* 1992; 327(8):524-528.

220. De Jonghe B, Lacherade JC, Durand MC, Sharshar T. Critical illness neuromuscular syndromes. *Crit Care Clin.* 2007;23 (1):55-69.

221. Angel MJ, Bril V, Shannon P, Herridge MS. Neuromuscular function in survivors of the acute respiratory distress syndrome. *Can J Neurol Sci.* 2007;34(4):427-432.

222. Garnacho-Montero J, Amaya-Villar R, Garcia-Garmendia JL, Madrazo-Osuna J, Ortiz-Leyba C. Effect of critical illness polyneuropathy on the withdrawal from mechanical ventilation and the length of stay in septic patients. *Crit Care Med.* 2005;33(2):349-354.

223. De Jonghe B, Bastuji-Garin S, Sharshar T, Outin H, Brochard L. Does ICU-acquired paresis lengthen weaning from mechanical ventilation? *Intensive Care Med.* 2004;30(6):1117-1121.

224. Latronico N, Shehu I, Seghelini E. Neuromuscular sequelae of critical illness. *Curr Opin Crit Care.* 2005;11(4):381-390.

225. Macciocchi S, Seel RT, Thompson N, Byams R, Bowman B. Spinal cord injury and co-occurring traumatic brain injury: assessment and incidence. *Arch Phys Med Rehabil.* 2008;89(7):1350-1357.

226. Ciesla N, Ridriequez A, Anderson P, Norton B. The incidence of extrapleural hematomas in patients with rib fractures. *Phys Ther.* 1987;67:766.

227. Imle P. Percussion and vibration. In: Mackenzie C, ed. *Chest Physiotherapy in the Intensive Care Unit.* 2nd ed. Baltimore, MD: Williams & Wilkins; 1989:141.

228. Kigin C. Advances in chest physical therapy. In: O'Donohue WJ, ed. *Current Advances in Respiratory Care.* Park Ridge, IL: American College of Chest Physicians; 1984:145.

229. Hopkins RO, Spuhler VJ, Thomsen GE. Transforming ICU culture to facilitate early mobility. *Crit Care Clin.* 2007;23(1):81-96.

230. Burns JR, Jones FL. Letter: Early ambulation of patients requiring ventilatory assistance. *Chest.* 1975;68(4):608.

231. King J, Crowe J. Mobilization practices in Canadian critical care units. *Physiotherapy Canada.* 1998(Summer):206-211.

232. Morris PE, Herridge MS. Early intensive care unit mobility: future directions. *Crit Care Clin.* 2007;23(1):97-110.

233. Stiller K. Physiotherapy in intensive care: towards an evidence-based practice. *Chest.* 2000;118(6):1801-1813.

234. Heyland DK, Groll D, Caeser M. Survivors of acute respiratory distress syndrome: relationship between pulmonary dysfunction and long-term health-related quality of life. *Crit Care Med.* 2005;33(7):1549-1556.

235. Dowdy DW, Eid MP, Dennison CR, et al. Quality of life after acute respiratory distress syndrome: a meta-analysis. *Intensive Care Med.* 2006;32(8):1115-1124.

236. Stevens RD, Dowdy DW, Michaels RK, Mendez-Tellez PA, Pronovost PJ, Needham DM. Neuromuscular dysfunction acquired in critical illness: a systematic review. *Intensive Care Med.* 2007;33(11):1876-1891.

237. MacIntyre N. Evidence-based guidelines for weaning and discontinuing ventilatory support. *Chest.* 2001;120(6):375S-395S.

238. De Jonghe B, Lacherade JC, Durand MC, Sharshar T. Critical illness neuromuscular syndromes. *Crit Care Clin.* 2006;22(4):805-818.

Physical Therapy Associated with Ventilatory Pump Dysfunction and Failure

Mary Massery & Lawrence P. Cahalin

INTRODUCTION

The physical therapy examinations and interventions presented in this chapter focus on the patient with cardiopulmonary dysfunction fitting the model of preferred Practice Pattern 6E: *Impaired Ventilation and Respiration/Gas Exchange Associated with Ventilatory Pump Dysfunction or Failure.*[1] In the first edition of the *Guide to Physical Therapy Practice* in 1997,[2] this pattern was separated into two different practice patterns to distinguish ventilatory pump dysfunction (PPP 6F) from ventilatory pump failure (PPP 6H). However, the main difference between the dysfunction and the failure is the

severity and/or acuity of the dysfunction; thus, it is more appropriate that they be grouped into one practice pattern. In this way, particular levels of impairment or function may be used to specifically distinguish ventilatory pump dysfunction from ventilatory pump failure using identifiable characteristics within a continuum of ventilatory pump function. As we shall see, several specific patient characteristics can be used to distinguish ventilatory pump dysfunction from failure that will enable more specific and appropriate physical therapy interventions.

VENTILATORY PUMP DYSFUNCTION

Ventilatory pump dysfunction can be caused by a wide variety of pathologies and impairments. Identifying the primary pathology or impairments is critical to the physical therapist for planning and implementing an effective intervention plan. In the *Guide,* four broad categories of pathologies and impairments were identified to help the physical therapist categorize their patient's primary impairment pattern.[1] These pathology and impairment categories are (1) musculoskeletal, (2) neuromuscular, (3) cardiopulmonary, and (4) integumentary. Practice Pattern 6E would include patients who frequently come from the cardiopulmonary impairment category and may include patients with a number of different primary pulmonary disorders such as asthma, emphysema, chronic bronchitis, and restrictive lung disease, among others. In other words, if the lung disorder causes a patient to work harder than a normal person for their next breath, then the ventilatory pump will be impaired secondary to the lung disorder.[1] **The primary goal of the physical therapist should be to identify the degree of impairment and functional capacity, regardless of the pathology.**

Ventilatory pump dysfunction can originate from any of the other pathology and impairment categories (musculoskeletal, neuromuscular, cardiopulmonary, or integumentary). These pathologies and impairments are listed under the

"Patient/Clients Diagnostic Classification" section of each practice pattern.[1] For example, "severe kyphoscoliosis" is listed under Pattern 6E as a cause for ventilatory pump dysfunction. Why? Because, pump dysfunction will occur where there is a restriction to the mobility of the chest wall and/or spine (ie, with arthritis, scoliosis, kyphosis, traumas). The resultant restriction will decrease the efficiency and/or the potential for optimal function of the ventilatory muscle pump.

Likewise, patients with "neuromuscular disorders" are also listed as patients with potential ventilatory pump dysfunction. Neurologic disease or trauma can affect the strength and motor control of the trunk as well as the respiratory muscles, which may cause ventilatory pump dysfunction (ie, spinal cord injury, brain injuries, cerebral palsy, multiple sclerosis, or Parkinson disease).

Last, patients with integumentary disorders, in whom the movement of skin or other connective tissue over the spine, rib cage, and proximal extremity joints (such as the upper extremities, lower extremities, or neck) is limited, may also present with ventilatory pump dysfunction. Patients with burns and connective tissue disorders may have such a ventilatory pump dysfunction. Thus, simply because the practice pattern states that the problem is "ventilatory pump dysfunction," the cause of that dysfunction may not initially stem from the cardiopulmonary system (Table 20-1).

TABLE 20-1 Impairment Categories from the *Guide to PT Practice*: A Sampling of Diagnoses Associated with Ventilatory Pump Dysfunction or Failure Originating from That Category

Cardiopulmonary	Asthma, emphysema, chronic bronchitis, pneumonia, pulmonary fibrosis, pulmonary hypertension, cystic fibrosis, etc. Any primary lung dysfunction that results in impaired mechanics of the ventilatory pump.
Musculoskeletal	Arthritis, scoliosis, kyphosis, other disorders of the spine or rib cage, etc. Any musculoskeletal disorder or trauma that results in impaired mechanics of the ventilatory pump.
Neuromuscular	Spinal cord injury (SCI), brain injuries, cerebral palsy, muscular dystrophy, multiple sclerosis, cerebral vascular accidents (CVA), Parkinson, etc. Any neuromuscular disease or trauma that results in impaired mechanics of the ventilatory pump.
Integumentary	Burns, connective tissue disorders, etc. Any integumentary disease or trauma that results in impaired mechanics of the ventilatory pump.

VENTILATORY PUMP FAILURE

Ventilatory pump failure occurs when the demands placed on the ventilatory muscles prevents adequate ventilation and respiration. Ventilatory pump failure is commonly diagnosed by an elevation in partial pressure of carbon dioxide (PCO_2) and reduction in partial pressure of oxygen, arterial (PaO_2). Ventilation is also reduced.

Ventilatory pump failure can result from abnormal lung tissue or poor ventilatory muscle performance. Abnormal lung tissue from a variety of lung disorders may impose a significant workload on the ventilatory muscles that along with poor ventilation and respiration may eventually cause them to fail. It has been suggested that ventilatory pump failure can be recognized by a paradoxical breathing pattern. There are several different paradoxical breathing patterns, and the paradoxical breathing pattern most often associated with ventilatory pump failure (and likely most often observed) is an abdominal paradoxical breathing pattern that is seen in patients with severe chronic obstructive pulmonary disease (COPD). The patient with neuromuscular pathology will often show a different paradoxical pattern where the belly rises and the chest falls (upper chest paradoxical breathing).

The effects of severe COPD and hyperinflated lungs as well as limited diaphragmatic excursion appear to produce a less efficient diaphragmatic descent during breathing. The inefficient diaphragmatic descent and subsequent ineffective ventilation of the lungs stimulate the accessory muscles of breathing to play a more active role in breathing. As such, patients often exhibit a breathing pattern that is characterized by an inward movement of the abdomen and outward movement of the upper chest during inspiration rather than by the normal breathing pattern of simultaneous outward movements of the abdomen and upper chest during inspiration.

FACTORS ASSOCIATED WITH NORMAL AND PARADOXICAL BREATHING

Two factors that appear to be associated with development of an abdominal paradoxical breathing are hyperinflation of the lungs and the subsequent flattening of the diaphragm. The flattening of the diaphragm is likely to produce two specific changes including (1) a greater use of accessory muscles for inspiration and (2) an inward pull on the lower ribs when the flattened and shortened costal diaphragmatic muscle fibers contract with a different angle of inclination. The greater use of the accessory muscles generates a negative pressure in the upper chest area rather than the normal generation of negative pressure in the abdominal area from the downward descent of the diaphragm. If the diaphragm is unable to generate adequate negative intrathoracic pressure, the abdominal area may actually be sucked in from the negative pressure generated in the upper chest area (producing an abdominal paradox) from the increased activity of the accessory muscles.

Under normal conditions, the muscles of the diaphragm contract and pull the central tendon and the dome of the diaphragm caudally. The descending diaphragm increases the volume of the thorax. According to Boyle's law, the increased volume in the thorax decreases the intrathoracic pressure, which facilitates inspiration. These particular changes are shown in Fig. 20-1. It is important to note that the biomechanical changes occurring as a result of increased intra-abdominal pressure (letters a and b in Fig. 20-1) are due to specific

Diaphragmatic contraction
↓
Compression of abdominal contents, thus increasing intra-abdominal pressure causing:
(a) Lateral transmission of pressure to the lower ribs = expansion of lower rib cage
(b) Upward and outward motion of lower ribs = bucket handle motion
(c) Anterior/posterior motion of upper ribs = pump handle motion
↓
Increase in thoracic volume vertically and transversely
↓
Decrease in intrathoracic pressure
↓
Facilitates inspiration

FIGURE 20-1 Biomechanics of breathing.

changes in the costal diaphragmatic fibers upon the inner aspect of the lower rib cage (the zone of apposition). The costal diaphragmatic fibers at the lower rib cage within this zone of apposition produce (1) a cranially oriented force on the lower ribs, (2) outward motion of the lower ribs, and (3) separation of the lower ribs, as the abdominal viscera (with adequate abdominal muscle support) opposes the descent of the diaphragmatic dome.

Hyperinflation of the lungs and flattening of the diaphragm shorten the muscle fibers of the diaphragm providing it (1) little to no room to descend downward, (2) an inadequate length–tension relationship, and (3) less activity at the zone of apposition. The aforementioned changes may result in the development of inadequate intrathoracic pressure in the abdominal area and inadequate ventilation of the lungs. As a result, the accessory muscles become more active and generate the needed negative pressure to ventilate the lungs. Therefore, the pump handle motion of the upper chest referred to in Fig. 19-1 may become greater than the bucket handle motion of the lower ribs, resulting in a paradoxical breathing pattern.

In the same manner, excessive bucket handle motion with accompanying lack of structural support in the upper chest may produce an upper chest paradoxical breathing pattern that is characterized by an inward motion of the upper chest and profound outward motion of the abdominal area. Such a breathing pattern is occasionally seen in patients with spinal cord injury or other neurological disorders. It appears to be less often associated with ventilatory pump failure, but may contribute to ventilatory pump failure if the inward upper chest motion is excessive and contributes to an increased work of breathing and decreased degree of lung ventilation.

It is hopefully apparent from these examples that the topic of ventilatory pump dysfunction and failure is so extensive that it would be impossible to discuss every possible patient scenario. Hence, this chapter will focus on one case at length to illustrate cardiopulmonary preferred Practice Pattern 6E. The case presented is the result of a neuromuscular disorder, an SCI, and is the patient case presented in Chapter 18. Why is a spinal cord injury a good example for Pattern 6E? Following an SCI, the mechanics of breathing are compromised because of the weakness and paralysis of the chest wall muscles, thus impairing the ventilatory pump. In fact, these impairments can be so significant that respiratory problems have consistently been identified as the major cause of death in America for this population.[3-5] Therefore, a patient with an SCI shows both ventilatory pump dysfunction and the potential for pump failure. This chapter will follow a patient with a cervical SCI who was first described in the acute phase of injury in Chapter 19 (Practice Pattern 6F). He will be used to illustrate the cardiopulmonary risks, examinations, and interventions associated with patients who have ventilatory pump dysfunction.

MICROANATOMY AND PHYSIOLOGY

The biomechanics of breathing were described in detail in Chapters 4, 5, and 9 and will now be reviewed in respect to the musculoskeletal support that is necessary to prevent ventilatory pump dysfunction. Following this review of both inhalation and exhalation, the case study introduced in Chapter 19 will be presented with emphasis on the biomechanics of breathing following an SCI.

Normal Skeletal Support for Breathing

The rib cage is an inherently mobile structure designed to move three-dimensionally, freely, and efficiently via skeletal support from the thoracic spine and muscle support from the respiratory and postural muscles.[6-10] Without muscle support, the skeletal structure of the rib cage would collapse anteriorly, particularly in an upright posture. This would occur because the only significant stabilization of the thoracic cage is derived from its posterior attachment to the thoracic spine through the costotransverse ligaments. This leaves the anterior chest wall particularly vulnerable to external forces. The costotransverse ligaments, 3 per spinal segment, are aligned in three different planes of movements and overlap the thoracic segment above and below them (see Chapter 4). This provides a very stable posterior junction, limiting chest wall movements and making dislocations or subluxations of the costotransverse joints a rare event (rib shaft fractures are far more common than rib shaft dislocations). On the other hand, the anterior chest wall is attached only to the sternum, which has no inferior bony attachment and superiorly is only attached to the clavicle. This provides little structural support, but maximizes mobility potential. In fact, the lowest rib segments, ribs 8 to 12, are often called "false ribs" because they do not insert into the sternum at all (ribs 10–12), or they insert into the sternum via the seventh rib's cartilage (ribs 8–10), giving these rib segments even greater potential for mobility than ribs 1 to 7.

Clinically, we see these skeletal facts played out when a therapist examines a patient's breathing pattern. The therapist will find greater anterior chest movement and less posterior chest movement during inhalation. Hence, the rib cage's structural support significantly influences breathing in the anterior and posterior chest (see Chapter 9).

Normal Muscle Support for Breathing: A "Triad" of Support for Inhalation

How do the muscles of the trunk allow optimal mechanical alignment of the thoracic cage and thoracic spine in stationary, static postures while still allowing the active movements of breathing and dynamic trunk movements? Here we will discuss the most significant muscle groups involved in the dual role of providing trunk stability and trunk/respiratory movement.

Recall that the diaphragm is the major muscle of inspiration. Add to that, the importance of two other muscles, the intercostals and the abdominal, which provide the proper pressure support necessary for the diaphragm to move optimally and efficiently, creating a "triad of muscles" for optimal quiet breathing (Table 20-2). The diaphragm provides the

TABLE 20-2   **Muscle Support Necessary for Optimal Inspiratory Function: A "Triad" of Support**

Diaphragm	Provides approximately 75% of the effort during normal inspiratory lung volume. Shape allows for three-dimensional movement that optimizes the potential inspiratory lung volume. Innervated by C3–C5
Intercostals	Necessary to stabilize the inherently mobile rib cage to prevent the chest wall from collapsing inward toward the negative pressure created during inhalation, thus maximizing the diaphragm's effectiveness Innervated T1–T12
Abdominals	Provides abdominal wall support to maintain visceral position up and under the dome of the diaphragm. Also serves to stabilize the descending central tendon to stimulate diaphragm's peripheral fiber contractions and intercostal contractions Innervated T5–T12

greatest volume displacement, whereas the intercostal muscles stabilize the chest wall, and the abdominal muscles provide visceral support for the descending fibers of the diaphragm's central tendon.[11] This results in an increase in circumferential expansion of the chest which is noted as a "positive" chest wall expansion measurement when assessed with a tape measure during inspiration (see Chapter 9).[12,13]

The contraction of the diaphragm initiates the inhalation phase by essentially creating a vacuum, a negative inspiratory force (NIF), within the chest cavity. The NIF facilitates the movement of air from the atmosphere (positive pressure) into the lungs (now a negative pressure system). Air in the atmosphere rushes into the lungs because of the development of this area of negative pressure during inspiration (movement from a high-pressure to low-pressure area is common in this and many other similar pressure systems). This creates positive pressure within the lungs and chest cavity and therefore forces air out during exhalation. Without the active participation of the intercostal muscles to lift the upper chest upward and outward, the anterior chest wall would collapse inward during inhalation, toward the negative pressure.[14–16] This abnormal type of breathing pattern is called an *upper chest paradoxical breathing pattern* and is characterized by the excessive rising of the abdomen and the simultaneous collapse of the anterior rib cage. Frequently this collapse is seen near the junction of the xiphoid process and the corresponding ribs because without the intercostal muscle's support, this area of the chest wall has the greatest potential mobility and the least anatomical stability. Clinically, this is seen in patients with spinal cord injury and may result in the development of a pectus excavatum, otherwise known as a concave deformity along the lower sternum.

The importance of the stabilizing function of the intercostal and abdominal muscles was noted while taking chest wall expansion measurements of patients with complete cervical

SCIs.[13] While measuring inspiratory expansion at the xiphoid process in supine, every patient in the study demonstrated paradoxical or inward movements of the upper chest. Measurements with a tape measure revealed negative upper chest wall movements of one-fourth in or more of upper chest wall depression during inspiration. The expected positive upper chest wall expansion of resting (or quiet) inspiration did not occur and was replaced with an inward paradoxical motion of the upper chest. The reason that this was observed was likely due to a lack of intercostal muscle contraction that left the upper chest unsupported during inspiration. As the descending diaphragm created greater negative pressure, the upper chest simply fell into the vacuum created by the descending diaphragm.

Worse yet, when the patients were asked to take a deep breath (or vital capacity breathing), creating an even greater negative inspiratory pressure, the inward paradoxical movement of the upper chest wall became more severe with as much as two in of depression in many of the patients. Can patients with SCI generate the kind of negative pressure gradients that would cause a collapse of the rib cage? Yes. As long as their diaphragm remains functional, patients with SCI can still generate significant negative inspiratory mouth pressures (PI_{max}). A study by Gounden[17] found that patients with cervical SCI could generate a mean PI_{max} of -65 cm H_2O (see Chapter 9 for normal values and methods of measuring PI_{max}; normal PI_{max} for this patient population was between -75 and -100 cm H_2O). Thus, patients must have adequate function of the intercostal muscles to support the negative inspiratory pressures necessary for effective breathing strategies.

The last muscle group in the normal triad of breathing is the abdominal muscles. These muscles provide positive-pressure support on the viscera in order to maintain their placement up and under the dome of the diaphragm in upright postures. The abdominal muscles also provide positive-pressure support for the diaphragm to help stabilize the central tendon during the initial phase of inhalation. Without functional abdominal muscles, the abdominal contents will rest too low in the abdominal cavity in upright positions and produce a classic "beer belly" appearance which is frequently seen in patients with spinal cord injury (Fig. 20-2A). The lack of abdominal muscle support and lower resting position of the abdominal contents places the diaphragm's resting position very low in the thoracic cavity which reduces its length–tension relationship and mechanical efficiency. In addition, without abdominal muscle support (as in spinal cord injury), the central tendon of a descending diaphragm moves excessively in an inferior plane because of the absence of positive abdominal pressure. This excessive movement in the inferior plane produces paradoxical breathing characterized by greater lower abdominal protrusion and simultaneous flattening of the upper abdominal wall.[16,18] This paradoxical breathing pattern is also referred to as "belly breathing" (see Chapter 9). This paradoxical breathing can be reversed, or at least minimized by the use of an abdominal binder in upright.[19] Finally, a classic study by McCool[20] showed that providing a "substitute"

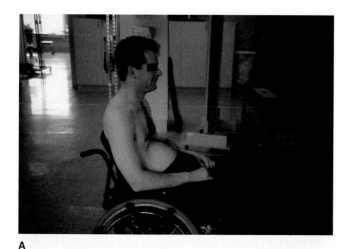

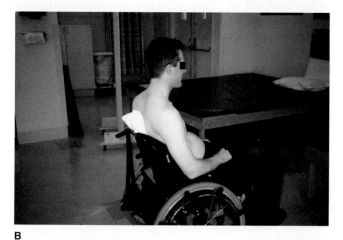

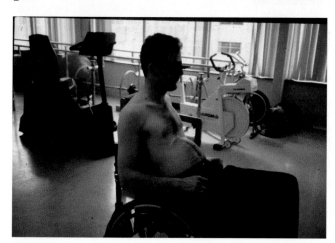

FIGURE 20-2 (**A**) Typical posture of a patient with cervical spinal cord injury in sitting. Lee demonstrates inadequate muscle strength to mechanically hold the trunk and vertebrae in proper alignment. Note the appearance of a "beer belly," protracted scapulae, internally rotated shoulders, and a mid-trunk fold between the ribs and abdomen. (**B**) Use of a towel roll as a temporary seating position adjunct: placed vertically along thoracic and lumbar spine to provide posterior mechanical stabilization. (**C**) Note the improvement in trunk alignment compared to "A": expansion of anterior chest wall, shoulder external rotation, scapular retraction towards neutral, and a reduced mid-trunk fold between ribs and viscera. Lee would also benefit from an abdominal binder to support the viscera.

abdominal muscle support through the use of an abdominal binder for patients with tetraplegia resulted in greater total lung capacity and greater chest wall excursion than that without the binding.

Abdominal muscle support also appears necessary to provide the stimulation to activate the intercostal muscles during normal chest wall development in the first 12 months of life.[21] If the child is hypotonic, that is, congenital hypotonia, Down Syndrome, and so forth, the diaphragm will continue to move primarily in an inferior plane as a newborn does, rather than recruiting its peripheral fibers and the intercostals at around 6 months of age. This results in a similar muscle imbalance as seen in adult patients with weak or paralyzed intercostals, but the resultant chest wall deformities (usually a pectus excavatum, rib flares, and concave anterior ribs around ribs 6–8) tend to be more extreme in the child. The irony is that the child may actually have innervation to the intercostal musculature but was never given the correct environmental cues to stimulate his or her development.

For all of the previously cited reasons, the primary muscles of inspiration appear to exist as a "triad" of coordinated muscle contractions among the diaphragm, intercostals, and abdominals, rather than as a sole diaphragmatic contraction.[22–24] Together, these muscles support the function and efficiency of the inspiratory effort in both normal quiet breathing and vital capacity maneuvers.[25] Other muscles assist in ventilation and are referred to as "accessory muscles of ventilation." A summary of the most significant accessory muscles is listed on Table 20-3.

TABLE 20-3   Significant Accessory Muscles of Ventilation

Erector spinae	Stabilizes thorax posteriorly to allow normal anterior chest wall movement to occur. Innervated at T_1–S_3
Pectoralis muscles	Provides upper chest anterior and lateral expansion. Innervated C_5–T_1 Can be taught to stabilize rib cage following paralysis of the inter-costal muscles. Can be recruited as an expiratory muscle.
Serratus anterior	Provides posterior expansion of rib cage when upper extremities are fixated. Innervated C_5–C_7 Only inspiratory muscle that is paired with trunk flexion movements rather than trunk extension movements.
Scalenes	Provides superior and anterior expansion of the upper chest. Innervated C_3–C_8
Sternocleidomastoid	Same as scalenes Innervated C_2–C_3 and accessory cranial nerve
Trapezius	Provides superior expansion of the upper chest Innervated C_2–C_4 and accessory cranial nerve

Examples of Inspiratory Pump Dysfunction

What happens to the ventilatory pump when the muscles of the trunk can no longer support an ideal skeletal alignment to facilitate proper biomechanics of breathing? Does it only pertain to patients with neuromuscular weakness? No. Ventilatory biomechanical dysfunction can stem from any impairment category. An example from each of the *Guide*'s four major impairment groups will demonstrate this dysfunction.

Neuromuscular—When a patient with weak or paralyzed trunk muscles attempts to assume an independent sitting posture, the patient's spine collapses into a kyphotic posture, the chest collapses forward, and the abdominal contents protrude anteriorly and inferiorly ("beer belly" impression).[26] Mechanically, the rib cage is then "blocked" from expanding in the anterior and lateral plane, thus markedly restricting inspiratory potential. In addition, this same patient also loses expiratory

potential because of paralyzed intercostal and abdominal muscles. Consequently, 1-single injury can cause the patient to lose both inspiratory and expiratory lung function, creating ventilatory pump dysfunction or failure. To give the reader even more detailed examples, Table 20-4 presents specific respiratory muscle impairments as it relates to patients with spinal cord injuries.

Cardiopulmonary—Consider the child with significant asthma. From a young age, the child learns to excessively recruit his accessory muscles to meet the increased workload associated with "pulling air" into the lungs. This will result in abnormal development of the respiratory muscles and an abnormal appreciation of what "normal breathing" should be. The child may present to the clinician with elevated shoulders, an elevated sternal angle, a pectus excavatum, a thoracic kyphosis, excessive inferior descent of the diaphragm, and

TABLE 20-4   Functional Limitations to Breathing Secondary to Spinal Cord Injury

Paraplegia Primarily T1–T5	Weakened and/or absent
	  Abdominals
	  Intercostals
	  Erector spinae
	Planes of ventilation limited
	  Slight decrease in anterior and lateral expansion
	Resulting in
	  Slight to moderate decrease in chest expansion and vital capacity (VC)
	  Decreased ability to build up intrathoracic and intra-abdominal pressures
	  Decreased cough effectiveness
	  May show paradoxical breathing

Tetraplegia C5–C8	Missing aforementioned muscles and weakened
	  Pectoralis
	  Serratus anterior
	  Scalenes
	Planes of ventilation limited
	  Marked decrease in anterior and lateral expansion
	  Slight decrease in posterior expansion
	Resulting in
	  Significant decrease in chest expansion and VC
	  Significant decrease in forced expiratory volume
	  Significant decrease in cough effectiveness
	  Paradoxical breathing in acute phase and perhaps longer

Tetraplegia C4	Missing aforementioned muscles and weakened
	  Scalenes
	  Diaphragm
	Planes of ventilation limited
	  Marked decrease in anterior and lateral expansion
	  Slight decrease in inferior and superior expansion
	Resulting in
	  Limitations mentioned previously but now more pronounced
	  May show decrease in tidal volume (TV)
	  May need mechanical ventilation

Tetraplegia C3–C1	Missing aforementioned muscles and weakened and/or absent, the last of the
	  remaining accessory muscles
	  Sternocleidomastoid (SCM)
	  Trapezius
	Planes of ventilation limited
	  All severely limited
	Resulting in
	  Significant decrease in TV
	  Most will require mechanical ventilation 20–24 h/d

excessive recruitment of the trapezius and sternocleidomastoid muscles. Thus, although asthma caused the initial muscle pump dysfunction, poor neuromuscular recruitment of respiratory muscles, and the resultant imbalance in the strength and length–tension relationships of these muscles, exacerbates the pump dysfunction.[27,28]

Musculoskeletal—Consider the teenager with idiopathic scoliosis or the geriatric patient with spontaneous collapsed vertebrae.[29] These musculoskeletal pathologies will likely produce mild to moderate pulmonary impairments due to pain and poor spinal alignment which will limit breathing and subsequent chest wall movement. Patients with such pathologies and impairments are frequently treated with a thoracic brace, such as a total contact thoracic-lumbar-sacral-orthosis (TLSO), to stabilize the spine and thoracic cavity. However, most TLSOs are provided to patients without an abdominal cutout that may have adverse pulmonary effects. In fact, patients may begin to complain of shortness of breath almost immediately after the TLSO is applied. Patients may be told that "it is in their head" because they have a skeletal problem not a cardiopulmonary problem. However, the only ventilatory muscle really capable of assisting with breathing for a person in a TLSO without an abdominal cutout is the trapezius muscle (which has limited respiratory muscle function because it only expands the chest in the superior plane). The trapezius is the only muscle capable of assisting with breathing, because the diaphragm's inspiratory descent is limited by the TLSO that does not allow for adequate forward displacement of the viscera. Therefore, the diaphragm is essentially locked into a very limited "range of motion." Likewise, the TLSO also limits the ability of the intercostals, sternocleidomastoid, and scalene muscles from expanding the upper chest. The limited upper chest motion and diaphragmatic descent will result in less generation of negative pressure necessary for ventilation and will ultimately produce increased dyspnea, work of breathing, and oxygen consumption.[30]

Therefore, a TLSO with an abdominal cutout will allow for optimal visceral displacement during the diaphragm's inspiratory descent. Thus, the initial musculoskeletal problem that produced a mild to moderate pulmonary impairment was exacerbated from the application of a TLSO without an abdominal cutout that restricted diaphragmatic descent and optimal biomechanics of breathing.

Integumentary—Consider the patient with chest and upper extremity burns.[31] Initially, pain would limit chest wall excursion, but as the scars heal and the resultant skin tissue and grafts become more fibrotic, the connective tissue itself may limit chest wall excursion and cause muscle imbalances from disuse atrophy or poor length–tension relationships for the anterior chest wall musculature. If this patient develops a significant kyphotic posture as a result of an extensive burn, it is possible that a posterior chest wall breathing pattern will emerge. As presented earlier, there is limited natural excursion posteriorly because of the stability provided by the rib cage

with the thoracic spine, so each posterior inspiration would require a much greater effort for the patient, thus adding to his ventilatory pump dysfunction.

Normal Muscle Support for Breathing: Exhalation

Not only is inspiration compromised from a variety of different disease/trauma situations, but also exhalation and its many functions can become compromised. Classically, exhalation is described as a passive activity caused by the release of the diaphragmatic contraction and by the natural elastic recoil properties of the lungs.[32] This makes exhalation very energy efficient, consuming very little if any oxygen in the process. However, exhalation can also be active for normal activities, such as in coughing or talking. The change in the expiratory process is described here first for normal function and then for those patients with ventilatory pump dysfunction resulting in poor expiratory maneuvers. Active exhalation is achieved by either an eccentric or a concentric contraction of the respiratory muscles. The process is distinctly different and will be discussed in the following section.

Eccentric Exhalation

In eccentric exhalation, the expiratory phase is prolonged by slowly releasing (eccentric contractions) the inspiratory muscles until the chest wall and lungs are near functional residual capacity (FRC), at which time the expiratory muscles become active.[33–35] Prolonged controlled exhalation is necessary for speech production or for gentle pursed-lip breathing.[36] For speech, the use of eccentric expiration allows for precisely controlled volume and flow rates through the vocal folds for the optimal production of vocal sounds. For normal adults, a typical vocalization of a vowel sound can be sustained for 15 seconds,[34] but it is not uncommon for the trained individual (ie, singers, wind-instrument players, long-distance athletes) to sustain a vowel sound for 30 to 60 seconds.

If, instead of eccentrically releasing the air, the air is allowed to passively escape during exhalation, the speech pattern will sound very breathy, the vocalization will be sustained for only a brief period of time (often only 1–3 seconds), and there will be markedly fewer syllables per breath (often only 1–3 rather than the normal of 8–10). There will also be a notable "falling" of the chest wall during exhalation, as the patient cannot slow down the expiratory maneuver. This undesired passive exhalation may be a result of (1) poor motor control, (2) weakness or paralysis of the respiratory muscles, (3) pain, (4) vocal fold dysfunction, or (5) the presence of a tracheostomy tube which prevents the patient from using his or her glottis to aid in the eccentric maneuver. This results in the patient inhaling larger inspiratory volumes prior to talking in order to sustain their expiratory effort, or in the patient learning to talk by forcefully (concentrically) contracting the expiratory muscles.[37] Both compensations lead to greater energy expenditure.[38]

Consequently, many patients who present with poor eccentric control of their respiratory muscles will complain of fatigue when talking, especially on the phone. To compensate, they may withdraw socially or respond to questions with short answers. Inevitably, if respiratory muscle dysfunction limits a patient's social interactions, it may contribute to the development of depression.[39]

Concentric Exhalation

The other type of active exhalation pattern is a concentric exhalation pattern. This occurs when the air is forcibly expelled (ie, coughing or yelling), calling into action a concentric contraction of the expiratory muscles. The intercostals and abdominal are the primary muscles recruited for this activity, although the pectoralis and latisimus dorsi muscles can also be recruited. When these muscles contract, they apply significant positive pressure on the thoracic cavity to assist in fast and forceful expirations. These expiratory flow rates, which are termed *peak expiratory flow rates* (PEFR), are generally between 6 and 12 L/s as determined by the individual's sex, height and age.[40,41] However, in patients who are unable to adequately contract the above expiratory muscles beneath a functional glottis (because of paralysis, weakness, pain, or a tracheostomy tube), the PEFR may be so low that forceful, concentric exhalation becomes ineffective for expelling particles from the airway.[41-43] This would obviously impair the patient's ability to cough or clear their airways, as well as impair their ability to talk loudly.

Examples of Inspiratory/Expiratory Pump Dysfunction and Failure Stemming from Primary Lung Disease

Primary lung diseases can also result in secondary dysfunction of the inspiratory and expiratory muscles. The muscles themselves may be functional and capable of demonstrating passive, concentric, and eccentric patterns, but the disease process demands that the expiratory muscles are activated with every expiratory effort, causing the patient significant fatigue. For example, the patient with a COPD, such as emphysema, may report of greater difficulty with expiratory maneuvers than with inspiratory maneuvers. An extended example of how obstructive and restrictive lung disease can adversely affect the normal biomechanics of breathing is presented in the following paragraphs.

Emphysema causes destruction to the alveolar sacs, resulting in the creation of large bulbous distal air sacs which in turn creates (1) excessive compression forces on the conducting airways, especially during exhalation, and (2) abnormal increases in the overall inspiratory lung volumes. Over time, this change in lung structure pushes outward on the chest wall, changing the length–tension relationship of the respiratory muscles and changing the alignment of the ribs to the spine. The resultant changes produce the characteristic "barrel chest" appearance of COPD, which adds a significant musculoskeletal impairment to an often-profound lung pathology.[44]

Early in COPD, patients have minimal impairments to the inspiratory muscles in spite of the underlying lung changes. In fact, the pulmonary function test results of patients with early COPD may be 100% of their predicted vital capacity values. However, as COPD advances, many pulmonary function test values become less of a percentage of the predicted value. Forced vital capacity [FVC] and forced expiratory volume in 1 second [FEV_1] in advanced COPD will often be 30% to 60% of the predicted value. Such values demonstrate that the ability to exhale air from the lungs is markedly diminished (only 30%–60% of the expected volume is expelled; see Chapter 9). The diminished ability to exhale air from the lungs is due to the alveolar damage, which traps air within the lungs. During exhalation, the pressure within the thorax, lungs, and airways becomes less negative (possibly even positive), which further increases the already positive pressure within the lungs of a patient with advanced COPD. As the pressures continue to increase within the lungs during exhalation, the distal and proximal airways may become compressed and narrowed which will limit the amount of air moving out of them. This makes patients with advanced COPD forcefully exhale, rather than passively exhale during quiet breathing, to get rid of excessive CO_2. Thus, even though the muscles and skeletal structures are technically intact, the biomechanics of their breathing is now altered, resulting in an increase in their work of breathing and ventilatory pump impairment. As their disease progresses, the chest wall itself is pushed outward by air trapped in destroyed alveoli and compressed airways, decreasing the efficiency of the diaphragm and accessory muscles of inspiration. Eventually, the resting position of the diaphragm itself will be pushed down by the ever-enlarging lung tissue, which will decrease the dome shape of this muscle and render the length–tension relationship of diaphragm less efficient. At the end stage of the disease, the diaphragm's dome may become completely flattened, which would render it ineffective in its ability to increase the chest wall dimensions for inspiration. At this point, the mechanics of both inspiration and exhalation are significantly impaired.

A different presentation is noted in the patient presenting with a restrictive lung disorder such as pulmonary fibrosis or pulmonary hypertension.[45] In this case, the lung tissue resists expansion, hence the term *restrictive lung disease*. The patient must generate a larger than normal NIF to ventilate the lungs. Thus, even though the muscles are neurologically intact, they must use greater force to generate the same inspiratory lung volumes as patients without restrictive lung disease. Unlike the patient with COPD, these patients will show a significant decrease in vital capacity and inspiratory capacity volumes. However, the patient with a restrictive lung disorder can exhale relatively more comfortably than patients with COPD. Patients with obstructive and restrictive lung disease will show an increase in the overall mechanical work of breathing. However, patients with restrictive lung disease will demonstrate more biomechanical impairments to inspiration, and the patients with obstructive lung disease will demonstrate more impairments to the expiratory mechanics until obstructive lung disease becomes more severe.[32,46] Patients with severe end-stage COPD experience marked biomechanical impairments to inspiration and expiration.

The remainder of this chapter will focus on a lengthy illustration of ventilatory pump dysfunction and potential for failure as it pertains to a patient with SCI. Applying these concepts extensively to a single case study will allow a more detailed depiction of how ventilatory pump dysfunction and the potential for failure occurs and what clinicians can do to minimize their impact on patient function. **However, it is important to keep in mind that the examinations and interventions presented in the following case study of a patient with SCI can and should be applied to a patient with ventilatory pump dysfunction or failure from any etiology. Therefore, these same examinations and interventions will likely apply to a patient with COPD, pulmonary fibrosis, or even CVA.**

CASE STUDY

This case study was introduced in Chapter 18 in the ICU setting, where the patient's case was applied to Practice Pattern 6F. It will now be continued into a new setting: the rehabilitation hospital. The patient, Lee, is a 38-year-old male Caucasian postal worker who sustained a motor-complete C5-SCI secondary to a motor vehicle accident (see Chapter 18 for a full detailed description of his ICU experience). The summary report sent to the rehabilitation hospital from his physical therapy (PT) in the ICU states the following:

> On day 20 (in the ICU setting), the patient had increased the periods of spontaneous ventilation to 18 hours per day, using the mechanical ventilator for 6 hours during sleep. The physicians decided to monitor the patient during the night while spontaneously breathing on a continuous positive airway pressure (CPAP) of 8 cm H_2O pressure. The patient tolerated this final step in weaning for the next 48 hours, no longer requiring mechanical ventilation. [See Table, Respiratory Parameters, Day 16, in Chapter 19.] When the patient was weaned from the ventilator, he was tolerating sitting out of bed in a wheelchair with his legs dependent twice daily for 90-minute sessions with the abdominal binder and ace wraps. The nursing and physical therapy staff assisted the patient with pressure relief every 15 to 30 minutes while sitting. He was participating in active and active-assistive ROM [range of motion] exercises to the upper extremities and able to sit on the edge of the bed supported by both upper extremities for 10 minutes. He was able to assist the nurses and therapists with applying abdominal pressure to cough. Although he remained dependent in bed mobility, he could roll side to side and transfer supine to sitting with moderate assistance from a caregiver. The patient was discontinued from this practice pattern due to successful separation from the mechanical ventilator.

This chapter begins with the patient 3 weeks after his SCI accident, as he is transferred to the acute rehabilitation hospital. He was weaned from a mechanical ventilator and was just discontinued from CPAP and O_2 support. He is still paralyzed secondary to the C5–SCI and consequently demonstrates neuromuscular impairments to the ventilatory pump. Upon review of his admitting paperwork, the doctors determine that he is currently medically stable. For these reasons, as he begins his rehabilitation phase, he clearly falls into Practice Pattern 6E: *Impaired Ventilation and Respiration/Gas Exchange Associated with Ventilatory Pump Dysfunction or Failure.*

What will be the overriding cardiopulmonary concerns and risks for this young man as he begins the rehabilitation phase? Will they be different from those in the ICU? One major concern does not change following a patient with SCI regardless of whether he is in the ICU or at home: impaired respiratory mechanics leading to potential respiratory complications/failure.[3,4] Therefore, from the initial admission onward, the entire team will be closely monitoring the patient's respiratory status and determining the degree of ventilatory pump dysfunction or failure.

CARDIOPULMONARY RISKS FOLLOWING A SCI

Table 20-5 lists a summary of many cardiovascular and cardiopulmonary risks for patients with an SCI.[47–49] These risks are then explored specifically as they apply to our patient as he enters the rehabilitation phase of his recovery.

Impaired Respiratory Mechanics

Lee was found to have paralysis of the intercostal and abdominal muscles, which means that, of the core "triad" respiratory muscle groups, only the diaphragm is spared. However, without the muscle support above and below the diaphragm from the intercostals and abdominal muscles, the diaphragm will not be capable of contracting at its highest level of function. In addition to paralysis, his spinal shock is now resolving and spasticity is beginning to develop in his trunk musculature.[50,51] Lee is finding that when he takes in a quick deep breath, it causes spasms and spasticity, which limits his ability to perform a maximal inspiratory effort. He says this shortness of breath is particularly evident when he is telling a story, laughing, or any other "breathing activity" that causes him to spontaneously take quicker inspiratory efforts. He also says that his Halo fixation device (cervical fixation device attached to a trunk vest that restricts cervical motion) restricts his chest causing him to feel confined when he tries to inhale. In fact, between his Halo device and the tracheostomy tube, Lee states that he is finding it impossible to bend forward and tuck his chin to cough, making him sense that he "cannot get the secretions out of his lungs." He also states that his cough is "wimpy."[52] To complicate the matter, he says that he is now experiencing right shoulder

TABLE 20-5   Cardiopulmonary Risk Factors Following an SCI

Impaired respiratory mechanics	• Paralysis/weakness of respiratory/trunk muscles • Abnormal tone: spasms, spasticity, flaccidity. May limit potential inspiratory/expiratory efforts • Posture: thoracic kyphosis, shoulder protraction with internal rotation. May limit chest expansion • Decreased ROM of spine, rib cage, shoulders or pelvis, caused by spinal fixation devices, spasticity, immobility, etc • Decreased cough effectiveness caused by weakness, poor posture, etc • Poor breath support for speech • Presence of a tracheostomy tube or cervical fixation devices such as a Halo or Somi brace • Pain: limiting motion or force
Sleep dysfunction	• Impaired respiratory mechanics. May result in retention of CO_2 at night • Potentially fatal if not detected and attended to
Autonomic dysfunction and cardiovascular dysfunction	• Autonomic dysreflexia: potentially severe cardiopulmonary responses. Can be fatal. • Inability to regulate body temperature • Inability to regulate sweating • Orthostatic hypotension • Significant bradycardia • Risk for development of deep vein thrombosis (DVT) and potential for pulmonary embolus (PE)
Increased risk of infections	• Ongoing risk for urinary tract infections: foley catheter, dehydration, inadequate or infrequent voiding, etc • Ongoing risk for respiratory infections: dehydration, secretion retention, hypoventilation, etc • Ongoing risk for septicemia: unhealed or infected skin injuries/bed sores, loss of sensation (possibly not aware of injury), etc
Heterotopic bone formation	• Limitations in ROM which could limit chest movements and inspiratory efforts
Decubiti (bed sores)	• Skin breakdown which could limit postural changes and secretion mobilization • Invites infections
Poor nutrition/hydration	• Swallowing dysfunction (secondary to tracheostomy tube, cervical fixation device, trauma to vocal folds, etc) • Gastrointestinal bleeds/ulcers, irregularities, etc • Inadequate caloric intake: reduce energy level • Inadequate liquid intake: dehydration
Other inherent risks	• Age: older patients carry higher respiratory risks • Obesity • Other medical history concurrent with SCI • Other past medical/social history • Previous lifestyle

pain. When he recruits his trapezius to take a deep breath, it exacerbates his shoulder pain.

Sleep Dysfunction

Because of impaired respiratory mechanics and the inability to counteract gravity due to weak or paralyzed respiratory muscles, patients with SCI will often develop secondary sleep dysfunction, especially chronic nighttime hypoxemia. If the patient is using a compensatory breathing pattern during the day to maintain his or her lung volumes, but does not spontaneously use this pattern at night, the patient may retain CO_2 during sleep. This may cause the patient's respiratory centers in the brainstem to "wake them up" in order to get

the patient to take a deep breath to blow off CO_2, or else the patient will wake up "groggy and disoriented" from inadequate gas exchange all night (hypoventilation). This may go undetected unless the clinician is aware of its symptoms: nocturnal desaturation (O_2 saturation below 90%), morning headaches, insomnia or frequent "wakeups" during the night, nocturnal restlessness, nightmares of suffocation, difficulty concentrating during the day, falling asleep during the day. This can be serious and even fatal if not diagnosed and treated.[53,54]

Patients with SCI are often reported to have obstructive sleep apnea secondary to supine positioning.[53] Lee reports that he always slept prone or three-fourth prone before his injury, but that now nurses position him supine. He hates sleeping on his back and has increasingly complained of headaches first thing in the morning.

Autonomic Dysfunction and Cardiovascular Dysfunction

Because of the disruption of the autonomic nervous system after a C5–SCI, numerous dysfunctions may occur.[48] During his stay in the ICU, Lee was complaining about being cold (normal hypothermic response immediately following SCI due to excessive peripheral vasodilation), but now he says he is more likely to feel too warm (after a few weeks, reflexive tone returns to peripheral vasculature, and the hypothermia usually resolves, but because the ability to sweat is lost below the level of lesion causing patients with SCI to overheat more easily in the chronic phase). He also stated that other "weird things happened in the ICU": His heart rate ran really low (typical bradycardic response in the acute phase) and he became easily dizzy when they sat him upright (orthostatic hypotension secondary to excessive peripheral vasodilation); but now all that seems better (these abnormal cardiovascular response effects generally resolve approximately 2 to 3 weeks after an SCI).

However, the most frightening incident that he described was his first bout of autonomic dysreflexia which was short lived, but very disturbing. Autonomic dysreflexia is caused by the disruption of the autonomic nervous system below the level of the SCI causing unbalanced sympathetic input. A noxious stimulus below the level of lesion, such as a full bladder, a urinary tract infection, constipation, or even an ingrown toenail, to name a few, starts a whole chain of cardiovascular responses.[48,55] These responses present quickly and often include marked increase in blood pressure (hypertension), marked decrease in heart rate (bradycardia), profuse sweating (above the level of lesion), intense headaches (secondary to the hypertension), flushing (vasodilation above the level of lesion), and anxiety (Table 20-6). This can be life-threatening because of the extreme hypertension. Autonomic dysreflexia, sometimes called hyperreflexia, does not occur until after spinal shock has resolved; thus, it is more commonly seen in the rehabilitation setting or later.[47,48,56]

The last cardiovascular abnormality that may affect our patient is the risk of developing deep vein thrombosis (DVT). During spinal shock, the patient experiences peripheral vasodilation, poor reflexive vascular tone, general immobility, a transient hypercoagulable state, and flaccid paralysis of the lower extremity musculature, all which lead to venous stasis and the potential development of a blood clot (DVT).[48,57] If the blood clot is released into the circulatory system, the patient may develop a pulmonary embolus (PE), which can be fatal. The risk for DVTs and PEs is highest for the first few months following their SCI; hence, thromboprophylaxic measures are aggressively pursued in this population starting in the ICU. Lee reports that his doctors in the ICU put him on a thromoboprophylactic program to minimize this risk, the physical therapists ace-wrapped his legs, and luckily he has not had any problems.[56,58]

TABLE 20-6 Autonomic Dysreflexia

Causes	• Disruption of the autonomic nervous system following SCI • Occurs most frequently above T6 lesion
Progression of episode	• *Starts* with a noxious stimulus: full bladder, rectal distention, or constipation, urinary tract infection, ingrown toenails, or other infections in the body • *Then* profuse sweating, increased blood pressure, and headache (excessive sympathetic response with increased cardiac output and peripheral vasoconstriction) • *Followed by* bradycardia and flushing (secondary increase in parasympathetic activity resulting in decreased heart rate and vasodilation above SCI level)
Signs and symptoms	• Increased blood pressure with resultant pounding headaches • Bradycardia • Facial flushing • Profuse sweating above level of lesion • Anxiety and fear, especially after they have experienced one attack and know the symptoms
Most serious consequence	• Stroke or death due to extreme hypertension

Increased Risk of Infections

In the ICU, our patient had a right lung atelectasis with possible pneumonia, both of which resolved prior to his discharge. However, lately he has not been drinking adequate fluids due to pain, vocal fold irritation (from being intubated initially after the accident), and depression. He is currently slightly dehydrated which dramatically increases his risk for respiratory, urinary, and blood infections, as well as an increased risk for DVTs and poorer overall healing capabilities. It is important to note that respiratory, urinary, and blood infections are some of the most common causes of morbidity in this population.[3,4] This means that an intervention as simple as maintaining adequate hydration levels can have a tremendously positive impact on the patient's successful recovery. It can improve pulmonary secretion mobility, decrease toxic concentrations in the blood, flush bacteria out of the urinary system, and decrease potential noxious stimuli that may trigger autonomic dysreflexia. Hearing this information, Lee declares that he will definitely drink more water now.

Heterotopic Bone Formation

For reasons not yet clear, ectopic bone is often laid in the muscles or other soft tissue beneath the level of lesion of injury following an SCI.[48,59] So far, our patient has not had any signs of heterotopic bone formation, but the staff will be watching for it. If it forms around the spine, shoulder, or pelvis and causes our patient to assume a more kyphotic posture, he will compromise the mechanics of his ventilatory pump, which would cause a decrease in inspiratory lung capacity.

Decubiti (Bed Sores)

Immobility, skin collagen degradation, circulatory changes, dehydration, and decreased sensation all contribute to an increase potential for skin breakdown, especially around bony prominences.[60] Lee preferred to lie on his left side in the ICU, and the nurses' discharge report indicated that he had increased redness around his left greater trochanter. This will have to be watched carefully to make sure the connective tissue does not break down completely and cause an open sore. This opening would invite infections and the potential development of septicemia, as well as limit his available options for positioning.

Poor Nutrition/Hydration

A secondary complication that has only more recently been recognized is poor nutrition and underhydration. Many patients are initially intubated following their SCI, and may develop transient vocal fold dysfunction after they are extubated. In addition, patients may find swallowing difficult due to cervical bracing, or other traumas that occurred with their injury. These oral-motor deficits will increase the risk of aspiration and aspiration pneumonia, as well as decrease the patient's willingness to eat and drink. Furthermore, gastrointestinal (GI) ulcers, bleeds, gastroesophageal reflux (GER), or other GI disorders are not uncommon following SCI.[61,62] Consequently, many SCI acute care facilities are now taking a prophylactic approach and surgically inserting a gastrostomy tube (G-tube) early in the acute phase to ward off these problems and guarantee the delivery of adequate nutrition and hydration. According to his family, our patient's appetite has recently been returning and he has even asked for "Chicago-Style Pizza," so adequate caloric intake no longer appears to be a problem. He has already pledged to increase his hydration level following our discussion noted previously.

Other Inherent Risks

Numerous other cardiopulmonary risks exist, such as advanced age, obesity, other medical problems accrued during the accident,

past medical problems, previous lifestyles, etc. These additional factors all play a role in the patient's potential for a successful rehabilitation. In particular, the patients' outlook following the injury and their outlook on life prior to the injury will influence their outcome. It is not surprising that the most well-adjusted, healthy persons, prior to the SCI, report the highest satisfaction level long after the SCI.[63-65] Our patient comes from a well-grounded family with strong support within both the family and the postal service communities. He was healthy prior to the accident, and had no other medical "risks" to potentially complicate his recovery from the SCI.

SUMMARY OF CARDIOPULMONARY RISKS FOLLOWING A SCI

In light of the preceding information, is our patient at risk for developing secondary cardiopulmonary complications? Yes. Even though he survived the acute phase of his injury and was successfully weaned from the ventilator, he still carries a risk for developing cardiopulmonary problems as long as his paralyzed state remains (Table 20-7). Because the research shows that this risk is higher with a complete SCI injury, and even higher with a cervical rather than a thoracic lesion, our patient and the medical team will need to monitor and reevaluate his cardiopulmonary status on an ongoing basis.[49,66] Also, the often fluctuating status of this patient's and many other patients' ventilatory pump (moving from ventilatory pump dysfunction to the potential for failure and back to dysfunction or even failure) requires frequent examination to determine the degree of dysfunction, potential for failure, or failure.

Examination and Evaluation

What tests and measures are important to consider for this patient or for other patients with ventilatory pump dysfunction, and how do you prioritize your examination to ensure

TABLE 20-7   Lee's SCI Cardiopulmonary Risk Factors

Impaired respiratory mechanics	Yes—*current problem*
Sleep dysfunction	Yes—*current problem*
Autonomic dysfunction and cardiovascular dysfunction	• Autonomic dysreflexia—*1 episode so far, current problem* • Inability to regulate body temperature—*current problem* • Inability to regulate sweating—*current problem* • Orthostatic hypotension—*resolved* • Bradycardia—*resolved* • Risk for development of DVT and PE—*managed with medication*
Increased risk of infections	Yes—*current problem*
Heterotopic bone formation	No—*not a problem at this time*
Decubiti (bed sores)	Fragile site over left greater trochanter—*current problem*
Poor nutrition/hydration	Inadequate caloric intake—*resolved* Inadequate liquid intake—*resolving*
Other inherent risks	None

TABLE 20-8 Appropriate Tests and Measures: Assessing the Cardiopulmonary Status and Function of a Patient with SCI

Medical tests	• Vital signs • ABGs[a] • Oximetry • PFTs • Sputum • X-rays • Cardiac test (ECG) • Renal/urinary tests • Nutrition/hydration/reflux/swallowing dysfunction
Physical tests	• ROM • mmt/muscle tone • Sensation • Skin • Gross motor skills/ADLs • Postural assessment • Breathing pattern assessment • Cough assessment • Breath support for phonation • Sleep assessment • Equipment

[a]ABG, arterial blood gases; ECG, electrocardiogram; PFT, pulmonary function test; ROM, range of motion; MMT, manual muscle test; ADL, activities of daily living.

that the most important tests are completed? In a perfect world, every single possible test would be performed for every single patient. However, this is not realistic. Priorities must be made because of time, money, available resources, patient's fatigue factor, etc. In this section, numerous different assessment tests will be presented with their relative value of information given our particular patient and 6E Practice Pattern. A review of the literature suggests that the following tests and measures are the most important evaluative tools to assess ventilatory pump dysfunction.[32,41,61,62,67,68] They are summarized in Table 20-8 and will be discussed in detail in the following section.

Medical History

A complete medical history is especially important when assessing the complex medical patient. The medical history for this patient can be found in Chapter 19. Our patient was healthy prior to his injury; thus, his medical history does not add complicating factors. However, other patients may have serious extenuating circumstances such as congestive heart failure, emphysema, asthma, hypertension, etc, which will significantly impact the patient's potential progress and functional outcomes relating to their current crisis. For example, let us say that instead of a young, healthy, college student sustaining an SCI, our patient was a 75-year-old sedentary gentleman with a history of emphysema (adding more respiratory compromise) and diabetes (adding more cardiovascular compromise). This past medical/social information would have a significant impact on which test procedures the clinician chose for that patient, what medical/social concerns the clinician would have for that patient, what interventions would be appropriate and effective,

and what outcome would be realistic to project. With our young relatively healthy patient from the case study in mind, we review possible tests and measures to be performed by the physical therapist and/or the entire medical team.

A pharmacological history is also noted during the history. There are a wide range of medications that may be appropriate for our patient or other patients with ventilatory pump dysfunction, potential for failure, or failure. Our patient is currently on antireflux medications, vitamins, a muscle tone relaxant for his spasticity, and a stool softener.

Medical Tests and Measures

Vital Signs—Heart Rate, Blood Pressure, Respiratory Rate, and Temperature

Heart rate (HR), blood pressure (BP), respiratory rate (RR), and temperature are meant to give the clinician a quick, inexpensive look into the patient's current medical status, and is seen as the "first line of attack" in performing a cardiopulmonary assessment. For example, if our patient showed a significant drop in HR accompanied by a significant elevation of his BP and an increase in RR, it could be indicative of the onset of autonomic dysreflexia. An increase in RR and temperature could be signaling the onset of pneumonia or other respiratory infection. A drop in BP with a change in posture, particularly a change from a recumbent to an upright posture, could indicate that our patient was experiencing orthostatic hypotension. Thus, vital signs are helpful for assessing stability at rest and with activity. Because of its ease of application, low cost, and valuable information, all patients should have ongoing assessments of their vital signs. Vital signs are assessed by any and all of the medical staff. Our patient's vital signs were stable, but BP tended to be on the low side (see Table 20-9).

Arterial Blood Gases (ABGs)

Patients who fall into Practice Pattern 6E are already identified as having ventilatory pump dysfunction. This means that they will have trouble providing the exterior support (optimal respiratory biomechanical support) for optimal gas exchange. They may have problems efficiently removing CO_2 and subsequently ABGs would be observed to have an elevated P_{CO_2} (normal is 35–45 mm Hg) and a resultant drop in pH (normal pH 7.35–7.45).[32] **Each patient and each facility may have a slightly different threshold that indicates acute ventilatory pump failure, but the generally accepted threshold value for a patient with ventilatory pump dysfunction (without lung**

TABLE 20-9 Lee's Vital Signs in Two Different Postures

Position	HR	BP	RR	Temperature
Supine	86	100/65	16	98.6
Sitting	92	85/60	19	98.6

disease) is a P_{CO_2} of greater than 50 mm Hg and a pH of less than 7.30.[67,69] However, observation of a paradoxical breathing pattern should alert the clinician that (1) the ventilatory pump has the potential to fail and (2) judicious administration of a variety of interventions may correct the paradoxical breathing pattern and prevent the aforementioned changes in ABGs.

Patients with SCI generally do not have a problem with their P_{aO_2} level except when developing an acute respiratory infection. This value is then particularly important when the patient is acutely ill and the doctor needs to decide if the patient's gas-exchange efficiency is so compromised that mechanical ventilation and/or oxygen support is needed. Generally a P_{O_2} less than 60 mm Hg would indicate the need for supplemental oxygen.[67,69] Consequently, ABGs are an essential evaluative tool during the acute phase and during changes in the patient's medical status, but are not necessary on a daily basis for the patient who is medically stable. Our patient, who is clearly in Practice Pattern 6E, is entering the rehabilitation center in stable condition with relatively normal ABGs; thus, there would be no reason to repeat the test unless his condition changed for the worse or if a paradoxical breathing pattern were observed. The nursing staff or physicians generally perform this test in the United States.

Oximetry (O_2 sat/Sao_2)

A normal oxygen saturation (O_2 sat) level is between 96% and 100%. A level of 90% or less is often used as a threshold value to indicate inadequate oxygenation and the need for supplemental oxygen. Clinicians can also use this test to determine how well the patient is tolerating a particular activity and examine the O_2 sat in contrast to the breathing pattern and RR. For example, a clinician may choose to monitor the O_2 sat, RR, BP, and breathing pattern when our patient moves from a reclining chair to a fully upright chair. A drop in O_2 sat and BP accompanied by an increase in RR and paradoxical breathing pattern indicates that the patient is presently unable to tolerate movement from a reclining position to a fully upright position. In view of the results of these tests and measures, the clinician knows that his physiologic state is not quite ready for a fully upright position without the use of some other intervention such as an abdominal binder or elevated footrests or simply less of an upright position (45-degree upright position using the reclining chair or a specialized bed).

Because oximeters are noninvasive, easy to apply, and easy to transport, and can give immediate feedback to the clinician, it can be a valuable ongoing evaluation tool. Like ABGs, once the patient is medically stable and the clinician knows that the patient's saturation level is stable in a variety of physical activities, then his oximetry level no longer needs to be monitored. Oximetry can be assessed by any and all of the medical staff. Our patient's O_2 sat values were stable at rest, but dropped to 86% to 88% when sitting fully erect and when transferring without his abdominal binder. Thus, his O_2 sat should continue to be monitored until no sign of desaturation is observed.

Pulmonary Function Tests (PFT)

Pulmonary function tests inform the clinician about lung volumes and flow rates for both inhalation and exhalation maneuvers. A few pertinent tests will be discussed here, and Chapter 9 can be reviewed for further material on PFTs.

Vital Capacity

One of the simplest and most readily available tests is the VC maneuver. It can tell the clinician about the patient's voluntary ability to move maximal volumes of air in and out of the lungs. The patient inhales and then blows out as hard and as long as he can. The expired volume is called VC. In general, when a patient's VC is less than 60% of the predicted value, it is generally indicative of inadequate lung volume. **If VC falls to less than 25% of the predicted value, it is generally indicative of the patient's inability to support adequate gas exchange (ventilatory failure) and the need for mechanical ventilation.[32]**

Tidal Volume

TV is a normal quiet breath and should be approximately 10% to 20% of the predicted VC.[32,70] This shows that the person has adequate respiratory reserves to meet the oxygen demands of activities that demand a greater inspiratory or expiratory effort, or both. When TV becomes a higher percentage of VC (because VC is shrinking or TV is increasing), it tells the clinician that the patient's respiratory reserves are lower, thus potentially limiting the patient's physical potential. If the patient cannot transport oxygen to the muscles because of limited reserves, he or she will not have the "energy" to perform physical tasks.

Flow Rate Measurements

Flow rates are also important to determine cough effectiveness as well as to detect any obstructive lung impairments. Two different methods of assessing flow rates will be presented. **According to Bach,[41,71] normal peak cough flow rates (PCFR) are between 6 and 12 L/s, and that any rate less than 2.7 L/s will clearly result in a nonproductive expectoration.**

Another way of measuring ineffective rates necessary for cough would be to test FEV_1. Normal FEV_1 is 80% of the actual VC. **Like a PCFR of less than 2.7 L/s, a FEV_1/actual VC below 60% indicates inadequate flow rates for cough.**

During acute episodes, PFTs may need to be taken daily or even more frequently to detect an improving or worsening situation. This is particularly true of the patient with neuromuscular impairments such as Guillian–Barré syndrome, amyotrophic lateral sclerosis, muscular dystrophy, or other progressive disorders. For a stable patient, PFTs may be rechecked periodically to make sure that the patient's functional lung capability has not changed. Portable models are available that are simple, relatively inexpensive, and usually available in the hospital setting. They are often not available in the home or community setting. The downside to PFTs is that they require the full cooperation of the patient; thus, their value is determined by

TABLE 20-10 Lee's Pulmonary Function Tests with Tracheostomy Tube Capped

PFT Maneuver	Amount Measured	Predicted Value	Percentage of Predicted Value
VC	2.2 L	5.0 L	44%
TV	0.8 L	0.5–1.0 L	WNL
TV/VC	36%	10%–20%	1.8–3.6 times higher
PCFR	2.2 L/s	6–12 L/s	18%–36%

L, liters; s, seconds; WNL, within normal limits.

the patient's ability to consistently give their maximal effort to the test. PFTs cannot be performed with the patient who is cognitively impaired, or with the patient with oral motor dysfunction who cannot make and maintain a good lip seal over the mouthpiece. PFTs can be performed by any and all of the medical staff.

Our patient's PFT results are summarized in Table 20-10. **The results show a significant decrease in VC and PCFR, which indicates an impaired cough. Other PFT results show a higher TV/VC ratio than normal, indicating that he may not be capable of meeting the ventilatory demands of activities that require greater levels of oxygen consumption due to decreased ventilatory reserves.** Obviously, these test results are important to the physical therapist whose activities often demand the greatest amount of oxygen consumption of any of the medical disciplines. These tests should be repeated periodically during his rehabilitation stay in order to see if they are improving or worsening with time.

Sputum—Sputum is cultured if an infection is detected or suspected in the lungs, or it can be done prophylactically for patients with a history of repeat infections. Our patient did not have an infection upon discharge from the acute care; thus, no sputum culture was ordered. Nursing, respiratory therapy, or PT performs this test.

Chest radiographs (X-rays)—Chest X-rays can tell a clinician about the current condition of the lung such as the presence of a pneumonia, atelectasis, or disease processes such as emphysema (see Chapter 9 for a more detailed review of radiographic techniques). Past X-rays may show a pattern of problems that would influence the clinician's future interventions. Our patient had an atelectasis in the acute care hospital so that X-ray would be compared to the admitting X-ray at the rehabilitation hospital to make sure that there was no residual deficit or new problem. Acute lung problems, such as atelectasis, can quickly occur so it is important to "treat the patient," not "the X-ray report." Contact the physician about any suspected changes. Only X-ray technicians perform X-rays. Our patient's admitting X-ray showed no residual atelectasis.

Cardiac/circulation tests—Patients with ventilatory pump dysfunction or failure may also have a history of cardiac dysfunction, or may be at risk for developing problems. An ECG may be performed to rule out any cardiac problems. Our patient's doctor decided that an ECG was not necessary. His HR was normal and his distal pulses were present. All cardiovascular tests were within normal limits (WNL) for our patient.

Renal/urinary tests—Because urinary tract infections (UTIs) are common complications following a spinal cord injury, periodic urine tests will be performed to monitor this possibility. Our patient's test returned negative, but all disciplines need to be trained to watch for signs of UTIs because of their quick onset and their potential trigger for autonomic dysreflexia and possibly death. Nursing typically performs this test in the United States.

Nutrition/hydration/reflux/swallowing dysfunction—The patient with ventilatory pump dysfunction may be expending a significant amount of their energy on breathing and may decide that eating "takes too much effort," as our patient did in the acute care setting. Nutrition can be assessed by weight loss/gain, gastrointestinal status, and the patient's report. Likewise, hydration is critical to his health and can be monitored by fluid intake/urine output, the color of the urine, the thinness of lung secretions, complaints of dry mouth and sore throat, to name a few. Our patient was determined to be slightly dehydrated upon admission. He also recently started taking in adequate calories to maintain his weight.

Occasionally, patients will develop reflux or other gastric dysfunctions secondary to SCI.[61,62] Reflux can be dangerous because of its potential for aspiration pneumonia as well as poor nutrition. Upon pH test, our patient was determined to have a slight case of reflux. This may have contributed to his poor appetite in the acute care. The patient will be started on antireflux medication to control the reflux. If our patient were also suspected of aspirating his food, fluids, or saliva, then a swallow study would be performed by a speech pathologist to determine if the patient's swallowing mechanism was impaired. Our patient showed no sign of aspiration; therefore, the test was not ordered.

Physical Tests and Measures

Tests and measures that are more specific to physical therapy will now be presented, as it would pertain to our patient Lee.

Range of Motion

Relatively good ROM with mild limitations only in shoulder flexion (right more than left), finger flexion, and ankle dorsiflexion were observed.

Manual Muscle Tests/Muscle Tone

Motor complete C5-SCI with no voluntary motion below C5 was observed. His key C5 muscles are 3/5 bilaterally (deltoids, biceps, brachioradialis). Above his lesion, his muscles are 4/5. Lee has mild spasticity in the trunk extensors, leg extensors, and biceps, and he complained to the physical therapist that his spasticity was making it hard for him to use his biceps functionally.

Sensation

Sensation was observed to be intact above C5 dermatome, somewhat spotty within C5–C6, and absent below C6.

Skin

Lee's skin was observed to be intact but shows an increased redness over the left greater trochanter. Surgical scar from liver laceration repair on right upper abdomen is healing well, but therapist suspects tightening onto underlying connective tissue. Restrictions to scar tissue movements noted superiorly and inferiorly. Chest tube scars healing well with no noted restrictions.

Gross Motor Skills/ADLs

Lee was just beginning to relearn gross motor skills when he was discharged from the acute care setting. Upon admission to rehabilitation he needed:

- Moderate assistance to roll to both sides, with the therapist noting poor coordination of breathing and movement.
- Maximal assistance to assume supine to sitting, demonstrating a "breath-holding" pattern when he assisted the therapist with elbow flexion maneuvers.
- Maximal assistance with sliding board transfers. Has not been instructed yet in how he can assist and direct the transfer.
- Moderate assistance for balance short-sitting on a mat table with right foot on the ground for 10 minutes. Left leg elevated due to long leg cast.
- Tolerating fully upright posture in wheelchair up to 30 to 60 minutes before complaining of fatigue. In addition, notes: pressure hose on his right lower extremity, long leg cast on left lower extremity, abdominal binder.

Postural Assessment

Lee is of moderate stature (5 ft 8 in. tall, 150 lb) with a flat anterior chest wall (normal for him) and no noted spinal abnormalities (other than surgical site). No abnormality noted over right rib fracture sites. Surgical scar on right upper abdomen is taut, pulling abdomen into a slightly "flexed" posture even in supine. Sitting with therapist's support in short-sitting posture without an abdominal binder, the therapist notes a midchest fold line between the chest and abdominal area, an excessive anterior and inferior displacement of the abdominal viscera (a "beer-belly" look in spite of his moderate frame), internal rotation of the shoulders, an excessive kyphotic posture in the lower thoracic/lumber spine area (just below the base of support for the Halo vest), and an increase in posterior tilting of the pelvis (see Fig. 20-2). When the therapist reapplied the abdominal binder, (1) the midchest fold and the poor visceral alignment were corrected, (2) the upper extremities assumed a less internally rotated posture, (3) the pelvis was less posteriorly tilted, (4) and the functional kyphotic posture improved but was not eliminated. These observations will be considered in relationship to Lee's positioning and support in a wheelchair. BP was taken in upright when he first went upright and 30 minutes later to test his cardiovascular tolerance of the posture. Supine: BP 110/75. Upright initial: BP 90/60. Upright 30 minutes: BP 100/65. No signs of dysreflexia.

Breathing Pattern Assessment

Lee was observed to be spontaneously breathing, but complains that with talking or eating, he becomes more easily short of breath. He reports a perceived exertion rating of 8 out of 10 (8/10) during these activities. Other activities: quiet breathing in bed 4/10, sitting in wheelchair with a binder 5/10, without binder 7/10. His breathing pattern in supine with the Halo vest opened reveals an excessive rise of the abdomen, and a slight collapsing of the anterior chest (paradoxical or "inward" breathing). In the wheelchair with the Halo vest tightened and the abdominal binder applied, his breathing pattern demonstrates less abdominal excursion and a significant increase in superior or trapezius breathing. Patient is primarily a diaphragmatic breather with little upper chest support in any posture. See Table 20-11 for circumferential chest wall excursion measurements in supine and wheelchair sitting.[12] **Note the increase in paradoxical breathing while Lee was in supine.[13] The RR was 16 in supine with vest opened, 20 in upright with vest and binder, 28 in upright without the binder.** Auscultation revealed decreased breath sounds in basal segments, but no adventitious sounds, indicating hypoventilation, but not secretion retention.

TABLE 20-11 Lee's Circumferential Chest Wall Excursion Measurements

	Upper Chest	Midchest	Lower Chest/Abdomen
Measurement site	Level of third rib	Xiphoid process	1/2 Distance between xiphoid and umbilicus
Supine TV maneuver	+ 1/16 in.	− 1/8 in.	+ 3/4 in.
Supine VC maneuver	+ 3/8 in.	− 1/2 in.	+ 1 in.
Sitting TV maneuver	Not possible due to Halo vest	Not possible due to Halo vest	1/2 in.
Sitting VC maneuver	Not possible due to Halo vest	Not possible due to Halo vest	+ 3/4 in.

in., inches.

TABLE 20-12   Lee's Cough Assessment

Phases	Description of the Four Phases of Cough	Patient's Cough Assessment
1	**"Inspiratory"** phase Threshold: >60% of predicted VC	**Impaired** VC 44% of predicted value
2	**"Hold"** phase Glottal closure Necessary for increasing intrathoracic and intra-abdominal pressures	**Impaired** Tracheostomy tube prevents use of the glottis
3	**"Force"** phase Creation of subglottal pressure via contraction of expiratory muscles	**Impaired** Paralyzed expiratory muscles
4	**"Expulsion"** phase Timing the opening the glottis and expulsion of air Threshold: FEV_1/actual VC > 60% and/or PCFR > 2.7 L/s	**Impaired** PCFR 2.2 L/s

VC, vital capacity; FEV_1, forced expiratory volume in 1 second; PCFR, peak cough flow rate; s, seconds; L, liters.

Cough Assessment

There are four phases to a normal cough which are described in Table 20-12.[41,71,72] Phase 1 is the inspiratory phase, phase 2 is considered a hold phase, and phases 3 and 4 are the force and expulsion phases, respectively. Lee stated that he has trouble coughing. Examination of the patient's cough and pulmonary function revealed inadequate inspiratory volume for phase 1 and an inability to use phases 2 and 4 effectively due to his tracheostomy. Phase 3 was also markedly impaired because of abdominal and intercostal paralysis. The cough was quiet and high pitched, and the patient was only able to produce two "weak and breathy" coughs per breath. In summary, Lee demonstrated significant impairments at every phase of cough and the PFTs confirmed these suspicions (Table 20-12).

In addition, during these coughs, Lee did not show any spontaneous incorporation of natural ventilatory strategies with the maneuver (ie, trunk/head extension with the inspiratory phase 1, and trunk/head flexion with the expiratory phases 3 and 4). For all of these reasons, our patient is classified as "at risk" for developing respiratory complications secondary to secretion retention unless his neurologic condition improves or an adequate intervention program is implemented. At this moment, he does not have a secretion problem, but his airway clearance assessment shows that he will be unable to effectively clear secretions when he needs to, such as when he develops a cold. Obviously, resolution of this problem is paramount to his successful rehabilitation outcomes, because pulmonary infections are the primary cause of death in patients with SCI and are likely the result of suboptimal secretion clearance due to a poor cough.

Breath Support for Phonation

Lee can sustain a vowel sound (ah) for 4.5 seconds (normal 15 seconds),[34] and uses 4 to 5 syllables per breath (normal 8–10) in upright with an abdominal binder on and a cap over his tracheostomy site. Without the binder, he sustains a vowel sound for 3.1 seconds and uses 2 to 3 syllables/breath (see Table 20-13). Patient states that he prefers to have the binder on in upright.[37] He tries to use an eccentric pattern for voicing (normal breath support pattern for quiet breathing), but he will move into a residual volume (RV) speech pattern, which uses a concentric pattern (utilizing his pectoralis, bicep, and neck flexors) when he wants to finish a sentence before taking another inspiratory effort. This is most likely a significant contributing factor to his complaint of dyspnea with conversations. The patient is a good candidate for a speaking valve or a tracheostomy button to facilitate speech prior to decannulation.

Sleep Assessment

Because of the patient's compliant of headaches in the morning, and a "poor night's sleep" in general, Lee had a sleep study screening test performed with nursing and PT during a daytime nap session. While the patient was supine, his O_2 sat level dropped to 89% and his RR increased to 24. The patient was then turned one-fourth off of supine with his uppermost

TABLE 20-13   Lee's Phonation: Sustained Vowel Sound Production

Position and Equipment	Length of Vocalization (Normal 15 s)	Syllables per Breath (Normal 8–10 syl/br)
Sitting in w/c—with binder[a]	4.5 s	4–5 syl/br
Sitting in w/c—no binder	3.1 s	2–3 syl/br

[a]w/c, wheelchair; s, seconds; syl/br, syllables/breath.

TABLE 20-14 Lee's Screening Test for Sleep Dysfunction

Sleep Posture	O$_2$ Saturation	RR
• **Threshold**	>90%	10–20 breaths/min
• **Supine**	89%	24
• **1/4 off supine with UE in extension**[a]	96%	16
• **3/4 prone**[b]	95%	18

UE, upper extremity.

[a]patient lies halfway between supine and sidelying with his arm pulled back toward his spine.

[b]patient lies halfway between sidelying and prone with his arm pulled forward towards his belly.

upper extremity positioned in extension against a pillow to maximize the upper chest opening. His O$_2$ sat and RR improved. The patient was also evaluated on his side and three-fourth prone with similar positive results[73] (Table 20-14).

Equipment

The Halo vest was observed to be restricting head, neck, and upper chest movements, and consequently impairing inspiratory maneuvers. However, the Halo vest provides much-needed spinal support and will remain in place until spinal precautions are removed (anticipated date: 3 months postinjury). Several studies show that the Halo vest has the potential to decrease VC.[74] A fenestrated tracheostomy, right lower extremity cast, and an abdominal binder were provided to the patient. Bilateral hand splints were provided to maintain ROM and bilateral nighttime ankle splints were applied to maintain ankle ROM.

PHYSICAL THERAPY DIAGNOSIS AND IMPRESSION

Diagnosis

The patient was a previously healthy young male who is now stable and recovering from an SCI 3 weeks ago. Lee is spontaneously breathing, but not as efficiently as he can or needs to be in order to maximize his function and minimize his long-term respiratory risk. (Common respiratory complications associated with SCI are chronic hypoventilation leading to atelectasis and/or pneumonia, chronic nighttime hypoxemia, and increased risk of infection.) He demonstrates a paradoxical breathing pattern at rest that worsens with increased effort and his O$_2$ sat decreases with upright body positions. He has poor respiratory endurance and resulting poor functional endurance. His cough is weak and ineffective, rendering secretion management ineffective. His breath support for speech is poor, hampering his communication efforts. Lee's nocturnal ventilation is inadequate in supine, contributing to his daytime fatigue level and poor concentration. His musculoskeletal

alignment in upright is faulty and could have long-term effects on the continued development of his spine, chest, shoulders, and pelvis. His nutritional and hydration state is improving from the acute care, but not yet adequate.

Impression

Lee's impairments demonstrate ventilatory pump dysfunction with the potential for ventilatory pump failure due to the presence of a paradoxical breathing pattern and desaturation with upright body positions. It is important for the physical therapist to identify specific signs and symptoms to distinguish among ventilatory pump dysfunction, the potential for ventilatory pump failure, or true ventilatory pump failure. This information can then be used to maximize ventilatory pump function and prevent ventilatory pump failure.

Figure 20-3 highlights the importance of distinguishing between ventilatory pump dysfunction and failure. Identifying the absence or presence of a paradoxical breathing pattern can be used to direct the interventions most appropriate for a particular patient. This hypothesis-oriented algorithm can be applied to patients with ventilatory pump dysfunction and the potential for failure due to a variety of etiologies.

For example, the upper chest paradoxical breathing pattern observed in the patient in this case is due to inadequate biomechanics of breathing. The inward movement of the upper chest during inspiration is because the upper chest wall structural support system (the muscles) is paralyzed and the contracting and descending diaphragm creates a sufficient negative pressure to pull (or actually suck) the upper chest inward (see Chapter 9). **Continued upper chest paradoxical breathing may place other patients at risk of developing ventilatory pump failure. The upper or middle chest paradoxical breathing pattern that is common in patients with SCI is more often an indication of significant ventilatory pump dysfunction, rather than ventilatory pump failure.**

Nonetheless, sitting the patient with an upper or middle chest paradoxical breathing pattern upright and leaning them forward (or giving them an abdominal binder) may provide them with greater abdominal support and decrease the effects of gravity on the upper or middle chest which should decrease the upper chest paradoxical breathing pattern (Fig. 20-3).

An abdominal paradoxical breathing pattern, as seen in patients with severe COPD, appears to be much more strongly associated with the potential for ventilatory pump failure. The abnormal biomechanics of breathing in COPD are characterized by excessive accessory muscle activity and diminished diaphragmatic activity because of hyperinflation of the lungs and subsequent flattening of the diaphragm. Flattening of the diaphragm places the muscle fibers of the diaphragm in a shortened and suboptimal position for contraction and relaxation. This suboptimal position decreases the diaphragm's ability to produce the much-needed bucket-handle motion of the lower ribs and subsequent generation of negative pressure to ventilate the lungs.

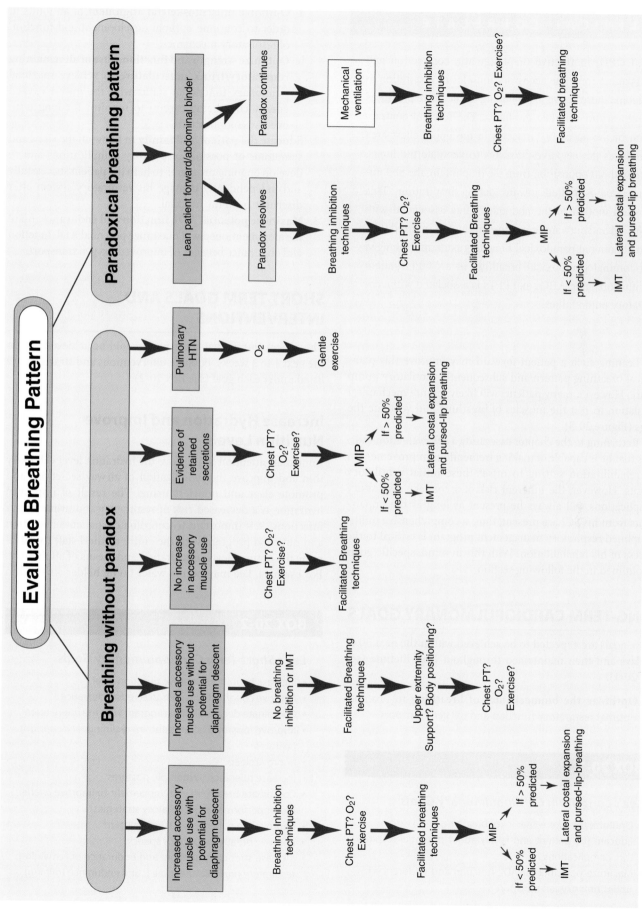

FIGURE 20-3 A hypothesis-oriented algorithm for patients with ventilatory pump dysfunction and the potential for ventilatory pump failure.

Leaning such a patient forward may improve this paradoxical breathing pattern and subsequently ventilatory pump failure. However, many patients will likely require mechanical ventilation to rest the muscles of breathing and ventilate the lungs (Figure 20-3).

Returning to the chapter case study, Lee's evaluation indicates that he is capable of making tremendous improvement in the rehabilitation setting to offset these initial ventilatory deficits. However, the inherent risk of secondary respiratory complications will always be present as long as the impairments from his SCI are present; thus, a comprehensive multidisciplined respiratory management program is critical to the success of his rehabilitation. With this in mind, specific goals are outlined in the following section.

LONG-TERM CARDIOPULMONARY GOALS

These goals are expected to be achieved within the next 30 to 60 days and then maintained throughout Lee's lifetime (see Box 20-1).

1. **Optimize the biomechanics of breathing** to promote optimal respiratory function and oxygen transport.

BOX 20-1

Lee's Long-Term Cardiopulmonary Goals

- Optimize the biomechanics of breathing
- Educate the patient and family about potential respiratory complications
- Maximize potential for ADL function and endurance by optimizing oxygen transport

   a. **Optimize musculoskeletal alignment** of all joints in order to continue optimal development and function of respiratory mechanics.
   b. **Optimize strength and functional use of all remaining respiratory/trunk musculature** to achieve maximal pulmonary functional status with the lowest oxygen energy cost, being careful to monitor for long-term overuse complications.

2. **Educate the patient and family** to know all the signs and symptoms of possible respiratory complications and to develop ongoing programs to help the patient successfully and independently manage his respiratory system after discharge from the hospital.

3. **Maximize potential ADL function and endurance.** All of the aforementioned will maximize potential ADL function and endurance because of improved oxygen transport.

SHORT-TERM GOALS AND INTERVENTIONS

The expectation is that these goals could be achieved within the next 1 to 3 weeks. Possible interventions and strategies are listed under each goal (see Box 20-2).

Increase Hydration and Improve Nutrition Levels

Immediate attention to improve the hydration level will likely thin and improve the mobilization of airway secretions and promote clear and odorless urine. The result of improved hydration is a decreased risk of respiratory and urinary tract infections. It is important to coordinate a patient's hydration and nutrition program with the entire medical staff to determine the optimal level of hydration and means of attainment. For example, Lee may need a water bottle holder attached to

BOX 20-2

Lee's Short-Term Cardiopulmonary Goals

- Increase hydration/improve nutrition level
- Improve cough effectiveness/secretion clearance
- Coordinate decannulation program with the entire team
- Improve postural alignment in reclining and upright postures
- Improve sleep
- Increase tolerance to multiple postures
- Coordinate breathing with movement to improve overall motor performance (ventilatory strategies)
- Improve the patient's breathing pattern
- Improve breath support for speech
- Increase strength, function, and endurance of remaining respiratory musculature (power and endurance training)

his arm rest, or a "camel pack" system (used by bicyclists for long-distance rides) attached to the back of his wheelchair, etc, so he can readily and independently maintain adequate hydration levels. This is important for both short-term and long-term respiratory management strategies. The patient must be educated about the respiratory and renal risks associated with dehydration to promote long-term carryover into his home life after discharge.

Improve Cough Effectiveness/Secretion Clearance

It is important to place a high priority on determining the best method of secretion mobilization and of airway clearance to prevent hypoventilation and atelectasis, thus reducing his chance of developing an acute respiratory infection. This section will focus on describing options for Lee's immediate airway clearance needs, but we will keep in mind that his needs may change with time and with the environmental setting (acute care, rehab hospital, home, work, etc).

Secretion Mobilization

In order to get secretions to the level where they can be expectorated, they must first be mobilized, or moved, from the periphery of the lungs to the proximal airways. Thus, an effective airway clearance program focuses initially at mobilizing secretions. Box 20-3 lists various strategies that can be used to accomplish this goal. Many studies have been done to evaluate the efficacy of mobilizing secretions with each of these techniques.[75-79] In particular, Hardy's 1994 article[78] details a comparison of approximately 40 different studies evaluating the effectiveness of airway clearance interventions. The conclusion drawn from this and other articles is that no single mobilizing or expectorating technique is "the most effective." All the methods demonstrate advantages and disadvantages. A clinician must decide which intervention works best for each particular patient based on the availability of an intervention, therapist's skill, time factors, finances, patient comfort, patient fatigue, and independent airway clearance effectiveness. With all things considered, the best combination for the patient in our case would probably be (1) an adequate humidification program, (2) the implementation of postural drainage positions in his recumbent positioning program, (3) the purposeful timing of his medications to coincide with therapy sessions, (4) improving his overall hydration level, and (5) possibly the use of a PEP device if needed. Percussion and vibration can be added if this initial treatment was ineffective. Finally, the costly *Vest* could be used if it was available and the other methods failed.

Expectoration

Now Lee is ready for us to help him expectorate his secretions more effectively. He showed impairments at all four phases of cough (expectoration). He cannot inhale deep enough to have an adequate inspiratory volume for coughing (impaired phase 1), he cannot close his glottis due to the tracheostomy (impaired

---

BOX 20-3

Possible Secretion Mobilization Strategies

- Using a humidification system at the level of the tracheostomy to thin the secretions and keep them mobile
- Increasing systemic hydration level to thin secretions
- Incorporating postural drainage positions into recumbent positioning
- Adding percussion and vibration if necessary to loosen tough secretions
- Changing the timing of medications such as nebulizing medications (secretion thinning) or tone reduction medications (spasticity management) to occur 30 to 60 minutes prior to physical therapy to maximize secretion mobilization
- Implementing the use of PEP (positive expiratory pressure) devices such as the Ther-a-PEP, Flutter, or Acapella to mobilize secretions
- May not be capable of generating the expiratory pressure necessary to benefit from a PEP device
- Using the pneumatic vibrating vest (the Vest) which mechanically vibrates the entire chest wall while the patient is sitting

(Effective, but very expensive. Currently about $16,000.)

---

phase 2), he cannot build up intra-abdominal or intrathoracic pressures due to intercostal and abdominal paralysis (impaired phase 3), and he cannot forcefully open his glottis and cough due to the tracheostomy (impaired phase 4). Thus, Lee needs assistance at all four levels.[53]

Start simply (Box 20-4). Begin with educating the patient on the importance of avoiding a secondary respiratory complication and about the lifelong risk he has for acquiring a respiratory complication secondary to paralysis. After his tracheostomy tube is removed, Lee will regain normal control of his glottis (phases 2 and 4), but he will always have significant impairments with phases 1 and 3 if his paralysis remains.

At this point of his rehabilitation, part of the patient's education involves teaching him to use independent ventilatory strategies (see the section on coordinating breathing with movements later) to augment the phases of cough. For example, teaching him to use trunk extension (or at least shoulder/scapular movements); eye gaze up, and a quick, long inspiratory effort before coughing should augment phase 1. Then, instruct him to look down, bring his shoulders/trunk forward into flexion (as far as he can safely control the motion), while he coughs or huffs through his tracheostomy, to augment phases 3 and 4. The one phase that he cannot assist at this point is phase 2 (closing the glottis) because the tracheostomy tube allows the air to escape below the level of the glottis. Patients with cervical SCIs appear to be able to increase their PCFR by using these ventilatory strategies during independent coughing. This early, simple education assists the patient in developing

Possible Secretion Expectoration Strategies

Education
Educate the patient about secondary respiratory complications due to inadequate airway clearance.

Instruction
Instruct the patient to utilize ventilatory strategies with coughing to improve phase 1 (inspiration) and phase 3 (building up intrathoracic pressure).

Instruct the patient in active cycles of breathing (ACB) with or without forced expiratory technique (FET).

Manual Assistive Cough Techniques
Use assistive cough techniques, such as costophrenic assist, anterior chest compression, Heimlich-type assist (aka quad cough or abdominal thrust), counterrotation assist (see CD-ROM), etc.

Mechanical Devices
Use mechanical assistive devices such as suction machines or the cough assist (aka *Cof-flator, mechanical in-exsufflator*) to physically remove secretions.

lifelong skills that will be necessary for effective management of pulmonary secretions.

Another type of independent airway clearance strategy was developed for patients with cystic fibrosis, but can sometimes be adapted for some patients with neuromuscular impairments or other diseases. This independent airway clearance strategy is called the *active cycle of breathing* (ACB) with forced expiratory technique (FET or "chicken wings").[80] ACB involves varying inspiratory lung volumes in an attempt to mobilize secretions from peripheral to proximal airways (secretion mobilization). It is then followed up by FET, which uses ventilatory strategies and chest wall compression to aid in expectoration.[80,81] Theoretically, the patient with SCI can follow the instructions necessary for ACB and FET, but they may not have the potential to sufficiently increase inspiratory lung volumes adequately to effectively mobilize their secretions. Additionally, if SCI patients lack adequate trunk support, they may be unable to raise both upper extremities at the same time to perform the FET technique. Therefore, the compressive force on their chest wall may not be adequate to aid in expectoration. At this point in his rehabilitation, ACB is probably not a realistic intervention for our patient. However, as his lung volume potential increases, and his sitting balance gets better, it may become a viable option.

If independent strategies do not work well enough, the therapist can try manually assisted cough techniques. Many different assistive cough techniques are available and the majority of them appear to quite effective.[41,53,82,83] Several are demonstrated on the accompanying CD-ROM.[84] Each of these assistive cough techniques addresses all four components of

effective coughing, so how do you decide which assistive cough technique is the most effective for our patient? Several assessment methods are available, such as production of secretions, changes in breath sounds, improvement in ABGs or PFTs, or PCFR during an independent cough effort and during a cough while assisting the patient (see Chapter 9). The intervention that produces the greatest PCFR is the most effective and should be used with that particular patient. **The minimal threshold PCFR for an effective cough appears to be 2.7 L/s.**[70]

Thus, any intervention that produces a PCFR of at least 2.7 L/s can be considered a viable choice of interventions. The peak flow meter can measure the PCFR and is an inexpensive, readily available device.[85] In addition to objective data, the therapist also needs to consider which technique is (1) the most comfortable to the patient, (2) the most effective from the patient's perspective, (3) the one the patient is willing to have performed on him, and (4) the easiest and safest one to use by different staff or family members.

If secretion mobilization, independent strategies, or manually assisted cough techniques cannot adequately clear secretions, then mechanical assistance can be added or substituted for the less effective intervention. The most common mechanical device is a suction machine (tracheal suctioning). A sterile catheter is introduced into the patient's airway through the tracheostomy down to or near the level of the carina (second rib). The secretions in the mainstem bronchus and trachea can then be suctioned out through this catheter (see Chapter 19). The advantage of this technique is that it is completely passive for the patient (however, it can also be seen as a disadvantage in terms of learning independent strategies to clear secretions). It is an extremely effective intervention for clearing secretions in the large airway.[86] However, it is an invasive procedure and complications can arise, such as (1) transient oxygen desaturation, (2) soft tissue damage to the airway from the catheter, and (3) secondary increase in secretion production, in response to the introduction of a foreign object in the airway.[86]

Another mechanical device that has been reintroduced as an airway clearance device is the *Cough Assist* (or the *Cofflator* or *Mechanical In-Exsufflation* by JH Emerson, Cambridge, MA). This device delivers a positive-pressure cycle (inspiration) to the patient through an upper airway mask, or in our patient's case, through his tracheostomy, tube, to augment phase 1. It is followed by a negative-pressure cycle (exhalation) to pull the secretions out. This device was originally developed in the 1950s for patients with polio and was almost completely abandoned in the 1960s when tracheotomies became commonplace.[87] It was modified and reintroduced as a noninvasive means to mechanically assist expectoration in the 1990s. Thus far, the literature has shown it to be as viable as suctioning in expectorating secretions from patients with neuromuscular impairments.[53,88–90] In addition, the *Cough Assist* has been successfully used to combat chronic hypoventilation (micro- and macroatelectasis) that often occurs secondarily to a decreased inspiratory lung capacity following a neuromuscular impairment such as a SCI. Complications of the *Cough Assist* noted in literature include (1) complaints of musculoskeletal pain along the chest wall due to the passive expansion of the chest during the inspiratory cycle, (2) dry mouth, and (3) nose bleeds.

No single intervention will work for every patient, and often several can be incorporated during physical therapy. It is important to note that finding and implementing an effective strategy to prevent secondary pulmonary complications is not the sole responsibility of any one medical discipline; rather it is the responsibility of the entire team, including the patient and his family. If the patient needs assistance with clearing his secretions, every team member shares a part of the responsibility in helping the patient. Thus, once an effective program has been developed, every team member, perhaps most significantly the family members and caretakers, needs to be educated about the best interventions. They also need to show competence in performing these interventions. Methods of evaluating competence should be based on the desired goals and the methods of examination that family members and caregivers feel most comfortable in using.

Coordination of the Decannulation Program with the Entire Team

It is imperative to work with the entire team to assist in a speedy and effective decannulation program (see Chapter 19 for further information on decannulation). Regardless of the method of decannulation, the patient will demonstrate a readiness for decannulation by demonstrating (1) his ability to breathe adequately through his upper airway; (2) his ability to clear his airways independently, or with assist, through his upper airway; and (3) his ability to safely swallow and protect his lower airway from aspiration. Closing off the tracheostomy site will allow the patient to use his upper airway to assist in cleansing, heating, and humidifying the inspired air before it reaches the lungs, thus helping to reduce the risk of further respiratory complications. In addition, removal of the tracheostomy tube allows the patient to use his glottis for functional tasks such as (1) coughing, (2) talking, (3) valsalva maneuvers for bowel and bladder management, and (4) the generation of subglottal pressures utilized for fine gradations of trunk movement necessary for upright posture control and balance.

Decannulation programs may include the use of one-way tracheostomy valves that allow for unrestricted inhalation through the tracheostomy site, but prevents exhalation through the site, thus forcing exhalation through the upper airway. These are also called "speaking valves" (ie, Passy Muir valves) because the exhalation volume passes through the vocal folds.

Another option to foster decannulation would be to place a "trach-cap" or a "trach-button" in the tracheostomy tube. The tracheostomy cap literally prevents any air from entering or exiting the tracheostomy tube, thus forcing inspiration and expiration through the upper airway. Because the resultant blocked tracheostomy tube is simply taking up space in the trachea, creating an obstruction and not assisting with ventilation, the trach-cap inadvertently makes it harder for the patient to breathe. Additionally, the patient cannot have an inflated cuffed tracheostomy tube with any of these valves because the cuffed tube prevents air from entering the upper airway; thus, the patient would have no method of exhaling.

Perhaps a better method to progress the patient with a tracheostomy toward decannulation is to use a "trach-button." The tracheostomy button also forces upper airway breathing for both inhalation and exhalation, but the tracheostomy tube is removed and is replaced with a button at the level of the tracheostomy stoma. The patient still relearns to breathe through his upper airway, but the obstruction in the trachea from a tracheostomy tube is no longer present.

There are multiple methods to decannulate a patient. The type of decannulation program that Lee would utilize depends on the type of institution, as well as on personnel and equipment resources. The physical therapist generally plays a supportive rather than a leading role in this process.

Improve Postural Alignment in Reclining and Upright Postures

It appears to be critically important to develop and implement a program for the whole team that maintains an optimal alignment of the chest wall and spine to facilitate efficient and effective ventilation.[91] In order to maximize the biomechanical properties of the diaphragm and other accessory muscles, passive alignment of our patient should include (1) opening his anterior chest wall to facilitate use of the pectoralis muscle as a substitute for the paralyzed intercostal muscles and to maximize the recruitment of the upper accessory muscles to counteract the paradoxical forces on his chest caused by gravity and an unopposed diaphragmatic contraction, (2) positioning his shoulders in relative external rotation, again to facilitate pectoralis activation, to improve the length–tension relationship of the long neck flexors and to promote scapular adduction which supports more thoracic spine extension, and (3) positioning his pelvis in a relative anterior tilt to take advantage of the mechanical stacking of the vertebral spine to minimize the potential for a secondary scoliosis and/or kyphosis. Obviously, maintaining ROM of all joints will aid in his positioning options. The physical therapist will also need to focus on reducing the adhesions from the scar tissue around his liver laceration, which is preventing his trunk from being positioned in a full-extension posture. If the scar is allowed to heal with limited mobility, it may secondarily contribute to the development of a spinal deformity (pulling him into kyphosis), thus limiting his respiratory mechanics.

In the short term, Lee still has a Halo vest on for cervical spine fixation; therefore, his spine will stay in a more optimal alignment during his acute rehabilitation. However, he needs to be educated about the need for continued optimal spinal positioning once the Halo is removed in order to prevent the development of adverse spinal curves over the long term.[92]

These concepts can and should be applied in both the upright and the reclining postures and can often be accomplished through the use of simple supports such as towel rolls or pillows (Figs. 20-2B and 20-2C). Of course, as with any assistive device used for positioning, the patient's skin tolerance must be closely monitored to watch for any breakdown areas. However, because of his abdominal paralysis, Lee will always need an abdominal binder to help maintain visceral alignment under the dome of the diaphragm in upright posturing.[37,53,93,94] This "need" for an abdominal binder will continue as long as his abdominal muscles are paralyzed. He will not "outgrow" it simply because he had his SCI a long time ago or because he has achieved cardiovascular stability.

Consideration for the mechanics of breathing, and the maintenance of the spine, pelvis, and chest wall alignment, can and should be adapted into a patient's personal seating system. The seating system is normally designed and ordered along with a personal wheelchair during the patient's rehabilitation phase. Long-term positioning management may also include a medication regimen (coordinated with the doctor) to help regulate our patient's spasticity levels if they become so significant as to limit ROM and positioning options.

Improve Sleep

It also appears important to develop and implement a positioning plan with nursing to optimize our patient's ability to get a good night's sleep in order to function more effectively during the day. In addition to making sure that the patient can breathe effectively in a particular sleep posture, several other aspects need to be considered for nighttime positioning including (1) airway protection—Can he safely swallow or spit his saliva/secretions in a particular posture; (2) joint alignment—Are his joints positioned safely and effectively considering his long-term ROM maintenance; and (3) skin tolerance—Does his skin tolerate weight bearing without breakdown in that position? His sleep evaluation showed several possible alternative postures to supine to improve his respiratory support (see Table 20-14).

If these simple positioning changes are unable to adequately support nocturnal ventilation, then he could be evaluated for use of a positive pressure device, most commonly a CPAP or a BiPAP (bilevel positive airway pressure) system (see Chapter 19). Through the use of continuous positive pressure during exhalation, these devices help to prevent hypoventilation during sleep that results from shallow breathing. Both systems can be used with a tracheostomy attachment, or with a nasal or face mask attachment, and can be used if needed during the day as well. A modification of nocturnal nasal CPAP that automatically fine-tunes the level of positive pressure support while the patient is sleeping is currently being evaluated clinically and shows an improvement in patient comfort. One recent study showed that breathing could be well supported by both CPAP and the autoadjusting model (APAP), but that the APAP could accomplish this task with significantly less positive pressure and greater report of patient comfort.[95]

Increase Tolerance to Multiple Postures

It also appears to be very important to monitor patient's cardiovascular response to different postures and activities and implement changes where necessary to increase the patient's tolerance to postures that improve cardiopulmonary function and functional activities. Lee's BP tends to be low, especially in upright postures (orthostatic hypotension); thus, the team will continue with periodic BP checks, especially if the patient complains of lightheadedness. The patient's BP improved following the application of his abdominal binder and should therefore continue to be used. The patient also needs to be educated about the importance of the abdominal binder for both cardiovascular and pulmonary reasons. If the binder alone did not work, "pressure support hose" on his lower extremities could be continued to help increase the BP. Within a few weeks our patient should be able to tolerate sitting in a wheelchair for most of the day without the support hose, but the binder should always be worn for favorable cardiovascular, pulmonary, and postural adaptations.

A significant rise in BP will often accompany autonomic dysreflexia, which Lee has experienced. The patient must be educated about the signs and causes of dysreflexia and what to do during an episode. He should be told to instruct those around him to elevate his head, drop his legs down, open his binder (anything to decrease the hypertensive response caused by the dysreflexia), and to immediately check for a full bladder or impacted bowel which are often the precipitating causes.[48,56]

Tolerance to postures may also be determined by noncardiovascular responses, such as skin tolerance, painful joints, scar tissue adhesions, abnormal tone (spasms/spasticity), and restricted ROM. The entire team should be checking for signs of skin breakdown along weight-bearing points in both upright and reclining postures. Our patient has had signs of skin intolerance along the left greater trochanter, so left sidelying should be closely monitored. The patient's position should be modified (such as upper extremity positioning) within each posture in response to pain or joint limitations.

Coordinate Breathing with Movement to Improve Overall Motor Performance (Ventilatory Strategies)

Teaching a patient to breathe in coordination (using ventilatory strategies) with all motor tasks appears to be important for all patients with ventilatory pump dysfunction and failure. Our patient has limited muscular resources due to paralysis, thus learning to purposely coordinate his breathing with these movements can help to augment his functional motor skills.[93] The common theme of ventilatory strategies is to match the type of thoracic spine movement inherent in a particular motor task (extension vs flexion), and the type of muscular contraction needed to perform that task (concentric, eccentric, or isometric contractions), to the same type of movement associated within a specific breathing pattern (inhalation, exhalation, slow-, or fast-breathing patterns) and specific sensory cues (visual, auditory, manual, or others). By doing so, Lee can take advantage of well-established motor plans to assist in maximizing his motor response. Breaking this concept down into four component parts is helpful to understanding its global application.[96]

Thoracic Spine/Cage

Similar musculoskeletal movements can be paired with similar respiratory movements for efficiency of movement. Trunk extension is associated with inspiration (thoracic spine/thoracic cage complex expands), whereas trunk flexion is associated with exhalation (thoracic spine/thoracic cage complex compresses).

Muscle Contractions

Pair similar types of muscle contractions: concentric trunk/limb movements with concentric respiratory movements, eccentric with eccentric.

Breathing Patterns

Inspiration is always a concentric muscle contraction regardless of which muscles are used to inhale, whereas exhalation can be (1) passive, (2) eccentric (speech or controlled slow exhalation maneuvers), or (3) concentric (yelling, coughing, sneezing).

Sensory Patterns

Loud, fast commands tend to recruit the fast-twitched, power-oriented, accessory muscles (upper chest breathing). Slow, softer commands tend to recruit the slow-twitched, endurance-oriented diaphragm. Thus, audible cues can be used to encourage a specific type of breathing pattern. Likewise, the eyes tend to follow respiratory patterns. Eye-gaze-up is associated with inspiration (learned synergistic pattern through normal development), whereas eye gaze down is associated with exhalation.

Last, manual cues make use of the muscle spindle and joint receptor responses to facilitate specific muscle (breathing pattern) responses.

By combining all four components, the therapist can teach any patient to move more efficiently combining the musculoskeletal, neuromuscular, cardiopulmonary, and sensory systems as an integrated, dynamic system, rather than looking at these systems as isolated, independent systems.[96] For example, early in the rehabilitation program, Lee will begin to learn bed mobility skills to increase his independence. Rolling from supine to side-lying can be achieved with either trunk flexion (the most common method) or with trunk extension (a less common method). Because our patient has a Halo cervical fixation device restricting his neck motion, and because of the weight of this device, he will likely find it easier to attempt rolling with a trunk extension pattern.

How should he breathe when rolling in this scenario? Analyzing this movement, the therapist would note that his rolling required trunk extension and concentric muscle contractions. Thus, according to the principles of ventilatory strategies stated earlier, our patient should pair rolling with (1) inhalation, (2) upward eye gaze, and (3) a loud command to roll. If, 3 months later, when the Halo is removed, he finds trunk flexion to be a more natural trunk pattern to use for rolling, he would switch to another strategy. Rolling for him would then utilize a trunk flexion/concentric pattern, and as a result, he would then pair rolling with (1) exhalation, (2) downward eye gaze, and (3) a loud command (because he still needs to recruit accessory neck flexors). Using the concepts of ventilatory strategies, each movement is separately analyzed according to how a patient actually moves, not according to what is supposed to happen. This individualized approach encourages the most optimal pairing of breathing and movement for each individual patient based on their own motor planning and performance. Examples of ventilatory strategies are illustrated on Table 20-15.

TABLE 20-15 Examples of Pairing Ventilatory and Sensory Strategies with Movement

Activity	If the Movement Pattern Analysis Shows This…		Then Add These Ventilatory and Sensory Strategies to Improve the Motor Response		
	Thoracic Spine	Primary Muscle Contraction	Inhalation/Exhalation	Eye Gaze	Audible Cues
Rolling—supine to side-lying	Flexion	Concentric	Forceful exhalation (combining trunk flexion and concentric patterns)	Down	Strong, loud cues
Rolling—supine to side-lying	Extension	Concentric	Quick upper chest inhalation (combining trunk extension and concentric patterns)	Up	Strong, loud cues
Reaching up to get glass of water	Extension	Concentric	Quick upper chest inhalation (combining trunk extension and concentric patterns)	Up	Strong, loud cues
Lowering the glass to avoid spilling	Flexion	Eccentric	Slow, prolonged exhalation such as talking, singing, or humming (combining trunk flexion and eccentric patterns)	Down	Slow, soft cues, ie, "count outloud from 1 to 5"

Ventilatory strategies are based on normal anatomic alignments, the normal biomechanics of movement and breathing, and the normal development of motor plans. If a particular pattern does not work for your patient, do not force the issue. Rather, find a pattern that does work to maximize that patient's motor response. Once a patient learns the basics of applying ventilatory strategies to movement, they appear to spontaneously carry it over to new motor activities because they find it more efficient.

Improve the Patient's Breathing Pattern

Teaching a patient to recruit accessory muscles to compensate for paralyzed intercostal muscles, thereby preventing or minimizing paradoxical chest wall movements, should improve breathing, ventilation, and functional abilities. The goal of this intervention is to create an efficient balance of the utilization of the respiratory muscles to maximize inspiratory volumes with a minimal "energy cost" of breathing and to simultaneously minimize the muscle imbalance (paradoxical breathing) that leads to the development of a pectus excavatum (or other musculoskeletal deformities) and smaller inspiratory volumes. The goal is not to prevent the diaphragm from participating in inspiratory maneuvers. The goal is to balance the diaphragm's role with the other remaining respiratory muscles.[19]

It is important for the reader to realize that for this particular patient learning to activate the upper accessory muscles of ventilation is exactly what he needs to create a balanced inspiratory force with a minimum of unwanted side effects. However, for many patients with ventilatory pump dysfunction, the exact opposite may be true. For a wide variety of diagnoses stemming from primary pulmonary disorders such as COPD or asthma to secondary ventilatory dysfunction resulting from neuromuscular or musculoskeletal limitations, many patients overly recruit the upper accessory muscles and underutilize the diaphragm. For those patients, the goals of facilitation techniques would be to promote greater participation of the diaphragm and lessen the excessive activation of the upper accessory muscles. Lee needs a relatively greater amount of upper accessory muscle activity to counter the predominant diaphragmatic contraction. Thus, the techniques described here are appropriate only for the patient who needs to learn to recruit the accessory muscles. In this case study, our patient does not have functional abdominal or intercostal muscles and must therefore substitute the task of stabilizing the anterior chest wall with the utilization of his remaining respiratory musculature.

How quickly and effectively a patient with SCI learns to modify his breathing pattern depends on the individual patient. Breathing is a motor activity with a certain degree of volitional control that will require an active learning process. The patient in our case could learn it as quickly as 1 session or as slowly as 20 sessions or longer. Breathing retraining appears to be possible and beneficial.[97,98] It is up to the therapist to find the most effective training method for their patient based on the disease process, patient and physical therapist skill level, costs, time availability, and available equipment. Examples of

manual techniques that can be utilized successfully to facilitate upper chest expansion are demonstrated in the accompanying CD.[84,99] They primarily utilize the principles and practice of PNF (proprioceptive neuromuscular facilitation) techniques.[100] In order to take full advantage of the therapist's manual input, the therapist must be sure to position the patient successfully first (optimize the length–tension relationship of the muscles to be facilitated) and to utilize appropriate ventilatory strategies during the technique.[97] This will facilitate quicker success and carryover into function.

Success of these techniques is easily assessed by (1) repeating PFTs taken pre- and posttraining sessions, (2) measuring chest wall excursion pre- and posttraining, (3) timing phonation length or noting a change in number of syllables/breath, and/or (4) noting the patient's report of shortness of breath using a dyspnea scale,[100] Borg scale,[101] or fatigue level (see Chapter 9).

Immediately following successful activation of the desired breathing pattern, activities must be used that promote a direct incorporation of this new breathing pattern into functional tasks in order to promote a functional carryover. In other words, breathing retraining cannot take place in a vacuum, or the patient will learn that proper breathing is only done in "therapy sessions," but not in "real life." For example, for our patient, a progression of the manual intervention could include, initially using manual, visual, and audible cues. This could be progressed to giving less audible, visual, or manual input to the patient's chest wall and observing whether the patient could maintain the proper activation of the accessory muscles. Once positive results are observed, a therapist could use different postures and body positions to examine whether the desired pattern of breathing is maintained. Finally, the therapist could demand more functional use of the breathing pattern by incorporating it into tasks such as bed mobility, dressing, ROM exercises, and strengthening exercises. By this point, the pattern should become so well ingrained into the patient's daily movement patterns (a result of active motor learning) that it would become his "preferred breathing pattern" and not just a therapeutic intervention.

Other training methods can be utilized in addition to manual facilitation techniques such as air stacking, biofeedback, and visualization.[94] The important factor is to find an intervention that hastens the patient's learning curve to achieve competency with upper chest muscle recruitment for both quiet breathing and deep breathing to achieve ventilatory efficiency. See Box 20-5 for a summary of possible breathing retraining methods.

If our patient had a higher cervical SCI, it may have been necessary to teach him glossopharyngeal breathing (GPB).[102] This technique was developed during the polio epidemics, by patients themselves, to develop spontaneous breathing independent of a ventilator (iron lung), in spite of diaphragmatic, intercostal, and abdominal muscle paralysis. Using the innervation of the upper accessory muscles via the cranial nerves, the patient learns to draw air into his or her mouth and then "push" it down into his or her lungs. They do not actually push the air down, but that is a common description of the

BOX 20-5

Strategies to Facilitate Breathing Retraining

"Positioning for success"—to facilitate the likely activation of a particular breathing pattern

Ventilatory strategies—to maximize a desired breathing pattern response via the purposeful coordination of trunk movements, breathing, and sensory input

Manual facilitation techniques—to facilitate specific muscle spindle and joint receptor responses of the desired respiratory muscle

Air stacking—to add the effort of numerous smaller inspiratory efforts into 1 larger inspiratory volume

Biofeedback—to provide visual and/or audible feedback

Visualization—to provide internal feedback training

Training in tai chi or other Eastern modalities—to improve breath control

Glossopharyngeal breathing—to maximize voluntary inspiratory efforts in spite of devastating respiratory muscle impairments

technique. The patient actually increases the size of his or her oral cavity, which creates a negative inspiratory pressure, thus facilitating inspiration. Second, they pull their chin and tongue back toward their neck causing positive pressure in the mouth, which forces the air down the trachea into the lung.[99] This sequence, or *stroke* as it is called, is repeated numerous times per breath ($\sim$3–12 strokes per inspiratory effort) and can result in dramatic increases in vital capacity.[103] Learning this technique can result in successful time off the ventilator for patients who would otherwise be completely ventilator dependent.[104,105] In some cases, the learner has been so successful as to be off the ventilator during all wakeful hours. For other patients, it may simply represent a life-saving technique that would help them ventilate independent of a ventilator for a few minutes. A patient with a C4-SCI demonstrates the GPB technique on the accompanying CD.[106]

Improve Breath Support for Speech

Teaching the patient to utilize expiratory breath support for speech with a more controlled pattern will likely improve the disablement of cardiopulmonary disorders. This would require our patient to learn to use his inspiratory muscles eccentrically during phonation in order to elongate the expiratory phase for phonation. Refining breath support for phonation is a natural continuation of the patient's breathing retraining program. Here our patient is asked to refine his breath control at a fine motor skill level, which is the production of speech. This does not require strength, but rather control. It will be much easier to accomplish once Lee is decannulated or at least once he is using a speaking valve, trach cap, or trach button. Decannulation or one of the aforementioned devices provides a closed system in which the

glottis is able to alter (open and close) the entrance into the lungs. A tracheostomy tube without a speaking valve, trach cap, or trach button does not allow the glottis to control air leaving the lungs. Consequently, the air just "falls out" of the open airway, making one unable to use the slow expiratory volumes and flow rates generated during eccentric exhalation patterns that are necessary for speech.[33,34]

Because breathing retraining at any level requires the development of a new motor plan, success may be accomplished very quickly or slowly depending on the patient's ability to learn motor tasks. It appears that patients who are relatively athletic tend to learn these maneuvers quickly ($\sim$1–4 sessions, with independent follow-up practice), whereas people who are less athletic and relatively clumsy tend to be slower in learning new breathing techniques (>6 sessions and follow-up practice). It appears to be related to their general ability to plan and learn new motor tasks.

Several approaches to phonation breathing retraining can be taken. All of the approaches focus on refining the length and control of expiratory maneuvers. Common recreational activities such as singing, humming, choral readings, blow toys that require prolonged exhalation, and/or wind and brass instrument playing demand refinement of expiratory control in order to be successful, thus directly improving breath support for phonation. Using these types of activities also provide the repetition that is necessary for the development of a new motor plan.

If the patient needs more sensory or motor input to develop adequate breath support for speech, then manual techniques can be employed. These techniques are demonstrated on the accompanying CD and all focus on developing better kinesthetic awareness of the chest wall movements during exhalation in order to assist the patient in better eccentric motor planning.[99,107]

A final suggestion for assisting the patient in developing a more refined breathing pattern comes from the incorporation of ventilatory strategies with movement. Because quiet everyday speech is primarily an eccentric contraction, the patient can be taught to purposely combine eccentric movements with speech. Thus, if the patient's trunk or limb muscles have better eccentric control than his breath support, he can use his limb or trunk musculature to facilitate the ventilatory muscles. The reverse is also true. If the patient has better phonation breath support than eccentric control of the limb or trunk muscles, he can be taught to use his phonation to augment other motor responses. Let us say, for example, that our patient wants to reach up to the top of his dresser from his wheelchair to pick up a comb and bring it down to his lap. According to ventilatory strategies described earlier in this section, the patient uses trunk extension and shoulder flexion (both concentric contractions) to reach the comb; thus, an upper chest inspiratory pattern and upward eye gaze would be the natural corresponding ventilatory pattern. On the way back down, he must use eccentric contractions of his shoulder flexors and trunk to slowly lower (not drop) the comb in his lap; thus, the natural corresponding ventilatory pattern would be eccentric exhalation, or speech. Lee could easily be instructed to inhale and look up while reaching for the comb to augment his reach through the chest and spine position associated with inhalation, and then to count outloud or hum and watch the comb (downward glance) while he lowers the comb to his lap. If his phonation skills are better developed than his shoulder muscle skill, then his voice can be used to facilitate better shoulder control. However, if his shoulder skill is better developed than his phonation skills, then his shoulder movements can be used to facilitate better breath control.

Like the interventions described in the previous section on improving breathing patterns, effectiveness of any particular technique or activity can be immediately assessed by pre- and posttesting such as (1) length of a vocalization, (2) number of syllables per breath, (3) loudness of vocalization, and (4) report of fatigue. It is not unusual for a patient to double or even triple their length of phonation following specific retraining programs because it appears to improve control, not strength. Thus, the effort it takes to implement a program for improved phonation is well worth the investment in terms of potential benefit in functional abilities.

Increase Strength, Function, and Endurance of Remaining Respiratory Musculature (Power and Endurance Training)

Development and implementation of a program to strengthen remaining respiratory muscles and develop the necessary endurance of those muscles to support maximal gross motor activity are of great importance for patients with ventilatory pump dysfunction and the potential for failure. In other words, even though our patient may now be capable of breathing properly (a good motor plan), he may still have weakness within that pattern. Second, once he develops some strength or power with this breathing pattern, he may not have the necessary endurance to use the power functionally. Consequently, even though our patient can now properly activate his ventilatory musculature, he still needs a basic strengthening/ endurance program.

Endurance

Respiratory muscles normally become stronger in response to a physiologic demand. For example, running a marathon is a high-oxygen-consuming task, which requires higher TVs and RRs over a prolonged period of time, to meet the physiologic need. As a result, the body secondarily builds strength and endurance of the respiratory muscles to be able to consistently supply the inspiratory volume needed. However, how do you get patients with SCI to strengthen their respiratory muscles if they cannot sustain a gross motor activity, like pushing the wheelchair, long enough to demand a greater physiologic response from the respiratory system? How will they ever build endurance? For patients like Lee, the therapist will need to bypass the large muscle groups and go straight to the respiratory muscles themselves. Creating an artificial demand for greater inspiratory and/or expiratory muscle contraction like

that demanded when running, the respiratory muscles can be specifically targeted for strengthening and endurance training. Ventilatory muscle trainers (VMTs) were designed to accomplish such a goal.

VMTs can be either inspiratory muscle trainers (IMT) or expiratory muscle trainers (EMT). Both work by creating resistance to inspiration or expiration, thereby forcing the patient to create a stronger muscle contraction to exchange their ventilatory volumes. It is similar to breathing in or out through your mouth with a straw, while wearing a nose clip to prevent cheating via nasal breathing. VMTs focus on improving the strength and endurance of the ventilatory muscles because they offer resistance to muscular contraction. There are several devices to choose from such as the *P-flex* or *Threshold* devices (Respironics/ Healthscan Products in Cedar Grove, NJ). Numerous recent studies have shown the efficacy of such programs with both primary and secondary lung dysfunction populations[108-111]; hence, every patient with respiratory muscle weakness or poor endurance, who has the capability to use a VMT, should be started on a program. Most programs last 4 to 6 weeks for 15 to 20 minutes per session, 5 to 7 days/wk. The instructions are to breathe in or out against resistance, not at a maximal level, but at a level the patient can sustain. The patient progresses to greater levels of resistance as he can tolerate it during the 4- to 6-week period. In the most recent studies, all groups show improvement in inspiratory muscle strength (PI_{max}) and endurance (minute ventilation) regardless of whether their condition was acute, chronic, primary lung dysfunction, or ventilatory pump dysfunction.[108-111] More specific methods to perform IMT and EMT are provided in Box 20-6, and methods to measure ventilatory muscle endurance are presented in Chapter 9.

Strength and Power

Similarly, our patient should start a power (strengthening) program. In order to focus on strength and power, Lee needs to work at higher resistance levels with shorter repetitions, generally 3 sets of 10 repetitions (or modified per patient). The patient can use the same IMTs with the resistance increased and the time decreased. Inspiration strengthening can also be achieved through the use of incentive spirometers with specific target ranges. The patient is asked to give a maximal effort and sustain the inspiration for a few seconds (if possible) before releasing the breath. Expiratory muscles can be strengthened using a peak flow meter or an EMT with target ranges. The patient is instructed to take a deep breath first and then to blow hard and fast. Lee should show significant gains in both respiratory strength and endurance, as measured by ventilatory muscle strength and PFTs following completion of this program (see Chapter 9 for methods to measure ventilatory muscle strength).

Endurance and strengthening programs overlap in their application and choice of assistive devices. The main objective, regardless of the chosen intervention, is to improve the respiratory muscle "strength and endurance" enough to provide the maximal benefit to the patient in terms of oxygen delivery for functional ADL use and reducing the work of breathing and the "risk" for acute pulmonary complications.

Methods to Perform Inspiratory and Expiratory Muscle Training

Measurement

Measurement device: Several different types of devices are used to measure ventilatory muscle strength. The methods to measure the positive and negative pressure (in centimeters of water) generated by the patient during such testing is by using a manometer or pressure transducer. When using a manometer, a needle is deflected to the point of maximal generated pressure after which the needle may fall back to the resting level of 0. Such devices typically have poorer resolution and reliability. Newer devices have an internal pressure transducer that provides a digital display, which remains illuminated and as a result has desirable resolution and reliability.

Body position: During the measurement of ventilatory muscle strength the patient should wear a noseclip and be seated with the trunk at a 90-degree angle to the hips.

1. Maximal inspiratory pressure (MIP):
   a. Have patient expire fully (near residual volume).
   b. Motivate patient to inspire as forcefully as possible.
   c. Document the MIP and repeat the aforementioned until a stable baseline is observed.
2. Maximal expiratory pressure (MEP):
   a. Have patient inspire fully (total lung capacity).
   b. Motivate patient to exhale as forcefully as possible.
   c. Document the MEP and repeat the aforementioned until a stable baseline is observed.

Administration of ventilatory muscle training

Ventilatory muscle training should be administered by using the aforementioned results.

Inspiratory muscle training: Begin breathing with one of several available devices at 20% to 40% of MIP for 5 to 15 minutes, 2 to 3 ×/day. Increase resistance to 40% to 60% of MIP based on patient tolerance.

Expiratory muscle training: Begin breathing with one of several available devices at 5% to 10% of MEP for 5 to 15 minutes, 2 to 3 ×/day. Increase resistance to 10% to 15% of MEP based on patient tolerance.

MEDICAL INTERVENTIONS FOR VENTILATORY PUMP DYSFUNCTION AND POTENTIAL FOR FAILURE

Medical Interventions for Ventilatory Pump Dysfunction

The medical interventions for ventilatory pump dysfunction include many of the interventions presented in Chapters 7 (Pulmonary Pathophysiology) and 8 (Medications). These interventions are summarized in Table 20-16 with focus on the correction of ventilatory pump dysfunction and failure. The primary methods to correct ventilatory pump dysfunction or failure appear to be risk factor reduction and pharmacologic, mechanical, surgical, and pulmonary rehabilitation. All of the interventions listed in Table 20-16 have the potential to (1) decrease the amount of bronchospasm in the bronchials, (2) decrease the work of the breathing, or (3) improve the length–tension relationships of ventilatory muscles. It is important to note that pharmacologic agents combined with optimal pulmonary rehabilitation services have the potential to decrease the amount of bronchospasm and work of breathing and possibly improve the length-tension relations of the ventilatory muscles.[112–114]

The primary goals of medical treatment for persons with ventilatory pump dysfunction are to decrease bronchospasm and the work of breathing. Pharmacologic agents such as bronchodilators and glucocorticoids are the primary methods to achieve the aforementioned goals. Mechanical interventions such as CPAP or BiPAP may be used either in conjunction with pharmacologic agents or alone to also achieve the aforementioned goals. The provision of these noninvasive positive-pressure mechanical ventilators often decrease bronchospasm, the work of breathing, and may provide the ventilatory muscles an improved length–tension relationship.[110–113] Brief to prolonged use of CPCP or BiPAP may improve the breathing of patients with ventilatory pump dysfunction or the potential for ventilatory pump failure and improve exercise and functional abilities.[115–118] If the previous methods of treatment are ineffective at improving ventilatory pump dysfunction or failure, surgical techniques may be employed. Several surgical techniques that appear to be beneficial for select patients include volume-reduction surgery and lung transplantation. Administration of supplemental oxygen appears to improve most of the previous goals of medical treatment and often improves the dyspnea associated with ventilatory pump dysfunction or failure. Finally, optimal pharmacologic therapy in conjunction with a comprehensive pulmonary rehabilitation program appears to improve the disablement of ventilatory pump dysfunction and failure.[112–118]

MEDICAL INTERVENTIONS FOR VENTILATORY PUMP FAILURE OR THE POTENTIAL FOR VENTILATORY PUMP FAILURE

The medical interventions for patients with ventilatory pump, failure, or the potential for ventilatory pump failure are also listed in Table 20-16. The methods to attain these goals are similar to the medical interventions for ventilatory pump dysfunction. Furthermore, the goals of treatments for ventilatory pump failure are similar to those presented in Chapter 18 (Physical Therapy Associated with Cardiovascular Pump Dysfunction or Failure) for cardiovascular pump failure but are directed at the ventilatory pump. For example, the goals of most interventions for ventilatory pump failure or the potential for failure are to decrease the work of breathing and improve the work performed by the ventilatory muscles, whereas the goals of most medical treatments for cardiac pump failure are to decrease the work of the heart and improve the work of the heart.[112–118]

TABLE 20-16   Medical Interventions for Ventilatory Pump Dysfunction and Failure

Medical Interventions for Ventilatory Pump Dysfunction and Failure	Description	Outcome
Pharmacologic agents 　Anticholinergics 　Anti-inflammatory agents (Corticosteroid) 　Antihistamines 　Antileukotrienes 　β_2 agonists 　Methylxanthines 　Nonselective β agonists 　Phosphodiesterase inhibitors 　Potassium-channel agonists 　Prostaglandin inhibitors	Blocks parasympathetic activity Decrease inflammation Blocks histamine receptors Decrease inflammation Stimulates β_2 receptors Inhibits phosphodiesterase and 　stimulates diaphragm contraction Stimulates β_1 and β_2 receptors Inhibits the degradation of camp Promotes smooth muscle relaxation Decrease inflammation	Bronchodilation ↓ Improve ventilation ↓ Improve O_2 and CO_2 exchange ↓ Decrease work of breathing ↓ Improve functional abilities
Supplemental oxygen	Increases oxygenation	Decreases bronchoconstriction and functional limitations
Comprehensive pulmonary rehabilitation	Ex., psych, social, and dietary interventions	Risk-factor reduction with possible decrease in morbidity and mortality
Abdominal pneumobelt	Corset with an inflatable bladder (via a positive-pressure delivery device) worn over the abdominal area; inflation and deflation of the bladder are easily synchronized with a patient's respiratory rate.	Inflation and deflation of the bladder assists breathing by providing positive pressure in the abdominal area when the bladder is inflated (which is believed to push the abdominal contents and diaphragm cranially), and deflation of the bladder removes abdominal pressure and allows the diaphragm and abdominal contents to descend (from gravity—**patients must be upright**) and generate negative pressure necessary to ventilate the lungs.
Noninvasive CPAP or BiPAP	Noninvasive positive-pressure ventilation	Improved ventilation of the lungs and decreased work of breathing
Noninvasive negative-pressure ventilation devices (eg, iron lung or chest cuirass)	Noninvasive negative-pressure ventilation synchronized with a patient's respiratory rate which is provided by a shell that encloses the thorax and allows negative ("sucking") pressure to be generated which pulls the chest wall outward when the machine is on (thus creating the negative pressure necessary to ventilate the lungs). When the machine is off, the chest wall falls inward because of gravity and subsequently generates a positive pressure in the intrathoracic area which expels air from the lungs.	Improved ventilation of the lungs and decreased work of breathing
Invasive mechanical ventilation	Invasive positive pressure ventilation	Improved ventilation of the lungs and decreased work of breathing
Lung volume reduction surgery (LVRS)	Removal of 20%–30% of the volume of one or both lungs	Improved ventilation and perfusion of the lungs and length–tension relationship of the diaphragm
Lung transplantation	Diseased lungs are excised and replaced with donor lungs (single or double) or donor segments (eg, living related donor)	Provides "new" lungs without apparent disease which improves ventilation and perfusion of the lungs and length–tension relationship of the diaphragm

OUTCOMES—UTILIZATION OF THRESHOLD BEHAVIORS FOR IMPROVEMENTS IN EXERCISE AND FUNCTIONAL ABILITIES FROM AEROBIC EXERCISE TRAINING: IDENTIFICATION OF RESPONDERS VERSUS NONRESPONDERS TO PULMONARY REHABILITATION

The identification of patients with ventilatory pump dysfunction or the potential for failure who are likely to respond to pulmonary rehabilitation is critical to allocate optimal pulmonary physical therapy.[119-123] **A recent study by Troosters, Gosselink, and Decramer found that patients with reduced exercise capacity, maximal inspiratory strength, and peripheral muscle strength (handgrip and quadriceps strength) who experience less ventilatory limitation to exercise are most likely to improve from exercise training.[121] Table 20-17 lists these and several other threshold behaviors associated with improvements in disablement from pulmonary rehabilitation for patients with a variety of pulmonary disorders.[119-123]**

Tables 20-18 through 20-20 provide an overview of the literature by providing select studies of aerobic and

TABLE 20-17   Possible Predictors of Success or Failure of Patients With Ventilatory Pump Dysfunction or the Potential for Ventilatory Pump Failure in Pulmonary Rehabilitation[a]

Author	Sample Size	Baseline Study Predictor	Possible Threshold for Success	Rationale
ZuWallack et al.[119]	50	FEV_1	?[b]	Patients with more preserved pulmonary function have a greater capacity for improvement
ZuWallack et al.[119]	50	Baseline 12′ walk test	≤2000 ft	Patients with a poorer exercise tolerance have a greater capacity for improvement
ZuWallack et al.[119]	50	$\dot{V}_E$/MVV	?[b]	Patients with less of a ventilatory limit (a greater ventilatory reserve) to exercise have a greater capacity for improvement
ZuWallack et al.[119]	50	$\dot{V}_{O_{2peak}}$ and O_2 pulse	?[b]	Patients with a lower peak $\dot{V}_{O_2}$ and O_2 pulse have a greater capacity for improvement
Maltais et al.[120]	42	FEV_1	≥40% of Predicted	Patients with better pulmonary function have a greater capacity for greater levels of exercise
Maltais et al.[120]	42	$\dot{V}_{O_{2max}}$ and % predicted FEV_1 and training intensity	Greater% predicted $\dot{V}_{O_{2max}}$ and% predicted FEV_1	Patients with a greater% predicted $\dot{V}_{O_{2max}}$ and FEV_1 have a greater ability to exercise at a greater intensity
Troosters et al.[121]	49	$\dot{V}_E$/MVV	≤90%	Patients with less of a ventilatory limit to exercise have a greater capacity for improvement
Troosters et al.[121]	49	MIP	<80% of Predicted	Patients with a lower MIP have a greater capacity for improvement
Troosters et al.[121]	49	Handgrip strength	≤82% of Predicted	Patients with lower handgrip strength have a greater capacity for improvement
Troosters et al.[121]	49	Quadriceps strength	≤76% of Predicted	Patients with lower quadriceps strength have a greater capacity for improvement
Morgan[122]	126	Dyspnea	≤Moderate dyspnea	Patients with ≤ moderate dyspnea have greater capacity for improvement in walking and quality of life
Senjyu et al.[123]	116 Elderly patients with emphysema requiring oxygen therapy	Participation in pulmonary rehabilitation	Participation in pulmonary rehabilitation	Improved survival in patients participating in pulmonary rehabilitation (RR = 4.5)

PFTs, pulmonary function tests; VE/MVV, ventilatory reserve; MIP, maximal inspiratory pressure; RR, relative risk.

[a]Success, improvement in disablement (cardiovascular or pulmonary function, exercise tolerance, aerobic capacity, functional performance, disability), completion of cardiac rehabilitation program, and absence of complications.

[b]?, Unknown.

TABLE 20-18   **Aerobic Exercise Training of Patients With Ventilatory Pump Dysfunction due to Asthma or COPD–Results of Meta-Analytic Studies**

Outcome Measure	Number of Studies	Effect	95% CI[a]	p Value
Maximal exercise capacity	11	0.3	0.1–0.6	0.85
6-min walk distance	11	0.6	0.3–1.0	0.0008
Dyspnea[b]	6	0.8	0.5–1.2	0.12
Fatigue	4	0.6	0.3–0.8	0.36
Emotion	4	0.5	0.2–0.8	0.68
Mastery[b]	4	0.6	0.4–0.9	0.77
Maximal exercise capacity[c]	12	0.4	0.2–0.6	<0.0001
Endurance time	7	1.2	0.9–1.5	<0.0001
Walking distance[c]	15	0.5	0.3–0.7	<0.0001
Dyspnea	5	0.7	0.4–1.0	<0.0001
Fatigue	4	0.6	0.3–0.9	0.0001
Emotion	4	0.5	0.2–0.7	0.001
Mastery	4	0.6	0.3–0.9	<0.0001
Total score	11	0.6	0.5–0.7	<0.0001

[a]CI, confidence interval.

[b]A minimum clinically important difference (MCID; defined as the smallest difference perceived as important by the average patient) was calculated for each of the aforementioned outcome measures, and the overall effect of treatment was compared to the MCID. Dyspnea and mastery of health-related quality of life were both larger than the MCID. Maximal exercise capacity and the 6-minute walk test improved by 8.3 W and 55.7 m, respectively.

[c]The raw mean differences in these outcome measures reveal an overall improvement in maximal exercise capacity of 26 W, whereas the improvement in walking distance was categorized for the duration of the walk test (4-minute walk test improved 30 m, 6-minute walk test improved 49 m, and 12-minute walk test improved 133 m).

From (top half) Lacasse Y, Wong E, Guyatt GH, King D, Cook DJ, Goldstein RS. Meta-analysis of respiratory rehabilitation in chronic obstructive pulmonary disease. *Lancet*. 1996;348:1115-1119.

From (bottom half) Cambach W, Wagenaar RC, KoelmanTW, Ton van Keimpema ARJ, Kemper HCG. The long-term effects of pulmonary rehabilitation in patients with asthma and chronic obstructive pulmonary disease: a research synthesis. *Arch Phys Med Rehabil*. 1999;80(1):103-111.

strengthening exercise studies (Table 20-18),[124,125] IMT studies (Table 20-19),[126–134] and diaphragmatic breathing studies (Table 20-20) for patients with ventilatory pump dysfunction and potential for failure.[134] The information provided in these Tables appears to support the clinical utility of the threshold behaviors provided in Table 20-17 and reveals the beneficial effects of these interventions in the majority of patients enrolled in aerobic/strengthening exercise and breathing exercise programs. Identification of optimal patients for specific interventions should enable even greater improvements in the disablement of patients with ventilatory pump dysfunction, potential for ventilatory pump failure, or even ventilatory pump failure.

Boxes 20-7 and 20-8 provide specific methods to perform aerobic or strength training and Box 20-9 provides important methods to administer diaphragmatic breathing exercises to patients with ventilatory pump dysfunction or the potential for failure. The methods to perform aerobic and strength training in patients with ventilatory pump dysfunction and the potential for failure are similar to the methods of training patients with cardiac pump failure, except that patients with ventilatory pump dysfunction or the potential for failure often have more of a ventilatory limitation to exercise. In view of this, more emphasis should be placed on attempting to decrease the ventilatory limitation to exercise via medications, body positions, ventilatory muscle training, and airway clearance techniques when needed. Patients who are unable to decrease ventilatory constraints to exercise training likely require noninvasive mechanical ventilation like CPAP and BiPAP.

One potential method to train the ventilatory muscles is diaphragmatic breathing. Diaphragmatic breathing may be beneficial for select patients, and an extensive review of diaphragmatic breathing in COPD revealed that patients who have elevated respiratory rates, low tidal volumes that increase during DB, and abnormal arterial blood gases with adequate diaphragmatic movement are most likely to benefit from diaphragmatic breathing.[135] Administering diaphragmatic breathing to such patients while using the methods described in Box 20-9 should optimize efforts to administer diaphragmatic breathing. Furthermore, administering inspiratory and expiratory muscle training as described in Box 20-6 with the methods of diaphragmatic breathing presented in Box 19-9 should enable patients with ventilatory pump dysfunction and

TABLE 20-19 Select Studies of Inspiratory Muscle Training in Patients With Ventilatory Pump Dysfunction

Author	Sample Size	Type of Breathing Exercise	Study Measurements	Study Outcomes
Chen et al.[126]	13	PFLEX-like inspiratory muscle training program at 35% of MIP	Ventilatory muscle strength and endurance; exercise tolerance; pulmonary function	Improved ventilatory muscle strength and endurance, but no change in exercise tolerance or pulmonary function
Larson et al.[127]	22	Threshold IMT,[a] 15% of MIP (group 1) or 30% of MIP (group 2)	Ventilatory muscle strength and endurance; dyspnea; 12-min walk test; pulmonary function; quality of life	Improved ventilatory muscle strength and endurance and 12-min walk test in group 2
Harver et al.[128]	19	Threshold IMT at 5 cm H_2O (group 1) or 5–35 cm H_2O (group 2)	Ventilatory muscle strength and dyspnea	Improved ventilatory muscle strength and dyspnea in group 2
Dekhuijzen et al.[129]	40	Threshold IMT at 70% of MIP	Ventilatory muscle strength and endurance; 12-min walk test	Improved ventilatory muscle strength and endurance and 12-min walk test
Weiner et al.[130]	36	Progressive threshold IMT from 15% to 80% of MIP	Ventilatory muscle strength and endurance; 12-min walk test; pulmonary function	Improved ventilatory muscle strength and endurance, 12-min walk test, and pulmonary function
Weiner et al.[131]	30	Progressive threshold IMT from 15% to 80% MIP	Ventilatory muscle strength and endurance; pulmonary function; symptoms; hospitalizations, ER visits, medication use, and absence from school/work	Improved ventilatory muscle strength and endurance, pulmonary function, symptoms, and hospitalizations, ER visits, medication use, and absence from school/work
Suzuki et al.[132]	12	Threshold IMT at 30% of MIP	Ventilatory muscle strength	Improved ventilatory muscle strength after only 2 weeks
Nomori et al.[133]	100	Diaphragmatic breathing with 2 kg on abdomen and expiratory muscle training	Ventilatory muscle strength and postoperative complications	Improved ventilatory muscle strength with fewer postoperative complications
Preusser et al.[134]	20	Threshold IMT at 22% of MIP (group 1) or 52% of MIP (group 2)	Ventilatory muscle strength and endurance; 12-min walk test	Improved ventilatory muscle strength and endurance and 12-min walk test

[a]Threshold IMT, inspiratory muscle training with a portable handheld device through which a patient can breathe only when they overcome the threshold resistance (provided via a calibrated spring) of the device.

the potential for failure to develop improved ventilatory pump function.

SUMMARY AND APPLICATION TO THE DISABLEMENT MODEL

The Disablement Model by Nagi (pathology, impairments, functional limitations, disability) was described in Chapter 2 and has been applied to a patient with SCI throughout the chapter. In this chapter, the focus has been on identifying the long-term impairments and risk factors associated with cardiopulmonary dysfunction following an SCI (ventilatory pump dysfunction/failure, preferred Practice Pattern 6E) and the potential for decreasing the resulting functional limitations based on successful cardiopulmonary management of these impairments and risks.

The management of the patient with ventilatory pump dysfunction, and the ongoing risk for ventilatory pump failure, is complicated and unending. All team members need to be part of the evaluation process, the development and implementation of a successful cardiopulmonary program, and the continuing reassessment of its effectiveness. Perhaps the most important component of the program in the rehabilitation setting versus the acute ICU setting is the education of the patient and his family. Although our patient, Lee, was in the ICU, the emphasis of his medical intervention was to "save his life." In the rehabilitation setting, the emphasis switches to helping the patient regain and maintain a "quality to his life," thus focusing on minimizing his long-term disability. The patient and his family must know how to continue these programs after discharge from the hospital setting in order to foster a lifelong successful management of his cardiopulmonary risks. If well managed, this patient should encounter fewer respiratory complications.[4,63,136,137] This will result in minimizing his long-term functional limitations and resultant disability level. However, if he fails to be vigilant about managing his impairments, they can result in acute pulmonary problems and secondary functional limitations with potential for greater physical disability.

Close examination of the case study presented in this chapter should make it clear that the proposed examinations

TABLE 20-20 **Studies of Diaphragmatic Breathing in COPD**

Author	Study Type	N^a	FVC % Predicted	FEV$_1$	DB Instruction	DB Training (Days)	DB Competency
Becklake et al.	QE	15	74	NR	Improve diaphragmatic movement, the expiratory phase, and general relaxation, aradic muscle F stimulation was applied to 9 patients	80	NR
Miller	PE	24	69	NR	Poorly reported	42–56	NR
Campbell, Friend	PE	12	NR	NR	Relaxation of neck and upper thorax muscles, prolonged expiration, diaphragmatic movement and "controlled even breathing"	28–42	NR
Sinclair	PE	22	NR	NR	Correcting uncoordinated breathing patterns by increasing abdominal breathing and eliminating upper chest breathing	21–84	NR
McNeill, McKenzie	TE	33	NR	NR	Asthma Research Council	28–84	NR
McKinley et al.	PE	6	NR	NR	Practice DB repeatedly during the day and to "correlate breathing with walking, stairclimbing, etc"	28	NR
Cole et al.	QE	31	NR	NR	NR	336–448	NR
Sackner et al.	PE	11	NR	NR	Relaxed sitting with auditory, tactile, and visual stimulation	NR	NR
Grimby et al.	PE	6	74	58	NR	NR	NR
Johnston, Lee	PE	12	NR	NR	NR	NR	NR
Brach et al.	PE	6	46–94	NR	NR	NR	NR
Tandon	TE	22	NR	NR	NR	252	NR
Sergysels et al.	QE	20	67	45	Low-frequency breathing (often accomplished with pursed-lip breathing) with high tidal volume and adequate abdominal motion was emphasized.	56–168	NR
Ambrosino et al.[b]	TE	51	NR	NR	"Consisted of relaxation and slow breathing, diaphragmatic breathing and pursed-lip breathing"	28	NR
Williams et al.	QE	8	NR	NR	"Move lower chest and abdomen"	21	NR
Willeput et al.	PE	11	89	75	6 Different breathing techniques taught by a physical therapist	5 min	Visual observation
Sackner et al.	PE	9	NR	NR	NR	NR	NR
Holliday, Ruppel	PE	8	NR	NR^	Keep the rib cage and abdominal RIP and EMG feedback in phase to reduce asynchrony	?[c]	NR
Gosselink et al.	PE	7	88	34	NR	21	Doubling of abdominal tidal excursion with reduced upper chest wall excursion
Kanamori, Okubo	QE	43	55	37	Patient education	56	Movement of weight on abdomen

(continued)

TABLE 20-20 **Studies of Diaphragmatic Breathing in COPD** *(Continued)*

Author	Study Type	N^a	FVC % Predicted	FEV₁ % Predicted	DB Instruction	DB Training (Days)	DB Competency
Onodera, Yazaki	PE	16	NR	NR	Semi-Fowlers with patients hands on upper chest and abdomen with tactile stimulation if needed	21	NR
Vitacca et al.	PE	25	NR	NR	Semirecumbent with tactile stimulation and instructions to "inspire maximally with abdominal motion"	3	Visual observation
Ito et al.	PE	16	87	42	Supine with 1-kg weight on abdomen	NR	NR
Pasto et al.	PE	10	NR	33	? Body position with tactile stimulation to increase abdominal and decrease upper chest wall motion	NR	Visual observation

Author	Study Measurements	Study Outcomes
Becklake et al.	Symptoms; PFTs[a]; and oximetry	DB produced no substantial improvement in any of the study measurements except for symptoms
Miller	PFTs; ABGs; diaphragmatic excursion via fluoroscopy; resting and exercise (undefined 1-min exercise test) calculated respiratory gas analyses and ventilation via respirometry and ventilographic attachment	DB produced a decrease in resting respiratory rate and arterial carbon dioxide levels and an increase in diaphragmatic excursion, tidal volume, maximal expiratory pressure, inspiratory capacity, maximal breathing capacity, arterial oxygen saturation, and calculated oxygen consumption. Despite these improvements there was no significant change in resting ventilation. However, exercise oxygen consumption was calculated to increase after DB.
Campbell, Friend	PFTs; oxygen consumption; EMG	DB produced no substantial effect on pulmonary function, lung volumes, oxygen consumption, or EMG activity acutely or chronically
Sinclair	PFTs; subjective report (via personal reporting), and diaphragmatic excursion	DB improved symptoms and diaphragmatic excursion (with the improvement likely due to increased spinal movement), but without change in pulmonary function
McNeill, McKenzie	Dyspnea at rest, walking on a flat surface, and walking up stairs or a hill; PFTs	No significant change in pulmonary function while change in dyspnea was not reported in the paper
McKinley et al.	PFTs; transpulmonary pressures; and Symptoms	Improved symptoms and an increased work of breathing both acutely and chronically
Cole et al.	PFTs; Subjective report (via daily patient report and monthly interview)	No significant difference in subjective report, pulmonary function, or lung volumes between the medical therapy group versus the medical therapy combined with DB group
Sackner et al.	Distribution of ventilation via nitrogen wash-out and [133]xenon distribution; and chest wall motion	DB did not alter any of the indices of distribution of ventilation via the nitrogen washout analyses in persons with COPD. Likewise, analysis of [138]xenon distribution revealed no difference in the topographic distribution of [138]xenon during thoracic breathing compared to DB in persons with COPD. However, in five of the eight normal subjects,[138]xenon distribution was directed to the lower lung zones during DB, whereas thoracic breathing directed [138]xenon distribution to the upper lung zones.
Grimby et al.	[133]xenon distribution and chest wall motion	Improvement in the relative contribution of the abdomen to ventilation during DB, but no difference in ventilation distribution between DB and spontaneous breathing.
Johnston, Lee	Spirometry and EMG	Continuous audio- and visual feedback of EMG from abdominal muscles improved DB learning with fewer instructional sessions.
Brach et al.	[133]xenon distribution, tidal volume, and ventilation	No difference in clearance indices for any region of the lung in the normal subjects or persons with COPD between NB and DB. Overall washout of [138]xenon from the lungs was more rapid during DB in all normal subjects and in three persons with COPD (who also demonstrated increased tidal volumes during DB compared to NB). The three other persons with COPD were observed to have no difference in tidal volumes or overall washout of [138]xenon during NB or DB.
Tandon	Symptoms, ABGs, PFTs, and maximal cardiorespiratory cycle ergometry exercise testing	No difference in arterial blood gases or pulmonary function after training in either group, but peak workload and symptoms were observed to be improved after yogic breathing.

(continued)

TABLE 20-20   Studies of Diaphragmatic Breathing in COPD *(Continued)*

Author	Study Measurements	Study Outcomes
Sergysels et al.	PFTs, DLCO, and respiratory gases during submaximal and maximal exercise testing	Significant improvements in total lung capacity, vital capacity, diffusion capacity for carbon monoxide, and resting partial pressure of arterial carbon dioxide after DB and similar improvements after DB combined with bicycling exercise training as well as significant improvements in resting partial pressure of arterial oxygen, peak oxygen consumption, and pulmonary hypertension.
Ambrosino et al.	PFTs, ABGs, exercise tolerance via cycle	Improved ABGs, PFTs, and exercise tolerance in the medical therapy combined with DB group compared to improved pulmonary function in the medial therapy group.
Williams et al.	PFTs, 12-minute walk test, and Borg rating of perceived exertion (RPE)	PFTs, 12-minute walk test, and Borg RPE were unchanged after DB.
Willeput et al.	PFTs and chest wall motion	Decreased respiratory rates and increased tidal volumes for all breathing techniques, but substantial paradoxical movements of the chest including an outward movement of the rib cage or abdomen during expiration and an inward movement of the rib cage or abdomen during expiration.
Sackner et al.	PFTs and chest wall excursion	Healthy subjects increased ventilation during DB without improvement from visual feedback. Persons with COPD were observed to have a greater inspiratory time and tidal volume during DB without visual feedback, but DB with visual feedback produced greater abdominal movement compared to DB without visual feedback. Patients with COPD were observed to have a variable amount of paradoxical chest wall motion during spontaneous breathing, which worsened during DB. Paradoxical chest wall motion was observed to decrease when the COPD patients were moved (via tilt table) from supine to upright postures.
Holliday, Ruppel	PFTs; symptoms; chest wall motion; EMG	Significant improvements in symptoms and abdominal breathing with less asynchrony between the rib cage and abdomen.
Gosselink et al.	Chest wall motion, mechanical efficiency, and dyspnea during normal breathing, loaded breathing, and DB	DB in patients with severe COPD worsened the coordination of chest wall movement and mechanical efficiency and increased dyspnea sensation. Also, there were no significant differences in many respiratory variables between loaded and unloaded NB and DB.
Kanamori, Okubo	PFTs, ABGs, and 12-minute walk test	12MD increased significantly in both groups (group A = $Spo_2 < 90\%$ and group B = $Spo_2 \geq 90\%$), but Pao_2, vital capacity (VC) and forced expiratory volume for a second (FEV_1) increased only in group A.
Onodera, Yazaki	PFTs, Visual Analog Scale at the end of 6-minute walk distance (6MD) test, 6MD, maximum exercise tolerance on a treadmill	Dyspnea decreased significantly at the end of 6MD test after the rehabilitation program and a significant increase in the 6MD. Endurance time during an incremental treadmill exercise test and spirometric pulmonary function test results did not change after the study. However, total lung capacity (TLC), functional residual capacity (FRC), and residual volume (RV) decreased significantly after the program.
Vitacca et al.	ABGs, transcutaneous partial pressure of carbon dioxide, and inspiratory muscle strength	DB (in severe COPD patients with chronic hypercapnia and reduced inspiratory muscle strength recovering from acute respiratory failure) improved blood gases and ventilation, but increased inspiratory muscle effort and dyspnea.
Ito et al.	PFTs, oxygen consumption, and carbon dioxide production; end-tidal oxygen and carbon dioxide fraction, and chest wall excursion	DB decreased ventilation, tidal diaphragmatic volume, carbon dioxide production, respiratory exchange ratio, and end-tidal oxygen and carbon dioxide fraction.
Pasto et al.	PFTs, maximal inspiratory mouth pressure, and transdiaphragmatic, abdominal, and intrathoracic pressures; ABGs; and continuous spirometry during 2 minutes of NB and DB	DB produced significantly greater tidal volumes and esophageal, transdiaphragmatic, and abdominal pressures in the supine position and significantly greater transdiaphragmatic pressure in sitting. Although it was not presented or discussed (analyses between NB and DB did not appear to be performed) tidal volume, inspiratory time/total respiratory time, and esophageal pressure appeared to be significantly greater during DB compared to NB in both supine and sitting positions. No significant change in respiratory rate was observed between NB and DB and between DB and a maximal inspiratory effort. However, the lower Vt/Pdi during DB suggests that the mechanical efficiency of the diaphragm was less during DB compared to a maximal inspiratory effort, but mechanical ventilation was slightly greater during DB compared to NB.

FVC, forced vital capacity; FEV_1, forced expiratory volume in 1 second; DB, diaphragmatic breathing; QE, Quasi-experimental study; PE, Pre-experimental study; TE, trueexperimental study; NR, not reported; RIP, respiratory inductive plethysmography; EMG, electromyography; PFTs, pulmonary function tests; ABGs, arterial blood gases; NB, normal breathing; Spo_2, oxygen saturation; DLCO, pulmonary diffusing capacity for carbon monoxide, arterial blood gases; RPE, rating of perceived exertion.

[a]*N*, sample size.

[b]Ambrosino evaluated the effects of medical therapy (bronchodilators, mucolytics, and antibiotics, if necessary; *N* = 28) and medical therapy combined with DB (*N* = 23).

[c]Holliday and Ruppel reported a mean $FEV_1/FVC = 49\%$ and provided 12 sessions of DB, but the time period was not reported.

BOX 20-7

Exercise Training Methods for Patients with Ventilatory Pump Dysfunction and the Potential for Failure

1. Perform an exercise test or utilize recent exercise test results—**6- or 12-minute walk tests may be substituted for a structured exercise test (see Chapter 9)***
2. Determine whether the cardiovascular and pulmonary response during the exercise test is adaptive
3. If exercise test results are adaptive without signs or symptoms of myocardial ischemia or cardiac arrhythmias, the exercise prescription should be developed via one of several methods including:
   a. Karvonen method
   b. 60% to 85% of peak heart rate or peak oxygen consumption
   c. Rate of perceived exertion corresponding to optimal training heart rate or level of oxygen consumption
   d. Heart rate or rate of perceived exertion just below the ventilatory threshold/anaerobic threshold
   e. **Level of dyspnea**
4. If exercise test results are not adaptive and show signs of signs or symptoms of myocardial ischemia, cardiac arrhythmias, desaturation, excessive accessory muscle with or without a paradoxical breathing pattern, or a marked ventilatory limit to exercise (see Chapters 9 and 10), the exercise prescription should be developed via one of several methods including:
   a. Ischemic threshold via heart rate
   b. Ischemic threshold via rate pressure product (double product)
   c. Ischemic threshold via electrocardiographic evidence of myocardial ischemia or cardiac arrhythmias
   d. **Heart rate or rate of perceived exertion/dyspnea just below the threshold for maladaptive cardiovascular or pulmonary exercise test results**
5. Perform physical exercise using the most appropriate mode, duration, frequency, and duration based on exercise test results, **the level of dyspnea and resting and exercise breathing pattern, and patient goals/enjoyment.**
6. Begin with gentle stretching and aerobic exercise and progress to a greater exercise duration and intensity as exercise training continues.
7. Set realistic goals for exercise with a range of 20 to 45 minutes exercise duration, 3 to 5 ×/wk frequency, and at an appropriate training intensity based on numbers 3 and 4 above.
8. Monitor patient during exercise using the methods described in Chapters 9 and 10 and determine the frequency of monitoring during an exercise training session based on the exercise test results, level of dyspnea, resting and exercise breathing patterns, and other patient signs/symptoms.
9. Reexamine the patient during each exercise session using the methods described in Chapters 9 and 10.
10. Perform a second exercise test after 1 to 3 months of exercise training to establish safety of *progressive exercise training and develop a new exercise prescription.*

*Bolded sections identify key concerns for patients with ventilatory pump dysfunction or the potential for failure.

BOX 20-8

Criteria for the Initiation and Progression of Exercise Training in Patients with Ventilatory Pump Dysfunction or the Potential for Ventilatory Pump Failure (Compensated Ventilatory Pump Failure)

I. **Relative criteria** necessary for the initiation of an aerobic exercise training program—**Compensated ventilatory pump failure**
1. Ability to speak **relatively** comfortably without signs or symptoms of marked dyspnea (able to (1) vocalize and sustain vowel sounds like "ah" for ≥5 seconds before taking a breath, (2) ≥5 syllables per breath, or (3) loudly with a RR < 40 breaths/min)
2. ≤Moderate fatigue
3. Breath sounds present in one-half of the lungs
4. No paradoxical breathing pattern or a paradoxical breathing pattern is resolved with forward leaning.
5. Ability to increase tidal volume above a reliable (repeatedly stable) baseline value via change in body position, breathing pattern, or other perturbation/intervention
6. Oxygen saturation level >90%

II. Relative criteria indicating a need to modify or terminate exercise training
   a. Marked dyspnea or fatigue (eg, Borg rating > 4–5/10)
   b. Oxygen saturation < 88%
   c. Respiratory rate > 50 breaths/min during exercise
   d. Development of S_3 or pulmonary crackles
   e. Increase in pulmonary crackles
   f. Significant increase in the intensity of the second component of the second heart sound (P_2)
   g. Poor pulse pressure (<10 mm Hg difference between the systolic and diastolic blood pressures)
   h. Decrease in heart rate or blood pressure of >10 bpm or mm Hg, respectively, during continuous (steady-state) or progressive (increasing workloads) exercise
   i. Increased supraventricular or ventricular ectopy
   j. Increase of >10 mm Hg in the mean pulmonary artery pressure (for invasively monitored patients)
   k. Increase or decrease of >6 mm Hg in the central venous pressure (for invasively monitored patients)
   l. Diaphoresis, pallor, or confusion

Adapted with permission from Cahalin LP. Heart failure. *Phys Ther.* 1996;76:529.

BOX 20-9

Specific Methods to Instruct and Perform Diaphragmatic Breathing—A Literature and Research Synthesis[130]

1. Comfortable body position—sitting, semi-Fowler's position (sitting at a 45-degree angle), side-lying, or sitting with trunk flexion if marked hyperinflation of the lungs and a paradoxical breathing pattern are present at rest or during diaphragmatic breathing. Measure tidal volume before beginning instruction in DB.

2. Appropriate position of the pelvis, neck, eyes, and upper and lower extremities—posterior pelvic tilt, neck extension, upward position of the eyes, upper extremities in external rotation and flexion, and lower extremities in external rotation and flexion may improve diaphragmatic breathing.

3. Tactile stimulation—placement of patients hand and therapists hand on the abdomen (level of the umbilicus) and the upper chest (level of the manubrium) with a quick stretch inward and upward at end exhalation at the abdominal area.

4. Auditory stimulation—Therapist loudly inspires with the inspiratory maneuver of the patient and loudly exhales with the expiratory maneuver of the patient.

5. Visual stimulation—Patient instructed to observe increased motion of hand over the abdomen and decreased motion of hand over the upper chest; biofeedback of respiratory maneuvers via electromyography of respiratory muscles, oxygen saturation, or a mirror may be useful.

6. Breathing instruction—Request patient to "breathe into my hand" during inspiration while instructing the patient to inspire through the nose and exhale orally with pursed lips.

7. Provide supplemental oxygen, bronchodilator therapy, and secretion removal if needed.

8. Breathing instruction—Request patient to "sniff" to promote a diaphragmatic contraction and then to "breathe into my hand" during inspiration.

9. Evaluate competency in diaphragmatic breathing—Doubling of abdominal tidal excursion with reduced upper chest excursion. Measure tidal volume during DB.

10. Possibly use an abdominal–diaphragmatic breathing pattern which incorporates an *abdominal* contraction at end-expiration followed by DB.

and interventions can be applied to a patient with ventilatory pump dysfunction or failure from any etiology. These same examinations and interventions likely apply to a patient with COPD, pulmonary fibrosis, or CVA and should enable optimal physical therapy to patients with ventilatory pump dysfunction or failure. One important behavior that appears to be capable of differentiating between ventilatory pump dysfunction and the potential for failure is a paradoxical breathing pattern.[138–144] Identification of the absence or presence of a paradoxical breathing pattern may be helpful in allocating physical therapy interventions.[138–144]

The primary domains of disablement most affected in patients with ventilatory pump dysfunction or failure are similar to those of patients with cardiac pump failure which are listed in Table 18-20. Subtle differences exist, but the methods to manage these domains of disablement are very similar for patients with cardiac pump failure and for patients with ventilatory pump dysfunction and failure.

LIMITS OF OUR KNOWLEDGE

Significant research on SCI and resultant ventilatory pump dysfunction and on secondary respiratory complications has already been conducted, but more research is needed on the effectiveness of current physical therapy interventions in minimizing these risks. Which interventions, or combination of interventions, are the most effective and efficient? Airway clearance interventions are probably the best studied area of intervention within the physical therapy realm, with good

evidence-based data to assist the therapist in planning a plausible intervention. More clinical research is needed in evaluating the effectiveness of interventions such as using ventilatory strategies with movement, improved breath control for speech, and the best methods for successful breathing retraining and carryover into function. Furthermore, further investigation of the clinical utility of paradoxical breathing patterns in physical therapy examinations and allocation of specific interventions is needed.[138–144] Other areas worthy of further investigation include patient motivation, family support, and financial issues which should assist the physical therapist's clinical decision-making skills and optimal allocation of physical therapy interventions.

Heads Up!

This chapter contains a CD-ROM activity.

REFERENCES

1. American Physical Therapy Association. Guide to Physical Therapist Practice. 2nd ed. *Phys Ther.* 2001 Jan;81(1):9-746.
2. American Physical Therapy Association. Guide to Physical Therapist Practice. *Phys Ther.* 1997;77(11).
3. DeVivo MJ, Black KJ, Stover SL. Causes of death during the first 12 years after spinal cord injury. *Arch Phys Med Rehabil.* 1993;74:248-254.
4. Frankel HL, Coll JR, Charlifue SW, et al. Long-term survival in spinal cord injury: a fifty year investigation. *Spinal Cord.* 1998; 36(4):266-274.

5. DeVivo MJ, Krause JS, Lammertse DP. Recent trends in mortality and causes of death among persons with spinal cord injury. *Arch Phys Med Rehabil.* 1999;80(11):1411-1419.

6. Amonoo-Kuofi HS. The density of muscle spindles in the medial, intermediate and lateral columns of human intrinsic postvertebral muscles. *J Anat.* 1983;3:509-519.

7. Flynn TW. *The Thoracic Spine and Rib Cage: Musculoskeletal Evaluation and Treatment.* Newton, MA: Butterworth-Heinemann; 1996.

8. Dean E, Hobson L. Cardiopulmonary anatomy. In: Frownfelter DL, Dean E, eds. *Principles and Practice of Cardiopulmonary Physical Therapy.* 3rd ed. St Louis, MO: Mosby-Year Book; 1996: 23-51.

9. Takeuchi T, Abumi K, Shono Y, Oda I, Kaneda K. Biomechanical role of the intervertebral disc and costovertebral joint in stability of the thoracic spine: a canine model study. *Spine.* 1999;24(14): 1414-1420.

10. Bouisset S, Duchene JL. Is body balance more perturbed by respiration in seating than in standing posture? *Neuroreport.* 1994;5(8):957-960.

11. Flaminiano LE, Celli BR. Respiratory muscle testing. *Clin Chest Med.* 2001;22(4):661-677.

12. LaPier TK, Cook A, Droege K, Oliverson R, et al. Intertester and intratester reliability of chest excursion measurement in subjects without impairment. *Cardiopulm Phys Ther.* 2000;11(3):94-98.

13. Massery MP, Dreyer HE, Bjornson AS, Cahalin LP. Chest wall excursion and tidal volume change during passive positioning in cervical spinal cord injury [Abstract]. *Cardiopulm Phys Ther.* 1997;8(4):27.

14. Sumarez RC. An analysis of action of intercostal muscles in the human rib cage. *J Appl Physiol.* 1986;60(2):690-701.

15. Han JN, Gayan-Ramirez G, Dekhuijzen R, Decramer M. Respiratory function of the rib cage muscles. *Eur Respir J.* 1993;6(5): 722-728.

16. Lissoni A, Aliverti A, Tzeng AC, Bach JR. Kinematic analysis of patients with spinal muscular atrophy during spontaneous breathing and mechanical ventilation. *Am J Phys Med Rehabil.* 1998;77(3):188-192.

17. Gounden P. Static respiratory pressures in patients with post-traumatic tetraplegia. *Spinal Cord.* 1997;35(1):43-47.

18. DeTroyer A, Estenne M, Vincken W. Rib cage motion and muscle use in high tetraplegics. *Am Rev Respir Dis.* 1986;133: 1115-1119.

19. Perez A, Mulot R, Vardon G, Barois A, Gallego J. Thoracoabdominal pattern of breathing in neuromuscular disorders. *Chest.* 1996;110:454-461.

20. McCool FD, Pichurko BM, Slutsky AS, Sarkarati M, Rossier A, Brown R. Changes in lung volume and rib cage configuration with abdominal binding in quadriplegia. *J Appl Physiol.* 1986;60(4):1198-1202.

21. Massery MP. Chest development as a component of normal motor development: implications for pediatric physical therapists. *Pediatr Phys Ther.* 1991;3(1):3-8.

22. Chen CF, Lien IN, Wu MC. Respiratory function in patients with spinal cord injuries: effects of posture. *Paraplegia.* 1990;28:81-86.

23. Cala SJ, Edynean J, Engel LA. Abdominal compliance, parasternal activation, and chest wall motion. *J Appl Physiol.* 1993;74(3):1398-1405.

24. Kondo T, Kobayashi I, Taguchi Y, Ohta Y, Yanagimachi N. A dynamic analysis of chest wall motions with MRI in healthy young subjects. *Respirology.* 2000;5(1):19-25.

25. Wilson TA, Angelillo M, Legrand A, de Troyer A. Muscle kinematics for minimal work of breathing. *J Appl Physiol.* 1999; 87(2):554-560.

26. Massery MP. The patient with neuromuscular or musculoskeletal dysfunction. In: Frownfelter DL, Dean E, eds. *Principles and Practice of Cardiopulmonary Physical Therapy.* 3rd ed. St Louis, MO: Mosby-Year Book; 1996:679-702.

27. Cserhati EF, Gregesi KA, Poder G, Mezie G, et al. Thorax deformity and asthma bronchial. *Allergo Immunupathol (Madr).* 1984;12(1):7-10.

28. Fonkalsrud EW, Salman T, Guo W, Gregg JP. Repair of pectus deformities with sternal support. *J Thorac Cardiovasc Surg.* 1994;107(1):37-42.

29. Leong JC, Lu WW, Luk KD, Karlberg EM. Kinematics of the chest cage and spine during breathing in healthy individuals and in patients with adolescent idiopathic scoliosis. *Spine.* 1999;24(13):1310-1315.

30. Gonzalez J, Coast JR, Lawler JM, Welch HG. A chest wall restrictor to study effects on pulmonary function and exercise; the energetics of restrictive breathing. *Respiration.* 1999;66(2): 188-194.

31. Alpard SK, Zwischenberger JB, Tao W, Deyo DJ, Traber DL, Bidani A. New clinically relevant sheep model of severe respiratory failure secondary to combined smoke inhalation/cutaneous flame burn injury. *Crit Care Med.* 2000;28(5):1677-1678.

32. Cherniack RM, Cherniack L. *Respiration in Health and Disease.* 3rd ed. Philadelphia, PA: WB Saunders; 1983.

33. Hixon TJ. *Respiratory Function in Speech and Song.* San Diego, CA: Singular Publishing Group; 1991.

34. Deem JF, Miller L. *Manual of Voice Therapy.* 2nd ed. Austin, TX: PRO-ED Inc; 2000.

35. Moore CA, Caulfield TJ, Green JR. Relative kinematics of the rib cage and abdomen during speech and nonspeech behaviors of 15-month-old children. *J Speech Lang Hear Res.* 2001;44(1): 80-94.

36. Hoit JD, Lohmeier HL. Influence of continuous speaking on ventilation. *J Speech Lang Hear Res.* 2000;43(5):1240-1251.

37. Hoit JD, Banzett RB, Brown R, Loring SH. Speech breathing in individuals with cervical spinal cord injury. *J Speech Hear Res.* 1990;33(4):798-807.

38. Chung F, Dean E, Ross J. Cardiopulmonary responses of middle-aged men without cardiopulmonary disease to steady-rate positive and negative work performed on a cycle ergometer. *Phys Ther.* 1999;79(5):476-487.

39. Lundqvist C, Siosteen A, Blomstrand C, Lind B, Sullivan M. Spinal cord injuries: clinical, functional, and emotional status. *Spine.* 1991;16(1):78-83.

40. Leiner GC, Abramowitz S, Small MJ, Stenby VB, Lewis WA. Expiratory peak flow rate: standard values for normal subjects. *Am Rev Respir Dis.* 1963;88:644-651.

41. Bach JR. Mechanical insufflation–exsufflation: comparison of peak expiratory flows with manually assisted and unassisted coughing techniques. *Chest.* 1993;104:1553-1562.

42. Wang AY, Jaeger RJ, Yarkony GM, Turba RM. Cough in spinal cord injured patients: the relationship between motor level and peak expiratory flow. *Spinal Cord.* 1997;35(5):299-302.

43. DeTroyer A, Estenne M. The expiratory muscles in tetraplegia. *Paraplegia.* 1991;29(6):359-363.

44. Haas F, Fain R, Salazar-Schicchi J, Axen K. Pathophysiology of chronic obstructive pulmonary disease. In: Bach JR, Haas F, eds. *Physical Medicine and Rehabilitation Clinics of North America.* Vol 7. Philadelphia, PA: Saunders; 1996:205-223.

45. Aggarwal AN, Gupta D, Behera D, Jindal SK. Analysis of static pulmonary mechanics helps to identify functional defects in survivors of acute respiratory distress syndrome. *Crit Care Med.* 2000;28(10):3480-3483.

46. Papastamelos C, Panitch HB, Allen JL. Chest wall compliance in infants and children with neuromuscular disease. *Am J Respir Crit Care Med.* 1996;154:1045-1048.

47. Nixon V. *Spinal Cord Injury: A Guide to Functional Outcomes in Physical Therapy Management.* Gaithersburg, MD: Aspen Publishers Inc; 1985.

48. Somers MF. *Spinal Cord Injury: Functional Rehabilitation.* Norwalk, CT: Appleton & Lange; 1992.

49. Coll JR, Frankel HL, Charlifue SW, Whiteneck GG. Evaluating neurological group homogeneity in assessing the mortality risk for people with spinal cord injuries. *Spinal Cord.* 1998;36(4): 275-279.

50. Shepherd Spinal Center. *C4–C5 Complete Tetraplegia Non Vent-dependent Critical Pathway.* Atlanta, GA: Shepherd Spinal Center; 1999.

51. Illis L. Clinical evaluation and pathophysiology of the spinal cord in the chronic stage. In: Illis L, ed. *Spinal Cord Dysfunction: Assessment.* New York, NY: Oxford University Press; 1988.

52. Atkinson PP, Atkinson JL, eds. Spinal shock. *Mayo Clin Proc.* 1996;71(4):384-389.

53. Bach JR. Update and perspective on noninvasive respiratory muscle aids: Part 2: the expiratory aids. *Chest.* 1994;105: 1538-1544.

54. Burns SP, Little JW, Hussey JD, Lyman P, Lakshminarayanan S. Sleep apnea syndrome in chronic spinal cord injury: associated factors and treatment. *Arch Phys Med Rehabil.* 2000;81(10): 1334-1339.

55. Klefbeck B, Sternhag M, Weinberg J, Levi R, Hultling C, Borg J. Obstructive sleep apneas in relation to severity of cervical spinal cord injury. *Spinal Cord.* 1998;36(9):621-628.

56. Consortium for Spinal Cord Medicine. *Clinical Practice Guidelines. Acute Management of Autonomic Dysreflexia: Adults with Spinal Cord Injury Present to Health-Care Facilities. J Spinal Cord Med.* 1997 Jul;20(3):284-308.

57. Consortium for Spinal Cord Medicine. *Clinical Practice Guidelines. Prevention of Thromboembolism in Spinal Cord Injury. J Spinal Cord Med.* 1997 Jul;20(3):259-83.

58. Cook D, Attia J, Weaver B, McDonald E, Meade M, Crowther M. Venous thromboembolic disease: an observational study in medical–surgical intensive care unit patients. *J Crit Care.* 2000;15(4):127-132.

59. Lal S, Hamilton B, Heinemann A, Betts H. Risk factors for heterotopic ossification in spinal cord injury. *Arch Phys Med Rehabil.* 1989;70(5):387-390.

60. Celani MG, Spizzichino L, Ricci S, Zampolini M, Franceschini M. Spinal cord injury in Italy: a multicenter retrospective study. *Arch Phys Med Rehabil.* 2001;82(5):589-596.

61. Kao CH, ChangLai SP, Chieng PU, Yen TC. Gastric emptying in male neurologic trauma. *J Nucl Med.* 1998;39(10):1798-1801.

62. Rodriguez DJ, Benzel EC, Clevenger FW. The metabolic response to spinal cord injury. *Spinal Cord.* 1997;35(9):599-604.

63. McColl MA. Expectations of health, independence, and quality of life among aging spinal cord-injured adults. *Assist Technol.* 1999;11(2):130-136.

64. DeVivo MJ, Richards JS. Community reintegration and quality of life following spinal cord injury. *Paraplegia.* 1992;30:108-112.

65. Whiteneck GG, Charlifue MA, Frankel MB, Fraser BM, et al. Mortality, morbidity and psychosocial outcomes of persons spinal cord injured more than 20 years ago. *Paraplegia.* 1992; 30:617-630.

66. Tator CH, Duncan EG, Edmonds VE, Lapczak LI, Andrews DF. Complications and costs of management of acute spinal cord injury. *Paraplegia.* 1993;31:700-714.

67. Frownfelter D. *Arterial Blood Gases.* 3rd ed. St Louis, MO: Mosby-Year Book; 1996.

68. Shapiro BA. Evaluation of blood gas monitors: performance criteria, clinical impact, and cost/benefit. *Crit Care Med.* 1994; 22(4):546-548.

69. Frownfelter D. Pulmonary function tests. In: Frownfelter DL, Dean E, eds. *Principles and Practice of Cardiopulmonary Physical Therapy.* 3rd ed. St Louis, MO: Mosby-Year Book; 1996:145-152.

70. Bach JR, Saporito L. Criteria for extubation and tracheostomy tube removal for patients with ventilatory failure: a different approach to weaning. *Chest.* 1996;110:1566-1571.

71. Bach JR, Ishikawa Y, Kim H. Prevention of pulmonary morbidity for patients with Duchenne Muscular Dystrophy. *Chest.* 1997; 112:1024-1028.

72. Primiano FP Jr. Theoretical analysis of chest wall mechanics. *J Biomech.* 1982;15(12):919-931.

73. Trottier SJ. Prone position in acute respiratory distress syndrome: turning over an old idea. *Crit Care Med.* 1998;26(12):1934-1935.

74. Lind B, Bake B, Lundqvist C, Nordwall A. Influence of Halo vest treatment on vital capacity. *Spine.* 1987;12(5):449-452.

75. Wong WP. Physical therapy for a patient in acute respiratory failure. *Phys Ther.* 2000;80:662-670.

76. Dallimore K, Jenkins S, Tucker B. Respiratory and cardiovascular responses to manual chest percussion in normal subjects. *Aust J Physiother.* 1998;44(4):267-274.

77. App EM, Kieselmann R, Reinhardt D, et al. Sputum rheology changes in cystic fibrosis lung disease following two different types of physiotherapy: flutter vs. autogenic drainage. *Chest.* 1998;114:171-177.

78. Hardy KA. A review of airway clearance: new techniques, indications, and recommendations. *Respir Care.* 1994;39(5):440-451.

79. Kluft J, Beker L, Castagnino M, Gaiser J, Chaney H, Fink RJ. A comparison of bronchial drainage treatments in cystic fibrosis. *Pediatr Pulmonol.* 1996;22(4):271-274.

80. Webber B, Pryor JA. Active cycle of breathing techniques. Bronchial Hypersecretion: Current Chest Physiotherapy in Cystic Fibrosis. International Physiotherapy in Committee for CF. Tokyo, Japan; 1993.

81. Downs AM. Physiologic basis for airway clearance techniques and clinical applications of airway clearance techniques. In: Frownfelter DL, Dean E, eds. *Principles and Practice of Cardiopulmonary Physical Therapy.* 3rd ed. St Louis, MO: Mosby-Year Book; 1996:321-366.

82. Massery MP, Frownfelter DL. Facilitating airway clearance with coughing techniques. In: Frownfelter DL, Dean E, eds. *Principles and Practice of Cardiopulmonary Physical Therapy.* 3rd ed. St Louis, MO: Mosby-Year Book; 1996: 367-382.

83. Kirby NA, Barnerias MJ, Siebens AA. An evaluation of assisted cough in quadriparetic patients. *Arch Phys Med Rehabil.* 1966; 47:705-710.

84. Massery MP, Schneider F. *Ventilatory Management Program for the Patient with Quadriplegia (Video).* Chicago: The Rehabilitation Institute of Chicago; 1999.

85. Massery M, Dreyer H, Borjenson A, Cahalin L. A Pilot Study Investigating the Effectiveness of Assisted Cough Techniques and the Clinical Utility of a Peak Flow Meter to Measure Peak Cough Expiratory Flow in Persons with Spinal Cord Injury

[abstract]. In: Proceedings for the World Congress for Physical Therapy. May 1999:30.

86. Wood CJ. Endotracheal suctioning: a literature review. *Intensive Crit Care Nurs.* 1998;14(3):124-135.

87. Beck GJ, Barach AL. Value of mechanical aids in the management of a patient with poliomyelitis. *Ann Intern Med.* 1954;40: 1081-1094.

88. Sammon K, Menon S, Massery MP, Cahalin L. A pilot clinical investigation comparing the effects of the mechanical inexsufflator to suctioning and chest physical therapy in persons with difficulty mobilizing pulmonary secretions [Abstract]. *Cardiopulm Phys Ther.* 1998;9(4):22-23.

89. Brinkrant DJ, Pope JF, Eiben RM. Management of the respiratory complications of neuromuscular diseases in the pediatric intensive care unit. *J Child Neurol.* 1999;14:139-143.

90. Garstang SV, Kirshblum SC, Wood KE. Patient preference for in-exsufflation for secretion management with spinal cord injury. *J Spinal Cord Med.* 2000;23(2):80-85.

91. Landers M, et al. A comparison of tidal volume, breathing frequency, and minute ventilation between two sitting postures in healthy adults. *Physiother Theory Pract.* 2003;19:109-119.

92. Brown JC, Swank SM, Matta J, Farras DM. Late spinal deformity in quadriplegic children and adolescents. *J Peditar Orthop.* 1984;4(4):456-461.

93. Goldman JM, Rose LS, Williams SJ, et al. Effect of abdominal binders on breathing in tetraplegic patients. *Thorax.* 1986; 41(12):940-945.

94. MacLean D, Drummond G, Macpherson C, et al. Maximum expiratory airflow during chest physiotherapy on ventilated patients before and after the application of an abdominal binder. *Intensive Care Med.* 1989;15(6):396-399.

95. Randerath WJ, Schraeder O, Galetke W, Feldmeyer F, Ruhle KH. Autoadjusting cpap therapy based on impedance efficacy, compliance and acceptance. *Am J Respir Crit Care Med.* 2001;163(3):652-657.

96. Massery MP. What's positioning got to do with it? *Neurol Rep.* 1994;18(3):11-14.

97. Gallego J, Perez de la Sota A, Vardon G, Jaeger-Denavit E, Jaeger-Denavit O. Learned activation of thoracic inspiratory muscles in tetraplegics. *Am J Phys Med Rehabil.* 1993;72: 312-317.

98. Estenne M, Knoop C, Vanvaerenbergh J, Heilporn A, De Troyer A. The effect of pectoralis muscle training in tetraplegic subjects. *Am Rev Resp Dis.* 1989;139(5):1218-1222.

99. Massery MP, Frownfelter DL. Facilitating ventilatory patterns and breathing strategies. In: Frownfelter DL, Dean E, eds. *Principles and Practice of Cardiopulmonary Physical Therapy.* 3rd ed. St Louis, MO: Mosby-Year Book; 1996:383-416.

100. Sullivan PE, Markos PD, Minor MA. *An Integrated Approach to Therapeutic Exercise: Theory and Clinical Application.* Reston, VA: Reston Publishing Co; 1982.

101. Frownfelter D, Ryan J. Dyspnea: measurement and evaluation. *Cardiopulm Phys Ther J.* 2000;11(1):7-15.

102. Zumwalt M, Adkins H, Dail C, Affeldt J. Glossopharyngeal breathing. *Phys Ther Rev.* 1956;36(7):455-460.

103. Mazza FG, DiMarco AF, Altose MD, Strohl KP. The flow-volume loop during glossopharyngeal breathing. *Chest.* 1984;85(5): 638-640.

104. Warren VC. Glossopharyngeal and neck accessory muscle breathing in a young adult with C2 complete tetraplegia resulting in ventilator dependency. *Phys Ther.* 2002;82(6):590-600.

105. Moloney E, et al. A case of frog breathing. *Irish Med J.* 2002; 95(3):81-82.

106. Massery MP. *Glossopharyngeal Breathing Demonstration (Video).* Glenview, IL: Massery Physical Therapy Video Collection; 1979.

107. Massery MP. *Enhancing Phonation Skills with Manual Techniques (Video).* Glenview, IL: Massery Physical Therapy Video Collection; 1997.

108. Gosselink R, Kovacs L, Ketelaer P, Carton H, Decramer M. Respiratory muscle weakness and respiratory muscle training in severely disabled multiple sclerosis patients. *Arch Phys Med Rehabil.* 2000;81(6):747-751.

109. Rutchik A, Weissman AR, Almenoff PL, Spungen AM, Bauman WA, Grimm DR. Resistive inspiratory muscle training in subjects with chronic cervical spinal cord injury. *Arch Phys Med Rehabil.* 1998;79(3):293-297.

110. Weiner P, Magadle R, Berar-Yanay N, Davidovich A, Weiner M. The cumulative effect of long-acting bronchodilators, exercise, and inspiratory muscle training on the perception of dyspnea in patients with advanced COPD. *Chest.* 2000;118(3):672-678.

111. Liaw M, Lin M, Cheng P, Wong MA, et al. Resistive inspiratory muscle training: its effectiveness in patients with acute complete cervical cord injury. *Arch Phys Med Rehabil.* 2000;81:752-756.

112. American Thoracic Society. Standards for the diagnosis and care of patients with chronic obstructive pulmonary disease (COPD) and asthma. *Am Rev Respir Dis.* 1987;136:225-244.

113. Guyatt GH, Townsend M, Pugsley SO, et al. Bronchodilators in chronic airflow limitation: effects on airway function, exercise capacity, and quality of life. *Am Rev Respir Dis.* 1987;135: 1969-1974.

114. Persson CGA. Some pharmacological aspects of xanthines in asthma. *Eur J Respir Dis.* 1980;61(suppl):7-16.

115. Henke KG, Regnis JA, Bye PTP. Benefits of continuous positive airway pressure during exercise in cystic fibrosis and relationship to disease severity. *Am Rev Respir Dis.* 1993;148:1272-1275.

116. Maltais F, Reissmann H, Gottfried SB. Pressure support reduces inspiratory effort and dyspnea during exercise in chronic airflow obstruction. *Am J Resp Crit Care Med.* 1995;151:1027-1032.

117. O'Donnell DE, Sanii R, Younes M. Improvement in exercise endurance in patients with chronic airflow limitation using continuous positive airway pressure. *Am Rev Respir Dis.* 1988; 138:1510-1515.

118. Cahalin L, Cannan J, Prevost S, et al. Exercise performance during assisted ventilation with bi-level positive pressure airway pressure (BiPAP). *J Cardiopulm Rehabil.* 1994;14:323.

119. ZuWallack RL, Patel K, Reardon JZ, Clark BA, Normandin EA. Predictors of improvement in the 12-minute walking distance following a six-week outpatient pulmonary rehabilitation program. *Chest.* 1991;99:805-808.

120. Maltais F, Leblanc P, Jobin J, et al. Intensity of training and physiologic adaptation in patients with chronic obstructive pulmonary disease. *Am J Respir Crit Care Med.* 1997;155:555-561.

121. Troosters T, Gosselink R, Decramer M. Exercise training in COPD: How to distinguish responders from nonresponders. *J Cardiopulm Rehabil.* 2001;21:10-17.

122. Morgan MDL. The prediction of benefit from pulmonary rehabilitation: setting, training intensity, and the effect of selection by disability. *Thorax.* 1999;54:S3-S7.

123. Senjyu H, Moji K, Takemoto T, Kiyama T, Honda S. Effects of pulmonary rehabilitation on the survival of emphysema patients receiving long-term oxygen therapy. *Physiotherapy.* 1999;85(5):251-258.

124. Lacasse Y, Wong E, Guyatt GH, King D, Cook DJ, Goldstein RS. Meta-analysis of respiratory rehabilitation in chronic obstructive pulmonary disease. *Lancet.* 1996;348:1115-1119.

125. Cambach W, Wagenaar RC, Koelman TW, Ton van Keimpema ARJ, Kemper HCG. The long-term effects of pulmonary rehabilitation in patients with asthma and chronic obstructive pulmonary disease: a research synthesis. *Arch Phys Med Rehabil.* 1999;80:103-111.

126. Chen H, Dukes R, Martin BJ. Inspiratory muscle training in patients with chronic obstructive pulmonary disease. *Am Rev Respir Dis.* 1985;131:251-256.

127. Larson JL, Kim MJ, Sharp JT, et al. Inspiratory muscle training with a pressure threshold breathing device in patients with chronic obstructive pulmonary disease. *Am Rev Respir Dis.* 1988;138:689-694.

128. Harver A, Mahler DA, Daubenspeck JA. Targeted inspiratory muscle training improves respiratory muscle function and reduces dyspnea in patients with chronic obstructive pulmonary disease. *Ann Intern Med.* 1989;111:117-123.

129. Dekhuijzen R, Folgering HTM, van Herwaarden CLA. Target-flow inspiratory muscle training during pulmonary rehabilitation in patients with COPD. *Chest.* 1991;99:128-134.

130. Weiner P, Azgad Y, Ganam R. Inspiratory muscle training combined with general exercise reconditioning in patients with COPD. *Chest.* 1992;102:1351-1356.

131. Weiner P, Azgad Y, Ganam R, et al. Inspiratory muscle training in patients with bronchial asthma. *Chest.* 1992;102:1357-1342.

132. Suzuki S, Yoshike Y, Suzuki M, et al. Inspiratory muscle training and respiratory sensation during treadmill exercise. *Chest.* 1993;104:197-203.

133. Nomori H, Kobayashi R, Fuyuno G, et al. Preoperative respiratory muscle training: assessment in thoracic surgery patients with special reference to postoperative pulmonary complications. *Chest.* 1994;105:1782-1788.

134. Preusser BA, Winningham ML, Clanton TL. High- vs low-intensity inspiratory muscle interval training in patients with COPD. *Chest.* 1994;106:110-115.

135. Cahalin LP, Braga M, Matsuo Y, Hernandez ED. Efficacy of diaphragmatic breathing in persons with chronic obstructive pulmonary disease—A review of the literature. *J Cardiopulm Rehabil.* 2002;22(1):7-21.

136. McColl MA, Walker J, Stirling P, Wilkins R, Corey P. Expectations of life and health among spinal cord injured adults. *Spinal Cord.* 1997;35(12):818-828.

137. Krishnan KR, Nuseibeh I, Savic G, Sett P. Long-term survival in spinal cord injury: a fifty year investigation. *Spinal Cord.* 1998;36(4):266-274.

138. Cohen CA, Zagelbaum G, Gross D, et al. Clinical manifestations of inspiratory muscle fatigue. *Am J Med.* 1982;73:308-313.

139. Tobin MJ, Perez W, Guenther SM, Lodato RF, Dantzker DR. Does rib cage-abdominal paradox signify respiratory muscle fatigue? *J Appl Physiol.* 1987;63(2):851-860.

140. Agostoni E, Mognoni P. Deformation of the chest wall during breathing efforts. *J Appl Physiol.* 1966;21(6):1827-1832.

141. Ashutosh K, Gilbert R, Auchincloss JH, Peppi D. Asynchronous breathing movements in patients with chronic obstructive pulmonary disease. *Chest.* 1975;67(5):553-557.

142. Sampson MG, DeTroyer A. Role of intercostal muscles in the rib cage distortions produced by inspiratory loads. *J Appl Physiol.* 1982;52(3):517-523.

143. Polkey MI, Moxham J. Clinical aspects of respiratory muscle dysfunction in the critically ill. *Chest.* 2001;119:926-939.

144. Tobin MJ, Chadha TS, Jenouri G, Birch SJ, Gazeroglu HB, Sackner MA. Breathing patterns—Diseased subjects. *Chest.* 1983;84(3):286-294.

CHAPTER 20
An International Perspective: Japan

Yoshimi Matsuo

Physical therapy (PT) enjoys widespread utilization within the Japanese health care system. There are currently about 31,000 practicing physical therapists who are members of our professional organization, the Japanese Physical Therapy Association (JPTA). Japanese physical therapists practice in a wide variety of practice settings, including hospitals, outpatient facilities, rehabilitation centers, and many long-term care facilities. We practice in many other areas, including home care, acute care, orthopedics, neurology, and sports. Japanese physical therapists can obtain board certification as clinical specialists in one of seven specialty areas of practice, of which cardiopulmonary physical therapy is one. To date there are around 38 cardiopulmonary clinical specialists. In Japan, physical therapists must practice with a doctor's prescription. There are no licensed PT assistants.

Cardiopulmonary physical therapy is an important, though relatively small, specialty area of practice in Japan. Nonetheless,

cardiopulmonary physical therapists may be found in intensive care units, outpatient facilities, wellness programs, and acute care hospitals. They are an integral part of cardiac and pulmonary transplant teams and open heart surgical teams, among others. Currently there is a measure of competition and overlap of service provision to patients with cardiovascular and pulmonary disease. Nursing may provide "chest physical therapy" in some hospitals; exercise physiologists may provide exercise programs; and nursing may oversee cardiac rehabilitation programs and monitor the patient during exercise. Currently, cardiopulmonary physical therapists are actively engaged in reducing hospital stay through the prevention of pulmonary complications. Also, cardiopulmonary physical therapists in Japan are developing evidence-based models of practice in order to improve PT outcomes in all practice settings.

Development of evidence-based practice in physical therapy is much needed in Japan. The American Association of

Cardiovascular and Pulmonary Rehabilitation (AACVPR) guidelines have the potential to promote change in Japanese clinical settings.[1] Japanese physical therapists need evidence in order to select the most effective methods to examine and treat patients. The Japanese Respiratory Society and Japan Society for Respiratory Care have both produced statements for respiratory rehabilitation in 2001.[2] The latter published "A Manual for Respiratory Rehabilitation—Therapeutic Exercise" in 2003.[3]

The medical payment system in Japan is presently changing, with the Japanese government adopting a DPC (diagnostic procedure combination) system, which is somewhat different from the DRG-PPS methods employed in the United States. As a result, the number of days that patients are in-hospital after an acute event is rapidly decreasing. Japanese physical therapists treat a wide variety of patients during the hospitalization period including patients with acute myocardial infarction or those with angina, those with thoracic and abdominal surgery including transplantation, those with chronic obstructive pulmonary disease (COPD) or other type of restrictive lung disease, those with neuromuscular disease or spinal cord surgery, and those in the intensive care unit. Although only a moderate number of Japanese physical therapists currently practice in the cardiopulmonary environment, more are showing interest. This greater interest in cardiovascular and pulmonary physical therapy in Japan may be due to recent advances in treatment techniques developed by Japanese physical therapists. However, the language barrier between Japan and other countries limits what Japanese therapists can learn about cardiovascular and pulmonary physical therapy in the United States, and what American therapists or physical therapists from other countries can learn about Japanese cardiovascular and pulmonary physical therapy. The role of respiratory physical therapy in Japan will be described in the following sections.

PULMONARY REHABILITATION PROGRAM CHARACTERISTICS: AN INTERNATIONAL SURVEY

Kida et al. surveyed pulmonary rehabilitation programs in Tokyo, Japan, and compared them to similar programs in North America and Europe.[4] The survey instrument was a 13-item questionnaire sent in December 1994 to institutions in North America (n = 178), Europe (n = 179), and Tokyo (n = 399). Response rates were 51%, 40%, and 51%, respectively. Survey results showed that pulmonary rehabilitation programs (PRP) were available at 56% of hospitals in North America and at 74% of hospitals in Europe, but at only 20% of hospitals in Tokyo. Most pulmonary rehabilitation programs existed as outpatient clinics in North America (98%), whereas both outpatient (55%) and inpatient programs (65%) were found in Europe. Although COPD was the predominant type of lung disease for which patients in both North America and Europe were referred, this accounted for only 34% of referrals in Tokyo.

Referrals for primary tuberculosis sequelae ($p = 0.028$) and bronchiectasis ($p = 0.021$) were more common in Tokyo, as well as in Europe. Table 1 shows that many of the program components available in North America were less available in Europe; most were unavailable in Tokyo. These included family education, psychological support, nutritional instruction, treadmill and bicycle ergometry, gait training, and activity of daily living sessions. The survey showed that pulmonary rehabilitation programs in North America are more multidimensional. However, target diseases differ between North America, Europe, and Tokyo. Problems common to all three regions included a lack of staff and insufficient reimbursement. In summary, these findings demonstrate a need for Japanese physical therapists to have a greater role in the care provided to patients enrolled in Japanese respiratory programs.

DIFFERENCES IN INTERVENTION EFFECT IN PATIENTS WITH COPD BETWEEN JAPAN AND OTHER COUNTRIES

Many investigations in the United States and Europe have reported that respiratory rehabilitation does not improve pulmonary function. However, Gimenz et al. reported that endurance training in patients with COPD improved maximum inspiratory and expiratory pressures.[5] Furthermore, some Japanese investigators emphasize that physical therapy and respiratory rehabilitation *do* improve pulmonary function.[6,7] Taniguchi et al.[8] found that the percentages of vital capacity (VC), forced expiratory volume (FEV), residual volume (RV), functional residual capacity (FRC), and the ratio of residual volume (RV) to total lung capacity increased with pulmonary physical therapy. The authors hypothesized that physical therapy decreased FRC and improved ventilatory efficacy.[8]

Watanabe et al.[9] evaluated the effects of pulmonary rehabilitation on pulmonary function in 15 patients with chronic emphysema who underwent pulmonary rehabilitation for 6 weeks as inpatients. Pulmonary rehabilitation consisted of relaxation techniques, breathing retraining, thoracic massage, therapeutic exercise, and walking. In 8 of the 15 patients, vital capacity increased by more than 200 mL (over 10%; Table 2), and in 7 of the 15 patients maximum exercise capacity increased by more than 5 watts (over 10%). Increases in vital capacity were not associated with increases in maximum exercise capacity. The percentage of change in vital capacity associated with pulmonary rehabilitation correlated significantly with the percentage of change in tidal volume and the percentage of change in expiratory minute ventilation at the maximum workload. The percentage of change in tidal volume at maximum workload correlated significantly with the percentage of change in maximum oxygen uptake. The increase in vital capacity was attributed to an improvement in thoracic cage movement. These findings suggest that pulmonary rehabilitation can increase vital capacity in some patients with chronic pulmonary emphysema, and that such an increase is not directly connected to increases in exercise capacity.

TABLE 1   **Comparison of Pulmonary Rehabilitation Program Content in North America, Europe, and Tokyo**

Content Item	North America ($n = 50$)%	Europe ($n = 51$)%	Tokyo ($n = 202$)%	North America vs Europe	North America vs Tokyo	Europe vs Tokyo
Education about pulmonary disease	98	86	20	$p < 0.05$	$p < 0.0001$	$p < 0.0001$
Medication	92	90	20	NS	$p < 0.0001$	$p < 0.0001$
Breathing retraining	90	80	47	NS	$p < 0.0001$	$p < 0.0001$
Oxygen	86	78	84	NS	NS	NS
Walking	86	61	39	$p < 0.005$	$p < 0.0001$	$p < 0.005$
ADLs[a]	84	28	20	$p = 0.000$	$p < 0.0001$	NS
Nutrition	84	55	36	$p < 0.005$	$p < 0.0001$	$p < 0.05$
Upper and lower extremity exercise	82	61	24	$p < 0.05$	$p < 0.0001$	$p < 0.0001$
Relaxation	78	65	13	NS	$p < 0.0001$	$p < 0.0001$
Phychosical support	78	59	1	$p < 0.05$	$p < 0.0001$	$p < 0.0001$
Family education	76	33	20	$p = 0.000$	$p < 0.0001$	$p < 0.05$
Pulmonary hygiene	74	59	42	NS	$p < 0.0001$	$p < 0.05$
Bicycle ergometer	72	45	6	$p < 0.01$	$p < 0.0001$	$p < 0.0001$
Smoking cessation	70	69	66	NS	NS	NS
Treadmill	68	33	6	$p < 0.01$	$p < 0.0001$	$p < 0.0001$
Respiratory muscle training	58	49	47	NS	NS	NS

[a]ADL, activity of daily living; NS, not significant.

Kida K, Jinno S, Nomura K, Yamada K, Katsura H, Kudoh S: Pulmonary rehabilitation program survey in North America, Europe, and Tokyo. *J Cardiopulmo Rehabil.* 2003;8:304.

TABLE 2   **Outcomes of a Pulmonary Rehabilitation Program**

	Mean ± SE		
	Pre	Post	P
VC (L)	2.55 ± 0.09	2.65 ± 0.09	0.0423[a]
VC (%)	83.3 ± 2.1	86.7 ± 2.2	0.219[a]
FVC (L)	2.34 ± 0.08	2.58 ± 0.14	0.0012[b]
FVC (%)	76.4 ± 2.1	80.7 ± 2.1	0.0013[b]
FEV_1 (L)	0.80 ± 0.04	0.85 ± 0.05	0.0225[a]
FEV_1 (%)	38.4 ± 1.9	40.8 ± 2.0	0.0162[a]
FEV_1 (%)	34.4 ± 1.2	34.3 ± 1.2	NS
FRC (%)	113.3 ± 4.7	108.2 ± 4.7	0.0145[a]
RV (%)	171.6 ± 6.1	163.0 ± 6.1	0.0287[a]
RV/TLC (%)	158.3 ± 4.6	151.9 ± 4.5	0.0205[a]
DLCO/VA (%)	76.8 ± 4.4	76.8 ± 4.4	NS
pH	7.403 ± 0.005	7.404 ± 0.005	NS
Pao_2 (torr)	80.4 ± 1.5	78.4 ± 2.0	NS
$Paco_2$ (torr)	37.8 ± 0.8	37.6 ± 0.9	NS

[a]$p < 0.05$.

[b]$p < 0.01$.

Reprinted with permission from Watanabe F. Effect of a pulmonary rehabilitation program in our outpatient with chronic obstructive pulmonary disease. *J Jpn Soc Respir Care.* 2000;10:251.

An important goal of Japanese physical therapist interventions is to mobilize the chest wall of patients with COPD. The techniques used to mobilize the chest include relaxation and stretching of the respiratory muscles and arthrokinematic intervention for the synovial joints. For example, Japanese physical therapists have started to mobilize the costovertebral and costosternal joints, meeting with apparent success. This type of arthrokinematic intervention appears to reduce chest wall size on forced expiration and may be useful in improving the elasticity of the chest wall. These mobilization techniques, however, require further investigation in treating various pulmonary disorders.

CHANGES IN PULMONARY FUNCTION FOLLOWING SURGERY

Postoperative pulmonary complications are still a major cause of postoperative mortality in Japan, especially in elderly patients. Toyota and his colleagues reported on the change in pulmonary function after surgery and an adequate period of intervention for chest physical therapy.[10] They performed pulmonary rehabilitation in 98 patients who had undergone surgery using general anesthesia. Lung function (%VC and %FEV$_1$) was measured via spirometry preoperatively and weekly for 3 weeks following surgery. Patients were divided into four groups: thoracotomy incision with lung lobectomy, thoracotomy incision without lung lobectomy, upper abdominal incision, and lower abdominal incision. The changes in %VC relative to preoperative values were significantly reduced within 7 days after surgery in all groups (Figs. 1 and 2). This finding was most remarkable in the lung lobectomy group. The second most remarkable response was in thoracotomy; the third was in upper abdominal incision, the fourth was in lower abdominal incision. The incidence of postoperative pulmonary complication was 13.8% in lobectomy, 4.0% in thoracotomy, 3.0% in upper abdomen, 0% in lower abdomen. These data identify areas of need for physical therapy services in patients who undergo thoracoabdominal surgery.

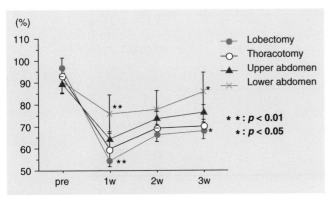

FIGURE 1 Changes of %VC following surgery. (Reprinted with permission from Toyota A. Pulmonary rehabilitation and the changes of pulmonary function after surgery. *Jpn J Rehabili Med.* 2001;38:771.)

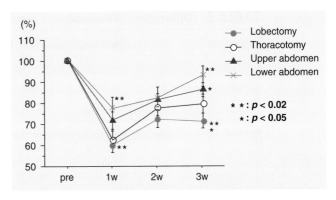

FIGURE 2 Changes of % VC recovery rate following surgery. (Used with permission from Toyota A. Pulmonary rehabilitation and the changes of pulmonary function after surgery. *Jpn J Rehabil Med.* 2001;38:771.)

SOME INTERESTING PHYSICAL THERAPY THERAPEUTIC INTERVENTIONS IN JAPAN

Most Japanese physical therapists believe percussion is not an effective manual technique for bronchial hygiene. They prefer squeezing with postural drainage and breathing-assist techniques.

Squeezing

In Japan, squeezing is performed by the physical therapist in order to facilitate inspiration and exhalation and consists of manually compressing different areas on the thorax during expiration. The therapist pushes into areas of the thorax which have limited motion or under which retained secretions lie. Squeezing appears to increase both expiratory flow and expiratory pressures. As a result, passive inspiration and sputum clearance is facilitated. Miyagawa and Kaneko[11] showed bronchoscopic evidence of improved sputum clearance from squeezing compared to percussion.

Okumura and Sakata[12] reported on the efficacy of squeezing and postural drainage for children with asthma. A total of 21 chest physiotherapy treatments were performed on 10 children hospitalized for acute asthma attacks between June and November 1999. Ages of the patients ranged from 1 to 4 years. All patients received standardized basic treatment with administration of bronchodilators as a continuous infusion of aminophylline and inhalation of disodium cromoglycate and salbutamol 3 times a day. In 13 out of 21 treatments O$_2$ saturation by pulse oximetry was significantly elevated from 0.8 to 3.8% after chest physiotherapy. However, O$_2$ saturation by pulse oximetry decreased in two cases. Overall, chest physiotherapy was generally well tolerated by these infants based on their cardiovascular response and O$_2$ saturation. The authors state that chest physiotherapy may be a useful adjunctive treatment for children with asthma attack.

Miyagawa[13] analyzed several research reports published from 1966 to 1997 related to respiratory physical therapy. His

TABLE 3   **Differences of Pulmonary Complication Between Squeezing and Percussion**

Objectives	Squeezing Group	Percussion Group	Odds-ratio	95% CI
Emergency	80	81	0.62	0.33–1.16
Intensive care unit	32	29	0.21	0.06–0.68
Total	112	110	0.48	0.28–0.84

Reproduced, with permission, from Miyagawa T. Science in respiratory physical therapy. *Jpn J Respir Care*. 1998;15:97.

meta-analysis revealed that squeezing was often used in Canada, but not in the United States. He compared squeezing and percussion for pulmonary complications. Table 3 shows the odds ratios for acute respiratory failure in emergency rooms and intensive care units, revealing that pulmonary complications were similar among patients who received squeezing or percussion in both emergency rooms and intensive care units. Additionally, Uzawa and Yamaguchi[14] described beneficial changes in lung mechanics during application of chest physical therapy techniques, which included squeezing, percussion, and vibration. See Table 4. In summary, it appears that squeezing may be an important adjunctive treatment for a variety of patients with respiratory disorders.

Breathing-Assist Technique

The breathing-assist technique (BAT) is often used in Japan for patients with respiratory disorders. The BAT assists the patients' ventilation by passive or active-assist maneuvers per-formed by the physical therapist (Fig. 3).[15] This technique facilitates air entry into the thoracic cavity. Improved air entry promotes airway hygiene by mobilizing sputum from peripheral to central airways. This technique may improve ventilation and possibly reeducate breathing control. We often use BAT during the extubation process while patients are still in the intensive care unit. Patients appear to more easily shift to natural breathing after being extubated and receiving BAT. Furthermore, Ihashi and his colleagues[16] found that BAT improved arterial blood oxygenation and assisted with general conditioning exercises in 12 patients with dyspnea.

Mechanical external chest compression (MECC) has been used in Australia and is similar to BAT, but is mechanical rather than manual.[17,18] Both MECC and BAT have been used to suppress asthmatic attacks. The technique of external chest compression to assist expiration has been used in asthmatic patients for some years. Fisher et al.[18] described a method similar to MECC and BAT that assisted expiration and reported on its apparent value in the emergency treatment of asthma.

TABLE 4   **The Change in Lung Mechanics During Application of Chest Physical Therapy Techniques**

	Mean ± SD		
	Squeezing	Percussion	Vibration
Tidal volume (mL)	70.5 ± 44.3	6.7 ± 22.3	13.0 ± 35.1
Expiratory flow speed (mL/s)	76.4 ± 31.0	31.2 ± 33.0	31.1 ± 33.3
Dynamic compliance (mL/cm H$_2$O)	7.9 ± 9.7	0.8 ± 4.3	2.7 ± 4.9
Airway resistance (cm H$_2$O/L/s)	1.1 ± 3.2	0.5 ± 1.7	−20.2 ± 1.7

[a] $p < 0.01$.

[b] $p < 0.05$.

Data from Uzawa Y, Yamaguchi Y. Change in lung mechanics during application of chest physical therapy techniques. *J Jpn Phys Ther Assoc*. 1998;25:222.

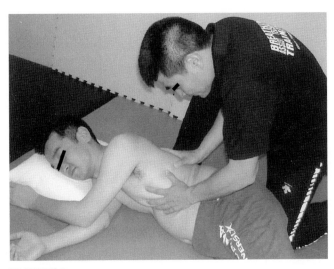

FIGURE 3 Breathing-assist technique.

These techniques require further evaluation to determine their role in the resuscitation of patients with asthma. Although the MECC or BAT techniques are not discussed in the *Resuscitation Guideline 2000,* the need for it within the intensive care unit may be less than it is outside of specialized units where acute respiratory disorders require immediate attention. MECC or BAT will likely have its greatest impact when initiated in the prehospital setting for patients suffering from severe, sudden-onset, asphyxic anthma. Fukada and co-workers[19] reported MECC improved hypoxemia due to asthma when administered in the ambulance and prevented deaths in Japan. BAT has been used in emergency vehicles and on transport carts for patients with acute asthmatic attacks. Shigemoto and colleagues[20] have educated paramedics in the use of BAT with patients on emergency transport carts and suggest that physicians, physical therapists, and emergency medical technicians should initiate BAT immediately to improve outcomes of acute asthmatic attacks (Fig. 4).

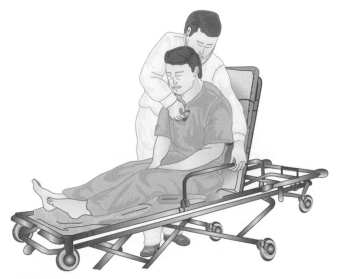

FIGURE 4 BAT in an emergency car. (Modified with permission from Nakano T. Breathing assist technique. *Emerg Nurs.* 2003;16:63.)

However, It is controversial whether we can actually control chest wall motion and subsequent ventilation during asthmatic attacks; therefore, further investigation on the use of these techniques is needed.[21,22]

Respiratory Muscle Stretch Gymnastics

Respiratory muscle stretch gymnastics (RMSG) have been designed to stretch and condition the respiratory muscles, mainly the chest wall muscles, and to decrease chest wall elasticity. Several Japanese researchers have studied the use of RMSG.[23–26] Kakizaki and colleagues[26] reported the effects of RMSG on chest wall mobility, pulmonary function, and dyspnea during activities of daily living in 22 patients with COPD who were regularly treated in an outpatient clinic of a university hospital. The patients did not have severe limitations in shoulder range of motion and were unfamiliar with RMSG. Chest wall mobility (difference of chest circumference during deep expiration and that during deep inspiration), pulmonary function tests (forced expiratory volume in 1 second (FEV_1) and VC), and dyspnea in daily living (Fletcher's rating) were measured before and after 4 weeks of RMSG. Four RMSG patterns were demonstrated to each patient to ensure that they could perform the gymnastics without assistance. The patients were instructed to perform each pattern four times during each session (3 sessions per day) for 4 weeks, at which time the patients were asked to return for reevaluation. Chest wall expansion and reduction increased at both the upper (0.8 ± 0.2 and 1.3 ± 0.2 cm, respectively) and the lower (0.4 ± 0.2 and 0.7 ± 0.2 cm, respectively) chest walls (Figs. 5 and 6). Vital capacity increased 1019 ± 43 mL, whereas FEV_1 remained unchanged (Fig. 7). Fletcher's rating improved in 12 patients and remained unchanged in 10; it did not worsen in any of the 22 patients. RMSG, therefore, appeared to increase chest wall mobility by improving chest wall elasticity in patients with COPD.

Muscle Relaxation Technique— The Designed Plate Method

It has been suggested that respiratory muscle dysfunction plays a major role in the development of acute respiratory failure in patients with COPD. Because of this, Fujimoto et al.[27] created a specially designed plate method to treat spasm of the respiratory muscles and other muscles (Fig. 8). This tool is curious in appearance and the therapist uses it like a carpenter, with the anticipated goal of decreasing muscle spasm or muscle tone. Fujimoto et al. devised this method, which combines respiratory muscle relaxation exercises and the use of wedge-shaped wooden plates with which pressure is applied to the intercostal and accessory respiratory muscles. The specific techniques of the designed plate method includes placing a wooden plate on a hypertonic muscle and applying pressure either by hand or by tapping the wooden plate with a light hammer for 15 to 20 minutes twice a day. The effects of this muscle relaxation maneuver with designed plates on pulmonary

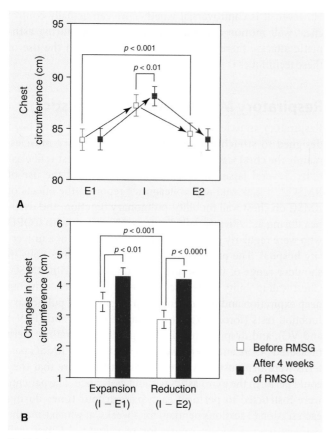

FIGURE 5   (**A**) Mean $\pm$ SE of upper chest circumference during deep expiration (E1), deep inspiration (I), and subsequent expiration (E2) before and after respiratory muscle stretch gymnastics (RMSG) in 22 patients with chronic obstructive pulmonary disease. (**B**) Upper-chest expansion and reduction. (Used with permission from Kakizaki F. Preliminary report on the effects of respiratory muscle stretch gymnastics on chest wall mobility in patients with chronic obstructive pulmonary disease. *Respir Care.* 1999; 44:412-413.)

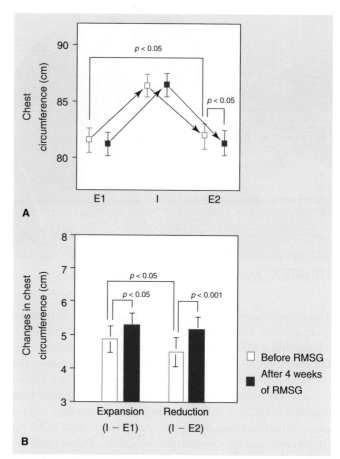

FIGURE 6   (**A**) Mean $\pm$ SE of lower-chest circumference during deep expiration (E1), deep inspiration (I), and subsequent expiration (E2) before and after respiratory muscle stretch gymnastics (RMSG) in 22 patients with chronic obstructive pulmonary disease. (**B**) Lower-chest expansion and reduction. (Used with permission from Kakizaki F. Preliminary report on the effects of respiratory muscle stretch gymnastics on chest wall mobility in patients with chronic obstructive pulmonary disease. *Respir Care.* 1999;44:412-413.)

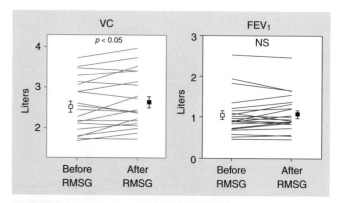

FIGURE 7   Vital capacity (VC) and forced expiratory volume in 1 second (FEV_1) before and after 4 weeks of respiratory muscle stretch gymnastics (RMSG) in 22 patients with chronic obstructive pulmonary disease. Lines indicate individual results; boxes indicate group mean $\pm$ SE. NS, not significant. (Used with permission from Kakizaki F. Preliminary report on the effects of respiratory muscle stretch gymnastics on chest wall mobility in patients with chronic obstructive pulmonary disease. *Respir Care.* 1999;44:412-413.)

function was examined in five patients with moderate-to-severe pulmonary emphysema for 4 weeks and in seven patients with mild to moderate emphysema for 6 weeks. After the specially designed plate therapy, inspiratory capacity (IC) and vital capacity (VC) increased in both the 4-week and the 6-week-treated groups, and the (FEV_1) increased in the 6-week-treated group. Furthermore, CO_2 retention was also improved and daily peak expiratory flow (PEF) showed significant increases from 2 weeks until the end of therapy. These results suggest that the respiratory muscle relaxation maneuver with specially designed plates is an effective method to improve pulmonary function of patients with pulmonary emphysema.

Upper Limb Exercise Test

Patients with emphysema frequently have dyspnea during upper limb exercise alone or combined with lower limb exercise. Several investigators have explored the role of upper limb exercise tests, which appear to be helpful in identifying dyspnea and determining treatment effects from pulmonary rehabilitation

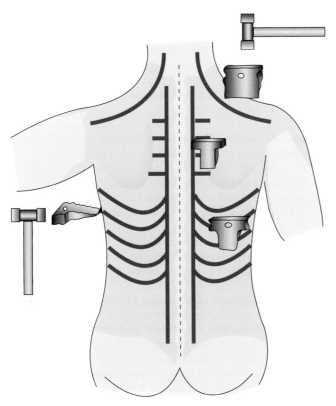

FIGURE 8 Schema for procedure of the respiratory muscle relaxation maneuver. A wedge-shaped wooden plate of appropriate size was placed on each bilateral intercostal, trapezius, scalenes, and antigravity muscles, and pressure was exerted by hand or by tapping the plate with a wooden hammer. (Used with permission from Fujimoto K. Effect of muscle relaxation therapy using specially designed plates in patients with pulmonary emphysema. *Intern Med.* 1996;35:756-763.)

programs.[28–31] Several upper-limb exercise tests have been described including a supported test, an arm ergometry test, an unsupported test, and a test of simulated activities of daily living. Each of these tests has advantages and disadvantages. Takahashi et al. have described an unsupported and dynamic progressive exercise test for upper-limb performance in patients with emphysema, during which a patient sits against a wall and elevates 200 g of weight to a low target and then repeats the lift to a progressively higher target.[32] This progressive lifting protocol is performed 30 times per minute and has been found to be more strongly correlated with ($\dot{V}O_{2peak}$) and maximum voluntary ventilation than static-upper-limb exercise testing. Therefore, dynamic upper-limb exercise testing appears to be an important test to include in the examination of patients with emphysema and with possibly other respiratory disorders.

ORGAN TRANSPLANTATION

In March of 1999 the *Boston Globe* ran a headline stating, "Heart transplantation ends old taboo in Japan." Organ transplantation from brain-dead donors began in 1999 under a new law of organ transplantation in Japan. Some physical therapists in Japan are now treating patients before and after trans-

plantation. The Japanese government has approved lung transplantation in four Japanese medical institutions and cardiac transplantation has been approved in three institutions. To date, there have been 17 cardiac and 14 lung transplantations from brain-dead donors from 1999 to October, 2003. As of October 2003, 32 living-donor lung transplants have been performed.

Living-Donor Lobar Lung Transplantation

Lung transplantation has not been reported in Japan until recently when Shimizu and his colleagues performed the 1st successful bilateral living-donor lobar lung transplantation.[33,34] A 24-year-old woman with primary ciliary dyskinesia began experiencing severe respiratory insufficiency and required mechanical ventilation. On October 28, 1998, she underwent bilateral living-donor lobar transplantation, receiving her sister's right lower lobe and her mother's left lower lobe under cardiopulmonary bypass. The patient was discharged from the hospital 61 days after transplantation. Six months postoperatively, she has returned to a normal life and is able to perform daily activities comfortably. She is currently in good physical condition and has a vital capacity of 1770 mL. One year after transplantation, her forced vital capacity was 2160 mL (73.2% of her predicted forced vital capacity). The recipient's sister was observed to have a decrease in forced vital capacity of 410 mL, and her mother had a decrease in forced vital capacity of 440 mL. Both donors have since returned to normal, unrestricted lives.

In Japan and internationally, patients undergo lung transplantation when a recipient's chest size and donor lung size do not match. We have found that patients who have undergone lung transplantation often demonstrate excessive work of breathing which we attempt to manage using many of the techniques described within this Chapter 20, "Physical Therapy Associated with Ventilatory Pump Dysfunction and Failure." We also focus on maintaining and improving the functional status and cardiorespiratory capacity of patients before and after transplantation.[35]

Lung Transplantation from Brain-Dead Donor

Miyoshi et al. reported on the results of two single-lung transplants from a single cadaveric donor that were successfully conducted at two different institutions on March 29, 2000. This was the 1st such procedure in Japan under newly introduced legislation.[36] One of the patients was a 48-year-old woman with idiopathic pulmonary fibrosis who underwent left single-lung transplantation under cardiopulmonary support at Osaka University Hospital. The postoperative course was uneventful. The patient was discharged on postoperative day 62 with satisfactory respiratory function. Several physical therapists have been engaged in the patients preoperative and postoperative care. The other patient suffered from end-stage emphysema and expired shortly after the transplantation.

Cardiac Transplantation

Cardiac transplantation began in 1968 and has been established as a therapeutic strategy for patients with end-stage heart failure throughout most of the world. In Japan, however, cardiac transplantation has been performed only occasionally. Although legislation for its approval was passed in 1997, it was not until February of 1999 that Japan experienced its first cardiac transplantation.[37] This was the result of long and steady efforts to enlighten Japanese society about the concept of brain death and the importance of organ transplantation. The patient was 47-year-old male with a dilated hypertrophic cardiomyopathy who had been supported with an implantable left ventricular assist device (LVAD). At present, several physical therapists work with cardiac surgeons and a transplantation coordinator to allocate care to patients before and after heart transplantation. We have successfully treated many patients awaiting cardiac transplantation (with and without LVADs) and one additional patient after cardiac transplantation. The fifth cardiac transplant patient was a 24-year-old patient who was in Osaka University Hospital with LVAD over 500 days and subsequently received a donor heart. She has returned to her home and is independent and preparing to return to her job.

SUMMARY

This International Perspective has presented the strengths and weaknesses of "Physical Therapy Associated With Ventilatory Pump Dysfunction and Failure" and has highlighted several Japanese issues that demonstrate the similarities and differences of physical therapy in Japan and around the globe. Many similarities exist between the physical therapy examination and management techniques of Japan and those of other countries, but differences also exist. The major differences between the physical therapy practiced in Japan and that practiced in other countries may be the primary focus on manual techniques to treat patients with ventilatory pump dysfunction and failure and on the relationship of medical practices to society at large in Japan. The key similarities between physical therapy in Japan and that in other countries is the continued search for evidence to support physical therapy care and the increasing role of physical therapy in many novel areas.

REFERENCES

1. Association of Cardiovascular and Pulmonary Rehabilitation. *Guidelines for Pulmonary Rehabilitation Programs.* 2nd ed. 1998. Champaign, IL: Human Kinetics; 1998.
2. The Japanese Respiratory Society/Japan Society for Respiratory Care. The statement for respiratory rehabilitation. *J Jpn Soc Respir Care.* 2001;11:321-330.
3. Japan Society for Respiratory Care Respiratory Rehabilitation Guideline Panel, et al. *A Manual for Respiratory Rehabilitation Therapeutic Exercise.* Tokyo: The Japanese Respiratory Society, Japan Society for Respiratory Care and The Japanese Physical Therapy Association; 2003.
4. Kida K, Jinno S, Nomura K, Yamada K, Katsura H, Kudoh S. Pulmonary rehabilitation program survey in North America, Europe, and Tokyo. *J Cardiopulmonary Rehabil.* 2003;8:304.
5. Gimenez M, Servera E, Vergara P, Bach JR, Polu JM. Endurance training in patients with chronic obstructive pulmonary disease: a comparison of high versus moderate intensity. *Arch Phys Med Rehabil.* 2000;81:102-109.
6. Inoue M, Ohtsu I, Tomioka S, et al. Effects of pulmonary rehabilitation on vital capacity in patients with chronic pulmonary emphysema. *Nihon Kyobu Shikkan Gakkai Zasshi.* 1996;34:1182-1188.
7. Miyagawa T. Effects and future perspectives of pulmonary rehabilitation. *Jpn J Respir Care.* 2000;9:91-104.
8. Taniguchi H, Kondoh Y, Nishiyama O, et al. The role of community hospital as a center for pulmonary rehabilitation. *Kokyu.* 2001,20:1212-1221.
9. Watanabe F, Ogawa T, Taniguchi H, Kondoh Y, Mikawa K. Effect of a pulmonary rehabilitation program in our outpatient with chronic obstructive pulmonary disease. *J Jpn Soc Respir Care.* 2000;10:251.
10. Toyota A, Hiramatsu K, Kanazawa I, Fujimura T, Toba K. Pulmonary rehabilitation and the change of pulmonary function after surgery. *Jpn J Rehabil Med.* 2001;38:771.
11. Miyagawa T, Kaneko N. The findings of bronchoscopy on airway cleaning technique. *Rigaku Ryohogaku.* 1997;24:561.
12. Okumura K, Sakata H. Efficacy of chest physiotherapy for the hospitalized children with asthma. *Jpn J Pediatr Pulmonol.* 2000;1:133-137.
13. Miyagawa T. Science in respiratory physical therapy. *Jpn J Respir Care.* 1998;15:97.
14. Uzawa Y, Yamaguchi Y. Change in lung mechanics during application of chest physical therapy techniques. *J Jpn Phys Ther Assoc.* 1998;25:222.
15. Nakano T, Ochi T, Ito N, Cahalin LP. Breathing assist techniques from Japan. *Cardiopulm Phys Ther J.* 2003;14:19-23.
16. Ihashi K, Saito A, Ito N. Effect of manual breathing assist technique on patients with dyspnea of exertion. *J Jpn phys Ther Assoc.* 1990;17:83-90.
17. Fisher MM, Bowey CJ, Ladd-Hudson K. External chest compression in acute asthma: a preliminary study. *Crit Care Med.* 1989;17:686-687.
18. Fisher MM, Whaley AP, Pye RR. External chest compression in the management of acute severe asthma—a technique in search of evidence. *Prehospital Disaster Med.* 2001;16:124—127.
19. Fukada Y, Sakaida K, Kim H, Tajimi K. Prevention of death from asthma by doctor-car system. *Japanese Emerg Med J.* 1998;7:188-193.
20. Shigemoto T, Hayashimoto H, Ochi T, Nakano T. The introduction of breathing assist technique for pre-admission emergency treatment. In: *Proceedings Twenty-Fourth Meeting of Japan Society of Respiratory Care Medicine.* Tokyo, Japan;2002:84.
21. Van der Touw T, Tully A, Amis TC, Brancatisano A, Rynn M, Mudaliar Y, Engel LA. Cardiorespiratory consequences of expiratory chest wall compression during mechanical ventilation and severe hyperinflation. *Crit Care Med.* 1993;21:1908-1914.
22. Van der Touw T, Mudaliar Y, Nayyar V. Cardiorespiratory effects of manually compressing the rib cage during tidal expiration in mechanically ventilated patients recovering from acute severe asthma. *Crit Care Med.* 1998;26:1361-1367.
23. Kanamaru A, Sibuya M, Nagai T, Inoue K, Homma I. Stretch gymnastic training in asthmatic children. In: Kaneko M, ed. *Fitness for the Aged, Disabled, and Industrial Worker.* Champaign, IL: Human Kinetics; 1990:178-181.

24. Yamada M, Kakizaki F, Shibuya M, Nakayama H, Tsuzura Y, Tanaka K, et al. Clinical effects of four weeks of respiratory muscle stretch gymnastics in patients with chronic obstructive pulmonary disease. *Nippon Kyobu Shikkan Gakkai Zasshi.* 1996;34:646-652.

25. Yamada M, Shibuya M, Kanamaru A, et al. Benefits of respiratory muscle stretch gymnastics in chronic respiratory disease. *Showa Univ J Med Sci.* 1996;8:63-71.

26. Kakizaki F, Shibuya M, Yamazaki T, Yamada M, Suzuki H, Homma I. Preliminary report on the effects of respiratory muscle stretch gymnastics on chest wall mobility in patients with chronic obstructive pulmonary disease. *Respir Care.* 1999;44:412-413.

27. Fujimoto K, Kubo K, Miyahara T, et al. Effect of muscle relaxation therapy using specially designed plates in patients with pulmonary emphysema. *Intern Med.* 1996;35:756-763.

28. Celli B. The clinical use of upper extremity exercise. *Clin Chest Med.* 1994;15:339-349.

29. Ellis B, Ries AL. Upper extremity exercise training in pulmonary rehabilitation. *J Cardiopulm Rehabil.* 1991;11:227-231.

30. Martinez FJ, Vogel PD, Dupont DN, Stanopoulos I, Gray A, Beamis JF. Supported arm exercise vs unsupported arm exercise in the rehabilitation of patients with severe chronic airflow obstruction. *Chest.* 1993;103:1397-1402.

31. Lake FR, Henderson K, Briffa T, Openshaw J, Musk AW. Upper-limb and lower-limb exercise training in patients with chronic airflow obstruction. *Chest.* 1990;97:1077-1082.

32. Takahashi T, Jenkinns S, Adachi H, Taniguchi K. Upper limb exercise tests for chronic emphysema. *Lung Perspect.* 2001;9:166-170.

33. Shimizu N, Date H, Yamashita M, et al. First successful bilateral living-donor lobar lung transplantation in Japan Nippon Geka Gakkai Zasshi. 1999;100:806-814.

34. Date H, Yamamoto H, Yamashita M, Aoe M, Kubo K, Shimizu N. One year follow-up of the first bilateral living-donor lobar lung transplantation in Japan. *Jpn J Thorac Cardiovasc Surg.* 2000;48:648-651.

35. Matsuo Y, Inoue S, Minami M, et al. Physical therapy before and after lobar lung transplantation—an experience in the second case of bilateral living-donor lobar lung transplantation in Japan. *J Jpn Soc Respir Care.* 2001;10:370-375.

36. Miyoshi S, Minami M, Ohta M, Okumura M, Takeda S, Matsuda H. Single lung transplantation from a brain-dead donor for a patient with idiopathic pulmonary fibrosis. A breakthrough after new legislation in Japan. *Jpn J Thorac Cardiovasc Surg.* 2001;49:398-403.

37. Hori M, Yamamoto K, Kodama K, et al. Successful launch of cardiac transplantation in Japan. Osaka University Cardiac Transplant Program. *Jpn Circ J.* 2000;64:326-332.

Physical Therapy Associated with Respiratory Failure in the Neonate

M. Kathleen Kelly*

INTRODUCTION

The patient group that defines Practice Pattern G are those neonates who have impaired ventilation, respiration/gas exchange, and aerobic capacity/endurance associated with respiratory failure.[1] Patients are included in this practice pattern if they are younger than 4 months and present with the following risk factors or pathophysiologic processes:

- Abdominal thoracic surgeries
- Apnea and bradycardia
- Bronchopulmonary dysplasia
- Congenital anomalies
- Respiratory distress syndrome
- Meconium aspiration syndrome
- Neurovascular disorders

- Pneumonia
- Rapid desaturation with movement or crying and the following impairments, functional limitations, and disabilities:
  - Abnormal pulmonary responses to activity
  - Impaired airway clearance
  - Impaired cough
  - Impaired gas exchange
  - Intercostal or subcostal retraction on inspiration
  - Paradoxical or abnormal breathing pattern at rest or with activity
  - Physiological intolerance of routine care

Patients older than 4 months are excluded from this pattern.

ANATOMY AND PHYSIOLOGY

Fetal to Extrauterine Transition

The transition to extrauterine life presents one of the greatest anatomic and physiologic challenges faced by an infant. At birth, a series of events must occur in order to support adequate lung and cardiac function during the conversion from liquid to air breathing and to establish parallel pulmonary and systemic circulation.[2] Throughout fetal life, circulatory functions take place primarily in the placenta with relatively little blood flow through the lungs. During delivery, however, various bioch and structural changes must be initiated rapidly in order to ensure the transition from fetal to neonatal circulation. The key elements in the birth transition are the shift from maternally dependent oxygenation to continuous respiration; a switch from fetal circulation to mature circulation; the onset of independent glucose metabolism; the onset of independent oral feeding, thermoregulation, and the regulation of hormonal control of growth.[3]

At birth, the airways are partially filled with fluid that has been derived from the amniotic sac, tracheal glands, and lung tissue.[4] The presence of this fetal lung fluid is crucial to the development of the respiratory system; however, its clearance is equally essential for the respiratory adaptations to air breathing. Within seconds of emergence from the uterine environment and the initiation of breathing, air rapidly replaces the intra-alveolar fluid. Normally, newborns rapidly establish the critical negative pressure needed to expand the alveoli and then are able to maintain adequate respiratory function and good aeration. It is only during the last few weeks of prenatal development that the lung tissue becomes fully capable of autonomous respiration—that is, gas exchange (see Table 21-1). At this time in development, the alveolar–capillary membrane thins out enough to permit gas exchange. In addition, the process of alveolarization is initiated and continues to be completed postnatally. These structural changes in the lung result in increased lung volumes and increased surface area for gas exchange. During prenatal development, a number of factors can negatively influence or affect lung development resulting in *primary pulmonary hypoplasia*. *Secondary pulmonary hypoplasia,* which is seen more often than a primary pulmonary hypoplasia, may result from an absence of fetal breathing or any restriction in the chest wall space.

In addition to the structural changes in the lung tissue that contribute to neonatal viability, *surfactant* production is essential to neonatal viability and morbidity. Surfactant synthesis begins at approximately 20 weeks' gestational age and continues until the lungs are generally mature, around 35 weeks' gestational age. Several measures of lung maturity are available, but the most widely used is the lecithin/syphingomyelin

TABLE 21-1   Stages of Lung Growth

	Time
Embryonic	3–7 wk
Canalicular	7–16 wk
Pseudoglandular	16–26 wk
Saccular	26–36 wk
Alveolar	36 wk to 2 y
Postnatal growth	2–18 y

From Kotecha S. Lung growth: implications for the newborn infant. (Reprinted from *Arch Dis Child.* 2000;82:F69-F74, with permission from the BMJ Publishing Group.)

(L/S) ratio; a larger value is indicative of a more mature system. A deficiency of surfactant due to immature lungs is the hallmark of neonatal respiratory distress syndrome (RDS), a leading cause of neonatal deaths.[4]

During the transition from fetal to neonatal respiration, there is a large increase in pulmonary blood flow, a fall in pulmonary vascular resistance, and the establishment of lung volumes, all of which occur in the first few breaths after birth. The pressure gradient from the increased pulmonary blood flow causes the foramen ovale to close, which in turn causes right ventricular outflow to be directly diverted into the pulmonary circulation.[5] Three other major structures, the ductus venosus, ductus arteriosus, and umbilical vessels, also constrict soon after birth. These closures are functional at birth, with true anatomical closure typically occurring over the next several hours and days.[2]

The success of the transition to extrauterine life is captured in the *Apgar score* (Table 21-2). This scoring system is applied to newborns in the immediate postpartum minutes and is meant to be a predictor of neonatal survival. Five easily identifiable characteristics are scored on a scale of 0, 1, or 2. These include heart rate, respiratory rate, color, reflex irritability, and tone. An Apgar score of 0 to 3 indicates the need for immediate maximal intervention including intubation and oxygen therapy; a score of 4 to 6 indicates marginal adaptation and requires stimulation, oxygen by face mask, and possibly

other interventions as well as close observation; and an Apgar score of 7 to 10 indicates good adaptation to extrauterine life. At a minimum, the scores are determined at 1 minute and 5 minutes; in certain other situations an Apgar score is given at consecutive 5-minute intervals.[6]

Anatomic and Physiologic Features Affecting Cardiopulmonary Function in the Neonate

There are a number of age-related anatomic and physiologic differences which impact respiratory function in the neonate. These differences are most striking in premature infants and newborns and result in an increased vulnerability and susceptibility to respiratory dysfunction and cardiopulmonary compromise. Some of these differences include the following[7-9]:

- Small airways (increased predisposition to airway obstruction)
- Circular rib cage (decreased mechanical advantage of the diaphragm and less efficient ventilation)
- Decreased alveolar surface area
- Increased compliance of the airways (decreased bronchial stability)
- Decreased lung compliance (results in increased inflation pressures needed to maintain lung volume and resultant increased work of breathing)
- Immature neural respiratory centers (easily disrupted by drugs, sleep state, temperature)
- Susceptibility to diaphragmatic fatigue
- Irregular rate and rhythm of breathing (prone to apneic episodes)
- Compensation for respiratory insufficiency by increase in the rate, not the depth of breathing

For the otherwise healthy newborn, these developmental differences may not be problematic, but for the medically fragile or very immature infant, they can have serious consequences. There are a number of pathophysiologic processes that may result in placing a neonate in Practice Pattern 6G: *Impaired Ventilation, Respiration/Gas Exchange, and Aerobic Capacity/Endurance Respiratory Failure in the Neonate.* Some

TABLE 21-2   Apgar Scoring System for Newborns

Sign	Apgar Score		
	0 Points	1 Point	2 Points
Heart rate	Absent	<100 beats/min	>100 beats/min
Respiration	Absent	Irregular, shallow, gasping	Vigorous, crying
Skin color	Pale, blue	Acrocyanosis	Pink
Muscle tone/activity	Limp	Some flexion of extremities	Active movement
Reflex irritability (catheter in nostril)	Absent	Grimace	Active avoidance Cough/sneeze

Modified from Apgar V. Proposal for new method of evaluation of newborn infant. *Curr Res Anesth Analg.* 1953;32:260-267.

of the diagnoses and pathophysiologic processes that may result in respiratory failure are listed here:

- Primary lung disease
  BPD (bronchopulmonary dysplasia)
  Aspiration syndromes (eg, meconium aspiration)
- Persistent pulmonary hypertension
- Central nervous system disorders
  Central hypoventilation syndrome (aka Ondine's curse)
  Encephalopathy, hemorrhage
- Intrinsic muscle disease
  Congenital myopathies
  Congenital abnormalities of the rib cage
  Infantile botulism
  Infantile myasthenia gravis
- Apnea of prematurity
- Congenital organ anomalies
  Congenital diaphragmatic hernia
  Congenital heart disease
- Congenital airway abnormalities (eg, tracheoesophageal fistula [TEF], subglottic stenosis, laryngomalacia)

Case Studies

Neonatal physical therapy is a specialty area of practice and one that requires advanced skills and competencies beyond traditional physical therapy education. Given the high-tech characteristics of the environment coupled with the unique vulnerabilities seen in an immature and fragile human, this is a challenging, but exciting environment in which to work. In both of the following cases, the infants have respiratory failure as one of their primary diagnoses; however, there are distinct differences in the pathophysiologic processes and secondary problems that they may encounter. It is noteworthy to mention that these infants may have very different courses of physical therapy interventions as they get older. This will likely depend on the degree of recovery from the acute respiratory failure and subsequent chronic lung disease and the degree of brain damage that results from the hemorrhagic or hypoxic events.

These cases illustrate the types of infants seen by physical therapists working in a neonatal intensive care unit (NICU) (see Fig. 21-1).

Case 1: Bronchopulmonary Dysplasia Associated with Prematurity

Sara was the 750-g product (1 lb, 10 oz) of a 26-week gestation to a 38-year-old who experienced preterm labor due to toxemia. In the delivery room, the Apgar scores were 2^1 5^5 $5.^{10}$ Sara was intubated in the delivery room (DR), brought to the NICU, and stabilized. At that time umbilical artery lines were placed, a chest X-ray was taken, and surfactant was administered. After two doses of surfactant, Sara was eventually put on a ventilator because of poor oxygenation. A synchronized intermittent mandatory ventilation (SIMV) mode of mechanical ventilation was used with a rate of 25 breaths per minute;

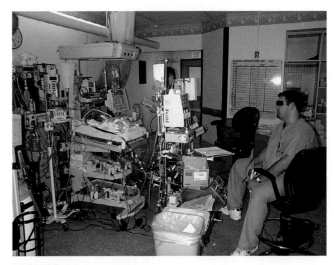

FIGURE 21-1   Infant in neonatal intensive care unit.

she was maintained at a SaO$_2$ (oxygen saturation, arterial) of 93% to 95%. At day of life 1 (DOL) total parenteral nutrition was started.

Sara's medical course was complicated by respiratory distress syndrome ultimately progressing to bronchopulmonary dysplasia. She was treated with diuretics, caffeine, inhaled aerosols, and steroids. Sara remained ventilator dependent until she was 4.5 months chronological age and was on supplemental oxygen for another 2 months. At 2.5 months of age she had a tracheostomy tube placed.

Nasogastric tube feedings were started when she was 30 weeks of gestational age (4 weeks of chronological age) and were administered until she was extubated. Nonnutritive sucking opportunities were provided while she was being fed. Once extubated, Sara began bottle-feeding, although with much difficulty secondary to decreased coordination with sucking and mainly due to poor endurance. It was noted that she desaturated during feedings and needed increased supplemental oxygen to maintain a SaO$_2$ of 93%.

Because of her prematurity, a head ultrasound was taken on DOL 14. The scan revealed a grade IV intraventricular hemorrhage on the left and grade II intraventricular hemorrhage on the right. Sara displayed some unusual movements at approximately 2 months of age, but a neurological consult determined that she was not having seizures.

A consult from the developmental pediatrician was made to physical therapy when Sara was 2 months of chronological age. Initially, the role of the physical therapist was to assist with creating the appropriate environmental modifications. This included consulting with the nursing staff to implement a *positioning program* for Sara. In addition, a major component of the intervention program was teaching both the nursing staff and Sara's parents to recognize and interpret her behavioral cues. For Sara's parents, this helped them to better understand Sara's physiologic status, but more importantly, they had fewer negative interactions because they could interpret her signs of "readiness" in terms of physical bonding and interactions.

Once Sara was physiologically stable during position changes, gentle movement and handling was introduced in order to acclimate her to movement in general, and movement against gravity. Throughout the entire session, she was constantly monitored to ensure physiologic stability. Sara was seen several times per week by physical therapy until she was discharged at 5.5 months' chronological age. Because of her birth history of prematurity, intraventricular hemorrhage, and bronchopulmonary dysplasia, Sara was at risk for an adverse neuromotor outcome. At the time of discharge, Sara was referred to her community-based early intervention program. The services through this program, developmental services, as well as other would be provided in her home and would include a continuation of physical therapy. The physical therapist also assisted with coordinating Sara's discharge plans and communicating the necessary information regarding Sara's medical issues and necessary precautions to the early intervention team. Because Sara's parents had learned the medical aspects of her care and were able to interpret her behavioral and physiologic cues, their transition to home was relatively smooth.

Sara returned to the hospital for her follow-up visits every 3 to 6 months, and at each visit she was evaluated by the child developmental team. Over time, she had demonstrated gradual improvements in her health status. She continued to require aerosols for reactive airway disease but has had no subsequent hospitalizations. There was some concern over her growth and nutritional status because she was gaining weight slowly and by report was a slow feeder. The physical therapy examination revealed that Sara exhibited significant delays in head control, reaching and grabbing, and sitting. She had muscle tone abnormalities, presence of primitive reflexes, decreased repertoire of movement, and abnormal postural control. Sara was ultimately diagnosed with cerebral palsy.

Case 2: Full-Term Infant with Persistent Pulmonary Hypertension and Meconium Aspiration Syndrome

Joshua was a 4,200-g baby boy born at 39 weeks' gestation via a vaginal vertex delivery to a 26-year-old. Labor lasted 24 hours, and the membranes ruptured approximately 21 hours prior to delivery. Joshua was resuscitated in the delivery room secondary to low Apgar scores of 2^1 2^5 4^{10} and 6^{15} after vigorous stimulation. He immediately presented with tachypnea and *expiratory grunting,* both of which are signs of respiratory distress. Grunting on expiration is thought to be a physiologic mechanism to prolong the expiratory phase and increase the functional residual capacity.[8] Joshua was subsequently placed on 100% O_2, and chest films were taken which revealed patchy infiltrates, indicative of aspiration syndrome. Pulse oximetry was 45% on room air and was unchanged on 100% O_2. Arterial blood gases were drawn, and the following results were obtained:

On room air: pH 7.22/32 $PaCO_2$/41 PaO_2

In 100% O_2: pH 7.23/32 $PaCO_2$/44 PaO_2

These results reveal a metabolic acidosis evidenced by the low pH, but more relevant was the failure to improve on 100% O_2. Because of the poor oxygenation, even in the presence of 100% O_2, an echocardiogram was taken to rule out congenital heart disease. The echo was negative for any cardiac abnormalities, and the diagnosis of persistent pulmonary hypertension (PPH) and meconium aspiration syndrome (MAS) was made. Joshua was sedated, intubated, and maintained on 100% O_2, with ventilator settings at a rate of 40 breaths/min, and pressor support (dopamine and dobutamine) was given in order to maintain blood pressure/peripheral perfusion. Neurologic examinations over the first several days were remarkable for seizures on DOL 2; lethargy and subsequent hypotonia were noted after the first week. He was weaned from the ventilator in 7 days and was on room air by DOL 12. Joshua remained hospitalized until he was 20 days old. The pediatric neurologist consulted physical therapy on DOL 10 because of Joshua's risk for neurologic dysfunction as a result of the hypoxia and also because of his respiratory status and ventilator dependence for a week.

EXAMINATION OF THE NEONATE WITH RESPIRATORY FAILURE

The physical therapy examination and evaluation of the neonate with respiratory failure needs to encompass a wide range of skills and observations. In addition to an understanding of cardiorespiratory anatomy and physiology in the neonate, one also needs to understand the implications of a compromise to those systems in the developing infant. In addition, knowledge of typical and atypical motor skill development is also necessary in order to interpret the examination results in light of potential functional limitations and disabilities.

The medically fragile neonate is unique with respect to anatomical, physiological, and behavioral characteristics. The immaturities in these systems and subsequent vulnerabilities related to physiologic and behavioral stability can result in the neonate easily becoming unstable during routine caregiving or social interactions. Therefore, the physical therapy examination process needs to take into account the multiple systems that interact to affect the neonate's status. For example, it is not unusual for the fragile neonate to show signs of physiologic instability such as desaturation and increased heart rate and respiratory rate in response to a rather benign interaction such as making eye contact, being handled, or being spoken to. Thus, although our efforts may be therapeutic by design, in this particular group of patients, well-intended examination or intervention methods may result in irreparable harm.

The complexity of the technical environment also makes this a challenging population; it is essential that the physical therapist be comfortable with all of the equipment (ventilators, intravenous lines, physiologic monitoring devices). Because an infant will not communicate directly, it is up to the therapist to interpret any signs of impending or actual distress. The essence of our intervention is to ensure that no harm be done

TABLE 21-3 **Normal Physiologic Parameters for Neonates**

Respiratory rate (bpm)	40–60
Heart rate (bpm)	120–200
P_{O_2} (mm Hg)	60–90
P_{CO_2} (mm Hg)	30–35
Blood pressure (mm Hg) Systolic Diastolic	60–90 30–60
Sa_{O_2} (%)	87–89 (low) 94–95 (high)

Data from Comer DM. Pulse oximetry: implications for practice. *J Obstet Gynecol Neonatal Nurs*. 1992;21:35-41.

Pagtakhan RD, Chernick V. Intensive care for respiratory disorders. In: Kendig EL, Cher-nick V. eds. *Disorders of the Respiratory Tract in Children*. 4th ed. Philadelphia, PA: WB Saunders; 1983:145-168.

in the delivery of services and to optimize the child's developmental potential. It is for this reason that physical therapists working with the medically fragile neonate have an advanced knowledge and understanding of the necessary competencies. Although it is outside of the scope of this chapter to cover in detail, more information on the recommended competencies for working with high-risk neonates can be found in the *Practice Guidelines for the Physical Therapist in the NICU*.[11]

Prior to beginning an examination or treatment session, the therapist should confer with the neonate's primary nurse or caregiver to determine their most recent medical status, in addition to their baseline physiologic parameters. Depending on the nature and severity of the predisposing condition, the cardiorespiratory parameters may vary from what is considered to be normal for an infant (see Table 21-3). It is always prudent to establish the "safe" physiologic parameters within which to work. Typically, the neonate's heart rate, respiratory rate, and oxygen saturation will be constantly monitored; **however, there is no substitute for the keen visual observation of signs of distress.**

History

The examination process consists of three major components: history, review of systems, and specific tests and measures. Typically, the physical therapist would use the pertinent history to identify impairments, functional limitations, and disabilities in order to establish a diagnosis/prognosis and ultimately to determine the intervention. Obtaining the initial data from the medical record is a crucial first step.

Relevant data for neonates include information about maternal health, pregnancy, and delivery—specifically the birthweight, length of gestation, and the status of the baby in the immediate perinatal period. Although physical therapists are not the ones who determine the infant's gestational age, that information is necessary for interpreting the physiologic, neurobehavioral, and musculoskeletal findings during the examination and evaluation. As well, a strong inverse correlation

exists between gestational age and respiratory disease, as well as other sequelae of preterm birth. Other relevant information includes the medical and/or surgical diagnoses, current level of respiratory support, level of physiologic monitoring, medications, feeding status, and general family support issues.

Systems Review

A review of the major systems in both cases would include a general screening to determine where examination and intervention efforts should be focused. Although there were no primary pathologies or impairments of the integumentary system in either case study, it cannot be overlooked in the examination. Preterm infants in particular are prone to skin breakdown due to their extremely fragile, thin skin that contains very little subcutaneous fat. Skin inspection should be a component of the PT examination. Especially prone to damage are the areas of skin underlying the adhesive pads placed for physiologic monitoring equipment. Also, in infants with tracheostomies, the stoma is vulnerable to trauma from the moisture and friction of the tube itself and from the ties, which secure it around the neck. General vigilance regarding skin breakdown is essential if an infant is not able or capable of much active movement.

The other major systems to screen prior to organizing the PT examination would be the neuromuscular and musculoskeletal systems. In both of the cases presented, the potential exists for neuromuscular impairments secondary to the documented brain hemorrhage in the case of Sara and the neurologic involvement secondary to hypoxia in Joshua. From a musculoskeletal perspective, it would be important to rule out any obvious joint or soft tissue impairments. Although neither infant had contractures or any type of musculoskeletal defect, they were at risk for contractures secondary to their relative immobility and the gravity-dependent position in which most nursing/medical care occurs. In both cases, positioning programs were recommended and carried out by the nursing staff.

Tests and Measures

The goal of the physical therapy examination process is to identify the "impairments, functional limitations, and disabilities and establish the diagnosis and the prognosis." The specific tests and measures are individualized with respect to the patient presentation and not to diagnosis alone. Although the diagnoses and other patient-related factors differ for the two cases presented, much is similar in terms of the tests and measures, indications for PT involvement, and expected outcomes.

One of the most important priorities and considerations when working with neonates, especially infants born prematurely like Sara, is recognition of their tolerance to handling. Thus, a critical part of the PT examination will be determining the infant's baseline physiologic stability. At any given time, this should be preceded by a discussion with the patient's primary nurse to determine that a true baseline is being obtained. If the baby has just had some medical intervention, for example,

TABLE 21-4   Sara and Joshua: Tests for Assessment of Aerobic Capacity and Endurance

Autonomic responses to positional changes	Look for color changes such as mottling of skin; changes in HR, RR, or Sao_2
Signs of respiratory distress	Increases in HR, RR (count by observing chest excursion; best to count for 1 minute to account for irregular rate and rhythm), increased retractions, asynchronous chest wall movement or paradoxical breathing, nasal flaring, expiratory grunting, color changes indicative of cyanosis. (Note: In neonates, clinical signs of hypoxia may be masked until low Pao_2 levels are reached.)
Standard vital signs at rest, during, and after activity (HR, BP, Sao_2)	Use of bedside monitoring and clinical observation

their physiologic status may have been affected, and the result of the PT test may reveal a "poststress" response, rather than a true baseline. This concept is not unlike that used in exercise testing, when the baseline measures are used to interpret the patient's exercise and postexercise recovery responses. The appropriate tests and measures for Sara and Joshua are presented in Tables 21-4 through 21-7; each is followed by the examination strategy and interpretation, when necessary.

Regardless of the reason for a neonate having respiratory failure, appreciation of the fact that the child is at a disadvantage in terms of developmental risks is a compelling reason to begin early intervention as soon as the infant or child is medically stable. Because of the risks for abnormal neurodevelopmental sequelae, physical therapists should be involved with providing developmental intervention early in the course of an infant's hospitalization. Delays in the initiation of rehabilitation or habilitation can place the child at risk for developing *preventable* secondary impairments and functional limitations.

INTERVENTIONS FOR NEONATES WITH RESPIRATORY DISTRESS

In a best-practice environment, neonates with respiratory failure are managed with a multidisciplinary approach. A unique role of the physical therapist on that team is to provide interventions that are physiologically and developmentally appropriate for infants who are at risk for delayed or abnormal motor development. Physical therapists are uniquely qualified to design and implement treatment plans with outcomes directed toward movement efficiency. Thus, in the patient cases presented here, the physical therapy interventions were developmentally appropriate motor activities that were

implemented and monitored in much the same way as one would monitor a cardiopulmonary rehabilitation exercise program. Tables 21-8 through 21-10 outline the various components of the physical therapy interventions for Sara and Joshua, the anticipated goals, and the specific strategies used to accomplish the goal. The anticipated goals served as a benchmark for the expected outcomes.

The direct interventions included goals from both the cardiopulmonary and the neuromuscular practice patterns (neuromuscular preferred Practice Pattern C: *Impaired Motor Function and Sensory Integrity Associated with Nonprogressive Disorders of the Central Nervous System—Congenital Origin or Acquired in Infancy or Childhood*). Activities were chosen that were developmentally appropriate while monitoring the physiologic cost to the infant. The concept of aerobic and endurance training was utilized with the strategies incorporating developmental motor skills typically acquired during the first few weeks of life.

During the initial examination, it was clear that both infants were medically fragile due to their behavioral instability and "time out" signs of stress. In both cases, the behavioral cues occurred concurrently with signs of a physiologic cost to the infant evidenced by changes in heart rate and oxygen saturation. There was constant vigilance of the physiologic monitors for both of the infants; and in fact, any changes indicative of increased stress or effort resulted in immediate modifications to the intervention.

A positioning program was instituted for both infants in which position changes were encouraged after every clustered caregiving episode. By incorporating this at a time when other caregiving occurs, the nursing staff did not feel overwhelmed with additional "duties." The positioning program included recommendations for prone positioning, supported side-lying, supported semisitting, and supine positioning with the

TABLE 21-5   Sara and Joshua: Tests for Assessment of Ventilation and Respiration/Gas Exchange

Thoracoabdominal excursions indicative of distress or increased effort with breathing	Observation of chest wall synchrony prior to and after handling
Evaluate physiologic responses to movement, handling, routine interventions	Ongoing use of bedside monitoring (HR, RR, and Sao_2); observe signs of distress, fatigue, or instability; as above, observation of cyanosis in neonates indicates low Pao_2 levels; observe for breathing irregularities or apneic episodes
Observe protective mechanisms	Observation of gag reflex; sneezing; ability to clear airway in prone
Auscultation of lung fields	Difficult in neonates because of easy transmission of sound, thus making it difficult to localize the involved segment; keep head in midline if possible; best to correlate findings with chest radiographs

TABLE 21-6 Sara and Joshua: Tests for Behavioral Responses and Stability[a]

General alertness and responsiveness	Note degree of alertness during awake periods; note ability to orient to face and voice

Observe and document signs of distress or "time-out"; note what event preceded these behaviors[12]	Physiologic signs of stress
	   Color change
	   Skin mottling
	   Change in RR or rhythm
	   Change in HR
	   Coughing, sneezing, yawning
	   Bowel movements
	   Hiccoughs
	Behavioral signs of stress
	   Gaze aversion
	   Staring
	   Diffuse sleep states
	   Irritability
	Motoric signs of stress
	   Stiffness
	   Flaccidity
	   Arching
	   Finger splaying
	   Grimacing
	   Jitteriness

Observe and document signs of physiologic instability; observe length of time for infant to "recover" to baseline values	Ongoing monitoring of vital signs and clinical signs of respiratory distress

[a]For more detailed information on neurobehavioral assessment of neonates, see Refs. 12,13–16.

TABLE 21-7 Sara and Joshua: Tests for Motor Function/Neuromotor Development/ Sensory Integration[a]

Reflex development	Note presence or absence of age-appropriate neonatal reflexes; note symmetry and robustness of response.
General movement and postural control (including assessment of muscle performance)[17]	Assess ability to move in various positions; ability to move against gravity and change position; degree of head control; quality of movement; quality of muscle tone; emergence of postural control; asymmetries in movement. May use standardized assessments to document degree of delay or deviation[a]

[a]For more detailed information on neuromotor and postural assessment of neonates, see Refs. 18 and 19.

TABLE 21-8 Sara and Joshua Interventions: Coordination, Communication, and Documentation

Anticipated Goals	Specific Interventions
Coordinated care (family, significant others, caregivers, other professionals)	Coordination of care with other NICU team members and the family; attendance at patient care conferences to discuss status Consultation with NICU staff to provide a nurturing environment that will support growth and development
Understanding of expectations, goals and outcomes	Use of a family-focused philosophy; therapist works with family to establish goals; examination and evaluation are discussed with family/caregivers as well as expected outcomes for the infant
Needs after discharge determined	Coordinating discharge planning with other team members; discussing Early Intervention services with family/caregivers

TABLE 21-9 Sara and Joshua Interventions: Patient/Client-Related Instruction

Anticipated Goals	Specific Interventions
Empowering parents with respect to knowledge of infant's condition, expected outcomes, environmental stressors and affordances	Ongoing communication with parents about infant's status; keeping them informed about changes that influence outcome
Decrease anxiety of parent interaction with infant	Parent teaching with respect to "reading" the infant's signs of stress; demonstrations of strategies for calming infant and handling and positioning strategies that are developmentally appropriate and physiologically safe; working with the infant while parents are present

TABLE 21-10 Sara and Joshua Interventions: Procedural Interventions[a]

Anticipated Goals	Specific Interventions
Improved physiologic response to increased oxygen demand	Developmentally appropriate motor activities emphasizing postural control and functional movement while monitoring HR, RR, and SaO_2
Improved tolerance for movement and developmentally appropriate activities (motor and behavioral)	
Decreased atelectasis	Positioning program to incorporate modified postural drainage positions On occasion, gentle percussion techniques followed by suctioning (done by nursing)[b]
Physiologic and behavioral stability during therapeutic activities	Constant monitoring of HR, RR, SaO_2 and behavioral signs of stress
Increased repertoire and quality of movement	Developmentally appropriate activities emphasizing functional movement and postural control; use of auditory and visual stimuli to increase interest in movement and activity
Increased strength	Developmentally appropriate motor activities emphasizing movement and control against gravity; prone positioning to encourage early weight bearing through UEs

[a]Interventions from neuromuscular Practice Pattern C were incorporated into the treatment plan for both infants.
[b]Only used with Case 2 (full-term infant with PPH and MAS).

use of blanket rolls to provide protraction and midline orientation for the upper extremities and to decrease the tendency toward abduction and external rotation in the lower extremities (Fig. 21-2). Prone positioning, in particular, has been recently discouraged as a position for babies to sleep because of the risk of *sudden infant death syndrome (SIDS)*; however, there are known benefits of its effects on oxygenation, heart rate, chest wall synchrony, and behavioral measures (for a review, see Refs. 8 and 19). In addition, the prone position is important for the infant to develop antigravity head control. Although there has not been evidence to support the effects of a positioning program on the musculoskeletal system, it was utilized with the assumption that it would decrease the effects of gravity on the soft tissue structures of the musculoskeletal system. For many reasons, in addition to their immature musculoskeletal systems, these infants lack strength, as evidenced by the paucity of movement against gravity.

Chest physical therapy techniques were limited to the use of positioning and gentle movement transitions to mobilize secretions.

Risk Factors

Efficient respiratory function requires an organ of gas exchange, that is, the lungs, and a "pump" mechanism consisting of the rib cage and respiratory muscles, in addition to an intact neural control mechanism for respiration.[20] Under normal conditions, the respiratory pump can adapt to satisfy the changing metabolic needs that may occur during exercise, hyperthermia, or other demands[21]; but when these systems are unable to deliver oxygen and remove carbon dioxide from the pulmonary circulation, respiratory failure ensues and gas exchange is impaired.[22] In the neonate, a number of anatomic and physiologic immaturities place them at risk for respiratory failure. Structurally, the infant is born with a compliant rib cage secondary to the lack of complete bony ossification. The latter, along with less

compliant lung tissue and decreased muscle mass, results in inefficient respiratory mechanics. **Infants also have a predisposition to diaphragmatic fatigue because of the decreased proportion of type I muscle fibers. Less than 10% of the diaphragmatic muscle fibers consist of high-oxidative and slow-twitch fibers, making them poorly equipped to handle high workloads.**[23]

Pathophysiology of Bronchopulmonary Dysplasia

These immaturities are exacerbated only in the infant born prematurely. One of the most common and most serious sequelae of preterm birth is RDS—the most common respiratory abnormality in the preterm infant, and the single most common cause of death in neonates.[4] The primary pathology in RDS is due to the decreased amount of surfactant. As a result, the infant's pulmonary status is characterized by an increase in alveolar surface tension, alveolar collapse, diffuse atelectasis, ventilation/perfusion mismatch, and decreased lung compliance. **Because of increased pulmonary artery pressures, a subsequent right-to-left shunt results in a ventilation–perfusion mismatch. Typical signs and symptoms of RDS include increased respiratory rate, retractions, nasal flaring, grunting, cyanosis, and an increased work of breathing.**

The introduction of surfactant therapy has made a significant difference in the outcomes of babies like Sara with RDS.[24] It is now standard practice for babies born less than 30 to 32 weeks GA to be given prophylactic surfactant administration in the delivery room within their first few breaths.[25] Numerous clinical trials have established evidence for surfactant's efficacy in improving gas exchange, reducing the severity of the acute disease and increasing survival in preterm infants.[25,26] Other management strategies for babies with RDS include steroid administration, supplemental oxygenation,

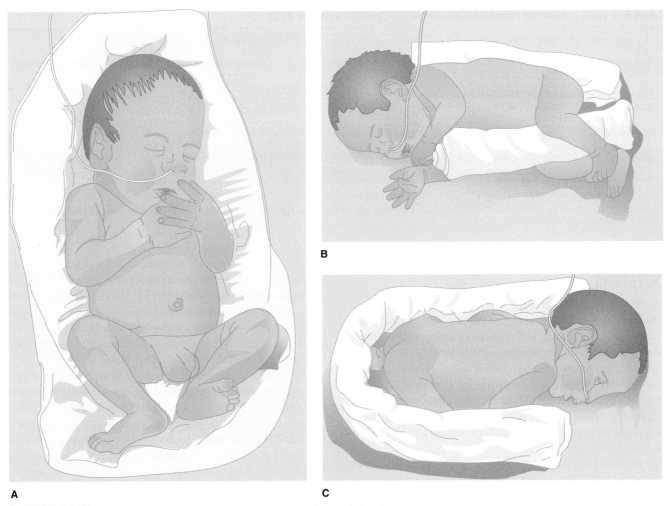

FIGURE 21-2 Positioning strategies for neonates. (**A**) supine, (**B**) side-lying, (**C**) prone.

assisted ventilation, and nutritional intervention. As a result of these interventions, the incidence and the profile of babies like Sara who develop a form of chronic lung disease known as BPD have changed.[27]

Bronchopulmonary dysplasia was first described by Northway and colleagues in 1967 as a disease of preterm infants characterized by both acute lung changes and chronic lung changes with resultant inflammation of the lung parenchyma, a combination of emphysema and fibrosis, and remodeling.[28] This classic form of BPD occurred primarily in preterm infants who required mechanical ventilation with high inspiratory pressures to maintain airway patency and high concentrations of supplemental oxygen, both of which were thought to contribute to its pathogenesis. The clinical diagnosis of BPD was made when the infant was oxygen dependent (greater than 30%) beyond 28 to 30 days and had accompanying radiographic changes in the lungs. The cohort of infants described in Northway's original work was over 31 weeks of gestational age and all but one weighed more than 1,500 g.

As a result of improved, less traumatic ventilation methods, antenatal steroids, and surfactant, it is now infrequent to see BPD in babies with birth weights greater than 1,200 g and gestational ages beyond 30 weeks.[29] Despite this, the incidence of BPD has not changed much because of the increased survival of smaller and more preterm babies. Similar to RDS, the risk of developing BPD increases linearly with decreasing gestational age and birth weight. Furthermore, BPD continues to be a major complication in preterm infants who require mechanical ventilation.[30]

More recent histopathologic findings from babies who die from respiratory complications of BPD have revealed a newer and different profile of BPD. No longer are the prominent findings related to airway and lung tissue trauma and inflammation; rather, less fibrosis and more uniform inflation are noted.[31] In addition, the major manifestation of lung injury seems to be an interruption in lung development. These very recent findings have forced a major reconsideration of the pathogenesis, diagnosis, management, and long-term outcomes of infants with BPD. As well, a newer clinical definition of BPD has emerged, as the original definition would only apply to a small number of babies. A very recent workshop on BPD summarized a new definition of BPD that also provides a classification of severity based on the need for supplemental oxygen and/or positive pressure ventilation[29] (Table 21-11).

TABLE 21-11   Newly Proposed Guidelines for Classification of BPD[a]

Gestational age	<32 weeks	≥32 weeks
Time point of assessment	36 weeks PMA or discharge to home, whichever comes first	>28 days but <56 days or discharge to home, whichever comes first
Treatment with oxygen >21 for at least 28 days plus		
Mild BPD	Room air at 36 weeks or discharge, whichever comes first	Breathing room air by 56 days or discharge, whichever comes first
Moderate BPD	Need for <30% oxygen at 36 weeks or discharge, whichever comes first	Need for <30% oxygen at 56 days or discharge, whichever comes first
Severe BPD	Need for ≥30% oxygen and/or positive pressure (PPV or NCPAP) at 36 weeks or discharge, whichever comes first	Need for ≥30% oxygen and/or positive pressure (PPV or NCPAP) at 56 days or discharge, whichever comes first

[a]NCPAP, nasal continuous positive airway pressure; PPV, positive-pressure ventilation.

Reprinted with permission from Jobe AH, Bancalari E, Bronchopulmonary Dysplasia. *Am J Respir Crit Care Med.* 2001;163:1723-1729. Official Journal of the American Thoracic Society. © American Thoracic Society.

Treatment of Bronchopulmonary Dysplasia

The treatment of BPD includes nutritional support to promote lung development and maturation, fluid management, pharmacologic management, and respiratory support. Commonly used pharmacologic approaches include bronchodilators and diuretics to improve airway conductance, decrease edema, and increase gas exchange; sedatives for persistent agitation; and high-dose corticosteroids to decrease inflammation of the respiratory tract. The respiratory management may range from supplemental oxygen given by nasal cannula to a tracheostomy and mechanical ventilation.

Because lung tissue continues to grow postnatally, most infants recover from BPD and eventually function independent of assisted ventilation and supplemental oxygen if conditions for growth are optimized. Nevertheless, a relatively small proportion of the infants who develop BPD will go on to require prolonged ventilation. As noted previously, the collective use of steroids, surfactant replacement, and fewer traumatic ventilatory strategies has contributed to improved outcomes seen in infants with BPD. Thus far, it appears that the best prevention of BPD is the ability to avoid prematurity, lung barotrauma, overuse of the ventilator, and the release of free oxygen radicals associated with the inflammatory process. **The decrease in barotrauma to the lungs is in large part due to the introduction of gentler methods of mechanical ventilation and the use of lower tidal volumes.**[32]

Neurologic Sequelae in Neonates with Chronic Lung Disease

Premature infants with chronic lung disease are at risk for adverse neurologic outcomes because of the exposure to hypoxic events and because of central nervous system immaturity. Together, these pathophysiologic processes may result in a number of impairments and put them at risk for having neurodevelopmental disabilities.[16,27,33] The smaller and more preterm the infant, the greater this risk is.

The two major types of brain injuries characteristic of premature infants are intraventricular hemorrhage (IVH) and periventricular leukomalacia (PVL). *Intraventricular hemorrhage* results from hemorrhaging into the delicate germinal matrix tissues—a fragile vascular bed seen in the developing brain. These delicate blood vessels are thought to be especially vulnerable to alterations in cerebral blood flow.[34] The incidence of IVH is greatest in infants of lower gestational age; however, regardless of gestational age, the greatest risk period for IVH is in the first 3 to 4 postnatal days. IVH is diagnosed using cranial ultrasonography and is classified from grade I through IV according to severity: Grade I is a germinal matrix bleed only and a grade IV signifies parenchymal involvement of the hemorrhage with accompanying ventricular enlargement.[34] Infants with the most severe IVH (grade IV) are at high risk for neurodevelopmental disabilities; however, recent data suggest that those with less severe involvement still may have learning difficulties.[35,36]

Periventricular leukomalacia is the major hypoxic brain injury seen in preterm infants and results in necrosis of the periventricular white matter. It generally occurs after the first week of life and is diagnosed using cranial ultrasonography. The evolution of PVL is of critical importance for its diagnostic and prognostic usefulness. The pathophysiologic mechanisms underlying this lesion continue to be investigated but are thought to be due to several factors. Traditionally it was thought that these lesions occurred in the arterial watershed zones due to the loss of cerebral autoregulation following an asphyxic event.[34] More recent evidence suggests that the white matter damage may be the result of systemic inflammatory responses in the absence of adequate neuroprotective factors.[34,37] Evidence also exists suggesting that the immature oligodendrocytes are metabolically vulnerable, thus making them susceptible to excitotoxicity.[37]

Persistent Pulmonary Hypertension and Meconium Aspiration Syndrome

As described earlier in the chapter, within the first few breaths, the vascular tone in the pulmonary circulation decreases, reducing the pressures on the right side of the heart. The foramen ovale closes functionally, followed within hours by functional closure of the ductus arteriosus; both of these structures undergo complete anatomic closure at a later time. Thus, normal postnatal circulation is established.

In PPH, pulmonary vasoconstriction occurs shortly after birth and results in extrapulmonary shunting of blood from the right to left side via the foramen ovale and/or ductus arteriosus. In addition to the increased pressures on the right side of the heart, the decreased flow through the lungs results in central hypoxemia and cyanosis that are not responsive to high concentrations of inspired oxygen. In the case of Joshua, his arterial blood gases remained abnormal in the presence of 100% oxygen, indicating that the inspired oxygen was not being picked up by the systemic circulation. The accepted clinical criteria for PPH are a PaO_2 of less than 70 torr in and FiO_2 of 1.0, absence of structural heart disease, and documented right to left shunting[38]; thus, it is essential to rule out congenital heart disease in an infant who is unresponsive to inspired oxygen.

Often associated with disorders of circulation or cord complications is meconium aspiration syndrome. MAS is defined by the presence of meconium below the vocal cords and occurs in up to 20% to 30% of infants with meconium stained amniotic fluid.[39] The development of the syndrome is thought to be due to airway obstruction, chemical injury to the respiratory epithelium, and a secondary surfactant deficiency due to its inactivation by the meconium.[40-42] In approximately 7% to 20% of all deliveries, meconium is passed in the amniotic fluid.[39,42] This phenomenon is rare before 34 weeks of age, and the risk of occurrence increases in relation to advanced gestation, with the greatest risk beyond 37 weeks' gestational age.

Infants born through meconium-stained fluid face a 100-fold risk of developing respiratory distress compared to infants born through clear amniotic fluid. The risks of morbidity and mortality also differ with respect to the timing and the quality of the meconium. Typically, the consistency of meconium is described as being thick or thin. The presence of meconium at the onset of labor indicates that some event occurred prenatally; meconium that is present during labor is indicative of a more acute event. There is a five- to seven fold increased risk of death when thick meconium is present at the onset of labor.

A strong association exists between MAS and PPH for reasons that are not completely understood. Whether and to what extent the aspiration occurs in utero as opposed to during delivery has not been resolved. Furthermore, there are debates as to whether MAS represents chronic hypoxia *in utero* or whether the aspiration sets up a sequence of events that directly result in acute distress. If the infant has suffered *in utero* hypoxia and hypercapnia, they are more likely to develop PPH. As well, both of those conditions can stimulate fetal gasping and meconium passage, in which case the aspiration occurs before the birthing process. In these infants, there is a greater likelihood of having more serious and long-term respiratory and neurologic complications.[39]

Early management of the infant with PPH and MAS is focused on clearance of the meconium from the pharynx, trachea,

and stomach, after which treatment is directed toward management of the acute distress. Strategies are typically directed at mechanical ventilation, circulatory support, and pulmonary arteriole vasodilation. The repertoire of treatment for PPH includes conventional therapies such as mechanical ventilation (to produce hyperoxia and hypocapnia), sedation, paralysis, alkali infusion, intravascular volume support, and normalization of serum electrolytes and glucose.[38,43,44] Despite often aggressive management of babies with PPH, the diagnosis was associated with high rates of mortality prior to the development and use of extracorporeal membranous oxygenation (ECMO) in the mid-1980s.[45] Currently ECMO is used as a rescue therapy of last resort in infants with PPH[38,46] (see Fig. 21-3). In addition, more recent treatment strategies that are widely available include inhaled nitric oxide, high-frequency mechanical ventilation, and exogenous surfactant administration.[47]

Inhaled nitric oxide is the newest of the aforementioned therapies and has been the subject of several clinical trials, because it was found to be a potent selective pulmonary vasodilator in both animals and patients with pulmonary hypertension. Prior to this, it had been difficult to obtain pulmonary vasodilation without widespread systemic hypotension.[48] To date, clinical trials have demonstrated its efficacy in improving oxygenation and reducing the need for ECMO in babies with PPH.[46] However, the optimal dose and timing of administration have yet to be agreed on, and it is not overwhelmingly clear whether the clinical improvements are always sustained long enough to reduce overall mortality.[18] Recent studies have shown that the effects of inhaled NO are enhanced when used in conjunction with high-frequency oscillatory ventilation (HFOV).[19,38,46]

Although PPH is a transient condition, it can have devastating consequences and long-term effects if the lung tissue is injured or if there is brain injury from the postnatal asphyxia. If severe enough, the result could be *hypoxic-ischemic encephalopathy* (HIE). Through various mechanisms, the

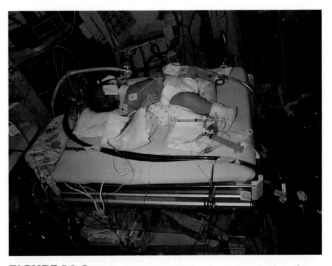

FIGURE 21-3 Infant in neonatal intensive care unit. Note the presence of the extracorporeal membranous oxygenation (ECMO) system.

brain undergoes metabolic and vascular changes in response to the oxygen deprivation and decreased perfusion. Tissue damage may also result from the excitotoxic cascade (due to extracellular glutamate accumulation) and the release of oxygen-free radicals. Whereas all regions of the brain are susceptible, the watershed regions of the cerebral vasculature are particularly vulnerable to the hypoxia-ischemia. Differential patterns of lesions occur in preterm (see previous discussion of PVL) and full-term infants due to the location of these watershed zones. In the full-term infant, these regions are at the base of the cortical sulci. As well, these babies also seem to be vulnerable to deep gray matter injury, which is associated with a poor outcome.[49]

Summary of Risk Factors

Despite the significant advances in the care of medically fragile preterm and full-term infants, these babies, like Sara and Joshua, still face an increased risk of neurologic and/or developmental impairments and disability. Regardless of the diagnosis, these infants typically experience a prolonged period of hospitalization, have limited endurance secondary to cardiopulmonary compromise, and are often constrained with technical support—all of which limit their opportunities for movement. Essentially these babies are products of a deprived environment in which the opportunities for experience and action are quite limited. Not only does this impact their motoric competencies, but also it severely limits their ability to attach meaning and relevance to their environment, a critical feature of early sensorimotor development. The result of such deprivation may lead to a documented developmental delay for reasons that may not necessarily be explained by an organic or pathophysiologic mechanism; however, for many there are known neurologic impairments associated with their primary pathology. For these reasons, physical therapy management of these patients should ideally focus on the infant's medical *as well as* on the developmental goals.

THRESHOLD BEHAVIORS

At this point, there is a lack of identified threshold behaviors shown to be useful predictors of physical therapy outcomes with this patient group. Patients who fall into Practice Pattern G are distinguished from those in other cardiopulmonary practice patterns essentially by virtue of their age. In this pattern, the patients are neonates—which, by formal definition is an infant who is 0 to 4 weeks of age—although the practice pattern extends the age group to 4 months. By virtue of their immaturity, these patients have unique characteristics that make them especially vulnerable to failure of the respiratory pump and to impaired gas exchange. As a group, infants who are high risk and medically fragile are overrepresented in the population of children who end up having neurodevelopmental impairments and disabilities. Thus, in a best-practice setting, physical therapy management would include strategies to address the acute medical issues as well as strategies to address

the neurodevelopmental consequences that the infant *is* or *may be* at risk for.

The most widely accepted framework for working with these vulnerable infants utilizes an individualized approach to care.[12,50,51] By observing each infant's behavioral and physiologic responses to interaction, an individualized care plan incorporates knowledge of the infant's stressors and thus limits unnecessary stimulation. This approach to care of infants in the NICU has been shown to have a number of positive effects such as a lower incidence of intraventricular bleeds, less severe chronic lung disease (less time on the ventilator, decreased need for supplemental oxygen), faster weight gain, and shorter hospital stays.[14,15] What is not known, however, are those critical behaviors or measures that can be of predictive or of prognostic value to physical therapy outcomes. Most would agree that there is paucity of such research and of studies that meet the rigorous criteria of best evidence.

LIMITS OF OUR KNOWLEDGE

It is well known that the human is capable of growth, repair, and regeneration in a number of systems. The last stage of lung development, for example, continues well into childhood. **Over 90% of the alveoli develop postnatally. For infants with chronic lung disease, this allows much of their growth and healing to occur with potentially new and healthier lung tissue.** In the central nervous system, there are also developmental changes in neuronal structure and function that occur postnatally. Recently there has been evidence from several studies demonstrating neuronal and functional plasticity in the central nervous system following damage.

These are but a few examples which highlight the capabilities of the human body. Our limits, as a profession, lie in our ability to exploit these "windows of opportunity" that exist and to better define how we can impact recovery and prevent secondary problems. Although there has been research examining different issues with respect to physical therapy evaluation and/or intervention with high-risk infants, to date, there is not strong evidence of its effectiveness in reducing or ameliorating the adverse pulmonary or neurodevelopmental impairments often seen in high-risk infants. The environment is ripe for our profession to lead the way in asking and answering the critical questions regarding the efficacy of our interventions.

In this group of patients, we have a unique opportunity to impact on their development almost from the beginning. The critical question though is, "Do we?" Does physical therapy intervention with neonates improve their cardiopulmonary status? Does a developmentally appropriate, functional movement program increase their "exercise" tolerance? What are the parameters for exercise training in a neonate? What is the cost–benefit ratio of exercise in an infant with chronic lung disease? What are the long-term effects of early intervention? How "early" is too early? The answers to these, and many other questions, are long overdue. Our challenge now and in the future will be to better define our roles and the expected outcomes in our care of high-risk neonates.

TABLE 21-12   The Nagi Model Applied to Respiratory Failure in the Neonate

Primary Pathology	Secondary Pathologies	Impairments	Functional Limitations	Disability
Bronchopulmonary dysplasia	Parenchymal damage to lung tissue	Decreased lung compliance Increased work of breathing	Decreased endurance for motor activity, social interaction, and feeding	Negative reinforcement during interaction with parents (affects parental bonding)
	Atelectasis	Decreased ventilation	Poor physiologic stability and behavioral organization	Failure to thrive
	Airway inflammation	Increased resistance to airflow; airway obstruction		
	Disrupted lung growth/ alveolarization			
	Intraventricular bleed bilaterally	Motor abnormalities	Delayed motor skill acquisition Paucity of movement	Behavioral instability
		Decreased strength	Disorganized movement patterns	Developmental delay
			Poor postural control	
			Decreased oral motor coordination	
Persistent pulmonary hypertension with MAS	Pulmonary vasoconstriction	L→R shunting Pulmonary hypertension	Decreased endurance for motor activity, social interaction, and feeding	Negative reinforcement during interaction with parents (affects parental bonding)
	Aspiration of meconium	Hypoxemia Cyanosis Tachycardia Increased respiratory effort Respiratory distress	Poor physiologic stability Poor feeding tolerance	Failure to thrive
	Airway inflammation	Increased resistance to airflow; airway obstruction		Developmental delay
	Hypoxic–ischemic insult	CNS depression Motor abnormalities Seizures Hypotonia	Decreased alertness Delayed motor skill acquisition Paucity of movement Disorganized movement patterns Poor postural control Decreased oral motor coordination	

NAGI MODEL

The disablement associated with respiratory failure in the neonate is outlined in Table 21-12. The two primary pathologies under which secondary pathologies, impairments, functional limitations, and disabilities fall are bronchopulmonary dysplasia and persistent pulmonary hypertension with meconium aspiration syndrome. Note that, even as a neonate, this child may be destined to develop disabilities related to parental bonding and developmental delays. Aggressive, early physical therapy interventions aimed at correcting impairments and functional limitations will hopefully minimize disabilities of the neonate in respiratory failure.

REFERENCES

1. American Physical Therapy Association. Guide to Physical Therapist Practice. 2nd ed. *Phys Ther.* 2001 Jan;81(1):9-746.
2. Moore KL, Persaud TVN. *The Developing Human: Clinically Oriented Embyrology.* Philadelphia, PA: WB Saunders; 1998.
3. Gluckman PD, Harding JE. Fetal growth retardation: underlying endocrine mechanisms and postnatal consequences. *Acta Paediatrica Suppl.* 1997;422:69-72.
4. Lee K, Khoshnood B, Wall SN, et al. Trend in mortality from respiratory distress syndrome in the United States, 1970–1995. *J Pediatr.* 1999;134:434-440.
5. Gluckman PD, Sizonenko SV, Bassett NS. The transition from fetus to neonate—an endocrine perspective. *Acta Pediatr Suppl.* 1999;428:7-11.

6. Apgar V. Proposal for a new method of evaluation of newborn infants. *Curr Res Anesth Analg.* 1953;32:260-267.

7. Kotecha S. Lung growth: implications for the newborn infant. *Arch Dis Child Fetal Neonat Ed.* 2000;82(1):F69-F74.

8. Crane LD. Physical therapy for the neonate with respiratory disease. In: Irwin S, Tecklin JS, eds. *Cardiopulmonary Physical Therapy.* St Louis, MO: Mosby; 1995:486-515.

9. Oberwaldner B. Physiotherapy for airway clearance in paediatrics. *Eur Respir J.* 2000;15:196-204.

10. Kornecki A, Frndova H, Coates AL, Shemie SD. A randomized trial of prolonged positioning in children with acute respiratory failure. *Chest.* 2001;119(1):211-218.

11. Sweeney JK, Heriza CB, Reilly MA, et al. Practice guidelines for the physical therapist in the neonatal intensive care unit. *Pediatr Phys Ther.* 1999;11:119-132.

12. Als H. A synactive model of neonatal behavioral organization: framework for the assessment of neurobehavioral development in the premature infant and for support of infants and parents in the neonatal intensive care environment. *Phys Occupat Ther Pediatr.* 1986;6(3/4):3-54.

13. Sweeney JK. Physiologic adaptation of neonates to neurologic assessment. *Phys Occupat Ther Pediatr.* 1986;6:155-169.

14. Als H, Lawhon G, Duffy FH, et al. Individualized developmental care for the very low birthweight preterm infant: medical and neurofunctional effects. *JAMA.* 1994;272:853-858.

15. Als H, Lawhon G, Brown E, et al. Individualized behavioral and environmental care for the very low birth weight preterm infant at risk for bronchopulmonary dysplasia: neonatal intensive care unit and developmental outcome. *Pediatrics.* 1986;76:1123-1132.

16. Campbell SK. The infant at risk for developmental disability. In: Campbell SK, ed. *Decision Making in Pediatric Neurologic Physical Therapy.* New York: Churchill Livingstone; 1999:260-332.

17. Einspieler C, Prechtl HFR, Ferrari F, et al. The qualitative asessment of general movements in preterm, term and young infants-review of the methodology. *Early Hum Dev.* 1997;50(1): 47-60.

18. Cheifetz IM. Inhaled nitric oxide: plenty of data, no consensus. *Crit Care Med.* 2000;28(3):902-903.

19. Kinsella JP, Abman SH. Clinical approach to inhaled nitric oxide therapy in the newborn with hypoxemia. *J Pediatr.* 2000;136(6): 717-726.

20. Watchko JF, Mayock DE, Standaert TA, Woodrum DE. The ventilatory pump: neonatal and developmental issues. *Adv Pediatr.* 1991;38:109-134.

21. Bureau MA, Begin R. Chest wall diseases and dysfunction in children. In: Kendig EL, Chernick V, eds. *Disorders of the Respiratory Tract in Children.* Philadelphia, PA: WB Saunders; 1983: 601-616.

22. Pagtakhan RD, Chernick V. Intensive care for respiratory disorders. In: Kendig EL, Chernick V, eds. *Disorders of the Respiratory Tract in Children.* 4th ed. Philadelphia, PA: WB Saunders; 1983:145-168.

23. Make BJ, Hill NS, Goldberg AI, et al. Mechanical ventilation beyond the intensive care unit: report of a Consensus Conference of the American College of Chest Physicians. *Chest.* 1998;113(5):289S-344S.

24. Halliday HL, Ehrenkranz RA. Early (<96 hours) postnatal corticosteroids for preventing chronic lung disease in preterm infants. *Cochrane Database Syst Rev.* 2000;(2):CD001146. http://www.ncbi.nlm.nih.gov/pubmed/10796252?itool= EntrezSystem2.PEntrez.Pubmed.Pubmed_ResultsPanel.Pubmed _RVDocSum&ordinalpos=11. Accessed January 1, 2010.

25. Rennie JM, Bokhari SA. Recent advances in neonatology. *Arch Dis Child.* 1999;81(1):1F-4F.

26. Gortner L, Wauer RR, Hammer H, et al. Early versus late surfactant treatment in preterm infants of 27 to 32 weeks' gestational age: a multicenter controlled clinical trail. *Am Acad Pediatr.* 1998;102:1153-1160.

27. Bancalari E. Changes in the pathogenesis and prevention of chronic lung disease of prematurity. *Am J Perinatol.* 2001;18:1-9.

28. Northway WH Jr, Rosan RC, Porter DY. Pulmonary disease following respirator therapy of hyaline-membrane disease. Bronchopulmonary dysplasia. *N Engl J Med.* 1967;276:357-368.

29. Jobe AH, Bancalari E. Bronchopulmonary dysplasia. *Am J Respir Crit Care Med.* 2001;163:1723-1729.

30. Eber E, Zach MS. Long term sequelae of bronchopulmonary dysplasia (chronic lung disease of infancy). *Thorax.* 2001;56:317-323.

31. Husain NA, Siddiqui NH, Stocker JR. Pathology of arrested acinar development in postsurfactant bronchopulmonary dysplasia. *Hum Pathol.* 1998;29:710-717.

32. Thome UH, Carlo WA. High frequency ventilation in neonates. *Am J Perinatol.* 2000;17(1):1-9.

33. Bregman J, Farrell EE. Neurodevelopmental outcome in infants with bronchopulmonary dysplasia. *Clin Perinatol.* 1992;19(3): 673-694.

34. Ment LR, Schneider KC, Ainley MA, Allan WC. Adaptive mechanisms of the developing brain. *Clin Perinatol.* 2000;27(2):303-323.

35. Ment LR, Vohr B, Allan W, et al. Outcome of children in the indomethacin intraventricular hemorrhage prevention trial. *Am Acad Pediatr.* 2000;105:485-491.

36. Whitaker AH, Feldman JF, Van Rossem R, Schonfeld IS, et al. Neonatal cranial ultrasound abnormalities in low birth weight infants: relation to cognitive outcomes at six years of age. *Pediatrics.* 1996;98(1):719-729.

37. Dammann O, Leviton A. Brain damage in preterm newborns: biological response modification as a strategy to reduce disabilities. *J Pediatr.* 2000;136(4):433-438.

38. Gross I. Recent advances in respiratory care of the term neonate. *Ann NY Acad Sci.* 2000;900:151-158.

39. Klingner MC, Kruse J. Meconium aspiration syndrome: pathophysiology and prevention. *J Am Board Fam Pract.* 1999;12(6): 450-466.

40. Meydanli MM, Dilbaz B, Caliskan S, Dilbaz AH. Risk factors for meconium aspiration syndrome in infants born through thick meconium. *Int J Gynaecol Obstet.* 2001 Jan;72(1):9-15.

41. Lotze A, Mitchell BR, Bulas DI, et al. Multicenter study of surfactant (beractant) use in the treatment of term infants with severe respiratory failure. *J Pediatr.* 1998;132(1):40-47.

42. Soll RF, Dargaville P. Surfactant for meconium aspiration syndrome in full term infants. *Cochrane Database System Rev.* 2000;4.

43. Paz Y, Solt I, Zimmer EZ. Variables associated with meconium aspiration syndrome in labors with thick meconium. *Eur J Obstetr Gynecol Reproduct Biol.* 2000;94:27-30.

44. Walsh-Sukys MC, Tyson JE, Wright LL, et al. Persistent pulmonary hypertension of the newborn in the era before nitric oxide: practice variation and outcome. *Pediatrics.* 2000;105(1): 14-20.

45. Hintz SR, Suttner DM, Sheehan AM, et al. Decreased use of neonatal ECMO: how new treatment modalities have affected ECMO utilization. *Pediatrics.* 2000;106(6):1339-1343.

46. Lemons JA, Blackmon LR, Kanto WP, et al. Use of inhaled nitric oxide. *Pediatrics.* 2000;106(2):344.

47. Christou H, Van Marter LJ, Wessel DL, et al. Inhaled nitric oxide reduces the need for extracorporeal membrane oxygenation in infants with persistent pulmonary hypertension of the newborn. *Crit Care Med.* 2000;28(11): 3722-3727.

48. Cornfield DN, Maynard RC, deRegnier RA, Guiang SF, et al. Randomized, controlled trial of low-dose inhaled nitric oxide in the treatment of term and near-term infants with respiratory failure and pulmonary hypertension. *Pediatrics.* 1999;104(5): 1089-1094.

49. Roland EH, Poskitt K, Rodriguez E, et al. Perinatal hypoxicischemic thalamic injury: clinical features and neuroimaging. *Ann Neurol.* 1998;44:161.

50. Als H, Lester BM, Tronick EZ, Brazelton TB. Toward a research instrument for the assessment of preterm infant's behavior (APIB). In: Fitzgerald HE, Lester BM, Yogman, eds. *Theory and Research in Behavioral Pediatrics.* New York : Plenum; 1982:63-65.

51. Lotas MJ, Walden M. Individualized developmental care for very low birth weight infants: a critical review. *JOGNN.* 1996;25: 681-687.

C H A P T E R   21

An International Perspective: Colombia— Physical Therapy Practice in Neonates from the Colombian Perspective

Adriana Yolanda Campos, Maria Fernanda Guzman, Edgar Debray Hernandez, & Gloria Amalfi Luna

Physical therapy in Colombia is considered a liberal arts profession within the area of human health. University training is required with emphasis on patient care in relation to his/her family and the community in which they develop. The objective of physical therapy practice is the study, understanding, and management of human physical movement—considered an essential element that contributes to optimun health. Physical therapy in Colombia is directed toward the maintenance and optimization of movement as well as prevention of, and recovery from, accidental injury. The habilitation and rehabilitation of patients is included with the purpose of optimizing the quality of life and of contributing to the social development of individuals. The foundation of physical therapy practice is knowledge of biological, social, and humanistic sciences, which are used to advance the profession's own theories and technologies (Law 528 of 1999).

Colombian physical therapists receive training in the conduction of scientific research and in strategies related to health and kinetic well-being. Physical therapists are also trained in health care policy and management, and in academic endeavors.

Presently, there are 26 physical therapy programs offering pregraduation university training in Colombia. In addition, there are six specialization programs in physical therapy— four of them related to the cardiopulmonary field.

In Colombia, provision of physiotherapy services to the neonate population is based on an integrated process recognizing normal human body motions called HBM. This approach requires measurements and assessments that are individuated to the patient. The results of these assessments can be used to categorize the neonate based on the complexity of their non-systemic interactions. Intervention strategies can then be implemented which will facilitate proper neonatal development. Appropriate interventions usually include motor activities, which are graduated from lowest to highest complexity. Those at the lowest level include activities designed to enhance force development, flexibility, speed, and cardiovascular endurance. The next level is perceptive motor activities, which include coordination. Coordination is subdivided into issues of equilibrium, perception, kinetics, and perceptions of time and space. Finally, resultant activities are at the highest level of complexity and include skills that require speed and agility.

A properly planned and executed physiotherapy assessment establishes the extent of involvement of the neonate while under stress and provides information on the real or possible impact that such findings may have on the future development of normal MCH.

At the Corporacion Universitaria Iberoamericana in Bogota, our neonatal assessment has three components: the anatomical status, the physiological status, and the motor status. The anatomical status is dependent on the biotype of morphological features of the neonate—its size, weight, cephalic and thoracic measurements, facial symmetry, skin condition (eg, vernix, color nails, lanugo), and gestational age.[1,2] The physiological status includes assessment of the current and potential capacity of the cardiovascular and pulmonary systems, both at rest and under stress. These tests include measurements of oxygen consumption, the anaerobic threshold, and the aerobic functional capacity. The motor status is understood to mean the set of attributes that are relevant to age-appropriate MCH and that are not necessarily dependent on the cardiovascular system. The purpose of such measurements is to determine the extent of neurophysiologic maturity of the neonate and his or her adaptability to the environment. Such adaptability is particularly important for the neonate, as it passes from a wet, warm, and dark environment to one that is cold, luminous, and noisy. It is this dramatic change that forces the newborn to develop adaptive psychophysiological responses as it struggles for survival.

At our institution, the physiotherapist would begin the plan of care with a thorough review of the clinical record in order to identify factors that may influence neonatal development. The therapist selects and applies appropriate tests that are then used to determine the maturity of sensory receptors and motor pathways.

- *Sensory organs.* It must be emphasized that high-risk neonates do not show sufficient neuroanatomic development and maturity for optimal kinetic function. It is essential that the physiotherapist establish the functionality of these elements, especially because they are the fundamental pillars upon which human kinetic diversity is built.
- *Motor activity.* This includes both involuntary and voluntary activity. Involuntary motor activity involves assessment of muscle tone and reflex development. Voluntary activity refers to the ability of the neonate to initiate spontaneous movement. It is particularly important to note the neonate's posture as a reflection of possible injury to the neuromuscular system.

Deterioration of functional aerobic capacity is one of the most common problems observed in neonates, particularly in preterm neonates. These individuals are particularly susceptible to functional aerobic impairments because of the lack of maturity of the cardiovascular and pulmonary systems, which render them maladaptive to a hostile and constantly changing environment. Cardiac pathologies observed among neonates in Columbia include cardiac pump dysfunction and failure. Pulmonary pathologies include both restrictive (eg, hyaline membrane disease) and obstructive phenomena (eg, bronchopulmonary dysplasia).

Identification of deficiencies in the cardiovascular and pulmonary systems allows the physiotherapist to link these systems to physical motor quality. This is accomplished by filling in data to the following assessment categories:

- Gas exchange, assessed through indexes of oxygenation (eg, PaO_2, SaO_2, PaO_2/FiO_2, shunt, interalia) and indexes of ventilation ($PaCO_2$, $PetCO_2$)
- Ventilation mechanics, assessed through calculations of distension of pulmonary parenchyma and/or thorax, strength

to flux in the airway, and the qualitative analysis (and if possible, the quantitative analysis) of respiratory load
- Hydroelectrolytic balance
- Acid–base balance
- Cardiac pump function, assessed through indirect inferences from calculations of preload, afterload, contractility, and chronotropy
- Tissue perfusion, assessed through clinical observation, or through the derivation of data from calculations of the a-$\dot{V}O_2$ difference and/or the rate of oxygen withdrawal
- Fluid input/consumption ratio

Using data obtained from tests and measures, and from direct observations of the neonate, the physiotherapist can determine a plan of care. The patient's current physical status will determine the appropriateness of interventions, goals, and therapeutic modes designed to enhance cardiovascular and pulmonary functions and promote kinetic development.

Therapeutic strategies that can improve and/or reverse pulmonary dysfunction range from position changes and oxygen supplementation to the use of ventilatory support (invasive or noninvasive) aimed at optimizing gaseous exchange and ventilation.

In Colombia, stimulation that is provided to the at-risk neonate usually takes the form of a set of interventions aimed at providing the neonate with experiences that stimulate body receptors from the time of birth in order to maximize kinetic potential. Thus, both sensory and motor stimuli are presented to the neonate during any given treatment session.[3]

Whether the stimuli are sensory or motor, the goal of treatment is to release motor responses. This approach provides the rationale for the use of tactile stimuli to release sucking or searching responses, the use of position changes to encourage physiological stability, and the stimulation of vestibular and kinetic receptors that will promote the development of basic motor patterns.[4]

REFERENCES

1. Cruz I. Guia del Manejo Fisioterapeutico Para la Atencion del Recien Nacido con Enfermedad de Membrana Hialina Grado II. 2000.
2. Manno R. *Fundamentos Del Entrenamiento Deportivo.* Barcelona, Spain: Paidotribo; 1994.
3. Correa A. *Recien Nacido Normal.* Medellin, Colombia: OID; 1997.
4. Diaz P. *Estimulacion Temprana.* Lidium: Buenos Aires; 1990.

Physical Therapy Associated with Lymphatic System Disorders

Kimberly D. Leaird

INTRODUCTION

This chapter will address lymphedema management and the evaluation and treatment of patients fitting the model of preferred Practice Pattern 6H: *Impaired Circulation and Anthropometric Dimensions Associated with Lymphatic System Disorders.*[1]

Knowledge of this practice pattern will enable therapists to effectively evaluate, differentiate between diagnoses, and provide appropriate intervention for patients with lymphatic system dysfunction.

This chapter provides a review of the anatomy and physiology of the lymphatic system, discussions of the stages of lymphedema, and evidence to refute and support current methods of treatment for lymphatic system disorders. It is imperative to have a basic understanding of the lymphatic system in order to deliver appropriate interventions.

PURPOSE OF THE LYMPHATIC SYSTEM

In addition to immune defense, the purpose of the lymphatic system is to drain substances that the venous blood circulation is unable to reabsorb. The lymphatic system functions like a "sweeper" to clear the interstitial space (also known as the third space or tissue space) of excess fluids, cellular debris, long-chain fatty acids (found only in the intestines), and protein molecules, otherwise known as the *lymphatic loads.*[2] There is a continual shift of fluids within the body at the microcirculatory level of the blood capillaries. It is the responsibility of the lymphatic system to facilitate the fluid movement from the tissues back into the bloodstream—to maintain a state of homeostasis. Under normal physiological conditions, this fluid management will "maintain blood volume and eliminate chemical imbalances in the interstitial fluid."[2-5]

OVERVIEW OF THE LYMPHATIC SYSTEM

Lymphatic vessels, lymph nodes, and other lymphoid organs and tissues comprise the lymphatic system. The lymph system represents an accessory route by which fluid can move from the tissue spaces into the blood. The lymph system protects the body by removing foreign material from the lymph fluid; that is, it filters lymph fluid and constantly surveys the body for the presence of foreign material. Lymph tissues contain macrophages, lymphocytes (T cells or B cells), plasma cells that produce antibodies, and reticular cells that form the lymphoid tissue stroma.[3,4]

The main organs of the lymph system are the lymph nodes, spleen, thymus, and tonsils. Lymph nodes appear in clusters or chains intermittently along lymphatic vessels, and their primary responsibility is to filter the lymph fluid. There are approximately 600 to 700 lymph nodes in an average-size person. A larger number of lymph nodes are strategically located in the cervical region (100–200) and in the mesentery (200). A fibrous capsule surrounds each lymph node that encloses the cortex and the medulla. The cortex of the lymph node contains mostly lymphocytes, which act in the immune response. The medulla contains macrophages, which engulf and destroy viruses, bacteria, and other foreign debris. Lymph moves quickly into the lymph node via afferent lymphatic vessels from the capsular side of the node and proceeds slowly through the chambered areas of the medulla. Lymph fluid leaves the nodes via the efferent lymphatic vessels from the hilus area of the node. There are more afferent vessels leading into the nodes than efferent vessels leaving the nodes. This causes lymph flow to almost stagnate in the lymph node, allowing time to cleanse the lymph fluid[2-4] (see Fig. 22-1).

The spleen provides a site for lymphocyte proliferation and immune function and destroys aged or defective red blood cells and blood-borne pathogens. The thymus is most functional during youth. Many of the thymus cells are inactive; however, some mature into T lymphocytes, which support immunity function. The tonsils and other lymph node aggregates known as *Peyer patches* (distributed throughout the mucous lining of the small intestines) function to prevent pathogens in the respiratory and digestive tracts from penetrating the mucous membrane lining.[4,6]

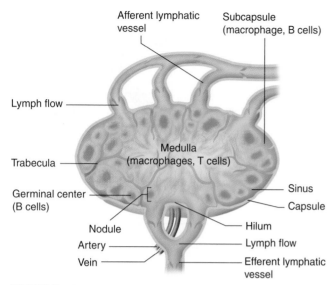

FIGURE 22-1   Lymph node. (Reprinted with permission from Shier D, Butler J, Lewis R. *Hole's Human Anatomy and Physiology*. 9th ed. Boston, MA: The McGraw-Hill Companies Inc; 2002.)

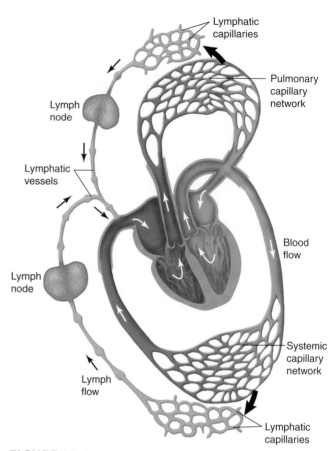

FIGURE 22-2   Schematic representation of lymphatic vessels transporting fluid from the interstitial spaces to the venous system. (Reprinted with permission from Shier D, Butler J, Lewis R. *Hole's Human Anatomy and Physiology*. 9th ed. Boston, MA: The McGraw-Hill Companies Inc; 2002.)

The lymphatic system is similar to the cardiovascular system in that it aids in the circulation of body fluids. The driving force behind the cardiovascular system is the heart muscle, which serves to propel the fluids. **However, there is no "central pump" for the lymphatic system.** Lymph return to the venous circulation occurs via the contraction of smooth muscles in the lymph collectors, the contraction of surrounding skeletal musculature, the pulsation of adjacent arteries and veins, and diaphragmatic breathing.[2–5]

The lymphatic system is not a closed system like the circulatory system, but a one-way system that starts in the interstitial spaces with initial lymph vessels (initial lymph capillaries) and ends in the venous part of the blood circulatory system. **One of the most important functions of the lymphatic system is its ability to remove proteins from the tissue spaces. Reabsorption of large, protein macromolecules will not occur at the blood capillaries.**[2–5] **The "removal of proteins from the interstitial spaces is an essential function, without which we would die in approximately 24 hours"**[4] (see Fig. 22-2).

ANATOMY OF THE LYMPHATIC SYSTEM

The lymphatic system is divided into the *superficial* and *deep* systems and separated by the fascia. There are many connections between the two systems; therefore, the transport of lymph occurs from distal to proximal and, in general, from superficial to deep. The purpose of the superficial lymphatic system is to drain the lymphatic loads of the skin: water, cells, and proteins. Fat is found only in the digestive system, cisterna chyli, and thoracic duct as a lymphatic load. The deep lymphatic system drains muscles, tendons, joints, inner organs, and so forth—everything but the skin. **Lymphedema presents more frequently in the superficial lymphatic system. The**

deep lymphatic system is often not involved because the fascia provides compression to resist swelling.[2–4]

Generally, there are no lymph vessels in areas without blood supply. The major exception to this is the central nervous system (CNS). Obviously, there is a blood supply to the brain and spinal cord, but there are no lymphatic vessels in the CNS to drain the lymphatic loads produced by the brain and spinal cord. There are no lymph vessels found in the nails, hair, dentin of the teeth, inside of the eyes, and bone tissue.[2–4]

Lymphatic Vessels

Lymphatic vessels are also referred to as *lymphatics*. The lymphatic vessels absorb interstitial fluid and return this fluid to the venous circulation. The lymphatics begin as *initial lymph vessels* and *initial lymph capillaries*. The initial lymph vessels represent the beginning of the one-way lymphatic system and begin "blindly" in the interstitium[2–4] (see Fig. 22-3).

Initial lymph capillaries are slightly larger than blood capillaries and are composed of a single layer of endothelial cells. Many of these cells do not connect end to end as with blood capillaries but actually *overlap* at their junction—with the potential to create large openings. The areas of overlap resemble a "swinging flap" and create the one-way opening for fluid—particularly

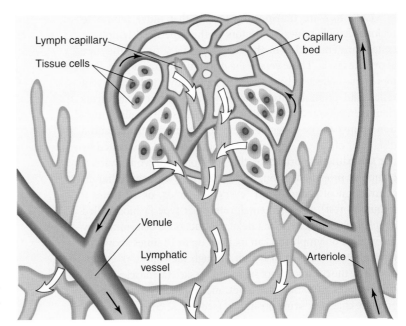

FIGURE 22-3 Initial lymph capillaries are microscopic, one-way vessels that begin "blindly" in the interstitial spaces. The black arrows indicate blood flow, and white arrows indicate lymph flow. (Reprinted with permission from Shier D, Butler J, Lewis R. *Hole's Human Anatomy and Physiology.* 9th ed. Boston, MA: The McGraw-Hill Companies Inc; 2002.)

large molecules like proteins and the other lymphatic loads—to enter the lymphatic system[2-4] (see Fig. 22-4).

Initial lymph capillaries of the skin are located just below the epidermis. These vessels are *valveless* and cover the entire body (excluding the previous areas identified that do not contain lymph vessels) to form a *plexus.* The lymph capillaries of the skin are responsible for draining an area 3 to 4 cm in circumference, which is called a *lymphatic area.* On the palms and soles of the feet, the lymphatic area is 1.5 to 2 cm in circumference.[2,7]

Endothelial cells that compose the initial lymph vessel connect to the cells and tissues in the surrounding interstitial space via semielastic *anchoring filaments.* If water increases in the tissues, an increase in pressure in the interstitial spaces will occur. Under normal physiological conditions, the continued water increase will cause a pull on the anchoring filaments and cause the overlapping junction areas to open. Pressure in the initial lymph capillary is lower than that in the interstitial spaces. This will cause the larger molecules of the lymphatic loads to move into the initial lymph vessels. *Lymph formation* occurs when the fluid from the interstitial spaces (containing the lymphatic loads) enters the initial lymph vessels.[2-4]

Precollectors connect the initial lymph capillaries to the lymph collectors of the superficial lymphatic system and are characterized by underdeveloped valves and muscles. The most numerous types of precollectors in the superficial system are previously described—those that connect the superficial lymph capillaries and collectors. The remainder of the precollectors provides a direct connection between the superficial lymph capillaries and the deep lymph collectors. These are called *perforating precollectors*—they perforate the fascia and provide a direct connection between the superficial and deep lymphatic system. Perforating precollectors are found in larger numbers in the parasternal, paravertebral, and intercostals areas.[2,7]

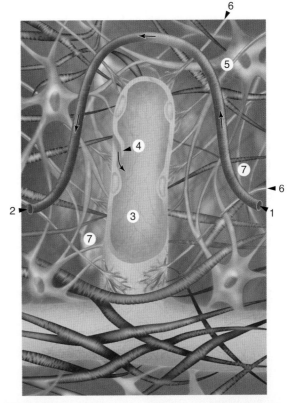

FIGURE 22-4 Initial lymph capillary in the interstitium. (1) Arterial blood capillary loop, (2) venous blood capillary loop, (3) lymph capillary, (4) opening between 2 lymph capillary endothelial cells: "swinging flap," (5) fibrocyte, (6) anchoring filament, (7) interstitial space. Small arrows indicate directional blood flow; large arrows indicate flow of interstitial fluid. (Reprinted with permission from Földi M, Kubik S. *Lehrbuch der Lymphologie.* 5th ed. Munich, Jena: Urban & Fischer; 2002. Copyright Urban & Fischer Verlag, Munich, Germany.)

Collectors are transporting vessels that move lymph to regional lymph nodes. Collectors of the superficial lymphatic system are embedded in the superficial fatty tissue; they are above the fascia. These vessels are distinguished from precollectors in that collectors have well-developed valves (which prevent reflux and promote directional flow) and distinct wall layers (intima, media, and adventitia). The *angion* is the smallest functioning unit of the collector located between a proximal and a distal pair of valves. Angions are smooth muscles innervated by the sympathetic portion of the autonomic nervous system. Lymph is propelled through the collectors with the inherent contraction of each angion (every 6 seconds, or 10 times a minute at rest) in a segmental, caterpillar-type fashion called *lymphangiomotoricity*. The rate of contraction is determined by the volume of lymph and can increase up to 10 times above the resting rate. Transport of lymph through the collectors is supported by the contraction of surrounding skeletal muscles, external pressures, pulsation of arteries, and respiratory and thoracic pressure changes during breathing[2] (see Fig. 22-5).

The lymph moves into the deep system and into larger collecting vessels called *lymphatic trunks*. Lymph from the upper extremities moves through collectors, to the regional lymph nodes (axillary lymph nodes), into their respective trunks, then into the left or right venous angle. From the lower extremities, lymph moves into the inguinal lymph nodes, pelvic nodes, and lumbar lymph nodes and then into their respective trunks. The *left and right lumbar trunks* converge from the lower extremities with the *gastrointestinal trunk* (long-chain fatty acids return to the venous system here), which comes from the intestines. These three trunks converge to form the *cisterna chyli* at the T12 through L2 levels. The thoracic duct originates at the cisterna chyli and runs anterior to the vertebrae, continues slightly left of the vertebrae (at the T7 level), and returns lymph to the venous circulation at the left venous angle. The junction of the internal jugular and subclavian veins forms the venous angles on both the right and left sides of the body. The venous pressure is lower at the

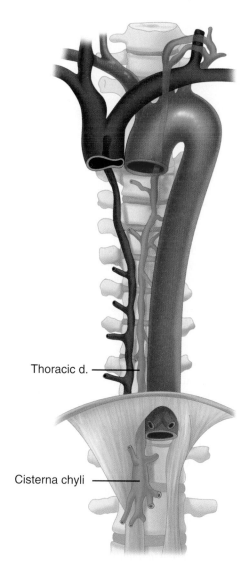

Thoracic d.

Cisterna chyli

FIGURE 22-6   Overview of thoracic duct and surrounding vessels. (1) left lumbar trunk; (2) right lumbar trunk; (3) cisterna chyli; (4) thoracic duct; (5) cervical part of thoracic duct; (6) esophagus; (7) trachea; (8) left venous angle; (9) right venous angle; (10) aorta; (11) azygos vein; (12) hemiazygos vein; (13) diaphram (a) medial portion, (b) Intermediate portion, (c) lateral portion; (14) right lymphatic duct; (15) superficial cervical artery. (Reproduced, with permission, from Brunicardi FC, Andersen DK, Billiar TR, et al. Schwartz's Principles of Surgery. 9th ed. New York: McGraw-Hill, 2010, Fig. 19-49.)

venous angles to allow for the return of lymph to the venous circulation. In a 24-hour period, 2 to 4 L of lymph is returned to the left venous angle by the thoracic duct, and approximately 300 mL (a 12-oz soda can) returns to the right venous angle[2,5] (see Figs. 22-6 through 22-9).

MICROCIRCULATION AND THE LYMPHATIC SYSTEM

The transfer of nutrients to tissues and the removal of cellular waste products occur at the blood capillary level. The blood

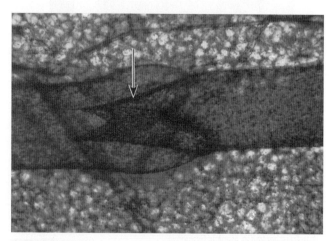

FIGURE 22-5   Light micrograph of valve in lymph collector (25×). (Reprinted with permission from Shier D, Butler J, Lewis R. *Hole's Human Anatomy and Physiology.* 9th ed. Boston, MA: The McGraw-Hill Companies, Inc.; 2002.)

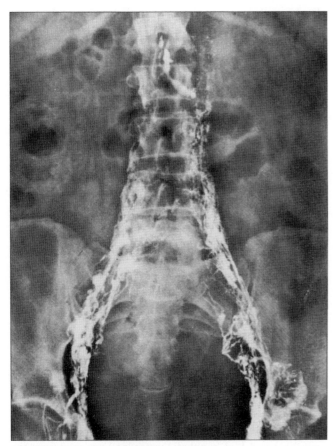

FIGURE 22-7 Lymphangiogram (radiograph) of the lymphatic vessels and lymph nodes of the pelvic region. (Reprinted with permission from Shier D, Butler J, Lewis R. *Hole's Human Anatomy and Physiology.* 9th ed. Boston, MA: The McGraw-Hill Companies, Inc.; 2002.)

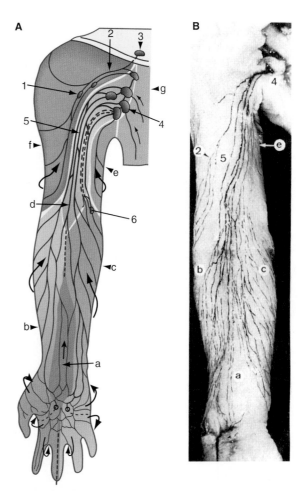

FIGURE 22-8 Schematic overview of lymphatic territories and watersheds of the upper extremity. (**A**) Schematic drawing. (a) Medial forearm territory with lymph vessels. (b) Radial forearm territory with lymph vessels. (c) Ulnar forearm territory with lymph vessels. (d) Medial upper arm territory with lymph vessels. (e) Dorsomedial upper arm territory with lymph vessels. (f) Lateral upper arm and shoulder territory with lymph vessels. (g) Right upper quadrant territory (anterior). (**B**) Cadaveric model. (1) Lymph nodes in deltopectoral groove. (2) Lymph vessels of upper arm territory (short type). (3) Supraclavicular lymph nodes. (4) Axillary lymph nodes. (5) Medial upper arm territory. (6) Anticubital lymph nodes. (Reprinted with permission from Földi M, Kubik S. *Lehrbuch der Lymphologie.* 5th ed. Munich, Jena: Urban & Fischer; 2002. Copyright Urban & Fischer Verlag, Munich, Germany.)

capillaries are located between the arterial (high-pressure) and venous (low-pressure) systems and are formed by a single layer of endothelial cells that are highly permeable to small molecules.[2,4,8]

The transfer of nutrients and gases and reuptake of waste products occur at the blood capillary level via a process called *diffusion*. Diffusion is the one-way movement of particles from a higher to a lower concentration. The hydrostatic pressure and colloid osmotic pressure (oncotic pressure) assist the diffusion process at the blood capillaries. In most areas of the body, the normal *diffusion distance* between the cells and the interstitial tissues is 1/10 mm. With a mere 1-cm increase in edema, the normal diffusion distance is increased by 100 times.[2,8]

Filtration occurs primarily at the arterial end of the blood capillaries. The driving force behind filtration is hydrostatic pressure, which normally measures 29 mm Hg. The colloid osmotic pressure at the arterial end measures 20 mm Hg. The hydrostatic pressure acts to push water and other nutrients from the arterial end of the blood capillaries and into the tissue spaces.[2,4,8]

Reabsorption occurs primarily at the venous end of the blood capillaries. The colloid osmotic force of the plasma proteins (20 mm Hg) will overcome the hydrostatic pressure

exerted at the venous end (14 mm Hg) to cause reuptake of waste products and water into the venous blood capillaries. These pressures were first measured by Dr. Ernest Starling and are known as Starling's law or Starling's equilibrium. For more detailed information on Starling's equilibrium, please refer to Chapter 16 of Guyton and Hall and to the Despopulos *Color Atlas of Physiology*.[2,4,8]

The number of blood capillaries in the human body would approximately cover the total surface area of a football field when placed end-to-end. Given this large surface area, and given that the average circulating blood volume is 4 to 6 L, there must be a mechanism to control the flow of blood into the capillaries.[4,8]

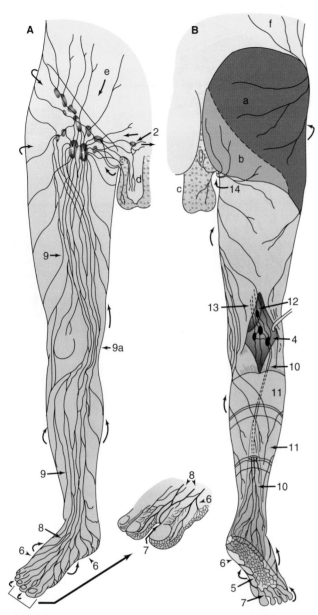

FIGURE 22-9   Schematic overview of lymphatic territories and watershed of the lower extremity. (1) Superficial inguinal lymph nodes; (2) prepubic lymph nodes; (3) lymph nodes of the penis; (4) popliteal lymph nodes; (5) plantar lymphatic plexus; (6) lymph vessels of medial sole of the foot; (7) interdigital lymph vessels; (8) lymph collectors on dorsum of foot; (9) ventromedial bundle (a) medial knee (bottleneck area); (10) dorsolateral bundle; (11) fascia; (12) adductor hiatus; (13) lymph vessels with femoral vein (deep); (14) gluteal-femoral sulcus (a) lymph vessels of gluteal area, (b) lymph vessels of gluteal area, (c) lymph vessels of the anus and scrotum, (d) lymph vessels of external genitalia, (e) lower anterior quadrant, (f) lower posterior quadrant. (Reprinted with permission from Földi M, Kubik S. *Lehrbuch der Lymphologie.* 5th ed. Munich, Jena: Urban & Fischer; 2002. Copyright Urban & Fischer Verlag, Munich Germany.)

The *precapillary sphincter* is a smooth muscle located in the precapillary arterioles. Contraction of the precapillary sphincter allows less blood into the capillaries. Less blood in the blood capillaries will register a lower blood capillary pressure (BCP). Dilation of the sphincter will increase the flow of

blood into the capillaries. The larger volume of blood in the capillaries will cause an increase in BCP. The higher BCP will ultimately lead to an increase in ultrafiltration. The amount of blood in the blood capillaries at any given time is due to the metabolic demand of the tissues.[2,4,8]

The Lymphatic Loads

Dr. Michael Földi coined the term *lymphatic loads* to describe the substances not reabsorbed by the venous system. The lymphatic loads include water, proteins, cells, and fat (in the digestive system). The following discussion will address each of the lymphatic loads and identify how each component becomes a lymphatic load.[2,7]

Water

Only a fraction of water becomes a lymphatic load. Water leaves the arterial end of the blood capillaries by filtration to supply the tissues with needed nutrients and water-soluble substances. Reabsorption returns water, solvents, lactic acid, and other cellular waste products to the venous circulation. **Only 80% to 90% of the water returns to the venous blood capillaries.** The 10% to 20% of water that remains in the interstitial spaces is termed the *net filtrate*. It is the responsibility of the lymphatic system to remove this 10% to 20%, which ultimately will become *part of the lymphatic load of water*. However, the total volume of the net filtrate equates much more than the 2 to 4 L of lymphatic water load returned from the interstitial space in a 24-hour period. The remaining filtrate is collected from the numerous blood capillaries at the lymph node level.[2,7]

Proteins

Blood is composed of roughly 52% to 62% of plasma and 38% to 48% of cells, which includes erythrocytes, leukocytes, and thrombocytes. There is approximately 3 L of plasma in an adult and 66 to 83 g/L of plasma proteins, which means there is approximately 200 g of protein molecules circulating in the plasma. Under normal physiological conditions, approximately half of the circulating proteins will leave the total blood capillary surface in 24 hours and go into the interstitial space for tissues repair, nourishment, and so forth. **It is the responsibility of the lymphatic system to remove these proteins from the interstitial spaces and return them to systemic circulation.** Proteins are macromolecules, and therefore physically too large to be reabsorbed at the venous blood capillaries.[2-4,7]

Cellular Components

All cells and macromolecular particles free in the interstitial space become a lymphatic load. Examples of these cells include cell fragments from hematomas, red and white blood cells, cancer cells, macrophages, pathogens (eg, silica dust, mites, or spores), either inhaled or ingested. All the aforementioned cells are macromolecules and the responsibility of the lymphatic system to return to the venous system.[2-4,7]

Long-Chained Fatty Acids

A large portion of the fat we ingest are *long-chained fatty acids* (LCFA), that is, composed of more than 16 carbon atoms. The LCFA enter the lymphatic system from the intestinal tract and are covered with a phospholipid coating to form a *chylomicron*. These chylomicrons are too large for reabsorption by the blood vessels of the small intestines and are absorbed by lymph vessels located in the intestines called *chylous vessels*.[2-4,7]

LYMPHEDEMA

Lymphedema is a high-protein edema that results from mechanical insufficiency of the lymphatic system. Lymphedema can occur anywhere in the body but occurs more frequently in the extremities. If left untreated, lymphedema can lead to significant pathological and clinical consequences for the patient.[2,5]

The *transport capacity* (TC) of the lymphatic system represents the maximum amount of lymph transported by the lymphatic system with the system working at its maximum frequency and amplitude. *Lymph time volume* (LTV) is the amount of lymph transported by the lymphatic system in a given unit of time. Normal values for LTV are 10% of the TC. The *lymphatic load* (LL) represents the normal amount of lymphatic load returning to the venous system in a 24-hour period, that is, 2 to 4 L[2] (see Table 22-1).

Under normal physiological conditions, the lymphatic system will respond to an increase in the LL with an increase in LTV. This is known as the *safety factor* or *safety valve function*. To increase LTV, the lymphatic system will increase the frequency and contraction of the collectors[2,7] (see Table 22-2).

Lymphatic System Insufficiencies

If the lymphatic system is healthy, the transport capacity is 10 times higher than the normal amount of LL (2–4 L). There is a built-in *functional reserve* (FR) to handle any increase in LL. In

TABLE 22-1   Normal Lymphatic System

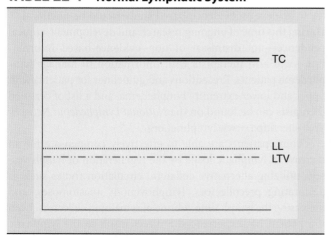

TABLE 22-2   Safety Factor or Safety Valve Function

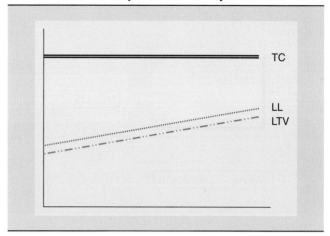

a high-volume or *dynamic insufficiency*, the LL exceeds the TC of the intact lymphatic system. *Edema* will result in this scenario and the edema can be protein rich (in response to the inflammatory response or traumatic edema) or low in protein in nature[2] (see Table 22-3).

A low-volume insufficiency or a *mechanical insufficiency* occurs when the TC drops below the normal amount of LL. Morphological and functional changes have occurred to the lymphatic system, which limits the ability to transport lymph fluid. The most common causes of a reduced TC are a surgical procedure involving the lymphatic system (eg, mastectomy with lymph node removal, prostectomy), radiation of lymph nodes, a congenital malformation of the lymphatic system, trauma, and chronic venous insufficiency. Once the TC is reduced, it can never be returned to its original levels—prior to disease. Swelling will result from a mechanical insufficiency, and this swelling is called *lymphedema*[2,5] (see Table 22-4).

Classifications of Lymphedema

Primary lymphedema results from a malformation or dysplasia of the lymphatic system that can be hereditary or congenital.

TABLE 22-3   Dynamic Insufficiency

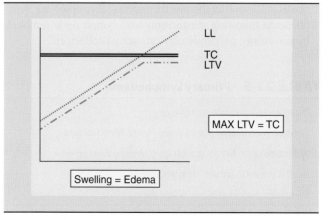

TABLE 22-4 Mechanical Insufficiency

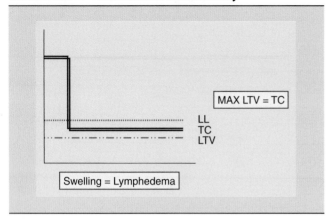

With primary lymphedema, development of the lymphatic vessels has been impaired. *Hypoplasia* is the most common type of dysplasia. Lymph vessels/collectors that are smaller than normal, or a lower number of lymph vessels in a given area, is characteristic of a hypoplasia. *Hyperplasia* means the lymph collectors are larger than normal, rendering their valves incompetent, and unable to transport lymph fluid effectively. An *aplasia* is the defective development or absence of lymph vessels in a given area. The most common area for an aplasia is the dorsum of the foot. *Inguinal node fibrosis* or *Kinmonth syndrome* is a dysplasia of the capsule and trabeculi area of the lymph nodes. Primary lymphedema can also be associated with *Klippel–Trenaunay syndrome*, which is a dysplasia of blood vessels, lymph vessels, and the skeletal system[2,5] (see Table 22-5).

Secondary lymphedema results from a known insult to the lymphatic system. Worldwide, secondary lymphedema is more common than primary lymphedema. Possible causes of secondary lymphedema include, in no particular order, the following:

- *Radiation therapy,* which can cause fibrosis to the involved tissues. Fibrosis in an area can reduce collateral circulation and inhibit the flow of lymph through tissues, for example, lymph nodes.[2,5]
- *Trauma* to a given area, which can reduce the TC below the normal level or LL, giving rise to early signs of lymphedema.[10]
- *Iatrogenic* lymphedema, which may result following diagnostic and/or therapeutic treatments. Examples are lymphedema following mastectomy with lymph node removal, hysterectomy, perpendicular cuts across collectors.[9]

TABLE 22-5 Primary Lymphedema[9]

More common in lower extremities
Symptoms occur after age 35 years—*lymphedema tardum*
Symptoms occur before age 35 years—*lymphedema praecox*
More common in females than in males
Symptoms present at birth—*Milroy disease*

- *Lymphatic filariasis,* which describes infection caused by filarial *Wuchereria bancrofti*. This nematode worm is transmitted by the bite of a mosquito and lives and grows in the lymphatic system—causing permanent damage. These infections are more common in subtropical and tropical regions of the world.[11]
- *Surgery* that directly involves the lymphatic system. There are numerous studies that support the fact that there is a high correlation between the degree of axillary node dissection and the degree of inguinal node dissection with higher incidences of developing lymphedema.[10,12–19]
- *Infection,* which will ultimately increase the lymphatic load by increasing blood flow and capillary permeability in the area, which creates a dynamic insufficiency and could precipitate lymphedema.[2,5]
- *Chronic venous insufficiency,* which can exacerbate or initiate the symptoms of lymphedema due to the chronic stress on the venous system.[2,5,11]
- *Benign or malignant tumors,* which can grow in the lymph vessels and clot/block the lymphatics. Tumors can also grow outside the lymphatics and cause damage to the vessels by blocking flow.[2,5,11]

Precipitating Factors for Lymphedema

Evidence-based research is slow in coming to the field of lymphedema management. At this time, researchers are unable to clearly identify who will develop lymphedema.[2,10,20] Because of this uncertainty, clinicians should work from a list of guidelines that suggest sensible and cautious practices to promote prevention.[2] Those clinicians not familiar with lymphedema, or those who do not understand its development due to the lack of evidence-based data, tend to prescribe rapid return to normal, daily activities. Rather, patients should take a gradual progression to the return of daily activities.[2]

In an article written for the *National Lymphedema Network* (NLN), Dr. Michael Földi addressed the concern of a lack of evidence-based research in the following statement: "There are cases in which anecdotal observations are in harmony with scientific fact and established knowledge. It is textbook knowledge that healthy elastic fibers are prerequisite for lymph formation and that sunshine can destroy those elastic fibers. To try to achieve an evidence-based study would be unethical."[10] During this time of ongoing research and development, clinical prudence—not dismissal of non–evidence-based information—will arm therapists with information to manage lymphedema patients. Precautions and guidelines for patients with upper and lower extremity lymphedema, and a list of certified therapists can be found on the *National Lymphedema Network* Web site: http://www.lymphnet.org.

Some patients are able to effectively compensate for an increase in lymphatic loads by the regeneration of lymph vessels, utilizing alternative collateral circulation routes such as perforating precollectors, lymphovenous anastomoses, and increasing the lymph time volume of remaining collectors. Even if a patient has experienced a direct insult to the lymphatic system via surgery or some primary cause (eg, hypoplasia), the patient may not exhibit signs or symptoms of lymphedema if the lymphatic system has found a way to compensate for an increase in lymphatic loads.[2,5,7]

There are certain "initiating factors" that can trigger lymphedema, or place a further stress on the already impaired transport capacity. The *change* in cabin pressure during an airline flight coupled with inactivity may trigger the onset of lymphedema. The reduced cabin pressure may allow more fluid into the tissue spaces as a result of decreased hydrostatic pressure. Inactivity allows for venous pooling, which will eventually cause an increase in pressure at the blood capillary level, therefore increasing ultrafiltration and the lymphatic loads. For a more in-depth review of how airline travel can affect patients with lymphedema, please refer to the "Taking Flight" article in the July 7, 2003 (Vol. 14, No. 15), *Advances for Physical Therapists and PT Assistants.*[2,21]

Any *fluctuation in weight gain and fluid volumes* such as pregnancy, congestive heart failure, or obesity can add further stress to an impaired lymphatic system. Medications that cause sudden fluctuation in body fluids can also be detrimental.[2]

Active hyperemia that results from local or systemic application causes an increase in blood flow, which ultimately will increase the lymphatic load of water, and stress a compromised lymphatic system. Examples of active hyperemia include local hot pack, massage, vigorous exercise, or infection to the limb at increased risk; hot tubs/saunas, hot weather and high humidity; and sprains/strains.[2–5]

With a *passive hyperemia*, swelling may result from "some other problem," for example, from chronic venous insufficiency (CVI) or hypoproteinemia (liver dysfunction). In CVI, the prolonged venous pooling affects venous return and eventually the blood capillary level. An increase in ultrafiltration will occur at the blood capillaries, and the lymphatic system will try to compensate with an increase in lymph time volume (as a safety factor). If the lymphatics are able to compensate, no edema will result.[2]

Hypoproteinemia results from a decreased colloid osmotic pressure (COP) of the plasma due to an increase in protein loss through the urine and the inability of the liver to produce adequate protein synthesis for the body's demands. The lymphatic system will increase the lymph time volume but may become overwhelmed. Edema will initially begin as the result of a high-volume or dynamic insufficiency. This edema will be systemic in nature and begin at the scrotum or eyelids.[2,5]

Stages of Lymphedema

Lymphedema is a progressive condition—There is no cure for lymphedema. If not managed, lymphedema will progress.[2]

Stage 0 (Prestage)

Anyone who has had surgery directly affecting the lymphatic system, but does not present with swelling, is considered to be in a prestage. The best example of this is a woman who has undergone a mastectomy, but does not develop lymphedema. She is considered to be in a prestage, because the surgery (mastectomy with lymph node removal and possibly radiation to the axillary nodes) decreases the transport capacity of the lymphatic system, yet the TC remains high enough to take care of the normal amount of lymphatic loads produced.[2,22]

There are two "subcategories" in a prestage: *lymph angiopathy* and *latency stage.* A decline in the TC due to a congenital malformation or dysplasia (as in primary lymphedema) of the lymphatic system is known as a lymph angiopathy. Any patient who has undergone surgery directly involving the lymphatic system, for example, mastectomy with lymph node removal, hysterectomy, or trauma directly involving the lymphatic system, is considered to be in a latency stage. Again, when a patient is in a prestage, **the TC remains high enough to take care of the normal amount of lymphatic load produced.** The onset of lymphedema correlates to the ability of the lymphatic system to compensate for any added stress to the system, or the frequency of the occurrences that may cause a dynamic insufficiency in the limb at high risk to develop lymphedema.[2]

Stage I (Reversible Lymphedema)

In stage I, it is possible for the swelling that typically presents at the end of the day to recede overnight. The involved extremity is soft, and pitting is easily induced. With proper management in stage I, it is possible for the patient to expect complete reduction of the involved limb (when compared to the normal limb).[2,7]

Stage II (Spontaneously Irreversible Lymphedema)

Progression from stage I to stage II is primarily identified by an increase in fibrotic tissue. Pitting is more difficult to induce and the patient is at a higher risk for frequent infections due to the increased diffusion distance, that is, the increased size of the limb.[2,7]

Stage III (Lymphostatic Elephantiasis)

Without management, lymphedema will progress. In stage III, a further progression of skin changes occurs, for example, lymphostatic fibrosis, sclerosis, and papillomas (benign skin tumors).[2] In most cases, an extreme increase in swelling develops in stage III, but this does not always occur[2,7] (see Fig. 22-10).

Patients do not remain in a particular stage for a given amount of time. For example, a patient will not be in stage I for 2 months, then progress to stage II for 3 months before moving to stage III. *Tissue changes,* or the progression of fibrosis, remains the clinical trait that distinguishes the stages of lymphedema. Tissue changes commonly seen in the progression of lymphedema include proliferation of connective tissue cells, production of collagen fibers, an increase in fatty deposits, and fibrotic changes. These changes initially become evident at the distal end of the extremities, that is, the fingers and toes. A *Stemmer sign* is positive for lymphedema—the inability or difficulty in lifting the skin from the dorsum of the fingers or toes. The absence of a

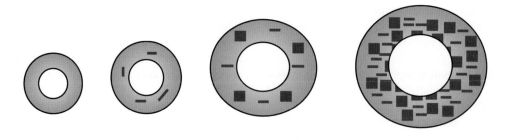

| Normal | Stage I | Stage II | Stage III |

FIGURE 22-10   Stages of lymphedema. Edema mainly located above the fascia. Increased interstitial protein concentration marked by dashes; fibrosis marked by squares.

Stemmer sign **does not exclude** the presence of lymphedema. In some cases—for example, in primary lymphedema—the patient may be able to keep their shoes on, which provides compression and retards the progression of swelling.

DIAGNOSTIC TESTING

Diagnostic testing specifically for lymphedema is not routinely performed to determine the stage of lymphedema or the type of malformation present that may have caused the lymphedema. Imaging techniques are used only if there is question regarding the origin of the swelling, for example, tumor (benign or malignant), and are rarely used to determine a treatment plan or the response to a treatment. It should be noted that any diagnostic testing that involves the injection of a substance, that is a dye, or a radiographic tracer, could contribute to further destruction and compromise of the lymphatic system.[2,5,7,11]

- **Indirect lymphangiography:** A contrast medium is injected subepidermally into the dorsum of the hand or toes. Serial X-rays are taken 3 minutes after the first injection, then at 3- to 5-minute intervals. When the superficial lymphatics are visualized, the test is terminated.[2,5,7,11]
- **Direct lymphography:** An imaging medium is injected directly into the lymphatic vessels of the dorsum of the hand or foot. Patients who have had this test will often present with a perpendicular scar over the dorsum of their hand or foot. Again, serial X-rays are performed to visualize the collectors and nodes. This direct method is used to closely examine the pelvic and retroperitoneal regions; but today, less invasive measures are preferred: MRI, computed tomography (CT), and ultrasound for example.[2,5,7,11]
- **Fluorescent microlymphography:** A fluorescent microscope and video camera are used to visualize the superficial lymphatic vessels.
- **Magnetic resonance imaging (MRI):** This is a noninvasive method used to visualize the lymphatics. Patients are placed in a magnetic field in order to measure the "relaxation of hydrogen protons (eg, in water, fat, etc) as a function of their location."[11]

EXAMINATION

As with any good evaluation, a thorough history and review of the systems are necessary for patients with lymphedema. *Social history,* to include favored activities and *family/caregiver resources,* are discussed in order to work toward discharge goals. Current job/work status assessment will determine the potential for return to work goals/criteria. *Other criteria* to include in the patient history are duration of swelling (years, months, or weeks); reason for swelling (testing procedures, vigorous activity, infection); other conditions present (arthritis, CVI, CHF); history of other treatments for the swelling and the outcome. It is important to identify if any diagnostic testing has been performed to identify the type of lymphedema or to rule out tumor progression or cancer reoccurrence. *Integumentary review* should include skin integrity, presence of scars, presence of wounds, and degree of pitting. Included in this category are evaluation for the presence of lymphatic cysts (outgrowth of lymph capillaries or collectors) and/or fistulas (abnormal connections between the skin and the superficial lymph vessels, ie, ruptured cysts), papillomas (benign skin tumors), and the presence of a *Stemmer's sign.* A positive Stemmer's sign results in the inability or difficulty lifting the skin folds at the base of the second finger or toe. However, a negative Stemmer's sign does not exclude the presence of lymphedema.

Clinically, it is imperative to assess for the presence of adequate *circulation* and the appropriateness of applying compression. An ABI or ankle–brachial index is helpful to determine the presence of adequate arterial blood flow. This is a comparative value of a peripheral to a more central blood pressure that identifies arterial patency or sufficiency. A value of 1.0 signifies normal arterial flow, that is, safe for compression. A value between 0.5 and 0.8 identifies moderate arterial impairment, and a value below 0.5 identifies severe compromise of arterial blood flow. Compression is not recommended for ABI measurements in the moderate and severe ranges.[2]

Musculoskeletal and *neuromuscular deficits* may also accompany lymphedema due to the increased size and weight

TABLE 22-6   Classification for Lymphedema[1]

Mild: Less than 3 cm difference between affected and unaffected limb.

Moderate: Between 3 and 5 cm difference between affected and unaffected limb.

Severe: 5+ cm difference between affected and unaffected limb.

of the limb with chronic postural compensations to deal with the added size of the limb. Subjectively, patients will often report a feeling of heaviness, fatigue, fullness, and, initially, pain (mild aching or tightness). Benign lymphedema is not painful, but the patient may initially experience some pain from the stretching of the skin's elastic fibers. A review of patient's *medications* should also be included. The patient's *balance* and the need for *assistive devices* are evaluated to consider the patient's safety. Patient compliance and follow-through with the *self-management* phase are imperative—Assessment of *cognition* level and *mentation* are also important.[2,4]

Anthropometric measurements of the involved and uninvolved limbs are necessary to have baseline comparative values. There is currently no standardization in the methods of obtaining anthropometric measurements. Several current clinically accepted methods include specified point circumferential measurements, volumetric measurements, and water displacement methods. Recent research has compared the calculation of limb volume measurements using the water displacement and circumferential measurements derived from a truncated cone formula. These results determined that either method could be used with confidence to calculate volumes of fluid, but the two methods were not interchangeable.[23] Another study showed that the 6-cm frustum method for the arm and the frustum method for the hand "correlated strongly" with volume determined by water displacement, but that the two methods produced dissimilar results.[24]

There are limitations to all of the aforementioned methods. Water displacement methods are often time-consuming and messy; the patient may have difficulty lifting the involved limb to place it correctly in the water-holding vessel; the water-holding vessel may not be large enough to accommodate the involved limb; and finally, total limb volume measurements by circumferential measurements and water displacement methods require standardization using a measurement from the uninvolved limb. Bioelectric impedance analysis (BIA) has gained popularity for its ability to determine both intracellular and extracellular fluid content. "The reference value used in this index is that of the intracellular fluid within" the measured area. BIA can be used in calculating the volume with bilateral lymphedema. BIA appears to be more sensitive to slight increases in volume, and therefore may detect lymphedema earlier.[25,26]

There is no consensus in the literature on the degree of enlargement that identifies lymphedema. The most common figures are a 2- or 3-cm difference between four comparative points of the involved and uninvolved extremities: metacarpal-phalangeal joints, the wrist (smallest point), 10 cm distal and 15 cm proximal to the lateral epicondyle.[5,27,28] In some cases, a 2-cm difference can normally occur between the dominant and nondominant extremities.[27] A 2-cm difference can be nonsignificant in larger, more muscular upper extremities, but very significant in smaller upper extremities[29–32] (see Table 22-6).

The entry-level clinician may experience difficulty in differentiating lymphedema from regular edema. Table 22-7 presents clinical findings that may be used to differentiate one from the other.

INTERVENTIONS

Therapeutic nihilism (ie, no treatment at all) for lymphedema is deplorable, although quite common. All too often, a woman is told that she "should be thankful to be alive" and that she must "learn to live with it." The fact that the average clinician is ill prepared to both detect and recognize early signs of lymphedema must be remedied, as data suggest that the sooner the treatment is started, the smaller the amount of treatment required to prevent further progression, and the better the ultimate result.[27]

Moist Heat and Cryo Modalities

CLINICAL CORRELATE

Ice, heat, hydrotherapy (hot packs), saunas, contrasts baths, and paraffin are all contraindicated for the involved limb for lymphedema management. Basic and advanced physiology identifies that vasodilation occurs with any of these modalities. This vasodilation increases blood capillary pressure and, in turn, will increase the lymphatic load of water—overloading an already-stressed or impaired lymphatic system. Any modality that causes vasodilation to the involved limb and/or ipsilateral trunk quadrant should be avoided.[2–5]

Ultrasound

Because of its thermal affects, ultrasound should only be used in lymphedema management at a setting that significantly minimizes the heating effect. Suggested parameters for ultrasound are 3 MHz (50% pulsed) at 0.1–0.3 W/cm^2 for 5 to 8 minutes with a dynamic head movement. This setting minimizes heating effects on the tissues that will avoid increasing blood flow in the area—avoiding the increase in the lymphatic load of water. Pulsed ultrasound at a lower intensity will produce mechanical or nonthermal effects that will soften fibrotic tissues. Ultrasound may be used for its fibrinolitic effects on lymphostatic fibrosis, but not on radiation fibrosis.[2,33]

TABLE 22-7   Edema Versus Lymphedema

Edema	Lymphedema
Increased water in the interstitial space	Increased water and protein in the interstitial space
Improves with elevation	*Initial stage*—may improve with elevation *Chronic stages*—no improvement with elevation
Usually, symmetrical appearance except with posttraumatic edema	Asymmetrical appearance
Can be localized or systemic presentation	Localized presentation-never generalized
Dynamic insufficiency of the lymphatic system	Mechanical insufficiency of the lymphatic system
Usually bilateral—except posttraumatic	Usually unilateral—can present bilateral
Pitting always present	Pitting only present in stages I and II

Electrotherapeutic Modalities

No electrotherapeutic modalities greater than 30 Hz should be used on the involved lymphedematous extremity or in the ipsilateral adjacent quadrant. Electrotherapeutic current greater than 30 Hz will create erythema under the pads, which will increase blood flow, increase BCP, and ultimately increase the lymphatic load of water.[2,4,7]

Medications

Frequently, patients are given *diuretics* to manage lymphedema without success. The diuretics will help decrease the size of the limb for 1 to 2 days and do an effective job of removing water from the interstitial spaces. However, diuretics fail to remove proteins from the interstitial spaces; frequently there is a rapid return of swelling. Often, the involved limb is larger than it was before the patient began taking the diuretics.[2,4]

Topical and oral *benzopyrones* are a group of drugs that include flavonoids and coumarins. Flavonoids occur frequently in nature, particularly in vegetables and fruits. Studies have shown that benzopyrones may improve chronic lymphedema by stimulating macrophage proteolysis to remove excess proteins in the interstitial spaces.[34,35] Benzopyrones are a standard of care in Australian and some European lymphedema management programs. Reduction of limb volumes in patients who combine benzopyrones and other lymphedema management strategies is slow—at least 6 months.[34–39] In the United States, benzopyrones are not used. High liver toxicity and morbidity are associated with the use of benzopyrones. Loprinzi et al.[39] performed a study that treated 140 women with 200 mg of oral coumarin or placebo twice daily for 6 months, followed by another commonly used treatment for the following 6 months. They found that coumarin was tolerated well, but there was no difference in the volumes of the involved arms and hands after 12 months of treatment. The researchers also found serologic evidence of liver toxicity in 6% of the women.[2,7,34,37,39]

Surgery

The best summative statement about surgical attempts to repair the lymphatic system and surgical correction for lymphedema is from Goldsmith and De Los Santos: "The large number of operations devised for improving lymphatic drainage from a chronically lymphedematous limb indicates the lack of a surgical procedure which is consistently effective."[40] Various types of surgical repairs for the lymphatic system include lympholymphatic repair, lymphovenous repair, collector replacement, and the use of enteromesenteric bridge. To date, surgical attempts to increase the transport capacity (the maximum carrying capacity) of the lymphatic system have failed. Földi asserts, "The use of prosthetic material (eg, nylon threads) with hopes of reestablishing lymph flow simply disregards the fact that the propulsive force of the lymph flow is furnished by the pulsation of the lymphangions. A blood vessel may readily be replaced by a tube because the heart pumps the blood through it, but there is no force that could propel lymph through an artificial, valveless tube."[22] Transplanted areas of tissue from the deep lymphatic system to the superficial lymphatic system are not successful in removing lymph stasis because the deep system is usually also involved with lymphedema (recall that lymph flow is from superficial to deep).[22]

Debulking procedures open the skin, remove all of the superficial tissues, and then close the skin via incision or graft skin over the remaining tissue. Another option for debulking is to remove the skin and the superficial tissues, and then place skin grafts over the fascia. One can only imagine the grotesque appearance of the residual limb. These operations are not as common as they were in the late 1980s and early 1990s; however, they were considered successful when the swelling was removed. This procedure does not prevent the reaccumulation of lymph fluid and does nothing to repair or improve the function of a compromised lymphatic system.[2]

Patients may seek help following a failed attempt at *liposuction* to "cure" lymphedema or debulk an involved area. Liposuction removes the superficial fatty tissues and destroys any remaining intact lymph collectors. However, because the extra fatty deposits are removed, lymphedema can still reoccur, and lymphatic microcirculation will be significantly disturbed. The long-term effects of liposuction on patients with lymphedema are still an enigma.[2,7,41–43]

Brorson, from Sweden, supports the use of liposuction to correct a "physical and psychological handicap" for post–breast cancer patients. He advocates the use of liposuction combined with compression over the use of compression alone to reduce the size of the involved limb. Brorson notes that liposuction does not improve lymphatic system function but does increase "skin microcirculation."[44]

In a second study, Brorson and Svensson performed liposuction combined with compression on 28 patients and compared them to 28 patients who only received compression to manage their lymphedema. One-year postoperation, the liposuction group had maintained their decreased arm size results. On the 1-year postoperative follow-up, the researchers recommended that six participants (who achieved full reduction) remove their garments for 1 week. "A marked increase in arm volume was observed, which was immediately remedied by reapplying the garments."[45]

Clinically, liposuction is considered a major surgery for some patients. It can be costly and very invasive. In lymphedema, the elastic fibers of the skin are destroyed, necessitating the use of compression for lifelong management of lymphedema. However, there are less invasive options with minimal to no side effects to effectively manage lymphedema.

Massage

Massage has traditionally been used to treat edema, but is *not* recommended to manage lymphedema. As previously mentioned, *lymphedema* is a high-protein edema due to the accumulation of protein in the interstitial spaces. It is the sole responsibility of the lymphatic system to remove the proteins from the interstitium. If the lymphatic system is compromised, protein removal will not occur, and a high oncotic pressure will form in the interstitial space.[2–5,46] *Edema* of the superficial tissues can become manifest from a variety of conditions or situations: prolonged sitting or standing, insufficient venous return (incompetent valves), pregnancy, heart failure, liver disturbances in renal function, fluid and electrolyte imbalances, inflammations, and infections. Edema results when the *intact* lymphatic system is overwhelmed or overloaded (dynamic insufficiency), which results in an accumulation of water in the tissues.[2,5,46]

Massage (Greek: *massain*) means, "to knead" and describes the forms of "classical" or "Swedish" massage.[47] Massage triggers the release of histamines from mast cells, which produce an active hyperemia in the tissues. This ultimately causes an increase in blood capillary pressure and ultrafiltration. More water accumulates in the interstitial spaces, which overloads an impaired lymphatic system. Superficial lymphatics of the skin are located in the subepidermal layer and are extremely vulnerable to high pressures from massage or trauma.[46] Research has shown that a 3- to 5-minute massage affects the endothelial lining of the initial lymphatics and causes artificial cracks that develop from injury to the lymphatic wall.[48]

Pneumatic Compression

The use of pumps for lymphedema management and decongestion continues to be a topic of frequent discussion. Compression pumps consist of a single sleeve or a multichambered sleeve that uses rubber tubing to connect to a pump that moves compressed air into the sleeve. Single sleeves fill uniformly, where multichambered sleeves fill sequentially from distal to proximal. Newer versions of compression pumps offer "on/off" cycles with variation. Pumps do an effective job at removing water from the interstitial spaces but do nothing to remove proteins. Proteins that remain in the tissues continue to attract fibroblasts and generate new connective tissue, which creates more scar tissue.[2,5,7]

Disadvantages of Compression Pump Therapy for Lymphedema Management2

- Remaining/intact functioning lymph collectors may be destroyed.
- Trunk quadrants previously not involved may fill with fluid.
- Pumps have no effect on fibrotic tissue and may worsen fibrotic areas.
- Pumps push fluid into the ipsilateral trunk quadrant, which may be congested.
- Pumps can cause genital swelling.
- Length of treatment time is long and questionable (minimum of 4 hours; some protocols suggest 8 hours).
- Patients are immobile during pump sessions.

Segers et al. investigated multichambered pumps to determine whether the pressure set on the dial was the actual pressure produced in the chamber "on the skin."[49] He found that even though the dial was set at 30, 60, 80, and 100 mmHg, respectively, the pressure applied to the skin in each chamber actually reached 54, 98, 121, and 141 mmHg.[49]

Boris et al.[50] performed a retrospective analysis and found that 53 of 128 patients with lower-extremity lymphedema used a compression pump during their course of lymphedema management. It was not stated whether the pump was used during the initial decongestive stages of therapy, but it was noted that 23 of the 53 patients who used the pump developed genital edema, and only 2 of the 75 patients who did not receive pump therapy experienced genital edema. This study concluded that the "incidence of genital edema after pump therapy was unaffected by age, sex, grade, or duration of lymphedema; whether lymphedema was primary or secondary; whether a single or sequential pump was used; and by the pressure level applied or duration or hours per day of pump therapy. It was concluded that compressive pump therapy for lower limb lymphedema produces an unacceptably high incidence of genital edema."[50]

Miranda et al.[51] performed a prospective, blind study protocol with sequential intermittent pneumatic compression (SIPC), which they suggested was an accepted treatment method for lymphedema. The study evaluated 11 patients that underwent an isotope lymphography before SIPC and 48 hours following a 3-hour session of SIPC. Measuring the lower extremities at six designated points revealed that there was a significant reduction after SIPC below the knee, but not in the thigh. They concluded that "compression increased transport of lymph fluid (ie, water) without comparable transport of macromolecules (ie, protein). Alternatively, SIPC reduced lymphedema by decreasing blood capillary filtration (lymph formation) rather than by accelerating lymph return thereby restoring the balance in lymph kinetics responsible for edema in the first place."[51]

Some patients who attempt to use pneumatic compression eventually realize the transitory or limited benefits and discontinue its use. A survey conducted by the Greater Boston Lymphedema Support Group in 1998 revealed that 48 (78%) of their 56 members discontinued use of the pump because (1) no further results were gained, (2) pain increased in adjacent areas to the involved limb, and (3) swelling of previously uninvolved areas began.[52]

At the 1993 International Congress of Lymphology, it was determined that *if pumps were used at all,* the adjacent trunk area and base of the involved limb should be cleared first. Specific manual techniques—manual lymph drainage—should be taught by certified instructors and specialized programs, which are listed at the end of this chapter.[53]

Manual Lymph Drainage with Complete Decongestive Therapy

As early as 400 and 500 BC, Hypocrates and Aristotle discussed vessels containing "white blood" or "white milky fluid." These early findings were forgotten for nearly 2,000 years after the death of these early pioneers—Anatomical studies were considered sinful by the early Catholic Church. Nothing was documented on the lymphatic system again until the early 17th century by Caspare Asselli—an Italian anatomist—who primarily performed research on cadavers and animals. During a vivisection of a dog, Asselli discovered "cords" in the digestive system. He initially believed these cords to be nerves, but a "milky, creamlike substance escaped" from the cords when cut.[2]

In the 1800s, Dr. Alexander von Winiwarter, a German physician, successfully treated elephantiastic limbs with compression, elevation, and a "special massage." Dr. von Winiwarter died in the 1890s, and his work was forgotten until Emil Vodder, PhD, MT, and his wife rediscovered the von Winiwarter techniques in the 1930s. Dr. Vodder and his wife ran a successful clinic on the French Riviera, where they treated patients with chronic colds and swellings of various origins. Treatment consisted of "intuitively manipulating" the patient's swollen cervical lymph nodes in order to "boost their immune system." The Vodders coined the term "manual lymph drainage" (MLD) to describe their techniques.[3]

In the early 1980s, Dr. Michael Földi noticed that many of his patients had swollen limbs. He heard about the success the Vodders had with their manual lymph drainage techniques and began to study the new method. Accepted treatment for elephantiastic limbs at that time was tight compression with

elastic bands, which often caused sores, skin breakdown, and eventually amputation of the swollen limb. Dr. Vodder and Dr. Földi met to discuss Vodder's new treatment but could not agree on the specific implications for the treatment. Vodder claimed his new therapy—MLD—could cure such things as hair loss and obesity. The more scientific-oriented Földi did not agree with these implications, but believed Vodder's techniques did have a scientific basis that effectively treated the lymphatic system. Much of Dr. Földi's work—along with that of his wife Dr. Ethel Földi—has produced significant research and laid the foundation for the advancement of MLD. Dr. Földi coined the term "complete decongestive therapy (CDT)" and realized that a *combination of treatments* should be employed to successfully treat lymphedema: MLD, skin care, compression, and exercise. Földi modified the manual lymph drainage techniques of Vodder to fit a more scientific profile, but to honor the work of Vodder, he refers to his techniques as "modified Vodder techniques." The Vodder techniques and modified Vodder techniques are the more popular methods used in North America today.[2]

Other professionals have made significant contributions to the field of lymphedema management over the years. Drs. John Casley-Smith and Judith Casley-Smith have added research, trained lymphedema therapists, and treated patients for more than 40 years. Albert Leduc and his son Oliver Leduc have used isotopic lymphography to establish standards and "efficacy of manual techniques" and also provided instruction and patient care. Joachim E. Zuther founded the Department of Lymphology in Ulm, Germany, in 1990 and offered the first certification classes in MLD/CDT (Vodder/Földi technique) in the United States through the Academy of Lymphatic Studies, which he founded in 1994. A list of the larger schools that teach scientific-based techniques can be found in Table 22-8. Please refer to the references listed at the end of this chapter for other noted contributors.[2,5]

CDT has been referred to by a variety of names from the different schools of lymphedema management that have developed over the years: complex physical therapy (Casley-Smith), combined decongestive therapy (Vodder), and complete decongestive physiotherapy or combined physiotherapy (Földi and Leduc). The 1998 American Cancer Society Workshop on Breast Cancer Treatment-Related Lymphedema included a review of the techniques from the major CDT methods (Vodder, Leduc, Casley-Smith, and Földi) and found that the "principles followed are the same for each school, the [MLD] techniques vary somewhat in terms of the degree of pressure, motion and the timing of strokes. Additionally, the Leduc technique uses low, intermittent pneumatic pressure [<40 mm Hg] pumps and the Casley-Smith group uses benzopyrone medications."[5,27,54–57]

Complete decongestive therapy (CDT) is a two-phased, noninvasive treatment approach, which recognizes that lymphedema also affects the ipsilateral body quadrant adjacent to the involved limb. The effects of lymphedema are most obvious in the involved limb. During phase I (treatment phase), the patient is given daily 45- to 75-minute treatments over a period

TABLE 22-8   Lymphedema Management Programs

Academy of Lymphatic Studies Office: 11632 High Street, Suite A 　　Sebastian, FL 32958 Phone: 1-800-863-5935 Fax: 772-589-0306 Web site: http://www.acols.com		
Casley-Smith Centers in North America Lymphedema Therapy Center, Inc. Office: Roswell, GA Phone: 770-518-4700 E-mail: CLTcourse@cs.com	and	Boris-Lasinski School Office: Woodbury, Long Island, NY Phone: 516-364-2200
Coast-to-Coast School of Lymphedema Management Leduc Method Office: Temecula, CA Phone: 909-600-0634 Web site: http://www.lymphedemamanagement.com The Földi School—Privateschule Földi GMBH Office: Merzhausen, Germany Phone (from United States): 011-49-761-406921 Fax: 01149-761-406983 Web site: http://www.foeldiklinik.de/engl/info.htm		
Klose Norton Training and Consulting, Inc. Office: Red Bank, NJ Phone: 877-842-4414 Fax: 732-842-5299 Web site: http://www.klosenorton.com Dr. Vodder School of North America Office: Victoria, BC, Canada Phone: 250-589-9862 Web site: http://www.vodderschool.com		

of 2 to 6 weeks (depending on the severity, this time frame could be longer or shorter) that includes MLD, decongestive exercises, education regarding skin and nail care, and compression (using short-stretch bandages). In phase II (self-improvement phase), the patient works to maintain and improve the effects gained in the treatment phase by continuing the skin care, exercises, bandaging, and self-MLD techniques learned in phase I. MLD may be performed 1 to 2 times a week or on an "as-needed" basis. The self-improvement phase is lifelong—There is no cure for lymphedema. All treatment options to date are symptomatic in nature.[2,5,7,27]

Components of Complete Decongestive Therapy

Meticulous skin and nail care utilizes basic hygiene principles—The patient needs to bathe and keep the limb clean as well as moisturized. Sweat and sebum (an oily secretion produced by sebaceous glands) mix to form a protective layer on the skin called the *acid mantle*. The pH of the acid mantle ranges between 4 and 5.5 (pH of 7 is neutral; above 7 is alkaline). Normal skin is mildly acidic in order to protect it from the elements of nature (pollutants and wind) and to inhibit the growth of harmful bacteria and fungi. If the acid mantle loses its acidity, the skin becomes more prone to damage and infection. A mild, neutral soap with minimal or no fragrance should be used to clean the involved limb. Moisturizing cream or lotion with a

low pH—such as *Eucerin* or *Aquaphor* (Beiersdorf, Inc)—should be used to maintain subtleness of the skin and the slightly acidic acid mantle. **Because the diffusion distance of the involved limb is increased (localized swelling if the involved limb), this puts the lymphedema patient at a higher risk for infections and dryer skin.**[2,58]

Fingernails and toenails should be monitored for nail infections and fungus. Patients with Lymphedema need to be reminded not to trim their nails too close on the involved limb. This will only serve as another possible avenue for infection due to the increased diffusion distance in the involved limb.[2,7]

MLD utilizes a special technique to manipulate and activate superficial lymphatic vessels, deep lymph nodes, and larger transport vessels; lympholymphatic anastomoses; perforating precollectors and lymph vasavasorum vessels (lymph vessels and nodes of larger veins). With correct pressure and timing, MLD stimulates lymph vessels to contract with greater frequency (increasing LTV or lymphangiomotoricity) and intensity. MLD techniques also reroute stagnant lymph fluid from a congested area into an adjacent body quadrant via anastomoses and then toward healthy lymphatics. The general principle of MLD is to begin centrally and then work distally toward the congested limb (ie, stimulate the cervical lymph nodes in the healthy quadrant, in order to create a suction effect on the plexus/collectors, then use modified techniques in the involved quadrant adjacent to the ipsilateral involved limb, then the involved limb). To be successful, it is essential to *first* decongest the involved trunk quadrant, before progressing to the involved extremity. MLD treatments should begin in the proximal body regions then progress distally.[2,7,22,48,59–61]

The elastic fibers of the skin are damaged in lymphedema patients. Therefore, *compression* using multilayered padding and short-stretch bandages is used to increase external tissue pressure to control ultrafiltration (retard swelling).[62–64] Short-stretch bandages have a high working pressure and a low resting pressure. They provide resistance against working muscles but relax to avoid arterial compromise when the patient is at rest (at night). Padding and bandages are generally applied over the entire limb from distal to proximal (ie, from fingers to axilla). The padding is used to distribute pressure and create a uniform surface for the bandages to compress—to eliminate areas of increased pressure or "hot spots." Consistent compression—during the day and night—can help the body absorb and break down lymphostatic fibrotic tissue. As a general rule, lymphedema patients require 24-hour compression[2,7,65–69] (see Figs. 22-11 and 22-12).

It is recommended that patients perform *decongestive exercises with compression in place*. Appropriate exercises can

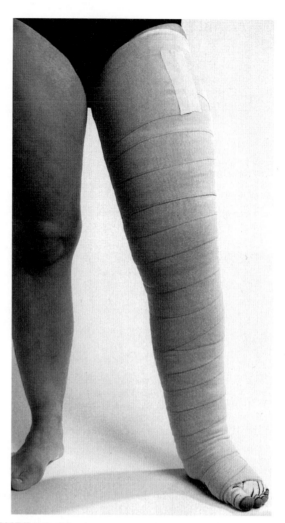

FIGURE 22-12 Lymphedema bandaging of a lower extremity. (Reprinted with permission from Lohmann and Rauscher, Inc., Topeka, Kansas.)

be any simple active exercise that addresses each joint to maintain range of motion and activate the muscle and joint pumps. Decongestive exercises improve the flow of lymph to the venous angle; deep breathing improves transport of lymph via the thoracic duct (the thoracic duct goes through the diaphragm at the aortic hiatus), helps to maintain normal hydrostatic pressure, varies tissue pressure, and prevents reaccumulation of lymph fluid. Of course, exercise helps to increase the patient's level of fitness, and improves self-perception, and increases their tolerance to daily activities. Patient constraints and ability levels govern exercise prescription.[2,7]

Physiologically, exercise increases active hyperemia, which in turn increases blood capillary pressure, ultrafiltration, and the lymphatic load of water. Under normal physiological conditions, an intact lymphatic system can handle this increase without difficulty. Vigorous exercise may trigger the onset of lymphedema or exacerbate current symptoms for patients with an impaired lymphatic system. How much exercise is too much? How can one patient return to playing golf and another patient play three rounds of nine holes and experience lymphedema? These questions remain unanswered.

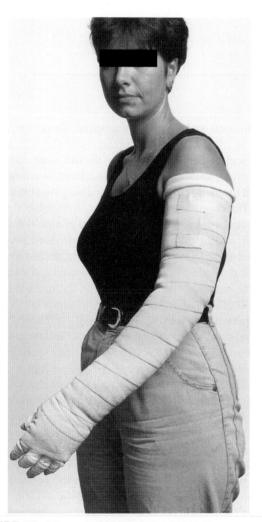

FIGURE 22-11 Lymphedema bandaging of an upper extremity. (Reprinted with permission from Lohmann and Rauscher, Inc., Topeka, Kansas.)

The lack of evidence-based research regarding specific exercise prescription for patients at a higher risk to develop lymphedema symptoms is due to the inability of clinicians to accurately predict which patients will develop lymphedema. Therefore, exercise prescription is based on the patient's fitness level and tolerance to activity. Even a more physically fit individual should be progressed through graded exercise programs (beginning at a lower intensity level) that focus on smooth, concentric activities with light resistance. Prudent clinicians and therapists will educate their patients about risk factors and precautions in an attempt to prevent against the onset of lymphedema. These precautions may be too conservative for some, but clinicians should be in a "conservative or prevention" mode, which may prevent the onset of lymphedema. This is not to say that certain patients should not be progressed above a minimal to moderate fitness level. Some studies refute the need to adhere to precautions, and support this claim by referencing data on participants who have performed strenuous activities and have not developed lymphedema or an exacerbation of symptoms.[70] This may be the case, but clinical prudence and precaution should take precedence until it can be determined who will develop lymphedema. Progression of exercise and appropriate exercise prescription should be issues determined by clinicians knowledgeable about the physiological aspects of exercise and the response of a lymphedematous limb to exercise.[2,5,7,28,70]

Phase I of treatment ends when measurements of the involved limb(s) plateau. In phase II, or the self-improvement phase, all components of phase I are continued. Patients adhere to the principles of skin and nail care. Once the limb size has plateaued, the patient can be measured for compression garments. (*Juzo* and *Beiersdorf-Jobst* are the largest manufacturers of lymphedema garments.) Garments are made of a special weave of fabric that prevent reaccumulation of fluid by increasing external tissue pressure to accommodate for destroyed elastic fibers of the involved limb(s). Compression should be maintained during the day with garments and at night with bandages and padding. Patients who have no lymphostatic fibrotic tissue may not be required to wear compression bandages at night.[2,7]

Compression garments are divided into compression classes (CC) I–IV. Generally, an uncomplicated arm should require a CC II, and a leg should require a CC III. Of course, there will be exceptions. An older individual with an arthritic hand or no assistance at home may not be able to donn a CC II for the arm or a CC III for the leg, and a lower class should be utilized to achieve some degree of compression[2] (see Figs. 22-13 to 22-15).

The involved limb should be monitored for response to exercise. It is important for the patient to recognize the signs and symptoms of an exacerbation (increase in swelling) and adjust their activity level appropriately[2,7] (see Table 22-9).

The patient can be taught basic self-MLD strokes to promote contraction of the lymph angions. It is imperative the patient learn the correct depth of the strokes—a light skin stretch is used versus a kneading motion as in traditional massage. Performing self-MLD should not take the place of exercises or bandaging.[2,7]

Continuation of the home exercise program helps to maintain the benefits of MLD, stimulates contraction of the lymph collectors, maintains joint range of motion, and increases the patient's tolerance to activity. Exercise for 10 to 15 minutes, 2 times a day, with a few simple exercises is more beneficial than no exercise.[2]

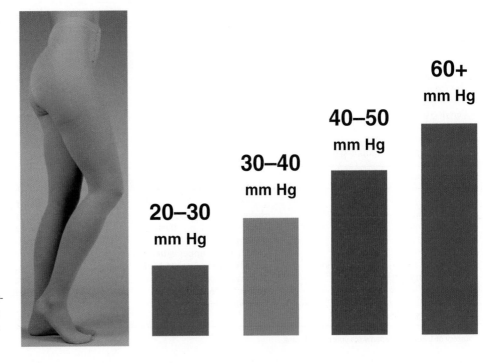

FIGURE 22-13 Example of lower-extremity pantyhose with compression classes. (Reprinted with permission from Juzo USA, Cuyahoga Falls, Ohio.)

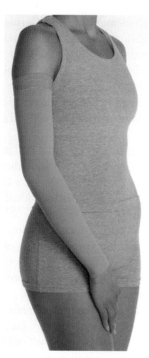

FIGURE 22-14   Example of upper extremity garment. (Reprinted with permission from Juzo USA, Cuyahoga Falls, Ohio.)

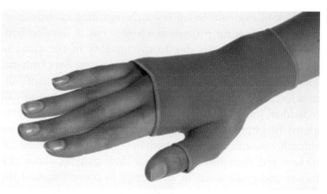

FIGURE 22-15   Example of hand garment. (Reprinted with permission from Juzo USA, Cuyahoga Falls, Ohio.)

It is recommended that a certified lymphedema therapist perform complete decongestive therapy. For certification, a therapist must complete a minimum of 135 hours of training, to include anatomy and physiology of the lymphatic system, bandaging techniques, and the correct manual techniques and principles of treatment. Specialized training is required to properly apply the manual lymph drainage techniques and the short-stretch bandages. Adequate education for lymphedema management cannot be accomplished in 4 days, a weekend, or even 7 days. A prevalent amount of anecdotal evidence has shown CDT to be successful for more than 50 years. Evidence-based

TABLE 22-9   Exercise Risk Classifications

Patient Education		
The list below is a general guideline of high-risk, medium-risk, and beneficial activities for upper and lower extremity lymphedema patients. Always take maximal precautions and discuss any planned activities you are unsure of with your therapist.		

Upper Extremity		
High Risk	**Medium Risk**	**Beneficial**
Gardening	Jogging/running	Swimming
Tennis/racquet sports	Biking (minimize grip)	Lymphedema exercise
Golf	Stairmaster program (grip bars for support)	Walking
Shoveling snow	NordicTrack	Stairmaster (no grip and elevate arm sometimes)
Moving furniture	General weight lifting of rest of body	Self-MLD
Carrying luggage	Easy horse riding (hold the reigns loose)	Yoga
Carrying grocery bags		Water aerobics
Scrubbing		
Weight lifting with arm		
Intense horse riding (gripping reigns)		

Lower Extremity		
Running	Light jogging	Walking
Intense hiking	Hiking longer than 30 min	Easy biking 10–20 min
Moving furniture	Skating longer than 20 min	Lymphedema exercises
Soccer	Golfing	Easy skating 10–15 min
Hockey	Weight lifting (upper extremity)	Swimming
Sitting or standing over long periods	NordicTrack longer than 15 min	Calf pumps
Weight lifting with legs	Stairmaster longer than 5 min	NordicTrack 5–10 min
Stairmaster longer than 15 min	Volleyball/tennis (easy)	Deep breathing exercises
Wrestling	Easy horse riding	Yoga
Intense horse riding		Water aerobics

Courtesy of J. Zuther/Academy of Lymphatic Studies.

literature is slowly accumulating to support the efficacy of this new intervention for patients with lymphedema.

CASE STUDY

Patient/Client Diagnosis Classification

In order to include patients in Pattern 6H of the *Guide*, a thorough history and review of the systems are necessary to identify risk factors and pathological or pathophysiological impairment of the lymphatic system. Lymphatic system impairment can result from surgical interventions directly involving the lymphatic system, trauma, filariasis, infection of lymph collectors (lymphangitis) or lymph nodes (lymphadenitis), complex regional pain syndrome, postradiation, frequent bouts of cellulitis (particularly in an immune compromised limb), and trauma. Regardless of the precipitating incident, lymphedema results from an abnormal accumulation of protein-rich edema due to the inability of the lymphatic system to remove this protein-rich swelling. Patients with severe impairments or multiple complicating factors are not excluded from the pattern; however, the frequency of visits and duration of care may require modification.[1,2,5,7]

Not all swellings or edemas are classified as lymphedema. Examination findings may support exclusion from this pattern, or the physical therapist may determine the patient/client may be managed more appropriately through (1) classification into another pattern, (2) classification in both Pattern 6H and another pattern, and (3) educated and objective inclusion of *selective portions* of Pattern 6H to appropriately manage the condition.[1]

Edema resulting from congestive heart failure (CHF) may require classification into a different pattern.

A vital part of lymphedema management is compression, which limits ultrafiltration and increases reabsorption. One should consider the added volume return to the heart and the integrity of the heart wall with compression and CHF patients. Patients with lymphedema may have comorbidities, for example, CHF that accompany lymphatic insufficiencies. A physician who understands the principles and components of lymphedema management should medically clear these patients.[1,2,7]

The swelling from *lipedema* is the result of an abnormal accumulation of adipose tissue. Lipedema is more common in women and may be caused by a genetic or hormonal component (specifics are still not known). There is a decrease in the transport capacity of the lymphatic system because the collectors must "cork-screw" and wind their way through adipose tissue versus running directly toward their regional lymph nodes. Over time, with the further proliferation of adipose tissue and increase of the lymphatic loads, further stress is placed on the lymphatic system that further decreases transport capacity. Initially, a full lymphedema management program may not be appropriate for these patients with lipedema (depending on the severity, because lymphedema can develop over lipedema; ie, *lipolymphedema*). A patient with lipedema can be effectively managed with compression that supports the venous return and the lymphatic system.[2,7]

Description of the Case

Rebecca is a 36-year-old, obese (5 ft 7.5 in.; 350 lb), white female who reports a long-standing, progressive history of increased swelling of her bilateral lower extremities. The swelling has gradually increased over the years. Her attempts to resolve the swelling with rest and elevation have failed.

History of Present Illness/ Past Medical History

The patient presents to therapy and reports that she has experienced swelling in both lower legs (below the knees) since the age of 13. She has wrapped her lower legs since that time with ace bandages (long-stretch bandages) in an attempt to prevent progression of the swelling. As a child, she was active and always enjoyed movement activities, but continued to experience a gradual increase in swelling of her lower extremities, which seemed to worsen without compression. Rebecca reports no history of CHF, diabetes, or deep vein thrombosis.

Rebecca states that over the last 3 to 4 years, she has experienced problems with chronic infections in her legs (left more than right). A small scratch from the family cat transformed into cellulitis for Rebecca 4 or 5 times over the last 2 years. She continues to wrap her lower legs but has "given up" with her thighs. A cat scratch on her left thigh 2 years ago resulted in her leg "weeping clear fluid for days." She went to her primary care physician at that time for help and suggestions without success. The weeping eventually stopped after 5 days. Following that incident, Rebecca noticed that lobes began to develop on her thighs. Both thighs have lobes at the medial aspects (left 50 lb; right 30 lb), and she reports difficulty finding appropriately sized clothing. One year ago, she noticed a lump at her left medial thigh. Her physician at that time suggested that it may be a fibrotic lymph node, and should be removed (she did not report any unusual swelling or soreness). After the removal of the benign, fibrotic lymph node, the lobes and her thighs further increased in size. Rebecca also states she has had a nonhealing wound on the medial aspect of her left lower leg for more than 3 years. She was prescribed wound care treatments at a local wound care center—3 times a week for 4- to 6-week intervals for more than a year. Rebecca expressed frustration in regard to her wound care experience, in that the wound did not heal. Rebecca is excited about her referral to physical therapy for lymphedema management and willingly accepts and agrees with her plan of care.

Examination
Social History/Family/Caregiver Resources

Rebecca has a degree in accounting and plans to continue working while undergoing treatment. She performs mainly deskwork, but can move about during the day as needed, and feels her employer will work with her to allow time for physical therapy appointments. Rebecca lives with her sister's family in an extended family situation. She is active with church activities and attends school- and church-sponsored activities with her niece and nephew. If she needs help with bandaging or donning garments, Rebecca feels her family will provide the necessary assistance.

Other Criteria

As previously mentioned, Rebecca has experienced swelling below the knee since age 13. The swelling has gradually progressed since that time. She experienced an increase in swelling following episodes of cellulitis and surgical removal of a benign, fibrotic lymph node on the left medial thigh.

General Health

Rebecca is obese and reports chronic back and hip pain from lifting her heavy lower extremities. A chronic leg wound is present on the left lower leg. Blood pressure is 138/85 mm Hg, and she is not currently taking blood pressure medications. Rebecca has no history of diabetes. She is able to care for herself and is oriented to person, place, time, and situation. She does not smoke or drink.

Integumentary Review

A chronic venous wound on the medial aspect of the left lower leg has been present for 3 years. No odor or drainage is noted, with good granulation tissue in the wound bed. Prior treatment for this wound included wet-to-dry dressing at a local wound care facility for almost 1 year. Rebecca has no other skin infections in the large skin folds or nail fungus. Pitting is difficult to induce at the distal lower extremities. Lymphostatic fibrosis is present—The skin is hard/firm to touch. *Hemosiderin staining* is present on both lower extremities below the knees, indicating a venous involvement (CVI). The Stemmer's sign is positive bilaterally.

Musculoskeletal/Neuromuscular Deficits

Rebecca has fair lower back range of motion, but is only able to achieve 70 degrees of left-hip active flexion and 20 degrees of left-hip abduction due to the weight of her left lower extremity and the ensuing pain with active range of motion. Strength measures 4+/5 for the upper extremities, 4+/5 for the right lower extremity, and 4/5 for the left lower extremity.

Pain

Rebecca reports a 5 for low back pain and an 8 for pain using the Visual Analog Scale. This pain subsides with rest and elevation of the lower extremities.

Medications

The only medication reported at this time is a diuretic for the swelling in Rebecca's legs. She has taken this medication for the last 6 months but experienced an increase in the size of her leg.

Balance and the Need for Assistive Devices

Rebecca demonstrates good dynamic and static sitting and standing balance. She does not use an assistive device for gait but reports she is always careful when stepping into the tub, negotiating stairs, and so forth.

Current Conditions/Chief Complaints

Rebecca is anxious to begin her course of treatment of lymphedema management. She understands the involvement and compliance she will need to gain optimal benefits and feels certain she will have support from work and family members at home. Rebecca's goals are to be able to decrease her back and hip pain, increase her mobility into and out of the tub/shower, fit into normal clothing without making alterations, and decrease the size of her legs.

Circulation

Capillary refill assessed at the nail beds of the toes is normal. Pedal pulses are normal. The ankle–brachial index measures one.

Anthropometric Measurements

This was documented using girth measurements every 4 cm to the groin (see Table 22-10).

Evaluation Summary

On the basis of the objective data and patient history, Rebecca can be classified as a primary lymphedema (lymphedema precox), in stage II or early stage III. She presents with a venous wound at the medial aspect of her left leg, and pitting is difficult to induce below the knees. The Stemmer's sign is positive at the skinfold of the second toe.

Treatment Summary

Because of the amount of lymphostatic fibrosis and the size of her lower extremities, Rebecca will require an extended treatment time. Two times a day would be preferred; however, insurance in the United States usually will not cover this (at least not in this case). In Europe, Rebecca would be able to receive treatment for her lymphedema in an inpatient setting, with at least two sessions of treatments a day by qualified manual lymph drainage therapists. Rebecca received MLD/CDT daily visits for 6 to 8 weeks. The continuous 6- to 8-week sessions continued for 5 months with 2- sometimes 3-week breaks between the sessions. Even during breaks from CDT, Rebecca continued to bandage herself independently and perform her home exercise program. A decrease in the volume of the left and right leg can be appreciated from the girth measurements every 4 cm up the leg beginning at the malleolus. When measurements plateaued, Rebecca was measured for a full pantyhose compression garment with closed toes. She was thankful for the garment, because this meant she would be able to wear the garment during the day, and only bandaged at night. Rebecca was required to bandage at night because of the amount of lymphostatic fibrosis present. She also required consistent compression to

TABLE 22-10   Rebecca's Before and After Anthropometric Measurements

Limb Measurement Date: 10/31/2000			Limb Measurement Date: 5/5/2001		
	Values			Values	
CM Mark	Right	Left	CM Mark	Right	Left
0 (Ankle)	10	20	0 (Ankle)	7	12
4	10	28	4	8	15
8	15	35	8	10	15
12	22	45	12	12	30
16	22	45	16	12	30
20	30	50	20	20	35
24	35	50	24	20	42
28	35	55	28	20	43
32	38	55	32	30	45
36	38	60	36	30	50
40	38	60	40	30	50
44	44	60	44	35	50
48	50	75	48	40	55
52	55	80	52	41	68
56	59	80	56	60	68
60	62	95	60	60	78
64	62	100	64	60	80
68	62	100	68	60	80
Volume difference (mL) = 14079.6			**Volume difference (mL) = 7836.616**		
Percentage difference = 140.1312			**Percentage difference = 105.5777**		

hold back the reaccumulation of fluid. With constant compression, the body is able to absorb scar tissue. Rebecca was not diagnosed with lymphedema when she was younger. This diagnosis would have been beneficial. She could have adhered to certain precautions for patients with lymphedema, and received education regarding the benefits of compression, skin care in combination with MLD. Tables 22-11 and 22-12 summarize Rebecca's physical therapy management while on program.

Limits of Our Knowledge

The field of lymphedema management has significantly evolved in the United States over the last 10 years. Clinically, a major limitation is that the signs and symptoms of lymphedema are not managed early enough. Unfortunately, patients with lymphedema are told they have to live with the swelling or the swelling is a side effect of surgery and it should resolve.

TABLE 22-11   Summary of Rebecca's Treatment Interventions

Treatment Intervention	Description	Duration
CDT		
MLD	45 min daily sessions	6–8 wk sessions
Compression	Specialized bandaging after Each MLD session	Ongoing
Exercise	See HEP	Ongoing
Skin and nail care	Hygiene, precautions	Ongoing
Address fibrotic tissue	US: pulsed, 0.1–0.3 W/cm^2, 5–7 min	1–2 wk
	Compression: bandages and Komprex material	3–4 wk
Wound care management	Application of topical agent to promote closure of chronic wound of 2–3 y	3 wk
MLD	45 min daily sessions	See above

TABLE 22-12   Rebecca's Home Exercise Program

Exercise	Repetitions
Aquatic exercise	20–30 min; 3–4 times a week
Walking	Total of one-fourth to one-fourth mile throughout the day
Seated leg extensions	10 repetitions—2 times a day
Seated ankle pumps	10 repetitions—2 times a day
Seated pillow squeezes	10 repetitions—2 times a day
Seated marching	10 repetitions—2 times a day

All exercises are performed with bandages in place with the exception of aquatic exercises.

There has been much anecdotal success with CDT. For some individuals, this is not satisfactory, and a resounding cry for more evidence-based research has evolved. More clinical research and evidence-based research are needed to support the efficacy of MDL/CDT and to prove that the inclusion of all components of CDT provides a more effective treatment than does just one component, which is, exercise or compression. Other areas worthy of investigation include patient well-being and financial issues.

REFERENCES

1. American Physical Therapy Association. Guide to Physical Therapist Practice. 2nd ed. *Phys Ther.* 2001 Jan;81(1):9-746.
2. Zuther JE. *Lymphedema Management: The Comprehensive Guide for Practitioners.* Stuttgart, NY: Thieme; 2005.
3. Williams P, Warwick R, Dyson M, Bannister LH. *Gray's Anatomy.* 37th ed. New York: Churchill Livingstone; 1993.
4. Guyton AC, Hall JE. *Textbook of Medical Physiology.* 9th ed. Philadelphia, PA: WB Saunders; 1996.
5. Kelly D. *A Primer on Lymphedema.* Upper Saddle River, NJ: Prentice Hall; 2002.
6. Shier D, Butler J, Lewis R. *Hole's Human Anatomy and Physiology.* 9th ed. Boston, MA: McGraw-Hill; 2002.
7. Földi M, Kubik S. *Lehrbuch der Lymphologie für Mediziner und Physiotherapeuten.* 4th ed. neubearbeitete Auflage, Ulm, Germany: Gustav Fischer; 1999.
8. Despopulos A, Silbernagl S. *Color Atlas of Physiology.* 4th ed. New York: Thieme Medical Publishers Inc; 1991.
9. Casely-Smith JR. Alterations of untreated lymphedema and its grades over time. *Lymphology.* 1995;28(4):174-185.
10. Földi M. Are there enigmas concerning the pathology of lymphedema after breast cancer treatment? *NLN Newsl.* 1998;10(4):1-4.
11. Weissleder H, Schuchhardt C. *Lymphedema Diagnosis and Therapy.* 3rd ed. Köln, Germany: Viavital Verlag; 2001.
12. Kissin MW, Querci della Rovere G, Easton D, Westbury G. Risk of lymphoedema following the treatment of breast cancer. *Brit J Surg.* 1986;73:580-584.
13. Rotmensche J, Rubin S, Sutton J, Javaheri G, et al. Preoperative radiotherapy followed by radical vulvectomy with inguinal lymphadenectomy for advanced vulvar carcinoma. *Gynecol Oncol.* 1990;36:181-184.
14. Martimbeau P, Kjorstad K, Kolstad P. Stage 1B carcinoma of the cervix, the Norwegian Radium Hospital, 1968–1970. Results of treatment and major complications. *Am J Obstet Gynecol.* 1978;131:389-394.
15. Karakousis C, Heiser M, Moor R. Lymphedema after groin dissection. *Am J Surg.* 1983;145:205-208.
16. Ko D, Lerner R, Klose G, Cosimi A. Effective treatment of lymphedema of the extremities. *Arch Surg.* 1998;133:452-458.
17. Wrone D, Tanage K, Cosimi A, Gadd M, et al. Lymphedema after sentinel lymph node dissection biopsy for cutaneous melanoma. *Arch Dermatol.* 2000;36:511-514.
18. Petereit DG, Mehta MP, Buchler DA, Kinsella TJ. A retrospective review of nodal treatment for vulvar cancer. *Am J Clin Oncol.* 1993;16(1):38-42.
19. Kavoussi L, Sosa E, Chandhoke P, Chodak G, et al. Complications of laparoscopic pelvic lymph node dissection. *J Urol.* 1993;149:322-325.
20. Rockson SG. Precipitating factors in lymphedema: myths and realities. *Cancer.* 1998;83(suppl 12B):2814-2816.
21. Zuther J. Taking flight: how airline travel can affect patients with lymphedema. *Adv Phys Ther PT Assist.* 2003;14(15):41-43.
22. Földi E, Földi M, Clodius L. The lymphedema chaos: a Lancet. *Ann Plast Surg.* 22:505-515.
23. Karges J, Mark B, Stikeleather SJ, et al. Concurrent validity of upper-extremity estimates: comparison of calculated volumes derived from girth measurements and displacement volume. *Phys Ther.* 2003;83(2):133-145.
24. Sander AP, Hajer NM, et al. Upper-extremity volume measurements in women with lymphedema: a comparison of measurements obtained via water displacement with geometrically determined volume. *Phys Ther.* 2002;82(12):1201-1212.
25. Cornish BH, Thomas BJ, Ward LC, et al. A new technique for the quantification of peripheral edema with application in both unilateral and bilateral cases. *Angiology.* 2002;53(1):41-47.
26. Cornish BH, Chapman M, Hirst C, et al. Early diagnosis of lymphedema using multiple frequency bioimpedance. *Lymphology.* 2001;34(1):2-11.
27. Petrek JA, Pressman PI, Smith RA. Lymphedema: current issues in research and management. *CA Cancer J Clin.* 2000;50(5):292-307.
28. Harris SR, Hugi MR, Olivotto IA, et al. Clinical practice guidelines for the care and treatment of breast cancer: 11. Lymphedema. *CMAJ.* 2001;164(2):191-199.
29. Kissin MW, Querci della Rovere G, Easton D, Westbury G. Risk of lymphedema following the treatment of breast cancer. *Br J Surg.* 1986;73:580-584.
30. Werner RS, McCormick B, Petrek J, et al. Arm edema in conservative management of breast cancer: obesity is a major predictive factor. *Ther Radiol.* 1991;180:177-184.
31. Lin PP, Allison DC, Wainstock J, et al. Impact of axillary lymph node dissection on the therapy of breast cancer patients. *J Clin Oncol.* 1993;11:1536-1544.
32. Brennan MJ. Lymphedema following the surgical treatment of breast cancer: a review of pathophysiology and treatment. *J Pain Symptom Manage.* 1992;7:110-116.
33. Prentice WE. *Therapeutic Modalities for Allied Health Professionals.* New York: McGraw-Hill; 1998.
34. Casley-Smith JR, Gaffney RM. Excess plasma proteins as a cause of chronic inflammation and lymphodema: quantitative electron microscopy. *J Pathol.* 1981;133:243-272.
35. Pecking AP, Fevrier B, Wargon C, Pillion G. Efficacy of Daflon 500 mg in the treatment of lymphedema (secondary

to conventional therapy of breast cancer). *Angiology*. 1997; 48:93-98.

36. Casley-Smith JR. There are many benzopyrones for lymphedema. *Lymphology*. 1997;30:38-39.

37. Burgos A, Alcaide A, Alcoba C, et al. Comparative study of the clinical efficacy of two different Coumarin dosages in the management of arm lymphedema after treatment for breast cancer. *Lymphology*. 1999;32:3-10.

38. Casley-Smith JR, Morgan RG, Piller NB. Treatment of lymphedema of the arms and legs with 5,6-benzo[alpha]pyrone. *N Engl J Med*. 1993;320:1158-1163.

39. Loprinzi CL, Kugler JW, Sloan JA, et al. Lack of effect of coumarin in women with lymphedema after treatment for breast cancer. *N Engl J Med*. 1999;340:346-350.

40. Goldsmith HS, De Los Santos R. Omental transposition in primary lymphedema. *Surg Gynecol Obstet*. 1967;125:607.

41. Miller TA. Surgical approach to lymphedema of the arm after mastectomy. *Am J Surg*. 1984;148(1):152-156.

42. Brorson H, Svensson H. Complete reduction of lymphedema of the arm by liposuction after breast cancer. *Scand J Plast Reconstr Surg*. 1997;31:137-143.

43. O'Brien BM, Khazanchi RK, Dumar PAV, Dviv E, Pederson WC. Liposuction in the treatment of lymphoedema: a preliminary report. *Br J Plast Surg*. 1989;42:530-533.

44. Brorson H. Liposuction gives complete reduction of chronic large arm lymphedema after breast cancer. *Acta Oncol*. 2000; 39(3):407-420.

45. Brorson H, Svensson H. Liposuction combined with controlled compression therapy reduces arm lymphedema more effectively than controlled compression therapy alone. *Plast Reconstr Surg*. 1998;102(4):1058-1067.

46. Zuther J. Is there a role for traditional massage therapy in the treatment and management of lymphedema? *NLN Newsl*. 2001:1-2.

47. Zuther J. Treatment of lymphedema with complete deconjestive physiotherapy. *NLN Newsl*. 1999;11(2):1-3.

48. Eliska O, Eliskova M. Are peripheral lymphatics damaged by high pressure manual massage? *Lymphology*. 1995;28(1):21-30.

49. Segers P, Belgrado JP, Leduc A, Leduc O, Verdonck P. Excessive pressure in multichambered cuffs used for sequential compression therapy. *Phys Ther*. 2002;82(10):1000-1008.

50. Boris M, Weindorf S, Lasinski BB. The risk of genital edema after external pump compression for lower limb lymphedema. *Lymphology*. 1998;31(1):15-20.

51. Miranda F, Perez MC, Castiglioni ML, et al. Effect of sequential intermittent pneumatic compression on both leg lymphedema volume and on lymph transport as semi-quantitatively evaluated by lymphoscintigraphy. *Lymphology*. 2001;34(3):135-141.

52. Lynnworth M. Greater Boston Lymphedema Support Group Pump Survey. *Newsl Natl Lymphedema Network*.1988;10:6-7.

53. Witte MH, Witte CL. The International Society of Lymphology, Zürich, Switzerland and Tucson, Arizona, USA. Progress in Lymphology—XIV. Proceedings of the 14th International Congress of Lymphology. *Lymphology*. 1994:27(suppl):1-893.

54. Kasseroller RG. The Vodder school: the Vodder method. *Cancer*. 1998;83(12 suppl American):2840-2842.

55. Leduc O, Leduc A, Bourgeois P, Belgrado JP. The physical treatment of upper limb edema. *Cancer*. 1998;83(12 suppl American):2835-2839.

56. Földi E. The treatment of lymphedema. *Cancer*. 1998;83(12 suppl American):2833-2834.

57. Casley-Smith JR, Boris M, Weindorf S, Lasinski B. Treatment for lymphedema of the arm—The Casley-Smith method: a non-invasive method produces continued reduction. *Cancer*. 1998;83 (12 suppl American):2843-2860.

58. Todorov G. *Sebum, Sweat, Skin pH and Acid Mantle*. Copyright 1998-2001. http://www.smartskincare.com/skinbiology/ sebum.html. Accessed December 31, 2009.

59. Franzeck UK et al. Combined physical therapy for lymphedema evaluated by fluorescence microlymphography and lymph capillary pressure measurements. *J Vasc Res*. 1997;34:306-311.

60. Hwang JH et al. Changes in lymphatic function after complex physical therapy for lymphedema. *Lymphology*. 1999;32:15-21.

61. Casley-Smith JR. Varying total tissue pressures and the concentration of initial lymphatic lymph. *Microvasc Res*. 1983;25: 369-379.

62. Mortimer PS et al. The measurement of skin lymph flow by isotope clearance—reliability, reproducibility, injection dynamics and the effect of massage. *J Invest Dermatol*. 1990; 95(6):677-682.

63. Olszewski WL, Engeset A. Intrinsic contractility of prenodal lymph vessels and lymph flow in human leg. *Am J Physiol*. 1980; 239(6):H775-H783.

64. Smith A. Lymphatic drainage in patients after replantation of extremities. *Plast Reconstr Surg*. 1978;79:163-168.

65. Hutzschenreuter P, Brummer H, Ebberfeld K. Experimental and clinical studies of the mechanism of effect of manual lymph drainage therapy [in German]. *Z Lymphol*. 1978; 13(1): 62-64.

66. Johansson K, Albertsson M, Ingvar C, Edkahl C. Effects of compression bandaging with or without manual lymph drainage treatment in patients with postoperative arm lymphedema. *Lymphology*. 1999;32:103-110.

67. Schmid-Schönbein GW. Microlymphatics and lymph flow. *Physiol Rev*. 1990;70(4):987-1028.

68. Brennan MJ, DePompolo RW, Garden FH. Focused review: Postmastectomy lymphedema. *Arch Phys Med Rehabil*. 1996;77: S74-S80.

69. Badger CM, Peackcock JL, Mortimer PS. A randomized, controlled, parallel-group clinical trial comparing multiplayer bandaging followed by hosiery versus hosiery alone in the treatment of patients with lymphedema of the limb. *Cancer*. 2000;88 (12):2832-2837.

70. Harris SR, Niesen-Vaertommen SL. Challenging the myth of exercise-induced lymphedema following breast cancer: a series of case reports. *J Surg Oncol*. 2000;74:95-99.

The Future of Cardiopulmonary Rehabilitation

CHAPTER

23

Barbara W. DeTurk

INTRODUCTION

As we move into the 21st century, much has been written about what the new millennium will bring. Forecasters have made detailed projections about world demographics and what the population will look like in terms of disease, activity levels, and health in the next quarter of a century. Dramatic changes are expected in the field of medicine that will impact the manner in which diseases are diagnosed and treated. There are large initiatives already in place in the United States, aimed at *prevention and wellness,* which project into the next decade. Information technology, an area where health care companies are beginning to invest heavily, will revolutionize how we communicate and utilize information.

This chapter will examine forecasts made for the next 20 years or so to create a picture of health care in the future and relate it to the practice of cardiopulmonary physical therapy. Many questions come to mind when one thinks so far into the future. What will the profile of a physical therapist look like in the year 2030? In what environments will therapy be practiced? How will physical therapists use new information technologies? There is no doubt that those just entering the field of cardiopulmonary physical therapy will witness a wide variety of change in the next 20 years. This chapter will attempt to prepare both the new and experienced therapist to meet the challenges of tomorrow's health care environment.

GLOBAL DEMOGRAPHICS

Let us begin by looking at the world at large, to examine the changes anticipated in the growth of the population. Most demographers agree that the population of the world will continue to grow from its present 6.6 billion people to approximately 9.4 billion in 2050. The incredible fact is that 212,036 people are being added to the world's population each day![1] United Nations forecasting predicts global population to peak at 11 billion in the year 2200. The total population in industrial countries is expected to decline, whereas 60% of the increases will take place in Asia, China, India, and Africa. Countries with the highest growth rate will feel the greatest impact on their public health system. Unfortunately, most of the world's population growth is projected to occur in the most distressed regions, where destruction of land, lack of food, and water will have a major impact on the health of the inhabitants.[2-5]

Aging Demographics in the United States

Age composition of the United States will change dramatically as we move further into the 21st century. By the end of the 1990s, one in every four persons was aged 50 years or older. The United States Bureau of the Census projects a moderate increase in the elderly population until 2010, then a rapid increase for the next 20 years to 2030, and then a return to a moderate increase in the years 2030 to 2050.[6] This is based on population momentum, more commonly referred to in the United States as the impact of the "baby boomers." Baby Boomers are considered to be those born between 1946 and 1964, after the end of World War II. Seventy-eight million

Indicator 1—Number of Older Americans

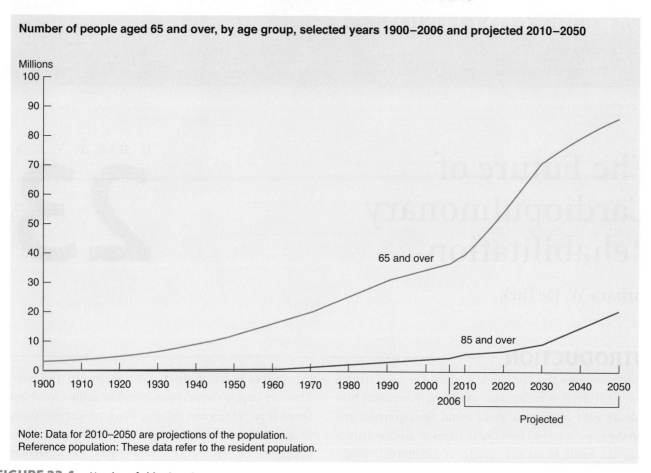

Number of people aged 65 and over, by age group, selected years 1900–2006 and projected 2010–2050

Note: Data for 2010–2050 are projections of the population.
Reference population: These data refer to the resident population.

FIGURE 23-1   Number of older Americans. (*Source: U.S. Census Bureau. http://www.agingstats.gov. Older American 2008.*)

baby boomers will turn 65 in 2011; an influx that will exceed the number of providers who can care for them.[7] This group will be responsible for the rapid rise in the elderly population between 2010 and 2030. The population will fall off again after 2030 because boomers have reproduced at a lower rate.[6] The population of the oldest old (85 years and older) is expected to grow by 56% between 1995 and 2010. From 2030 to 2050 the population of 85 years and older is expected to increase to a whopping 116%, as the baby boomers reach 85 years. **This means that a larger share of the elderly will be older than 85 years.** (See Fig. 23-1.)

It makes sense then that the number of elderly in poor health are projected to increase sharply from 1990 to 2030. Heart disease and stroke deaths rise significantly after age 65 years, accounting for more than 40% of all deaths among persons aged 65 to 74 years, and almost 60% of those aged 85 years and older. The number of people in nursing homes is projected to double and possibly triple by the year 2030. Also projected to increase are the numbers of people with disabilities, with greater than 19% of the population expected to have activity of daily living limitations (ADLs) by 2020.[6] (See Fig. 23-2.)

Racial and gender composition of the elderly in the next 50 years will undergo significant change. Elderly women

(85 years and older) will outnumber men by more than 4 million, or nearly 60%. Minority populations are projected to represent 25.4% of the elderly population in 2030. By 2050, **the United States will be more of a multicultural society** with Hispanic, African American, and Asian comprising the largest cultural groups (Fig. 23-3). As the racial ethnic ratios change, a greater proportion of our elderly will fall into a lower socioeconomic category, with fewer health benefits, access to health care, and less education on wellness and prevention.[6]

The need for rehabilitative health care services in the United States should escalate dramatically by 2011. As the baby boomers reach age 65 years, they will tend to have more health-related problems, and a higher incidence of disabilities. There will be greater numbers of Hispanic, African American, and Asian elderly, with different cultures and beliefs that therapists must be sensitive to in their patient management. Therapists may increasingly practice cardiopulmonary physical therapy in nursing homes, assisted living facilities, and home care environments due to the anticipated growth in the elderly population. By 2011 there should be tremendous opportunity for physical therapists in general and cardiopulmonary therapists in particular. Let us see why . . .

Indicator 20—Functional Limitations

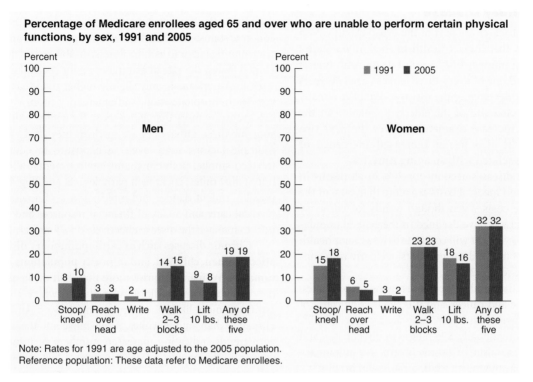

Percentage of Medicare enrollees aged 65 and over who are unable to perform certain physical functions, by sex, 1991 and 2005

Note: Rates for 1991 are age adjusted to the 2005 population.
Reference population: These data refer to Medicare enrollees.

FIGURE 23-2   Functional limitations. *(Source: Centers for Medicare and Medicaid Services, Medicare Current Beneficiary Survey.)*

Indicator 2—Racial and Ethnic Composition

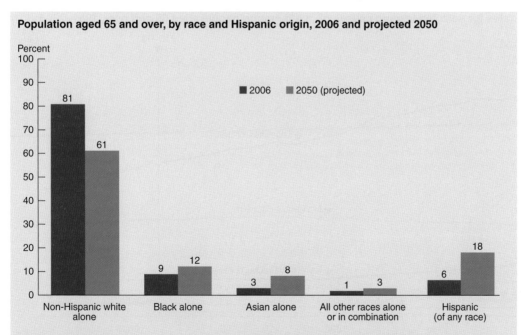

Population aged 65 and over, by race and Hispanic origin, 2006 and projected 2050

Note: The term *non-Hispanic white alone* is used to refer to people who reported being white and no other race and who are not Hispanic. The term *black alone* is used to refer to people who reported being black or African American and no other race, and the term *Asian alone* is used to refer to people who reported only Asian as their race. The use of single-race populations in this report does not imply that this is the preferred method of presenting or analyzing data. The U.S. Census Bureau uses a variety of approaches. The race group "All other races alone or in combination" includes American Indian and Alaska Native, alone; Native Hawaiian and Other Pacific Islander, alone; and all people who reported two or more races.
Reference population: These data refer to the resident population.

FIGURE 23-3   Racial and ethnic composition. *(Source: U.S. Census Bureau, Population Estimates and Projections.)*

Incidence/Trends for Cardiopulmonary Disease

Cardiopulmonary diseases are part of the broad classification of chronic diseases that impact health in the United States. Heart disease is the number one cause of death, with one of every two males and one of every three females aged 40 years and over at risk for developing the disease.[8] We have already seen that the projected size of the elderly population in the United States will increase dramatically over the next two decades. **There will also be an increased incidence of chronic disease associated with an aging America.**

Today chronic diseases account for 70% of all deaths in the United States, and medical costs are more than 60% of the nation's health care costs. Even though trends for coronary heart disease death rates have declined in the general population over the past 35 years, it will continue to be a major health problem due in part to the shear numbers of elderly who contract the disease.[9] (See Fig. 23-4.)

Lung disease is the number three killer in the United States, behind heart disease and cancer, and it is the leading cause of death in babies younger than 1 year. Lung disease costs the U.S. economy $154 billion annually, $95 billion in direct costs, and $59 billion in indirect costs.[10] Chronic obstructive pulmonary diseases are ranked as the fourth leading cause of mortality.[11,12] Asthma ranks highest in number of cases reported, as compared to bronchitis and emphysema. Although more adults have asthma, the incidence in children and adolescents has actually doubled in the time periods 1979–1980 to 1993–1995.[8] Socioeconomic status, particularly poverty, appears to be an important contributing factor to asthma illness, disability, and death. In the United States, the rate of asthma cases for Asian, Hispanic and African Americans is only slightly higher than that for whites; yet, death, hospitalization, and emergency room visit rates for this group are more than twice those for whites.[2] Although reasons for these differences are unclear, they likely result from multiple factors: high levels of exposure to environmental tobacco smoke, pollutants, and environmental allergens (eg, house dust mites, cockroach particles, cat and dog dander, and possibly rodent dander and mold); a lack of access to quality medical care; and a lack of financial resources and social support to manage the disease effectively on a long-term basis.[11]

Chronic diseases such as cardiopulmonary disorders will affect women, children, and minority populations disproportionately. Women comprise more than half of the people who die each year from cardiovascular disease, whereas death from asthma is more likely to occur among African Americans and Hispanics than among whites. As we move into the next decade, with trends indicating increased numbers of minorities and women in the population, we can project that chronic diseases will continue to be a major health and financial issue.[11,12]

Indicator 15—Mortality

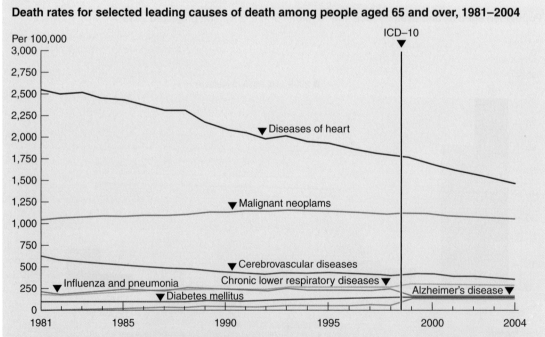

Death rates for selected leading causes of death among people aged 65 and over, 1981–2004

Note: Death rates for 1981–1998 are based on the 9th revision of the *International Classification of Diseases* (*ICD-9*). Starting in 1999, death rates are based on *ICD-10* and trends in death rates for some causes may be affected by this change. For the period 1981–1998, causes were coded using *ICD-9* codes that are most nearly comparable with the 113 cause list for the *ICD-10* and may differ from previously published estimates. Rates are age adjusted using the 2000 standard population. Reference population: These data refer to the resident population.

FIGURE 23-4   Mortality. (*Source: Centers for Disease Control and Prevention, National Center for Health Statistics, National Vital Statistics System.*)

MEDICAL CARE IN THE FUTURE

Wellness Revolution Merging of Eastern and Western Medicine

It has begun to happen. We are presently in a wellness revolution. What had been considered Eastern philosophy has begun to merge with concepts of Western medicine. Although scientists exclaim that there is little proof that Eastern techniques "work," the American public has begun to embrace herbs, massage therapy, acupressure, acupuncture, and meditation as accepted forms of alternative medicine.[13]

In a recent article by *The Journal of the American Medical Association,* Dr. S. Straus, the Director of the National Center for Complementary and Alternative Medicine projected that by 2020 medicine will be integrative. Dr. Straus believes rigorous scientific studies of alternative therapeutic and preventive modalities will prove some interventions to be effective, and they will be incorporated into conventional medical practice. Those that are not found to be effective will be discarded. The effectiveness of herbal and nutritional supplements will also be further researched and clarified. By 2020 the terms *alternative* and *complementary medicine* will be replaced by **integrative medicine.** This new field will embrace the best of Western and Eastern medicine philosophies and offer the patient a more holistic approach.[14]

As the mainstream medical approach becomes integrative, physical therapy practice may evolve and become more holistic. What might a holistic physical therapist be like? We know that holistic health principles focus on the interrelationships among the body, the mind, and the spirit. In addition, how different body parts react to one another is seen as an important component of the healing process.[15] Envision if you will, the therapist of the future routinely using a hands-on approach to not only unlocking muscle strain but also assisting in clearing mental and spiritual stressors as well. Some therapeutic techniques that are holistic in nature are already beginning to be integrated into physical therapy practice, such as acupressure, yoga, Feldenkrais, and t'ai chi chuan. Those who currently practice craniosacral therapy, for example, know that when the body begins to unwind, emotional feelings often accompany them as well. It is possible that therapists of the future will more frequently utilize their hands-on connection with the patient to improve functional status, while contributing to a more balanced spiritual state.[13,16,17]

Future Medical Advances

National Institute of Health Projections

The future of medical care will be characterized by dramatic change. Forecasters predict unprecedented medical innovations in the next few decades.

Dr. Claude Lenfant, NIH Director of The Heart, Lung, and Blood Institute, projects that coronary artery bypass operations will become mostly obsolete.[14] He believes favorable trends in coronary risk factors should reduce the need for surgical intervention. Those who still require bypass surgery will benefit from replacement vessels that behave more like arteries than like veins. Dr. Lenfant predicts that arteries will be grown in advance of the procedure from the patient's own cells. Dr. Anthony Fauci, NIH Director of the National Institute of Allergy and Infections, believes we will find new therapies and vaccines to fight chronic as well as infectious diseases. Chronic diseases such as cardiovascular disorders will be shown to have infectious etiologies and will be treatable with inexpensive antibiotics and vaccines.[14]

Advances in Pulmonary Care

Large organizations are stepping to the plate to conduct research leading to improved medical management of chronic disease. The American Lung Association has a network of 20 research centers currently conducting large clinical trials focused on the direct care of those with asthma. The most current clinical trial is a study of the connection between gastro esophageal reflux (GERD) and asthma. Other leading researchers are focused on genetic and molecular-level markers in relation to asthma, and bronchial thermoplasty.

Bronchial thermoplasty is now under clinical trial for consideration as a treatment for severe asthma. The theory is that asthma is caused by an overgrowth of smooth muscle tissue in the large airways. During asthma attack, the muscle contracts and narrows the passageway making breathing more difficult. In bronchial thermoplasty, heat is applied to the smooth muscle through a flexible tube during a bronchoscopy procedure. The heat causes the muscle to relax and keeps the airway open. Bronchial thermoplasty has been effective in reducing the number of asthma attacks, and reducing the use of rescue medication in patients with severe asthma.[18]

Of particular interest to physical therapists is the current research on the association of weight and asthma. In an analysis of seven studies those people who were considered overweight or obese had a 51% greater chance of having asthma than a person of normal weight. Physical therapists can have direct impact on this patient population through the use of weight reduction exercise programs, and referral for nutritional counseling.[18]

Innovations in modern medicine in the past had taken many years of research and clinical trials before treatments were introduced to the public. Now the development cycle has been greatly decreased because of the society's demand for short-term payoff.[19] In fact Cetron and Davies forecast that the **first decade of the 21st century will be one of the most productive in the history of medicine.**[19] There will be hundreds of new treatments and diagnostic advances available to patients in the areas of gene therapy, stem cell transplants, and nanotechnology. These new treatments and devices will lead to rapid diagnosis, help predict disease, provide relief to patients with chronic respiratory ailments, repair damaged heart muscle, and treat hereditary diseases. For our purposes, we will examine those innovations that impact the field of cardiovascular and pulmonary physical therapy.

Advances in Cardiac Care

As an example of the fast-paced development cycle for clinical products, the progress in creation of ventricular assist devices (VAD) has been remarkable. Over the last few years VADs have been used experimentally as a bridge to transplantation, recovery therapy, and most recently as destination therapy. On April 22, 2008, the FDA gave approval for the use of the first compact heart assist device to support the weakened heart of a small-sized adult man or woman with heart failure awaiting heart transplant. Previous models were too large to be placed in the abdomen of the patient, and required the patient to be tethered to an external power source. The HeartMate II is a mere 3 in. in length and weighs approximately 1 lb, and can operate on two external batteries worn at the waist, allowing the patient to move freely for up to 3 hours. In a clinical study at 26 transplant centers, 57% of patients with the HeartMate II survived to receive heart transplantation. This result is comparable to those patients treated with currently approved assist devices of larger size. By the year 2020, who knows what the VAD will look like, perhaps technology will progress to the point where it will be completely internal.[20]

The Human Genome Project

The Human Genome Project, a publicly funded, international effort, has completed one of its primary goals: to map the human genome. This represents one of the most significant medical achievements in our time, and has far-reaching potential to improve health over the next decade! Begun in 1990, the project was originally slated to last 15 years, but because of rapid technological advances, some of its goals were completed ahead of schedule. The goals of the Human Genome Project were to identify all 30,000 genes in human DNA, determine the sequences of the 3 billion chemical bases that make up DNA, and store the information on databases.[21]

A mutation of a single gene has been known to cause as many as 4,000 rare diseases, such as cystic fibrosis, sickle cell anemia, and Tay-Sachs disease. The causes of heart disease, diabetes, hypertension, and hypercholesterolemia, from a genetic point of view, are considered more complex. These diseases are thought to be caused by multiple gene mutations, or be the result of a combination of environmental factors, such as diet and gene mutation. Gene alteration may also influence an individual's ability to respond to viruses, bacteria, and toxins.[21–23] Dr. Francis Collins, the Director of the National Human Genome Research Institute, likes to paraphrase Churchill when he says, "Sequencing the genome is not the end, or the beginning of the end, but simply the end of the beginning."[22] **Unlocking the genetic code is the first step in understanding the nature of disease and may lead toward more effective treatments, possible cures, or ways to prevent thousands of diseases.[23]**

Genetic Effect on Medicine

What do scientists project will be the effect of genetics on the practice of medicine by the year 2020? A complete list of the human genome will give rise to a vast number of new medications. Drell and Adamson predict the number of new drugs tested and released for consumer use will increase sixfold from 500 new drugs in 2,000 to 3,000 in 2020.[24] Consumers of health care will have a record of their genome available during routine medical visits, and it will be used to predict which medications will most closely align with their body to minimize side effects and maximize treatment. Drugs will be prescribed more accurately for each patient based on information from their genome, and from knowledge of environmental factors that may also play a role in the disease process. Knowledge of specific gene abnormalities, which predispose a person to, for example, high cholesterol, will allow that person to make lifestyle changes prior to the development of active disease. By 2020 neonatal genetic testing will be routine and single gene related disorders will be readily treated.[24]

Gene Therapy

At present the Food and Drug Administration (FDA) in the United States has not approved any gene therapy product for sale. Gene therapy is still considered very experimental in nature; however, gene-related research and development continues to grow at a rapid pace.[25]

Gene therapy works by the insertion of a normal gene into the genome to replace an abnormal disease-causing gene. To get the gene into the body, a vector molecule is used, most commonly a virus. Viruses are used because of their capacity to encapsulate a molecule and then deliver it to a targeted cell. Different types of inactive viruses are used for their ability to deliver molecules to various areas of the body. One example is the adenovirus, the virus that causes the common cold. It has been used to deliver genetically repaired cells to cardiac muscle in gene therapy studies for patients with congestive heart failure.[26]

In 1990, 4-year-old Ashanti DeSilva was the first recipient of gene therapy with an infusion of white blood cells carrying synthetic DNA. Ashanti suffered from severe combined immunodeficiency disorder, or SCID, which left her without a functioning immune system. Doctor W. French Anderson, formerly of the U.S. National Institutes of Health, treated Ashanti with her own genetically altered cells. They were administered through her bloodstream and produced the missing enzyme, the lack of which had caused her disease. In subsequent months she received four more cell infusions. Since then she has required booster shots but has regained her health through the use of gene therapy, and medication.[19]

Use of Gene Therapy in Congestive Heart Failure

Prospects for the use of gene therapy in the treatment of congestive heart failure are very real indeed. Scientists have begun basic investigative studies on rodents and on isolated cardiomyocytes from failing human hearts. The interventions that were studied focused on enhancing sarcoplasmic calcium transport, which is decreased in patients with congestive heart failure. Disturbances in calcium metabolism have been shown to contribute significantly to the contractile dysfunction observed in heart failure. In these studies the subject was "infected" with sarcoplasmic reticulum Ca^{2+} ATPase (*SERCA2a*). In other words, the *SERCA2a* gene was carried by an adenovirus to targeted cells in the rodent or cardiomyocyte. The results showed that gene transfer of *SERCA2a* improved left ventricular function. Scientists are quick to point out that these are preliminary studies, and further experimentation is needed before this form of gene therapy is ready for use in humans.[27–29]

First Commercial Gene Therapy Product for Humans

In October 2003, China became the first country in the world to produce a commercial gene therapy product called Gendicine for use in the treatment of head and neck squamous cell carcinoma. In 2005, a second product called Oncorine was also approved for use of head and neck cancer in China. Gendicine is delivered by an adenovector virus. Eight weeks of injections of this gene therapy product are used in conjunction with radiation treatments. After 5 years of clinical trials with Gendicine on 26 patients, 64% of late stage tumors showed regression, and 32% of tumors demonstrated partial regression. So far the only side effect seems to be self-limited fever.[30] Five-year survival rates show 17 of 26 patients surviving, 16 without reoccurrence of disease. In the control group of 26 patients, 14 have survived for 5 years and 10 remained cancer-free.

In the United States and other countries around the world, an experimental sample size of 26 patients is considered too small to reach a credible level of statistical significance. In addition, the combined therapies, genetic and radiation, make it difficult to discern how much gene therapy contributed to patient improvement.[31]

Stem Cell Research—The Body's Self-Repair Kit

Human stem cell research, like gene therapy, is another important area in the medical field that holds great promise. Research in human developmental biology has led to the discovery of human *stem cells* (precursor cells that can give rise to multiple tissue types), including embryonic stem cells, embryonic germ cells, fetal stem cells, and adult stem cells. Embryonic (pluripotent) stem cells are harvested from 7-day-old embryos or aborted fetuses. These cells are used because they have the unlimited capacity to divide. In fact pluripotent stem cells can become any tissue in the body, including muscle, nerve, heart, and blood cells. Adult stem cells; however, appear to be restricted in what they can become. For example, adult stem cells in bone marrow give rise to blood cells, whereas those that are from muscle seem to create only new muscle cells. Pluripotent stem cells hold the most promise for treatment of disease but are controversial in nature due to their origin. In 2000, it was reported that scientists at the University of Wisconsin and Johns Hopkins University were able to isolate and successfully grow pluripotent human stem cells. The University of Wisconsin has been able to establish a stem cell bank so that new embryos are no longer needed, thus avoiding some of the controversy involved with this research.[32,33]

Scientists believe stem cells have the potential to cure disease, reverse the advance of chronic disorders, and heal injuries. These cells will be able to generate tissue for transplantation and replace damaged tissue such as myocardium. Stem cells also have the potential to assist in the way we currently develop new drugs. The drugs will be tested on stem cells first, then later on humans. Researchers project that patients with heart disease, Parkinson's disease, severe combined immunodeficiency (SCID), diabetes, and spinal cord injuries will be some of the few that may be helped with this type of treatment.[32,33]

Scientists have begun to study the use of stem cells for patients with congestive heart failure. Preliminary work in mice and other animals has demonstrated that healthy heart muscle cells transplanted into the heart successfully repopulate cardiac tissue, without rejection from surrounding tissue. Use of stem cell transplants has the potential to overcome the problem of tissue incompatibility and the need to use immune-suppressing drugs currently used during cardiac transplantation. The challenge now is to develop heart muscle cells from *human* pluripotent stem cells and transport them into failing heart muscle in order to support cardiac function.[34]

Telomerase Activation—The Fountain of Youth?

Telomeres form the ends of human chromosomes, like the plastic caps on the end of a shoelace. The telomeres function to maintain chromosome stability, and require a minimum length. Telomeres shorten with each round of cell division, and this mechanism limits proliferation of human cells to a finite number of cell divisions. There is growing evidence indicating that telomere shortening also limits stem cell function, regeneration, and organ maintenance during ageing. Moreover, telomere shortening during aging and disease is associated with a 3.18-fold higher mortality rate from heart disease. Telomeres have emerged as crucial cellular elements in the aging process and in various diseases including cardiovascular and chronic obstructive pulmonary disease.[35]

Since 1995, scientists have been working on ways to activate telomerase, which functions to repair and lengthen the telomere. They have already accomplished this in both mice and humans. T.A. Sciences Center in New York Center, New York, now offers a telomerase-activating product called TA-65, as part of a 12-month protocol. TA-65 is produced by a company called Geron and is administered in tablet form like a supplement. In clinical trials 2 to 4 daily doses of 10-mg tablets of TA-41 (a precursor to TA-65) were given to men aged 60 to 85 years for 12 weeks in a double-blind study, and the condition of their immune system, eye sight, sexual function, and skin improved dramatically. As a result of these human trials, T.A. Sciences now offers a 1-year supply of TA-65 at the low price of $25,000.00! The fountain of youth may be here, but it comes with a hefty price tag![36]

Nanotechnology: The Doctor That Floats in Your Bloodstream

Molecular nanotechnology is a field of research aimed at the manipulation of atoms and molecules into nanometer size (a nanometer is 1 billionth of a meter).[37] All manufactured products are made from atoms manipulated in simple ways. "Nanoscience and nanoengineering—the ability to manipulate and move matter—are leading to unprecedented understanding of the fundamental building blocks of all physical things."[38] **President Obama's fiscal year 2010 budget requests $7 billion for the National Science Foundation, to support scientific research in the United States. It remains to be seen what portion of that scientific funding will go toward the National Nanotechnology Initiative.[39]** It is expected that nanotechnology will impact the way vaccines, medical-testing devices, computers, and even automobile tires are made.

An article in *The New York Times* relates a futurist episode where a person has an episode of chest pressure at lunch. Instead of rushing to the emergency room, the person injects themselves with minuscule cylinders called *respirocytes* packed with pressurized oxygen, designed to mimic the function of red blood cells. Aboard each respirocyte is a tiny computer that gives the command to deliver oxygen when the distressed cells are reached. Instead of collapsing, the person finishes lunch and goes for a checkup with their doctor.[37] Ralph Merkle, a nanotechnology engineer, foresees a time when patients with cardiac and respiratory disorders will carry respirocytes like diabetics carry insulin. This technology may be 30 years in the future, but less fantastic medical applications may be only a few years away.[40]

The first medical applications of nanotechnology will probably be in the field of screening and diagnostic tools. *The New York Times* reports that a Palo Alto–based company called Quantum Dot Corporation is developing nanoscopic crystals to be used in basic genetic screening and detection of disease. These nanosensors will greatly enhance tools such as CAT scans, MRIs, and catheter tips that will allow physicians a better view of a patient's anatomy. Within a decade we may see passive *nanobots* that can be inserted into the bloodstream to study internal organs. Beyond that, some predict that we will be able to create self-replicating nanobots, which will actually follow directions. They can be programmed to seek out viruses or cancer cells and destroy them before they have impact on the body.[37]

HEALTH CARE POLICY

Healthy People 2010

Did you know that *the United States has an agenda for a health wellness and prevention program?* Healthy People is a national program that sets the agenda for managing preventable threats to health and focuses public and private sector efforts in order to address those threats.[8] The purpose of Healthy People is to improve health, not only of individuals but also of communities and the nation. It began in 1979 from the Surgeon General's report entitled "Healthy People," and has blossomed into the Healthy People Consortium. The consortium is a user alliance of 350 national membership organizations and 250 state health, mental health, substance abuse, and environmental agencies (with input from the American Physical Therapy Association [APTA]). Every 10 years new objectives and goals

are determined for the health of the nation. These goals serve as a *guide* for developing a set of objectives, which focus on determinants of health. Three of the Healthy People goals pertain to cardiovascular and pulmonary physical therapy: heart disease and stroke, physical activity, and respiratory disease. Ultimately the success of the goals is measured by the health status of the target population.[8]

Healthy People 2020 Guidelines were due to be released in the fall of 2008, but due to a reevaluation of the goal-setting process, the publishing date has been pushed back. It was felt that the goals and objectives were too lengthy, and needed revision. A midcourse review was conducted in 2003 that evaluated the progress towards those goals. It is interesting to note that some physical activity goals set by Healthy People 2010 have been partially met, while others have fallen below previous health levels. For example, the objective for moderate activity in children between the ages of 9 and 12 moved away from its target. In 1999, 27% of children participated in moderate physical activity, but by 2003 that level had dropped to 25% instead of rising to the target of 35%.[41]

Using Healthy People Objectives

Healthy People materials are in the public domain and posted on their extensive Web site (http://www.healthpeople.gov) to encourage groups to integrate their objectives into health care programming. Cardiovascular and pulmonary therapists should review the objectives that pertain to their patient populations, and incorporate them into daily practice where appropriate (Box 23-1). For example, to apply Healthy People leading indicators to physical activity and obesity, therapists might conduct screenings of body mass or monitor heart rate and blood pressure before and after exercise. Therapists may find that they already inadvertently participate in Healthy People through data collection projects such as the Health Plan Employer Data and Information Set (HEDIS). Healthy People is an excellent example of a far-reaching public health policy that sets the standard for health care in the future. As health care practitioners, we should join in this national effort to prevent cardiovascular and pulmonary disorders and promote wellness of our communities.[8,42]

COMMUNICATION TECHNOLOGY OF THE FUTURE

Online Medical Records

There are now a number of online Web sites that provide storage for medical records. Google and General Electric to name just two, have started secure Web sites for online medical records.[43] The online site allows patients to organize health information all in one place, gather medical records from doctors, hospitals, and pharmacies, and share that information securely with doctors and caregivers.[43]

The Obama Administration in its economic stimulus legislation entitled the American Recovery and Reinvestment Act of 2009, incorporated payment incentives to Medicare and

BOX 23-1

Healthy People 2010 Goals and Objectives Pertaining to Cardiovascular and Pulmonary Physical Therapy Practice

1. *Heart Disease*

   Goal—Improve cardiovascular health and quality of life through the prevention, detection, and treatment of risk factors; early identification and treatment of heart attacks and strokes; and prevention of recurrent cardiovascular events.

   Objectives (health determinants for cardiovascular disease)—coronary artery disease (CAD) deaths, knowledge of symptoms of heart attack and importance of dialing 911, artery-opening therapy, bystander response to cardiac arrest, out-of-hospital emergency care, and heart failure hospitalizations.

2. *Respiratory Disease*

   Goal—Promote respiratory health through better prevention, detection, treatment, and education.

   Objective—The health determinant objectives are deaths from asthma, hospitalizations for asthma, hospital emergency department visits for asthma, activity limitations, school or workdays lost, patient education, appropriate asthma care, and surveillance systems.

   Example—An example of a specific goal for respiratory disease is to slow the rise in deaths from chronic obstructive pulmonary disease to achieve a rate of no more than 25/100,000 people.

3. *Physical Activity*

   Goal—Improve health, fitness, and quality of life through daily physical activity.

   Objective—The objectives monitor the degree of physical activity, muscular strength, flexibility, endurance, physical education requirements in schools, and television viewing.

   Example—A more community-minded objective reads as—increase community availability and accessibility of physical activity and fitness facilities as follows: hiking, biking, and fitness trail miles: 1/10,000 people. Of the 13 physical activity and fitness objectives, only worksite fitness programs have met the year 2000 targets.

Medicaid programs that utilize health IT (information technology). Health IT includes online medical records, computerized medical records, and telehealth to name a few types of technology. The Congressional Budget Office, which advises congress on the cost of legislation, expects that the increased utilization of health IT would reduce total spending on health care by decreasing inappropriate tests, paperwork, and medical errors.[44]

Physical therapists working in all types of environments now and in the future will benefit from online medical records. There are many instances in current practice when a therapist must evaluate a patient with little or no medical history other than what a client is able to relate. Therapists with online capabilities in their workplace will have a tremendous advantage if they are able to tap into the online medical record for information. Communication with other professionals working with the client may also improve, if their reports are included in the online medical record.

Communication Technology and Physical Therapy

Communication technology in the form of handheld computers is reaching out to the field of home care practice. Federal requirements now demand home care evaluation and discharge paperwork to be "locked and loaded," as it is called, into a computer system within a short-time frame. Traditional paper-driven home care agencies are struggling to meet these strict time deadlines, as it is difficult to get paperwork data entered this quickly. Forward-thinking agencies are turning to handheld or laptop computer technology that allows staff to document care directly into a relatively small unit that is connected to a centralized server. There is no paper, and the documentation is available to the home care agency and payer source with little turnaround time.

In the future, handheld computerized documentation devices or laptops will probably become the norm in home care and in other practice environments. Technology may even advance to the point where all communication takes place via an *all-in-one watch*,[37] a wristwatch-sized cell phone, with a keyboard and Internet access that will provide a direct link to the patient's online medical record. For those who dread documentation, hang in there; future technology may solve your problems!

Telemedicine

Advances in telecommunication technology have now made it possible to link hospitals, medical centers, and patients in the home, for the purpose of providing support and clinical care at a distance. Telehealth has been defined as the use of electronic communication to provide and deliver health-related information and health care services. Those services include patient evaluation, education, medication reminders, and monitoring of interventions, performed by doctors, nurses, radiologists, physical therapists, and others. The benefit of telehealth is that it can be utilized over large distances, providing medical management to those who might not have access to care.[45]

East Carolina University School of Medicine (ECU), a leading center for telecommunications in the United States, began conducting telemedicine consultations in 1992. To date they have completed more than 3,000 consultations in 34 different specialties of medicine. ECU has integrated a hybrid network of telecommunication technology to link approximately 40 sites with 3 discrete channels of audio, video, and data. The ability to telecommunicate is dependent on the "lines" (ie, wires, cables, optical fibers, and microwaves) that connect 1 station to another.[46–48]

In the home care setting, there are various products available today that link the patient via a phone line to a centralized station that monitors the data transmitted. One such product called the *AlereNet System* is being used with congestive heart failure patients to help recognize the *early* signs of cardiac failure. Because daily monitoring by home care personnel is prohibitively expensive ($132/d), utilization of a telecommunication device allows for the necessary monitoring at a lower cost ($13/d).[48]

The *AlereNet System* is placed in the patient's home and establishes an audio/visual link with the patient. The monitor asks the patient physician-specified questions about their symptoms, via an audible voice and visual display. The patient answers the questions by pressing yes or no keys and then uses a biometric measurement device to record their weight. The information obtained is then stored and forwarded to the home care agency or MD for interpretation. Health care practitioners can access the patient's entire history of symptoms and weight, as well as their medical history and medications[49] (Fig. 23-5).

Another telehealthcare system called The *Viterion 500 Telehealth Monitor* uses store-and-forward technology to relay vital sign measurements and personalized questions or advice, as well as digital video technology and Web access. Depending on the specific needs of the patient, this telehealth device can be set up to monitor blood pressure, heart rate, breath sounds, heart sounds, ECG, weight, glucose levels, O_2 saturation, and temperature. The video component allows a health care practitioner to have a two-way interaction with the patient, to answer patient questions and provide a supplement to in-home visits. Web access can link patients to specific disease management education programs that offer beginner through advanced information on topics related to the patient's medical regime.

The *Viterion 500* has been utilized in Veterans Administration Hospitals to assist in caring for patients with chronic disease. One such patient was the subject of an article in the *Boston Globe* on September 23, 2003. Richard Keirsead, a 72-year-old Air Force veteran, used to rush to the hospital at least 10 times a month for medical problems caused by diabetes, multiple sclerosis, and advanced heart disease. Since he started using a The *Viterion 500,* he has been able to manage his health at home through frequent monitoring of his vital signs. If there is a problem he can "meet" a nurse or physican at the Veterans Hospital via live video. Mr. Keirsead has only been hospitalized once since 2001 when he began using this telehealth device, a savings in travel time for him, and dollars for the VA Hospital.[50]

The American Physical Therapy Association's stance on telehealth has evolved to now include the use of this technology in the practice of physical therapy. APTA guidelines have been revised to indicate that telehealth must adhere to basic assurances of quality and professional health care. Telehealth must be in accordance with the Guide to Physical Therapist Practice, and the laws of the jurisdiction in which the care is rendered. Services via telehealth must ensure that patient safety is comparable to the physical therapist being physically present.[45]

Physical therapists have just begun to interact with telehealth devices in the home care setting in the management of patients with chronic disease such as asthma, CHF, diabetes, and COPD. The therapist has improved capability to monitor patients through the use of ECG, and O_2 saturation levels, as well as blood pressure, heart rate, and respiratory rate that are traditionally monitored. Therapists can utilize these units to relay vital signs taken pre- and postexercise, where they can be compared with previous readings. This allows closer patient monitoring during exercise and tighter control of medication regimes. In the future physical therapists may supplement home visits with the use of the video component of a telehealth device to monitor home exercises from the home care agency office. This might be particularly useful for patients located in remote areas, where travel time is an issue.

Kenneth Sparks, PhD of Cleveland State University, sees the use of telemedicine in outpatient cardiac rehabilitation. He studied 400 patients from five hospitals in Cleveland, Ohio, to determine if patients enrolled in cardiac rehabilitation would self-pay (because insurance does not yet pay for telemedicine) for rehabilitation services if they were more convenient. Apparently there were a number of patients who could not enter programs because of scheduling difficulties or distance. Eighty-four of 206 (40%) patients responding indicated that they would be willing to pay for more convenient cardiac rehabilitation services. From this study, Dr. Sparks developed a model for the use of telemedicine for monitoring patients with heart disease. He believes that a viable self-pay model can be established to bring cardiac monitoring to patients via telemedicine.[51]

PROFILE OF A PHYSICAL THERAPIST IN THE FUTURE

At the June 2000 annual APTA conference, the House of Delegates endorsed a vision statement describing the future of

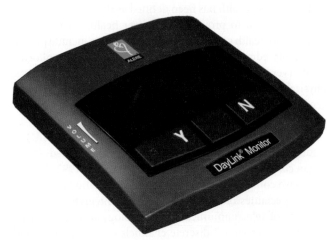

FIGURE 23-5 The *AlereNet System*: an audiovisual device that links the home-bound patient directly to the health care provider. (Reprinted with permission from Alere Medical, Inc., Reno, Nevada.)

physical therapy and the characteristics of the physical therapist and physical therapy assistant. It so clearly defined the focus of strategic planning for the growth of the profession, the text is quoted directly:

> By 2020, physical therapy will be provided by physical therapists who are doctors of physical therapy, recognized by consumers and other health care professionals as practitioners of choice to whom consumers have direct access for the diagnosis of, interventions for, and prevention of impairments, function limitations, and disabilities related to movement, function, and health.
>
> Physical therapy, by 2020, will be provided by physical therapists who are doctors of physical therapy and who may be board-certified specialists. Consumers will have direct access to physical therapists in all environments for patient/client management, prevention, and wellness services. Physical therapists will be practitioners of choice in clients' health networks and will hold all privileges of autonomous practice. Physical therapists may be assisted by physical therapist assistants who are educated and licensed to provide physical therapist-directed and supervised components of interventions.
>
> Guided by integrity, life-long learning, and a commitment of comprehensive and accessible health programs for all people, physical therapists and physical therapist assistants will render evidence-based service throughout the continuum of care and improve quality of life for society. They will provide culturally sensitive care distinguished by trust, respect, and an appreciation for individual differences. While fully availing themselves of new technologies, as well as basic and clinical research, physical therapists will continue to provide direct care. They will maintain active responsibility for the growth of the physical therapy profession and the health of the people it serves.[52]

Many Catherine Worthingham Fellows share the APTA's vision of the future. Their thoughts have been recorded in a special section of *PT Magazine* titled Forecast 2000. When asked the question "What does the profession of physical therapy need to do to thrive in the new millennium?" one of the most common replies centered on evidence-based research. In the words of Beverly Schmoll, PT, PhD, FAPTA, "As we enter the new millennium, the profession of physical therapy must be grounded in clinical research, emphasize the behavioral sciences, and become 'other' oriented through effective advocacy for those whom we serve."[53] Other common themes included the idea that physical therapists must be seen as diagnosticians, that therapists must position themselves in the area of prevention and wellness, and that therapists must have direct access to the patients they serve. Arthur Nelson, PT, PhD, FAPTA, makes note of stem cell research and genetic manipulations that make it possible to rebuild components of the nervous system. He projects that physical therapists will be the clinicians who will design exercise programs to relearn movement![54]

The Scientific Practitioner

Physical therapists of the future will be able to rely on a growing scientific base of knowledge for diagnosis and treatment of their patients. In the last 10 years, therapists have been challenged more and more frequently to justify the effectiveness of their treatment. Insurance companies have denied coverage of some traditionally used treatments because their efficacy had not been proven through clinical research. The physical therapy profession has been in a conundrum: They could not suspend certain physical therapy treatments until they could be scientifically supported, nor could they recommend continuing to practice without systematic inquiry and empirical justification. In response to this dilemma, in November 1999, APTA's Board of Directors adopted a clinical research agenda that would provide scientific data to support clinical practice.[55]

The APTA's Agenda for Clinical Research will project out at least 5 years, if not more. This group plans to rely on the resources of the Foundation for Physical Therapy to implement research, but will need additional funding sources to complete the proposed agenda. It is the goal of the Research Agenda to bring time-tested physical therapy practice into a full-blown science of physical therapy. Completion of the Research Agenda will modify physical therapy practice into evidence-based care. This will strengthen the profession's standing with insurance providers, as well as with other practitioners in the community. The APTA projects that in the future physical therapists will be seen as *scientific practitioners.*[55]

PRACTICE SETTINGS OF THE FUTURE

Physical therapists have a long track record for effectively treating a "core" group of patients with functional limitations, disabilities, and changes in physical function and health status resulting from injury, disease, or other causes. Traditionally, therapists have practiced in setting locations that are often part of a continuum of care: from the acute hospital environment, to a postacute facility, to home care services, and finally to an outpatient clinic. Within the current health care revolution, these traditional settings will continue to demand the services of physical therapists; however, new avenues for practice may open up as well.

Today's health care consumer has greater access to medical information and is more assertive about their care. In a sense *the consumer is driving a health care revolution.* They demand quality services, reasonable prices, and convenience. The health care consumer has learned that they must be their own advocates.[56] As such, demand for convenient quality health care has created a new supply of treatment locations and options. *Integrative outpatient centers* have emerged to provide a variety of services in a convenient "one-stop shop" atmosphere. Corporations have opened their own employee fitness/wellness centers for the benefit of their staff and for lower health insurance premiums. Let us examine the opportunities that new practice environments present.

Longevity/Wellness Centers

Although the concept of a *longevity* or *wellness center* has just recently gained recognition, the *Pritikin Longevity Center*, one of many longevity centers in the United States, has treated patients for the past 25 years. They are particularly well known for their work with cardiac disorders.[57] Wellness centers such as the *Cardiovascular Wellness Center* in Westbury, New York, utilize traditional noninvasive diagnostic tests (stress tests) along with careful analysis of blood chemistry, vitamin and mineral assay, body composition, and digestive analysis as part of their standard evaluation. A personalized program is recommended from the results of the comprehensive evaluation that incorporates proper nutrition, diet, exercise, and an integrated approach to medicine using essential drugs with natural therapies.[58] Physical therapists can play a role in this setting by designing appropriate exercise programs and participating in wellness education.

Some longevity/wellness centers now offer a new nonsurgical therapy called enhanced external counterpulsation (EECP). This new treatment is indicated for patients with stable angina and utilizes a series of three compressive air cuffs wrapped around the legs to increase blood flow to the heart. A typical program calls for 30, 1-hour treatments over the span of 7 weeks. The increased blood flow to the heart causes the development of coronary artery collaterals that replace compromised vessels. Multicenter clinical research studies show EECP to reduce anginal pain, improve exercise treadmill time, and improve coronary blood flow as documented by thallium stress testing.[59,60] EECP has a promising future as a noninvasive treatment for patients with angina, perhaps administered in conjunction with an exercise program provided by a physical therapist.

The Henry Jackson Foundation for the Advancement of Military Medicine and Walter Reed Army Medical Center has developed an intensive lifestyle change program for military health care beneficiaries with coronary artery disease. In a study they conducted, 144 participants with a mean age of 61 participated in lifestyle changes for 1 year (lacto-ovo vegetarian diet, exercise, stress management, group support). Study participants were measured at baseline, 3 months, and 1 year with significant results. Fiber intake rose from 35% at baseline to 94% at 1 year, exercise levels greater than or equal to 150 min/wk increased from 31% to 79% at 1 year. Other parameters such as low-density lipoprotein levels, body mass index, and blood pressure also showed improvement. Study participants who were compliant with the program achieved improvement in at least three of the five heart health characteristics. The authors concluded that intensive lifestyle changes can promote improvement in health characteristics that, if maintained, may lead to reduced cardiovascular events.[61]

Health Clubs and Fitness Centers

Physical therapy practices have begun to emerge in health clubs and fitness centers. These clubs offer convenient locations for exercise during a lunch hour or after work, and do not evoke feelings associated with a medical office visit. Fitness programs are now being offered for those who are postsurgery, and for special populations such as seniors with cardiopulmonary disorders. Cardiac programs located in fitness centers can offer monitoring by telemetry, as well as blood pressure and heart rate response. Educational sessions on risk-factor management are also frequently available in these settings. As the patient improves, they require less monitoring, and can exercise in other parts of the facility.[62,63]

In the future, the health club or fitness center may be more frequently utilized as the site for *primary prevention programs* for families. In this setting the cardiovascular and pulmonary therapist would promote healthy exercise programs not only for adults but also for their children. Inactive lifestyles, an indicator that is currently tracked by Healthy People 2010, can put children at risk for cardiopulmonary disease later in life. Who would better serve the community than the physical therapist to establish movement and activity programs for people of all ages?[64]

Occupational Health

A number of physical therapists have identified the area of *occupational health* as a practice setting of great potential.[65] They see this as an opportunity to provide on-site immediate care for disorders such as repetitive strain and acute injuries. Occupational health physical therapy can also play a role in employee asthma management, wellness and prevention education, preemployment screening, and on-site cardiac monitoring. As more studies document the effectiveness of moderate activity in the reduction of heart disease, the corporate world must be educated on the cost-effectiveness of programs like cardiac rehabilitation. Physical therapists may also play a larger role in primary prevention of cardiopulmonary disorders through promotion of employee wellness programs. Experience shows that penetration into the field of occupational health in corporations requires high-quality, comprehensive services that are marketed effectively. This relatively new practice environment offers exciting challenges for cardiopulmonary physical therapy![64,65]

Integrative Outpatient Practice

Integrative outpatient practices that combine alternative and traditional medical practice techniques are beginning to emerge. These practices may employ many different types of practitioners such as physical therapists, acupuncturists, chiropractors, podiatrists, and massage therapists. The practices are designed to be one-stop shops where patients can get complete medical care under one roof. The additional benefit of alternative or integrative medicine in the form of acupuncture, chiropractic, or perhaps Chinese herbal medicine offers choice to consumers who are seeking out this form of therapy with increasing frequency. In this setting, physical therapists may find greater freedom to integrate nontraditional skills they have learned (shiatsu, craniosacral, Feldenkrais) to progress their patients to their highest level of function.[56,58]

Home Care Setting

As the population in the United States continues to age, we know that by 2030 all baby boomers will be 65 years or older representing a huge cohort of people seeking health care services. Ninety percent of adults older than 50 years have indicated they want to age at home rather going to a nursing home.[66] We also know that when costs are compared, services provided in the home are considerably less expensive than a hospital ($5,765/d), or skilled nursing facility ($544/d) with homecare costing only $132/d.[67] As health care costs rise with the volume of baby boomers seeking services, our health care system is already seeking the lowest cost environment to care for our elderly. Physical therapists will play an integral role in providing care in the home, by working for various types of home care agencies such as certified, hospice, and long-term agencies. Certified agencies are able to provide care for Medicare and Medicaid patients. Hospice agencies are the fastest growing segment of home care services, and physical therapists play an important role in family education. Long-term agencies are primarily focused on care of the patient with a chronic disease process like multiple sclerosis.

In the future another type of home care service will gain an important niche in communities around the United States. Naturally occurring retirement communities (NORC) have begun to spring up in areas where there is a concentrated group of people 60 and older. NORC provide supportive services to help older people stay in their own homes. At present there are approximately 80 NORC programs in 25 states, and they are part of a national trend to encourage aging in place. Typically NORC use the services of existing home care agencies, volunteers, and businesses to provide low-cost services. A University of California survey of 530,000 elderly on Medicaid found that Medicaid saved an average of $15,000 a year for each person served at home as opposed to a nursing home.[66] Fall risk prevention is a key educational activity provided by many NORC, due to the high health care costs associated with falls in the elderly. Physical therapists will have an important role in this setting in evaluating the home environment for safety, instructing in fall prevention, and providing exercises to improve balance and strength.

Focused Factories

How many of you have eaten a McDonald's hamburger in your life? Admit it; probably most of us have. By doing so you have eaten at one of the best known *focused factories* in the service industry. Focused factories are facilities that concentrate their efforts on one type of service for the purpose of improving the relationship between cost and output. They are common in the restaurant service sector but are an emerging breed in health care. In the case of McDonalds, they have perfected every operating procedure involved in the production of a fast, good-tasting meal.[56]

Health care–focused factories function in a similar way. Take, for example, Shouldice Hospital in Toronto, Canada, a hospital that performs only abdominal hernia operations. They are so good at what they do, and so successful in creating a social experience, that patients come back yearly to celebrate the repair of their hernias. Because care is focused on one surgery, each step in the process is carefully scrutinized until the best possible operating procedure is determined. The components of the Shouldice system not only create patient satisfaction but also result in lower cost and fewer surgical revisions than regular hospitals.[56]

St. Francis Hospital on Long Island, NY, is another example of a focused factory, in this instance in the field of cardiac care. Over the past 20 years St. Francis has performed more than 40,000 open-heart surgeries with excellent success rates. Studies demonstrate that patients benefit when hospitals and surgeons perform a high volume of procedures. In the case of St. Francis, the focus on cardiac care has allowed them to be leaders in the innovation of new techniques and procedures. They are now using robotically assisted surgery to repair heart valves on patients who qualify for this minimally invasive procedure. A patient who has undergone cardiac valve replacement using this technique may find themselves out to dinner within 1 week of the procedure, and 4 weeks later back to work full-time and working out at the gym! Dr. Alan Guerci, President and CEO of St. Francis, predicts by 2029 advances in medical technology and expertise will mean increased comfort, shorter stays and improved quality of life for patients. According to Michael Dowling, CEO of North Shore-LIJ Health System, most future health care will be delivered in outpatient settings, with hospitals serving as centers for wellness related activities.[68]

The financial community views focused factories as the next wave of transformation in health care. Venture capitalists have poured millions of dollars into focused factory services, especially those that target diabetes, asthma, and congestive heart failure. These venture capitalists observed that a small percentage of asthma patients (33%) accounted for 73% of the costs of treating the disease. They also found that a small portion (37%) of patient's with chronic obstructive pulmonary disease caused 86% of the costs for one large employer. The venture capitalists concluded that a relatively small number of focused factories aimed at high-cost diseases could provide enormous health care benefits.[56]

Physical therapists may find that they will utilize their cardiovascular and pulmonary skills in focused factories that handle all aspects of care of one of the high-cost diagnoses, such as asthma or congestive heart failure. A limited choice of patients allows for more intense scrutiny of therapeutic procedures and techniques. Patients will benefit from specialized care, delivered by experts in their condition. If the success of the Shouldice system is replicated, the quality of care will be high, and the cost for management will be less. Due to the health care revolution currently in progress, physical therapists should anticipate changes to their practice environment. Therapists need to "think out of the box" and open their eyes to the needs of the health care consumer. By following those needs, the successful therapist will create new and exciting practice locations.

Demand for Physical Therapists in the Future

Historically, physical therapists have been in short supply. Therapists have enjoyed strong increases in salary, high job placement rates, and a choice of job opportunities. At the close of the 1990s the job opportunities for physical therapists began to diminish. This has been attributed to greater numbers of physical therapy graduates as education programs have increased over the past 10 years, the influence of managed care, and the health care cost controls implemented by the federal government. As a result, the APTA commissioned a study in 1997 on the supply of and demand for physical therapists for the years 1995, 2000, and 2005.[65] The most recent data collected by this study was in November 2001.[69]

In order to make accurate forecasts, the study considered a wide variety of factors that would influence the outcome of both the supply and the demand for therapists. For instance, managed care penetration, increased competition from alternative providers such as chiropractors, athletic trainers, and occupational therapists were all taken into consideration. Forecasts were also estimated using a synthesis of information from a broad and comprehensive search of available survey databases, published and unpublished reports, and phone interviews with those knowledgeable in the field.

The initial projections of the Workforce Study have come to pass. We have moved from a shortage of physical therapists and through a period of increased unemployment in the late 1990s, and now are emerging with an improved job outlook for therapists.[70] In fact The Bureau of Labor Statistics expects the employment of physical therapists to grow 27% from 2006 to 2016, much faster than the average occupation. Demand will be spurred by increasing numbers of patients with disabilities.[71]

As we approach the year 2011, when the baby boomers begin to reach 65, there will be a resurgence in demand for therapy services. As Jules Rothstein so aptly put it in the March 2000 issue of *Physical Therapy*, "Americans in the next two decades will go from being the baby boomer generation to being the largest geriatric population our nation has ever seen. Maintaining the status quo will not be enough when the boomers begin to devour health care resources like locusts devouring wheat."[72] Remember, cardiovascular and pulmonary disorders are in the top diagnostic categories for the elderly, and qualified therapists will be needed to utilize the most advanced means of treatment available.

SUMMARY

Step into the future, if you will, to the year 2030. We observe a physical therapist trained at the DPT level working in a facility that specializes in management of chronic cardiovascular and pulmonary disorders. Although most of the patients are 65 years and older, there is a fairly large contingency of children and adolescents with asthma. Women comprise 60% of the older population, and the ethnic composition of the clinic is multicultural, with high proportions of white, Hispanic, African American, and Asian clients. Coronary artery disease and chronic obstructive pulmonary disease are still major health problems for those seen in the facility, but they are being diagnosed and treated in different ways. Genetic testing is used routinely to determine who is predisposed to cardiopulmonary disorders. Nanotechnology has been incorporated into sophisticated diagnostic equipment to allow better visualization of internal human anatomy. New vaccines and gene therapy have been developed to ward off the onset of chronic disorders. Cardiac open-heart surgery, once performed routinely, is now done only rarely.

As a student entering the world of physical therapy today, it is essential to stay current with the changing face of American health care. Students should read from a broad spectrum of resources not only health-related journals but also current affairs, scientific research, and health policy. They should approach the workplace in a creative, imaginative way, perhaps pushing the field of physical therapy to places it has not been before. They should embrace technological advances that may allow one to practice without ever *writing* a note, or may allow monitoring of a patient in the next town, instead of in the next room. Students should use their knowledge of scientific research to expand the application of physical therapy practice into areas such as stem cell transplants and gene therapy. With a flexible, creative mind, the future practice of cardiopulmonary physical therapy will be rewarding indeed!

As a new therapist moving into the job market, be sensitive to consumer demands for convenient health care services, and consider employment in new environments. Recognize that health care costs will continue to be carefully controlled, and work with evidence-based treatments that will support the provision of physical therapy services. By "*Catching the Age Wave*," forward-thinking physical therapists can ensure that our profession will lead in the provision of cardiovascular and pulmonary rehabilitative services in the future.[72]

REFERENCES

1. World Population Demographics. http://www.xist.org. Accessed December 30, 2009.
2. Mitchell JD. Before the next doubling. *World Watch*. January/February 1998:20-27.

3. Hollingsworth W. Population explosion: still expanding. *USA Today*. July 1998:28-29.

4. McRae H. *The World in 2020*. Boston: Harvard Business School Press; 1994.

5. Swanson S. Global population will peak at eleven billion, U.N. forecasting unit says. *Chicago Tribune*. February 1998:16.

6. Siegel J. Aging into 21st Century. Special Report for Administration on Aging HHS-100-95-001. http://www.aoa.dhhs.gov. Accessed September 22, 2003.

7. Boomers, 65, in Search of Medical care. *Time Magazine*. April 2008:19-22.

8. Healthy People 2010. http://www.health.gov. Accessed December 16, 2003.

9. Seeman T, Adler N. Older Americans: who will they be? *Natl Forum*. 1998;78:22-25.

10. American Lung Association. Data and statistics. http://www.lungusa.org. Accessed June 16, 2008.

11. Cardiovascular Statistics. http://www.lungusa.org. Posted March 2003.

12. National Center for Health Statistics. Data warehouse on trends in health and aging. http://www.cdc.gov/nchs. Accessed September 22, 2003.

13. Galantino M, Kane R. Evidence based complementary therapy interventions for the elderly. *Gerinotes*. 2001;8:10-13.

14. Goldsmith MF. 2020 Vision: NIH heads foresee the future. *JAMA*. 1999;282:2287.

15. New York College and FAIM Ed team-up for 10th health care symposium. *Health Waves Newsletter*. 2000;4:1.

16. Johnson J, Yu T. T'ai Chi for the elderly. *Gerinotes*. 2001;8:21-23.

17. Taylor M. Yoga for the elderly. *Gerinotes*. 2001;8:25-28.

18. American Lung Association Web site. What is new in asthma research? http://www.lungusa.org/site. Accessed June 16, 2008.

19. Cetron M, Davies O. *Probable Tomorrows. How Science and Technology will Transform Our Lives in the Next Twenty Years*. New York: St Martin's Press; 1997.

20. FDA approves first compact heart assist device. http://www.fda.gov/bbs. Accessed June 16, 2008.

21. *Human Genome Project*. http://www.ornl.gov/hgmis. Accessed December 16, 2003.

22. Mestel R. Beyond the DNA map. *Newsday*. May 2000:C3.

23. Casey D. Genes, dreams, and reality. *Judicature*. 1999;183:3.

24. Drell D. Fast forward to 2020: what to expect in molecular medicine. http://www.ornl.gov/hgmis. Accessed May 5, 2008.

25. Human gene therapy. http://www.fda.gov/consumer/update. Accessed May 5, 2008.

26. Human genome project. http://www.ornl.gov/sci/rechresources/human genome. Accessed May 9, 2008.

27. del Monte F, Harding S, Schmidt U, et al. Restoration of contractile function in isolated cardiomyocytes from failing human hearts by gene transfer of SERCA2a. *Circulation*. 1999;100(23):2308-2311.

28. Miyamoto M, del Monte F, Schmidt U, et al. Adenoviral gene transfer of SERCA2a improves left-ventricular function in aortic-banded rats in transition to heart failure. *Proc Natl Acad Sci U S A*. 2000;97(2):793-798.

29. Hajjar R, del Monte F, Matsui T, et al. Prospects for gene therapy for heart failure. *Circ Res*. 2000;86(6):616-621.

30. China Approves First Gene Therapy. Nature Biotechnology 22, 3-4 (2004). http://www.nature.com/nbt. Accessed May 9, 2008.

31. China's Gene Therapy Cancer Drugs. http://www.seekingalpha.com/article/58759. Accessed May 5, 2008.

32. U.S. Department of Health and Human Services. *Stem Cell Research Fact Sheet*. U.S. Department of Health and Human Services. http://www.hhs.gov. Accessed December 16, 2003.

33. Gorman C. Brave new cells. *Time Magazine*. May 2000:58-60.

34. National Institutes for Health. *Stem Cell Information*. http://stemcells.n.h.gov. Posted September 2002.

35. Jiang H, Ju Z. Telomere shortening and aging. *Z Gerontol Geriatr*. 2007;40:314-324.

36. Prenatt D. Ending Old Age Through Telomerase Activation. http://www.netesq.com. Accessed June 3, 2008.

37. Breslau K, Jones M, Webster D. A catalog of the near future. *New York Times*. June 11, 2000:80-102.

38. The White House Office of the Press Secretary. National Nanotechnology Initiative: leading to the next industrial revolution. http://www.whitehouse.gov. Accessed June 5, 2000.

39. National nanotechnology initiative. http://www.whitehouse.gov/omb/budget. Accessed March 8, 2009.

40. Merkle RC. Nanotechnology Web site. http://www.zyvex.com/nano. Accessed June 6, 2000.

41. Health People Web site. http://www.healthypeople.gov/data/midcourse. Accessed March 15, 2009.

42. Bainbridge D. Working for a healthier America. *PT Magazine*. October 2000:50-57.

43. Google health. On-line medical records. http://www.google.com/health. Accessed April 11,2009.

44. Schwartz R. *Health IT Boosted in Economic Recovery. Remington Report*. March/April 2009.

45. Telehealth holds to same standards as all PT care. http://apta.org/AM. Accessed May 9, 2008.

46. Telemedicine: statement of experience. http://www.telemed.med.ecu.edu. Accessed September 23, 2003.

47. Dansky K, Palmer L, Shea D, et al. Cost analysis of telehomecare. *Telemed J E Health*. 2001;II(3):225-232.

48. Kinsella A. Chronic disease management and telehealthcare. Telemedicine Information Exchange. March 23, 1999. http://tie.telemed.org/articles/article.asp?path=articles&article=diseaseManagement_ak_tie99.xml. Accessed January 1, 2010.

49. AlereNet System. http://www.alere.com. Accessed September 24, 2003.

50. Dember A. Keeping patients connected, technology helps VA reduce hospital visits. *The Boston Globe*. September 23, 2003:1.

51. Sparks K. Efficacy of telemedicine self-pay cardiac rehabilitation clinics. Lecture at American Association of Cardiovascular and Pulmonary Rehabilitation; September 23, 2000; Tampa, FL.

52. American Physical Therapy Association Vision Statement for the Future. http://www.apta.org/news. Accessed September 23, 2003.

53. Schmoll B, Wolf S, Sahrmann S, et al. Forecast 2000. *PT Magazine*. January 2000:38-42.

54. Nelson A, Harris S, et al. Forecast 2000. *PT Magazine*. September 2000:12-15.

55. Guccione AG, Goldstein M, Elliott S. Clinical research agenda for physical therapy. *Phys Ther*. 2000;80:499-513.

56. Herzlinger RE. *Market Driven Health Care*. New York: Harper-Collins; 1997.

57. Pritikin Longevity Center. http://www.pritikin.com. Accessed April 11, 2009.

58. Cardiovascular Wellness Center. http://www.vagnini.com. Accessed April 12, 2009.

59. Arora R, Nesto R, Chou T, et al. Results of the multicenter study of enhanced external counterpulsation (MUSTEECP): EECP reduces anginal episodes and exercise-induced myocardial ischemia. *J Am Coll Cardiol.* 1999;33(7):1833-1840.

60. Lawson W, Hui J, Zheng Z, et al. Improved exercise tolerance following enhanced external counterpulsation: cardiac or peripheral effect? *Cardiology.* 1996;87(4):271-275.

61. Marshall D, Walizer E, et al. Achievement of heart health characteristics through participation in an intensive lifestyle change program. *J Cardiopulm Rehabil Prev.* 2009;29:2.

62. Highlighted physical therapy practice settings. http://www.apta.org/career center. Accessed July 30, 2003.

63. Francis K. Fitness Watch. *PT Magazine.* October 1999:53-59.

64. Tepper S, Kovacek P, Morris D, et al. Challenges 2000. *PT Magazine.* January 2000:43-47.

65. Wicken A. The reliable resource. *PT Magazine.* June 1999:30-32.

66. Amon R. No place like home. *Newsday.* May 10, 2008.

67. National Association of Home Care Web site. http://www.nahc.org. Accessed April 11, 2009.

68. Hanc J. Hospitals of tomorrow on the drawing board today. *Newsday.* April 7, 2009.

69. Workforce study. Vector Research, Inc. 1997. http://www.apta.org/research. Accessed December 16, 2003.

70. APTA employment survery. http://www.apta.org/research/survey. Accessed July 25, 2003.

71. Bureau of Labor Statistics. *Occupational Outlook Handbook 2008-09.* http://www.bls.gov.oco. Accessed April 7, 2009.

72. Lewis C, McAndrew JM. Catch the age wave. *Adv Phys Ther.* 2000:45.

Index

Note: Page numbers followed by the letter "*t*" indicate tables; those followed by the letter "*f*" indicate figures.